Patient Care
STANDARDS
Collaborative Planning
& Nursing Interventions

with 466 illustrations

Seventh Edition

Patient Care STANDARDS
Collaborative Planning & Nursing Interventions

Susan Martin Tucker, MSN, RN, PHN, CNAA
Healthcare Consultant
Quality Management and Perinatal Systems
Roseville, California

Mary M. Canobbio, MN, RN, CNS, FAAN
Cardiovascular Clinical Specialist
Lecturer, School of Nursing
University of California, Los Angeles
Los Angeles, California

Eleanor Vargo Paquette, BS, RN, PHN
Holistic Healthcare Consultant
The Paquette Group
Raleigh, North Carolina

Marjorie Fyfe Wells, BS, RN, PHN
Home Health Care Specialist
MEW Consulting
Dexter, Michigan

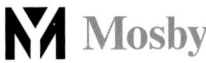

An Affiliate of Elsevier

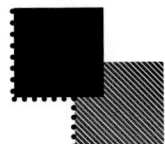

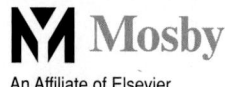

Mosby

An Affiliate of Elsevier

Vice President, Nursing Editorial Director: Sally Schrefer
Executive Editor: N. Darlene Como
Senior Developmental Editor: Laurie Sparks
Project Manager: John Rogers
Senior Production Editor: Beth Hayes
Designer: Kathi Gosche

7th EDITION

Copyright © 2000 by Mosby, Inc.

NOTICE

Pharmacology is an ever-changing field. Standard safety precautions must be followed, but as new research and clinical experience broaden our knowledge, changes in treatment and drug therapy may become necessary or appropriate. Readers are advised to check the most current product information provided by the manufacturer of each drug to be administered to verify the recommended dose, the method and duration of administration, and contraindications. It is the responsibility of the treating provider, relying on experience and knowledge of the patient, to determine dosages and the best treatment for each individual patient. Neither the publisher nor the editor assumes any liability for any injury and/or damage to persons or property arising from this publication.

Mosby, Inc.
An Affiliate of Elsevier
11830 Westline Industrial Drive
St. Louis, Missouri 63146

Printed in China

Library of Congress Cataloging in Publication Data

Patient care standards : collaborative planning and nursing interventions / Susan Martin Tucker ... [et al.].—7th ed.
    p.cm.
    Includes bibliographical references and index.
    ISBN 0-323-00996-4
        1. Nursing care plans.   2. Nursing—standards.   I. Tucker, Susan Martin
    [DNLM: 1. Nursing Care—standards.   2. Critical Pathways—standards.   3. Patient Care
Planning—standards. WY 100 P297 2000]
    RT49 .P38 2000
    610.73 02 18 21—dc21   99-043230

04 CL/KPT 9 8 7 6 5 4 3

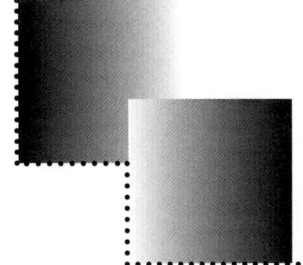

Contributors

Beth Bandy, MSN, ARNP
Clinical Director
Via Christi Regional Medical Center
Wichita, Kansas
  Chapter 7, Endocrine System

Mary M. Canobbio, MN, RN, CNS, FAAN
Cardiovascular Clinical Specialist
Lecturer, Acute Care Section,
UCLA School of Nursing
Los Angeles, California
  Chapter 3, Cardiovascular System
  Chapter 14, Immune System
  Chapter 12, Integumentary System

Deborah Caswell, MN, RN, ANP-C
Assistant Director
UCLA Gunda Vascular Center
UCLA Medical Center
Los Angeles, California
  Chapter 3, Cardiovascular System

Elizabeth Cattell, MN, RN, CNS, CCRN, ACNP
Lecturer
School of Nursing/Acute Care Section
University of California, Los Angeles
Los Angeles, California
  Chapter 9, Neurologic System

Patricia Coleman, PhD, RN, ANP
Medicine Nurse Practitioner
Crouse Hospital
Syracuse, New York
  Chapter 8, Musculoskeletal System

Donna L. Cramer, BS, BA, RN
Clinical Analyst/Patient Care Consultant
Kaiser Permanente Medical Center
Sacramento, California
  Chapter 4, Hematologic System

Caroline L. Dettbarn, MS, ARNP, CCRN
Clinical Nurse Specialist/Education Coordinator
Critical Care
Via Christi Regional Medical Center
Wichita, Kansas
  Chapter 7, Endocrine System

Karon Giles, MSN, ARNP, CCRN
Clinical Nurse Specialist
Critical Care
Via Christi Regional Medical Center
Wichita, Kansas
  Chapter 7, Endocrine System

Bonni Lapp Horwitz, MSN, RNC
Nursing Coordinator
Hartford Hospital
Hartford, Connecticut
  Chapter 6, Digestive System

Sandra Green Lobdell, BSN, MPA, RN, PHN,
  CPHQ, CETN
Wound, Ostomy, Continence–Enterostomal Therapy Nurse
Kaiser Permanente Medical Center
Walnut Creek, California
  Chapter 6, Digestive System

Marvel Logan-Darrough, MN, RN, MSFT
Advanced Registered Nurse Practitioner
Clinical Nurse Specialist—Diabetes
Licensed Marriage and Family Therapist
Certified Sex Therapist
Clinical Director, Pulsatile Intravenous Insulin Therapy
  Program
Via Christi Regional Medical Center
Wichita, Kansas
  Chapter 7, Endocrine System

Mei-Sheng Lu, MSN, RN, ACNP
Acute Care
Vencor Hospital
Los Angeles, California
Researcher
Department of Neurology
UCLA Medical Center
Los Angeles, California
   Chapter 9, Neurologic System

Marise C. Magsarili, MN, RN, ACNP
Regional Department of Cardiac Surgery
Kaiser Permanente Medical Center
Los Angeles, California
   Chapter 5, Respiratory System

Michele Mair, MSN, RN, C, CCRN, RCIS
Cardiac Catheterization Lab and Cardiac Recovery Unit
Educator
St. Luke's Hospital
Bethlehem, Pennsylvania
   Chapter 3, Cardiovascular System

Margaret A. Marinow, BSN, RN
Commander USN, Retired
Seal Beach, California
   Chapter 13, Optic and Auditory Systems

Lucille C. Mertel, BS, RN
Clinical Supervisor
Pinnacle Home Care
Sherman Oaks, California
   Chapter 2, Dimensions of Nursing

Robyn J. Parker, MN, ARNP, CS, FNP, CDE
Diabetes Nurse Practitioner
Via Christi Regional Medical Center
Wichita, Kansas
   Chapter 7, Endocrine System

Leah Ann Phillips, BSN, RN, PHN
Case Manager
Providence Home Hospice
Burbank, California
   Chapter 2, Dimensions of Nursing

Carol Reed, BS, RN
Clinical Director
Via Christi Regional Medical Center
Wichita, Kansas
   Chapter 7, Endocrine System

Laura S. Rogers, MSN, RN
Oncology Research Nurse Coordinator
St. Joseph Mercy Hospital
Ann Arbor, Michigan
   Chapter 11, Female Reproductive System/Women's Health

Cynthia A. Serway, MPA, RRT
Director of Health and Services Outcomes
Quality Management Department
Napa-Solano Area
Kaiser Foundation Hospital
Vallejo, California
   Chapter 5, Respiratory System

Carol S. Smith, MSN, ARNP
Critical Care Education Coordinator
Clinical Nurse Specialist
Via Christi Regional Medical Center
Wichita, Kansas
   Chapter 7, Endocrine System

Valerie A. Sweig, BSN, RN, CCRN
Clinical Resource Nurse
Regional Burn Center
University of California at Davis Medical Center
Sacramento, California
   Chapter 12, Integumentary System

Susan M. Tucker, MSN, RN, PHN, CNAA
Healthcare Consultant
Roseville, California
   Chapter 1, Introduction: Guides for Collaborative Patient Care
   Chapter 2, Dimensions of Nursing
   Chapter 10, Genitourinary/Renal System
   Chapter 11, Female Reproductive System/Women's Health

Ellen R. Whalen, MS, RN, CNA
Senior Director, Clinical Services
USC Care Medical Group, Inc.
Los Angeles, California
   Chapter 15, Cancer

Marge Zerbe, BS, RNC
President
Obstetrical Seminars and Consulting
Clermont, Florida
   Chapter 11, Female Reproductive System/Women's Health

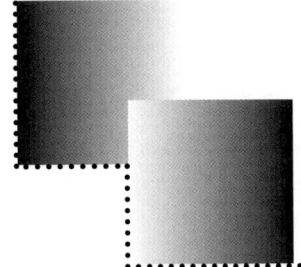

Reviewers

Judith Albers, RN, CRRN
Rehabilitation Intake Coordinator
Forest Park Hospital
St. Louis, Missouri

Patricia Bates, BSN, RN, CURN
Staff Nurse, Urology
Kaiser Permanente
Portland, Oregon

Judith A. Csokasy, PhD, RN
Associate Professor
College of Nursing
Indiana University Kokomo
Kokomo, Indiana

Ellen Stoetzner Duke, MSN, RN
Instructor of Nursing
Angelina College
Lufkin, Texas

Debra Hagler, MS, RN, CS, CCRN
Clinical Associate Professor
College of Nursing
Arizona State University
Tempe, Arizona
Critical Care Resource Team
Desert Samaritan Medical Center
Mesa, Arizona

Bette Hammond, MSN, RN
Assistant Professor (Retired)
St. Charles County Community College
St. Peters, Missouri

Mary Hirsch, MSN, RN, CETN
Director, Medical Services
St. Louis Medical Supply, Inc.
St. Louis, Missouri

Judy Kaye, PhDc, ARNP, CNRN, CCRN, GNP, ANP, CS
Research Specialist/Adult Nurse Practitioner
University Hospital
Augusta, Georgia

Christine Miaskowski, PhD, RN, FAAN
Professor and Chair
Department of Physiological Nursing
University of California
San Francisco, California

Nursing Practice Council
St. Luke's Hospital and Health Network
Bethlehem, Pennsylvania

Barbara Solomon, MSN, DNSc, RN
Nurse Researcher
Walter Reed Army Medical Center
Washington, D.C.

Laurel Wiersema-Bryant, MSN, RN, CS
Clinical Nurse Specialist and Adult Nurse Practitioner
BJC Health System, Barnes-Jewish Hospital
St. Louis, Missouri

Preface

At one time nurses were not allowed to take blood pressures, offer opinions on care, or discuss treatment plans with their patients because these were functions performed only by physicians. Patients were medicated and treated but not always told the exact purpose. Patients were admitted to hospitals for routine checkups and stayed several days. Well, times have changed, practice patterns have changed, and we've all come a long way!

The majority of health care now takes place in the outpatient/ambulatory setting. Patients who were once routinely managed in the acute inpatient setting now receive care in short-stay or observation units, skilled nursing facilities, and extended-care facilities. Others have their care managed at home with the support of public health or home health care nurses. Patients who are admitted to acute inpatient facilities are generally very ill or in need of a surgical procedure or other treatment.

In the past decade, hospitals that once competed with each other have now consolidated into larger systems to achieve economies of scale. Some have closed altogether. The length of stay has diminished markedly over the last several years and is still decreasing in many facilities. Care has become less provider oriented and more patient centered. Multidisciplinary team members have learned to appreciate the unique contributions that others make toward moving the patient to the conjointly agreed upon goals and expected outcomes. Developing mutually agreed upon goals among the members of the health care team is critical to ensuring their engagement in a successful plan of care.

At the same time, patients have become partners with health care professionals in managing their own health care needs. The public is increasingly more knowledgeable about their bodies, their health care needs, and healthy practices. Information is obtained from health care providers, educational forums, printed and televised communication media, and the Internet. Patients want and have the right to know, to understand, and to make informed choices.

With the multitude of changes, one thing has remained constant—the need to provide safe, comprehensive, and quality patient care in a seamless manner across the health care continuum. This book, *Patient Care Standards,* has set the standard of care for more than the past two decades and will continue to do so into the new millennium.

The seventh edition of *Patient Care Standards* has been revised and updated to reflect the dynamic changes in the delivery of patient care. The content is organized by body systems and uses a patient-centered, collaborative approach to over 300 patient care plans. New 1999-2000 NANDA nursing diagnoses have been incorporated where appropriate into existing care plans. The purpose continues to be to assist in the planning, implementation, and evaluation of comprehensive patient care and nursing interventions with the multidisciplinary health care team in a patient-focused environment in a variety of settings.

Each chapter begins with an assessment of the designated body system and includes geriatric considerations as part of this assessment. This is followed by medical conditions, surgical interventions, diagnostic studies, procedures, and treatment regimens. These are described and followed by subjective and objective assessment data, diagnostic tests, multidisciplinary management, patient problems/NANDA nursing diagnosis statements, nursing interventions, measurable expected outcomes for outcome evaluation, patient/family teaching, and discharge/home care planning. The chapter format is described in greater detail in the Guidelines for the Use of This Book. Topics in this book include care of patients with interventional cardiac procedures, special equipment, rehabilitation guides, symptom management for patients on chemotherapy, substance abuse, death and dying/end-of-life care, guidelines for culturally sensitive patient care, and care of patients with behavioral problems who can present in any health care setting. In addition, several timeline-based care plans, often termed "care paths," are provided at the end of each chapter as examples, to demonstrate the variety of formats that may be useful to the reader for developing these documents for specific patient populations.

Patient Care Standards can be used for planning and delivering care to the hospitalized patient by bedside nurses, case managers, discharge planners, charge nurses, and advanced practice nurses such as clinical nurse specialists and nurse practitioners. Nurse executives, nurse managers, or quality performance improvement staff members can use these standards as the basis for evaluating the provision of care and patient outcomes and identifying opportunities for systems improvement. Students will find these standards invaluable as an instant reference for the planning, implementation, and evaluation of care, as well as for patient teaching and discharge planning. In addition, brief rationales are provided where they are most helpful.

Care delivered to patients in skilled nursing facilities, extended-care facilities, and assisted living centers and by public and home health nurses can be guided by these standards, especially those that pertain to patients with chronic conditions. Discharge planners, case managers, utilization managers, patient educators, and ambulatory care professionals will find these standards helpful in providing a seamless approach to patient care by promoting consistency and continuity of care across all health care settings.

Patient Care Standards has been revised to support the provision of patient care within the context of the current health care environment. It is provided to ensure that those who depend on us receive a planned, safe, comprehensive, and compassionate standard of quality care across the health care continuum.

Susan Martin Tucker
Mary M. Canobbio
Eleanor Vargo Paquette
Marjorie Fyfe Wells

Guidelines for the Use of This Book

The first chapter of the book provides guidelines for the planning of patient care and demonstrates the use of this book as an as-is, single source of patient care plans. In addition, the content can be used as a tool for the creation of multidisciplinary timeline plans of care known as "care paths." The second chapter of the book focuses on dimensions of patient care. This includes aspects of care that may be applied as appropriate to any patient, such as perioperative care, variations of and care of the aging patient, death and dying, management of behavior problems, nutritional support, and special equipment such as PICC lines, PCA pumps, and subclavian catheters. Care of patients based on several of the NANDA (1999-2000) nursing diagnoses is included, as well as a new care plan for Latex Allergy response.

The subsequent chapters are divided into body systems, and each chapter begins with extensive assessment guidelines for that body system. The following describes the components of the standards of patient care.

TITLE

The medical condition, surgical intervention, procedure, or treatment regimen that is the basis for the standard of care is identified.

DEFINITION

A brief description of the medical condition, surgical procedure, diagnostic procedure, pharmacologic agent, or supportive equipment is given.

ASSESSMENT

SUBJECTIVE DATA

Descriptive terms used by patients are listed and are based on the patient's perception of the problem.

OBJECTIVE DATA

Observable signs and symptoms are listed from the viewpoint of the nurse or health care provider to guide ongoing assessment.

DIAGNOSTIC TESTS

Condition-appropriate imaging, laboratory, and other diagnostic tests and studies are identified.

POTENTIAL COMPLICATIONS

These are potential condition/procedure-related complications that the nurse should consider and monitor as indicated as part of the patient assessment. Nursing interventions are directed toward preventing these complications.

MULTIDISCIPLINARY MANAGEMENT

This section includes therapeutic management as provided by nonnursing multidisciplinary health care providers. These include the physician, physician assistant, nutritionist, respiratory therapist, physical therapist, social worker, spiritual counselor, speech/language pathologist (speech therapist), occupational therapist, and others.

PATIENT PROBLEMS—NURSING DIAGNOSES/INTERVENTIONS

Problems and diagnoses are listed in a priority sequence and are those most commonly associated with the condition. They are related to the etiologies or other factors from the assessment data to assist in understanding the reason or rationale for performing the intervention. Interventions are listed in priority sequence and are directed toward reducing, correcting, or eliminating the patient problem or nursing diagnoses. In addition, intervention-specific rationales are provided and italicized for easy identification. This is important to the student population but also serves to support the practicing nurse in providing explanations to the patient for the purpose of the intervention.

EXPECTED OUTCOMES

This section serves three purposes: as goals, expectations, and an evaluation of the efficacy of the interventions. If the statements were reworded prospectively, these phrases would be goal statements. As currently worded they are expected outcomes and in addition provide an evaluation mechanism by which the success of the interventions can be measured for quality/performance improvement purposes.

ADDITIONAL NURSING DIAGNOSES TO CONSIDER

This list includes problems or diagnoses that should be kept in mind when assessing and managing the patient's care, because they are possible but not highly probable.

PATIENT/FAMILY TEACHING

This section provides the educational component. Education is a nurse-sensitive indicator of the success of the patient's outcome. The patient and/or family (which may include a significant other in the absence of family) should be able to articulate the information and understand their role in engaging in or complying with the plan for continuing care in the outpatient setting. The articulation of information learned by the patient and family is important and indicates that they have the knowledge about the patient's condition and plan of care. However, mere possession of information does not necessarily mean that the information will be used appropriately or at all. Some individuals are simply noncompliant, whereas others may not value the information or find it contrary within their cultural context.

It is the nurse's role to identify sources of discrepancy between the patient's and health care provider's conception of the information, especially that which is related to cultural factors, and to identify any barriers that can be accommodated, adjusted, or removed. Follow-up may be indicated to determine the patient's engagement in care by post-discharge phone calls or home health visits, as necessary.

DISCHARGE/HOME CARE PLANNING

These are factors that the nurse should consider to help the patient transfer to another level of care or get ready for going home. These could include things to anticipate at home or potential problems that might be encountered, such as stairs, privacy, a place to store dressings or supplies, security, and telephone access. In addition, community service agencies may be identified for further support. Generally this section should be reviewed upon the patient's admission, because the content is an integral component in preparing the patient and in maintaining an appropriate standard of care.

Contents

Contents **xv**

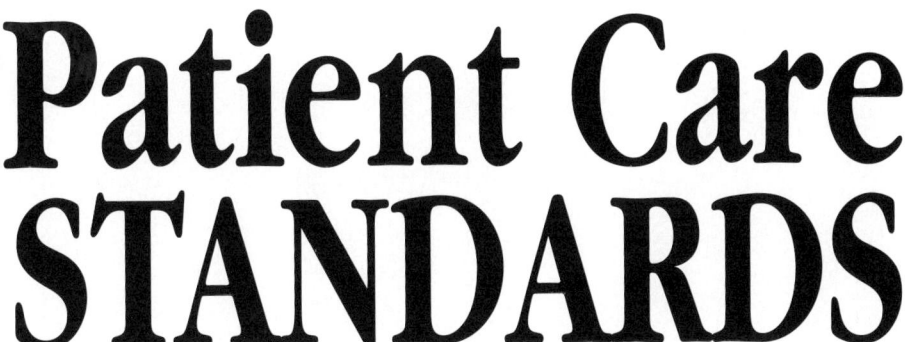

Patient Care
STANDARDS
Collaborative Planning
& Nursing Interventions

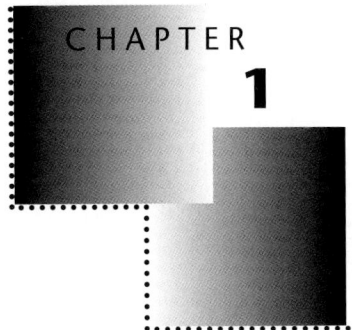

Introduction: Guides for Collaborative Patient Care

Patient care standards are plans for multidisciplinary practice representing the predicted care requirements for patients. They are based on an analytical and problem-solving sequence of assessment, planning, intervention, and evaluation. Expected outcomes, patient/family teaching, and home care considerations are delineated. At one time, planning for patient care was done exclusively by nurses, based on requirements and standards of licensing and accrediting bodies and taught in the curriculum of nursing education programs. The nursing process (assessment, diagnosis, planning, intervention, and evaluation) has been successfully used by nurses to plan patient care for years. Now that patient care is more patient centered rather than provider centered, and because patients and their families/significant others are involved as partners in the planning and often the provision of patient care, it has become imperative to provide a more collaborative approach to the provision of care.

The goal of patient care is to provide individualized, planned, and appropriate care in settings that support the patient's care, treatment, rehabilitation goals, and specific needs. The patient's individualized plan of care must be consistent with the medical plan for care, as well as the therapeutic plans of the multidisciplinary healthcare team. Patient care standards focus on the recipient of care, the patient, and provide the framework for effecting multidisciplinary care.

Many healthcare organizations use published references, such as *Patient Care Standards,* on each patient care unit for guiding patient care and nursing interventions. Others create their own institution-specific plans of care for their patients via preprinted care plans, computer-based online plans of care, or multidisciplinary care pathways. The requirements and standards of licensing and accrediting bodies such as the Joint Commission on Accreditation of Healthcare Organizations (JCAHO) accept a variety of means for patient care planning. The JCAHO does not prescribe any particular format for the planning of care but evaluates compliance with the standards of the *Accreditation Manual for Hospitals* based on the scoring guidelines. A clear understanding of the standard, associated intent language and scoring guidelines is all that is necessary to ensure that the patient care delivered at the institution is congruent with JCAHO standards.

Critical paths, care paths, and clinical maps have provided a more consistent timeline methodology to plan for patient care. The timeline is viewed from left to right and divided into days, periods, or hours depending on the condition or diagnosis. Variation exists among institutions in the categories of care that are delineated across the course of time. The content of *Patient Care Standards* can be used to create a timeline care path by denoting the particular assessment, diagnosis/patient problem, intervention, and expected outcomes in the appropriate category identified by the institution. A variety of timeline care paths are provided as examples to the user of *Patient Care Standards* in this chapter, as well as in most of the other chapters. There is no right or wrong means to the development and use of timeline care paths. Variations in format will and should occur in different institutions in order to meet the particular needs of patients and multidisciplinary providers of care in a particular facility.

It is important for any institution creating timeline care paths to list the items that are important to include, and the examples herein should provide a springboard for discussion of these items. Chart reviews of the past several patients with a particular diagnosis (DRG) may be helpful if there is no consensus as to when an activity should occur. Significant learning can be gleaned from plotting out the activities in a timeline format on the same diagnosis of multiple patients, especially when managed by multiple providers. Physicians and other healthcare providers are often surprised at the differences in managing the same type of condition, and this data-driven approach is more objective than unsupported subjective comments as to the appropriate time frame for the management of patient care.

In summary, the strides being made in providing a multidisciplinary approach to patient-centered care can only enhance the well-being of the population and better use our precious and limited resources. *Patient Care Standards* guides multidisciplinary practice whether used exclusively or as a source for creating a timeline-based plan of care.

page 1 of 2

Interdisciplinary Care Path:

UNCOMPLICATED MI CARE PATH

Expected Length of Stay: 4.5

This Plan of Care has been discussed with patient/significant other. Date: _____
Signature: _____, RN
If discussed with someone other than the patient, specify.
Name: _____ Relationship _____
If "NA," explain: _____

Addressograph

Patient Care Problems	Patient Outcomes	Emergency Dept. Date:	Day 1 Date:	INTERVENT Day 2 Date:	Day 3 Date:	Day 4 Date:	D/C Date:
1. Alteration in comfort related to anginal pain/myocardial hypoxia.	1. The patient will report pain level of 0 on a scale of 0-10. Date: _____ *If not achieved, a narrative note must be written.*	— BR — O_2 — Cardiac monitor — IV access — RN cardiac assessment — Discuss plan of care	— BR — O_2 — ASA — NTG SL ordered — MS IV ordered — Cardiac monitoring — IV access — RN cardiac assessment — Obtain rhythm strip — Assess CP q4 hrs Scale 0-10	— BR with BRP — O_2 — Cardiac Monitoring — IV access — RN cardiac assessment — Obtain rhythm strip — Assess CP q4 hrs Scale 0-10	— Ambulate — DC O_2 — Telemetry Monitoring — RN cardiac assessment — Obtain rhythm strip — Assess CP q4 hrs Scale 0-10	— Ambulate — DC Telemetry Monitoring — O_2 — RN cardiac assessment — Obtain rhythm strip — Assess CP q4 hrs Scale 0-10	— DC Saline Lock
2. Alteration in tissue perfusion related to cardiac ischemia/damage and dysrhythmia.	2. The patient will be hemodynamically stable with a MAP≥60 Date: _____ *If not achieved, a narrative note must be written.*	— ECG — CXR — CBC — LYTES	— CPK#1 with ISOS on admission — CPK#2 8 hours after admission — CPK#3 16 hours after admission — Continue CPK every 8 hours until CPK is normal	— ECG	— ECG	— ECG	

INSTRUCTIONS FOR USE: *Initial* if intervention *initiated* Leave blank if intervention *not initiated* Write NA if intervention *not applicable*	If the intervention is not initiated within 24 hours, document a narrative note. A narrative note is not required for NA (not applicable).	Staff assures that the care path is reviewed and variances are documented.	Discharge to: Home ☐ SNF ☐ HH ☐ SOC ☐ Date: _____ Time: _____ SOC: _____

Used by permission of Kaiser Permanente Medical Center; Kaiser Foundation Hospital, Martinez, California.

INTERVENTIONS

Patient Care Problems	Patient Outcomes	Emergency Dept. Date:	Day 1 Date:	Day 2 Date:	Day 3 Date:	Day 4 Date:	D/C Date:
2. continued			— Chest pain ☐ None ☐ Relieved with medication ☐ ECG done with persistent chest pain	— Chest pain ☐ None ☐ Relieved with medication ☐ ECG done with persistent chest pain	— Chest pain ☐ None ☐ Relieved with medication ☐ ECG done with persistent chest pain — ETT ☐ Scheduled ☐ Not indicated ☐ Not available	— Chest pain ☐ None ☐ Relieved with medication ☐ ECG done with persistent chest pain — ETT ☐ Scheduled ☐ Not indicated ☐ Not available	
3. Knowledge deficit related to disease process, prescribed regimen, and diagnostic tests.	3. The patient/ significant other will communicate understanding of diet, activity, and disease process. Date: ___ If not achieved, a narrative note must be written. 4. The patient will be provided with referrals, resources, and teaching. Date: ___ If not achieved, a narrative note must be written.		— Discuss Plan of care with patient and/or family. — Assessment of discharge needs. — Patient copy of care path given to patient and/ or family.	— Implement cardiac patient learning checklist — Review patient copy of care path with patient and/or family — Give patient *An Active Partnership for the Health of Your Heart* book	— Continue patient learning checklist with patient and/ or family.	— Continue patient learning checklist with patient and/ or family.	— Complete patient learning checklist — Review discharge instructions — Review discharge medication — Schedule return appointment — Give patient copy of discharge instructions
		GRASP: 8 am-4 pm ___	GRASP: 8 am-4 pm ___	GRASP: 8 am-4 pm ___	GRASP: 8 am-4 pm ___	GRASP: 8 am-4 pm ___	GRASP: 8 am-4 pm ___
		Admission Shift	#2 Shift	#3 Shift	DC		

Emergency Dept.				Admission Shift			#2 Shift			#3 Shift			DC		
INIT	PRINT NAME	TITLE	INIT	PRINT NAME	TITLE	INIT	PRINT NAME	TITLE	INIT	PRINT NAME	TITLE	INIT	PRINT NAME	TITLE	

All assigned registered nurses are responsible to update/review and sign the patient care path each shift.

*6/94 This care path is to be used as a guideline only and does not necessarily imply a standard of care.

PATIENT STANDARD OF CARE
Chest Pain

page 1 of 2

1. We will make a plan of care to meet your basic care needs.
2. It is important that you and your family let us know about any questions or concerns.
3. We will provide a safe and clean environment.
4. We will help you understand your condition and treatments.
5. You will be asked to participate in your care.
6. We will help you plan for your continued care.

PATIENT CARE ISSUES	WHAT WE WILL DO	WHAT YOU CAN DO	EXPECTATIONS
You need information about your condition.	Health care team members will provide you with information about your condition. We will tell you about treatments, medicines you receive, and follow-up care.	Please ask any questions about your treatment and follow-up care. Let us know if you do not understand something we say or if you still have questions.	You will have the information you need and want about your treatment plan.
What will happen to you during your hospitalization?	We will take your temperature, pulse, and blood pressure as needed. We may need to wake you up at night. We may keep track of how much you eat and drink and how much you urinate. You may be on a special diet. It may be difficult for you to rest as a result of lights, noise, and treatments. We will control these as much as we can.	If you are able, help us keep track of what you eat, drink, and urinate. Ask us any questions you have about your diet. Check with the nurse before you eat or drink anything that we have not brought to you. Let us know if there is something we can do to help you rest.	You will understand the treatments and activities you experience in the hospital.

Used by permission of Kaiser Permanente Medical Center, Kaiser Foundation Hospital, Martinez, California.   *Continued*

PATIENT CARE ISSUES	WHAT WE WILL DO	WHAT YOU CAN DO	EXPECTATIONS
(During your hospitalization, cont.)	You will have tests that have been ordered by your physician such as blood samples, x-rays, and ECGs. You may have tests done while you are uncomfortable to help us diagnose or treat your problem.	Ask us if you have questions or concerns about these tests.	
	We will watch your heart rhythm continuously, through the small sticky patches we put on your chest. The signal from them appears on a special monitor screen at the nurses' station.	Try not to pull on the patches or wires.	
	We will let you know how active you can be while hospitalized and will gradually increase your activity level.	Remain in bed until instructed by staff to get up. Rest between activities.	You will be up and about with no chest discomfort or new shortness of breath.
You may experience discomfort or shortness of breath.	We may give you medicines under your tongue, on your skin, by pill, or through your IV. Oxygen, if used, will be stopped when you no longer have any discomfort and are up and around.	Tell your nurse if you have any body symptoms that make you uncomfortable or uneasy. Do not wait to see if the sensations go away on their own.	Your discomfort will be controlled or relieved to a level acceptable to you.
Plan for your continued care.	We will ask you about any special needs you have at home. We will give you written instructions about diet, activity, medications, and things you need to tell your physician. We will help you to schedule your follow-up vists with your physician.	Tell us about any concerns or needs you have. Review the instructions we give you; ask about anything that is unclear before you leave. Follow instructions closely. Before discharge, confirm the name of your physician. Arrange for someone to drive you home before 11 AM.	You will be able to care for yourself at home and gradually increase your activity to prehospitalization levels.

NOTES:

_____

_____

PATIENT LEARNING CHECKLIST   page 1 of 2

DIAGNOSIS: **MI, R/O MI, UNSTABLE ANGINA, CAD, ANGINA**
(Circle appropriate diagnosis)

INTERVENTION CODES	PATIENT / SIGNIFICANT OTHER CODES
A. Questions answered **B.** Information provided; list written materials **C.** Task demonstrated **D.** Multidisciplinary referrals; specify **E.** Refer to class	**A.** Needs instruction/reinforcement **B.** Demonstrates verbal understanding **C.** Returns demonstrations **D.** See flow record

TEACH / DEMONSTRATE	INTERVENTION				PATIENT/SIGNIFICANT OTHER RESPONSE				COMMENTS
	CODE	DATE	TIME	INITIAL	CODE	DATE	TIME	INITIAL	
A. Patient has been oriented to plan of care									
• ECG									
• Enzymes									
• Activity restriction									
• Oxygen									
• Reportable symptoms									
• Report chest pain using 0-10 scale									
B. Patient has reviewed *Take Heart* packet									
C. Patient has been referred to *Take Heart* class									
D. Teach/Demonstate									
• Anatomy and Physiology: Video 1									
• Signs and Symptoms: Videos 1, 2, and 7									
• Risk Factors: Videos 1 and 2									
• Sexual Activity: *Sensuous Heart* (Binder)									
• Diet: Video 4									
• Emotional Health: Video 6									
• Activity Programs: Videos 2 and 5									
• Quitting Smoking: Video 3									
• Other_____									

Used by permission of Kaiser Permanente Medical Center, Kaiser Foundation Hospital, Martinez, California.   *Continued*

TEACH / DEMONSTRATE	INTERVENTION				PATIENT/SIGNIFICANT OTHER RESPONSE				COMMENTS
	CODE	DATE	TIME	INITIAL	CODE	DATE	TIME	INITIAL	
E. Tests									
• Stress tests									
• Cardiac catheterization									
• Other _____									
F. Notify advice nurse of the following									
• Shortness of breath									
• Unrelieved chest pain or pain level/ patterns new to the patient									
• Fainting									
G. Discharge									
• Medications reviewed with patient									
• Instructions reviewed with patient									

INITIAL	SIGNATURE	TITLE	INITIAL	SIGNATURE	TITLE

CHAPTER
2

Dimensions of Nursing

As a science and an art, nursing is multidimensional. Patients are admitted to acute care facilities for the care and management of medical conditions and surgical and diagnostic procedures. Skilled nursing or extended care facilities care for patients with rehabilitative, convalescent, or ongoing care needs. As clinical standards of care guide the care of these patients there are other factors that require the attention of the nurse in order to provide a holistic and comprehensive approach to patient care. These aspects of care may be pertinent at any point in the continuum of care, that is, during hospitalization, postdischarge in the ambulatory setting, or in the home care environment.

This chapter focuses on those dimensions of patient care that are not related to any particular medical diagnosis or surgical procedure. These aspects of care include care of the patient with special needs, including general pre- and postoperative care, care of the aging patient, behavior problems that can occur in any environment, care of the dying patient, transcultural patient care, nutritional support, care of the patient with special equipment, and care related to patient problems or nursing diagnoses.

The last section of this chapter contains planning guides related to nursing diagnoses, to assist the nurse in selecting appropriate interventions on which to act independently. They are divided into Functional Health Patterns (Gordon, 1997). The interventions under each diagnosis are not meant to be all inclusive. The nurse must select the appropriate interventions based on the related factors, the risk factors, and the defining characteristics. The nursing diagnoses included are based on those published by the North American Nursing Diagnosis Association (NANDA). Several but not all of the NANDA diagnoses are included.

In summary, the content within this chapter should be integrated as appropriate into the patient's primary clinical standard of care. This will provide a comprehensive approach to the patient's care.

CARE OF PATIENT WITH SPECIAL NEEDS

■ GENERAL PERIOPERATIVE CARE AND EDUCATION

PREOPERATIVE ASSESSMENT
  SUBJECTIVE AND OBJECTIVE DATA
  Psychologic Status
Understanding of operative, preoperative, and postoperative procedures
Ability to verbalize fears and anxieties
Ability to concentrate
Past successful coping behaviors
Previous experience with pain relief measures
Relationship, response, and behavior of patient and family
Family's knowledge of operative procedure

  Physical Status
Nutritional and hygienic state
Elimination habits
Medication history
Medical background
    Preexisting diseases (e.g., diabetes, hypertension, bleeding disorders)
    Prior surgery
    Anesthesia history
    Substance abuse history
Allergies
Physical handicaps and other limitations
Signs of infection
Mental, visual, and auditory acuity

  Legal Status
Informed consent signed for procedure
Physician's preoperative orders complete
Identification bands on and correct
Patient's willingness to receive blood documented
Environmental orientation recorded
    Use of equipment in room
    Use of call bell
    Purpose and use of side rails

INTERVENTIONS

Maintain nothing by mouth (NPO) after midnight or according to policy

Take and record patient's baseline blood pressure (BP), temperature (T), pulse (P), respiration (R), and weight; report any abnormalities to physician

Check for and record any allergies

Monitor laboratory work; report any abnormalities to physician

Assess surgical preparations for completeness

Monitor for electrocardiogram (ECG) and chest x-ray examinations

Assess patient's skin for baseline color

Assess patient's history, physical, and anesthesia records for completeness

Assess patient's blood type and cross match results; note number of units of blood available

Administer preoperative medications; make sure that side rails are up

Insert nasogastric tube and/or indwelling bladder catheter according to policy

Initiate parenteral fluids

Encourage patient to void before leaving for operating room

Ensure that patient removes dentures, contact lenses, nail polish, makeup, prosthesis, and/or valuables before leaving for operating room; religious medals may be pinned to gown

Identify and note presence of dental implants and capped teeth

PREOPERATIVE EDUCATION

PSYCHOLOGIC STATUS

Reinforce physician's explanation of surgical procedure

Answer any questions as honestly as possible

Allow time for and encourage verbalization of fears and anxieties

Avoid standard clichés such as "Don't worry," "Everything is just fine," or "I know how you feel"

Listen to and *hear* patient

Avoid rushing through explanations

Accept patient's behavior unless it is unsafe; avoid judging patient's behavior or trying to change it

Involve family or significant other in patient's care and instructions when possible

Explain pain management plan: using patient controlled analgesia (PCA), determining pain scale, asking for medication before pain becomes severe

PHYSICAL STATUS

Explain all procedures and their reasons and importance
Preoperative
Intravenous (IV) line, indwelling urethral catheter
Skin preparation
Nothing by mouth (NPO)
Laboratory work
Bispectral index monitor to assess depth of anesthesia during procedure, as appropriate

Postoperative
Parenteral fluids
Vital signs
Dressings
Pain and availability of medications
Nasogastric and other tubes
Indwelling urethral catheter
PCA pump
Sequential compression device (pneumatic compression stockings)
Pulse oximeter
Incentive spirometer, oxygen therapy
Not touching the incision

Teach patient, using return demonstration, how to do the following:
Turn, cough, and deep breathe, depending on surgical procedure
Use spirometer
Support incision during coughing
Breathe deeply every hour after surgery
Exercise lower extremities actively
Sit up, get up, and ambulate; prolonged chair sitting should be avoided

Explain importance of progressive care
Early ambulation
Self-care encouraged as soon as patient is able

Discuss purpose of recovery room with patient and family
Visiting policies
Type of care
Length of stay if applicable
Possibility of placement in intensive care unit (ICU) if indicated

Explain other hospital policies as indicated
Visiting hours
Number of visitors
Location of waiting rooms
How physician will contact visitors after operation

■ IMMEDIATE POSTOPERATIVE CARE

ASSESSMENT

SUBJECTIVE AND OBJECTIVE DATA
General Anesthesia

Level of consciousness (LOC)
Unconscious state
Absence of cough or gag reflex
Presence of endotracheal tube or airway
Semiconscious state
Absence of endotracheal tube
Presence of oral or nasal airway
Partial return of all reflexes
Conscious state
Return of all reflexes

Respiration: rate, rhythm, depth, quality

Laryngospasm

Endotracheal tube or airway present
Position
Adequate ventilation

Pulse: rate, rhythm, quality

Blood pressure: hypotension, hypertension, normal

Parenteral infusion: flow rate, type of solution, site, patent vein, medications; observe for infiltration

Pain: location, amount, severity, type, tolerance of

Skin

    Color: normal, flushed, cyanotic, pallid

    Condition: dry, moist, hot, cold

Nail beds: color, pink, cyanotic, purple, dark brown

Return of reflexes

Type of surgery performed

Site of incision: dry, bleeding, drainage, drains

Dressing: dry, intact

Drainage tubes: patency and connections

Past and current medical problems

Spinal Anesthesia

Monitor each item under the general anesthesia section and check the patient's legs for the following:

    Mobility

    Color in dependent and independent position

    Temperature, pedal pulses

    Return of sensation

INTERVENTIONS

Maintain patent airway

    Maintain endotracheal tubes; nasal or oral airway

        Suction prn

    For an inadequate airway

        Hyperextend neck

        Bring chin forward

        Turn head to one side

        Insert oral or nasal airway

        Notify anesthesiologist of respiratory impairment

Take initial BP, P, and R and report findings to anesthesiologist

Monitor patient q15min and prn until stable

    BP, R, and apical pulse

    Pulse oximetry if applicable

    LOC

    Return of reflexes

    IV site

    Site of incision

    Drainage tubes and equipment

    Movement of extremities

Monitor rectal or axillary temperature q1h to 4h

Auscultate chest for breath sounds q30min

Administer oxygen, or incentive spirometer

Maintain NPO

Maintain parenteral fluids

Review fluid intake during operative procedure

Measure intake and output; report less than 30 ml/hr of output to physician

Reinforce dressing prn; notify physician if drainage is excessive

Administer blood and blood components as indicated

Administer all medications as ordered

Encourage patient to move his or her legs and feet, if not contraindicated

Position patient to maintain optimal ventilation and comfort

Use pain scale to assess need for analgesia

Maintain pain management; administer narcotics in one-fourth, one-third, or one-half doses until patient has reacted fully

Monitor PCA or continuous epidural anesthesia (CEA) as warranted

Keep patient warm and dry; cover him or her with warm blankets if necessary

Remain with patient if he or she is restless

Turn patient's head to one side at first sign of vomiting; suction as needed

Administer oral hygiene q1h to 4h; keep patient's mouth and tongue moist

Assist patient to turn, cough, and deep breathe q1h to 2h when reactive; provide support to incision as needed

Monitor traction equipment for accurate placement and weights

Monitor casts for position and body alignment

Maintain quiet environment; avoid discussions over patient's bed

Transfer from recovery/post anesthesia care unit to postoperative patient care unit occurs when:

    Patient is fully reactive

    Patient is moving extremities well

    Patient's vital signs have been stable for 1 hour

    Patient is medicated for pain and vital signs are stable

    Dressings have been checked and no bleeding or excessive drainage is noted

    All drainage tubes are functioning

Notify unit of patient's arrival and any equipment needed.

Accompany patient to unit and give receiving nurse a comprehensive report of his or her condition, including type of surgery, last time he or she was medicated for pain, and his or her latest vital signs

■ CARE OF THE AGING (OLDER ADULT, ELDERLY) PATIENT

DESCRIPTION

Aging: part of the continuum of life; effects vary widely from one individual to the next; does not progress at a uniform rate, and at any given time the patient may exhibit only a few of the characteristics (disease should not necessarily be equated with aging; however, when one health problem is identified, others must be suspected because multiple disease conditions are a primary characteristic of advancing years); classification of aging has changed in recent years because of increasing longevity—65 to 75 years: older adult; more than 75 years: elder-older adult

NORMAL VARIATIONS DURING THE AGING PROCESS

ASSESSMENT
SUBJECTIVE AND OBJECTIVE DATA

Eyes
- Dry and lusterless
- Discoloration of sclera, conjunctiva
- Arcus senilis (opaque ring near edge of cornea)
- Diminished pupil size, which may be opaque
- Pale brown discoloration in iris
- Diminished peripheral vision
- Decreased lens accommodation, tearing

Ears
- Hearing loss
- Initial loss of high-frequency tones

Mouth
- Loss of taste perception; dry mucous membranes
- Recession of gums if not edentulous
- Reduced acuity of taste buds
- Decreased mastication
- Increased difficulty in swallowing

Respiratory system
- Decreased tidal volume
- Decreased peripheral perfusion
- Tracheal deviation if upper dorsal scoliosis present
- Increased rigidity of chest wall
- Decreased pulmonary elasticity

Cardiovascular system
- Decreased resting heart rate and cardiac output
- Easily palpable peripheral pulse
- Decreased arterial circulation
- Increased BP; orthostatic hypotension

Gastrointestinal system
- Diminished salivation and gastric acid secretion
- Reduced gastrointestinal motility
- Decreased esophageal peristalsis
- Weight gain in women; weight loss in men
- Constipation

Renal/genitourinary system
- Decreased renal blood flow
- Frequent nocturnal micturition
- Incontinence
- Difficulty in initiating and ending the stream in male (caused by prostatic hypertrophy)

Female reproductive system
- Narrowing and shortening of vagina
- Diminished vaginal lubrication
- Dyspareunia
- Decreased estrogen production
- Decreased libido in some women
- Uterine contractions with orgasm may be uncomfortable
- Pendulous, elongated, and/or flaccid breasts

Male reproductive system
- Decrease in size and firmness of testes
- Enlarged prostate gland
- Decrease in amount and viscosity of seminal fluid
- Increased diameter of penis

- Longer duration of excitement and plateau of orgasmic phases; resolution phase may last 12 to 24 hours
- Libido and sense of satisfaction usually do not change
- Decreased testosterone production

Musculoskeletal system
- Decrease in quick voluntary movements
- Decrease in muscle mass (not necessarily associated with loss of strength)
- Diminished height, 2.5 to 10 cm
- Osteoarthritic changes in joints
    - Heberden's nodes at distal finger joints
    - Bouchard's nodes at proximal finger joints
- Dupuytren's contracture of lateral fingers, preventing full extension
- Osteoporosis (kyphosis may be an early indication)
- Broad-based stance; flexion of hips and knees

Integumentary system
- Thinning of skin over back of hands
- Decreased activity of sebaceous and sweat glands, which may result in "dry skin"
- Thinning and/or loss of scalp, pubic, and axillary hair
- Small, scattered scarlet growths (senile telangiectasis)
- Paler skin with increased pigment deposition (freckles)
- Local or general skin areas lacking pigmentation (vitiligo); increases with age
- Hyperkeratosis, or warts with raised pale, brown, or black epidermal overgrowth usually located over long axis of skin creases
- Cutaneous skin tags (acrochordons) around lower neck, axillary area; usually soft, flesh colored, and on pedicles
- Ears and nose appear large in relation to face
- Dry, wrinkled, and sagging skin
- Loss of hair and pigmentation

Neurologic system
- Decrease in conduction velocity of some nerves
- Diminished sense of smell
- Diminished sense of position
- Decreased tactile sense
- Deep tendon reflexes may be decreased
- Diminished sensitivity to hot and cold extremes in temperature
- Altered sleep patterns
- Decreased range, duration, intensity of voice

INTERVENTIONS

Assess support systems and recent changes in patient's life that may have bearing on his or her ability to meet own needs

Monitor fluid and nutritional intake
- Observe for retention, dehydration, malnutrition, or overhydration
- Assess skin turgor
- Provide fluids and food within parameters of disease process
- Assess patient's ability to chew and swallow; check for the presence of dentures
- Assess patient's food likes and dislikes
- Allow patient time to finish his or her meals

Monitor elimination patterns
    Observe for incontinence, constipation, or diarrhea;
        note frequency
    Provide bedpan or urinal within easy reach
Maintain safe environment
    Adequate lighting
    Clear passage for moving about
    Use of canes, walkers
    Assist with activities as needed
Monitor patient's activity and rest
    Observe patient's ability to perform activities of daily
        living (ADLs) and range-of-motion (ROM) exercises
    Provide balance between activity and rest
Monitor communication and social skills
    Provide alternative means of communicating as needed
    Involve patient in his or her care plan
    Encourage family or significant other to support patient
Monitor medications
    Administer medications judiciously
    Absorption, detoxification, and excretion of drugs is
        diminished; lower dosage levels and decreased
        frequency of administration may be indicated
    Assess need for analgesia carefully because sensitivity
        to pain is usually decreased
    Monitor side effects carefully
Monitor vital signs to assess cardiopulmonary function
Monitor patient's skin for redness and/or broken areas
    Provide support and frequent position changes to
        prevent pressure ulcers
    Encourage and teach good physical hygiene
    Avoid dryness by applying lanolin-based lotions on
        patient's skin

■ VOIDING MEASURES

Measures to induce voiding may be needed in any patient
    population. The following interventions have proven
    helpful.
Encourage fluids to maximum allotted for patient's
    condition
Ensure privacy
Place in proper position to urinate
    Sit upright in bed
    Use bedside commode
    Stand at bedside
    Sit on toilet with urine collection device
    Lean forward slightly if on commode or toilet
Run tap water near patient
Offer fluids: warm water, tea, or coffee
Blow bubbles in glass of water through straw
Place hands in warm water
Apply heat to suprapubic area
Pour warm water over perineum
Administer warm tub bath
Relaxation techniques
Apply oil of peppermint (a few drops in bedpan/urinal or
    on cotton ball in front of urinary meatus)
Stroke inner aspect of thigh gently with ice
Offer analgesic

Void every hour or two after fluid intake
Initiate voiding by manual stimulation
    (Crede's maneuver)
    Exert manual pressure over suprapubic region
    Contract abdominal muscles and strain down
Pull pubic hairs gently
Stroke inner aspect of thigh gently

Expected Outcomes
Voids without difficulty and does not experience urinary
    retention

■ CARE OF THE DYING PATIENT

DEATH
*An unavoidable part of life and the part most difficult
to accept; each person dies uniquely and therefore must
be cared for uniquely; that is, the nurse must develop and
maintain a positive needs-perceptive relationship with
the patient and family that will allow the patient to die
in comfort and with dignity*

NURSE SELF-ASSESSMENT/INTERVENTIONS
To care for the dying patient, you must:
    Learn about yourself and your own feelings
        concerning dying
    Look at your own ethnocultural background
    Examine your own exposure to death
        Family and friends
        Reactions to these experiences
    Be honest about your own feelings (anxiety,
        depression, avoidance, coping mechanisms)
    Examine how you view your own death
    Share your feelings about death with others; initiate
        open discussion to better understand behavior
    Learn to listen; realize that all of patient's questions do
        not require answers; often patient will answer his or
        her own questions if you do not provide "pat" answers
    Explore your feelings about life (respect, discontent)
    Recognize your own power in controlling patient and
        his or her responses to care
        Avoid using this power as threat to patient
        Use it to give respectful, humane care
        Respect patient's own plan of care
    Consider effect patient has on you; examine how you
        see patient as an individual human being
Consider the following in caring for the dying patient:
    Be aware of what physician has told patient; avoid
        conflicting statements
    Realize that decision to tell patient of outcome of
        disease lies with physician, patient, and family
    Be honest in dealing with patient who has not been
        told of impending death; ask patient what he or she
        thinks or feels about his or her question, "Am I
        going to die?"
Communicate situations and conversations with patient
    to others on the staff; provide continuity and avoid
    discrepancies in emotional care

Involve all multidisciplinary healthcare team members when
  preparing the plan of care with the patient and family

FAMILY ASSESSMENT/INTERVENTIONS
Realize that family or significant other will need support
  during patient's illness
Be aware of cultural differences as part of assessment and
  intervention process
Assess and evaluate patient's and family's feelings about
  death and work within the framework of those feelings
Identify the presence of an advance directive and power
  of attorney for health care
Do not judge actions or behavior of family
  Realize that family members may have gone through a
    lot with a long illness and are no longer able to cope
  Understand that a change in family structure is occurring
    Emotional: loss of a loved member
    Financial: long illnesses become a burden
  Be aware that preillness relationships and/or problems
    will continue
Encourage family to be involved with patient's care
  Frequent visits and telephone calls
  Staying with patient
  Bringing valued objects to patient
  Providing home-cooked meals
  Bringing children and pets for visits
Assist family in grieving process
  Understand that they also will go through the stages of
    dying
  Be aware that timing of stages is very often not the
    same as the patient's timing
  Understand that family very often may not reach stage
    of acceptance
  Work with family members so that they can let patient
    know the truth, thus permitting open and frank
    communication with patient past denial stage
Assist family in making both intermediate and long-term
  plans
Help family see patient's need to live as normally as
  possible for as long as possible
Assist family in making arrangements for home care when
  it is possible and desirable for patient
  Teach methods of care that will be required
  Arrange for help through social service department
    and community resources
  Explore possibility of hospice care

PATIENT ASSESSMENT/INTERVENTIONS
Realize that patient needs compassionate, consistent, and
  realistic care during terminal illness
Be aware that he or she is sensitive to feelings of others
  Understand that patient will avoid discussing his or
    her death and feelings if he or she senses others are
    unable to talk of dying
  Be aware that patient will often discuss feelings with
    nursing staff rather than with the physician
Provide needed hope, human contact, and caring
  Understand that hope must be realistic; patient needs
    treatment for alleviation of pain rather than getting
    well

Do not avoid patient during any of the stages of dying
  Realize that patient needs continuous caring by all
    members of staff
Support patient in understanding that his or her needs
  and those of the family will vary at a different pace as
  the patient and family progress through the stages of
  dying
Be aware that patient has many fears
  Encourage expression of feelings
  Provide an accepting environment
  Demonstrate warmth and friendliness
  Encourage use of spiritual resources
  Explore past coping strengths
  Explain all procedures and nursing functions
  Discuss patient's fears with him or her
    Fear of the unknown
    Loss of control of body and behavior
    Pain: Patient needs explanation of availability of
      different drugs and therapies, such as radiation
      or surgery
    Understand that patients who are restless, upset,
      anxious, fearful, angry, or depressed have a lower
      threshold and thus feel more pain
    Helplessness: Patient needs general nutrition, some
      activity, and deep breathing every day, which
      usually helps initially
Understand that patient needs to have each day be as
  comfortable, positive, and productive as possible
Promote self-care and diversional activities
Help patient to maintain a normal lifestyle for as long
  as possible

■ CARE DURING THE STAGES OF DYING

▌ DENIAL AND SHOCK

ASSESSMENT
SUBJECTIVE AND OBJECTIVE DATA
Ignoring or distorting reasons given for illness
Refusal to participate in care
Refusal to follow directions of physician or staff

INTERVENTIONS
Recognize that denial and shock may be used by the patient
  after he or she is told of his or her impending death
Do not interfere with this mechanism unless it becomes
  destructive (e.g., patient refuses further treatment and
  care)
Spend time with patient to show that he or she will not
  be left alone
Do not support denial; conversations should include reality
Continue to teach and encourage self-care and activities

▌ ANGER

ASSESSMENT
SUBJECTIVE AND OBJECTIVE DATA
Abusive language
Refusal of care

Refusal of nutrition and self-care
Negative criticism of staff
Striking out
> Not permitting others to be close to him or her
> Throwing objects
> Removing IV needle, leads
> Calling for nurse and then asking why nurse is there

INTERVENTIONS
Recognize that patient is not angry with you personally
Do not allow physically harmful behavior to continue
> Spend time with patient and discuss his or her anger
> Encourage verbalization of anger; be empathetic
Plan patient's care with him or her and encourage mutual problem solving
Question how patient evaluates care being given
Continue to question and discuss patient's anger
Assess need for social services

BARGAINING

ASSESSMENT
OBJECTIVE DATA
Statements such as "I hope I live until . . . ," "If only I could . . ."

INTERVENTIONS
Realize that patient needs time to accept his or her impending death
Spend time with patient
Discuss importance of valued objects and people
Set small, realistic, attainable goals
Provide praise for goals reached or attempted

DEPRESSION

ASSESSMENT
SUBJECTIVE AND OBJECTIVE DATA
Apathy
Decreased ability to concentrate
Insomnia
Inability to wake up
Crying
Constant fatigue
Poor appetite
Lack of interest in people or environment
Sitting alone

INTERVENTIONS
Recognize that patient is beginning to separate himself or herself from life
Do not attempt to cheer patient
Be available to sit quietly and, if appropriate, to hold patient's hand
Accept crying; do not interrupt
Realize that patient may only want his or her most beloved person to be with him or her
Promote positive relationships to maintain patient's dignity
Soothe patient with gentle back care and oral hygiene

ACCEPTANCE

ASSESSMENT
SUBJECTIVE AND OBJECTIVE DATA
Devoid of feelings
Absence of emotional affect
Peacefulness
Less pain and discomfort (usually)
Less anxiety

INTERVENTIONS
Plan patient's care to allow person with whom patient is comfortable to care for patient
Realize that patient may not want to be alone

■ TRANSCULTURAL PATIENT CARE*
The health care provider must focus on the way in which people of different cultures and ethnicities perceive life events and the healthcare system. To be effective, patient care must be provided in a culturally sensitive manner

SELF-ASSESSMENT
Identify your personal beliefs about persons from cultures different from your own
Review your personal beliefs and past experiences
Set aside any values, biases, ideas, and attitudes that are judgmental and may negatively affect care

PATIENT ASSESSMENT
Assess communication variables from a cultural perspective
Determine the ethnic identity of patient, including generations in this country
Use the patient as a source of information when possible
Assess cultural factors that may affect your relationship with the patient and respond appropriately

INTERVENTIONS
Plan care based on patient's communicated needs and cultural background
> Learn as much as possible about patient's cultural customs and beliefs
> Encourage patient to reveal cultural interpretation of health, illness, and healthcare
> Be sensitive to the uniqueness of patient
> Identify sources of discrepancy between patient's and your own conceptions of health and illness
> Communicate at the patient's personal level of functioning
> Evaluate effectiveness of patient care actions and modify care plan when necessary
Modify communication approaches to meet cultural needs
> Be attentive to signs of fear, anxiety, and confusion
> Respond in a reassuring manner in keeping with the patient's cultural orientation

---

Modified from Giger J, Davidhizar R: Transcultural nursing, ed 2, St Louis, 1995, Mosby (pp 19-38).

Be aware that in some cultural groups discussion concerning the patient with others may offend and impede patient care activities

Understand that respect and communicated needs are central to the therapeutic relationship

Communicate respect by using a kind and attentive approach

Learn how listening is communicated in the patient's culture

Use appropriate active listening techniques

Adopt an attitude of flexibility, respect, and interest to help bridge barriers imposed by culture

Communicate in a nonthreatening manner

Conduct verbal interactions in an unhurried manner

Follow acceptable social and cultural amenities

Ask general questions during the information gathering stage

Be patient with a respondent who gives information that may seem unrelated to the current health problem

Develop a trusting relationship by listening carefully, allowing time, and giving the patient your full attention

Use validating techniques in communication

Be alert for feedback that the patient is not understanding

Do not assume meaning is interpreted without distortion

Be considerate of reluctance to talk when the subject involves sexual matters

Be aware that in some cultures sexual matters are not discussed freely with members of the opposite sex

Adopt special approaches when the patient speaks a different language

Use a caring tone of voice and facial expression to help alleviate the patient's fears

Speak slowly and distinctly, but not loudly

Use gestures, pictures, and play-acting to help the patient understand

Repeat the message using different words

Be alert to words the patient seems to understand and use them frequently

Keep messages simple and repeat them frequently

Avoid using medical terms and abbreviations that the patient may not understand

Use an appropriate language dictionary

Use interpreters to improve communication

Ask the interpreter to translate the message, not just the individual words

Obtain feedback to confirm understanding

Use an interpreter who is culturally sensitive

Provide caregivers with a common cultural background and language if at all possible

Refer to references on cultural variations for general guidelines

Validate information with patient/family and adjust before applying the information to the patient's individualized plan of care

Communicate cultural variation information with members of the multidisciplinary healthcare team

Adjust patient care to accommodate cultural preferences as much as possible

Involve patient in adjusting environment to meet cultural needs

Obtain consultation from nutritional services to adjust meal plans to accommodate dietary preferences

Maintain flexibility in scheduling of activities

Support routines of spiritual practices

Partner with the patient's family/significant others in planning care, provision of care, education, and home care planning

Involve members of multidisciplinary care team in adjusting activities to meet cultural preferences, as appropriate

Expected Outcomes

Verbalizes feeling understood

Relates that patient care activities were adjusted to accommodate cultural needs as much as possible

Demonstrates satisfaction with healthcare providers

Experiences a satisfying therapeutic milieu in the healthcare setting

CARE OF THE PATIENT WITH BEHAVIOR PROBLEMS

■ MANIPULATIVE BEHAVIOR

DESCRIPTION

Manipulative behavior involves two ways of controlling the behavior of others to achieve one's goals: passive behavior gets needs met indirectly through others; aggressive behavior is directed against or toward others in an attempt to get one's own needs met; these two ways of interacting are used when an individual feels powerless to meet his or her own needs through assertive interaction

DESCRIPTIVE CHARACTERISTICS

Lack of insight toward problems and/or denial of problems

Inability to express anger openly

Changing subject of conversation or activity of group

Crying or acting helpless when confronted

Attention-seeking behavior such as monopolizing conversations in both social and therapeutic interactions

Constantly seeking approval and recognition

Being overly solicitous and ingratiating

Attempting to gain special attention or privileges

Demonstrating anger and feeling hurt, deserted, and unworthy when above attempts are denied

Reporting confidential information to others

Attempting to use others' weaknesses against them; playing one person against the other

Consistently breaking rules and routines and disrupting procedures

Intellectualizing and rationalizing problems away

Projecting blame onto others

Viewing self as uniquely special and deserving

Attempting to get others to rescue him or her by being helpless and boosting others' self-esteem by relying on them to fix the problem

INTERVENTIONS

Assess needs that patient is trying to meet through manipulation

Decrease patient's manipulation of staff

Avoid discussing yourself and other staff members with patient

Assign consistent staff when possible

Develop plan of care with other staff members and communicate with everyone involved with patient's care

Communicate often with other staff members to ensure continuity and consistency of approach

Point out manipulative behavior to patient if he or she states:

"You're the only one who understands . . ."

"You're the only one who cares about me"

"You're the only one I can talk to"

Caution staff not to attempt to be liked or to be patient's favorite nurse

Do not accept favors as gifts; this fosters a personal relationship

Be matter of fact in any interactions with patient

Avoid angry, negative, and punitive responses to patient when patient is being manipulative

Offer limited choices (e.g., "Would you like to ambulate now or at 9 o'clock?")

Be direct in your interactions; do not bargain or rationalize

Assist patient in recognizing his or her own patterns of manipulative behavior by providing nonthreatening similar examples

Point out relationship between need to control and inability to achieve self-control

Encourage identification of alternative and appropriate behaviors for meeting needs; use role playing

Give verbal and nonverbal positive reinforcement when patient functions without being manipulative

Encourage and support patient to verbalize his or her feelings, medical conditions, and/or surgery and current treatment; listen nonjudgmentally

Build trust through consistency and keeping promises

Assure patient that if limits are set, it is because you care and that caring and limit setting are neither mutually exclusive nor opposites

Involve patient in his or her own plan of care without allowing patient to dictate aspects of care

Expected Outcomes

Verbalizes satisfaction with improved social interaction

Demonstrates ability to define and meet needs without manipulative behavior

Participates actively in planning own care

■ DEMANDING BEHAVIOR

DESCRIPTION

Demanding behavior occurs in syndromes involving anxiety, fear, helplessness, inadequacy, inferiority, hostility, manipulation, and dependent behavior; the individual believes he or she is incapable of fulfilling own needs or having his or her needs met by making requests in a direct, matter-of-fact manner; attempts are then made to coerce others to meet these needs by making requests with forceful and manipulative behavior with implied threat

DESCRIPTIVE CHARACTERISTICS

Making frequent requests

Constant attention seeking

Attempting to coerce others to meet needs

Asking others to do what he or she is capable of doing

Displaying helplessness when making requests

Displaying anger when requests are not met immediately

Detaining staff with subsequent requests after initial request has been met

Domineering, sarcastic, or ridiculing behavior

Using threats if requests are not met

Not using proper channels of communication (e.g., goes over nurses' authority by talking to supervisors)

INTERVENTIONS

Be aware that dynamics between staff and patient can create and maintain the problem situation

Be aware that staff's responses to patient will influence whether or not patient continues to be demanding; avoid displaying annoyance or anger with patient's request; understand that such a display perpetuates patient's demands

Be aware that depersonalization caused by hospitalization promotes anxiety and contributes to patient's perception of lack of control and self-esteem

Assess patient's unfilled needs

Involve patient in deciding how his or her needs will be met

Assist patient with identifying demanding behaviors

Relate to patient your own responses to demanding behavior in nonemotional tone of voice

Assist patient with developing alternative behavior by the following actions:

Asking directly for what is wanted

Taking responsibility for behavior by using the personal pronoun "I" before a request

Becoming more aware of responses and associated feelings when requests are not met immediately

Reinforcing independently made direct questions

Do not refuse or ignore patient's request

Give reasons why requests cannot be met

Anticipate realistic requests and meet them rapidly

Allow patient as much control in his or her own care as possible

Spend time with patient when he or she is not demanding; set up a regular schedule of checking in with patient that is independent of call light usage

Give patient your full attention during verbal interactions and recognize positive qualities to promote self-esteem

Demonstrate interest and be attentive to patient as a person

Allow opportunity for appropriate ventilation of feelings regarding annoyances, restrictions, and feeling of powerlessness

If you tell patient that you will return in 20 minutes, be sure that you do

Avoid withdrawing from patient by insensitive mechanistic actions

Expected Outcome

Demonstrates ability and willingness to learn to meet needs without having to resort to demanding behaviors

■ WITHDRAWN BEHAVIOR

DESCRIPTION

Withdrawn behavior is an attempt to avoid interaction with others and thus avoid relatedness; it is a defense against anxiety that is related to a stressor or threat; the range of behavior can be from disinterest in others to severe withdrawal with an accompanying increase in primary process thinking; this may ultimately lead to autistic behavior or delusions and hallucinations as the individual withdraws more from the environment and attends to internal thoughts and stimuli

DESCRIPTIVE CHARACTERISTICS

Dull, flat, or inappropriate affect/mood

Apathy

Depression

Absence of spontaneity

Inappropriate response to environmental stimuli

Excessive fear and increasing levels of anxiety

Decreased or absent verbalization

Decreased motor activity or agitation

Lack of awareness of surroundings

Inattention to grooming and personal habits

Inappropriate social behavior, including open masturbation, obscene language, handling of excreta

Regression (the patient may assume the fetal position)

Disturbance in thought content, such as delusions

Disturbance in perception, such as hallucinations

INTERVENTIONS

Communicate with patient in a positive, accepting manner

Plan time to sit with patient

Make sure that you have patient's attention before speaking or giving directions on care

Avoid attempts to ououtverbalize with patient

Remain comfortable during silent periods

Ask open-ended questions, not "yes" or "no" questions

Expect patient to respond to conversation

Provide reality-oriented conversation focusing on the here and now; avoid generalizations and abstract concepts

Allow sufficient time for patient to respond

Avoid placing patient in a private room

Administer psychotropic medications and antidepressants as ordered

Measure intake and output if indicated

Assist with meeting patient's basic needs (e.g., eating, drinking, elimination, bathing, and ambulation)

Assist and teach range-of-motion (ROM) exercises; turn patient q2h if bedridden

Maintain skin integrity

Use television and/or radio in room

Provide newspapers and magazines

Involve patient in his or her plan of care

Assist patient with identifying alternative and appropriate behaviors

Orient patient to time, place, and person; use clock and calendar in room

Provide positive reinforcement for self-care activities

Be aware that logical arguments only increase delusional thought content

Encourage and support verbalization of feelings about concrete issues (e.g., medical condition, menu)

Decrease anxiety level (see anxiety care plan, p. 56)

Provide a regular schedule of activities (routines)

Use empathy (e.g., "That must be frightening.")

Gradually introduce patient to more people in environment

Expected Outcomes

Exhibits a decrease in withdrawn behavior, depression, and social isolation

Demonstrates an increase in social interactions

Exhibits an increase in self-care and other functional task activities

■ DEPENDENT BEHAVIOR

DESCRIPTION

Dependent behavior includes impaired decision making; a tendency to lean on others for guidance, direction, support, protection, and advice; and a compelling need to relate to a stronger person in coping with stressors

DESCRIPTIVE CHARACTERISTICS

Constant attention seeking

Whining

Helplessness when making a request

Refusing to make decisions

Asking others to do what he or she could do himself or herself

Feeling no responsibility for the following:

Decisions

Behaviors

Feelings

Thoughts

Lack of initiative

Low self-esteem

Procrastination

Passiveness

Low frustration tolerance

Lack of social skills
Few adaptive coping skills
Lack of problem-solving skills
Moderate interpersonal anxiety
Moderate-to-severe depression
Covert expressions of anger
Repeated hospitalizations; many physical complaints
Substance abuse and/or dependency
Inability to define or express needs appropriately

INTERVENTIONS
Assess for suicidal thoughts and behaviors
Assess patient's dependence on drugs and/or alcohol
Maintain consistent approach
  Set limits for unrealistic and inappropriate requests
  Use calm, firm tone of voice when speaking
  Do not display anger or frustration toward patient
  Do not reward attention-seeking behavior
  Meet patient's dependency needs at first, then
    gradually assist patient to become more
    independent in stages: (1) do for patient; (2) do
    with patient; (3) allow patient to take lead while
    you provide support; (4) provide positive
    reinforcement for independent behaviors
  Avoid making simple decisions for patient
  Offer alternative choices
  Investigate physical symptoms reported by patient, but
    do not encourage "sick role" behavior
  Assist patient with verbalizing and identifying strengths
  Do not be the only person with whom the patient can
    talk; involve other staff with patient
  Avoid feelings of sympathy; do not give your phone
    number to patient or allow patient to call you at
    work or home
  Assist patient with identifying consequences of
    behavior, including indecisiveness
  Assist patient with expressing anger in open and direct
    manner when his or her demands or requests are
    not met
  Positively reinforce expression of genuine feelings
  Refer patient to self-help groups when appropriate
  Teach patient about physical and/or psychologic
    dependency that occurs with continued use of
    tranquilizers and/or alcohol

Expected Outcomes
Assumes responsibility for major areas of life
Resumes appropriate role functioning
Reports satisfying social interactions
Makes decisions independently
Copes with stressors without using tranquilizers and/or
  alcohol

■ ASSAULTIVE BEHAVIOR

DESCRIPTION
*An unlawful act that places another person, without
that person's consent, in fear of immediate bodily harm
or battery. The act must be apparently possible, thus*
*causing well-founded apprehension in the victim. Health-
care personnel and visitors can be the victims in the
healthcare setting*

DESCRIPTIVE CHARACTERISTICS
Actual threats of harm
Screaming, yelling
Actual grabbing, hitting, scratching, or kicking
Spitting or biting
Throwing object at someone
Refer to Risk for violence directed at others for other
  descriptive characteristics (p. 63)

INTERVENTIONS
Intervene to protect the patient and others from harm
Speak in calm, firm manner
Obtain assistance from other staff members
Defuse hostility when patient has legitimate complaint
Do not touch patient
Do not invade personal space
Give patient as much control over his or her own area as
  is safely possible
Offer medication early in preescalation phase
Administer chemical restraint (medications) according to
  orders and policy
Be aware of own feelings in response to patient's behavior
Refer to Risk for violence directed at others for other
  interventions (p. 63)

Expected Outcomes
Does not commit battery
Uses alternative ways to manage expression of anger
Displays effective coping strategies in reducing anxiety
  and resolving issues with healthcare team
Develops increased self-awareness and increased self-esteem

■ DISORIENTATION

DESCRIPTION
*Disorientation is the inability to correctly identify self
in relation to time, place, or person*

DESCRIPTIVE CHARACTERISTICS
Chronic dementia
Acute delirium
Psychomotor agitation
Insomnia
Excessive fear
Visual or auditory hallucinations
Aggressive behavior
Purposeless or repetitive activity
Reversible causes (e.g., alcohol intoxication, altered
  cerebral blood flow, dehydration, electrolyte
  imbalance, high fever, infection, metabolic disturbance,
  sleep pattern disturbance, toxic reactions, head
  trauma, malnutrition, sensory deprivation or overload,
  overmedication)
Irreversible causes (e.g., senile dementia [Alzheimer's
  disease], AIDS dementia, chronic progressive neurologic

conditions, neoplasms that are present with the following behaviors: psychomotor agitation or retardation, disinterest in personal care, confabulation, "sundowner's" syndrome [extreme nocturnal agitation], short-term memory loss, inability to concentrate, loss of intellectual abilities, delusions, lability of affect and concrete thinking)

INTERVENTIONS

Assess causative factors and possible etiology of disorientation (acute and reversible delirium versus chronic and irreversible dementia)

Treat acute delirium as a medical emergency

Protect patient from self-injury with attention to equipment at bedside

Provide soft restraints or restraint jacket to prevent unescorted wandering

Cover patient adequately to avoid unintentional physical exposure

Wear clearly visible name tag

Orient patient to place and time before giving him or her care

Speak in kind tone; use short and simple sentences

Give one direction at a time

Adjust lighting to prevent shadows and distortions

Leave on a night light

Assist patient in self-care activities

Maintain a therapeutic environment; orient patient to room: display familiar items, place personal items in accessible place, display clock and calendar, and keep equipment and possessions in same place

Post list of daily activities in clear view

Label bathroom and other areas with large-lettered signs or use a color code to help patient identify personal items and room

Encourage ambulation when possible

Encourage socialization

Provide radio, television, or newspapers

Address patient by name

Tell patient when you do not understand his or her statements

Do not point out deficits of behavior

Do not laugh at misinformation or misperceptions

Provide repetitive schedules

Encourage independence

Encourage visits from family and significant others

Assess patient's response to visitors

    Assist family with its emotional reactions

    Help family to set realistic goals

Provide patient with tasks that do not require new learning

Give positive reinforcement for participation in activities

Provide same staff when possible

Expected Outcomes

Demonstrates reality testing

Dismisses internal voices

Demonstrates increased cognitive functioning

Controls inappropriate and impulsive behaviors

Demonstrates ability to function in a structured setting

Interacts with environment

NUTRITIONAL SUPPORT

■ ENTERAL NUTRITION

Provision of nutritional support to meet nutritional requirements via a nasogastric tube, orogastric tube, esophagostomy, gastrostomy, duodenostomy, or jejunostomy; preferred for the patient who has a functional gastrointestinal (GI) tract but is unable to consume an adequate nutritional intake or when oral intake is contraindicated; may be indicated in the following clinical conditions: physical impairments (e.g., obstructive lesions of the esophagus or pharynx, following radical head and neck surgery, following fracture of facial bones); neurologic conditions associated with impaired swallowing and oropharyngeal trauma; increased metabolic needs caused by trauma, burns, or sepsis; or the presence of an endotracheal tube. Lactose-free nutritional support should be provided for patients with a lactase deficiency

ASSESSMENT
SUBJECTIVE DATA

Abdominal cramping, pain, feeling of fullness

Nausea

Dry mucous membranes

Constipation

OBJECTIVE DATA

Dietary history

Lactose intolerance

Food allergies, dietary restrictions

Medical history

    Chronic renal disease

    Liver disorders

    Diabetes mellitus

    Heart disease

Cerebrovascular accident (CVA)

    Coma

Respiratory problems

    Respiratory distress

    Aspiration

    Coughing

    Choking

    Cyanosis

    Increased respiratory rate

    Decreased breath sounds

    Rales at lung bases

Skin and mucous membranes

    Skin irritation and/or breakdown, nares, ostomy tube

    Poor skin turgor

    Diaphoresis

Level of consciousness

    Coma

    Change in mental status

Gastrointestinal system

    Vomiting

    Diarrhea

    Abdominal distention, delayed gastric emptying

Decreased or absent bowel sounds
Esophageal reflux
Gastric residual
Tube placement: nasogastric, nasoduodenal,
    nasojejunal, gastrostomy, jejunostomy, percutaneous
    endoscopic gastrostomy (PEG)

DIAGNOSTIC TESTS

Serum electrolytes, complete blood count (CBC)
Serum osmolality
Serum glucose
Urine glucose
Urine specific gravity
Blood urea nitrogen (BUN)
Serum creatinine
Serum albumin
Serum transferrin

POTENTIAL COMPLICATIONS

Hypernatremia
Hyperchloremia
Azotemia
Dehydration
Tube feeding syndrome
Hyperglycemia
Nausea
Vomiting
Pulmonary injury during insertion
Aspiration/pneumonia
Diarrhea
Constipation
Gastric retention
Fluid overload
Gastric rupture
Dumping syndrome
Weakness
Diaphoresis
Light-headedness
Tachycardia
Cramping
Tube displacement
Tube obstruction
Intraperitoneal leakage and leakage of fluid around
    catheter (associated with gastrostomy and jejunostomy
    tubes)

MULTIDISCIPLINARY MANAGEMENT
THERAPEUTIC MANAGEMENT

Treatment of underlying disease process
Desired route (e.g., ostomy, PEG)
Tube selection (small-bore tubes generally used)
Type of formula (concentration and rate)
Intermittent or continuous feeding
Antidiarrheal agents
Laxatives
Insulin
Intake and output
Daily weights
Daily laboratory studies
Formula preparation and distribution

PATIENT PROBLEMS—NURSING DIAGNOSES/INTERVENTIONS

▼ Diarrhea related to altered dietary intake, malabsorption, concomitant drug therapy, type of formula, bacterial contamination, stress/anxiety

Record color, odor, amount, and frequency of stool
    every day
Monitor intake and output q8h
Monitor stool for occult blood
Weigh patient daily at same time and in same clothing,
    using same scale
Assess for signs and symptoms of dehydration
    Poor skin turgor
    Decreased urine output
    Increased urine specific gravity
    Dry mucous membranes
Monitor laboratory results; report any abnormalities to
    physician
Review current medications, antibiotics, cimetidine, other
    H_2 blockers, electrolyte elixirs, and antacids for
    possible side effects such as diarrhea
Assess for intolerance to feeding solution q4h
Report untoward reactions to physician immediately:
    Abdominal distention, delayed gastric emptying
    Nausea
    Vomiting
    Cramping
Auscultate bowel sounds q4h
Report hyperactive or hypoactive bowel sounds to physician
Assess for gastric residual q4h
If gastric residual is greater than 100 ml, discontinue
    feeding and notify physician (replace residual)
Avoid rapid rate of infusion
    Initiate tube feeding slowly at half-strength
        concentration or as ordered by physician
    Increase rate according to patient tolerance
    Regulate flow rate using enteral pump (some IV infusion
        pumps can be adapted to deliver enteral feedings)
    Place time tape on formula bag or bottle; monitor rate q1h
    Give formula at room temperature
    Administer antidiarrheal agents as ordered
Avoid formula with high osmolality and high fat content
    Contact physician regarding change in formula
    Administer enteral feedings at approximate serum
        osmolality
    Administer dilute strength and/or decrease volume as
        ordered by physician
Intervene for lactose intolerance
    Contact physician regarding change to lactose-free formula
    Delete all dairy products from patient's diet
Avoid bacterial contamination
Wash hands thoroughly before preparing and handling
    formula
Use ready-mix formula whenever possible
Allow formula to hang for no longer than 8 to 12 hours;
    nocturnal feedings are best because they interfere less
    with daily activities
Refrigerate unused formula

Rinse feeding container and gavage set between feedings
Flush tube with water when feeding tube is disconnected
Change feeding container and gavage set daily

Expected Outcomes
Tolerates tube feeding volume, concentration, and
formula type
Evacuates soft-formed stool every other day
Maintains hydration and weight

▼ Risk for aspiration related to reduced level of consciousness, diminished or absent cough and gag
reflexes, incompetent esophageal sphincter, delayed gastric emptying, displaced feeding tube

Use small-bore feeding tubes: less likely to disrupt the
esophageal sphincter and cause reflux
Ensure correct placement of tube in stomach q4h; with
small-bore tube, an x-ray examination may be
necessary to confirm tube's placement
Confirm placement of all intestinal tubes by x-ray
examination
Keep head of bed elevated at 30 to 45 degrees during
feeding periods and 1 hour after feedings
Clamp feeding tube when patient must be placed flat
Check for gastric residual q4h for continuous feeding and
before each intermittent or bolus feeding
Report to physician if gastric residual is 100 ml or more;
discontinue feeding
Replace aspirate: prevents loss of gastric juices and
electrolytes
Assess patient for cramping, bloating, nausea, and
abdominal distension
Auscultate bowel sounds q4h
Monitor BP, T, P, and R, q4h
Inflate cuff for cuffed tracheostomy tube or endotracheal
tube; keep it inflated for 1 hour after feeding
Assess for signs and symptoms of aspiration; report any
findings to physician
    Shortness of breath (SOB)
    Fever
    Cough
    Discolored tracheal aspirate
    Increased respiratory rate
    Cyanosis
    Diminished breath sounds
    Rales/rhonchi
Before removal of orogastric or nasogastric tube, irrigate
and clamp or pinch tube to minimize risk of aspiration
when tube is withdrawn

Expected Outcomes
Breath sounds are normal as evidenced by
    No rales or rhonchi
    No cough
Temperature is within normal limits

▼ Fluid volume deficit related to insufficient fluid intake and abnormal fluid loss associated with high
osmolality of enteral feeding

Assess patient q8h for signs and symptoms of fluid
volume deficit
Report the following to physician
    Poor skin turgor
    Decreased urine output
    Dry mucous membranes
    Weight loss greater than 0.5 kg/day
    Decreased BP
    Increased urine specific gravity
Measure intake and output q8h
Weigh patient daily (same time, clothing, scale)
Increase free water administration via feeding tube as
prescribed; thereafter flush feeding tube with 30 to
50 ml of water q4h to 6h
Monitor urine specific gravity q8h
Administer hypertonic formulas using a half-strength
concentration
Change hypertonic formula to isotonic formula
Document patient's baseline mental status
Assess patient's mental status q4h; report any changes to
physician
Monitor continuous feedings qh
Use enteral pump to regulate rate of feedings
Monitor urine or serum glucose levels q6h or as ordered

Expected Outcomes
Maintains good skin turgor and color
Maintains moist mucous membranes
Maintains weight
Maintains urine specific gravity within normal limits

▼ Constipation related to formula composition, inadequate water intake, and immobility

Ensure administration of high-residue formula
Increase free water administration via feeding tube as
prescribed
Flush feeding tube with 30 to 50 ml of water q4h to 6h
Administer stool softener as prescribed
Administer 4 to 6 oz of prune juice daily through tube, if
prescribed
Monitor medications (e.g., narcotics) for their possible
side effects
Encourage physical activity within limits
    Assist with ambulation
    Assist patient to chair twice a day
    Change patient's position q2h
    Monitor for fecal impaction
    Allow patient adequate time in bathroom or with
        commode or bedpan
    Provide privacy
    Monitor patient's bowel elimination pattern

Expected Outcomes
Tolerates tube feeding and maintains weight
Evacuates soft, formed stool every day

▼ Impaired tissue integrity related to pressure from
feeding tube and/or drainage from ostomy tube
insertion site

Use small-bore feeding tube when possible

Position tube to prevent undue pressure on nares

Cleanse and lubricate nares q4h and prn

Provide oral care q4h and prn

Provide skin care at insertion site of ostomy tube

Encourage nasal breathing, rather than oral, to prevent dry mouth

Provide lozenges or hard candy, if allowed

Assess tube insertion site q8h for tenderness, redness, and drainage

Report any abnormalities to physician

Change ostomy/PEG site dressing q2h and prn

Cleanse site with soap and water and allow it to air-dry

Apply stoma adhesive around tube at insertion site

Cover site with transparent or similar dressing

Secure ostomy/PEG tube

Report any continuous leakage around tube to physician

Expected Outcome

Skin around the tube insertion site is clean and dry

▼Body image disturbance related to change in appearance resulting from nasal or ostomy tube

Assess patient's level of anxiety and understanding of need for tube feedings; if feasible, select and/or change to a feeding tube that patient tolerates physically and psychologically

Encourage patient to express his or her feelings about the way he or she feels and looks

Reassure patient that his or her feelings are appropriate

Continue to be sensitive to patient's needs and feelings

Assess for patient's readiness to begin self-care

Instruct patient and/or significant other regarding feeding procedure

Provide emotional support and positive feedback for patient's participation in his or her feeding

Provide opportunity for questions and reinforce instructions as necessary

Continue to support coping efforts

Provide referrals (e.g., social service, nutritionist or registered dietitian, support groups, clergy) as necessary

Encourage ambulation if not contraindicated

Provide small amounts of patient's favorite foods orally, if allowed

Expected Outcomes

Expresses understanding of need for tube feeding

Copes with imposed restrictions

Participates in own care

Shares feelings about how he or she views himself or herself

Additional Nursing Diagnoses to Consider

Perceived constipation related to belief that lack of daily bowel movement indicates constipation

Fatigue related to nutritional deficiencies

PATIENT/FAMILY TEACHING
PURPOSE AND ADMINISTRATION OF TUBE FEEDINGS

Explain that all necessary nutrients—protein, fats, carbohydrates, vitamins, and minerals—will be supplied by tube feeding

Discuss formula selection and reason for its choice

Instruct patient and/or significant other in formula preparation, storage, feeding schedule, and proper cleaning of equipment

Instruct patient and/or significant other how to administer formula and medications via feeding tube; administer only prescribed medications

COMPLICATIONS

Discuss signs and symptoms of feeding intolerance (e.g., nausea, vomiting, diarrhea, cramping, bloating, flatulence); discuss importance of reporting any signs and symptoms to physician

Explain reasons for administering feeding with patient in an upright position

Demonstrate procedure for checking placement of feeding tube to patient and family or significant other

Discuss signs and symptoms of possible aspiration (e.g., coughing, choking, difficulty in breathing, elevated temperature); discuss importance of reporting any signs and symptoms to physician

Discuss importance of flushing tube with water after each feeding and after administration of medications

Demonstrate urine and/or serum glucose checking procedure; discuss importance of reporting any abnormalities to physician

Discuss measures to prevent constipation

Contact home health nurse if tube is clogged, broken, or dislodged

NASAL, PEG TUBE, AND ENTEROSTOMY CARE

Demonstrate proper taping of tube to prevent slipping

Demonstrate cleansing and lubrication of nares; explain that this should be done q4h and prn

Teach importance of maintaining good oral hygiene

Demonstrate ostomy/PEG care

Discuss importance of reporting any redness, drainage, foul odor, or tenderness around stoma to physician

Teach patient how to remove and insert ostomy feeding tube per physician order (esophagotomy and gastrostomy tubes may be removed after several weeks and inserted only for feedings)

Demonstrate use of flow sheet for record keeping

ACTIVITY

Instruct patient to increase activity/exercise as desired and tolerated

Discuss benefits of exercise

    Promotes feeling of well-being

    Increases gastric motility

DISCHARGE/HOME CARE PLANNING

Assess and continue with patient and family education; monitor following:

    Caregivers' ability to prepare and administer tube feedings

Purchasing of needed supplies
Use of flow sheet
Ability to care for tube/PEG
Activity tolerance
Rest and exercise
Urine, serum glucose testing
Presence of telephone and numbers of home health
  team

■ TOTAL PARENTERAL NUTRITION

Infusion of necessary nutrients—amino acids, fat, trace elements, carbohydrates, vitamins, and electrolytes—through a peripheral or central vein; peripheral or central venous nutrition may be chosen when the enteral route is not available because of mechanical or functional abnormalities of the GI tract; clinical conditions that may indicate the need for parenteral nutrition are short bowel syndrome, ileus, malabsorption, pancreatitis, hypermetabolic states (trauma, sepsis), altered metabolic states (acute renal failure, hepatic insufficiency), burns, and cancer

ASSESSMENT
SUBJECTIVE DATA
Pain, discomfort at insertion site

OBJECTIVE DATA
Insertion site
  Warmth
  Redness
  Edema
  Drainage at insertion site
  Leakage at insertion site
Fever
Leukocytosis
Glucose intolerance

DIAGNOSTIC TESTS
Potassium
Phosphorus
Magnesium
Blood glucose
Calcium
Sodium
Chloride
BUN
Prothrombin time (PT)
White blood cell (WBC) count, urinalysis
Liver enzymes
Bilirubin
Serum albumin
Transferrin

POTENTIAL COMPLICATIONS
Mechanical complications
  Pneumothorax (with subclavian vein catheterization)
  Air embolism
  Catheter and venous thrombosis
Septic complications
  Catheter sepsis (bacterial or fungal)
Metabolic complications
  Hyperglycemia
  Hyperosmolar nonketotic coma
  Hypoglycemia
  Fatty acid deficiency
  Electrolyte abnormalities
  Liver dysfunction
  Mineral and trace elements deficiency

MULTIDISCIPLINARY MANAGEMENT
THERAPEUTIC MANAGEMENT
Route of administration; peripheral or subclavian
X-ray to determine placement of central line
Keeping vein open with isotonic solution until catheter
  placement is confirmed
Rate of flow
Increase or decrease in rate of solution
Lipid emulsion
Daily weights
Urine glucose
Blood glucose monitoring
Administration of insulin, glucose
Intake and output
Daily laboratory studies (see above)
Preparation, storage, and/or dispensing of formula

PATIENT PROBLEMS—NURSING DIAGNOSES/INTERVENTIONS

▼ Risk for infection related to invasive procedure and delivery of high concentrations of glucose parenterally

Peripheral venous nutrition
Wash hands thoroughly before inserting IV needle or
  catheter
Wear gloves per Standard Precautions
Select distal veins in upper extremities
Clip or shave any hair at site according to policy
Prepare site with povidone-iodine swab and allow site to
  air-dry
Cover site with occlusive dressing
Monitor for signs and symptoms of phlebitis and/or
  infiltration
Remove catheter or needle if phlebitis or infiltration is
  present
Rotate catheter insertion site according to policy
Tape IV tubing securely
Monitor catheter site every hour
Change IV tubing q24h or according to policy
Use strict aseptic technique when assembling and
  changing administration set
Monitor vital signs T, P, and R q4h; report elevation of
  temperature to physician
Monitor blood glucose as ordered
Monitor urine for glucose as ordered, usually q6h; glucosuria may indicate impending sepsis

Ensure that final amino acid concentration does not exceed 10% dextrose

Ensure continuous infusion of lipid emulsion when 10% dextrose is infused

Refrigerate total parenteral nutrition (TPN) solution until it is ready to use

Allow solution to hang for no longer than 24 hours

Never piggyback medications other than lipid emulsion via TPN line

Securely tape needle used for piggybacking lipid emulsion

Central venous nutrition

Assist physician with inserting central line catheter

Ensure that catheter insertion is completed under sterile conditions

Ensure proper site preparation

Change central line dressing using sterile technique

Prepare site with povidone-iodine and allow it to air-dry

Apply povidone-iodine ointment to catheter site

Cover site with sterile occlusive dressing

Observe site for signs of sepsis (e.g., erythema, swelling, tenderness, drainage at insertion site)

Monitor vital signs T, P, and R q4h; report temperature elevation to physician

Monitor blood glucose

Monitor urine for glucose as ordered, usually q6h; glucosuria may indicate impending sepsis

Monitor catheter site q1h

Tape tubing securely

Do not use stopcocks on TPN line

Change IV tubing q24h or according to policy

Use strict aseptic technique when assembling and changing administration set

Allow solution to hang no longer than 24 hours

Never use line for piggybacking medications, taking central venous pressure (CVP) readings, or aspirating blood for laboratory studies

Expected Outcomes

Temperature is within normal limits

Catheter insertion site is clean, dry, and intact with no sign of redness, edema, or drainage

Laboratory values are within normal limits

▼Altered protection related to inadequate nutrition, age, anorexia, adverse reaction to therapy, surgery

Metabolic abnormalities

Monitor for signs and symptoms of hyperglycemia
- Polyuria
- Glycosuria: elevated blood sugar
- Polydipsia, polyphagia
- Dimmed, blurred vision

Monitor for signs and symptoms of hypoglycemia
- Tachycardia
- Cold sweat
- Posterior occipital headache
- Irritability, jitteriness
- Lethargy
- Blood glucose level of less than 60 mg/dl

Perform urine and/or serum testing q6h

Monitor vital signs and electrolytes q4h

Assess patient's neurologic status q8h

Monitor intake and output q8h

Weigh patient daily (same time, scale, clothing)

Initiate TPN solution slowly

Increase rate per patient's tolerance and physician's order

Do not increase rate to "catch up"

Monitor flow rate of solution, using infusion control device

Do not interrupt infusion for more than 1 hour q8h

Ensure patency of line

For hyperglycemia, administer insulin

For hypoglycemia, administer IV 50% dextrose

Taper solution before discontinuing

Review medications that may affect glucose metabolism

Assess for possible sepsis

Monitor for signs and symptoms of fluid overload
- Pedal or sacral edema
- Rapid weight gain: 1 lb (0.45 kg) or more a day
- Pitting edema
- Increased BP
- Bounding pulse

Monitor for signs and symptoms of fluid deficit

Review all routine laboratory tests for any abnormalities

Assess for signs and symptoms of fatty acid deficiency, alopecia, brittle nails, desquamating dermatitis, decreased immunity, thrombocytopenia, and delayed wound healing

Report any abnormalities to physician

Pneumothorax

Auscultate patient's chest for breath sounds q1h

Assess patient's respiratory status q1h and report any signs and symptoms to physician
- Sudden onset of sharp chest pain
- Coughing secondary to pleural irritation
- Dyspnea, cyanosis, hypotension

Obtain baseline BP, apical pulse, T, and R

Keep vein open with isotonic solution until chest x-ray examination confirms correct placement of central line

Air embolism

Assess for signs and symptoms of air embolism, dyspnea, tachycardia, cyanosis, and hypotension

Place patient in head-down position during subclavian or jugular vein insertion

Use locking-type connections on all central line tubing

Securely tape all tubing connections

Use air-eliminating filters when possible

Clamp catheter or assist and teach patient to perform Valsalva's maneuver during tubing changes

Reaction to total parenteral nutrition

Assess patient for dyspnea; chest, abdominal, or back pain; fever; flushing; chills; headache; decreased BP; cyanosis; diaphoresis; and/or urticaria

Stop infusion and report any of above reactions to
physician
Monitor and report elevated triglyceride levels and/or
elevated liver function tests

Expected Outcomes
Central line is patent
Laboratory results are within normal limits
Weight is stabilized and/or progressing toward his or her
ideal
Skin turgor is good
Cardiopulmonary status is within normal limits

Additional Nursing Diagnosis to Consider
Fatigue related to increased psychologic, physical
demands, and/or discomfort

PATIENT/FAMILY TEACHING
Provide patient and/or significant other with instructions
regarding the following:
Reasons for TPN
Importance of therapy
Expected outcome
Need for protection of IV site
Need for prevention of tension on central venous
catheter
Importance of intake and output measurement
(provide flow sheet)
Explain signs and symptoms to report to nurse and/or
physician, including the following:
Excessive urination
Chills
Elevated temperature
Feeling of warmth
SOB
Excessive thirst
Leakage of fluid at catheter site
Pain or tenderness at catheter site
Swelling and/or redness at catheter site
Instruct patient about the following:
Amount of physical activity allowed
Need to keep follow-up appointments
Poor skin turgor
Dry mucous membranes
Tachycardia
Hypotension
Weight loss or gain
Ensure that patient and/or significant other understands
the following:
Resources for assistance as needed
Importance of avoiding crowds and persons with
infections
How to recognize and handle possible complications
(e.g., air embolism, blood backup, catheter injury)
Ensure that patient and/or significant other demonstrates
the following:
Proper handwashing technique
Preparation and infusion of TPN solution
Use of infusion pump

Clamping catheter
Flushing catheter
Changing injection site cap
Central line dressing change
Care of catheter insertion site
Measuring and recording intake and output
Testing urine for sugar and acetone
Taking and recording temperature

DISCHARGE/HOME CARE PLANNING
Assess and continue with patient and family education
and monitor the following:
Type of solution
Schedule of infusion
Obtaining the solution
Storage of solution
Inspection of solution
Procedure for changing central line dressing
Frequency of dressing change
Supplies needed
Where to obtain supplies
Cleansing of site
Observation of site
Procedure for flushing catheter
Purpose of flushing
Frequency of flushing
Solution used for flushing
Changing injection site cap
Frequency of change
Clamping of catheter before cap change
Signs and symptoms to report to physician
Elevated temperature
Rapid weight loss or gain
Increased fatigue
SOB
Tightness in chest
Redness, swelling, or drainage at insertion site
Glucose present in urine
Presence of telephone and emergency phone
numbers, as well as those of home care team

■ ELECTROLYTE, FLUID, AND ACID-BASE BALANCE (TABLE 2-1)
Electrolytes are substances that have been dissolved in the body fluids; they are potassium, sodium, chloride, calcium, soda bicarbonate, magnesium and phosphate; the fluid concentration of these electrolytes must be maintained at a very narrow margin of normal; many diseases, conditions, and/or medications can cause an imbalance

Fluid in the body accounts for about 60% of body weight and is found in two areas: in the cells (intracellular/ICF) and between the cells and blood vessels (extracellular/ECF); it is also located in the GI tract and the CSF; an increase/decrease of the ECF can cause a fluid imbalance.

Acid-base balance is regulated by the concentration of the hydrogen ion in the body fluids; pH *is the term used*

Text continued on p. 34

Table 2-1	**Observation of Electrolyte, Fluid, and Acid-Base Imbalances**

Causes	Affected Systems	Interventions

ELECTROLYTE IMBALANCES

Hyperkalemia (Potassium Excess): Normal Values, 3.5-5.0 mEq/L; Critical Values, >6.5 mEq/L

Causes	Affected Systems	Interventions

Excessive administration of potassium chloride
Decreased renal excretion, as in renal failure, hypovolemia, potassium-sparing diuretics
Trauma to tissues such as burns and crushing injuries (will release intercellular potassium and result in hyperkalemia)
Aldosterone insufficiency
Respiratory or metabolic acidosis
Banked blood
Medications, including aminocaproic acid (Amicar), antibiotics, antineoplastic, Captopril (Capoten), epinephrine, heparin, histamine, isoniazid (INH), lithium, mannitol, potassium-sparing diuretics, succinylcholine (anectine)
Hemolysis
	Neuromuscular
	  Weakness
	  Flaccid paralysis
	  Twitching
	  Hyperreflexia
	  Paresthesia or numbness and tingling sensations, (usually affect the face, tongue, hands, and feet)
	  Apathy
	  Confusion
	Gastrointestinal
	  Diarrhea
	  Intestinal colic
	  Nausea
	  Vomiting
	Respiratory
	  Paralysis and involvement of muscles of phonation
	Cardiovascular
	  Bradycardia
	  Lethal dysrhythmias
	  Cardiac arrest
	  ECG changes
	    Tall peaked T waves
	    Shortened QT interval
	    Disappearance of P waves
	    Widening of QRS complex
	    Flat-to-absent P wave and asystole
	    Prolonged PR interval
		Observe patient for changes in heart rate, rhythm, and ECG pattern
		Be aware cardiac arrest can occur
		Restrict potassium-containing foods, fluids, and salt substitutes
		Monitor serum potassium levels
		Do not give calcium if patient is on digitalis because calcium potentiates the effect of digitalis
		Avoid potassium-containing medications such as potassium penicillin
		Administer IV glucose, insulin, and sodium bicarbonate as ordered (helps shift potassium into the cells)
		Administer cation-exchange resins as ordered (helps to remove potassium by way of GI tract)
		Peritoneal or hemodialysis may be ordered if other therapy fails

Hypokalemia (Potassium Deficit): Normal Values, 3.5-5.0 mEq/L; Critical Values, <2.5 mEq/L

Causes	Affected Systems	Interventions

Increased renal loss (diuretics; diuresis phase after burns; diabetic acidosis, Cushing's syndrome; nephritis)
Hypomagnesemia
Inadequate intake of potassium
Acid-base imbalance: alkalosis; loss from vomiting, diarrhea, excess use of laxatives, GI suction or fistulas, steroid administration, anorexia, starvation
Medications, including acetazolamide (Diamox), aminosalicylic acid (PAS), amphotericin D, carbenicillin, cisplatin (Platinol), diuretics (potassium wasting), glucose infusions, insulin, lithium carbonate, penicillin G sodium (Bicillin), salicylates (aspirin), sodium polystyrene sulfonate (Kayexalate)
	Neuromuscular
	  Muscular cramps
	  Paresthesias
	  Muscular weakness to flaccid paralysis
	  Fatigue
	  Mental confusion
	  Hyporeflexia
	  Drowsiness
	  Apathy
	  Irritability
	  Tetany
	  Coma
	Gastrointestinal
	  Anorexia
	  Nausea and vomiting
	  Abdominal distension
	  Paralytic ileus
		Monitor serum potassium and report significant changes
		Observe for signs and symptoms of metabolic alkalosis
		Watch for signs of toxicity in patient receiving digitalis (blurred vision, nausea, and vomiting)
		Monitor rate of IV administration of potassium
		Monitor intake and output (report changes)
		Encourage intake of food and fluids rich in potassium (orange juice, bananas, bouillon, meat broths, colas, tea, leafy vegetables)
		Observe for changes in heart rate, rhythm, and ECG pattern
		Determine source of potassium losses

Continued

Table 2-1	**Observation of Electrolyte, Fluid, and Acid-Base Imbalances—cont'd**	
Causes	**Affected Systems**	**Interventions**

ELECTROLYTE IMBALANCES—cont'd

Hypokalemia (Potassium Deficit): Normal Values, 3.5-5.0 mEq/L; Critical Values, <2.5 mEq/L—cont'd

	Respiratory	
	Muscle weakness	
	Paralysis of the diaphragm	
	Shallow respirations	
	Apnea	
	Death may result	
	Cardiovascular	
	Irregular rhythm	
	ECG	
	Flat or inverted T wave	
	Appearance of U wave	
	Short and depressed ST segment	
	Peaking of P waves	
	QT interval prolonged	
	Circulatory failure, hypotension, and systolic arrest;	
	Effectiveness of digitalis enhanced (to the point of toxicity)	

Hypercalcemia (Calcium Excess): Normal Values, 9.0-10.5 mg/dL (Total), 4.5-5.6 mg/dL (Ionized); Critical Values, >13 mg/dL (Total)

Causes	Affected Systems	Interventions
Hyperparathyroidism	Neuromuscular	Assess for causes
Prolonged immobilization (causes calcium displacement from bone to blood)	Generalized muscle weakness	Administer loop diuretics to increase excretion of calcium
Hypophosphatemia	Depressed or absent deep tendon reflexes (DTRs)	Administer corticosteroids and mithramycin as ordered (lowers serum calcium concentration)
Metastatic carcinoma	Drowsiness	
Alkalosis	Lethargy	Administer antacids cautiously: some contain calcium
Thyrotoxicosis	Headaches	
Vitamin D overdose	Loss of muscle tone	Position and move patient carefully to prevent pathologic fractures
Addison's disease	Ataxia	
Multiple myeloma	Mental confusion	Administer isotonic fluids as ordered
Skeletal muscle paralysis	Impairment of memory	Encourage fluid intake of 2000 to 3000 ml a day
Cardiac failure	Slurred speech	
Prolonged thiazide diuretic therapy	Personality or behavior changes	Monitor intake and output
Excessive calcium intake	Stupor or coma	Avoid dietary intake of calcium (dairy products and green leafy vegetables)
Parathyroid tumor	Pathologic fractures may occur	
Sarcoidosis	Flank or deep bone pain	Monitor serum calcium levels
Medications, including hydralazine (Apresoline), lithium, parathyroid hormone	Gastrointestinal	Observe for changes in heart rate, rhythm, and ECG pattern
	Anorexia	Observe for digitalis toxicity
	Nausea	
	Vomiting	
	Constipation	
	Epigastric pain	
	Polydipsia	
	Increased thirst	
	Cardiovascular	
	Bradycardia	
	Hypertension	
	ECG	
	QT interval shortened	
	T waves inverted	
	Ventricular dysrhythmias	
	Enhanced effectiveness of digitalis	
	Renal	
	Development of renal calculi, kidney stones	
	Polyuria	

Table 2-1	**Observation of Electrolyte, Fluid, and Acid-Base Imbalances—cont'd**		
Causes	**Affected Systems**	**Interventions**	

ELECTROLYTE IMBALANCES—cont'd

Hypocalcemia (Calcium Deficit): Critical Values, <6 mg/dL (total)

Causes	Affected Systems	Interventions
Inadequate intake of calcium	Neuromuscular	Monitor rate, rhythm, and ECG
Decreased absorption from intestine	Muscle tremors	pattern
Hypoparathyroidism	Paresthesias, especially numbness	Administer calcium gluconate or
Vitamin D deficiency	or tingling	calcium chloride 10% as ordered
Rapid dilution of the plasma by	Skeletal muscle cramps	Monitor serum calcium levels every
intravenous calcium-free	Abdominal spasms and cramps	12-24 hr
solutions	Hyperactive reflexes	Report calcium deficit to physician
Chronic renal failure	Convulsions	Monitor PT and platelet levels
Chronic malabsorption syndrome	Positive Trousseau's sign	Observe for signs and symptoms of
Neoplastic diseases	Positive Chvostek's sign	tetany
Hypomagnesemia	Emotional depression or confusion	Provide dietary calcium (e.g., cheese,
Cushing's syndrome	Anxiety, irritability	cream, milk, yogurt)
Acute pancreatitis	Gastrointestinal	Administer vitamin D as ordered
Hyperphosphatemia	Paralytic ileus	Monitor prothrombin and platelet
Extreme stress situations	GI bleeding	levels
Excessive citrated blood, alkalosis	Cardiovascular	Check for bleeding from any source
Medications, including	Dysrhythmias	(calcium aids in blood clotting)
acetazolamide, anticonvulsants	Hypotension	Monitor use of laxatives and antacids
(Dilantin), asparaginase,	Prolonged QT interval with normal	(those containing phosphate
aspirin, calcitonin, cisplatin	T wave on ECG	affect calcium metabolism)
(Platinol), corticosteroids,		
heparin, laxatives, oral		
contraceptives		

Hypernatremia (Sodium Excess): Normal Values, 136-145 mEq/L; Critical Values, >160 mEq/L

Causes	Affected Systems	Interventions
Primary aldosteronism: excessive	Neuromuscular	Sodium ↑, water ↓:
steroids (Cushing's disease)	Sodium ↑, water ↓	Increase PO fluid intake
Excessive IV administration of large	CNS depression (lethargy to coma)	Administer IV fluids as ordered
amounts of sodium chloride	Muscle weakness	Instill water with or between tube
solution without water replacement	Muscle rigidity	feedings
Renal failure (with sodium retention	Muscle tremors	Sodium ↑, water ↑:
Neurohypophyseal dysfunction (as in	Restlessness, agitation	Administer diuretics as ordered
diabetes insipidus)	Gastrointestinal	Restrict sodium intake
High-protein diets with minimal	Intense thirst	Restrict fluid intake
fluid intake	Respiratory	Monitor intake and output q8h
Diabetes mellitus	Sodium ↑, water ↑ (increase in	Weigh daily
Excessive ingestion of sodium	extracellular fluid volume) may	Monitor vital signs q8h
chloride	cause pulmonary edema:	Check urine for specific gravity
Decreased water intake, severe	shortness of breath, coughing,	
vomiting or diarrhea	cyanosis, increased respiratory	
Inadequate circulation of blood to	rate	
the kidneys (congestive heart	Cardiovascular	
failure [CHF])	Sodium ↑, water ↓: postural	
Cirrhosis of the liver	hypotension	
Recent trauma, surgery, shock	Sodium ↑, water ↑: elevated blood	
Medications, including anabolic	pressure; pitting edema	
steroids, antibiotics, clonidine	Skin and mucous membranes	
(Catapres), corticosteroids, cough	Increased sodium with decrease in	
medicines, laxatives, methyldopa	fluid intake: observe for signs	
(Aldomet), NSAIDS, oral	and symptoms of dehydration	
contraceptives	(dry mucous membranes,	
	flushed skin, elevated	
	temperature)	

Continued

Table 2-1	Observation of Electrolyte, Fluid, and Acid-Base Imbalances—cont'd	
Causes	**Affected Systems**	**Interventions**
ELECTROLYTE IMBALANCES—cont'd		
Hyponatremia (Sodium Deficit): Critical Values, <120 mEq/L		
Inappropriate ADH syndrome	Neuromuscular	Administer IV normal saline solution
Excessive intake of hypotonic fluids	Headache	as ordered (monitor rate carefully)
Severe malnutrition	Vertigo	Monitor serum sodium and potassium
Vomiting	Anxiety	levels
Diarrhea	Muscle weakness and cramps	Administer sodium orally as ordered
GI drainage from suction or fistulas	Lassitude, apathy, confusion	Maintain intake and output q8h
Severe diaphoresis	Hyperreflexia	Weigh daily
Trauma such as surgery or burns	Irritability	Encourage foods and fluids high in
Small bowel obstruction and	Tremors	sodium (milk, meat, eggs, fruit
peritonitis	Gastrointestinal	juices, bouillon)
Renal disease	Anorexia	Use normal saline for all irrigations
Administration of sodium-removing	Nausea and vomiting	
diuretics	Diarrhea	
Water intoxication (IV therapy, tap	Cramping	
water enemas)	Respiratory	
Medications, including carbamazepine	Hyperpnea	
(Tegretol), sulfanylureas,	Cardiovascular	
triamterene (hydrochlorothiazide),	Hypotension	
vasopressin	Orthostatic hypotension	
	Tachycardia	
	Thready peripheral pulse or loss of	
	peripheral pulse, collapsed neck	
	veins	
	Renal	
	Decreased urine output	
	Oliguria to anuria	
	Skin and mucous membranes	
	Flushed, dry, hot skin	
	Fever	
	Loss of skin turgor	
	Dry mucous membranes	
Hypermagnesemia (Magnesium Excess): Normal Values, 1.5-2.5 mEq/L; Critical Values, >3.0 mEq/L		
Renal failure	Neuromuscular	Avoid use of all magnesium-
Adrenal insufficiency	Drowsiness	containing medications (Maalox,
Excessive ingestion of magnesium-	Lethargy	Mylanta, and Milk of Magnesia)
containing medications	Loss of deep tendon reflexes	Monitor vital signs and level of
Diabetic ketoacidosis (with severe	Respiratory depression, coma, and	consciousness q1h
water loss)	cardiac arrest	Encourage fluid intake
Hyperparathyroidism	Gastrointestinal	Administer calcium as ordered
Excessive magnesium for	Nausea	Monitor serum magnesium levels q6h
treatment of preeclampsia	Respiratory	Observe for flushing of skin and
	Decreased respirations	diaphoresis
	Cardiovascular	
	Hypotension	
	Bradycardia	
	Weak pulse	
	Prolonged QT interval on ECG	
	Heart block	
Hypomagnesemia (Magnesium Deficit): Critical Values, <0.5 mEq/L		
Acute pancreatitis	Neuromuscular	Administer magnesium sulfate as
Malabsorption syndrome	Neuromuscular irritability	ordered
(nontropical sprue or	Tremors, tetany, increased reflexes,	When administering IV magnesium
steatorrhea)	clonus	sulfate, observe patient carefully

Table 2-1	Observation of Electrolyte, Fluid, and Acid-Base Imbalances—cont'd		
Causes	**Affected Systems**	**Interventions**

ELECTROLYTE IMBALANCES—cont'd

Hypomagnesemia (Magnesium Deficit): Critical Values, <0.5 mEq/L—cont'd

Causes	Affected Systems	Interventions
Prolonged malnutrition	Convulsions	Monitor for signs and symptoms of high serum magnesium
Diarrhea, vomiting	Disorientation	Check for loss of patellar reflex q5min
Excessive calcium intake	Agitation, depression	Monitor respiratory rate q5min
Primary hyperparathyroidism and other hypercalcemic states	Hallucinations	Observe for increased thirst, flushing of skin, diaphoresis, anxiety, or drowsiness
Alcoholism	Athetoid or choreiform movements	
Bowel resection, small bowel bypass, or inherited intestinal defects	Convulsions	Notify physician immediately if patient develops loss of patellar reflex, hypotension, or flushing of face
GI fistulas	Clonus	
Excessive renal secretion	Positive Babinski's sign	
Nasogastric suctioning	Positive Chvostek's sign	Take precautions against seizures
Diabetic ketoacidosis	Positive Trousseau's sign	Monitor blood pressure, pulse, and neurologic signs q4h
Preeclampsia	Paresthesias of feet and legs	Watch for signs and symptoms of digitalis toxicity (a deficit in magnesium may precipitate or aggravate digitalis toxicity)
	Gastrointestinal	
	Anorexia	
	Nausea	
	Dysphagia	
	Cardiovascular	Monitor serum magnesium levels q6h
	Tachycardia	Observe for diarrhea
	Hypotension	
	Atrial or ventricular premature contractions	
	Nonspecific T wave changes	

ACID-BASE IMBALANCES

Respiratory Alkalosis (Deficit of H_2CO_3, Decreased Pco_2)

Causes	Affected Systems	Interventions
Fever, bacteremia, shock	Neuromuscular	Implement measures to treat underlying problem
Hyperthyroidism	Syncope	If alkalosis is caused by anxiety, attempt to calm and reassure patient
Severe pain	Vertigo	
Hyperventilation caused by hysteria, intentional overbreathing, brain trauma, or ventilators	Headache	
	Muscle spasm	Encourage breathing into a paper bag and/or other breathing techniques
Overdose of epinephrine or salicylates	Weakness	
CNS disturbances (meningitis, encephalitis, brainstem injury)	Tingling in fingers and face	Administer sedatives as ordered
	Tetany, convulsions, or coma may develop	
Pulmonary embolism	Respiratory	
Interstitial lung diseases, CHF	Rapid respirations	
Hypoxia caused by high altitude or severe anemia	Cardiovascular	
	Dysrhythmias may occur	
	Blood gas values	
	pH: increased	
	Pco_2: decreased	
	HCO_3: normal	

Respiratory Acidosis (Excess H_2CO_3, Elevated Pco_2)

Causes	Affected Systems	Interventions
Hypoventilation	Neuromuscular	Maintain patent airway
Emphysema	Anxiety	Place patient in semi-Fowler's position
Chronic obstructive pulmonary disease (COPD)	Weakness	Suction nasal and/or pharyngeal airways and trachea as necessary
Pneumonia	Headache	Avoid sedation
Asthma	Depression of CNS	Monitor heart rate and rhythm
Pickwickian syndrome	Disorientation and coma	Administer oxygen at flow rate ordered
Barbiturate poisoning	Gastrointestinal	Monitor fluid and electrolyte levels
Brain trauma with pressure on medulla	Nausea and vomiting may occur	
	Respiratory	
	Distressed respirations	
	Cyanosis	

Continued

Causes	Affected Systems	Interventions

ACID-BASE IMBALANCES—cont'd

Respiratory Acidosis (Excess H_2CO_3, Elevated Pco_2)—cont'd

Causes	Affected Systems	Interventions

Neuromuscular disorder (Guillan-Barré, myasthenia gravis)
Spinal cord trauma
Airway occlusion
Pneumothorax
Atalectasis
Postanesthesia
Inadequate mechanical ventilation
	Cardiovascular
	  Rapid pulse
	  Ventricular fibrillation may occur
	Blood gas values
	  pH: decreased
	  Pco_2: increased
	  HCO_3: increased
		Monitor ABGs
		Assess for signs and symptoms of respiratory distress
		Administer sodium bicarbonate as ordered
		Maintain mechanical ventilation as ordered
		Perform chest physiotherapy and postural drainage as ordered

Metabolic Alkalosis (Base Bicarbonate Excess)

Causes	Affected Systems	Interventions

Ingestion of large amounts of sodium bicarbonate (e.g., baking soda or antacids)
Vomiting
Prolonged gastric suction
Diarrhea
Potassium-free IV solutions
Transfusion
Alkalosis
Adrenocortical hormone use
Excess infusion of parenteral bicarbonate
	Neuromuscular
	  Hypertonicity
	  Tetany
	  Tremors
	  Convulsions
	  Sensorium changes
	  Irritability
	  Disorientation
	Respiratory
	  Shallow, slow respirations
	Cardiovascular
	  Sinus tachycardia
	  Dysrhythmias
	Blood gas values
	  pH: increased
	  Pco_2: normal or slightly increased
	  HCO_3: increased
		Monitor accurate intake and output
		Monitor vital signs q8h
		Perform neurologic check q8h
		Take seizure precautions
		Irrigate gastric suction with isotonic solutions
		Avoid excessive amounts of $NaHCO_3$
		Avoid sedatives or hypnotics
		Administer medications, treatments, and fluids as ordered by physician

Metabolic Acidosis (Base Bicarbonate Deficit)

Causes	Affected Systems	Interventions

Diabetic ketoacidosis
Prolonged starvation
Alcohol abuse
Renal failure
Vomiting of GI contents
Systemic infections
Salicylate intoxication
Severe diarrhea
Abnormal intake of exogenous acids (e.g., ammonium chloride and ferrous sulfate)
	Neuromuscular
	  Muscle weakness
	  Headache
	  CNS depression, disorientation, stupor, coma
	Gastrointestinal
	  Nausea, vomiting, diarrhea
	Respiratory
	  Kussmaul's respirations (rapid, deep breathing)
	  Shortness of breath on exertion
	Cardiovascular
	  Cardiac dysrhythmias
	  Bounding pulse
	  Increased blood pressure
	Blood gas values
	  pH: decreased
	  Pco_2: normal
	  HCO_3: decreased
		Monitor accurate intake and output
		Monitor serum electrolyte levels
		Monitor blood gas levels
		Observe for signs of hyperkalemia
		Monitor vital signs q4h
		Perform neurologic checks q4h
		Take seizure precautions
		Administer medications, treatments, and fluids as ordered by physician

FLUID IMBALANCES

Hypervolemia (Extracellular Fluid Volume Excess)

Causes	Affected Systems	Interventions

Excess sodium intake
Malnutrition
Excessive ADH secretion
	Neuromuscular
	  Behavior change
	  Loss of attention, confusion
	  Aphasia
	  Convulsions
	  Coma and death may follow
		Monitor accurate intake and output
		Weigh daily
		Monitor vital signs q4h

Causes	Affected Systems	Interventions
FLUID IMBALANCES—cont'd		
Hypervolemia (Extracellular Fluid Volume Excess)—cont'd		
Oliguria phase of renal disease	Gastrointestinal	Monitor IV fluid rate carefully
Excessive administration of IV fluids	Anorexia	Explain reason for restricted fluid
CHF	Nausea and vomiting	intake
Chronic liver disease with portal	Constipation	Observe for signs and symptoms of
hypertension	Thirst	CHF
	Respiratory	Restrict sodium intake
	Dyspnea	Administer diuretics as ordered
	Orthopnea	
	Rales	
	Productive cough	
	Cardiovascular	
	Observe for symptoms of	
	pulmonary edema: dyspnea,	
	orthopnea, coughing, cyanosis	
	Increased respiratory rate	
	Edema	
	Distended neck veins	
	Increased CVP readings	
	Auscultation of S_3	
	Renal	
	Oliguria	
	Skin and mucous membranes	
	Skin warm, moist, and flushed	
Hypovolemia (Extracellular Fluid Volume Deficit)		
Decreased fluid intake	Neuromuscular	Monitor intake and output
Anorexia	Behavior change	Monitor vital signs q8h
Excessive output: vomiting, diarrhea,	Apathy	Administer IV fluids as ordered
wounds, burns, excessive	Restlessness	Encourage PO intake, if allowed
diaphoresis	Disorientation	Set up 24-hr schedule for fluid intake
Uncontrolled diabetes leading to	Lethargy	Administer plasma or albumin as
osmotic diuresis	Muscle weakness	ordered
Antidiuretic hormone (ADH)	Tingling of extremities	Assist patient when moving from
insufficiency	Gastrointestinal	lying to sitting or standing position
Diuretic phase of renal disease	Anorexia	
Excessive use of diuretics	Nausea and vomiting	
	Diarrhea	
	Constipation	
	Abdominal cramps and distention	
	Thirst	
	Cardiovascular	
	Hypotension (postural systolic	
	hypotension)	
	Rapid heart rate	
	Collapsed neck veins	
	Decreased CVP readings	
	Renal:	
	Oliguria	
	Concentrated urine	
	Skin and mucous membranes	
	Poor skin turgor	
	Flushed skin	
	Dry mucous membranes	
	Furrows on tongue	

to represent this concentration; as the concentration increases, the pH decreases, causing acidosis; as the concentration decreases, the pH increases, causing alkalosis; the pH normal range in the plasma is 7.35 to 7.45

CARE OF PATIENT WITH SPECIAL EQUIPMENT

■ CENTRAL LINES

A venous catheter inserted into the superior vena cava through the subclavian, internal, or external jugular vein; can be used for monitoring of venous pressure, infusion of medications and TPN, rapid infusion of fluid and blood products, and blood withdrawal

INSERTION OF CATHETER
Auscultate chest for breath sounds
Obtain baseline BP, T, R, and apical pulse
Provide emotional support
 Explain procedure to patient
 Reinforce physician's explanation of procedure
Prepare to assist physician with inserting central venous catheter
 Maintain sterile technique
 Remove any hair from insertion site with razor or depilatory agents
 Prepare skin around insertion site with povidone-iodine solution
 Establish and maintain a sterile field throughout insertion procedure
Place patient in supine or Trendelenburg position if subclavian or jugular vein is chosen as insertion site
Administer isotonic IV solution at a keep-open rate until position of catheter is verified by chest x-ray examination
Apply sterile occlusive dressing to catheter insertion site; label dressing with date and time of insertion
Obtain chest x-ray film

POSTINSERTION ASSESSMENT
SUBJECTIVE DATA
Chest, shoulder, or neck pain

OBJECTIVE DATA
Edema in catheterized arm
Neck vein distention
Redness, swelling, or drainage at insertion site
Temperature elevation
Elevated WBC count
Occlusion of central line
Rejection of catheter
Air embolization
Accumulation of serous fluid around site

POTENTIAL COMPLICATIONS
Infection at site
Venous thrombosis
Catheter migration
Catheter embolus
Occlusion of catheter
Extravasation
Septicemia
Pneumothorax
Hemothorax
Hematoma
Cardiac tamponade
Cardiac dysrhythmias

POSTINSERTION CARE
IMMEDIATE INTERVENTIONS
Observe patient for signs of pneumothorax until chest x-ray film is read
 Auscultate chest for breath sounds q15min × 4 and then q1h; report diminished or absent breath sounds to physician
 Report any respiratory distress and presence of chest pain to physician
Prepare to insert chest tubes if pneumothorax is present

INTERVENTIONS
Check BP, T, P, and R q4h
Avoid using arm with line for BP
Auscultate chest for breath sounds q8h
Monitor parenteral fluids
 Maintain a closed system
 Keep system free of air
 Have a rubber-tipped hemostat available to clamp catheter if necessary
 Maintain a continuous drip of parenteral solutions at all times unless obtaining a CVP reading or aspirating a blood specimen
Change dressing daily
 Inspect catheter insertion site for any signs of infection, redness, tenderness, drainage, and edema
 Cleanse skin around insertion site with povidone-iodine solution
 Apply bacteriostatic ointment to catheter insertion site; avoid antibiotic ointment
 Apply sterile occlusive dressing
 Secure tubing to patient's skin to prevent tension on catheter
Measure intake and output q8h
Send tip of catheter to laboratory for culture when catheter is removed, according to institutional policy

PATIENT/FAMILY TEACHING
Ensure that patient and/or significant other describes and understands the following:
 Purpose of central catheter
 Importance of not touching catheter and tubing
 Importance of reporting any difficulty in breathing, sudden chest pain at insertion site, or fever to nurse
 When to flush catheter
 When to change dressing

Type and amount of parenteral solutions to be infused daily

Where to purchase solution and supplies needed

Need to keep solution refrigerated (bring to room temperature before administration)

Name of medication, dosage, time of administration, and side effects

Need to avoid crowds and persons with infections

Ensure that patient and/or significant other demonstrates the following:

Proper handwashing technique

Dressing change

    Inspect catheter insertion site for redness, tenderness, drainage, or swelling

    Inspect catheter for any damage or leakage

    Clean skin around insertion site with povidone-iodine solution

    Apply bacteriostatic ointment to insertion site

    Apply sterile occlusive dressing

Flushing catheter

Administration of parenteral solutions and/or medications as ordered by physician

Use of infusion pump if necessary

■ MULTILUMEN SUBCLAVIAN CATHETERS

Three separate subclavian catheters contained in one sheath; allows infusion of incompatible drugs simultaneously—the solutions do not mix but exit via separate lumens; the catheters vary in length, gauge, and volume (Fig. 2-1)

POSTINSERTION ASSESSMENT
SUBJECTIVE AND OBJECTIVE DATA
See Central Lines (p. 34)

POTENTIAL COMPLICATIONS
See Central Lines (p. 34)

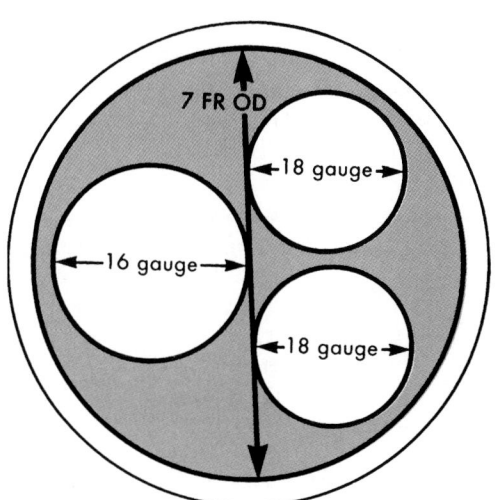

Fig. 2-1 *Multilumen Catheter* French polyurethane catheter featuring three internal lumens: 18-gauge proximal, 18-gauge middle, and 16-gauge distal.
(Redrawn from Recker DH, Metzler DJ: Crit Care Nurse 4[3]:92, 1984.)

INTERVENTIONS
POSTINSERTION CARE
Use large-gauge lumen for administration of blood products or blood withdrawal (e.g., 16-gauge CVP readings can be taken from distal lumen only)

Reserve one lumen for TPN use only

Keep occlusive clamp available at bedside

SITE CARE
Observe site qh

Inspect site for redness, pain, drainage, swelling, leakage of fluid, or loose sutures; notify physician if any of these occur

Change gauze dressing daily or whenever soiled; and transparent dressing q5d to 7d when wet, or incompletely adherent

Cleanse site with povidone-iodine solution

Apply povidone-iodine ointment to catheter insertion site

Apply occlusive gauze or transparent dressing

MAINTAINING PATENCY OF LUMENS
Flush each catheter lumen with heparin q12h or according to departmental policy if catheter lumen is not in use

Flush lumens after each intermittent medication infusion or blood sampling

Change injection site cap q3d or according to policy

Cap change should coincide with heparin flush

BLOOD WITHDRAWAL
Collect blood specimen for laboratory studies as ordered

Stop infusion through other lumens

Perform procedure using sterile technique

Aspirate and discard the first 3 ml of blood

Withdraw amount of blood needed for laboratory studies

Flush lumen with normal saline, then with 3 ml heparin solution

Resume infusion through other lumens

PATIENT/FAMILY TEACHING
See Central Lines (p. 34)

■ SILASTIC ATRIAL CATHETER

A central line catheter (single or double lumen) tunneled subcutaneously and inserted by cutdown into the central venous system by way of the cephalic or internal jugular vein; procedure is performed under fluoroscopy using sterile technique; a Dacron cuff anchors catheter subcutaneously

POSTINSERTION ASSESSMENT
SUBJECTIVE AND OBJECTIVE DATA
See Central Lines (p. 34)

POTENTIAL COMPLICATIONS
See Central Lines (p. 34)

INTERVENTIONS
POSTINSERTION CARE
Clamp catheters with occlusive clamp only

Administer TPN as ordered by physician

Administer prescribed parenteral fluid

Administer antibiotics as ordered by physician
Administer blood and blood products as ordered by
physician

BLOOD WITHDRAWAL
Collect blood specimen for laboratory studies as ordered
Stop infusion through both lumens
Perform procedure using sterile technique
Aspirate and discard first 5 ml of blood (adults) and 3 ml
of blood (children)
Aspirate amount of blood needed for laboratory studies
Flush lumen with normal saline, then with 5 ml heparin
solution
Resume infusion through other lumen

SITE CARE
Change transparent dressing or a nonocclusive dressing
according to departmental policy
Inspect catheter insertion site for redness, drainage, or
edema
Cleanse insertion site with povidone-iodine solution
Apply povidone-iodine ointment to catheter insertion site
Apply sterile transparent dressing, noting date and time
Secure IV tubing to prevent tension on catheter
Obtain order to remove site sutures within 7 days

MAINTAINING PATENCY OF CATHETER LUMENS
Flush each catheter lumen with heparin q24h or
according to departmental policy if lumen is not in use
Flush lumens after each intermittent medication infusion
or blood sampling
Change injection site caps q3d or according to policy
Use small-gauge (25-gauge or 22-gauge, 1-inch) needle
when entering injection site caps for flushing, and so
on

PATIENT/FAMILY TEACHING
See Central Lines (p. 34)
Ensure that patient and/or significant other demonstrates
the following:
Proper handwashing technique
Method of changing dressing
Technique for heparinizing the catheter
Method of changing injection site caps
Administration of prescribed medications and
parenteral solution
Use of infusion pump
Ensure that patient and/or significant other describes and
understands the following:
Need to notify physician if any of the following occur:
Inability to flush catheter
Broken catheter
Swelling, redness, drainage at insertion site
Dislodged catheter
Burning sensation during flushing
Fever of 100°F (37.8°C) or above
Instructions regarding activity
Resume activity as tolerated
Shower daily

Change transparent dressing after shower if wet
May swim, if allowed

■ IMPLANTED PORT
*Implantation of an infusion port under the skin to pro-
vide vascular access for patients requiring repeated infusion of drugs, TPN, blood products, and other fluids; the
system consists of an implantable silicone catheter and
an implantable stainless steel portal with a self-sealing
septum; the IV system is inserted into the superior vena
cava or right atrium via the subclavian or internal jugular vein with the portal placed over the third or fourth rib
(Figs. 2-2 and 2-3)*

POSTINSERTION ASSESSMENT
SUBJECTIVE DATA
Pain, tenderness at infusion site

OBJECTIVE DATA
Accumulation of serous fluid around implant site
Aching discomfort to acute pain in shoulder, neck, or arm
on ipsilateral or contralateral side
Supraclavicular or neck swelling
Venous dilation
Redness, swelling, and drainage at site
Device rotation
Palpate skin over device and check for possible rotation
or migration of portal
Device extrusion

POTENTIAL COMPLICATIONS
See Central Lines (p. 34)

POSTINSERTION INTERVENTIONS
SITE CARE
Always access the device, portal septum area, using sterile
technique
Cleanse skin over portal septum area with povidone-
iodine solution

ACCESSING THE SYSTEM
Use special noncore needles to access the device; regular
needles cannot be used

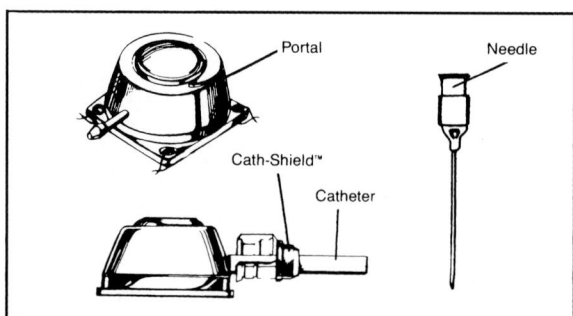

Fig. 2-2 Parts of Port-A-Cath implantable drug delivery system.
(Courtesy SIMS Deltec, Inc., St Paul, Minn.)

Do not leave needle open to air while it is in the portal, because it may cause air embolus

Attach extension tubing or stopcock to needle; this allows patient to move without dislodging needle, and it also facilitates changing of syringe or connections

Prime needle and extension tube with normal saline before use

MAINTAINING PATENCY OF THE DEVICE

Flush system with 10 ml of normal saline before administrating any drugs, then flush the heparin solution

Always leave system filled with heparinized saline after each use

For intermittent use, flush catheter every 4 weeks or according to departmental policy

Avoid reflux when withdrawing needle from septum; press down on portal and maintain positive injection pressure

DRESSING, TUBING, OR NEEDLE CHANGE

Change dressing and tubing q48h or according to policy

Provide site care

Apply povidone-iodine ointment to needle site

Place sterile, rolled gauze between skin and needle for support

Apply sterile transparent dressing over needle, gauze, and extension tube; note date and time on dressing

Tape needle securely to patient's skin

Administer prescribed parenteral fluids, TPN, antibiotics, and/or blood/blood components

Administer chemotherapeutic agents according to policy

BLOOD SAMPLING

Flush system with 5 ml of normal saline or according to departmental policy to ensure patency of line

Withdraw 10 ml of blood and discard

Aspirate amount of blood needed for laboratory studies

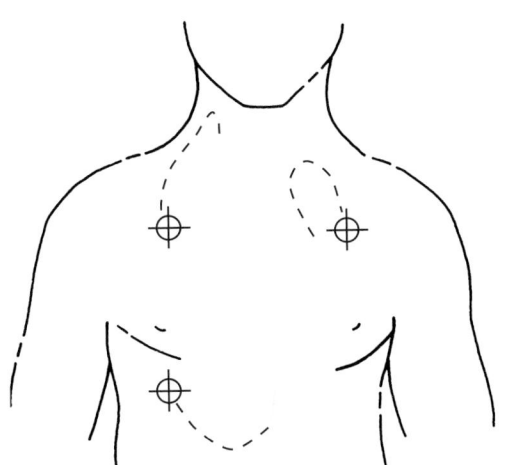

Fig. 2-3 Some commonly used locations for placement of Port-A-Cath portal and catheter.
(Redrawn from Patient information Port-A-Cath [booklet], SIMS Deltec, Inc., St Paul, Minn.)

Flush with 20 ml of normal saline, then flush with 5 ml of heparinized saline or according to policy

PATIENT/FAMILY TEACHING

See Central Lines (p. 34)

Ensure that patient and/or significant other demonstrates the following:

Proper handwashing technique

Technique for accessing the system (e.g., always cleansing skin around site with povidone-iodine solution)

Technique for expelling all air from syringe, tubing, and needle (Bandage or dressing on the site is not required.)

Technique for flushing the system

Administration of parenteral solution as ordered

Administration of medications as ordered

Use of infusion pump

Ensure that patient and/or significant other describes and understands the following:

Instructions regarding activity

Resume activity as tolerated

Shower daily

May swim, if allowed

Carry special identification card

Need to notify physician of any problems, including the following:

Inability to flush system

Movement of portal; appearance of bruising, swelling, redness, or tenderness at portal site

Fever of 100°F (37.8°C) or above

■ PERIPHERALLY INSERTED CENTRAL CATHETER

A peripherally inserted central catheter (PICC) is a radiopaque central catheter that is inserted peripherally, usually into a vein in the antecubital fossa through an introducer; the tip of the catheter is placed into the superior vena cava; it can be used for infusion of medications, TPN, fluids, or blood products

INDICATIONS

Venous access for intermediate-length infusion therapy

Eliminates the complications of neck and chest insertion

INSERTION

Obtain and record patient's baseline vital signs

Measure and record upper-arm circumference midway between shoulder and elbow of the arm to be used for insertion

Assist physician and/or certified PICC line nurse with insertion, providing a sterile field

Apply a sterile gauze dressing over insertion site

Obtain chest x-ray film

POSTINSERTION ASSESSMENT
SUBJECTIVE DATA

Shoulder, neck, or ear pain

OBJECTIVE DATA

Edema in catheterized arm

Neck vein distention

Redness, swelling, or drainage at insertion site

Occlusion of central line

Temperature elevation

Elevated WBC count

POTENTIAL COMPLICATIONS

Infection at site

Venous thrombosis

Catheter migration

Catheter embolus

Occlusion of catheter

Extravasation

Septicemia

INTERVENTIONS

Assess and record patient's vital signs every q4h to 8h

Administer fluids, blood products, or medications as ordered

Maintain scrupulous aseptic technique when manipulating catheter and fluid connections

Avoid use of multiple stopcocks to prevent contamination of IV system, potential blood loss, or air embolism

Use catheter tip syringe connections and tape all connections to prevent accidental opening of system

Administer one infusion at a time

Flush catheter between IV treatments to prevent particulate formation and/or clotting

Assess insertion site, arm, and neck daily for pain, redness, warmth, swelling, or leakage; notify physician if any of these are present

Measure circumference of upper arm weekly

Compare with baseline measurement

Notify physician if increase of 2 cm or more occurs

Change dressing

Remove gauze dressing 24 hours after insertion

Carefully handle tubing to prevent pulling on catheter

Clean skin at insertion site with povidone-iodine solution

Allow skin to dry at least 2 minutes to maximize action

Apply transparent dressing; date and initial tape

Change dressing and cleanse site per department policy or when dressing is moist or loose

Flush catheter and change cap

Flush catheter with normal saline after each infusion

Flush catheter with an intermittent motion (stop briefly after each millimeter of normal saline instilled) to ensure that blood or other substances clear valve

Flush catheter with 20 ml of normal saline (using intermittent motion) after blood administration

Use a 1-inch or shorter needle for flushing to prevent puncturing the catheter

Never use force when flushing catheter

Notify physician immediately if catheter ruptures and breaks

Seal catheter with a catheter tip syringe cap when it is not in use

Never use a clamp or hemostat; catheter is very soft and thin-walled and can be easily cut

Change catheter tip syringe cap when infusion is restarted or every 5 days or according to departmental policy when catheter is not in use

Collect blood samples

Do not use catheter to obtain routine blood samples because a lumen is too small

A single blood culture may be withdrawn if catheter-related sepsis is suspected

PATIENT/FAMILY TEACHING

Ensure that patient and/or significant other describes and demonstrates the following (when appropriate):

Purpose of central catheter

Importance of not touching catheter and tubing with hands

Need to report any pain in arm, neck, or ear; difficulty breathing; or fever

Need to avoid crowds and persons with infections

Handwashing technique, care of catheter, flushing method, dressing change, how to obtain supplies and solutions

Names of medications/solutions, purpose, dosage, side effects, and time and length of administration

DISCHARGE/HOME CARE PLANNING
FOR CENTRAL LINES

Assess and continue with patient and family education and evaluate the following:

Type of solution being used; importance of checking expiration date

Correct schedule, storage, and use of infusion pump

Procedure for dressing change

Handwashing technique

Available supplies

Condition of infusion site

Correct aseptic technique

Procedure for flushing catheter

Schedule, aseptic technique

Knowledge of where to purchase supplies

Signs of infection (e.g., fever, redness, swelling, drainage)

Signs of complications (e.g., weight loss or gain, dyspnea, glucosuria, tightness in chest)

Presence of telephone and emergency numbers, as well as those of home care team

Amount of rest and exercise

Intake and output flow sheet

■ INTRAVENOUS CONTINUOUS OPIOID INFUSION (ICOI)

A method of providing analgesia to the terminally ill and others with severe pain, such as burn, postoperative, and Crohn's disease patients; method of administration is usually PICC

INDICATIONS

Inability to provide pain relief by other routes

Bleeding, pain, or tissue damage from intramuscular or subcutaneous routes

Rectal and oral routes contraindicated

ASSESSMENT

SUBJECTIVE DATA

Nausea

Pain and/or tenderness at infusion site

Pain in neck, ear, chest

OBJECTIVE DATA

Dosage necessary for maximum pain relief and minimum side effects

Side effects

Drowsiness

Mood changes

Mental cloudiness

Respiratory depression

Increased $Paco_2$ (arterial carbon dioxide)

Decreased GI motility

Vomiting

Alterations of endocrine and autonomic nervous systems

Desired effects

Analgesia

Alertness

Increased coherence

Decreased anxiety

Improved coping ability

Improved relationships with others

Improved cardiac function

Decreased tachycardia

Modulation of BP

Regular respiratory rhythm

INTERVENTIONS

Choose opioid based on minimum toxicity; drug of choice is morphine or hydromorphine hydrochloride (Dilaudid)

Dilute solution based on dosage required for analgesia and amount of fluid per hour that is therapeutic for patient

Titrate hourly drip rate to level of analgesia desired without untoward effects

Regulate drip carefully with controller or pump as indicated (see Box 2-1)

Involve patient in his or her care plan; encourage patient to communicate how he or she feels

Monitor BP, P, R, and level of consciousness qh while dosage is being adjusted

Monitor BP, P, R, and level of consciousness q2h when optimum dosage is achieved

Check arterial blood gases (ABGs) as ordered

Initiate flow sheet and enter patient's vital signs and dosage per hour as indicated

Box 2-1	**Electronic Infusion Devices**		
Nonvolumetric devices	Deliver solution in drops/min	Drop rate—calibrated infusion pumps	Are designed to count drops and are set in terms of gtt/min; move solution through the line by application of positive pressure
Volumetric devices	Deliver a specific volume in a given time as shown in ml/hr	Volumetric infusion pumps	Have rate-setting adjustment calibrated in ml/hr rather than drops/min; pump output pressure limits are established by manufacturer and can range as high as 25 psi
Drop rate–calibrated infusion controllers	Regulate infusion rate via gravity by electronically counting or measuring drops (controllers that set the rate in drops/min are now considered obsolete)		
Volumetric infusion controllers	Count the volume in each drop; permit flow rate to be set in ml/hr rather than gtt/min (controllers *do not* add pressure to the line to overcome resistance to flow)	Variable pressure limit volumetric infusion pumps	Are designed to provide only the pressure needed for specific clinical situations; allow nurse to set pressure limit based on clinical considerations
Infusion pumps	Apply positive pressure to the line to overcome flow; most deliver solution to a vein at an average pressure of pounds per square inch (psi) (*pressure can increase if a line is occluded partially or totally*)		

PATIENT/FAMILY TEACHING

Ensure that patient and/or significant other knows and
understands the following:

Purpose of central catheter

Importance of not touching catheter and tubing

Importance of reporting any difficulty in breathing,
pain at insertion site, or fever to nurse

When to change dressing

Type and amount of solutions to be infused daily

Need to keep solution refrigerated (bring to room
temperature before administration)

Name of medication, dosage, time of administration,
and side effects

Need to avoid crowds and persons with infections

Ensure that patient and/or significant other demonstrates
the following:

Proper handwashing technique

Dressing change

Inspect catheter insertion site for redness,
tenderness, drainage, or swelling

Assess for catheter migration

Clean skin around insertion site with povidone-
iodine solution

Apply bacteriostatic ointment to insertion site

Apply sterile occlusive dressing

Use of infusion pump with alarm if necessary

Knowledge of side effects to report to physician

Respiratory distress

Drowsiness

Decreased mental acuity

Vomiting

DISCHARGE/HOME CARE PLANNING

Assess and continue with patient and family education
and evaluate for the following:

Ability of patient and caregiver to perform needed
tasks

Correct type and amount of infusion

Ability to care for insertion site and to change dressing

Knowledge and use of infusion pump

Use of flow sheet for record-keeping tasks

Mental acuity and signs of toxicity to opioid

Amount of rest and exercise

Intake and output

Elimination status

Nutritional status

Presence of telephone and emergency phone
numbers, as well as those of home health team

■ CONTINUOUS SUBCUTANEOUS OPIOID INFUSION

*An alternative method of administering opioids to the
terminally ill who have intractable pain when other ac-
cesses are not desirable*

INDICATIONS

Rectal and oral routes contraindicated

Intravenous sites not accessible or desirable

Intramuscular sites painful and/or damaged

ASSESSMENT

SUBJECTIVE DATA

Injection site pain

Nausea

OBJECTIVE DATA

Dosage necessary for maximum pain relief and minimum
side effects

Side effects

Drowsiness

Mood changes

Decreased mental acuity

Respiratory depression

Increased $Paco_2$—arterial carbon dioxide

Decreased GI motility, constipation

Nausea/vomiting

Desired effects

Analgesia

Alertness

Decreased anxiety

Improved interacting/coping ability

Improved vital signs

INTERVENTIONS

Choose opioid based on minimum toxicity; drug of choice
is morphine or hydromorphine hydrochloride (Dilaudid)

Dilute solution based on analgesic requirement and
hourly therapeutic intake

Select subcutaneous site using either abdominal, thigh, or
clavicular area

Using sterile technique, insert small-bore (27-gauge)
butterfly needle and connect it to a controller or
infusion pump

Titrate hourly drip rate to desired level of analgesia

Monitor BP, P, R and mental acuity qh until patient is
stable and then monitor them q4h

Monitor infusion site q8h for swelling and pain

Change site at least q6d to 7d and prn

PATIENT/FAMILY TEACHING

See ICOI (p. 38)

DISCHARGE/HOME CARE PLANNING

See ICOI (p. 38)

■ PATIENT-CONTROLLED ANALGESIA

*Patient-controlled analgesia (PCA) enables the patient
to self-administer a physician-prescribed dose of analgesia on demand; with PCA acute, as well as chronic, pain
can be managed; more severe pain such as that encountered by a patient with terminal cancer can be controlled
through the use of the continuous infusion feature; the
continuous infusion rate may also be used in conjunction with PCA to control severe chronic pain*

INDICATIONS

Acute postoperative pain

Laminectomy

Chest surgery

Major abdominal surgery
Orthopedic surgery
Acute pain in disease, such as sickle cell crisis
Chronic severe pain

ASSESSMENT
SUBJECTIVE DATA
Nausea
Constipation

OBJECTIVE DATA
Ability of patient, mentally and physically, to operate the
    device
Dosage adjustment for maximal pain relief with minimal
    side effects
Ability of patient and/or family to participate in his or her
    care
Side effects
    Respiratory depression
    Drowsiness
    Vomiting
    Mental cloudiness
    Increased $Paco_2$—arterial carbon dioxide
    Anxiety
    Decreased GI motility

INTERVENTIONS
Ensure completeness of physician's order
    Name of drug
    Concentration of drug
    Loading dose
    Lock-out interval
Program prescribed information into PCA unit
Verify accurate program entry with another registered
    nurse (RN)
Monitor patient's baseline vital signs and level of
    consciousness
Instruct patient about purpose of PCA and operation of unit
Stay with patient when first dose is administered
Be prepared to place the unit in stop mode if respiratory
    distress or change in sensorium is noted at any time
    during the infusion
Have naloxone hydrochloride (Narcan) available at all times
Monitor BP, P, R, and level of consciousness 30 minutes
    after the first dose and q4h thereafter
Monitor BP, P, R, and level of consciousness whenever a
    change in PCA dose occurs, when administering a
    loading dose, or when a change in the lock-out interval
    occurs
Monitor patient for adequate pain relief; use flow sheet
    and pain rating scale
Collaborate with physician to determine dosage needed if
    pain relief is not obtained
Monitor for side effects of the opioid drug

■ PERMANENT EPIDURAL CATHETER
*The placement of a radiopaque silicone catheter into
the epidural space for the administration of a narcotic
drug can be used as a method of pain control; the catheter*
*has two segments; the one with the smaller lumen is in-
serted at L1, and the proximal end is placed between T11
and C3 at the appropriate level to obtain pain relief; the
segment with the larger lumen is inserted in the abdomen, tunneled to the lumbar site, and joined to that
segment; a Dacron filter cuff is attached to the catheter 2
inches from the abdominal incision; subcutaneous tissue
adheres to the cuff, preventing bacterial entry*

INDICATIONS
Chronic pain such as that in the following conditions:
    Cancer
    Degenerative joint disease
    Spinal trauma
Pain not controlled by conventional therapy
Restriction of activity by usual pain therapy

ASSESSMENT
SUBJECTIVE DATA
Insertion site pain
Nausea

OBJECTIVE DATA
Severity of pain (rating scale)
Amount of pain relief (rating scale)
Dosage of opioid that will control pain with minimal side
    effects
Side effects
    Respiratory depression
    Drowsiness
    Vomiting
    Mental cloudiness
    Increased $Paco_2$
    Anxiety
    Decreased GI motility
    Constipation

POTENTIAL COMPLICATIONS
Infection
Displacement of catheter
Catheter malfunction

INTERVENTIONS
IMMEDIATE POSTOPERATIVE CARE
Obtain epiduragram to confirm placement and determine
    the spread of fluid in the epidural space
Maintain dressings at both lumbar and abdominal incision
    sites for the first 24 hours after operation
Assess for bleeding at sites
Reinforce dressings prn
If bleeding is noted, apply ice packs or apply pressure,
    using sand bags, to the subcutaneous tunnel
Catheter care
    Change dressings at both incision sites daily until
        sutures are removed from lumbar site
    Continue to change dressings at abdominal site on a
        daily basis
    Cleanse site with hydrogen peroxide followed by
        iodine solution
    Cover site with sterile occlusive dressing

Administration of drug
  Dilute prescribed drug with preservative-free normal
    saline solution to a volume of 5 to 10 ml because
    epidural space can safely handle only 15 ml/hr
  Stay with patient during first few infusions
    Monitor BP, P, and R q15 to 30min
    Keep injection of naloxone (Narcan) available
  Cleanse injection site of the catheter cap with iodine
  Inject the drug into the catheter as rapidly as is comfortable
  Change catheter filter daily for continuous infusion
    and q4d for intermittent infusion
Assess for signs and symptoms of infection at exit site
  q8h and report presence to physician
  Redness and edema
  Pain
  Seepage of fluid around catheter
  Fever of unknown origin
Assess severity of pain and pain relief q4h; use a rating scale
Monitor for medication side effects and toxicities q4h to 8h
  Assess BP, P, R, and LOC
If you are unable to inject medication into catheter, do
  the following:
  Change the filter
  Change patient position while trying to inject medication
  NOTE: If label on catheter indicates that it is not for IV
    access, and if IV is accidently infused, remove filter,
    aspirate as much of drug or solution as possible,
    attach a new filter, and notify physician *before*
    injecting any other drugs or solutions
  If previously mentioned interventions fail, report
    problem to physician

PATIENT/FAMILY TEACHING
Ensure that the patient and/or significant other describes
  and demonstrates the following:
  Purpose of epidural catheter
  Proper handwashing and sterile technique
  Method of dressing change
  Name, purpose, dosage, and frequency of medication
  Side/toxic effects of medication to report
  Need to notify physician if pain relief is not obtained
  Preparation of medication
  Administration of medication
  Method of changing filter and injection cap
  Symptoms of infection/inability to inject medication to
    report to physician

DISCHARGE/HOME CARE PLANNING
Assess and continue with the patient and family
  education and evaluate for the following:
  Proper handwashing and sterile technique
  Ability of caregiver(s) to perform tasks
  Preparation of opioid solution and administration
  Dressing change technique
  Mental acuity
  Response to infusion; decreased pain and discomfort
  Signs of side effects, toxicity of opioid infusion
  Presence of telephone and emergency phone
    numbers, as well as home care team
  Nutritional and elimination status

■ TRANSCUTANEOUS ELECTRICAL NERVE STIMULATION
*Transmission of an electrical impulse to the body from
a battery-powered device through electrodes attached to
the skin; pain is relieved by production of a pleasant
tingling, tapping, or massaging sensation*

INDICATIONS
Postoperative use
During labor and delivery
Acute injuries
Chronic conditions (herpes zoster, osteoarthritis, neuralgia)

CONTRAINDICATIONS
Cardiac pacemaker
Significant dysrhythmias
Myocardial infarction (MI)
Cardiac monitoring (creates artifact)
First trimester of pregnancy
Placement over carotid sinus nerve, eyes, laryngeal/
  pharyngeal muscles
Metastatic cancer

ASSESSMENT
SUBJECTIVE DATA
Muscle spasm
Increased pain
Nausea
Headache

OBJECTIVE DATA
Skin irritation
Sensations produced
  Tingling
  Pleasure
  Itching
  Burning
  Prickling
Unit function
  No stimulation
  Cuts in and out
Unit settings
  Rate: 2 to 200 pulses/min (hertz [Hz])
  Pulse width: 0 to 500 μsec
  Amplitude

INTERVENTIONS
Assist patient in placing electrodes according to the
  manufacturer's recommendations
Maintain electrodes in total contact with patient's skin
Change electrode positions prn to prevent skin irritation
Monitor patient for appropriate pain relief
Adjust rate and pulse width settings to prevent
  unpleasant sensations
Maintain electrodes in place
Activate unit in response to patient's pain
For skin irritation
  Remove electrodes
  Expose skin to air

Apply skin cream
Reposition electrodes away from irritation
Change type of electrode if necessary
For nausea
    Reposition electrodes
    Vary rate, pulse width, and amplitude
For headache
    Turn down pulse width dial
    Turn down amplitude
    Use shorter stimulation period
    Place electrodes farther apart
    Vary rate
If problems are not resolved
    Try different TENS device
    Discontinue using TENS device
Refer patient for assistance from a TENS specialist, if available
Refer patient to pain clinic

PATIENT/FAMILY TEACHING

Ensure that patient and/or significant other describes and demonstrates the following:
    Mechanisms of rate, pulse width, and amplitude adjustments
    Appropriate sensations to be achieved
    How to adjust settings to do the following:
        Achieve maximum pain relief
        Avoid unpleasant sensations
        Avoid muscle spasm and pain exacerbation
    Need to do the following:
        Change electrode placement prn
        Maintain skin integrity
        Wear TENS all day: on for 2 hours, off for 1 hour (total stimulation of 6 to 8 hours)
        Wear TENS all night if sleep is interrupted (turn unit on if awakened by pain)
        Maintain a record of settings that achieve desired effect

FUNCTIONAL HEALTH PATTERN I: HEALTH PERCEPTION AND MANAGEMENT

■ RISK FOR INFECTION

DEFINITION*

The state in which an individual is at increased risk for being invaded by pathogenic organisms

---

Definitions, risk factors, related factors, and defining characteristics in this section for NANDA nursing diagnoses are modified from NANDA Nursing Diagnoses: Definitions and Classifications 1999-2000, Philadelphia 1999, North American Nursing Diagnosis Association; and Kim MJ et al: Pocket guide to nursing diagnoses, ed 7, St Louis, 1997, Mosby.

RISK FACTORS

Inadequate primary defenses (e.g., broken skin, traumatized tissue, decrease in ciliary action, stasis of body fluids, change in pH secretions, altered peristalsis)
Inadequate secondary defenses (e.g., decreased hemoglobin, leukopenia, suppressed inflammatory response, immunosuppression)
Inadequate acquired immunity
Tissue destruction and increased environmental exposure to the sun, cold, or rain
Chronic disease
Invasive procedures
Malnutrition
Pharmaceutical agents and trauma
Rupture of amniotic membranes
Insufficient knowledge to avoid exposure to pathogens

INTERVENTIONS

Assess body systems for type, location, and cause of infections
    Wear gloves, gown, mask, goggles, as appropriate to procedure
    Wash hands after patient contact and before self-contact
Monitor vital signs
Monitor laboratory values (e.g., elevated WBC, urinalysis, positive blood culture)
Initiate cooling measures as prescribed
Administer antipyretics and antibiotics as indicated; assess for effectiveness and side effects
Discuss with and teach patient about adequate nutrition and fluid intake
Provide and review immunization requirements to help patient maintain his or her health
Discuss health practices and teach patient about hazards of substance abuse, unsafe sexual behaviors, and smoking
Integumentary system
    Maintain aseptic technique during dressing changes; change dressings prn
    Promote and provide skin care and oral hygiene daily
    Assess pressure points prn; apply lotion and protective covering as needed; massage skin only if it is not reddened
    Monitor intravenous insertion sites and central lines daily
    Maintain IV sites and dressings according to policy
    Discuss with and teach patient about principles of autocontamination and cross contamination
Respiratory system
    Assess for dyspnea, shortness of breath, and rales
    Assess frequency, color, and consistency of expectorate; culture as indicated
    Encourage coughing and deep breathing at least once q1h to 2h
    Assist patient with respiratory aids (e.g., incentive spirometer) and oxygen therapy
    Encourage ambulation or frequent position changes
    Elevate head of bed to promote more comfortable breathing
    Encourage fluid intake to liquefy sputum

Genitourinary system
    Maintain intake (oral/IV) at 2000 to 2500 ml/day, unless contraindicated
    Encourage fluids and foods high in acid content (e.g., cranberry, plum) to help prevent bacteria from adhering to bladder, wall where they can multiply and cause infection
    Maintain closed drainage system for urethral catheters as indicated
    Monitor intake and output
    Provide daily catheter care as indicated
    Culture urine as indicated
Gastrointestinal system
    Instruct patient to ingest only USDA-inspected meats
    Encourage patient to handle and store food properly

Expected Outcomes
Understands cause of infection
Expresses knowledge of methods of preventing further or recurring infections
Demonstrates ability to promote own wellness

■ RISK FOR INJURY

DEFINITION
The state in which an individual is at risk of injury as a result of environmental conditions interacting with the individual's adaptive and defensive resources

RISK FACTORS
Interactive conditions between individual and environment that impose a risk to defensive and adaptive resources of individual
Internal factors
  Biochemical factors
    Regulatory function
      Sensory dysfunction
      Integrative dysfunction
      Effector dysfunction
    Tissue hypoxia
    Malnutrition
    Immunity-autoimmunity
    Abnormal blood profile
      Leukocytosis or leukopenia
      Altered clotting factors
      Thrombocytopenia
      Sickle cell anemia
      Thalassemia
      Decreased hemoglobin
  Physical factors
    Broken skin
    Altered mobility
  Developmental factors
    Age
      Physiologic
      Psychosocial
  Psychologic factors
    Affective factors
    Orientation

External factors
  Biologic factors
    Immunization level of community
    Microorganisms
  Chemical factors
    Pollutants
    Poisons
    Drugs
      Pharmaceutic agents
      Alcohol
      Caffeine
      Nicotine
    Preservatives
    Cosmetics and dyes
    Nutrients (e.g., vitamins, food types)
Physical factors
  Design, structure, and arrangement of community, building, and/or equipment
  Mode of transport/transportation
  Nosocomial agents
People/provider
  Nosocomial agents
  Staffing patterns
  Cognitive, affective, and psychomotor factors

INTERVENTIONS
Assess patient's mental, visual, and auditory acuity
Review patient's neuromuscular status, age, medication history (including home remedies), and nutritional status
Assess patient's ability to perform ADLs, exercise, and ambulate
Maintain safe environment for patient
Orient patient to surroundings
Provide needed equipment and ensure patient's ability to reach it easily; avoid clutter
Maintain side rail, bed position, and use of restraints per policy
Remind patient about no smoking policy
Assist patient with ADLs; teach safe use of mobilizing devices as needed
Explain all treatments, procedures, and care; be aware of any language barriers
Provide adequate lighting
Ensure that electrical and hospital equipment is in good working condition
Practice safe medication administration
Monitor laboratory profiles for signs of impending problems
Administer medications according to policy
  Understand and monitor side effects
  Instruct patient to take medications as prescribed on discharge; explain that any side effects should be reported to physician
  Advise patient to avoid over-the-counter (OTC) medications unless advised by physician
Provide home safety teaching according to maturational age
  Avoid scatter rugs, icy steps or ramps, and wet or waxed floors

Avoid loose or flowing gowns near stove, use thick pot holders, and keep pan handles toward front of stove

Install handrails and antislip cover for bathtub or shower

Avoid heat or cold overexposure

Maintain adequate lighting for dispensing medications

Separate oral and eye medications from topical medications

Keep all medications out of reach of children

Expected Outcomes

Demonstrates understanding of potential health hazards

Practices injury prevention measures for self

Remains injury free

■ Latex Allergy Response

Definition

Allergic response to natural latex rubber products

Defining Characteristics

Type I reactions: Immediate

Type IV reactions: Eczema; irritation, reaction to additives causes discomfort, e.g., thiurams, carbamates, redness, delayed onset (hours)

Irritant reactions: Erythema, chapped or cracked skin, blisters

Interventions

In the presence of type IV or irritant reaction
  Change brand of gloves
  Change to a powder-free glove
  Avoid use of latex gloves and other products

Recognize signs/symptoms of a type I reaction
  Symptoms may be localized or systemic
  Hives, itching
  Generalized edema
  Wheezing, bronchospasm,
  Dyspnea, laryngeal edema
  Nausea, diarrhea
  Hypotension
  Tachycardia
  Dysrhythmias
  Feeling of faintness
  Respiratory or cardiac arrest

Remove cause immediately of type I reaction
  Use only nonlatex products or switch immediately to nonlatex products if there is a suspicion of a type I reaction
  Eliminate airborne latex allergens from environment
  Administer pharmacologic agents as ordered; antihistamines, epinephrine, intravenous fluids, corticosteroids
  Administer oxygen as indicated
  Assist with intubation as indicated

Avoid use of latex catheters

Use latex free IV tubing

Use caution with latex ports on IV tubing

Avoid "snapping" latex gloves *to prevent propulsion of latex-carrying powder into the air (aerosolization of latex); duration can last 5 to 12 hours*

Do not place balloons at patient's bedside

Refer to the institution's list of latex products to ensure that they are not present in the patient's immediate setting

Expected Outcomes

Does not experience skin integrity problems that result in infection

Does not experience anaphylaxis

Verbalizes understanding of risk factors and need to avoid latex products

FUNCTIONAL HEALTH PATTERN II: NUTRITIONAL AND METABOLIC

■ Altered Nutrition: More Than Body Requirements

Definition

The state in which an individual experiences an intake of nutrients that exceeds metabolic needs

Defining Characteristics

Weight 10% to 20% over ideal for height and frame

Triceps skinfold (TSF) greater than 15 mm in men and 25 mm in women

Sedentary activity level

Reported or observed dysfunctional eating patterns
  Pairing food with other activities
  Concentrating food intake at end of day
  Eating in response to external cues (e.g., time of day, social situation)
  Eating in response to internal cues other than hunger (e.g., anxiety)

Related Factor

Excessive intake in relation to metabolic need

Interventions

Assess patient for signs of fluid retention

Weigh patient daily (same time, scale, clothing)

Assess patient's desire for weight loss and his or her history of dieting

Obtain TSF measurements

Determine patient's height and ideal body weight (Tables 2-2 and 2-3)

Assess patient's dietary history, taking heredity, age, culture, religion, and medical problems into consideration; include laxative use

Collaborate with nutritionist or registered dietitian and patient. Help patient set realistic goals for weight loss; reward goals attempted and attained

Encourage patient to keep a diary of intake (i.e., what, when, and where food is eaten) and feelings at time of eating

Table 2-2	Height and Weight Table for Men and Women	
	Weight (Pounds)	
Height	Ages 19-34	Ages 35 and Older
5'0"	97-128	108-138
5'1"	101-132	111-143
5'2"	104-137	115-148
5'3"	107-141	119-152
5'4"	111-146	122-157
5'5"	114-150	126-162
5'6"	118-155	130-167
5'7"	121-160	134-172
5'8"	125-164	138-178
5'9"	129-169	142-183
5'10"	132-174	146-188
5'11"	136-179	151-194
6'0"	140-184	155-199
6'1"	144-189	159-205
6'2"	148-195	164-210
6'3"	152-200	168-216
6'4"	156-205	173-222
6'5"	160-211	177-228
6'6"	164-216	182-234

Source: Nutrition and your health: dietary guidelines for Americans, *Washington, DC, 1990, United States Department of Agriculture.*

Emphasize importance of a regular exercise program
Provide information on a reputable weight loss program
Refer patient for counseling as needed

Expected Outcomes
Expresses understanding of factors causing weight gain
Demonstrates desire to maintain normal weight for age and height

■ ALTERED NUTRITION: LESS THAN BODY REQUIREMENTS

DEFINITION
The state in which an individual experiences an intake of nutrients insufficient to meet metabolic needs

DEFINING CHARACTERISTICS
Loss of weight with adequate food intake (see Table 2-3)
Body weight 20% or more under ideal for height and frame
Reported inadequate food intake (i.e., less than the RDA)
Weakness of muscles required for swallowing or mastication
Reported or evidence of lack of food
Lack of interest in food
Perceived inability to ingest food
Aversion to eating
Reported altered taste sensation
Satiety immediately after ingesting food

Table 2-3	Height and Weight Assessment*
Females	45 kg (100 lb) for first 150 cm (5 ft), plus 2.25 kg (5 lb) for each additional 2.5 cm (1 inch)
Males	47.7 kg (106 lb) for first 150 cm (5 ft), plus 2.4 cm (6 lb) for each additional 2.5 cm (1 inch)

Yield ideal body weight + 10%.

Abdominal pain with or without pathologic conditions
Sore, inflamed buccal cavity

RELATED FACTOR
Inability to ingest or digest food or absorb nutrients because of biologic, psychologic, or economic factors

INTERVENTIONS
Assess patient's nutritional status, past eating patterns, and medications (Tables 2-4 and 2-5)
Assess causative factors (e.g., anorexia, bulimia, dysphagia, altered taste, age, unavailability of food)
Assess patient's cultural food preferences (i.e., likes and dislikes)
Monitor patient's intake and output; weigh patient weekly (same time, same scale, same clothing)
Monitor laboratory values (e.g., CBC, electrolytes)
Maintain calorie count chart
Establish rest/activity pattern
Encourage patient to keep a food intake diary
Encourage a well-balanced diet of 2400 calories every day
Provide four to six meals per day as needed
Encourage patient to establish regular exercise habits
Assess patient's oral cavity and ability to chew and swallow
Provide meals in a quiet environment; encourage patient to eat slowly and chew well
Help patient adjust to a comfortable position for meals
Encourage family or significant other to be involved with meals, eat with patient, and to bring food from home
Maintain clean environment to prevent nausea and anorexia
Collaborate with nutritionist or registered dietitian about cultural food preparation
Discuss and teach patient and significant other about nutritional guidelines, importance of eating regular meals, and appropriate foods to include
Refer patient for nutritional counseling as needed

Expected Outcomes
Expresses understanding of nutritional deficit
Demonstrates knowledge of adequate nutritional intake
Gains weight as needed to meet body needs

■ ALTERED ORAL MUCOUS MEMBRANE

DEFINITION
The state in which an individual experiences disruptions in the tissue layers of the oral cavity

Table 2-4	Effect of Drugs on Nutritional Status*	
Drug	**Effect**	
Antacids (aluminum)	Malabsorption of medications and some nutrients	
Aspirin	Malabsorption of folate	
	Excretion of vitamin C	
Barbiturates	Malabsorption of thiamin, vitamin B_{12}	
Corticosteroids	Malabsorption of calcium, zinc, phosphorus	
Hydralazine	Excretion of pyridoxine	
Laxatives	Loss of fluid/electrolytes	
Methotrexate	Malabsorption of vitamin B_{12}, folate, fat	
Mineral oil	Malabsorption of fat-soluble vitamins, calcium, phosphorus	
Neomycin	Malabsorption of major nutrients	
Oral contraceptives	Possible decreased absorption of vitamin C, B complex vitamins, magnesium, zinc	
Penicillin	Loss of potassium	
Tetracycline	Malabsorption of calcium, iron, magnesium, pyridoxine	
	Excretion of vitamin C, riboflavin, niacin, folic acid	
Thiazides	Excretion of potassium, magnesium, zinc, riboflavin	

Modified from Phipps WJ et al: Medical-surgical nursing: a nursing process approach, ed 4, St Louis, 1995, Mosby.

Table 2-5	Medications to Be Taken With Food*	
Aspirin	Nitrofurantoin (Macrodantin)	
Aminophylline	Phenylbutazone (Butazolidin)	
Chlorothiazide (Diuril)	Phenytoin (Dilantin)	
Ferrous sulfate	Prednisolone, Ibuprofen	
All nonsteroidal antiinflammatory drugs	Reserpine (Serpasil)	
	Triamterene (Dyrenium)	
Metronidazole (Flagyl)		

Updated from Phipps WJ et al: Medical-surgical nursing: a nursing process approaches, ed 6, St Louis, 1999, Mosby.

DEFINING CHARACTERISTICS
Coated tongue
Xerostomia (dry mouth)
Stomatitis
Oral lesions or ulcers
Lack of or decreased salivation
Leukoplakia
Edema
Hyperemia
Oral plaque
Oral pain or discomfort
Desquamation
Vesicles
Hemorrhagic gingivitis
Carious teeth
Halitosis

RELATED FACTORS
Pathologic conditions: oral cavity (radiation to head and/or neck)
Dehydration
Trauma
  Chemical (e.g., acidic foods, drugs, noxious agents, alcohol)
  Mechanical (e.g., ill-fitting dentures, braces, endotracheal tubes, nasogastric tubes, surgery in oral cavity)
NPO instructions for more than 24 hours
Ineffective oral hygiene
Mouth breathing
Malnutrition
Infection
Lack of or decreased salivation
Medication

INTERVENTIONS
Assess patient's mucous membranes, tongue, and gums daily
Observe for moisture, cleanliness, integrity, edema, color, bleeding, and odor
Assess patient's teeth for cleanliness, integrity, sensitivity to heat or cold, presence of dentures, and sores
Brush patient's teeth bid and prn with toothpaste, powder, baking soda, or mouthwash
Promote regular flossing
Advise patient to avoid foods that cause discomfort (e.g., hot, cold, and spicy foods)
Encourage adequate fluid intake
Advise patient to rinse with water or mouthwash after brushing
Apply petroleum jelly, lip balm, or glycerin-lemon mixture to patient's lips to prevent dryness and chapping
Remove patient's dentures (if applicable) and cleanse bid with toothpaste or powder and running water. Protect dentures from breaking by placing them in a marked denture cup when not in use
Cleanse patient's mouth with equal parts of hydrogen peroxide and water prn for crust removal
Perform oral cleaning as needed with toothettes or disposable foam swabs; avoid lemon-glycerine swabs because they can irritate the mucosa
Encourage routine dental checkups

Expected Outcomes

Demonstrates correct technique to promote proper oral care

Has oral cavity that is pink, clean, moist, and odor free

Reports a feeling of oral cleanliness

■ RISK FOR IMPAIRED SKIN INTEGRITY

DEFINITION
The state in which an individual's skin is at risk of being adversely altered

RISK FACTORS
External (environmental) factors
  Hypothermia or hyperthermia
  Chemical substance
  Mechanical factors
    Shearing forces
    Pressure
    Restraint
  Radiation
  Physical immobilization
  Excretions and secretions
  Humidity
  Moisture
  Extremes of age
Internal (somatic) factors
  Medication
  Alterations in nutritional state (e.g., obesity, emaciation)
  Altered metabolic state
  Altered circulation
  Altered sensation
  Altered pigmentation
  Skeletal prominence
  Developmental factors
  Alterations in skin turgor (e.g., change in elasticity)
  Psychogenic factors
  Immunologic factors

INTERVENTIONS
Assess causative factors and risk using an assessment tool (e.g., Braden scale)

Assess patient's bathing needs (e.g., complete or partial bed bath, tub or shower using warm water and mild superfatted soap)

  Provide privacy and ensure adequate temperature to avoid chilling

  Massage patient's skin gently with mild lanolin-based lotions to increase circulation and maintain integrity; never massage broken areas because it may provoke further ulceration

  Dry skin thoroughly

  Consider using "bagbath" method of bathing: place four washcloths in plastic baggies; add nonrinsable cleaner, such as Septisoft; and dilute according to directions; heat bag in microwave for 60 to 90 seconds; use one cloth for each part of body; allow patient to air-dry, which takes about 30 seconds; discard cloths in laundry hamper

Assess patient's skin for redness, lesions, blisters, swelling, or drainage; notify Wound, Ostomy, Continence/ET nurse if these conditions occur

Monitor for incontinence; cleanse area with mild soap and water prn

Encourage patient to ambulate; limit chair sitting to 1 hour

Assist with and/or teach ROM exercises

Provide nutritious diet and adequate fluid intake

Assess patient's perineal and perianal areas as needed; observe for excoriation, vaginal or penile discharge, and pain; apply lotions or cornstarch to area prn

Assess patient's feet and hands; observe nail beds and look for signs of rash, dryness, or skin breaks; use side lighting to assess rash

Soak patient's feet and hands in warm soap and water, dry well, and apply lotion prn

Cleanse and trim patient's nails as needed

Assess condition of patient's hair; observe for matting, tangles, signs of alopecia, lice, cradle cap scales, and dryness

  Comb hair daily and shampoo prn, with patient's permission; start with edges and work toward scalp, holding shaft of hair to prevent discomfort

  Apply baby oil and massage it into scalp; leave oil on for 1 hour to remove scales, then gently shampoo and comb

  Apply alcohol to release tangles

  Style patient's hair for attractiveness, comfort, and easy care

Assess male patient's shaving needs

  Apply warm towels to patient's face before shaving

  Rinse skin well and apply lotion after shaving

Maintain physical comfort

Change bed linen prn; keep linen neat, dry, wrinkle free, and clean

Provide adequate warmth

Change patient's position frequently to prevent pressure and fatigue

Expected Outcomes

Maintains skin integrity

Nails and hair are in optimal condition

Impairment is minimal if present

Maintains maximal circulation

Demonstrates optimal nutrition

■ RISK FOR ALTERED BODY TEMPERATURE

DEFINITION
The state in which an individual is at risk for failure to maintain body temperature within normal range

RISK FACTORS
Extremes of age

Extremes of weight

Exposure to cold/cool or hot/warm environments

Dehydration

Inactivity or vigorous activity

Medications causing vasoconstriction or vasodilation, altered metabolic rate, sedation

Inappropriate clothing for environmental temperature
Illness or trauma affecting temperature regulation
Altered metabolic rate

INTERVENTIONS

Hyperthermia
  Assess causative factors (e.g., heatstroke, lesions of
      anterior hypothalamus)
  Monitor patient's vital signs q1h
  Monitor patient's mental acuity
  Monitor intake and output; report output less than 30
      ml/hr to physician
  Monitor electrolytes, CBC, glucose, and liver function
  Monitor for tachycardia or tachypnea
  Maintain parenteral fluids as indicated
  Initiate cooling measures as indicated; cool slowly, and
      handle body gently
      Monitor patient's temperature q10min during
          procedure and q1h after procedure
      Discontinue cooling measures when temperature is
          1° F above normal
      Dry patient's skin thoroughly (avoid friction) and
          provide clean, dry linen
  Encourage patient to reduce physical activity and to
      drink plenty of fluids
  Administer prescribed antibiotics and antipyretics
  Reinstitute cooling measures as needed
  Maintain cool room temperature
Hypothermia
  Assess causative factors (e.g., accidental hypothermia,
      lesions of posterior hypothalamus)
  Monitor patient's vital signs q1h
  Monitor patient's mental acuity
  Initiate warming measures as prescribed; warm body
      slowly, and handle body gently
  Monitor for bradycardia or hypotension
  Monitor blood gases, electrolytes, and glucose; report
      any abnormal results to physician
  Monitor intake and output q1h. If urine output is less
      than 30 ml/hr, notify physician
  Maintain warm, comfortable environment

Expected Outcomes
Temperature is normal
Vital signs are normal
Skin is warm and dry

FUNCTIONAL HEALTH PATTERN III: ELIMINATION

■ CONSTIPATION

DEFINITION
*The state in which an individual experiences a change
in normal frequency of defecation characterized by a
decrease in frequency and/or passage of hard, dry
stools*

DEFINING CHARACTERISTICS
Change in bowel pattern
Bright red blood with stool
Presence of soft pastelike stool in rectum
Frequency less than usual pattern
Hard-formed stool; oozing liquid stool
Palpable mass
Reported feeling of rectal fullness
Straining at stool
Decreased or hyperactive bowel sounds
Reported feeling of abdominal fullness or pressure
Distended abdomen
Increased abdominal pressure
Percussed abdominal dullness
Indigestion
Severe flatus
Less than usual amount of stool
Nausea

OTHER POSSIBLE DEFINING CHARACTERISTICS
Abdominal pain
Back pain
Headache
Interference with daily living
Laxative use
Decreased appetite
Appetite impairment

RELATED FACTORS
Less than adequate intake
Less than adequate dietary intake and bulk
Less than adequate physical activity or immobility
Personal habits
Medications
Chronic use of medication and enemas
GI obstructive lesions
Neuromuscular impairment
Musculoskeletal impairment
Pain on defecation
Diagnostic procedures
Lack of privacy
Weak abdominal musculature
Pregnancy
Emotional status

INTERVENTIONS
Assess cause(s) of constipation
Determine patient's normal elimination pattern
Assess patient's daily defecation routine and encourage
    him or her to maintain pattern as much as possible
Provide natural stimulants (e.g., coffee, prune juice) as
    allowed
Provide privacy
Monitor and record patient's daily bowel movements;
    monitor for melena as needed
Initiate diet changes to maintain normal consistency;
    provide high-fiber foods (e.g., fruits, vegetables, whole
    grains)
Initiate high-fiber foods slowly to prevent intestinal
    distention and gas formation

Avoid excessive use of bran, which can increase gas formation

Increase activity, exercise, and fluid intake (six to eight glasses every day)

Provide natural laxatives initially (e.g., lemon juice in a glass of warm water, prune juice qAM) before administering laxative or enema

Instruct patient to avoid routine use of laxatives

Explain that medications often cause constipation

Explain importance of defecating as soon as urge occurs

Instruct patient to set schedule for defecating daily, such as after a meal

Initiate relaxing techniques to assist in defecation

Reduce rectal pain and discomfort from hemorrhoids through use of lubricants, cool compresses, stool softeners, and suppositories

Administer perianal care after each defecation

Expected Outcomes

Expresses understanding of causative factors of constipation

Demonstrates knowledge of the importance of diet, fiber, fluids, regularity, and exercise

Verbalizes need to avoid straining and using laxatives to defecate

■ DIARRHEA

DEFINITION
The state in which an individual experiences a change in normal bowel habits, which is characterized by the frequent passage of loose, fluid, and unformed stools

DEFINING CHARACTERISTICS
Abdominal pain
Cramping
Increased frequency of bowel movements
Increased frequency of bowel sounds
Loose, liquid stools
Urgency
Color changes

RELATED FACTORS
Stress and anxiety
Tube feedings
Medications
Inflammation, irritation, or malabsorption of bowel
Alcohol abuse
Toxins
Contaminants
Radiation

INTERVENTIONS
Assess causative factors, including impaction
Maintain NPO and parenteral fluids as indicated
Collaborate with physician; initiate fluids and progress to soft, bland diet as tolerated
Encourage dietary bulk in diet as soon as possible; psyllium (Metamucil) may be indicated

Avoid irritating foods (e.g., milk, caffeinated products, and raw fruits and vegetables)

Weigh patient daily (same time, scale, and clothing)

Assess usual elimination pattern

Monitor serum electrolytes

Monitor bowel sounds

Encourage patient to verbalize situations that cause stress

Assist and teach stress management techniques

Assess patient's perineal area for excoriation and irritation

Provide perineal skin care after each bowel movement; apply soothing ointments as indicated

Provide bedpan or commode, and place it within easy reach

Maintain uncluttered room for easy access to bathroom; provide a night-light

Allow for privacy

Suggest methods of eliminating odors

Expected Outcomes

Verbalizes causative factors of diarrhea

Reports improved frequency and consistency of stools

Presents normal electrolytes and fluid intake

■ ALTERED URINARY ELIMINATION

DEFINITION
The state in which an individual experiences a disturbance in urine elimination

DEFINING CHARACTERISTICS
Dysuria
Frequency
Hesitancy
Incontinence
Nocturia
Retention
Urgency

RELATED FACTORS
Sensory motor impairment
Neuromuscular impairment
Mechanical trauma
Urinary tract infection
Anatomic obstruction

INTERVENTIONS
Assess causative factors, including family history of kidney problems and peripheral edema
Determine patient's usual urinary pattern; inquire about any recent alterations in patient's pattern
Measure intake and output
Monitor urine for color, frequency, amount, odor, and consistency
Monitor urine for sugar, acetone, blood, and pH levels
Monitor for residual urine
Monitor for frequency, urgency, dysuria, and distension
Administer and teach female patient about perineal care after urination; explain correct wiping procedure

Provide privacy

Maintain uncluttered room for easy access to bathroom; provide a night-light

Increase fluid intake, if allowed, to maintain hydration

Institute voiding measures (e.g., running water, leaning forward, standing position, peppermint in bedpan) as needed

Maintain bedpan within easy reach

Monitor indwelling urethral catheters for patency, correct position of collection unit, and infection; teach self-catheterization as needed

Provide daily urinary meatal care according to policy

Monitor for incontinence

    Initiate voiding schedule q2h to 4h

    Provide protective padding as needed

Expected Outcomes

Expresses understanding of causative factors of altered urinary pattern

Verbalizes and demonstrates correct posturinating hygiene

Reports urination returning to a normal pattern

FUNCTIONAL HEALTH PATTERN IV: ACTIVITY AND EXERCISE

■ Activity Intolerance

Definition

The state in which an individual has insufficient physiologic or psychologic energy to endure or complete required or desired daily activities

Defining Characteristics

Verbal report of fatigue or weakness

Abnormal heart rate or BP in response to activity

Exertional discomfort or dyspnea

Electrocardiographic changes reflecting dysrhythmias or ischemia

Related Factors

Generalized weakness

Sedentary lifestyle

Imbalance between oxygen supply and demand

Bed rest or immobility

Interventions

Physical interventions

    Assess body systems for possible cause of inactivity

        Disturbance in oxygen maintenance

        Fluid or electrolyte imbalance

        Deficiencies in nutrition

        Neuromuscular disorders

    Observe patient for pain and insufficient rest or sleep

Monitor side effects of all medications and diagnostic studies

Collaborate with physical and occupational therapists as needed

Assess patient's tolerance of activity

    Assess past activity pattern

    Explain procedure, activity, or treatment

    Monitor resting vital signs

    Have patient perform activity at his or her own rate

    Monitor vital signs immediately and again in 3 minutes

    Discontinue activity if any of the following occur: chest pain, dyspnea, cyanosis, vertigo, confusion, hypotension, failure of systolic pressure increase, increased diastolic pressure, decreased respiratory rate, continuing tachycardia

    Reduce energy expenditure where possible

Increase activity slowly to increase patient's tolerance

    Assist as needed

Coordinate care and medication schedule to allow for rest periods

Maintain and increase strength with active or passive ROM exercises

Encourage self-care activities when patient is able

Provide adaptive devices, such as padded eating utensils and long-handled tongs, to assist in ADLs as needed

Psychologic interventions

    Assess patient for presence of depression or lack of incentive; assess for maladaptive behaviors

    Explain importance of activity to tolerance

    Involve patient in care plan and short-term goal setting

    Acknowledge and praise patient for attempting or completing tasks

    Discuss and assist patient with identifying possible incentives to increase activity

    Assist patient in identifying successful past coping behaviors

    Involve family or significant other in supporting and participating with patient in daily activities

Expected Outcomes

Participates in activities that increase ability to perform ADLs and other activities

Expresses understanding of a balanced rest/activity program

Seeks support of others to maintain optimal level of activity

■ Impaired Physical Mobility

Definition

The state in which an individual experiences a limitation of ability for independent physical movement

Defining Characteristics

Inability to purposefully move within physical environment, including bed mobility, transfer, and ambulation

Postural instability
Reluctance to attempt movement
Limited ROM
Limited ability to perform fine motor skills
Uncoordinated or jerky movements
Decreased reaction time
Gait changes
Slowed movement
Movement-induced tremor
Decreased muscle strength, control, and/or mass
Imposed restrictions of movement, including mechanical and medical protocol
Impaired coordination

RELATED FACTORS

Intolerance of activity (i.e., decreased strength and endurance)
Medications
Body mass index above 75th age-appropriate percentile
Sedentary lifestyle
Joint stiffness
Limited cardiovascular endurance
Pain and discomfort
Perceptual or cognitive impairment
Neuromuscular impairment
Musculoskeletal impairment
Depression or severe anxiety

INTERVENTIONS

Assess patient's mobility tolerance and motivation
Maintain circulatory function
    Encourage and teach arm and leg exercises to be performed q1h
    Apply antiembolic hose
    Monitor for thrombophlebitis; symptoms include pain, warmth, and edema of extremity
    Assist and teach patient turning techniques
Monitor patient's vital signs after activity at 3 minutes and 15 minutes
Observe for hypertension or hypotension, tachycardia, or bradycardia
Maintain respiratory function
    Encourage and teach deep breathing q1h
    Assist and teach patient how to use incentive spirometer
    Maintain patent airway
    Monitor respirations q1h to 2h
    Increase fluid intake to liquefy secretions
    Monitor vital signs after activity
    Observe for dyspnea, cyanosis, tachypnea, or bradypnea
Maintain normal elimination
    Increase fluid intake
    Encourage exercise and activity
    Provide diet that will promote elimination
        Bowel: high fiber, roughage, prunes
        Bladder: meat, fish, cereals
    Provide privacy
    Assist and teach perianal and perineal hygiene
    Provide bedpan within easy reach
Maintain musculoskeletal function
    Collaborate with physical and occupational therapist for supportive exercises

    Perform active exercises or assist with and teach passive ROM exercises q4h; note patient's tolerance and motivation
    Maintain bodily alignment while in bed
    Provide bed cradle as needed
    Prevent footdrop with foot board
    Support dependent limbs as needed with pillows or immobilizing devices; avoid placing pillow under knees
    Avoid letting patient remain in any one position for long periods; frequent small changes prevent pressure, discomfort, and fatigue
    Maintain casts, braces, traction, or prosthetic devices in correct position to avoid discomfort or pressure
    Help patient progress toward mobility slowly as tolerated
    Assist patient as needed with sitting up, dangling, standing, and ambulation
    Initiate and teach use of mobilizing devices (e.g., crutches, walker, wheelchair, sling) as needed
Maintain skin integrity
    Assess pressure points for signs of breakdown
    Administer gentle massage to pressure areas; apply lotion as needed
    Encourage activity as tolerated
    Prevent shearing force with use of turn sheet
    Provide nutritious diet of proteins and carbohydrates
    Increase fluid intake; monitor intake and output
    Change patient's position often if he or she is in wheelchair
Maintain psychologic integrity
    Encourage patient to express fears and anxieties
    Promote support of significant others
    Provide diversional activities
    Encourage patient to be involved in his or her care
    Maintain positive communication
    Reinforce positive coping patterns
    Provide and teach patient about available support resources; distribute handouts and telephone numbers of rehabilitation and social services

Expected Outcomes

Ability to interact with others, make own decisions, and use positive coping behaviors is increasing
Vital signs are normal
Elimination is normal
Activity is at optimal level
Skin integrity is maintained

FUNCTIONAL HEALTH PATTERN V: SLEEP AND REST

■ SLEEP PATTERN DISTURBANCE

DEFINITION

    A time-limited disruption of sleep amount and quality causes discomfort or interferes with desired lifestyle;

prolonged periods without sustained natural, periodic suspension of relative unconsciousness

DEFINING CHARACTERISTICS
Verbal complaints of difficulty in falling asleep
Awakening earlier or later than desired
Interrupted sleep
Verbal complaints of not feeling well rested
Changes in behavior and performance
    Increasing irritability
    Daytime drowsiness
    Decreased ability to function
    Forgetfulness
    Restlessness
    Disorientation
    Lethargy; malaise, tiredness
    Listlessness
    Lack of concentration
Physical signs
    Mild, fleeting nystagmus
    Slight hand tremor
    Ptosis of eyelid
    Expressionless face
    Slowed reaction
Thick speech with mispronunciation and incorrect words
Dark circles under eyes
Frequent yawning
Changes in posture

RELATED FACTORS
Sensory alterations
    Internal factors
        Illness
        Sleep apnea
        Psychologic stress
        Prolonged physical or psychologic discomfort
        Sustained circadian asynchrony
    External factors
        Environmental changes
            Sustained unfamiliar or uncomfortable sleep environment
        Social cues

INTERVENTIONS
Assess and identify causative factors
For patients with predetermined sleep apnea
    Provide and assist with application of CPAP machine
    Assist as indicated with oral retainer designed to improve airway opening
Assess patient's normal rest/sleep pattern
Control environmental disturbances, noise, and lighting
Maintain quiet environment; close doors and pull drapes and dividers; decrease incoming stimuli
Provide night lights and soft music
Coordinate nursing functions to allow for rest periods and fewer interruptions during night
Limit visitors during rest periods
Limit fluid intake where possible after 6 PM
Avoid stimulants such as coffee, cola, and tea
Maintain balance of daytime activity and rest
Increase activity to point of tolerance to promote tiredness
Limit sleep during daytime and stimulate wakefulness as required
Involve patient in unit and diversional activities
Provide comfort measures
Maintain warm, clean, and comfortable bed
Provide needed equipment within easy reach
Encourage usual sleeping aids
Administer hs care as close to bedtime as possible
Assess any sleep medication for effectiveness
Encourage patient to express fears and anxieties that may prevent or disrupt sleep
Monitor for pain or discomfort; administer analgesics if needed
Teach patient alternative pain/stress management techniques

Expected Outcomes
Expresses understanding of causative factors of sleep disturbance
Demonstrates optimal balance of rest and activity
Expresses increased ability to sleep

FUNCTIONAL HEALTH PATTERN VI: COGNITIVE/PERCEPTUAL

■ PAIN

DEFINITION
The state in which an individual experiences and reports the presence of severe discomfort or an uncomfortable sensation

DEFINING CHARACTERISTICS
  SUBJECTIVE DATA
Communication (verbal or coded) of pain descriptors
Self description of pain on pain scale

  OBJECTIVE DATA
Guarding behavior (i.e., protective)
Self-focusing behavior
Narrowed focus (altered time perception, withdrawal from social contact, impaired thought process, irritability, anxiety)
Distraction behavior (moaning, crying, pacing, seeking out other people and/or activities, restlessness)
Facial mask of pain (eyes lack luster, "beaten look," fixed or scattered movement, grimace)
Alteration in muscle tone, which may span from listless to rigid
Autonomic responses not seen in chronic, stable pain (e.g., diaphoresis, BP and P rate change, pupillary dilation, increased or decreased respirations)
Sleep disturbance

RELATED FACTORS

Injury agents
  Biologic factors
  Chemical agents
  Physical factors
  Psychologic factors

INTERVENTIONS

Assess location, type, duration, and frequency of pain
Assess intensity of pain using scale of 0 to 5 (0 being absence of pain and 5 being intense pain) or other standard pain scale
Assess causative factors
Discuss past effective and ineffective pain relief measures
Assess effect of pain on patient
  Altered sleep/activity pattern
  Decreased energy, sexual activity
  Reduced feelings of self-worth
Assess effectiveness of pain-relief measures
Encourage patient to keep a pain diary
Develop trusting relationship
  Encourage patient to talk about himself or herself
  Be a good listener
  Avoid making judgmental statements
  Be truthful and consistent
  Accept patient's view of pain
  Set realistic goals
  Assist patient in describing pain
  Explain relationship of pain to disease process
  Estimate duration of pain when possible
  Explain painful procedures realistically
Involve patient in his or her care; allow some control over his or her daily activities when possible
Encourage pain reduction techniques as appropriate: (e.g., rocking movements, external warmth, visual focal point with breathing patterns, imagery, relaxation techniques, touch)
Suggest self-help groups that assist in coping with pain
Administer analgesics as ordered
Collaborate with physician regarding indwelling lines for administration of analgesics; peripherally inserted central catheter (PICC) (see p. 37); intravenous continuous opioid infusion (ICOI) (see p. 38); continuous subcutaneous opioid infusion (CSI) (see p. 40); epidural analgesia (see p. 41); and patient controlled analgesia (PCA) (see p. 40).
Discuss alternative interventions such as biofeedback, TENS unit, hypnosis, and self-controlled pain procedure
Encourage support of family and significant others

Expected Outcomes

Expresses understanding of causative factors of pain
Demonstrates ability to reduce or control pain using learned skills

■ KNOWLEDGE DEFICIT

DEFINITION

Deficiency or lack of cognitive information related to a specific topic

DEFINING CHARACTERISTICS

Verbalization of the problem
Inaccurate follow-through of instruction
Inadequate performance of test
Inappropriate or exaggerated behaviors (e.g., hysterical, hostile, agitated, apathetic behavior)
Statement of misconception
Request for information

RELATED FACTORS

Lack of exposure
Lack of recall
Misinterpretation of information
Cognitive limitation
Lack of interest in learning
Unfamiliarity with information resources
Patient's request for no information

INTERVENTIONS

Establish patient's expected outcomes for learning
Use information obtained in assessment; be aware of any language or cultural barriers to information
Set patient's expected outcomes according to priority and to patient's needs and readiness to learn
Set small, specific, and realistic expected outcomes to provide patient with a sense of accomplishment
Reward goals that are attempted or completed
Write expected outcomes in patient's plan of care
Incorporate principles of learning and teaching
  Patient's desire to learn must be present before learning can take place
  Each individual learns at his or her own pace
  Environment must be free from stress, discomfort, pain, or distractions
  Information is best learned if it is meaningful, organized, and relevant
  Individual will learn only if he or she sees value in the information
Present information in small segments
Use language that is easily understood
Teach from a well-organized plan
Allow time for questions
Obtain feedback from patient after each segment is presented
Continue with teaching plan only when patient understanding is ensured
Maintain eye contact during discussions
Present information step by step and request a return demonstration when teaching a procedure
Present information using different techniques based on patient's learning preference and/or ability
Involve family and significant others in learning process
Use as many audiovisual aids as possible
  Films
  Slides
  Booklets
  Diagrams
  Procedure pictures
  Procedure equipment
Praise patient when learning takes place

Initiate teaching plan as soon as possible after admission, based on patient's condition, level of perception, and readiness to learn

Expected Outcomes
Verbalizes understanding of given instructions and information
Demonstrates learned procedure(s) correctly
Seeks assistance in clarifying misconceptions or misunderstandings

■ ALTERED THOUGHT PROCESSES

DEFINITION
The state in which an individual experiences a disruption in cognitive operations and activities

DEFINING CHARACTERISTICS
Inaccurate interpretation of environment
    Cognitive dissonance
    Distractibility
    Memory deficit or problems
    Egocentricity
    Hypervigilance/hypovigilance
    Decreased ability to grasp ideas
    Impaired ability to make decisions
    Impaired ability to solve problems
    Impaired ability to reason
    Impaired ability to abstract or conceptualize
    Impaired ability to calculate
    Altered attention span (i.e., distractibility)
    Obsessions, phobias
    Inability to follow commands
    Disorientation to time, place, person, circumstances, and events
    Changes in remote, recent, or immediate memory
    Delusions
    Illusions
    Ideas of reference
    Paranoid ideation
    Hallucinations
    Confabulation
    Inappropriate social behavior
    Altered sleep patterns
    Inappropriate affect
    Inappropriate or nonreality-based thinking

RELATED FACTORS
Physiologic changes
Psychologic conflicts
Loss of memory
Impaired judgment
Sleep deprivation

■ DECISIONAL CONFLICT

DEFINITION
A state of uncertainty about the course of action to be taken when choice among competing actions involves risk, loss, or challenge to personal life values (specify focus of conflict, [e.g., choices regarding health, family relationships, career, finances, or other life events])

DEFINING CHARACTERISTICS
Verbalized feeling of distress related to uncertainty about choices
Verbalization of undesired consequences of alternative actions being considered
Vacillation between alternative choices
Delayed decision making
Self-focusing behavior
Physical signs of distress or tension (e.g., increased heart rate, increased muscle tension, restlessness)
Questioning personal values and beliefs while attempting to make a decision

RELATED FACTORS
Unclear personal values and beliefs
Perceived threat to value system
Lack of experience or interference with decision making
Lack of relevant information
Support system deficit

INTERVENTIONS
Assess any physical condition that may affect decision making or cognition
Encourage patient not to make serious decisions while under severe stress
Practice relaxation techniques before decision making to decrease anxiety
Assist patient with clearly identifying a problem
Provide accurate data; be consistent to avoid misconceptions
Decrease anxiety (see anxiety interventions, p. 56)
Assist patient with identifying potential alternatives; encourage patient to write down pros and cons of each alternative
Assist patient with identifying previous successful decisions
Encourage verbalization and recognition of factors that hinder decision making
Reassure patient that it is acceptable to make mistakes
Remind patient that any decision will have negative aspects
Encourage patient to make simple choices first
Allow patient to make choices (e.g., select an item from menu or choose a time for a procedure)
Explain importance of not making decisions based on preference of others
Reinforce patient's verbalization of independent opinions, thoughts, and decisions
Assist and reinforce progression to more complex decision making
Point out available resources to assist in decision making
Teach assertive communication techniques
Assist with appropriate action once decision has been made

Expected Outcomes
Makes contribution to treatment plan
Seeks increasing responsibility for own activity and behavior

Verbalizes alternative solutions to problems
Involves others in decision-making process

FUNCTIONAL HEALTH PATTERN VII: SELF-PERCEPTION AND SELF-CONCEPT

■ ANXIETY*

DEFINITION
A vague, uneasy feeling, the source of which is often nonspecific or unknown to the individual

DEFINING CHARACTERISTICS
SUBJECTIVE DATA
Increased tension
Apprehension
Increased helplessness
Uncertainty
Fear
Feelings of being scared
Panic
Feelings of inadequacy
Shakiness
Fear of unspecific consequences
Regret, obsession, rumination
Guilt, shame
Overexcitement
Feelings of being rattled
Distress
Jitters
Nausea
Abdominal pain
GI discomfort
Sleep disturbance
Tingling in extremities
Headaches
Fatigue
Heart pounding, palpitations felt in throat
Dry mouth

OBJECTIVE DATA
Sympathetic stimulation (e.g., cardiovascular excitation, superficial vasoconstriction, pupil dilation)
Dizziness, hyperventilation
Restlessness
Insomnia, somnolence
Muscle tension
Glancing about
Poor eye contact
Trembling (especially hand tremors), twitching

All of the NANDA nursing diagnoses may be associated with anxiety in one of its levels.

Extraneous movements (e.g., foot shuffling, hand and arm movements)
Diarrhea
Expressed concern regarding changes in life events
Worried behavior
Inability to concentrate
Diminished productivity
Confusion
Preoccupation
Diminished learning ability
Crying, irritability
Anxiety
Facial tension, facial flushing
Voice quivering
Self-behavior focus
Increased wariness
Increased perspiration, sweaty palms, and/or flushing

RELATED FACTORS
Unconscious conflict about essential values and goals of life
Threat to self-concept
Threat of death, real or perceived
Threat to or change in health status
Threat to or change in socioeconomic status
Threat to or change in role functioning
Threat to or change in environment
Threat to or change in interaction patterns
Situational and maturational crises
Interpersonal transmission and contagion
Unmet needs
Exposure to toxins
Familial association/heredity
Substance abuse

■ MILD ANXIETY

DESCRIPTION
Mild anxiety is normal anxiety that motivates an individual on a daily basis to perform and problem solve

DEFINING CHARACTERISTICS
Slight discomfort
Restlessness
Mild insomnia
Mild change in appetite
Irritability
Repetitively questions
Attention-seeking behaviors
Increased alertness
Increased perception and problem solving
Easily angered
Focus on future problems
Fidgety movements

INTERVENTIONS
Watch for signs of increasing anxiety
Help patient channel energy constructively
Use prn medication sparingly

Provide supportive listening
Encourage problem solving
Provide accurate and factual information
Be aware of patient's defense mechanisms
Assist in identifying successful coping skills
Maintain a calm, unhurried manner
Teach patient that mild anxiety is a normal part of living
Teach relaxation exercises and techniques

Expected Outcomes
Identifies source of own anxiety
Employs stress management techniques
Modifies behavior related to anxiety stressors
Learns and employs relaxation techniques
Practices cognitive reframing of negative stressors
Works to achieve balance in life activities

■ MODERATE ANXIETY

DESCRIPTION
Moderate anxiety is anxiety that interferes with new learning by narrowing the perceptual field so that the individual grasps less but is able to attend with direction by others

DEFINING CHARACTERISTICS
Progression of mild anxiety
Selective attention to environment
Concentration on individual tasks only
Moderate subjective discomfort
Increase in amount of time spent on problem situation
Voice tremors
Change in voice pitch
Tachypnea
Tachycardia
Tremulousness
Increased muscle tension
Nail biting, finger drumming, toe tapping, or foot swinging
Increased obsessive, ruminating thoughts
Inability to concentrate
Panic, guilt, shame, crying, irritability

INTERVENTIONS
Maintain calm, unhurried manner when dealing with patient
Speak in calm, firm, reassuring manner
Use short, simple, and direct sentences
Avoid becoming anxious, angry, or defensive
Listen to patient with respect and interest
Offer physical touch or comfort only if patient desires it
Administer antianxiety medications as ordered
Assist patient with labeling and recognizing anxiety
Assist patient with identifying and describing feelings and the source of distress
Do not probe
Allow patient to cry
Allow for verbal expression of anger

Assist patient with correcting events that precipitated anxiety
Encourage participation in diversional activities
   Reading
   Watching television
   Listening to the radio
   Writing letters
   Walking and other physical activity
   Visiting with relatives or friends
Assist patient with identifying coping mechanisms that will reduce anxiety and with using those that have been successful in the past
Teach patient to use relaxation techniques
Encourage patient to engage in activities that use large muscle groups
Establish and maintain familiar routines
Teach patient the importance of establishing daily exercise to control stress level
Continue with mild anxiety care

Expected Outcomes
Has a decrease in anxiety symptoms
Is able to work on adaptive behaviors related to anxiety

■ SEVERE ANXIETY

DESCRIPTION
During an episode of severe anxiety, an individual's perceptual field is narrowed to the point that he or she is unable to problem solve or learn; the focus is on small or scattered details, and communication patterns are disrupted; the patient may exhibit many aborted attempts to reduce anxiety and usually verbalizes great subjective distress

DEFINING CHARACTERISTICS
Sense of impending doom
Excessive muscle tension (headache, muscle spasms)
Diaphoresis
Respiratory changes
   Sighing
   Hyperventilation
   Dyspnea
   Dizziness
GI changes
   Nausea, vomiting
   Heartburn
   Belching
   Anorexia
   Diarrhea or constipation
Cardiovascular changes
   Tachycardia
   Palpitations
   Precordial discomfort
Greatly reduced range of perception
Inability to learn
Inability to concentrate
Sense of isolation

Difficult or inappropriate verbalization
Purposeless activity
Hostility

INTERVENTIONS

Provide quiet and safe environment for patient
Provide frequent-to-constant contact and care
Administer medications as ordered
Assist and/or make decisions for patient; do not ask patient to do this entirely for himself or herself
Observe for signs of increasing agitation
Do not touch patient without his or her permission
Assure patient that he or she will be safe
Assess for safety in immediate environment

Expected Outcomes

Verbalizes decreased behavioral, affective, physiologic symptoms of anxiety
Demonstrates ability to concentrate and attends with assistance to immediate environment and care needs
Uses coping strategies to reduce anxiety
Identifies thoughts and perceptions that preceded anxiety

■ PANIC

DESCRIPTION

Anxiety has escalated to the level that the individual is now a danger to self and/or others and may become immobilized or strike out in a random fashion

DEFINING CHARACTERISTICS

Severe hyperactivity or immobility
Extreme sense of isolation
Loss of identity; personality disintegration
Severe shakiness and muscular tension
Inability to communicate in complete sentences
Distortion of perception and unrealistic appraisal of environment and/or threat
Disorganized behavior in attempting to escape
Assaultive behavior
Avoidant behavior, phobia, agoraphobia

INTERVENTIONS

Remain with patient; call for assistance
Remove as many physical and psychologic stressors from environment as possible
Speak in a calm, reassuring manner, using low voice tones
Tell patient that you (or staff) will not allow him or her to harm self or others
Isolate patient in quiet, safe area
Continue with severe anxiety care

Expected Outcomes

Does not harm self or others
Has a decrease in physiologic anxiety or panic symptoms
Has a decrease in anxiety or panic behaviors
Has regained some reality-oriented cognitive abilities

■ HOPELESSNESS

DEFINITION

Perception that one's own action will not significantly affect an outcome; the subjective state in which an individual sees limited or no alternatives or personal choices available and is unable to mobilize energy on own behalf

DEFINING CHARACTERISTICS

Passivity, decreased verbalization
Decreased affect
Verbal cues (indicating despondency, "I can't," sighing)
Lack of initiative
Decreased response to stimuli
Turning away from speaker
Closing eyes
Shrugging in response to speaker
Decreased appetite
Increased or decreased sleep
Lack of involvement in care (i.e., passively allows care)

RELATED FACTORS

Prolonged activity restriction creating isolation
Failing or deteriorating physiologic condition
Long-term stress
Abandonment
Loss of belief in transcendent values/supreme being

INTERVENTIONS

Maintain a kind but firm attitude in all patient care activities
Maintain adequate hydration and nutrition
Measure intake and output as ordered or if indicated
Allow patient to wear his or her own clothes when possible
Involve patient in decision-making process when formulating care plan
Help patient set small, realistic goals
Give positive reinforcement for independent functioning
Assess patient with identifying areas over which he or she has control
If patient's appetite is poor and he or she is eating insufficiently, offer soft, nutritious foods that are easily chewed; include high-protein, between-meal snacks and a variety of liquids such as milkshakes, custards, and eggnog
Maintain liquids and food within easy reach
Offer food in frequent small amounts
Discourage intake of nonnutritive items such as coffee and foods high in refined sugar
Encourage water intake
Serve food attractively and at proper temperature
Provide foods that patient prefers; assist with menu selection
Do not give patient choice of not eating by asking, "Do you feel like eating?" Offer foods and say, "I have something for you to eat"

Administer stool softeners or laxatives as needed

Encourage intake of foods rich in fiber

Reinforce and assist grooming efforts and personal hygiene; encourage male patients to shave and female patients to apply makeup and to style their hair

Encourage patient to do things for himself or herself in order to feel better rather than waiting to feel better first before doing things for self

Assist with positioning in bed, sitting, and ambulation

Offer positive recognition for increased activity level

Provide noncompetitive activities (e.g., handicrafts, sewing, simple puzzles) before progressing to competitive activities such as board games

Promote planned rest periods during the day based on patient's physical condition

Discourage patient from sleeping all day or remaining in bed

Decrease environmental and other stimuli at night to promote sleep

Promote bedtime rituals

    Avoid stressful conversation

    Discourage caffeine-containing substances

    Discourage exercise before bedtime

    Offer back rub and warm milk

    Do not encourage dependence on hypnotics, especially those that suppress rapid eye movement (REM) sleep

Continually assess for suicide potential

If patient expresses plan for suicide, ask for details of plan

Support all verbalization of feelings, especially anger

Report suicidal ideation to attending physician

Observe closely for any self-destructive behavior when mood-elevating medications take effect or if patient demonstrates a sudden change in affect or behavior

Plan time to sit with patient; do not act rushed and remain comfortable during silent periods; do not require patient to always talk

Do not discourage patient from crying; remain with and support patient unless he or she requests privacy

Do not belittle patient's statements or offer inappropriately cheerful remarks or platitudes such as "Everything's going to be all right"

Be sure that your reassurances are realistic and are meant for patient, not for yourself

Assess your own feelings of powerlessness and helplessness

Avoid agreement with self-deprecating statements and cast doubt on their validity, but do not argue with patient

Reinforce positive statements about self and others; do not be overcomplimentary

If patient expresses feelings of guilt, assist him or her with exploring its origin and with exploring associated feelings of anger and resentment

Respect denial of illness if patient is unable to accept it; do not force reality on patient

Assist and support gradually increasing amounts of independent self-care

Provide for physical exercise at patient's level of tolerance

Maintain a clean, orderly environment

Ask if visit by religious or spiritual support person is desired

Administer antidepressants as ordered

    Be aware of lag time of up to 2 weeks before they take effect

    Familiarize yourself with side effects; most common are anticholinergic effects

    Be aware of possible "cheeking" of medication or hoarding at bedside; antidepressants are lethal

Expected Outcomes

Identifies cause(s) of hopelessness and depressions

Reaches acceptance stage of death and dying if terminal illness is present

Develops and implements plan of adaptive behaviors for depression

Has reduction in the vegetative signs and symptoms of depression

Verbalizes no self-destructive thoughts

■ BODY IMAGE DISTURBANCE

DEFINITION

Disruption in the way one perceives one's body image/ physical self

DEFINING CHARACTERISTICS

Either of the following (A or B) must be present to justify the diagnosis of body image disturbance:

    A. Verbal response to actual or perceived change in structure and/or function

    B. Nonverbal response to actual or perceived change in structure and/or function

The following clinical manifestations may be used to validate the presence of A or B:

OBJECTIVE DATA

Missing body part

Actual change in structure and/or function

Not looking at body part

Not touching body part

Hiding or overexposing body part (intentional or unintentional)

Trauma to nonfunctioning part

Change in social involvement

SUBJECTIVE DATA

Negative feelings about body

Feelings of helplessness, hopelessness, or powerlessness

Preoccupation with change or loss

Emphasis on remaining strengths, heightened achievement

Extension of body boundary to incorporate environmental objects

Personalization of part or loss by name

Depersonalization of part or loss by impersonal pronouns

Behaviors of avoidance, monitoring, or acknowledgement of one's body

Refusal to verify actual change

It may be possible to identify high-risk populations such as those with the following conditions:

Missing parts

Dependence on machine

Significance of body part or functioning with regard to age, sex, culture, developmental level, or basic human needs

Physical change caused by biochemical agents (drugs)

Physical trauma or mutilation

Pregnancy and/or maturational changes

RELATED FACTORS

Biophysical factors

Cognitive perceptual factors

Psychosocial factors

Cultural or spiritual factors

Developmental changes

Illness, trauma, surgery

INTERVENTIONS

Determine patient's perception of change in body image and subsequent threat to self

Encourage verbalization of emotions such as anger, fear, frustration, and anxiety about altered functioning or lost body part

Encourage patient to look at and touch changed or lost body part

Assist family or significant other to adapt to change by providing resources, encouraging verbalization, and including them in care of patient

Encourage discussion of physical change in simple, direct, and factual manner

Assess your own attitudes and values related to wholeness and physical appearance

Give realistic feedback about loss or change

Discuss any sexual concerns openly and honestly

Encourage patient to participate in all therapeutic modalities offered in treatment

Give positive feedback for attempts to enhance and integrate new body image

Allow patient to progress at his or her own rate; do not force independent functioning or allow too much dependency

Help patient discriminate between internal stimuli and those that come from environment

Use active listening for nonverbal clues and verbal statements

Assess previous adaptive and maladaptive responses to stressors and illness

Assess for self-destructive behavior

Display empathy rather than sympathy

Provide patient and family/significant other with hospital and community resources

Discuss options available, such as cosmetic procedures, mechanical devices, and rehabilitative services

Teach patient and family/significant other the stages of grief and importance of grief work

Expected Outcomes

Progresses toward completion of grief work

Verbalizes an acceptance of altered body functioning or loss

Plans realistically for future role functioning

Incorporates prosthesis, stoma, or device into changed body image

Verbalizes an interest and willingness to rejoin and resume social interactions and activities

Uses hospital and community support systems

■ SELF-ESTEEM DISTURBANCE

DEFINITION

Negative self-evaluation or feelings about self or self-capabilities that may be directly or indirectly expressed

DEFINING CHARACTERISTICS

Self-negating verbalization

Expressions of shame and/or guilt

Evaluation of self as unable to deal with events

Rationalizing away or rejecting positive feedback and exaggerating negative feedback about self

Hesitancy to try new things and situations

Denial of problems obvious to others

Projection of blame and responsibility for problems

Rationalizing personal failures

Hypersensitivity to criticism

Grandiosity

RELATED FACTORS*

Loss of significant others

Change in body function or loss of part

Role change

Chronic illness

Aging

INTERVENTIONS

Provide for success experiences by introducing tasks at patient's level of functioning

Assess for possible alcohol or drug dependency

Communicate acceptance of patient and show genuine concern by spending unstructured, undemanding time

Explore patient's feelings and give validation for their expression

Provide for positive feedback on accomplishments

Explore alternative approach or coping strategies by giving observations; comment on positive attributes; avoid false praise

Explore with patient his or her current strengths

Encourage group interaction and explore possible support groups for aftercare

---

*Related factors in this section are not NANDA approved.

Assist with grooming and hygiene when necessary; promote attractiveness

Help patient list past success experiences

Teach assertive techniques (e.g., use of "I" statements, ability to say "no," body posture, eye contact, tone of voice, personal space, tactics for negotiation)

Teach difference between assertion and nonassertion, and aggressive and passive behaviors

Practice role playing and self-affirmation

Discuss activities that might increase self-esteem

Expected Outcomes

Verbalizes realistic appreciation of self, including attributes and limitations

Reframes losses or changes into opportunities for personal development

Presents a positive personal appearance that reflects good grooming and hygiene

Initiates approach strategies to potentially threatening events or changes in environment

Demonstrates appropriate assertive behavior in social interactions

Reports a minimal level of interpersonal anxiety

Displays no overt self-destructive behaviors

Communicates needs effectively

■ PERSONAL IDENTITY DISTURBANCE

DEFINITION

Inability to distinguish between self and nonself
Personal identity is the coherent sense of self as a unique and separate identity that develops through successful resolution of developmental issues; identity rests on the ability to distinguish self from nonself, others, and the environment

DEFINING CHARACTERISTICS*

Disturbance in body image

Sex role disturbance

Gender identity confusion

Pathologic symbiotic relationships

Undifferentiated or fused family

Dissociative states

Developmental crisis such as adolescence

Delirium or dementia

Functional psychotic states (e.g., schizophrenia, bipolar disorder)

Severe anxiety and/or panic

Hypnagogic states

INTERVENTIONS*

Assist patient with identifying actual threats to himself or herself from misinterpretation of perceived threat

Provide accurate information about threat

Provide calm, structured environment

Encourage self-care activities and taking responsibility for self

Direct activities that are simple and concrete and that support reality issues

Use simple, direct, and concise statements

Assess for altered homeostasis caused by physiologic disequilibrium

Assess developmental issues (e.g., age, crisis, regression)

Encourage verbalization of anxiety concerning sexual identity and sexual preference; be nonjudgmental

Assess for loss of contact with reality (i.e., for hallucinations and/or delusions)

Do not argue with delusions; do not reinforce them; look for needs patient might satisfy and find more appropriate manner of meeting them

Help patient to distinguish what is real and what is hallucination, delusion, or illusion; focus on here and now, decrease stimuli

Use anxiety-reducing interventions

Teach principles of normal growth and development

Refer patient to psychiatric unit or to psychotherapy as necessary

Expected Outcomes*

Distinguishes self from others

Engages in interpersonal relationships without egomerger or dissociation

Performs age-appropriate developmental tasks

FUNCTIONAL HEALTH PATTERN VIII: ROLE AND RELATIONSHIP

■ DYSFUNCTIONAL GRIEVING

DEFINITION

Extended, unsuccessful use of intellectual and emotional responses by which individuals, families, and communities attempt to work through the process of modifying self-concept based on the perception of loss.

DEFINING CHARACTERISTICS

Verbal expression of distress at loss

Denial of loss

Expression of guilt

Expression of unresolved issues

Anger

Sadness

Crying

Difficulty in expressing loss

Alterations in the following:

    Eating habits

    Sleep patterns

    Dream patterns

    Activity level

    Libido

These sections are not NANDA approved.

Idealization of lost object
Reliving of past experiences
Interference with life functioning
Developmental regression
Labile effect
Alterations in concentration and/or pursuits of tasks

RELATED FACTORS
Actual or perceived object loss
Thwarted grieving response to a loss
Absence of anticipatory grieving
Chronic fatal illness
Lack of resolution of previous grieving response
Loss of significant others, possessions, job, status, home, or ideals
Loss of physiopsychosocial well-being
Loss of parts and processes of the body

INTERVENTIONS
Identify significance of loss or multiple losses
Discuss ambivalence
Assess stage of grief and support patient's expression of grief
Use active listening and permit verbalization of anger
Observe for suicidal ideation
Facilitate discussion of positive and negative aspects of loss
Facilitate exploration of support groups
Provide opportunities for social interaction, especially with those who have coped successfully with similar loss
Teach patient and significant other about grief process
If patient attempts to consistently deny grief, plan to spend time each shift talking about loss, but avoid confrontation during discussion if patient changes subject and shifts reference; take cues from patient; be available to reopen subject when patient initiates conversation; use times of silence to convey support by offering your presence nonverbally.
Assure patient that all feelings are normal, including anger, hatred, and feelings of desertion, guilt, or betrayal
Expect patient to meet responsibilities; give positive reinforcement for resuming role responsibilities
Assist patient with identifying ways of adapting his or her lifestyle to accommodate the loss
Explore ways to assist patient to make new emotional investments
Be aware that it is acceptable to share your feelings with patient as long as these activities serve to support patient through his or her grief and are not expressions of unresolved loss on your part
If you become uncomfortable with your own unresolved feelings of loss, have another nurse who is comfortable talk with patient

Expected Outcomes
Demonstrates engagement in the first steps of the grieving process

Demonstrates ability to express feelings of anger, guilt, sadness, depression
Is able to talk about loss and its impact on own life situation
Resumes some before-loss role functions
Mobilizes network of supportive relationships
For anticipatory grief: patient maintains a constructive and meaningful relationship with the dying significant other without displaying characteristics of dysfunctional grief

■ ALTERED ROLE PERFORMANCE

DEFINITION
The pattern of behavior and self-expression do not match the environmental context, norms, and expectations; disruption in the way one perceives one's role performance

DEFINING CHARACTERISTICS
Change in self-perception of role
Denial of role
Change in others' perception of role
Conflict in roles
Change in physical capacity to resume role
Lack of knowledge of role
Change in usual patterns of responsibility

INTERVENTIONS
Assess nature and degree of disturbance in role performance
Assess patient's and significant other's perceptions of role disturbance
Assess cultural and economic factors
Determine number and types of roles within family structure
Assist patient and family with clarifying expected roles and those that must be relinquished or altered
Assist patient with verbalizing realistic expectations of role and concrete behaviors necessary to implement performance
Support grief work if role has been lost
Allow time for expression of fears and anxieties
Be nonjudgmental
Determine if patient is in role that is compatible with his or her sexual orientation, sexual functioning, and self-concept
Provide role model for patient or refer him or her to groups that supply new models
Assist in role rehearsal through role playing

Expected Outcomes
Verbalizes realistic perception and acceptance of new, lost, or altered role
Demonstrates role mastery
Develops with family or significant other specific behavioral strategies for assimilating role-specific changes in existing system

■ RISK FOR VIOLENCE: SELF-DIRECTED (SUICIDE)

DEFINITION
Behaviors in which an individual demonstrates that he/she can be physically, emotionally, and/or sexually harmful to self

RISK FACTORS
Ages 15 to 19 or over 45
Marital status: single, widowed, or divorced
Employment: unemployed, recent job loss/failure
Occupation: executive, administrator/owner of business, professional, semi-skilled
Conflictual interpersonal relationships
Family background: chaotic or conflictual, history of suicide
Sexual orientation: bisexual, homosexual
Physical health: hypochondriac, chronic or terminal illness, organic brain syndrome, major disability
Mental health: severe depression, psychosis, severe personality disorder, alcoholism or substance abuse
Emotional status: hopelessness, despair, increased anxiety, panic, anger, hostility
History of multiple suicide attempts
Suicidal ideation: frequent, intense, prolonged
Suicidal plan: clear and specific, lethality, method and availability of destructive means
Personal resources: poor achievement, poor insight, affect unavailable and poorly controlled
Social resources: poor rapport, socially isolated, unresponsive family
Verbal clues: talking about death, "better off without me," asking questions about lethal dosages of drugs
Behavioral clues: writing letters saying good-bye or asking forgiveness, directing angry messages at a person who has rejected the person, giving away needed personal items, taking out a large life insurance policy or checking on insurance status, making a will, refusing to spend money for new possessions, diminished ability to care for self, agitation, excessive guilt, moderate or extreme anxiety
People who engage in autoerotic sexual acts

INTERVENTIONS
Obtain psychiatric consultation for patient; active suicidal patients need to be seen daily by psychiatric consultant for evaluation and treatment
Administer antidepressant, antianxiety, and/or antipsychotic medications as ordered
   Administer prns as needed; watch for anticholinergic effects and extrapyramidal symptoms
Consider inpatient psychiatric hospitalization for moderate-to-severe depression
Refer patient to outpatient psychiatry for aftercare
Assess patient's suicidal ideation or plan each shift that patient is awake; note patient's sleep/wake patterns, ADLs, and eating behaviors

Assess patient for his or her level of agitation or energy to commit suicide
Assess environment for potential suicidal means such as sharp objects and remove them
Active suicidal patients require one-on-one staffing
Allow patient to talk about his or her depressed/suicidal feelings and respond with active listening
Discuss suicide alternatives and options with patient
Discuss past coping strategies that have lifted depression and ask why patient may want to go on living
Discuss anger management and thought-stopping techniques
Report any increase in suicidal ideation/plan or mood changes to physician; evaluate for use of medications
Engage patient in adaptive activities (e.g., exercise, expressive therapy [music/art/writing], talk therapy) to decrease depression

Expected Outcomes
Demonstrates ability to manage stressors without resorting to violence against self
Expresses satisfaction with current life situation
Demonstrates increased self-esteem
Develops discharge plans with staff

■ RISK FOR VIOLENCE: DIRECTED AT OTHERS

DEFINITION
Behaviors in which an individual demonstrates that he/she can be physically, emotionally, and/or sexually harmful to others

DESCRIPTION
A potential for violence directed at others is characterized by the acting out of anger, hostility, or resentment in such a manner that it brings threat or harm to others in a socially unacceptable context. Hostility may be considered different from anger in that it is viewed as destructive, whereas anger can be seen as constructive. Anger is often justified and can be a healthy response to threatening, fearful, or frustrating situations. Expressing anger may enhance self-esteem and give an individual a sense of power in a situation. Expressing anger appropriately involves the creative use of energy. Unexpressed anger tends to pile up and create a negative and resentful individual who often vents anger inappropriately or not at the original source. Aggressive behavior is hostility acted out and may involve significant danger to others. There are important ethical and legal issues involved in managing aggressive behavior. It is the responsibility of the nurse to become familiar with those issues within the institution. Aggression indicates that behavior is out of control, and it is the responsibility of the staff to protect the patient and others from harm, not to punish the patient

RISK FACTORS

History of violence

Against others (hitting, kicking, spitting, scratching, throwing objects, biting, attempted rape, rape, sexual molestation, urinating/defecating on a person)

Threats (verbal against property, against a person, social, cursing, threatening notes/letters, gestures, sexual threats)

Social (stealing, insistent borrowing, demands for privileges, interruption of meetings, refusal to eat, refusal to take medications, ignoring instructions)

Indirect (tearing off clothes, ripping objects off walls, writing on walls, urinating/defecating on floor, stomping feet, temper tantrum, running in corridors, yelling, throwing objects, breaking a window, slamming doors, sexual advances)

Other factors

Neurologic impairment (positive electroencephalogram [EEG], computerized axial tomography [CAT] scan, or magnetic resonance image [MRI], head trauma, positive neurologic findings, seizure)

Cognitive impairment (learning disabilities, attention deficit disorder, decreased intellectual functioning)

History of childhood abuse

History of witnessing family violence

Cruelty to animals

Firesetting

History of drug/alcohol/substance abuse

Pathologic intoxication

Psychotic symptomatology (auditory, visual, command hallucinations)

Paranoid delusions

Loose, rambling, or illogical thought processes

Motor vehicle offenses (frequent traffic violations, road rage)

Suicidal behavior

Impulsivity

Availability and/or possession of weapon(s)

Body language: rigid posture, clenching of fists and jaw, hyperactivity, pacing, breathlessness, and threatening stances

RELATED FACTORS

Antisocial character

Battered spouse/significant other/intimate partner

Catatonic excitement

Child abuse

Manic excitement

Organic brain syndrome

Panic states

Rage reactions

Suicidal behavior

Temporal lobe epilepsy

Toxic reaction to medications

INTERVENTIONS

Intervene early; prevention is the best strategy

Call patient by name; speak in calm, firm, manner and tell patient to stop his or her violent or assaultive behavior

Direct patient to calm and control himself or herself

Do not approach an openly hostile, aggressive patient by yourself; obtain assistance from other staff members

Listen to what patient has to say

Do not invade personal space

Do not touch patient

Remove others from immediate area

Do not threaten, argue, or respond with hostility

Do not approach patient who has a weapon by yourself or attempt to disarm him or her; get appropriate assistance

State that you cannot allow patient to harm himself or herself or anyone in environment

Do not leave patient alone

Be aware of your own feelings and behavior

Maintain and communicate control to patient

Do not become personally insulted or demonstrate anger at patient's behavior

Do not submit to patient's inappropriate demands

Have another nurse remain with patient if you become upset or defensive

Decrease environmental stimulation

Give patient as much control over his or her own area as is safely possible

Focus on patient's feelings

Avoid pat reassurances and overgeneralizations

Use the same terms that patient uses (e.g., "upset," "frustrated," "ticked off")

Make every attempt to talk patient out of intended assaultive behavior

Apply mechanical restraints only if absolutely necessary and according to policy; have a plan

Offer medication early in preescalation phase

Administer chemical restraint (medications) according to policy

When incident has passed, complete the following:

Assist patient with identifying and discussing his or her feelings

Assist patient with identifying what triggered loss of control

Assist patient with identifying alternative ways of expressing emotion and relieving tension

Be aware of importance of staff continuing with routine patient care activities

Manage emotional reactions of other patients to the incident

Involve patient in activities to promote release of energy and feelings (e.g., large muscle movement)

Understand that rejection of patient by staff can increase patient's anxiety and perpetuate anger

Teach difference between assertive and aggressive behavior

Expected Outcomes

Will not direct excessive hostility or assaultive behaviors toward others

Will use alternative ways to manage expression of anger

Displays effective coping strategies in reducing anxiety and in assessing potentially threatening situations

Develops increased self-awareness and increased self-esteem

■ DOMESTIC VIOLENCE*

DESCRIPTION
Physical or emotional harassment, assault and battery, including rape, between family members, significant others, or acquaintances; nearly 30% of all homicides in the United States occur among family members

ASSESSMENT
SUBJECTIVE DATA
Pain associated with physical trauma (including rape)

Anxiety, depression, apprehension, or hopelessness

Repetitive nightmares or reliving of event

Sleep pattern disturbances

Eating pattern disturbance

GI irritability

Sexual dysfunction

Depression

Fear of being indoors or outdoors

Fear of being with opposite gender, spouse, or lover

Suicide attempts

Describes typical behaviors of potential or actual batterer

　Actual injuries, including rape; injuries during pregnancy

　Controlling behavior; manages person's schedule, comings/goings, and decisions

　Jealousy of person's time with friends, family, and co-workers

　Isolation; cuts person off from supportive resources such as talking with friends on phone or socializing with co-workers

　Batterer blames others for personal problems; it is always someone else's fault; past history of battering with a list of excuses why someone else caused the battering behavior; disavows responsibility for personal actions

　Hypersensitive and easily upset by minor annoyances (e.g., criticism of any kind, request to assist with child care or chores)

　Cruelty to children and animals with seeming insensitivity to their pain and suffering; teases and/or hurts children and animals

　"Playful" use of force in sex; holding the person down or initiating sex when the person is asleep, sick, or tired

　Verbal abuse including degrading, cruel, and humiliating language; prevents person from going to sleep to argue or wakes person up to verbally abuse

　Mercurial behavior; sudden mood swings with unpredictability of demeanor, emotional outbursts

　Demonstrates loving remorse/sorrow and vows never to repeat the battering but does so

　Breaks or strikes objects, narrowly missing or actually hitting person or children; beats on furniture/table

　Threatens violence including threats to kill the person, hurt him or her, break his or her neck

　Uses physical force during an argument by holding person down or against a wall; pushes, hits, slaps, shoves, or kicks; chokes, stabs, or shoots

OBJECTIVE DATA
Injuries on face, neck, throat, chest, abdomen, or genitals

Multiple injuries in various stages of healing

History of injuries during pregnancy

Substantial delay between onset of injury and presentation for treatment

Minimization of the seriousness of the situation and the injuries

Flat affect; tearfulness; verbalization of hopelessness, helplessness, and apathy

Extent or type of injury inconsistent with explanation given

No verbalization of occurrence of assault, denial

Guilt, withdrawal

Sense of humiliation

Anxious

Evidence of alcohol or drug abuse

Partner appears to be overly (out of norm) concerned with patient's care; does not leave when requested; intrusive regarding patient's medical care

Evidence of nonspecific physical or psychologic complaints such as frequent headaches, nonorganic GI complaints, depression, anxiety, exhaustion, difficulty in concentrating

DIAGNOSTIC TESTS (FOR RAPE)
Cultures for gonorrhea and chlamydia

Microscopic examination of vaginal secretions for motile sperm

Baseline serologic tests for hepatitis B virus; human immunodeficiency virus (HIV), and syphilis

Pregnancy test

DIAGNOSTIC TESTS (FOR BATTERY)
Radiologic examination, including MRI, CT scans, and ultrasound

Endoscopic/laparoscopic procedures as indicated

Assessment for compartmental syndrome

CBC and coagulation factors

POTENTIAL COMPLICATIONS
Noncurable sexually transmitted disease (herpes, acquired immunodeficiency syndrome [AIDS])

Pregnancy

Intracranial bleed

Fractures

Internal bleeding

Hemorrhage, shock, death

MULTIDISCIPLINARY MANAGEMENT
THERAPEUTIC MANAGEMENT
Manage evident trauma: hematomas, fractures, lacerations

Photographs of injuries

Prophylaxis for sexually transmitted disease if raped

Postcoital hormonal prophylaxis to prevent pregnancy if raped

Not a NANDA-approved diagnosis.

Tetanus injection

Psychologic counseling

Notification of police department and/or child protective services

Forensic consultation

Referral to a "safe house" or shelter

Collection of evidentiary material for authorities, including pubic hair combings, samples of pubic and head hair, vaginal secretions, cultures, results of microscopic evaluation for motile sperm, and collection of patient's bagged clothing in rape cases

PATIENT PROBLEMS—NURSING DIAGNOSES/INTERVENTIONS

▼ Rape-trauma syndrome associated with attempted or actual attack

Provide safe and protected environment

Ensure considerate physical examination

Assist to establish a close relationship with a safe person *to ensure presence of an ongoing support person*

Assist patient and support person to discuss and focus on the subjective experience *to express feelings*

Discuss anger and related feelings *to avoid social withdrawal and isolation*

Assist patient to establish self-control over personal decisions

Counsel patient regarding stress response images, sounds, or sensations that provoke anxiety

Counsel immediate family about rape-trauma syndrome and how symptoms are manifested in patient and their response to the patient

Expected Outcomes

Verbalizes that support person has expressed concern and warmth

Verbalizes understanding of rape-trauma syndrome or retains document describing anticipated future reactions, signs, and symptoms

Verbalizes intent to adhere to decisions made about keeping follow-up appointments (medical, psychologic counseling, HIV results counseling, rape-support groups), taking of medications, and following through with legal authorities

▼ Powerlessness related to victimization by a violent individual

Encourage patient to identify the areas over which he or she has power, such as managing the care and nutrition for children, and reinforce those capabilities *to promote a sense of control and of capability*

Identify areas of perceived powerlessness and assist patient to consider alternatives and other courses of action

Assist patient to identify a resource person while he or she is safe; encourage patient to contact this person before leaving the health care provider's office *to ensure patient safety and security*

Provide opportunities to express feelings *to increase understanding of individual coping styles and mechanisms to provide a more objective perception of the violence/battering*

Encourage expressions of positive thoughts and emotions, including the will to live, hope and faith, and a sense of purpose

Assist patient to develop a "safety plan" for self and children in order *to be able to leave the home environment at any time day or night*

Expected Outcomes

Verbalizes positive feelings and confidence in ability to increase control over life circumstances

Demonstrates effective coping strategies based on realistic assessment of personal situation (e.g., seeks protective services for self or children and has a safety plan)

Acknowledges abilities for managing nutrition for self and children

PATIENT/FAMILY TEACHING AND DISCHARGE/HOME CARE PLANNING

Instruct patient to go to any emergency room if future injuries occur by calling an ambulance, friend, relative, or the police

Contact personal physician or other health care provider immediately if future injuries occur

Learn how to obtain a copy of patient's medical record, which will be needed when the district attorney files charges against the abuser

Develop a safety plan for self and children for leaving the abuser because this may need to occur during, after, or when anticipating a beating

A safety plan might include the following measures:

Pack an extra set of clothes, toilet articles, and necessary medications for self and children; store this with a friend or neighbor; include an extra set of keys to the house and car

Have extra cash, credit cards, checkbook, or savings account book hidden or with a friend; have identification for self and children such as birth certificates, Social Security cards, voter registration, marriage and/or driver's license, and children's immunization records, which may be required to enroll children in a school or to obtain financial assistance

Have a list of important phone numbers in a protected place, including police, attorney or legal aid, relatives, friends, social service agencies, crisis hotlines, or safe houses

Take something special or meaningful, such as a favorite toy, blanket, or book, for each child if possible

Take or have photocopies of important financial records, such as tax returns, grant deed, house payment or rent receipts, insurance, and title to the car, in a protected place

Have a plan and know exactly where to go and how to get there even if the battering should occur in the middle of the night

Explain that a period of loving remorse by the batterer who promises never to beat the victim again is a typical response of batterers who feel ashamed and horrified by their actions

Ensure that patient understands that remorseful batterers *do* typically repeat the battering and rarely discontinue battering without being brought into the legal system and that legal intervention *does* have a positive effect

◼ IMPAIRED SOCIAL INTERACTION

DEFINITION
The state in which an individual participates in an insufficient or excessive quantity or ineffective quality of social exchange

DEFINING CHARACTERISTICS
Verbalized or observed discomfort in social situations
Verbalized or observed inability to receive or communicate a satisfying sense of belonging, caring, interest, or shared history
Observed use of unsuccessful social interaction behaviors
Dysfunctional interaction with peers, family, and/or others
Family report of change in style or pattern of interaction

RELATED FACTORS
Knowledge/skill deficit about ways to enhance mutuality
  Communication barriers
  Self-concept or self-esteem disturbance
  Absence of available significant others or peers
  Limited physical mobility
  Therapeutic isolation
  Sociocultural dissonance
  Environmental barriers
  Altered thought processes
  Inadequate personality

FUNCTIONAL HEALTH PATTERN X: COPING/STRESS TOLERANCE

◼ INEFFECTIVE INDIVIDUAL COPING

DEFINITION
Inability to form a valid appraisal of stressors, inadequate choices of practiced responses, and/or inability to use available resources; impairment of adaptive behaviors and problem-solving abilities of a person in meeting life's demands and roles

DEFINING CHARACTERISTICS
Verbalization of inability to cope or inability to ask for help
Inability to meet role expectations
Inability to meet basic needs
Inability to problem solve
Alteration in societal participation
Destructive behavior toward self or others
Inappropriate use of defense mechanisms
Change in visual communication patterns
Lack of goal-directed behavior and problem resolution
Difficulty in organizing information
Poor concentration
Verbal manipulation
High illness rate
High rate of accidents
Overeating
Lack of appetite
Excessive smoking
Excessive drinking
Sleep disturbancc
Overuse of prescribed tranquilizers
Alcohol proneness
High blood pressure
Chronic fatigue
Insomnia
Muscular tension
Ulcers
Frequent headaches
Frequent neckaches
Irritable bowel
Chronic worry
General irritability
Poor self-esteem
Chronic anxiety
Emotional tension
Chronic depression

RELATED FACTORS
Situational crises
Maturational crises
Personal vulnerability
Inadequate level of confidence in ability to cope
Multiple life changes
No vacations
Inadequate relaxation
Inadequate support systems
Little or no exercise
Poor nutrition
Unmet expectations
Work overload
Too many deadlines
Unrealistic perceptions
Inadequate opportunity to prepare for stressor
Inability to conserve adaptive energies
Inadequate coping methods

INTERVENTIONS
Understand that patient may not know what the problem is
Assist patient with clearly identifying precipitating event
Explore major changes that have occurred in previous 2 weeks, past 6 months, or last year

Ask patient how he or she feels and help patient to put a label on emotion

Assist patient with identifying

How problem affects his or her life and future

How problem is affecting patient's family or significant other

If other factors could be influencing the way he or she sees problem

Assist patient with identifying his or her strengths and coping skills

Ask patient if anything like this has happened to him or her in past

Ask how past crises were handled

Inquire as to how patient usually decreases tension and anxiety

Ascertain whether patient has tried to use any of the same anxiety-reducing methods this time; if not, attempt to explore possible reasons or blocks to using prior coping skills

If anxiety-reducing methods were tried and were unsuccessful, ask what kept them from working

Assist patient with exploring and identifying what else he or she thinks might work

Assist patient with identifying nature and strength of situational supports; collect data about current and potential sources of support:

Persons with whom patient lives

Persons with whom patient is close

Friends or best friend

Persons available to help

Persons whom patient trusts and feels are understanding

Community services

Assist patient with planning alternative solutions using patient's own coping skills and situational and environmental supports

Offer suggestions of other adaptive coping strategies

Confront self-defeating and destructive behavior in a factual and nonjudgmental manner; make observations about amount of alcohol intake, use of tranquilizers, or overindulgence in food or smoking

Acknowledge patient's feelings about crisis

Assist patient with sorting out his or her feelings and validate them as acceptable and normal

Assist patient with exploring alternative coping skills

Assist patient with role playing or rehearsing new approaches to deal with problems

Present yourself as role model for open and direct communication, innovative thinking, flexibility, and self-awareness

Provide positive reinforcement for all adaptive coping skills used in situation

Teach relaxation techniques

Teach patient about psychologic and physiologic effects of chronic stress

EXPECTED OUTCOMES

Returns to precrisis level of functioning

Develops an adequate response repertoire

Displays no symptoms of excessive anxiety or lasting physiologic responses to stress

Increases self-esteem

Acknowledges increased confidence to solve future problems effectively

FUNCTIONAL HEALTH PATTERN XI: VALUE AND BELIEF

■ SPIRITUAL DISTRESS (DISTRESS OF THE HUMAN SPIRIT)

DEFINITION
Disruption in the life principle that pervades a person's entire being and that integrates and transcends one's biologic and psychosocial nature

DEFINING CHARACTERISTICS
Concern expressed regarding the meaning of life and death and/or belief systems

Anger toward supreme being (as defined by the person)

Questioning the meaning of suffering

Verbalizing inner conflict about beliefs

Verbalizing concern about relationship with deity/supreme being

Questioning meaning of own existence

Inability to choose or choosing not to participate in usual religious practices

Seeking spiritual assistance

Questioning moral and ethical implications of therapeutic regimen

Displacement of anger toward religious representatives

Description of nightmares or sleep disturbances

Alteration in behavior or mood evidenced by anger, crying, withdrawal, preoccupation, anxiety, hostility, apathy

Regarding illness as punishment

Not experiencing that God is forgiving

Inability to accept self

Engaging in self-blame

Denying responsibility for problems

Describing somatic complaints

RELATED FACTORS
Separation from religious and cultural ties

Challenged belief and value system (e.g., result of moral or ethical implications of therapy or result of intense suffering)

INTERVENTIONS
Assess cause(s) of spiritual distress

Assess patient's belief in divine power, its existence, and credibility

Meaning of religion; description or relationship of divine power

Means of communicating with divine power
Effect of beliefs on personal life
Sense of identity, worth, and purpose
Relationship with others: value, need, changes caused
    by illness
Meaning of illness or suffering in relation to belief
Important features of religious faith
    Assistance with fear, pain
    Source of strength, hope, love
Religious practices, symbols, medals, garments

Provide a quiet, private atmosphere for patient's
    expressions of faith, self, and meaning of life

Listen with attention, understanding, and compassion

Be available and sensitive to patient's needs to express his
    or her feelings

Talk *with,* not *at,* the patient

Be cognizant of your nonverbal behavior, biases,
    preconceptions, and judgments

Do not impose your beliefs on patient

Accurately interpret and clarify meanings expressed and
    behavior observed

Assist patient with facing reality; explore patient's
    experience with illness and meaning of suffering

Encourage self-awareness and mobilization of internal
    strengths and resources

Assist patient through uncompleted developmental stages
    to attain trust, hope, love, forgiveness, and purpose in
    life

Assist patient with exploring life situations and
    discovering practical solutions to problems

Allow and encourage free choice and decision making

Praise physical, emotional, and spiritual successes

Convey to patient that he or she is important and what
    he or she does with his or her life matters

Use touch therapeutically (e.g., stroking, holding hands,
    and grooming) when providing daily care if patient
    desires

Provide pleasant view and special pictures

Control odors and smoking as necessary

Provide articles necessary for religious practice (e.g.,
    special clothing, rosary, books)

Arrange patient's religious symbols for easy viewing

Arrange for patient's favorite music (i.e., obtain recordings)

Read favorite, comforting passages from Bible, Koran,
    Torah, Book of Mormon, poetry, or other meaningful
    works

Share in prayers or special practices when appropriate

Provide uninterrupted time for meditation, silence, and
    prayer

Arrange for communion, Holy Eucharist, anointment, and
    other practices

Arrange easy access for communication with loved ones,
    chaplain, priest, rabbi, or minister

Provide special foods, meals, and periods of fasting as
    needed

Consider needs in special situations
    Birth
        Baptism
        Circumcision

Medical procedures
    Amputation
    Burial
    Transfusions
Schedule for holy days
Religious observances
Anointment
Laying-on of hands
Healing services
Confession
Communion, Holy Eucharist
Restrictions or needs in diet or appearance
Not cutting or shaving of hair
Use of special clothing
Death
    Baptism
    Rite for anointing the sick
    Bathing and placement of body
    Positioning of extremities

Expected Outcomes

Expresses increase in spiritual wellness
Expresses increased sense of hope and well-being
Uses available religious resources

BIBLIOGRAPHY

Beare PG, Myers JL: *Adult health nursing,* St Louis, 1998, Mosby.

Braden GJ, Bergstrom N: Clinical utility of the Braden Scale for predicting pressure sore risk, *Decubitus* 2(3);44, 1987.

Crigger N, Forbes W: Assessing neurologic function in older patients, *AJN* 97(3):37, 1997.

Durham E, Weiss L: How patients die, *AJN* 97(12):41, 1997.

Eisenberg PG: A nursing guide to tube feeding, *RN* 57(10):62, 1994.

Gan TJ et al: Bispectral index monitoring allows faster emergence and improved recovery from propofol, alfentanil and nitrous oxide anesthesia, *Anesthesiology* 87(4):808, 1997.

Giger J, Davidhizar R: *Transcultural nursing,* St Louis, 1991, Mosby.

Glass PS et al: Bispectral analysis measures sedation and memory effects of propofol, midazolam, isoflurane and alfentanil in health volunteers, *Anesthesiology* 86(4):836, 1997.

Gordon M: *Manual of nursing diagnosis,* St Louis, 1997, Mosby.

Greene LM, Gerlach CJ: Central lines have moved out, *RN* 57(5):26, 1994.

Gritter M: The latex threat, *AJN* 98(9):26, 1998.

Isaacs A: Depression and your patient, *AJN* 98(7):26, 1998.

Kim MJ, McFarland GK, McLane AM: *Pocket guide to nursing diagnoses,* St Louis, 1997, Mosby.

Leuckenotte AG: *Gerontologic nursing,* St Louis, 1996, Mosby.

North American Nursing Diagnosis Association: *NANDA nursing diagnoses: definitions and classification, 1999-2000,* Philadelphia, 1999, The Association.

Phipps WJ et al: *Medical-surgical nursing: concepts and clinical practice,* ed 6, St Louis, 1999, Mosby.

Recker DH, Metzler DJ: Use of the multi-lumen catheter, *Critical Care Nurse* 4(3):92, 1984.

Shea CA, Mahoney M, Lacey JM: Breaking through the barriers to domestic violence intervention, *AJN* 97(6):26, 1997.

Swearingen PL, Ross DG: *Manual of medical-surgical nursing care,* St Louis, 1999, Mosby.

U.S. Department of Health and Human Services, Acute Pain Management Guideline Panel. *Acute pain management: operative or medical procedures and trauma:* *clinical practice guideline,* (AHCPR pub no 92-0032), Rockville, Md, Agency for Health Care Policy and Research, 1992.

Tellis-Nyak: The postacute continuum of care, understanding your patient's options, *AJN* 98(8):44, 1998.

Cardiovascular System

■ CARDIOVASCULAR ASSESSMENT

▌ SUBJECTIVE DATA

Pain
   Onset
   Duration
   Location
   Radiation
   Description
Indigestion
Weakness
Fatigue
Fainting
Dizzy spells, lightheadedness
Shortness of breath (SOB) with or without activity or on
   waking at night
Palpitations
Sudden awakening at night with SOB
Fever
Cough, wheezing, hemoptysis
Swelling of extremities
Blue discoloration of lips, fingers
Nausea
Numb, cold extremities
Changes in vision
Headaches

▌ OBJECTIVE DATA

Age
Sex
Weight/height
General appearance
   Color
   Assumed position
Vital signs
   Arterial pulses (P) (Fig. 3-1)
      Rate
      Rhythm
      Equality
      Presence
      Absence
   Respirations (R)
      Rate
      Character
      Type
      Temperature (T)

Neck veins
   Distension
   Venous pressure
   Pulsation
Blood pressure (BP)
   Position and extremity
   Pulse pressure
   Pulsus paradoxus
   Pulsus alternans
Urinary output
   Amount
   Character
   Color
Precordium (Fig. 3-3)
   Point of maximal impulse (PMI)
   Lifts
   Bulges
   Pulsations
   Thrills
Heart sounds (Fig. 3-4)
   Intensity
   Pitch
   Duration
   Timbre
   Origin
   S_1, S_2
   Presence of S_3, S_4
   Murmurs
   Pericardial friction rub
Breath sounds
   Location
   Description
      Normal
      Decreased
      Pleural friction rub
      Adventitious
      Rhonchi
      Crackles
Skin
   Color
   Temperature
   Turgor
   Diaphoresis
   Dryness

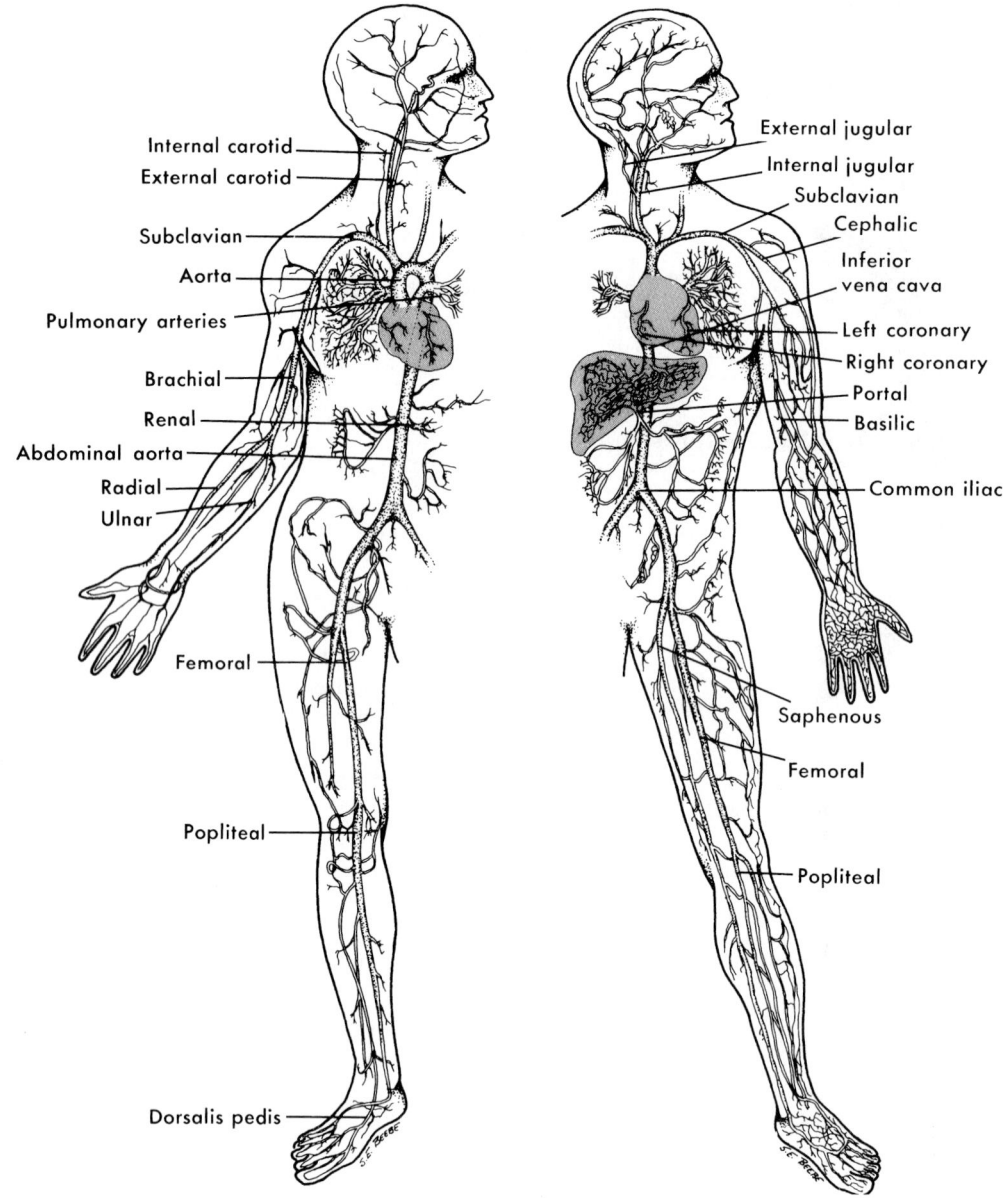

Fig. 3-1   Arterial system *(left)* and venous system *(right)*.

Extremities
  Appearance
  Color
  Temperature
  Edema
  Capillary filling time
  "Clubbing"
  Nail shape
  Description of lesions
Central nervous system (CNS)
  Level of consciousness (LOC)
  Neurologic signs
  Reflexes
  Response to pain
Gastrointestinal (GI) system
  Ascites
  Hepatomegaly

▌ PERTINENT BACKGROUND INFORMATION

CONCURRENT DISEASES OR CONDITIONS
Atherosclerosis
Hyperlipoproteinemia
Hypertension
Obesity
Diabetes
Pulmonary conditions
  Pneumonia
  Emphysema
  Cor pulmonale
Renal conditions

BEHAVIORAL RESPONSES
Response to stress
Methods of coping

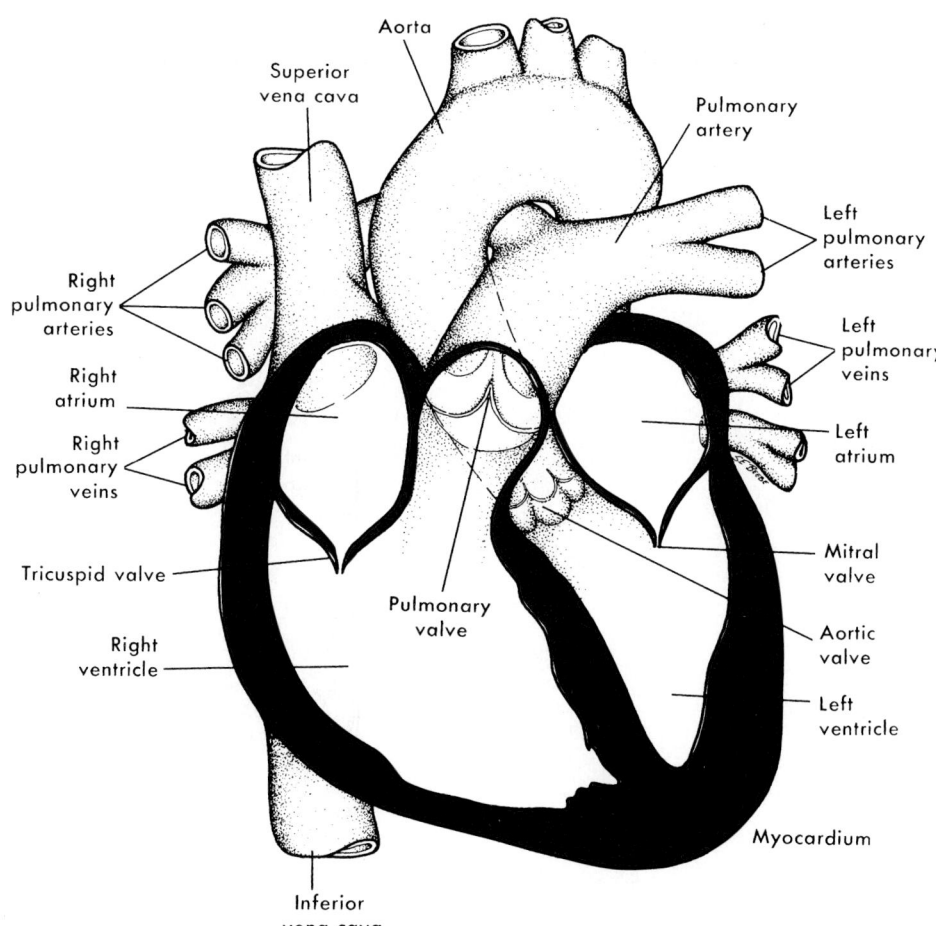

Superior
vena cava

Aorta

Pulmonary
artery

Left
pulmonary
arteries

Right
pulmonary
arteries

Left
pulmonary
veins

Right
atrium

Left
atrium

Right
pulmonary
veins

Mitral
valve

Tricuspid valve

Aortic
valve

Pulmonary
valve

Left
ventricle

Right
ventricle

Myocardium

Inferior
vena cava

Fig. 3-2   Circulatory system (heart).

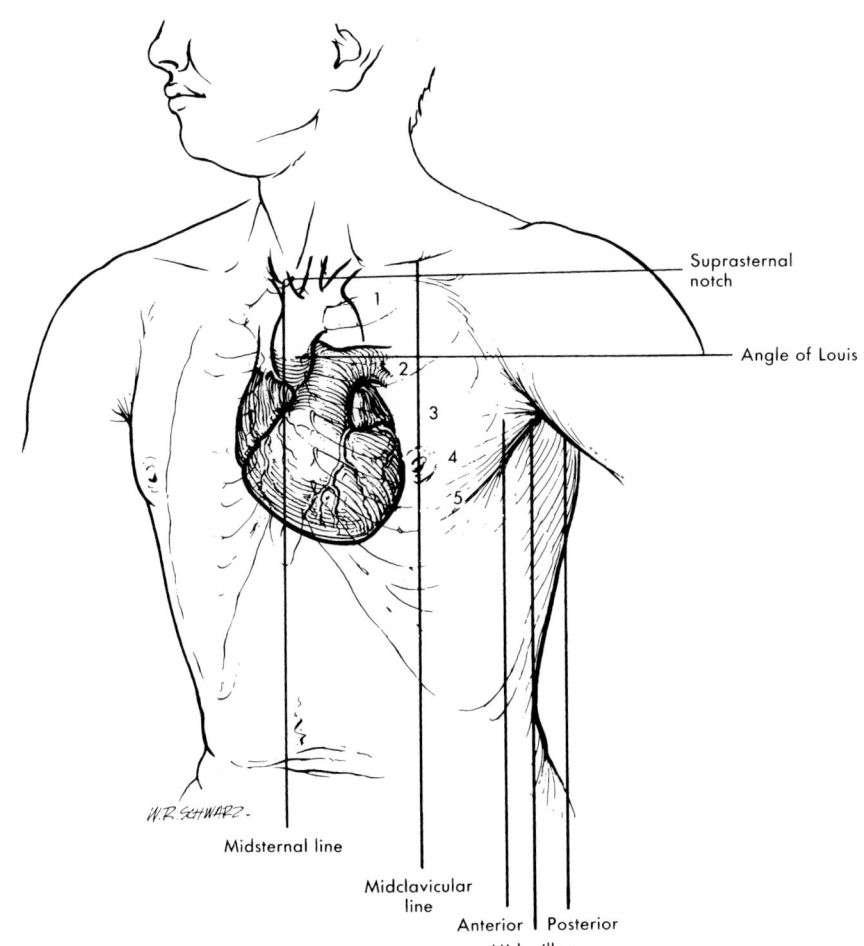

W.R. SCHWARZ

Suprasternal
notch

Angle of Louis

1

2

3

4

5

Fig. 3-3   Chest wall landmarks.
(From Malasanos L et al: Health assessment, *ed 4, St Louis, 1990, Mosby.)*

Midsternal line

Midclavicular
line

Anterior   Posterior

Midaxillary
lines

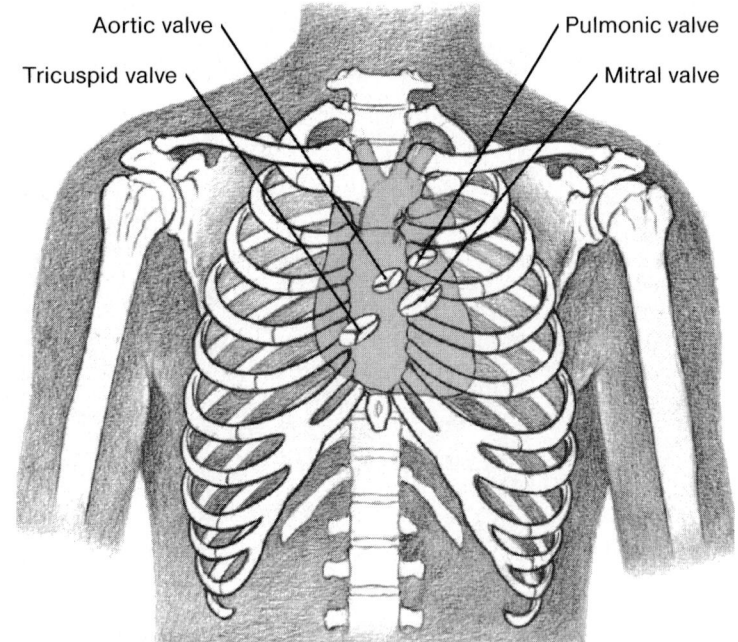

Aortic valve

Tricuspid valve

Pulmonic valve

Mitral valve

Fig. 3-4 Anatomic location of cardiac valves. *(From Canobbio MM: Mosby's clinical nursing series: cardiovascular disorders, St Louis, 1990, Mosby.)*

Response to pain
Relationships with others
Recent stressful life events

MEDICAL HISTORY
Infancy and childhood
   Cyanosis at birth
   Murmurs
Systemic infection
   Rheumatic fever
   Endocarditis
   Kawasaki disease
Coronary artery disease
   Myocardial infarction (MI)
   Angina
   Heart failure
Heart murmur
Congenital heart disease
Cardiovascular surgery
Thromboembolism
Occlusive vascular disease
Pulmonary conditions
Renal conditions

FAMILY HISTORY
Heart disease
Hypertension
Diabetes
Obesity
Arterial and venous diseases
Cerebrovascular accident (CVA)
Kidney disease

SOCIAL/CULTURAL HISTORY
Cultural orientation
Educational level

Smoking
Alcohol use
Exercise and activity levels
Nutritional status
   Height
   Weight
   Less or more than body requirements
Occupation (sedentary or active)
Sleep patterns
Leisure activities
Environmental factors
Economic resources
Insurability status
Social support resources
   Marital status
   Number of siblings, children

MEDICATION HISTORY
Prescription medications
   Digitalis preparations
   Antihypertensives
   Anticoagulants
   Beta blockers
   Angiotensin-converting enzyme (ACE) inhibitors
   Calcium channel blockers
   Vasodilators
   Diuretics
   Hormones: birth control pills, replacement therapy
   Other
Over-the-counter medications
   Aspirin
   Cold and influenza remedies
   Sleeping pills
Street or illicit drugs
   Cocaine
   Intravenous (IV) drug use

Gerontologic Considerations

- Changes in the cardiac musculature lead to reduced efficiency and strength, resulting in decreased cardiac output.
- Disorientation, syncope, and decreased tissue perfusion to organs and other body tissues can occur as a result of decreased cardiac output.
- Aging causes sclerotic changes in blood vessels and leads to decreased elasticity and narrowing of the lumen. Arterial pathology resulting from the aging process causes hypertension because of the increased cardiac effort needed to pump blood through the circulatory system.
- Progressive coronary artery changes can lead to the development of collateral coronary circulation. This can modify the severity of signs and symptoms seen in myocardial infarction. Angina symptoms may be less pronounced, and dyspnea may replace angina as a key symptom of acute infarction.
- Congestive heart failure can result from rapid intravenous infusion.
- Edema secondary to congestive heart failure may cause tissue impairment in the immobile older adult. Immobility leads to venous stasis and increases the risk of venous thrombosis and embolus formation.
- Older adults with cardiac disease often receive several medications, which are often prescribed at lower doses than for younger adults. Even with lower doses of medications, the older adult should be observed closely for signs of toxicity, because the rate of drug metabolism and excretion decreases with age.
- Independent older adults with cardiac conditions should receive adequate teaching regarding medication, diet, and warning signs of complications. They should be encouraged to maintain regular contact with the physician and to seek care at the first sign of problems.

From Christensen BL, Kockrow EO: Foundations of nursing, *ed 3, St Louis, 1998, Mosby.*

DIAGNOSTIC TESTS

Serum studies
  Enzyme profile
    Aspartate aminotransferase (AST)
    Creatine kinase (CK-MB), creatine phosphokinase (CPK-MB)
    Cardiac troponins (cTnT, cTnI)
    Lactic acid dehydrogenase (LDH)
  Electrolyte profile
  Cholesterol value
  Lipid levels; high-density lipoprotein (HDL) to low-density lipoprotein (LDL) ratio
  Triglyceride value
  Complete blood cell count (CBC)
  Erythrocyte sedimentation rate (ESR)
  Hemoglobin (Hgb)
  Hematocrit (Hct)
  Clotting profile
    Prothrombin time (PT)
    Activated partial thromboplastin time (APTT)
    International Normalize Ratio (INR)
    Heparin time
  Thyroid function tests (TFTs)
  Blood urea nitrogen (BUN), creatinine level
  Glucose level
  Urinalysis

ELECTROCARDIOGRAM (ECG)

P wave
P-R interval
QRS complex
Q-T interval
ST segment
T wave
U wave
Axis calculation
Rhythm identification
Chamber enlargement
Cardiac index (CI)
Cardiac output (CO)
Pulmonary artery pressure (PAP)
Pulmonary artery wedge pressure (PAWP)
Pulmonary vascular resistance (PVR)
Systemic vascular resistance (SVR)
Stroke volume index (SVI, SI)
Right atrial pressure (RAP)

OTHER PROCEDURES
NONINVASIVE
Radiologic studies
  Chest x-ray examination
Echocardiography
  M-mode
  Two-dimensional
  Doppler ultrasound
Transesophageal echocardiogram (TEE)
Exercise electrocardiography (exercise tolerance, stress test)
Ambulatory electrocardiography
  Continuous recording (Holter)
  Intermittent recording
    Transtelephonic
Signal averaging (SA) ECG
Atrial electrogram (AEG)
Head up–tilt table (HUTT)
Nuclear studies
  Thallium uptake
  Computed tomography (CT) scan
  Multigated cardiac blood pool imaging (MUGA)
  Magnetic resonance imaging (MRI)

INVASIVE
Arterial pressure
Digital subtraction angiography (DSA)
Digital vascular imaging (DVI)
Cardiac catheterization
Coronary arteriography

Coronary angiography
Ventriculography
Electrophysiologic (EP) studies
   His bundle recordings
   Programmed electrical stimulation (PES)
   Mapping (endocardial, epicardial)

■ PERIPHERAL VASCULAR ASSESSMENT

▌ SUBJECTIVE DATA

Limb pain
   Initiating factors: onset
      Sudden or chronic
      Continuous exercise
      Rest
      Amount of exercise tolerated
   Provoking factor: change in environmental
      temperature, exercise, position
   Alleviating factors
      Rest
      Exercise
      Repositioning of limb
      Effect of prescribed medication
   Location
      Buttock
      Thigh
      Calf
      Foot
Swelling of extremity
Skin discoloration: pale, red, blue tinged
Numb, cold extremities
Transient ischemic attack (TIA)
Abdominal or back pain

▌ PERTINENT BACKGROUND INFORMATION

CONCURRENT DISEASES OR CONDITIONS
Atherosclerosis
Hyperlipidemia
Hypertension
Diabetes
Obesity
Heart failure
Renal conditions
Collagen vascular disorder

MEDICAL HISTORY
Thrombophlebitis
Deep vein thrombosis (DVT)
Cerebrovascular disease
Coronary artery disease
Aneurysm
Previous surgeries (e.g., coronary artery bypass graft [CABG])

FAMILY HISTORY
Premature or sudden deaths
Cerebrovascular diseases
Atherosclerosis

Diabetes
Hypertension

MEDICATION HISTORY
Over-the-counter: aspirin
Prescribed medications
   Antihypertensives
   Anticoagulants
   Antiinflammatories
   Steroids
   Hormone therapy
   Fibrinolytics
   Vasodilators

SOCIAL HISTORY
Tobacco use; second-hand exposure
Alcohol and caffeine use
Occupation (sedentary or active)
Environmental factors
Exercise and activity levels: recent changes caused by
   increased symptoms
Leisure activities

▌ DIAGNOSTIC TESTS

NONINVASIVE
Ankle-brachial index (A-B index)
Segmental limb systolic pressure (SLP)
   Normal
      Lower extremities
         Midthigh: 16 mm Hg
         Upper third of leg: 3 to 12 mm Hg
         Above ankle: 1 to 18 mm Hg
         Foot: 0.2 to 1 mm Hg
      Upper extremities
         Upper arm: 4 to 16 mm Hg
         Elbow: 3 to 12 mm Hg
         Wrist: 1 to 10 mm Hg
         Hand: 0.2 to 2 mm Hg
Phlebography (venography)
Doppler flow velocity tracings
Plethysmography
Radioactive fibrinogen uptake
Infrared thermography (IRT)
Carotid phonoangiogram (CPG)
Stress testing
Allen test
   Radial
   Ulnar
CT scan
Magnetic resonance arteriogram (MRA)

INVASIVE
Digital subtraction angiography (DSA)
Angiography

OBJECTIVE DATA
General appearance
   Color
      Assumed position

Age
Vital signs: BP, T, P, and R
Pulses
  Rate
  Equality
  Rhythm
  Amplitude
    4+: strong, bounding (normal)
    3+: easily palpable
    2+: difficult to palpate
    1+: weak, thready
    0: absent
  Bruits
    Carotid
    Subclavian
    Abdominal
    Femoral
Skin
  Temperature
  Tissue loss
    Ulceration
    Gangrene
  Lesions
Color
  Pale: increased pallor of lower extremities with
    walking, with elevation
  Mottled
  Cyanosis
  Redness (rubor): increased in dependent position
Hair loss
Opacification of nails
Lower extremities
  Cold feet
  Intermittent claudication
    Pain: calves, thighs, buttocks
    Onset with continuous exercise
    Localized or radiates
    Relieved by rest or stopping activity
  Pain with rest
  Tissue loss
Upper extremities
  Digital ischemia
  Fingertip ulcerations
  Gangrene
  Positive Allen test
Abdomen
  Pulsatile abdominal mass
  Bruits
Capillary filling time
  Normal: <3 seconds
  Abnormal: >3 seconds

■ VENOUS THROMBOSIS

An abnormal vascular condition associated with thrombus formation within a blood vessel, which develops as a result of stasis, hypercoagulability, or damage to the internal lining of the vein; can occur in superficial or deep veins (Fig. 3-5); the following are terms used to describe venous disorders that reflect thrombus (clot) formation:

phlebitis: *Inflammation of a vein*

phlebothrombosis (venous thrombosis): *Intraluminal thrombus with minimal or no inflammatory component; these have a greater tendency to embolize*

thromboembolism: *Phenomenon of thrombus dislodgment and migration*

thrombophlebitis: *An acute condition characterized by thrombus and inflammation in deep or superficial veins*

ASSESSMENT
SUBJECTIVE DATA
Pain: ache, cramping, tenderness, heavy feeling over
  involved extremity
Swelling

OBJECTIVE DATA
Lower extremity (deep veins)
  Calf pain with dorsiflexion of foot (Homan's sign)
  Redness
  Taut, shiny skin
  Swelling and edema
  Increased size compared with nonaffected extremity
  Increased skin temperature
  Tenderness to palpation at calf
  Peripheral pulses: present, absent
Upper extremity (superficial veins)
  Redness
  Warmth
  Tenderness
Elevated temperature

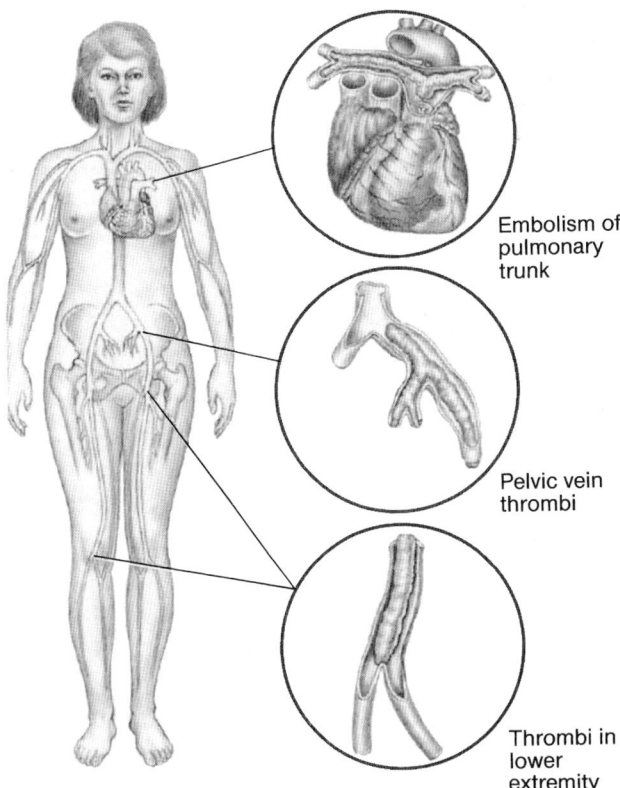

Embolism of pulmonary trunk

Pelvic vein thrombi

Thrombi in lower extremity

Fig. 3-5 Venous thrombosis.
(From Canobbio MM: Mosby's clinical nursing series: cardiovascular disorders, St Louis, 1990, Mosby.)

DIAGNOSTIC TESTS
Phlebography (venography)
Doppler ultrasound
Phlethysmography
Iodine-125 fibrinogen uptake test

POTENTIAL COMPLICATIONS
Venous ulcers
Pulmonary embolism
Chronic venous insufficiency
CVA

MULTIDISCIPLINARY MANAGEMENT
THERAPEUTIC MANAGEMENT
Medications
    Anticoagulant therapy: heparin, warfarin, enoxaparin
    Fibrinolytic agents: streptokinase, urokinase
    Antiplatelet agents
    Analgesics
Surgical management
    Iliofemoral thrombectomy
    Procedures to prevent distal embolization
        Extravascular vena cava interruption
        Intracaval filter (Mobin-Udden umbrella, Kimray-
           Greenfield filter)

PATIENT PROBLEMS—NURSING DIAGNOSES/INTERVENTIONS

▼Pain: peripheral related to inflammatory process

Assess quality and location of pain
Maintain bed rest; limit self-care activities
Elevate affected limb above level of right atrium
Apply warm, moist compresses as ordered; avoid burning
    edematous skin
Use bed cradle over affected extremity
Provide compression or antiembolic stockings
Administer analgesics as ordered

Expected Outcome
Verbalizes relief from pain and absence of swelling and
    redness

▼Altered peripheral tissue perfusion related to interruption of venous flow

Assess circulation of affected extremity q4h; measure and
    record size of affected limb qd
Assess pulses in all extremities q4h; use Doppler sensor if
    pulse seems absent
Maintain complete bed rest during acute phase (4 to 7
    days) *to prevent embolization*
Position patient comfortably; avoid *position that restricts
    venous blood flow by venous compression;* avoid use
    of pillows; never hyperflex knees without raising foot
    of bed
Elevate affected limb above the level of right atrium *to
    lessen venous stasis and improve venous flow*

Do not wash or massage affected extremity
Provide compression or antiembolic stockings
Administer anticoagulation and fibrinolytic therapy as
    ordered
Assess laboratory values as indicated *to reduce risk of
    bleeding*
    APTT: q4h to 12h to maintain 1½ to 2½ times control
        for heparin therapy
    PT; INR qd to maintain level between 2 and 3
Instruct patient *to avoid use of tobacco products to
    prevent vasoconstriction caused by tobacco*
Implement progressive exercise program as ordered *to
    improve venous return and avoid venous
    pooling*
    Ambulate as ordered
    Alternate with bed rest
    Never let legs dangle
    Ambulate 10 minutes qh while awake or as
        ordered
    Apply support stockings before ambulating
    Avoid having patient stand for long periods
    Have patient alternate position by standing on toes,
        then on heels
    Exercise toes and change weight distribution q10min
        to 15 min
Elevate legs 10 minutes qh when sitting
    Do not constrict circulation in groin area
    Flex calf muscles and perform quadriceps contractions
        10 minutes qh
    Avoid having patient cross legs at the knees
Advise patient to build exercise tolerance by increasing
    walking distance each day; continue after discharge,
    increasing distance to 1 to 2 miles
Refer to monitored exercise program

Expected Outcome
Demonstrates adequate tissue perfusion as evidenced by
    palpable pulses and warm extremities

▼Impaired gas exchange related to embolization of
thrombus

Assess for signs of pulmonary embolism: chest pain,
    dyspnea, tachypnea, tachycardia, hemoptysis, pallor,
    anxiety
Auscultate chest for breath sounds q4h
Maintain bed rest during acute phase
Avoid exercising and massaging affected extremity during
    acute phase
Administer anticoagulant therapy as ordered
Encourage patient to turn, cough, and breathe deeply q2h
    to 4h
Obtain and monitor Po_2 and Pco_2
Apply elastic support stockings when patient is
    ambulating or sitting for prolonged periods

Expected Outcome
Demonstrates effortless breathing and performs self-care
    activities without becoming short of breath

▼Risk for impaired skin integrity related to venous stasis and fragility of small blood vessels

Assess skin for redness, breakdown, or ulcerations
Administer daily hygiene measures
    Use small amount of mild soap
    Rinse well
    Dry gently but thoroughly; avoid vigorous rubbing
    Do not allow skin to remain wet
    Use bed cradle for affected extremity
    Do not wash or massage affected extremity
Assist and teach patient as appropriate to make small changes in position
Perform active or passive range-of-motion (ROM) exercises with unaffected extremities

Expected Outcomes
Demonstrates no signs of skin breaks or ulceration
Demonstrates management of home care

PATIENT/FAMILY TEACHING
Assess level of understanding
Discuss importance of not using tobacco products
Discuss symptoms of recurrence to report to physician (see Objective data, p. 77)
Review medications: name, dosage, time of administration, purpose, and side effects
Explain need to avoid taking over-the-counter medications without checking with physician
Discuss anticoagulant precautions if appropriate (p. 157)
Review dietary precaution if on anticoagulants (see p. 158)
Discuss symptoms of complications to report to physician
    Pulmonary emboli
    MI
    CVA
Explain importance of ongoing outpatient care

DISCHARGE/HOME CARE PLANNING
Explain skin care
    Avoid use of harsh soaps
    Do not rub or massage affected extremity
    Keep extremity warm and avoid exposure to temperature extremes
Discuss need to avoid use of constrictive clothing (garters, girdles, underwear with elastic groin bands, knee-high or ankle stockings with elastic tops)
Teach application of compression stockings
Review activity program
    Develop a planned exercise program that includes aerobic activities (e.g., swimming, progressive walking)
    Never let legs dangle; elevate legs when sitting
    Avoid standing for long periods

■ VEIN LIGATION AND STRIPPING
Ligation of the saphenous vein and its branches and stripping (removal) from the groin to the ankle to treat varicosities

ASSESSMENT
SUBJECTIVE DATA
Leg cramps when standing
Pain at night

OBJECTIVE DATA
Color, warmth, and sensation of affected extremity
Edema or heaviness of affected extremity
Dilation of leg veins

POTENTIAL COMPLICATIONS
Thrombophlebitis
Phlebitis
Hemorrhage
Infection

MULTIDISCIPLINARY MANAGEMENT
THERAPEUTIC MANAGEMENT
Medications: analgesics

PATIENT PROBLEMS—NURSING DIAGNOSES/INTERVENTIONS

▼Altered peripheral tissue perfusion related to inadequate venous return and/or immobility

Assess color, warmth, and sensation of affected extremity qh for 6 hours to establish a baseline; report any change to physician
Maintain bed rest
    Elevate legs as ordered
    Do not hyperflex knees
    Do not let legs dangle
Apply elastic bandages from toes to groin *to promote venous blood flow and decrease venous stagnation;* leave in place for 24 hours; remove elastic bandages or stockings as indicated
    Avoid constriction
    Keep bandages snug and wrinkle free
    Assess bandages frequently for slippage, especially after ambulation
Assist patient with ambulation within 24 hours as ordered
Have patient increase activity as ordered; ambulate with assistance
Do not allow chair sitting (patient must be either walking or in bed)
Perform active and/or passive ROM exercises to unaffected extremities q4h and dorsiflexion of foot of affected extremity

Expected Outcomes
Improved tissue perfusion
Peripheral pulses are palpable
Extremities are warm with normal color

▼Pain of lower extremities related to surgical incision

Assess quality and degree of pain
Determine source of pain
    Incision
    Constrictive dressings
    Bleeding
    Local site infection
Assess bandages for bleeding qh; report excessive
    bleeding to physician
Assess dressings for signs of wound infection; report to
    physician
    Low-grade temperature
    Swelling, redness, pain, purulent drainage
Reinforce and/or change dressings
Assess BP, T, P, and R q4h and as indicated
Administer analgesics as indicated

Expected Outcome
Verbalizes absence of pain

PATIENT/FAMILY TEACHING
Assess level of understanding
Discuss need to maintain normal weight for age and
    height and reduce if overweight
Explain need to check with physician before taking
    estrogen-based contraceptives
Discuss signs and symptoms of wound infection and
    bleeding to report to physician
    Redness, drainage
    Edema
    Pain
Explain importance of ongoing outpatient care
Discuss possibility of varicosities recurring

DISCHARGE/HOME CARE PLANNING
Explain importance of avoiding constriction of venous
    blood return in extremities
    Do not wear tight garters or girdles
    Avoid crossing legs
    Walk rather than sit or stand
    Wear compression stockings as ordered
    Elevate legs while sitting
    Sleep with legs elevated
Explain importance of skin care
    Keep legs and feet warm and dry
    Avoid chilling
    Avoid extreme temperatures
    Do not massage affected area

■ CHRONIC ARTERIAL INSUFFICIENCY
*Inadequate blood flow in arteries caused by occlusive
atherosclerotic plaques or emboli, damaged or diseased
vessels, aneurysms, hypercoagulability states, or heavy
use of tobacco*

*Progressive narrowing of the arterial tree gives rise to
collateral vessels to ensure adequate blood supply and
prevent peripheral ischemia. Progressive occlusion leads
to hypoperfusion and ischemia. The arms and legs are the
most vulnerable to ischemia*

ASSESSMENT
SUBJECTIVE DATA
Pain
    Foot, calf, thigh, or buttocks
    Sharp and viselike
    Cramping
    Tired feeling in legs
    Usually occurs during exercise; decreases when
        exercise stops (intermittent claudication)
    May occur at rest, especially at night, accompanied by
        very hot or cold feeling
    Increases with elevation of legs

OBJECTIVE DATA
Pulses: diminished-to-absent pedal and popliteal and
    femoral pulses
Extremities
    Numbness
    Hair loss
    Skin: glossy, thin, smooth, cold, discolored, atrophied
    Ulcerations, poor wound healing
    Nails thickened: accumulation of cornified material
    Pallor
        Increased with elevation of extremity
        Decreased with extremity below heart level
    Rubor
    Edema
    Delayed venous filling in dependent position

DIAGNOSTIC TESTS
Ankle-brachial index
Doppler ultrasonography
Angiography
Digit photo plethesmography

POTENTIAL COMPLICATIONS
Peripheral ischemia, necrosis
Cellulitis
Gangrene

MULTIDISCIPLINARY MANAGEMENT
THERAPEUTIC MANAGEMENT
Medications
    Antiplatelets: aspirin
    Pentoxifylline (Trental)
Regular walking program
Diet therapy
    Weight reduction
    Low-saturated-fat, low-cholesterol diet
Percutaneous or peripheral transluminal angioplasty (PTA)
Angiography with thrombolysis
Laser thermal angioplasty (LTA)
Surgical management
    Arterial reconstruction and/or revascularization with
        bypass graft
    Endarterectomy
    Lumbar sympathectomy
    Amputation of limb, digits
    Endovascular stenting

PATIENT PROBLEMS—NURSING DIAGNOSES/INTERVENTIONS

▼ Altered tissue perfusion related to interruption of arterial flow

Assess arterial pulses; determine pulse volume qid *to determine adequacy of peripheral circulation*

Elevate head of bed; use 4- to 6-inch block as ordered

Maintain extremity in dependent position *to maintain optimal and/or improve arterial blood flow;* avoid use of knee hyperflexion or other positions *that interfere with gravitational flow*

Protect affected extremity

    Place bed cradle over affected area

    Use heel guards (sheepskin) or white cotton socks

    Avoid use of heating devices on lower extremities

    Keep patient warm

    Have patient wear socks when in bed or walking

    Place cotton blankets next to patient

    Use flannel or cotton bedclothes

    Use extra blankets if required

Assist patient with getting out of bed as ordered; avoid one position, sitting or standing, for long periods

Initiate scheduled walking exercise program *to promote development of collateral flow;* with increased pain, have patient stand until pain eases, then continue walking

Have patient sit with feet dependent

Perform active or passive ROM exercises to all extremities q4h to 6h

Turn patient q2h while on bed rest

Change patient's position slightly q20min to 30min

Avoid raising lower extremity above heart level

Instruct patient to avoid use of nicotine

Administer medications as ordered

Expected Outcomes

Reports increased walking distances

Peripheral pulses are present, equal, and bilateral

Skin is warm with normal color

▼ Pain related to peripheral ischemia

Assess quality and degree of pain *to determine degree of claudication and exercise tolerance*

Assist patient with identifying activities that precipitate or aggravate pain and understanding nature of pain

Instruct patient to stand or dangle at side of bed *to obtain relief from ischemic pain*

Encourage regular exercise program with walking past point of claudication

Administer analgesics as indicated

Initiate alternative pain relief measures

    Relaxation techniques: meditation, deep breathing

    Guided imagery

    Biofeedback

Involve patient in decision making regarding measures to reduce pain

Assess effectiveness of pain relief measure(s)

Expected Outcomes

Reports relief or control of pain

Verbalizes and demonstrates a variety of strategies to reduce pain level

▼ Risk for impaired skin integrity, actual or potential, related to impaired circulation

Assess skin daily for signs of scaling, breaks, or cuts

Administer daily hygiene measures

    Use small amount of mild soap

    Rinse well

    Dry gently but thoroughly; avoid vigorous rubbing

    Apply lanolin-based lotions; do not allow skin to remain wet

Assess skin color and temperature in both legs qid

Treat ulcerated areas as they occur

    Administer soak, topical, and/or systemic antibiotics and dressings as ordered

    Avoid use of adhesive tapes directly on skin

    Avoid use of tight, constrictive socks or hose; use cotton socks; avoid use of knee hyperflex; reposition extremities frequently

Expected Outcomes

Shows no signs of skin breakdown

Demonstrates progressive healing of ulcerations

PATIENT/FAMILY TEACHING

Provide information regarding disease process and associated risk factors (see the box on p. 86)

Explain need to avoid using tobacco products

Discuss symptoms of recurrence to report to physician (see Subjective data, Objective data, p. 80)

Explain importance of maintaining diet (low calorie, low cholesterol, low fat) as ordered

Discuss medications: name, dosage, time of administration, purpose, and side effects

Explain need to avoid taking over-the-counter medications without checking with physician

Explain importance of ongoing outpatient care

DISCHARGE/HOME CARE PLANNING

Explain importance of care of legs and feet

    Inspect legs, feet, and toes daily for blisters, skin breaks, and discolored areas

    Wash daily with mild soap, dry well, and apply lanolin-based lotion; do not leave skin wet

    Clean small cuts or abrasions with soap and water; protect from further injury

    Report to physician cuts or skin breaks that do not begin healing in 2 to 3 days

    Trim toenails straight across; refer older or frail patients to podiatry department

    Do not cut, file corns or calluses or use over-the-counter medications on them

    Avoid exposing legs to temperature extremes; wear warm coverings in cold weather and avoid exposure to sunshine

Do not apply indirect heat to legs (e.g., hot water bottles or electric pads); wear cotton or woolen socks to warm feet

Avoid injury to legs and feet

Always wear well-fitting shoes or slippers; never go barefoot

Wear well-fitting, correct-size stockings

Avoid tight-fitting or constrictive clothing (garters, girdles, underwear with elastic legs, and knee-high or ankle stockings with elastic tops)

Avoid crossing legs

Avoid scratching legs or feet

Turn on lights when getting up at night to avoid bumps

Sleep with bed level or with head elevated

Avoid tight-fitting covers over legs and feet

Instruct and help patient plan a daily progressive walking program

Walk to tolerance; increase time each week until able to walk without pain for 30 to 60 minutes (may initially experience decreased ability)

Walk until pain increases, stop and stand still to decrease pain, then continue to walk

Do not sit or raise legs above heart level, to decrease pain

Remember that same distance walked in one direction must also be walked on return

■ CAROTID ENDARTERECTOMY

Surgical removal of atherosclerotic plaques or thrombus from the inner lining of the carotid artery to increase blood flow to the brain. Indicated for patient suffering from reversible ischemic neurologic deficit, TIAs, syncope, and dizziness or asymptomatic patients with carotid stenosis greater than 75%

ASSESSMENT
SUBJECTIVE DATA
Episodes of dizziness, amaurosis, paresthesias or paralysis, slurred speech, or memory loss

May be asymptomatic

OBJECTIVE DATA
Decreased temporal pulse, carotid pulse

Bruit over carotid pulse

Neurologic deficit
    Cerebral ischemia: TIAs
        Dizziness
        Confusion
        Disorientation
        Memory loss
    Altered speech
        Slurred
        Indistinct

DIAGNOSTIC TESTS
Duplex carotid ultrasound

Carotid angiogram

MRA/MRI

POTENTIAL COMPLICATIONS
Seizure activity

Hemorrhage

Shock

Embolism

Infection

CVA

Neurologic deficit

Hematoma

MULTIDISCIPLINARY MANAGEMENT
THERAPEUTIC MANAGEMENT
Parenteral fluids

Medications
    Antihypertensive
    Vasopressor

PATIENT PROBLEMS—NURSING DIAGNOSES/INTERVENTIONS

▼ Altered cerebral tissue perfusion related to interruption of arterial flow (see Care of patient in recovery room, p. 10)

Assess for changes in mental status

Assess and compare temporal pulses q15min × 4, then q2h to 4h

Mark pulse site on skin; note rate and volume

Assess neurologic signs q15 to 30min, increasing to qh

Assess BP, R, and apical pulse q1h to 2h for 24 hours; report increase or decrease to physician immediately

Maintain bed rest in quiet environment; position with head elevated 30 to 45 degrees

Check temperature q2h to 4h for 24 hours

Administer medications as ordered

Inspect incision qh *for bleeding and edema;* report excessive bleeding or edema to physician

Control pain as ordered; apply ice collar to neck as ordered

Provide emotional support
    Gentle reassurance

Continue with immediate postoperative care and decrease frequency of nursing functions as patient's condition improves

Ambulate as ordered; check and report any altered gait

Change dressing prn

Continue assessing neurologic signs q8h

Expected Outcomes
Demonstrates adequate cerebral blood flow as evidenced by the following:
    Mental alertness and orientation
    Absence of dizziness
    Equal and reactive pupils
    Normal sensorimotor function

▼ Risk for injury: respiratory distress, aspiration

Assess tracheal deviation, gag reflex and swallowing

Maintain patent airway

Perform oropharyngeal suctioning only if ordered

Assist and teach patient to turn and breathe deeply q1h to 2h

Avoid having patient cough

Auscultate chest for breath sounds q1h to 2h

Report complaints of severe hoarseness, sore throat, or dysphagia to physician

Monitor oxygen saturation via arterial blood gases (ABGs) or peripheral O_2 saturation as indicated

Expected Outcome
Demonstrates effortless breathing

PATIENT/FAMILY TEACHING
Assess level of understanding regarding disease process

Discuss diet restrictions as ordered; encourage low-fat, low-cholesterol diet

Explain importance of ongoing outpatient care

Explain importance of reporting sudden changes in vision, gait, speech or the experience of muscle weakness to physician immediately

DISCHARGE/HOME CARE PLANNING
Discuss risks associated with activities
　　Exercise to tolerance
　　Avoid bending from waist
　　Plan rest periods
　　Avoid lifting or straining
Demonstrate care of incision
Discuss signs of wound infection
　　Redness
　　Pain
　　Drainage
　　Edema

■ REVASCULARIZATION WITH BYPASS GRAFT
Insertion of prosthetic graft or vein graft to bypass arterial occlusion

ASSESSMENT
SUBJECTIVE DATA
Pain related to surgical incision versus pain related to development of graft thrombosis

OBJECTIVE DATA (POSTOPERATIVE FINDINGS)
Signs of arterial graft occlusion of lower extremities (lower limb ischemia)
　　Mottled or pale skin
　　Skin cool to touch
　　Absence of pulses
Site of incision
　　Redness
　　Pain
　　Swelling

DIAGNOSTIC TESTS
Doppler: systolic ankle pressure

White blood cell count (WBC), chemistries, electrolytes

POTENTIAL COMPLICATIONS
Cardiac complications
　　Congestive heart failure (CHF)
　　Dysrhythmias
　　Acute myocardial infarction (AMI)
Hemorrhage
Shock
Renal failure
Prosthetic graft infection
　　Purulent wound drainage
　　Low-grade fever without chills
　　Sepsis
　　Graft occlusion
　　Local hemorrhage
　　Septic embolization: cellulitis
　　Sinus tract infection

MULTIDISCIPLINARY MANAGEMENT
THERAPEUTIC MANAGEMENT
Medications
　　Antibiotic therapy
　　Vasodilators
Ankle-brachial index increased from pre-op

PATIENT PROBLEMS—NURSING DIAGNOSES/INTERVENTIONS

▼ Risk for altered tissue perfusion related to interruption of arterial flow secondary to development of graft thromboses

Assess affected extremity *to detect development of graft thromboses*

Assess swelling from reperfusion injury, which may cause compartment syndrome and constrict arterial flow

Compare pedal pulses q15min × 4 times, then q4h; mark pulse site on skin

Assess lower extremities for color, warmth, and sensation q15min for 4 hours

Assess and compare ankle-to-brachial index (ratio) as ordered; report if decreased

Maintain bed rest; elevate head 30 to 45 degrees (Fig. 3-6)
　　Do not hyperflex knees; avoid sharp hip flexion *to prevent graft pressure*

Do not massage or apply heat to lower extremities

Ambulate as ordered

Administer daily skin care
　　Observe for signs of breaks or drainage
　　Avoid use of adhesive tape on sensitive skin of distal lower extremity
　　Protect affected extremity
　　Place bed cradle over affected area
　　Use sheepskin heel protectors or lambs wool between toes

Expected Outcomes
Demonstrates improved tissue perfusion
　　Graft is patent
　　Peripheral pulses are palpable
　　Extremities are warm with normal color
　　Ankle-brachial index is normal or improved

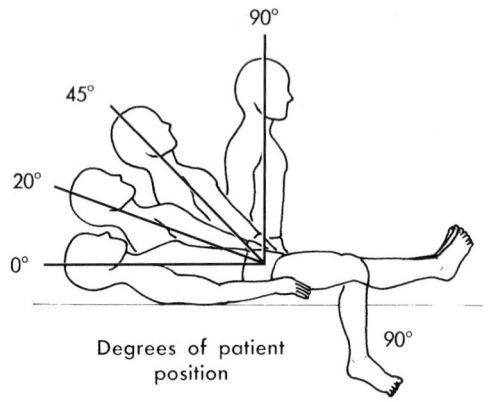

Fig. 3-6   Degrees of patient position.

▼Risk for infection related to arterial prosthetic graft procedure

Observe for signs of infection of incision (see Objective data, p. 83)
Check temperature q4h
Inspect dressing q1h to 2h
    Observe for healing process
    Reinforce dressing prn
    Report excessive drainage to physician
Administer prophylactic antibiotic as ordered
Avoid prolonged use of urinary catheters, nasogastric tubes, or pressure catheter, which may cause transient bacteremia
Use strict aseptic technique in dressing change, venipuncture, or suctioning procedures
If graft infection occurs
    Administer antibiotic therapy as ordered
    Perform irrigation of graft and wound as ordered
    Prepare for surgical intervention as ordered
        Graft removal
        Revascularization
        Amputation

Expected Outcomes
Demonstrates absence of graft infection
Temperature is normal
Graft is patent
Skin integrity is maintained

▼Risk for complications: myocardial ischemia, renal failure, hemorrhage

Cardiac complications
    Monitor ECG, arterial pressures, PAP, CVP qh
    Assess BP, R, and apical pulse q4h for 48 hours
    Auscultate heart and lung sounds q4h to 6h or as indicated
    Record description of chest pain; report increase or significant change to physician
    Obtain ECG rhythm strip during episodes of chest pain
    Obtain isoenzymes (CPK-MB) as indicated
    Monitor potassium levels

Bowel ischemia
    Maintain nothing by mouth (NPO), usually for first 12 hours or until bowel sounds are present
    Progress diet as tolerated and ordered after nasogastric tube removal
    Connect nasogastric tube to intermittent suction as ordered
    Auscultate abdomen q2h to 4h
    Measure abdominal girth for distension q8h
    Assess for and report increased distension to physician
Renal failure
    Administer parenteral fluids with electrolytes as ordered
    Measure intake and output
    Use indwelling urethral catheter as ordered
        Measure urine output qh
        Report urine output <30 to 50 ml/hr
Hemorrhage
    Assess for signs of bleeding q4h to 8h
        Hematoma in groin area
        Bleeding of skin incision
        Retroperitoneal bleeding: signs of hypovolemia— low CVP and pulmonary capillary wedge pressure (PCWP), decreased urine output, severe back pain
    Evaluate laboratory studies q4h to 8h

Expected Outcome
Demonstrates no signs or symptoms of complication

PATIENT/FAMILY TEACHING
Assess for level of understanding
Explain importance of not using tobacco products
Discuss symptoms of recurrence to report to physician
Explain importance of ongoing outpatient care

DISCHARGE/HOME CARE PLANNING
Explain importance of exercise and activity
    Avoid sitting or standing without moving for long periods
    Do not cross legs
    Exercise up to level of tolerance, with caution not to push beyond tolerance
    Discuss importance of maintaining planned rest periods
    Exercise feet and legs as ordered
Demonstrate correct application of antiembolic stockings or elastic bandages
Discuss care of legs and feet
    Do not wear constrictive clothing (e.g., girdles, garters)
    Avoid temperature extremes
    Keep feet warm
Demonstrate care of incision
Discuss signs of wound infection
    Redness
    Pain
    Swelling
    Drainage

■ ABDOMINAL AORTIC ANEURYSMECTOMY

Surgical resection of the aneurysm (local irreversible dilitation of the arterial wall at 150% of the normal aortic diameter) with insertion of graft into the aneurysmal defect

ASSESSMENT

SUBJECTIVE DATA (POSTOPERATIVE FINDINGS)

Pain at incisional site

OBJECTIVE DATA

Signs of arterial embolism
    Mottled skin distally
    Absence of distal pulses
    Decrease of ankle-brachial index
    Decreased or absence of movement to lower extremities
    Abdominal pain beyond incisional pain
    Melanotic stool
Incisional site
    Redness
    Pain
    Purulent drainage
    Induration
Vital signs
    Hypotension or hypertension
    Decreased or increased PAP, PCWP, CVP
    Tachycardia
Pulmonary
    Rales, ronchi
    Atelectasis
Urinary
    Decreased urinary output
    Hematuria
    Pyuria

DIAGNOSTIC TESTS

Doppler-systolic ankle pressure
CBC, electrolyte, creatinine, BUN, glucose, liver function tests, lactic acid, coagulation profile
CXR
ECG

POTENTIAL COMPLICATIONS

Embolism
Acute tubular necrosis (ATN)
Cardiac: MI, CHF, dysrhythmias
Hemorrhage
Shock
Graft infection

MULTIDISCIPLINARY MANAGEMENT

Hemodynamic monitoring
Cardiac monitor
Medications
    Antibiotic therapy
    Vasoactive drips
Ankle-brachial index

PATIENT PROBLEMS—NURSING DIAGNOSIS/INTERVENTIONS

▼ Risk for altered tissue perfusion related to interruption of arterial flow secondary to embolus or thrombosis (spinal, mesenteric, lower extremities)

Assess affected extremity *to detect development of embolus or thrombosis*
Assess vascular status of lower extremities including color, warmth, sensation and pulses q15 min for 4 hours, then q2h for 24 hours then q4h
Assess and compare ankle-brachial indexes
Assess urinary output q2h with specific gravity
Assess movement and sensation of lower extremities q2h

Expected Outcomes

Does not develop pathologic sequalae from embolic phenomenon
Peripheral pulses remain present
Urine output remains at 30 ml/hr or greater
Movement remains normal to lower extremities

▼ Risk for infection related to surgical incision, prosthetic graft

Observe for signs, symptoms of infection of incision
Check temperature q4h
Inspect dressing q1h to 2h
Administer antibiotics as ordered
Avoid prolonged use of urinary catheters, nasogastric tubes, or pressure catheter
Use aseptic technique in dressing changes, venipuncture, or suctioning procedures

Expected Outcomes

Demonstrates absence of graft infection
Temperature is normal
Skin integrity remains intact

▼ Risk for complications: cardiac, hemorrhage, pneumonia

Monitor ECG, arterial pressures, PAP, CVP qh
Assess BP, R, and pulse q4h after discharge from intensive care unit (ICU)
Auscultate heart, lung sounds q2h to 4h
If chest pain develops, record description and report to physician
Obtain ECG during episodes of chest pain
Obtain appropriate lab tests as indicated during episodes of chest pain
Administer medications as ordered for treatment of chest pain
Assess for signs of bleeding at incisional site or internal
Monitor oxygen saturation
Provide supplemental oxygen as needed
Pulmonary toilet every 4 hours

Expected Outcome
Demonstrates no signs or symptoms of complications

PATIENT/FAMILY TEACHING
Assess for level of understanding
Explain importance of not using tobacco products
Discuss symptoms to report to physician
Explain importance of ongoing outpatient care

DISCHARGE/HOME CARE PLANNING
Explain importance of exercise and activity
Demonstrate care of incision
Discuss actions, side effects of medications
Discuss signs of wound infection
  Redness
  Pain
  Swelling
  Fever
  Drainage

■ HYPERTENSION
Arterial hypertension is a persistent elevation of systolic BP greater than 140 mm Hg and diastolic pressure equal to or greater than 90 mm Hg. It is a major risk factor for coronary artery, renal cerebral, and peripheral vascular disease. It is classified according to cause, severity, and type

primary (essential, idiopathic): *Most common form constituting 90% to 95% of all cases. No single known cause but familial tendencies, race, and obesity are known risk factors. The disease begins insiduously and may be slow progressing. If uncontrolled or untreated, it may lead to serious complications such as malignant hypertension. Early detection and treatment can lead to good control and improved prognosis*

secondary: *Results from other diseases such as renal failure, dysfunction of adrenal medulla or cortex, coarctation of aorta, or other identifiable causes (e.g., estrogen-containing oral contraceptive)*

malignant: *Sudden severe elevation of BP (systolic greater than 200 mm Hg, diastolic greater than 140 mm Hg) with MAP greater than 150 mm Hg. This is a medical emergency necessitating aggressive therapy to prevent severe complications*

ASSESSMENT
SUBJECTIVE DATA
Symptoms range from no symptoms to the following:
  Morning occipital headaches
  Neck stiffness, soreness
  Dizziness, vertigo
  Nausea, vomiting
  Palpitations (heart pounding)

OBJECTIVE DATA
Arterial blood pressure (see Table 3-1)
Pulse
  Pulsus alternans
  Tachycardia
  Bounding
  Femoral delays

■ MALIGNANT HYPERTENSION

ASSESSMENT
SUBJECTIVE DATA
Severe suboccipital headache radiating frontally

OBJECTIVE DATA
Skin: pallor, diaphoresis
Hypertensive encephalopathy
  Confusion
  Irritability

Box 3-1	Cardiovascular Risk Factor Profile
Family history of heart disease	
Sex: Males (35-55)	
Females (>50 or	
after menopause)	
Hypertension	
Tobacco use	
Overweight/obesity	
Elevated serum level of lipids and cholesterol	
Diabetes mellitus	
Physical inactivity; sedentary lifestyle	
Stress	
For women <40 years: use of estrogen (i.e., birth control pills) and smoking	

Table 3-1	Classification of Blood Pressure for Adults Age 18 Years and Older	
Category	**Systolic (mm Hg)**	**Diastolic (mm Hg)**
Normal	<130	<85
High normal	130-139	85-89
Hypertension*		
Stage 1 (mild)	140-159	90-99
Stage 2 (moderate)	160-179	100-109
Stage 3 (severe)	180-209	110-119
Stage 4 (very severe)	≥210	≥120

From: Joint National Committee on Detection, Evaluation, and Treatment of High Blood Pressure: The Fifth Report of the Joint National Committee on Detection, Evaluation, and Treatment of High Blood Pressure, Arch Int Med *153:154-188, 1993.*
**Based on the average of two or more readings taken at each of two or more visits following an initial screening.*
NOTE: *In addition to classifying stages of hypertension based on average BP levels, the clinician should specify presence or absence of target-organ disease and additional risk factors. For example, a patient with diabetes and a BP of 142/94 mm Hg plus left ventricular hypertrophy should be classified as "stage 1 hypertension with target-organ disease (left ventricular hypertrophy) and with another major risk factor (diabetes)." This specificity is important for risk classification and management.*

Stupor
Somnolence
Coma
Eye signs and symptoms
    Diplopia
    Visual loss
    Optic fundi hemorrhage, cotton exudates,
      arteriovenous nicking papilledema
Cardiac symptoms
    Angina
    Dyspnea on exertion (DOE)
    Paroxysmal nocturnal dyspnea (PND)
    Orthopnea
    S_4 gallop
Renal symptoms
    Hematuria
    Nocturia
    Azotemia

DIAGNOSTIC TESTS
Blood
    Electrolytes, chemistries
    Aldosterone
    Cholesterol, triglycerides
Urine
    Steroids, catecholamines; renin
    Urinalysis: BUN, uric acid levels
    24-Hour VMA levels
    Aldosterone

Electrocardiogram (ECG)
    Left ventricular hypertrophy (LVH)
    Ischemia
Echocardiogram
    LVH with/without dilation
Chest x-ray examination
    Increased cardiothoracic ratio
CT scan
    Cerebral ischemia, infarct
    Encephalopathy

POTENTIAL COMPLICATIONS
Cardiac dysrhythmia
MI
Renal failure
Heart failure
CVA

MULTIDISCIPLINARY MANAGEMENT
THERAPEUTIC MANAGEMENT
For primary hypertension, a stepped approach to medical treatment is recommended (Box 3-2)
For malignant hypertension, admission to ICU (ICU with continuous arterial pressure and cardiac monitoring)
Oxygen therapy: 2 to 4L/min
Medications
    Vasodilators (nitroprusside, diazoxide)
    Beta blockers, short-acting (e.g., labetalol, esmolol)
    ACE inhibitors (e.g., captopril)

Box 3-2	**Stepped Care Approach for the Treatment of High Blood Pressure**

Step 0
Non-pharmacologic
Sodium restriction
Weight loss/exercise
Alcohol restriction
Smoking cessation
Relaxation/
  stress reduction

Step 1
Select an agent
Diuretic
  OR
Beta blocker
  OR
Calcium channel
blocker
  OR
ACE inhibitor

Step 2
Increase dose
  of first drug
  OR
Add a second drug
  of different class
  OR
Substitute a drug
  from another class

Step 3
Add a third drug
  OR
Substitute a
second drug

Step 4
Further evaluation
  and referral
  OR
Add a fourth drug

From Canobbio MM: Mosby's clinical nursing series: cardiovascular disorders, *St Louis, 1990, Mosby.*

Calcium channel blockers (e.g., nifedipine, diltiazem)
Adrenergic inhibitors (e.g., clonidine HCl)
Diuretics: loop (furosemide)
Diet: sodium restricted, fat reduced
Intake and output

PATIENT PROBLEMS—NURSING DIAGNOSES/INTERVENTIONS (FOR PATIENTS WITH MALIGNANT HYPERTENSION)

▼ Pain (headache) related to increased cerebral vascular pressure

Maintain bed rest; provide a quiet, low-lighted environment
Minimize environmental distractions and stimulations
Limit activities
Avoid use of nicotine products
Administer analgesia and sedation as ordered
Administer comfort measures as indicated
Apply ice packs
Give reassurance and frequent, simple explanations
Place patient in comfortable position; assist with turning gently, using pull sheet as indicated
Medications: vasodilators (nitroprusside, nitroglycerin)
Teach relaxation techniques
Suggest guided imagery
Explain need to avoid Valsalva maneuver
Explain need to avoid constipation

Expected Outcomes
Verbalizes absence of headache
Appears comfortable

▼ Risk for altered tissue perfusion: cerebral, renal, cardiac related to vasospasm, impaired circulation

Acute malignant hypertension
Maintain bed rest; elevate head of bed 30 to 45 degrees
Provide oxygen therapy *to improve and maintain oxygenation*
Assess BP on admission in both arms: lying, sitting, and with arterial pressure monitor if available
Assess BP, R, apical pulse, and neurologic signs q5min to 10min
Use same arm for BP reading each time
Use Doppler sensor if indicated
Monitor arterial pressure as ordered
Maintain parenteral fluids with medications as ordered
Administer medications as ordered
Antihypertensives: IV, IM
Observe for side effects or toxic effects of each medication
Monitor IV medications continuously
Titrate according to prescribed BP parameters as ordered
Place on cardiac monitor; monitor and record ECG rhythm strip q4h to 6h and prn for ST-T wave changes or dysrhythmia

Monitor hourly urine output; note color and presence of blood in urine; report urine output <30 ml/hr
Monitor electrolytes, BUN, creatinine levels as ordered
Check specific gravity and perform urinalysis as ordered
Keep NPO if nausea and/or vomiting is present
Restrict fluids as ordered
Ongoing care
Continue with immediate care and decrease frequency of nursing functions as patient's condition improves
Maintain progressive ambulation, observing at all times for orthostatic hypotension
Elevate head of bed slowly in beginning, then take BP reading
Progress to dangling for 10 minutes as ordered if BP is stable
Take BP reading while patient is sitting up
Take reading while patient is standing at bedside; then have patient take small steps when ordered
Ambulate to tolerance; avoid fatigue

Expected Outcomes
Demonstrates improved tissue perfusion as evidenced by BP within acceptable limits
No complaints of headache, dizziness
Laboratory values within normal limits
Urine output ≥30 ml/min
Patient's vital signs stable

Additional Nursing Diagnoses to Consider
Anxiety related to biologic psychosocial threat

PATIENT/FAMILY TEACHING
Explain nature of disease, associated risk factors, and means of reducing risk factors; describe and explain purpose of stepped-care treatment for hypertension
Discuss medications: name, dosage, time of administration, purpose, and side effects or toxic effects
Explain need to avoid taking over-the-counter medications without checking with physician
Discuss symptoms of recurrence or progression of disease to report to physician
Headache
Dizziness
Faintness
Nausea, vomiting
Bloody nose
Explain importance of not using tobacco products
Explain need to avoid constipation and straining

DISCHARGE/HOME CARE PLANNING
Diet
Sodium restriction (2 g sodium; 1 tsp salt = 2 g sodium), weight reducing (low fat, low calorie)
Discuss importance of decreasing weight or maintaining stable weight
Explain importance of maintaining proper fluid intake; amount allowed, limitations such as caffeinated beverages and alcohol

Activity

Discuss need to avoid fatigue and heavy lifting

Discuss importance of planned regular (3 to 5 times/wk) exercise (aerobic) program and rest periods

Demonstrate taking and recording of BP and P using home monitoring equipment

Discuss importance of using proper-size cuff; arm should be bare

■ ANGINA PECTORIS

Chest pain or discomfort caused by myocardial ischemia that occurs when myocardial oxygen demand exceeds the supply. Myocardial ischemia commonly occurs as a result of coronary atherosclerotic heart disease, although angina pectoris may occur in patients with normal coronary arteries. Classification of angina is found in Table 3-2

ASSESSMENT

SUBJECTIVE DATA

Chest pain or pressure: mild-to-severe aching; sharp, tingling, or burning sensation or pressure described as heavy, squeezing; heartburn or tight chest lasting 5 to 30 minutes

Complains of lightheadedness, palpitations, SOB

OBJECTIVE DATA

Precipitating factors

Physical or emotional stress

Exposure to temperature extremes

Eating a heavy meal

Table 3-2	Different Patterns of Angina		
Observations	**Stable Angina Pectoris**	**Variant (Prinzmetal's) Angina**	**Unstable Angina Pectoris**
CHEST PAIN			
Quality	Aching, sharp, tingling, or burning sensation or pressure	Similar to stable angina pectoris	Similar to stable angina pectoris but may be more severe
Location and radiation	Substernal with radiation to left shoulder, down inner aspect of left arm or both arms; neck, jaw, and scapula may be additional sites of radiation	Similar to stable angina pectoris	Similar to stable angina pectoris
Precipitating factors	Onset classically associated with exercise or activities that increase myocardial oxygen demand (e.g., physical exercise, heavy lifting, emotional stress, cold temperatures)	Onset at rest; pain is cyclic, often occurring during sleep (most common between midnight and 8 AM)	Pain may be brought on with less than usual exertion; may occur at rest
Duration and alleviating factors	3-15 min; relieved by rest, stopping pain-inducing activities, taking sublingual nitroglycerin (NTG) tablet	Characteristically, pain intensifies quickly, tends to last longer than angina, and subsides with exercise	Prolonged and not usually as quickly relieved by rest or taking NTG
Associated signs and symptoms	During anginal attack: dyspnea; anxiety; diaphoresis; cool, clammy skin	Similar to stable angina pectoris	Similar to stable angina pectoris but symptoms may be more prominent and may persist; may be associated with nausea
PHYSICAL EXAMINATION			
	Normal during asymptomatic periods; during anginal attacks, increased HR, pulsus alternans, and transient abnormal findings including precordial bulge and atrial and ventricular gallops (S_3, S_4)	Similar to stable angina pectoris	Similar to stable angina pectoris; may also demonstrate irregular pulse, hypotension, or signs of left ventricular dysfunction

From Canobbio MM: Mosby's clinical nursing series: cardiovascular disorders, St Louis, 1990, Mosby.

Alleviating factors
    Termination of precipitating factors
    Taking nitroglycerin (NTG) tablets
Diaphoresis
Anxiety
Indigestion
Skin: pallor, diaphoresis
Respiration: SOB
Cardiac: tachycardia, pulsus alternans, atrial and/or
    ventricular gallops (S_3, S_4)

DIAGNOSTIC TESTS (TABLE 3-3)

Cardiac enzymes: CK-MB, CPK-MB, LDH
Lipid profile: LDL, HDL, LDL : HDL ratio, triglycerides
ECG changes recorded during episodes of pain
Exercise stress test (EST): ECG changes recorded during
    chest pain
    Protocols: Bruce, Naughton
Echocardiography
Thallium-201 scintigraphy (viable myocardial cells extract
    thallium from blood)
Radionuclide blood pool imaging with technetium-99m
Coronary angiography

POTENTIAL COMPLICATIONS

Myocardial infarction
Heart failure

MULTIDISCIPLINARY MANAGEMENT

THERAPEUTIC MANAGEMENT

Medications
    Short- and long-acting nitrates
    Beta-adrenergic blocking agents
    Calcium antagonists
    Analgesics, sedatives
Oxygen therapy
Diet: low saturated fat, low cholesterol, low sodium
Interventional procedures
    Percutaneous transluminal coronary angioplasty (PTCA)
    Coronary stent procedure
Direct coronary atherectomy
Surgical management
    Minimally invasive coronary heart bypass (MIDCAB)
    Coronary artery bypass graft

PATIENT PROBLEMS—NURSING DIAGNOSIS/INTERVENTIONS

▼ Chest pain related to imbalance of myocardial oxygen supply and demand

Maintain rest during episodes of pain *to reduce myocardial oxygen demand*
Assess pain: location, duration, radiation, and onset of new symptoms
Administer oxygen as indicated *to increase oxygen supply to myocardium*
Assess and record description of pain *to establish baseline description and/or to detect extension of ischemia*

Obtain 12-lead ECG during anginal pain episodes *to document ischemic episodes; monitor RV leads*
Monitor for signs of associated symptoms
Monitor BP and apical pulse during episodes of pain
Administer medications as indicated; assess and record response
Maintain diet as ordered; if chest pain occurs during eating, advise small feedings rather than two or three large meals

Expected Outcomes

Verbalizes relief of pain
Appears relaxed and verbalizes a sense of calm

Additional Nursing Diagnosis to Consider

Anxiety related to perceived biologic threat and pain

PATIENT/FAMILY TEACHING

Assess level of understanding *to determine any misconceptions or areas of deficit*
Explain atherosclerotic process and its different clinical manifestations
Discuss contributing risk factors and importance of modification (see the box on p. 86)
Discuss management and nature of chest pain; assist in identifying precipitating factors
Discuss importance of avoiding use of all tobacco products
Explain importance of controlling any coexisting diseases that may aggravate atherosclerotic process: hypertension, diabetes, hyperlipidemia
Explain importance of weight control, avoiding obesity
Explain role that stress plays in aggravating heart disease; need to identify stress-producing factors; methods of stress management using relaxation techniques
Discuss medications: name, dosage, time of administration, purpose, and side effects
Instruct patient to carry NTG at all times; keep pills in dark dry container away from heat; replace pills every 3 to 4 months

DISCHARGE/HOME CARE PLANNING

Discuss activity allowances and limitations
    Avoid isometric-type activity: heavy lifting and pushing
    Exercise regularly; encourage regular home exercise program
    Avoid sexual activities when fatigued; if chest pain occurs during sexual activity, stop and take nitrates if ordered; if pain persists or extreme fatigue occurs, report symptoms to physician
Self-management during episodes of pain
    Stop activity and rest
    Take nitrates as ordered
Report to physician if pain persists longer than 15 minutes or diaphoresis and SOB appear
Discuss importance of maintaining diet that is low in saturated fats, cholesterol; avoid caffeine intake; refer to dietitian for counseling

Table 3-3	Diagnostic Tests

	Findings			
Diagnostic Test	Variant (Prinzmetal's) Stable Angina Pectoris	Angina	Unstable Angina Pectoris	Myocardial Infarction
Electrocardiogram (ECG)	Changes usually seen during anginal episodes; 50%-70% of patients have normal ECG during pain-free episodes; ischemia determined by horizontal ST segment or downsloping with depression of >1 mm; T wave inversion represents impaired repolarization caused by ischemia	Ischemia appears as ST elevation during anginal attack but regresses as pain subsides; ECG changes may be seen before patient complains of chest pain or may be recorded in absence of pain; A-V conduction defects may occur, particularly when right coronary artery is involved, and include Mobitz type II and complete A-V block; ventricular irritability such as premature ventricular contractions, ventricular tachycardia, or fibrillation can occur, particularly during ischemic attack	Ischemia determined by horizontal ST segment or downsloping with depression of >1 mm; T wave inversion represents impaired repolarization caused by ischemia; ventricular irritability such as premature ventricular contractions, ventricular tachycardia, or fibrillation	Changes are evolutionary and indicate progression of infarction; in acute stage, ST elevations with subsequent T wave inversion and Q wave formation; Q waves indicate necrosis and are considered pathologic if they are 0.04 seconds or greater in duration, 0.4 mm or greater in depth, or present in leads that do not normally have Q waves; ST elevations reflect myocardial injury that interferes with polarization of cells, are seen in leads facing injured area, and return to normal (isoelectric) within days; ST elevations beyond 4-6 wk should raise suspicion of ventricular aneurysm; infarction location determined by identifying leads that demonstrate characteristic ECG changes; such leads are those with positive terminals that face injured site of heart; reciprocal changes, seen in leads that face *opposite* surface of damaged heart, are absence of Q wave, increase in R wave amplitude, depressed ST segment, upright tall T wave *RV infarction:* ST elevation in right precordial leads (V_1, V_3R-V_6R). V_4R-V_6R may be more sensitive indicators
Laboratory tests Enzymes	No elevation; checked to rule out MI	No elevation; checked to rule out MI	No elevation; checked to rule out MI	
Complete blood count (CBC)	No elevation; checked to rule out anemia-induced angina	No elevation; checked to rule out anemia-induced angina	No elevation; checked to rule out anemia-induced angina	Elevated WBC and ESR reflect tissue necrosis

	Onset	Peak	Return to normal
AST	6-12 hr	24-48 hr	4-8 days
CK-MB	4-8 hr	24 hr	2-3 days
LDH_1	6-12 hr	24-48 hr	8-14 days
LDH_1 to LDH_2 ratio >1.0			

From Canobbio MM: Mosby's clinical nursing series: cardiovascular disorders, St Louis, 1990, Mosby.

Continued

Table 3-3   Diagnostic Tests—cont'd

Diagnostic Test	Variant (Prinzmetal's) Stable Angina Pectoris	Angina	Unstable Angina Pectoris	Myocardial Infarction
			Findings	
Glucose	No elevation	No elevation	No elevation	Transiently elevated owing to adrenergic response
Lipid levels (triglycerides, cholesterol, high- and low-density lipids)	Checked to determine any lipoprotein abnormalities	Checked to rule out presence of atherosclerotic process	Checked to determine any lipoprotein abnormalities	Checked to determine any lipoprotein abnormalities; total cholesterol and HDL may drop 48 hr after admission
Chest x-ray examination	Normal	Normal	Normal; may show signs of cardiomegaly or signs of left ventricular failure	Same as unstable angina
Exercise stress test (EST)	Chest pain; horizontal ST segment or downsloping of 1 mm or more; failure of systolic blood pressure to rise or drop; ST elevations	Normal stress test done to differentiate between variant and classic angina; ST elevation with or without associated chest pain occasionally develops	As in stable angina pectoris, should not be done until patient has been stable and pain free for 24 hr	Not done in presence of documented MI, low-level test may be performed before discharge from hospital
Echocardiography	Limited use, but performed after EST may detect wall motion abnormalities		Two-dimensional: may show transient abnormalities of ventricular wall motion	Identifies area of abnormal regional wall motion; aids in detecting complications associated with acute MI: papillary dysfunction, septal rupture; visualizes LV thrombus *Right ventricular (RV) infarction:* dilated RV, abnormal RV wall motion
Thallium-201 scintigraphy	Ischemic areas appear as "cold" areas, reflecting reduced thallium uptake; when ischemia relieved, "cold" areas show normal thallium uptake	Ischemic "cold" areas may be demonstrated once involved coronary artery has been identified	Similar to stable angina pectoris	Similar to stable angina pectoris

Test		
Radionuclide blood pool imaging with technetium-99m	Positive findings suggest recent (previous) minor degrees of subendocardial necrosis or infarction	Confirms myocardial damage by localizing and permitting estimation of size of transmural infarction; must be done within 2-6 days after acute infarction; determines wall motion abnormalities; permits estimation of ventricular function by determining ejection fractions
Magnetic resonance imaging (MRI)		Differentiates ischemic, infarcted, and normal myocardial tissue; used in early detection of MI to assess areas of perfusion and detect jeopardized or vulnerable tissue
Cardiac catheterization and coronary angiography	Determines number and location of obstructive lesions, "graftability" of artery distal to obstructive lesion, and ventricular function	As in stable angina pectoris, used in conjunction with percutaneous transluminal coronary angioplasty (PTCA)
	Distinguishes spasm in normal coronary arteries from those with severe obstructive lesions; IV injection of ergonovine maleate provokes coronary artery spasm in patients with variant angina	Generally not performed as diagnostic procedure during acute period unless done in conjunction with PTCA or thrombolysis

From Canobbio MM: Mosby's clinical nursing series: cardiovascular disorders, St Louis, 1990, Mosby.

■ ACUTE MYOCARDIAL INFARCTION (AMI)

Complete occlusion of the coronary artery and/or its branches, resulting in myocardial ischemia and necrosis (Fig. 3-7). It occurs as result of a sudden decrease in coronary perfusion or an increase in myocardial oxygen demand without adequate coronary perfusion. Two types of infarction are the following:

__subendocardial infarction (non–Q wave):__ Confined to a small area of myocardium, usually within the subendocardial wall of the left ventricle, ventricular septum, and papillary muscle

__transmural or full thickness (Q wave):__ Infarction is widespread myocardial necrosis, extending from the endocardium to the epicardium

ASSESSMENT

SUBJECTIVE DATA
Severe, crushing chest pain
    Precordial
    Substernal
    Unrelated to exertion or respiration
Dizziness, faintness
Indigestion, nausea

OBJECTIVE DATA
Diaphoresis
Skin
    Cold
    Clammy
    Pale
SOB
Decreased BP

Tachycardia
Elevated temperature
Anxiety
Restlessness
Behavioral responses
    Denial
    Depression
Heart sounds
    S_3 gallop
    Pericardial friction rub
    Murmurs
Right ventricular infarction
    Increased jugular venous distension
    Peripheral edema
    Liver tenderness

DIAGNOSTIC TESTS (SEE TABLE 3-3)
Serum studies
    Elevated enzymes: creatine kinase (CK-MB, CK), LDH, AST, cTnT, cTnI
    Elevated ESR
    Elevated WBC
ECG changes (Fig. 3-8)
    ST segment elevation
    T wave depression, inversions
    Q waves
    Dysrhythmias
Echocardiography: ventricular wall motion abnormalities
Radionuclide blood pool studies: thallium, technetium
    Localization of infarct area
    Ventricular function

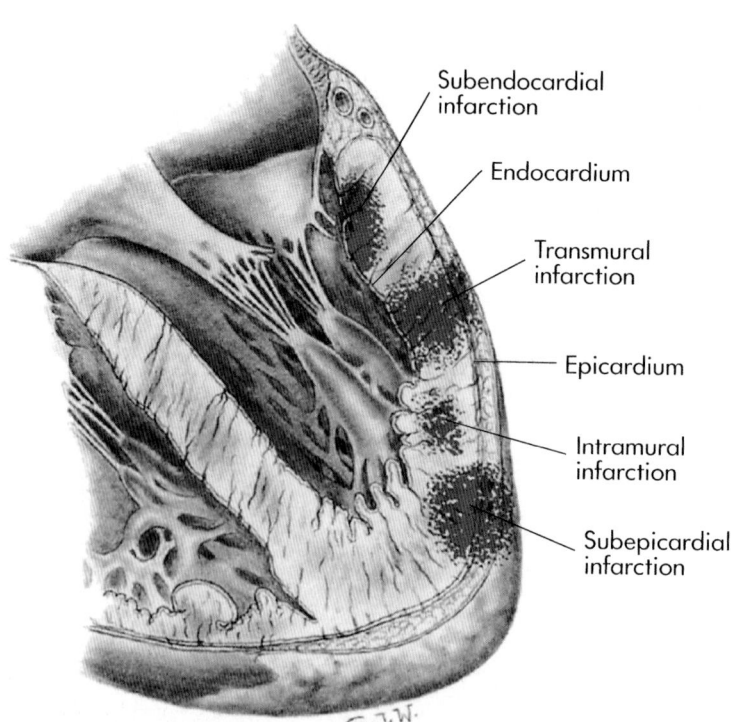

Fig. 3-7 Location of infarctions in the ventricular wall.
(From Thelan LA et al: Critical care nursing: diagnosis and management, *ed 3, St Louis, 1998, Mosby.)*

MRI
Cardiac catheterization: coronary angiogram,
    arteriogram

POTENTIAL COMPLICATIONS
Dysrhythmias
    Ventricular: PVCs, ventricular tachycardia, ventricular
        fibrillation
    Supraventricular ectopics (premature atrial
        contractions [PACs]), tachydysrhythmias
    Sinus bradycardia
    Conduction defects
Heart failure
Cardiogenic shock
Extension of MI or reocclusion of coronary artery
Pulmonary/systemic emboli
Pericarditis
Rupture
    Ventricular
    Papillary muscle
Sudden cardiac death (SCD)
Ventricular septal defect: systolic murmur left lower
    sternal border (LLSB)
Valvular dysfunction
Ventricular aneurysm
Postmyocardial infarction syndrome (Dressler's
    syndrome)

MULTIDISCIPLINARY MANAGEMENT
THERAPEUTIC MANAGEMENT
Coronary care unit (CCU) on admission with continuous
    cardiac monitoring
Oxygen therapy: 2 to 4 L/min by nasal cannula
Thrombolytic therapy: myocardial reperfusion within 4 to
    6 hours of onset of pain
Emergent procedures (within 4 to 6 hours of onset of
    chest pain)
    Percutaneous transluminal coronary angioplasty

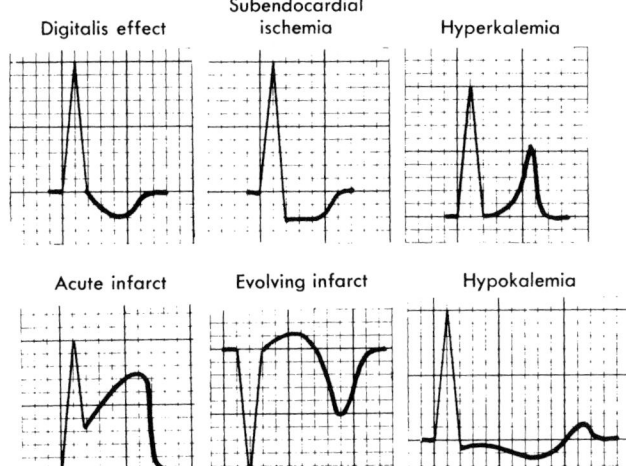

Fig. 3-8 ST-T segment changes.
*(From Goldberger AL: Clinical electrocardiography: a simplified ap-
proach, ed 6, St Louis, 1999, Mosby.)*

Coronary atherectomy
Coronary artery bypass graft surgery
Activity level
    Admission through day 2 to 3
        Bedrest until hemodynamically stable or free of
            chest pain
        Bedrest with bedside commode up to 12 hours
            from admission or until stable
        Bathing, toileting when stable
    Phase 1 rehabilitation begins on day 2 to 3 if stable
        (see p. 127)
Diet: NPO until stable, progressing to clear liquids, then
    low fat, low cholesterol, with no added salt
Parenteral fluids
Medications
    Pain management: morphine sulfate nitrates
    Sedation
    Antiarrhythmics
    Beta-adrenergic blocking agents
    Vasodilators
    Antiplatelets: low-dose aspirin
    Anticoagulants: heparin
    Calcium antagonist
Hemodynamic monitoring; SVo_2

PATIENT PROBLEMS—NURSING DIAGNOSIS/INTERVENTIONS

▼ Chest pain related to myocardial ischemia or
necrosis

Maintain bed rest with bedside commode for first 12 hours
    or 24 to 30 hours as indicated; position patient
    comfortably *to conserve myocardial oxygen
    consumption*
Using numeric rating scale (e.g., 0 to 10), assess and
    record description of pain and factors that aggravate
    pain; determine if influenced by respiration or body
    position
Administer oxygen *to ensure oxygen delivery to
    myocardium;* monitor oxygen saturation by pulse
    oximetry
Administer drug therapy as ordered; assess and record
    response
Obtain BP, P, and R during pain episode to monitor
    for signs of hypotension, *which may reflect
    hypoperfusion*
Initiate nonpharmacologic measures *to relieve pain* (e.g.,
    relaxation techniques, guided imagery; quiet, restful
    environment)

Expected Outcome
Verbalizes absence of pain and appears relaxed

▼ Decreased cardiac output related to alteration in
heart rate (dysrhythmia), decreased myocardial
contractility, and preload and afterload

Maintain bed rest for first 24 to 48 hours *to reduce
myocardial oxygen demand*

Maintain in upright position, which will *decrease venous return, lower preload, and decrease cardiac work*

Assess and report signs of decreased cardiac output; incidence of morbidity and motality are greatest in first 24 hours

    Decreased BP, increased heart rate

    Decreased urine output

    Fatigue and weakness

    Cool, pale, clammy skin

Assess and monitor BP, T, R, and apical pulse q2h to 4h or as indicated by clinical status

Monitor and record ECG continuously *to assess rate and rhythm* q2h to 4h or as indicated

Obtain and compare 12-lead ECG and/or right ventricular (RV) leads as ordered *to confirm and identify location of MI*

Administer oxygen therapy as ordered

Prepare and/or initiate thrombolytic therapy as ordered *to limit size of infarction by reperfusing ischemic heart muscle*

Auscultate breath and heart sounds q1h to 2h or as indicated

Monitor serial serum enzymes

Monitor PAP, PCWP, or CVP qhr if available or as indicated

Monitor intake and output q2h to 4h

Maintain parenteral fluids as ordered

Administer medications as ordered

Provide diet as tolerated

Instruct patient to avoid straining such as Valsalva's maneuver, which can cause *increased intraabdominal pressure;* use stool softeners or laxatives

Expected Outcomes

CO remains stable or improved

Demonstrates hemodynamic stability

Vital signs and urine output are within normal limits

Able to perform ADLs

▼Anxiety related to perceived or actual threat to biologic integrity

Assess for signs and verbal expressions of anxiety

Initiate comfort measures such as a quiet, restful environment and relaxation techniques (e.g., visual imaging, soft rhythmic music *to decrease unnecessary external stimuli that can stimulate sympathetic response*)

Minimize contact with stressful stimuli such as other anxious patients

Use calm, reassuring voice

Discuss and orient patient to ER/critical care environment and equipment

Administer sedation as indicated

Stay with patient during periods of highest anxiety and offer reassurance

Give simple explanations regarding care and procedures

Encourage expression of feelings; accept crying

Permit family member to assist patient whenever possible

Expected Outcomes

Anxiety level is reduced

Appears relaxed and verbalizes sense of calm

Additional Nursing Diagnoses to Consider

Activity intolerance related to cardiopulmonary dysfunction

Ineffective denial related to perceived life-threatening event

PATIENT/FAMILY TEACHING

Assess level of understanding and degree of readiness to learn

Review physician's explanation of heart condition

    Extent of infarction

    Associated complications

        Dysrhythmias

        Angina

        Postmyocardial infarction syndrome

        Heart failure

Describe the nature and course of coronary artery disease, including

    Risk factors involved and methods of modification (p. 86)

    Precipitating factors of angina

Discuss importance of controlling any coexisting disease that may aggravate recovery

    Hyperlipidemia

    Hypertension

    Diabetes

Explain importance of weight control

Explain stress management: need to control stress-producing events and activities

Discuss signs and symptoms of an extending MI reocclusion versus angina

    Extending MI reocclusion: chest pain, SOB, perspiration, weakness not relieved by medication or rest, pain not always associated with physical exertion

    Angina: chest pain or pressure is usually relieved by rest and/or vasodilators; pain is usually associated with physical or emotional strain

Using pain rating scale, explain importance of calling physician if there is a change in pain intensity, or if chest pain lasts longer than 15 minutes (if pain is associated with other symptoms, call physician immediately)

Explain names of medications, dosages, times of administration, purposes, and side effects

Explain need to avoid taking over-the-counter medications without checking with physician

Refer to cardiac rehabilitation program

DISCHARGE/HOME CARE PLANNING

Assist with development of exercise and activity plan

    Review limitations and allowances for walking and exercise limitations

    Instruct patient to avoid or modify activity after heavy meals, alcohol consumption, periods of emotional stress, or in temperature extremes

Explain importance of planned rest periods

Discuss importance of activity limitations as related to healing process (healing takes approximately 6 to 8 weeks)

Explain need to exercise at regular intervals; encourage home exercise program

Explain importance of checking with physician with regard to resuming sexual activity, travelling, and driving automobile

Explain need to avoid isometric-type activity (e.g., heavy lifting and pushing)

Explain need to monitor daily activities (space activities with periods of rest; stop when fatigued; avoid rushing)

Discuss importance of encouraging independence in self-care activities

Discuss importance of communication with significant other or family

Explain need to deal with feelings about possible role change and sexual activity

Explain importance of maintaining dietary restrictions, including low-cholesterol, low-fat, and low-calorie diet as ordered; refer to dietitian for education; if no specific diet is ordered, instruct to limit intake of eggs, cream, butter, and foods high in animal fat; modify or restrict salt intake

Explain need to rest after meals (avoid exercising up to 2 hours after having meals)

Explain need to avoid use of tobacco products such as cigarettes, cigars, and chewing tobacco; refer to smoking cessation program as needed

Explain need to avoid constipation and straining

Explain need to avoid sitting in same position for long periods

■ INFECTIVE ENDOCARDITIS

An inflammatory process involving the endothelium of the heart, including the cardiac valves (Fig. 3-9). Infective endocarditis begins as an infection that causes bacteremia. It is characterized by vegetations or thrombus composed of fibrin and platelets that form on valves and adjacent areas when endocardial tissue is damaged

Affected structures such as valves eventually become scarred, impeding function. The infection may also burrow into the myocardium, causing conduction defects, abscesses, and rupture of the chordae tendineae or ventricular septum

ASSESSMENT
SUBJECTIVE DATA
Complains of flulike symptoms: malaise, weakness, arthralgias

OBJECTIVE DATA
Recurrent temperature elevation
    Acute: 102° to 104° F (39° to 40° C)
    Subacute: 102° F (39° C)
Alternating chills and diaphoresis (may occur at night)
Signs of embolization
    Petechia
        Conjunctiva
        Palate, buccal mucosa
        Extremities
Osler's nodes
"Café-au-lait" complexion
Anorexia
Weight loss
Headache
Splenomegaly
Heart sounds
    Early: usually normal
    Late: murmurs

DIAGNOSTIC TESTS
Laboratory studies
    Positive blood cultures
    CBC
        Normocytic, normochromic anemia
        Elevated ESR
        Leukocytosis
    Rheumatoid factor: positive in patients with infection 6 weeks or longer
Echocardiogram: presence of vegetation or abscesses; valve involvement; LV dysfunction
Electrocardiogram: atrial fibrillation or flutter
Chest x-ray: normal to enlarged cardiac shadow, pleural effusion
Radionuclide studies
    Gallium-67 citrate

POTENTIAL COMPLICATIONS
Cardiac
    Abscesses
    Valvular heart disease
    Heart failure
    Myocarditis
Embolization: cerebral, renal, splenic, coronary
Mycotic aneurysms

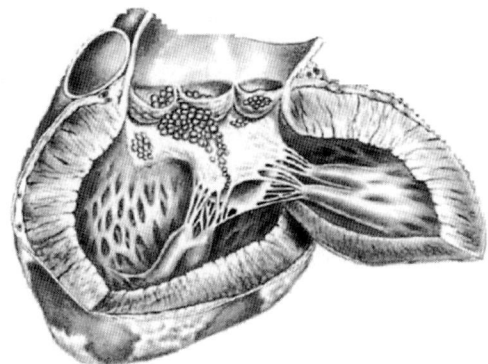

Fig. 3-9 Endocarditis.
(From Canobbio MM: Mosby's clinical nursing series: cardiovascular disorders, St Louis, 1990, Mosby.)

MULTIDISCIPLINARY MANAGEMENT

THERAPEUTIC MANAGEMENT

Parenteral therapy
Medications
    IV antibiotics
    Antipyretics: salicylates
    Analgesics
    Anticoagulation

PATIENT PROBLEMS—NURSING DIAGNOSES/INTERVENTIONS

▼ Altered nutrition: less than body requirements related to biologic factors (e.g., fever, infectious process)

Assess for progressive weight loss and signs of malnutrition *because infectious process increases metabolic* needs (chronic illness leads to anorexia)
Monitor daily caloric intake
Weigh daily *to determine amount of weight loss and need to add supplemental feedings*
Offer high-calorie and high-protein supplemental feedings *to ensure adequate intake of nutrients*
Consult with dietitian regarding nutritional requirements
Ensure patient comfort during meals

Expected Outcomes
Nutritional status is maintained or improved
Age-appropriate, sex-appropriate body weight is achieved or maintained
Verbalizes improved appetite

▼ Diversional activity deficit related to prolonged antibiotic therapy

Assess for diversional deficit; differentiate from progression of disease process
Encourage patient to explore diversional activities (e.g., reading, puzzles, and out-of-hospital passes) as indicated
Initiate occupational therapy if indicated
Encourage daily structured exercise program *to maintain muscle tone and promote sense of well-being*

Expected Outcome
Engages in identifiable inpatient diversional activities

▼ Altered body temperature related to infectious process

Assess for dehydration: diaphoresis, poor skin turgor, dry mucous membrane
    Obtain temperature q4h to 8h as indicated *to detect presence of infectious process*
    Monitor fluid intake and output q8h, noting water loss resulting from perspiration *to avoid negative fluid balance from dehydration*

Encourage fluid intake as tolerated *to maintain fluid balance*
    Administer antibiotics as ordered, ensuring they are given on time *to maintain consistent drug levels in blood*
    Administer antipyretics as ordered *to reduce temperature*
    Monitor laboratory reports on CBC with differential and blood cultures
    Monitor IV sites for redness and swelling; change site q48h *to reduce risk of infiltration and infection*

Expected Outcomes
Inflammatory process has cleared
Demonstrates normal body temperature
Skin is warm and dry

▼ Risk for altered cerebral tissue perfusion related to embolization

Assess for signs of embolization each shift and prn; report positive signs to physician immediately
Perform neurologic checks every shift or as indicated by patient's condition
Administer anticoagulant therapy as ordered
Instruct patient about need to continue with anticoagulants, if ordered, to prevent future embolic episodes

Expected Outcomes
Cerebral tissue perfusion is maintained
Alert and oriented
No signs of embolization are present

Additional Nursing Diagnoses to Consider
Risk for altered tissue perfusion (renal, pulmonary) related to embolization
Risk for decreased cardiac output related to mechanical factors secondary to heart failure

PATIENT/FAMILY TEACHING
Discuss symptoms of recurrence to report to physician
    Fatigue
    Elevated temperature
    Chills
    Weight loss
    Just not feeling well
Discuss need to avoid persons with infections, especially upper respiratory infection (URI), and to report symptoms (e.g., cold, influenza, cough) to physician
Explain importance of avoiding fatigue; need to plan rest periods before and after activity
Discuss importance of reporting to physician any event that may predispose to bacteremia
    Dental or gum therapy
    Surgical procedures
    Invasive medical procedures
    Childbirth

Trauma

Furuncles

Explain need to maintain good oral hygiene: daily care and regular visits to dentist

Explain importance of ongoing outpatient care

Discuss name of medication, dosage, times of administration, purpose, and side effects

Explain significance of prophylactic antibiotic therapy before procedures that predispose to bacteremia (Boxes 3-3 and 3-4, Table 3-4)

Box 3-3 | **Cardiac Conditions/Procedures for Which Endocarditis Prophylaxis Is Recommended/Not Recommended***

ENDOCARDITIS PROPHYLAXIS RECOMMENDED

High-Risk Category

Prosthetic cardiac valves, including bioprosthetic and homograft valves

Previous bacterial endocarditis

Complex cyanotic congenital heart disease (e.g., single ventricle, transposition of great arteries

Surgically constructed systemic pulmonary shunts or conduits

Moderate-Risk Category

Most congenital cardiac malformations

Acquired valvular dysfunction (e.g., rheumatic heart disease

Hypertrophic cardiomyopathy

Mitral valve prolapse with valvular regurgitation† and/or thickened leaflets

ENDOCARDITIS PROPHYLAXIS NOT RECOMMENDED

Negligible-Risk Category (No Greater Risk Than General Population)

Isolated secundum atrial septal defect

Surgical repair without residua beyond 6 months of secundum atrial septal defect, ventricular septal defect, or patent ductus arteriosus

Previous coronary artery bypass graft surgery

Mitral valve prolapse without valvular regurgitation†

Physiologic, functional, or innocent heart murmurs

Previous Kawasaki disease without valvular dysfunction

Previous rheumatic fever without valvular dysfunction

Cardiac catheterization, including balloon angioplasty

Cardiac pacemakers (intravascular and epicardial) and implanted defibrillators and coronary stents

Modified from The American Heart Association: JAMA 264, Dec 12, 1990.

*Cardiac conditions listed for which endocarditis prophylaxis is recommended/not recommended are not meant to be all-inclusive.

†Individuals who have a mitral valve prolapse associated with thickening and/or redundancy of the valve leaflets may be at increased risk for bacterial endocarditis, particularly men who are 45 years of age or older.

Box 3-4 | **Dental or Surgical Procedures for Which Endocarditis Prophylaxis Is Recommended/Not Recommended***

ENDOCARDITIS PROPHYLAXIS RECOMMENDED

Dental procedures known to induce gingival or mucosal bleeding, including professional cleaning

Tonsillectomy and/or adenoidectomy

Surgical operations that involve intestinal or respiratory mucosa

Bronchoscopy with a rigid bronchoscope

Sclerotherapy for esophageal varices

Esophageal stricture dilatation

Biliary tract surgery

Cystoscopy

Urethral dilatation

Urethral catheterization if urinary tract infection is present†

Urinary tract surgery if urinary tract infection is present†

Prostatic surgery

Incision and drainage of infected tissue†

Vaginal hysterectomy

Vaginal delivery in the presence of infection†

ENDOCARDITIS PROPHYLAXIS NOT RECOMMENDED‡

Dental procedures not likely to induce gingival bleeding, such as simple adjustment of orthodontic appliances or fillings above the gum line

Injection of local anesthetic (except intraligamentary injections)

Shedding of primary teeth

Tympanostomy tube insertion

Endotracheal intubation

Bronchoscopy with a flexible bronchoscope, with or without biopsy

Transesophageal echocardiography

Endoscopy with or without gastrointestinal biopsy

Cesarean birth

In the absence of infection for urethral catheterization, uterine dilatation and curettage, uncomplicated vaginal delivery, therapeutic abortion, vaginal hysterectomy sterilization procedures, or insertion or removal of intrauterine devices

The American Heart Association: JAMA 277:1799-1801, 1997. Copyright 1997.

*This table lists selected procedures but is not all-inclusive.

†In addition to prophylactic regimen for genitourinary procedures, antibiotic therapy should be directed against the most likely bacterial pathogen.

‡In patients who have prosthetic heart valves, a previous history of endocarditis or surgically constructed systemic-pulmonary shunts or conduits, physicians may choose to administer prophylactic antibiotics even for low-risk procedures that involve the lower respiratory, genitourinary, or gastrointestinal tracts.

Table 3-4	**Recommended Antibiotic Coverage for Endocarditis Prophylaxis**

Recommended standard prophylactic regimen for dental, oral, respiratory tract or esophageal procedures

Situation	Agent	Regimen*
Standard general prophylaxis	Amoxicillin	Adults: 2 g; PO 1 hr before procedure
Unable to take oral medications	Ampicillin	Adults: 2 g IM or IV within 30 min before procedure
Allergic to penicillin	Clindamycin or Cephalexin* or cefadroxil* or Azithromycin or clarithromycin	Adults: 600 mg; PO 1 hr before procedure Adults: 2 g; PO 1 hr before procedure Adults: 500 mg; PO 1 hr before procedure
Allergic to penicillin and unable to take oral medications	Clindamycin or Cefazolin*	Adults: 600 mg Adults: 1 g; children: 25 mg/kg IM or IV within 30 min before procedure

PROPHYLACTIC REGIMENS FOR GENITOURINARY/GASTROINTESTINAL (EXCLUDING ESOPHAGEAL) PROCEDURES

Situation	Agent	Regimen*
High-risk patients	Ampicillin plus gentamicin	Adults: ampicillin 2 g IM or IV plus gentamicin 1.5 mg/kg (not to exceed 120 mg) within 30 min of starting procedure; 6 hr later, ampicillin 1 g IM or IV or amoxicillin 1 g PO
High-risk patients allergic to ampicillin or amoxicillin	Vancomycin plus gentamicin	Adults: vancomycin 1 g IV over 1-2 hr plus gentamicin 1.5 mg/kg IV or IM (not to exceed 120 mg); complete injection or infusion within 30 min of starting procedure
Moderate-risk patients	Amoxicillin or ampicillin	Adults: amoxicillin 2 g PO 1 hr before procedure, or ampicillin 2 g IM or IV within 30 min of starting procedure
Moderate-risk patients allergic to ampicillin/ amoxicillin	Vancomycin†	Adults: vancomycin 1 g IV over 1-2 hr complete infusion within 30 min of starting procedure

From JAMA *277:1794-1801, 1997.*
IM, *intramuscularly;* IV, *intravenously.*
*Cephalosporins should not be used in individuals with immediate-type hypersensitivity reaction (urticaria, angioedema, or anaphylaxis) to penicillins.
†No second dose of vancomycin or gentamicin is recommended.

■ VALVULAR HEART DISEASE

An acquired or congenital disease involving the cardiac valves. The disorders fall into two classifications: insufficient (regurgitation), the inability to close sufficiently to permit blood flow, or stenosis, the inability to open sufficiently to permit blood flow. The most common forms of valvular heart disease (VHD) are aortic or mitral stenosis and aortic or mitral regurgitation (Fig. 3-10, Table 3-5)

ASSESSMENT
SUBJECTIVE DATA
General complaints
  Fatigue
  Malaise
  SOB
  DOE
  Anorexia
  Sleep disorders: PND, orthopnea, nocturnal sweats
  Palpitations

OBJECTIVE DATA
NOTE: Observations and care listed are for moderate-to-severe forms of valvular heart disease (see Table 3-5 for specific findings for most common forms of valvular heart disease)

DIAGNOSTIC TESTS
ECG
  Atrial, ventricular hypertrophy
  Dysrhythmias: atrial fibrillation, flutter
  Conduction defects: bundle branch blocks
Echocardiogram/TEE: decreased excursion of leaflets; chamber enlargement; dilation; presence of thrombus
Chest x-ray examination
  Cardiomegaly
  Pulmonary vascular congestion
  Valve calcification
Cardiac catheterization

POTENTIAL COMPLICATIONS
Infective endocarditis
Embolism
  Brain
  Lungs
Left ventricular (LV) failure
Right ventricular (RV) failure
Dysrhythmias
Rupture of papillary muscles or chordae tendineae
Pulmonary edema

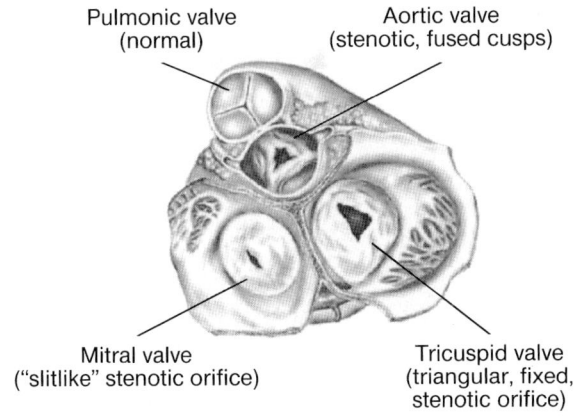

Pulmonic valve
(normal)

Aortic valve
(stenotic, fused cusps)

Mitral valve
("slitlike" stenotic orifice)

Tricuspid valve
(triangular, fixed,
stenotic orifice)

Fig. 3-10 Valvular heart disease.
(From Canobbio MM: Mosby's clinical nursing series: cardiovascular disorders, St Louis, 1990, Mosby.)

MULTIDISCIPLINARY MANAGEMENT
THERAPEUTIC MANAGEMENT
Medications
  ACE inhibitors
  Antibiotic prophylaxis
  Antidysrhythmics
  Diuretics
  Analgesics
  Anticoagulants
Diet: salt restriction
Cardioversion
Hemodynamic monitoring
Percutaneous balloon valvotomy
Surgical management
  Commissurotomy
  Valve repair
    Valvotomy
    Annuloplasty
    Valvuloplasty
  Valve replacement with either mechanical or biologic valve

PATIENT PROBLEMS—NURSING DIAGNOSES/INTERVENTIONS

▼Decreased cardiac output related to mechanical factors (preload, afterload) secondary to valvular dysfunction

Establish baseline assessment of cardiovascular status *to evaluate disease process and development of right or left ventricular failure*
Monitor BP, T, and R with apical pulse q4h or as indicated
Auscultate heart sounds q6h to 8h; record presence or absence of murmurs or gallop sounds *to determine progression in valve dysfunction or distention of heart chambers*
Monitor cardiac rhythm for changes from baseline; record any dysrhythmia (changes in rhythm *may reflect development of dysrhythmias, which can interfere with ventricular filling*)

Administer medications as ordered
Monitor intake and output
Restrict and monitor dietary intake of salt *to minimize sodium retention and excrete excess fluid*
Limit and/or modify activity during acute phase *to conserve energy and decrease myocardial oxygen demand*
  Avoid fatigue; maintain planned rest periods
  Perform active or passive ROM exercises to extremities qid

Expected Outcomes
Demonstrates stable or improved cardiac output
Reports improvement of symptoms
Lungs are clear
Vital signs and urine output are within normal limits
Able to perform ADLs

▼Fluid volume excess related to cardiac decompensation

Assess and monitor intake and output; report output <30 ml/hr or intake greater than output on daily basis
Assess and monitor for signs of fluid retention, increased congestion
  Auscultate for abnormal heart sounds (S_3, S_4) and breath sounds q4h to 8h
  Check for increase or decrease in jugular venous pressure
  Weigh daily (same time, scale, and clothing)
Administer diuretics and vasodilator therapy as ordered
Restrict sodium and fluids as indicated *to control sodium resorption and fluid retention*
Monitor electrolytes, chemistries, Hgb, and Hct

Expected Outcomes
Fluid balance is restored
Lung sounds clear
S_3, S_4 absent
Ideal body weight is achieved

▼Activity intolerance related to diminished cardiac reserve

Assess and monitor for signs of activity intolerance *as a result of an inability of myocardium to effectively increase stroke volume in response to increased demands*
Check BP, HR, and R before and after activity, report HR >20 bpm above resting HR, marked increase in BP, or complaints of dyspnea, chest pain, diaphoresis, or excessive fatigue
Maintain bed or chair rest as indicated
Identify factors known to cause fatigue *to promote energy conservation*
Space treatments and procedures *to allow for periods of uninterrupted rest to ensure periods of complete rest;* provide periods of rest throughout day and evening

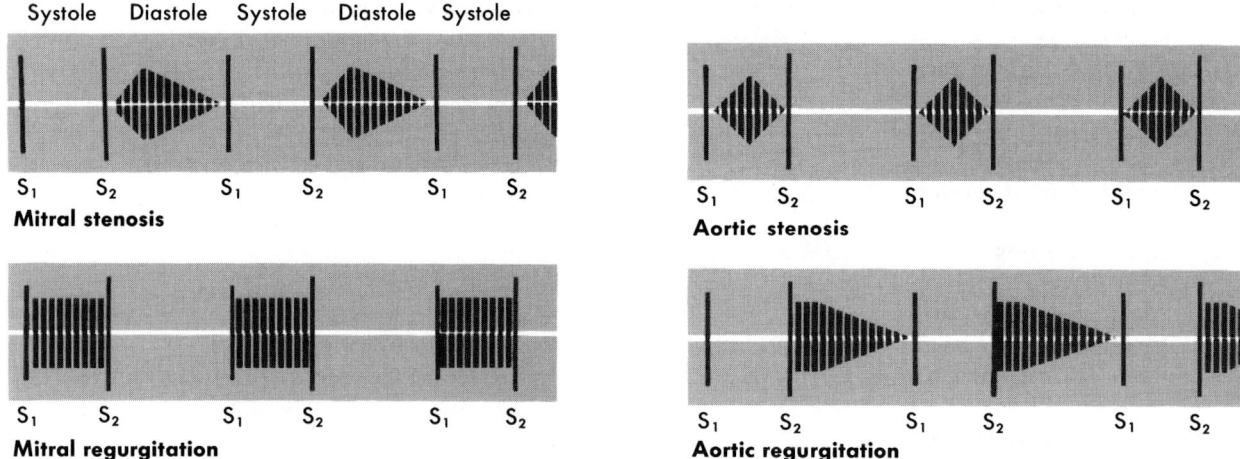

Fig. 3-11 Valvular heart disease murmurs.
(From Guzzetta C, Dossey B: Cardiovascular nursing: bodymind tapestry, St Louis, 1985, Mosby.)

Table 3-5	**Common Valvular Disorders: Adult Onset**		
Aortic Stenosis	**Mitral Stenosis**	**Aortic Regurgitation**	**Mitral Regurgitation**
OBSERVATIONS			
DOE	DOE	Dyspnea	Dyspnea
Syncope	Fatigue	Awareness of strong pulsations of heart	Fatigue
Fatigue	Decreased tolerance to exercise	Excessive sweating	Exercise intolerance
Angina pectoris	Orthopnea	Skin warm, flushed, and damp	Orthopnea
Decreased pulse pressure	PND	Dizziness	Palpitations
Carotid pulse	Cough	Neck pain	
Slow with long upstroke	Hemoptysis	Head bobbing (DeMusset's sign)	
Small quality to pulse		Pulses	
		Visible arterial pulsations in neck	
		Bisferiens pulse	
		Water-hammer (Corrigan's) pulse	
		Widened pulse pressure to >80 mm Hg	
Apical impulse: strong, sustained during systole	Apical impulse: tapping quality	Apical impulse: forceful, sustained, displaced downward and outward	Apical impulse; large, laterally displaced
Systolic thrill			
Heart sounds (Fig. 3-11)	Heart sounds (Fig. 3-11)	Heart sounds (Fig. 3-11)	Heart sounds (Fig. 3-11)
Moderate: crescendo-decrescendo, rough, harsh systolic murmur heard over aortic area	Loud first heart sound; low-pitched rumbling diastolic murmur with an opening snap heard at apex	Decrescendo: high-pitched blowing heard at left sternal border	Holosystolic systolic murmur heard at apex
Decreased aortic second sound		Systolic ejection sound	First heart sounds diminished
		Diastolic murmur	Splitting of second heart sound
			Third heart sound
POTENTIAL COMPLICATIONS			
Endocarditis	Endocarditis	Endocarditis	Endocarditis
Systemic emboli	Systemic emboli: brain, extremities, abdomen		Rupture of chordae tendineae; systemic emboli

Implement measures that will improve activity tolerance by minimizing fatigue (e.g., toileting via bedside commode rather than bedpan; up in chair with legs elevated rather than complete bed rest)

Increase activity level as indicated by condition; assess activity tolerance and activity progression *to evaluate improved myocardial performance*

Expected Outcomes

Activity level improved
Reports being able to participate in ADLs
Denies having SOB
HR, BP, R within normal limits

Additional Nursing Diagnoses to Consider

Risk for injury (cerebral) related to interruption of arterial blood flow secondary to embolization
Risk for infection

PATIENT/FAMILY TEACHING

Assess level of understanding
Explain nature and cause of disease process
Discuss importance of reporting signs and symptoms of heart failure
    Increased fatigue
    Tachypnea
    Orthopnea
    Cough
Infective endocarditis
    Elevated temperature
    Malaise and anorexia
    Chills alternating with diaphoresis
Discuss importance of reporting to physician any event that may predispose to bacteremia
    Dental or gum manipulation
    Genitourinary procedures
    Drainage of abscesses

Table 3-5	**Common Valvular Disorders: Adult Onset—cont'd**		
Aortic Stenosis	**Mitral Stenosis**	**Aortic Regurgitation**	**Mitral Regurgitation**
DIAGNOSTIC FINDINGS			
ECG Left ventricular hypertrophy (LVH) Conduction defects Left anterior hemiblock Left bundle branch block (LBBB) Complete heart block Dysrhythmias: atrial fibrillation	ECG P waves notched or peaked in I, II, III, and AV_F Atrial fibrillation Right ventricular hypertrophy (RVH)	ECG Normal Septal Q waves V_5, V_6 LVH	ECG Nonspecific ST segment and T wave abnormalities LVH P waves abnormalities Atrial dysrhythmias: premature atrial contractions (PACs), atrial fibrillation
Echocardiogram M-Mode, Doppler transesophageal electrocardiography (TEE) LV hypertrophy, valve calcification Pressure of transaortic valve gradient To identify other valve abnormalities mitral stenosis (MS), aortic regurgitation (AR)	Echocardiogram M-Mode, Doppler TEE: Enlarged left atria (LA); thickened mitral leaflets; valve calcification Presence of transmitral valve gradient (≥20 mm Hg) To detect/rule out presence of thrombosis	Echocardiogram M-Mode; Doppler TEE: Dilatation of aortic annulus thickening and failure of coaptation of leaflets Normal or supernormal velocity of LV wall	Echocardiogram M-Mode; Doppler: Enlarge LA; annular calcification, LV hyperdynamic To detect vegetation, incomplete coaptation of anterior and posterior mitral leaflets
Chest x-ray examination: enlargement of LV; calcification of aortic valve	Chest x-ray examination: enlargement of LA, RV, right atria (RA), and pulmonary trunk; calcification of mitral valve	Chest x-ray examination: enlargement of LV; dilation of aorta	Chest x-ray examination: enlargement of LA, LV
Hemodynamic changes: elevated left atrial (LA) and LV pressures	Hemodynamic changes: elevated pressures—LA, pulmonary artery (PA), and RV	Hemodynamic changes: elevated left ventricular end-diastolic pressure (LVEDP)	Hemodynamic changes: elevated LA and PA pressures and PCWP

Presence of skin boils
Gynecologic procedures
    Childbirth
    Dilation and curettage (D & C)
    Therapeutic abortion
    Tubal ligation

DISCHARGE/HOME CARE PLANNING

Explain importance of notifying dentist, urologist, and gynecologist of valvular heart disease before invasive procedure

For females, provide instruction regarding appropriate choice of contraceptives (i.e., to avoid estrogen-based contraceptives and intrauterine devices); explain importance of obtaining counseling regarding pregnancy before conception

Discuss name of medication, dosage, times of administration, purpose, and side effects

Explain need to avoid taking over-the-counter drugs without checking with physician

Explain importance of ongoing outpatient care

Instruct patient about importance of prophylactic antibiotic therapy to prevent endocarditis (see Table 3-4, Box 3-4)

Explain need to maintain good oral hygiene, daily care, and regular visits to dentist

Discuss activity allowances and limitations; assist to develop activity plan
    Explain need to avoid fatigue and to plan rest periods before and after activity
    Instruct patient in measures that will minimize fatigue
        Bathing: shower with chair rather than tub bath
        Avoid prolonged periods of standing; use stool to lean against when cooking, ironing

■ CONGENITAL HEART DISEASE

Structural or functional abnormalities or defects of the heart or great vessels existing from birth. With the advances in medical and surgical treatment, increasing number of persons are reaching adulthood. However, despite treatment, many of the defects continue to have residual problems that must continue to be monitored and treated

ASSESSMENT
SUBJECTIVE DATA
Dyspnea on exertion
Fatigue
Decreased exercise tolerance
Palpitations
Lightheadedness

OBJECTIVE DATA
See Table 3-6

DIAGNOSTIC TESTS
See Table 3-7
ECG
Chest x-ray

Echocardiogram
    Two-dimensional Doppler
    Transesophageal
Cardiac catheterization
Serum studies for patient with cyanotic congenital heart disease (CHD) (NOTE: Hct is normally elevated more than 45% with a range to 60%)
    Hct, Hgb, MCV, platelets
    Uric acid, BUN, creatinine levels

POTENTIAL COMPLICATIONS
Endocarditis
Dysrhythmias
Heart failure
Eisenmenger reaction

MULTIDISCIPLINARY MANAGEMENT
THERAPEUTIC MANAGEMENT
Medical
    Dictated by patient's clinical status
Surgery
    Palliative
        Systemic to pulmonary shunts (e.g., Blalock-Taussig, Glenn)
        Pulmonary artery banding
        Atrial septectomy
    Corrective (see Cardiac Surgery p. 119)
        Dictated by specific defect

PATIENT PROBLEMS—NURSING DIAGNOSES/INTERVENTIONS

▼ Anxiety related to threat to health status

Assess level of anxiety and determine primary cause *to determine patient's appraisal and perception of his or her clinical condition*

Assess usual coping mechanisms *to determine whether appropriate or sufficient to control anxiety and fear*

Provide and/or clarify information relative to condition *because anxiety can be result of misinterpretation of what congenital heart disease means*

Provide positive reinforcement about prognosis; assist patient in attaining realistic goals and lifestyle *to promote a sense of wellness and optimism about future*

▼ Risk for activity intolerance related to immobility, lack of knowledge, or progressive decreased cardiac reserve

Assess whether activity level is appropriate for medical condition because *patient may be misinformed about appropriate activity allowances and limitations*

Assess and monitor response to activity noting type, intensity, frequency, and type of symptoms that may develop

Implement measures that will improve activity tolerance if patient has reduced cardiac reserve *to limit myocardial oxygen demand*

Text continued on p. 109

Table 3-6 Congenital Heart Disease Objective Findings

Assessment	Patent Ductus Arteriosus	Atrial Septal Defect	Ventricular Septal Defect	Pulmonic Stenosis	Coarctation of Aorta	Ebstein's Anomaly	Tetralogy of Fallot
HISTORY	Small shunt: asymptomatic; large shunt: exertional dyspnea, decreased exercise tolerance	Small shunt: asymptomatic; moderate-to-large shunt: exertional dyspnea, decreased exercise tolerance, palpitations	Small-to-moderate shunt: asymptomatic, exertional dyspnea; large shunt: symptoms of failure	Asymptomatic; if develops symptoms: exertional dyspnea; decreased exercise tolerance	Asymptomatic; symptoms may be related to high BP or increased failure	Clinical symptoms vary from asymptomatic to mild-to-moderate exertional dyspnea and fatigue; complaints of palpitations and lightheadedness	In adulthood (following palliation): exertional dyspnea, cyanosis with clubbing
PHYSICAL EXAMINATION						Cyanosis: absent to moderate; mean jugular venous pressure (JVP)	
PALPATION	Neck vessels dilated and pulsating	Left parasternal lift	Large shunt: left parasternal lift	Left parasternal heave; subxiphoid pulsation	Delayed; diminished femoral pulsations; lag in timing of arterial pulses in lower extremities compared with upper extremities; presence of forceful carotid and suprasternal pulsations; visible collateral arterial pulses over scapula Precordium; suprasternal thrill, normal-to-sustained LV impulse	Normal; RV impulse absent	Precordial prominence; parasternal heave

Continued

From Canobbio MM: Mosby's clinical nursing series: cardiovascular disorders, St Louis, 1990, Mosby.

Table 3-6	Congenital Heart Disease Objective Findings—cont'd						
Assessment	Patent Ductus Arteriosus	Atrial Septal Defect	Ventricular Septal Defect	Pulmonic Stenosis	Coarctation of Aorta	Ebstein's Anomaly	Tetralogy of Fallot
AUSCULTATION	Systolic pressure normal; diastolic pressure low; wide pulse pressure; harsh, loud, continuous murmur in 1st, 2nd, 3rd intercostal space (ICS) at lower left sternal border (LSB); machinery-like murmur best heard when patient is lying, becoming fainter when patient is standing	Soft blowing systolic murmur at 2nd ICS at LSB	Small shunt: holosystolic at 3rd, 4th, and 5th ICS, systolic thrill; large shunt: holosystolic murmur at 3rd, 4th, and 5th ICS, splitting of S_2 during expiration, widening during inspiration, systolic ejection sound at 2nd ICS at LSB	S_1 normal; early systolic ejection click heard at base; midsystolic murmur at 2nd and 3rd ICS at LSB, radiates to suprasternal notch and to left side of neck; S_2 widely split	Systolic pressure > diastolic, wide pulse pressure, differences in arterial pressure between right and left arms; continuous murmur in interscapular area and/or over upper thorax anteriorly and posteriorly; S_2—normal with loud aortic component; with bicuspid aortic valve—a systolic ejection murmur	S_1 is widely split with a loud, delayed S_2; S_3 may be present because of abnormal filling of RV; early systolic or holosystolic murmur; short mid-diastolic murmur occurs, especially in prolonged P-R interval	Single S_2; systolic ejection murmur at 3rd ICS; may radiate upward to left side of neck

From Canobbio MM: Mosby's clinical nursing series: cardiovascular disorders, St Louis, 1990, Mosby.

Table 3-7 Diagnostic Tests

Diagnostic Test	Patent Ductus Arteriosus	Atrial Septal Defect	Ventricular Septal Defect	Pulmonic Stenosis	Coarctation of Aorta	Ebstein's Anomaly	Tetralogy of Fallot
ELECTROCARDIOGRAM (ECG)	Normal (small ductus); LVH; P-R interval may be prolonged; atrial fibrillation	Normal; RVH; RBBB; P-R interval may be prolonged; left axis deviation (ostium primum); normal or right axis (ostium secundum)	Normal if defect is small; if moderate to large, LVH; LVH/RVH in presence of pulmonary hypertension	Normal if stenosis is mild; if moderate to severe, RVH and right axis deviation; if severe, right atrial hypertrophy (RAH)	Normal; LVH (in older patients); T wave inversion, S-T depression (V_5V_6)	Normal; atrial flutter with one-to-one response or atrial fibrillation with rapid ventricular response via a right bypass tract; preexcitation (WPW) occurs in 20%-25% of patients	RVH
CHEST X-RAY	Normal; with moderate-to-large shunt, enlarged cardiac silhouette with enlarged LA, LV, and PA; enlarged aorta; enlarged pulmonary trunk and increased pulmonary flow	Enlarged RA, RV, PA; increased pulmonary vascular markings; LA, LV, and aortic knob may be small	Mild LVH with small shunt; with large shunt, increased LV, dilation of PA, increased pulmonary vascular markings, enlarged LA	Enlarged RV and PA; if severe, decreased peripheral pulmonary vascular markings	Normal; rib-notching caused by dilated intercostal collaterals; prominent ascending aorta; indentation below aortic knob at site of coarctation (3-sign); LV enlargement	Normal or cardiomegaly with enlarged RA; normal or decreased pulmonary vascularity	Small cardiac silhouette; small PA; prominent aorta (may arch to right in 25% of cases)
ECHOCARDIOGRAM	Ductus not visualized; enlarged LA and LV because of left-to-right shunt	With ostium secundum, enlarged RV, paradoxic movement of	Defect not visualized; large shunt; enlarged LA	Normal if stenosis is mild; if moderate to severe, enlarged RA and	Normal; confirms presence of bicuspid aortic valve; increased LV	12-dimensional: delayed closure and increased amplitude of	Overriding aorta visualized; pulmonary stenosis

From Canobbio MM: Mosby's clinical nursing series: cardiovascular disorders, St Louis, 1990, Mosby.

Continued

Table 3-7	Diagnostic Tests—cont'd						
Diagnostic Test	Patent Ductus Arteriosus	Atrial Septal Defect	Ventricular Septal Defect	Pulmonic Stenosis	Coarctation of Aorta	Ebstein's Anomaly	Tetralogy of Fallot
ECHOCARDIOGRAM—CONT'D		septum during systole; with ostium primum, mitral valve displaced inferiorly and anteriorly		RV thickness associated with bicuspid aortic valve	thickness associated with bicuspid aortic valve	anterior tricuspid leaflet and displaced septal leaflet; atrialized RV	visualized with degree of obstruction; enlarged ventricular septum (septal motion remains normal)
LABORATORY TESTS	No specific findings	No specific findings	No specific findings unless patient is cyanotic, then increased Hct value, decreased Hgb level and arterial oxygen saturation	No specific findings	No specific findings	No specific findings unless patient is cyanotic, then increased Hct	Increased Hct value; degree depends on amount of deoxygenated systemic blood
CARDIAC CATHETERIZATION	Increased pulmonary blood flow; increased oxygen saturation in PA; intracardiac pressures normal; RV and PA pressures may be slightly elevated	Left-to-right shunt; increased oxygen saturation in RA; RA pressure usually normal; mitral regurgitation	Left-to-right shunt; study determines degree of shunt; increased pulmonary blood flow, oxygen saturation in RV, and systolic pressure	Increased RA pressure, which determines systolic pressure gradient between RV and PA	Aortography confirms obstruction and determines pressure gradient	Done to evaluate degree of tricuspid regurgitation	RV outflow obstruction; increased RV pressure; RV-to-LV shunt; decreased PA pressure as catheter crosses obstruction

From Canobbio MM: Mosby's clinical nursing series: cardiovascular disorders, St Louis, 1990, Mosby.

Additional Nursing Diagnoses to Consider

Decreased cardiac output related to structural (defect), mechanical (preload, afterload, myocardial contractility), and electrical (dysrhythmias) factors

Ineffective individual and family coping related to incorrect information regarding clinical diagnosis or to progressive lifestyle and role changes imposed by disease process

PATIENT/FAMILY TEACHING

Ensure patient/family understand primary defect, and what (if any) palliative or corrective surgical interventions have occurred

Explain endocarditis, review preventive measures (see Infective endocarditis, pp. 97 to 100)

Explain importance of regular or periodic medical follow-up

DISCHARGE/HOME CARE PLANNING

Review activity allowances and limitations as indicated by clinical status, including recreational sports, ADLs

Provide counseling with respect to education, employment, and insurability

Discuss any dietary limitations

For adolescents and young adults, provide counseling concerning childbearing, genetics

For women, provide information regarding

Gynecology: report any signs of dysfunctional bleeding (e.g., heavy bleeding, irregular or missed periods)

Contraception: appropriate forms

Pregnancy and delivery, associated risk with type of defect, and current clinical status; discuss importance of obtaining prepregnancy counseling

For cyanotic patient

Describe signs of hyperviscosity: headaches, muscle aches, visual disturbances, lightheadedness, paresthesia of fingers and toes, and need to report to physician for laboratory evaluation

Discuss importance of avoiding dehydration and overexertion, particularly on hot days

Discuss importance of not using tobacco products

Discuss need to avoid aspirin and iron replacement without checking with physician

■ PERICARDITIS

An inflammatory process involving the parietal and visceral layers of the pericardium and outer myocardium. Pericarditis occurs as an acute process; an exudate of fibrin, WBCs, and endothelial cells is released. Chronic pericarditis, referred to as "constrictive pericarditis," is characterized by dense fibrous pericardial thickening

ASSESSMENT

SUBJECTIVE DATA

Chest pain

Precordial

May radiate to shoulder or neck

Severe, sharp

Dyspnea

Nausea

Muscle aches

OBJECTIVE DATA

Substernal chest pain

Increases with inspiration

Relieved by sitting up and leaning forward

Increased systemic venous pressure

Pericardial friction rub: scratchy sound in time with heartbeat

Elevated temperature

Chills alternating with diaphoresis

Restlessness

Anxiety

Fatigue

Orthopnea

DIAGNOSTIC TESTS

ECG

Elevated ST segment in LV leads: V_5, V_6, I, II, aV_L and aV_F

T wave inversion (late stage)

Low-voltage QRS complex in presence of pericardial effusion

Dysrhythmias

Blood studies

CBC: leukocytosis (increased WBC); increased ESR; elevated viral titers

Chest x-ray examination: normal or symmetrically enlarged cardiac silhouette

Echocardiogram: presence of pericardial effusion

Radionuclide blood pool scanning

Technetium label macroaggregated albumin and thallium (confirms presence of pericardial effusion)

MRI: visualizes pericardium

POTENTIAL COMPLICATIONS

Pericardial effusion

Cardiac tamponade

Heart failure

MULTIDISCIPLINARY MANAGEMENT

THERAPEUTIC MANAGEMENT

Medications

Nonsteroidal antiinflammatory drugs (NSAIDs): indomethacin

Analgesics, antipyretics: aspirin

Corticosteroids

Pericardiocentesis

Surgical procedures

Pericardial window

Pericardiectomy

PATIENT PROBLEMS—NURSING DIAGNOSES/INTERVENTIONS

▼ Chest pain related to pericardial inflammation

Assess and record quality of chest pain *to distinguish pericardial pain from myocardial ischemia*

Supervise activity

    Maintain bed rest, elevate head 45 degrees, position for comfort, provide padded overbed table *to minimize pain that is aggravated by movements*

    Administer pain medications *to provide relief and suppress inflammatory symptoms*

Expected Outcome

Chest pain is relieved

▼ Anxiety related to perceived or actual threat to biologic integrity

Assess level of anxiety and degree of understanding, noting verbal and nonverbal expressions, *to determine source of anxiety and identify any misunderstanding of disease process or treatment*

Provide supportive care *to ensure sense of trust, comfort, and reassurance*

Remain with patient if anxious

Encourage communication with significant other/family

Explain procedures and treatments thoroughly

Ensure quiet environment *to reduce external stimuli*

Use calm, reassuring voice

Expected Outcome

Anxiety level is reduced; appears calm

▼ Risk for decreased cardiac output related to reduced ventricular filling

Assess and monitor for signs of cardiac tamponade, which is a complication

Check for pulsus paradoxus, narrowing pulse pressure, respiratory filling of neck veins *to detect early signs of increasing intrapericardial pressure and development of tamponade*

Monitor BP, T, R, and apical pulse q4h as indicated *to detect pericardial restriction, hypotension, and tachycardia*

Place on cardiac monitor during acute phase, checking rhythm q1h to 2h *to detect nonspecific changes caused by superficial injury to epicardial surface of heart*

Obtain 12-lead ECG as ordered

Auscultate heart sounds for presence of pericardial friction rub, *which may reflect presence of pericardial effusion,* q6h to 8h

Administer medications as ordered

Prepare for pericardiocentesis when ordered

Expected Outcomes

Cardiac output and hemodynamic stability maintained

Vital signs within normal limits

Negative for pulsus paradoxus

PATIENT/FAMILY TEACHING

Discuss symptoms of recurrence to report to physician

    Increasing fatigue

    Elevated temperature

    Difficult respirations

    Chest pain

Explain that symptoms may continue up to 2 weeks, but notify physician if symptoms do not diminish or if they increase

Explain need to avoid persons with infections, especially URIs, and to report symptoms (e.g., cold, influenza, cough) to physician

Explain need to avoid overexertion and heavy lifting; alternate periods of activity with rest

Explain importance of ongoing outpatient care

Discuss medications: name, dosage, time of administration, purpose, and side effects

Explain need to avoid taking over-the-counter medications without checking with physician

CARDIAC TAMPONADE

Rapid accumulation of fluid or blood within the pericardial cavity that results in restriction of diastolic filling and causes decrease in the stroke volume and cardiac output

ASSESSMENT

SUBJECTIVE DATA

Pain or discomfort in chest, abdomen

Dyspnea

Restlessness

OBJECTIVE DATA

Distended neck veins with inspiratory rise in venous pressure (Kussmaul's sign)

Decreased systolic BP; narrowing pulse pressure; pulsus paradoxus >10 mm Hg

Decreased and/or distant heart sounds

Pericardial friction rub

Anxiety

Tachypnea

Tachycardia: weak, absent peripheral pulses

Skin

    Cyanotic

    Dusky

    Pale

Posture: Patient sits upright or leans forward

Hemodynamic findings

    Decreased CO

    Elevated RAP

    Elevated CVP

    Lowered left atrial pressure (LAP)

DIAGNOSTIC TESTS

Echocardiogram: pericardial effusion; paradoxic septal motion

ECG

    Tachycardia

    Nonspecific ST and T wave changes

    Diminished voltage, altering voltage of both P wave and QRS complex

    Dysrhythmias

Chest x-ray examination: enlarged cardiac silhouette (globular shape); lung fields clear

Blood pooling scanning
MRI: to show loculated effusions
Right heart catheterization: decreased ventricular filling
    pressures, elevated RAP

POTENTIAL COMPLICATIONS
Heart failure
Cardiogenic shock
Cardiac arrest

MULTIDISCIPLINARY MANAGEMENT
THERAPEUTIC MANAGEMENT
NPO
Parenteral fluids: volume expanders
Pericardiocentesis
Medications
    Inotropic, chronotropic
    Corticosteroids
    Antiarrhythmics
12-Lead electrocardiogram
Maintain defibrillator and emergency drugs at bedside
Surgery: pericardiectomy

PATIENT PROBLEMS—NURSING DIAGNOSES/INTERVENTIONS

▼ Decreased cardiac output related to restricted ventricular filling

Assess for and estimate degree of pulsus paradoxus and
    increased JVP *to confirm presence of tamponade and
    increased intrapericardial pressure*
Maintain bed rest; elevate head of bed 45 degrees (see
    Fig. 3-6)
Place patient on cardiac monitor; check rhythm strip qh
Monitor arterial pressure, pulse pressure, pulse volume,
    ECG, and level of consciousness q5min to 15min *to
    evaluate signs of progressive impairment of
    ventricular filling*
Administer parenteral fluids and medications as ordered
    to maintain hemodynamic stability
Assist with pericardiocentesis *to relieve compression*

Expected Outcomes
Demonstrates hemodynamic stability
Tests negative for pulsus paradoxus
Vital signs within normal limits
Jugular venous distension decreases
Skin warm and dry

▼ Anxiety (moderate to severe) related to perceived
and/or actual threat to biologic integrity

Assess level of anxiety, noting both verbal and nonverbal
    expressions
During this period, remain with patient and offer realistic
    assurances; use simple explanations *to ensure sense of
    trust and comfort*
Ensure quiet environment *to reduce external stimuli as
    much as possible*

Expected Outcome
Anxiety level is reduced (i.e., patient appears relaxed)

■ PERICARDIOCENTESIS
*Withdrawal of blood or fluid from the pericardial sac via
percutaneous needle puncture (Fig. 3-12)*

PREPARATION AND PATIENT TEACHING
Reinforce physician's explanation of procedure
Obtain signed consent
Maintain NPO 4 to 6 hours before procedure when possible
Elevate head of bed 20 to 30 degrees as ordered (see Fig. 3-6)
Obtain 12-lead ECG and rhythm strip; connect ECG
    unipolar lead to needle using alligator clip
Obtain laboratory studies as ordered: CBC, PT, PTT, platelets
Administer oxygen by mask or cannula as ordered
Obtain and record baseline arterial pressures, paradoxic
    pulse, and pulse pressure
Maintain parenteral fluids as ordered
Obtain equipment as ordered
    ECG machine
    Needles: No. 16 spinal
    Syringes: 30 ml and 50 ml
    Three-way stopcock
    Sterile drapes
Administer medications as ordered
    Atropine
    Lidocaine
    Sedatives
Maintain defibrillator and emergency drugs at bedside
Provide emotional support

ASSESSMENT DURING AND AFTER PROCEDURE
OBJECTIVE DATA
LOC
ECG
    ST elevations
    Increased P-R interval

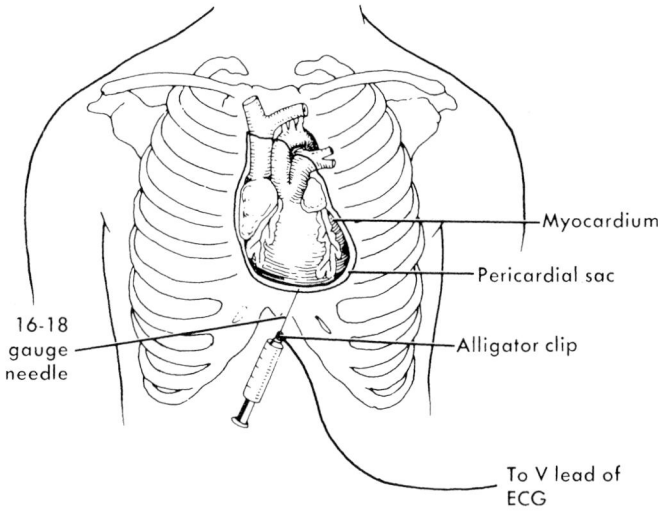

Fig. 3-12 Pericardiocentesis.
(From Sheehy SA: Emergency nursing: principles and practice, *ed 3,
St Louis, 1992, Mosby.)*

Arterial pressure
RAP
Pericardial aspirate
  Amount
  Color
  Turbidity
  Presence/absence of blood

POTENTIAL COMPLICATIONS
Puncture of coronary artery, ventricle, or lung
Dysrhythmias
Ventricular fibrillation
Laceration of lung
Pneumothorax
Recurring cardiac tamponade

POSTPROCEDURE CARE AND PATIENT TEACHING
Maintain bed rest
Assess BP, R, and apical pulse q15min for 1 hour, then q4h
  as ordered
Monitor arterial pressures; check for decreased pulse
  pressure or pulsus paradoxus q15min for 1 hour, then
  q4h as ordered
Maintain NPO as ordered
Auscultate heart sounds q2h to 4h
Observe for recurrence of tamponade; be prepared to
  repeat pericardiocentesis or surgical intervention
Continue ongoing care for specific disease process

■ HEART FAILURE
Clinical syndrome characterized by signs and symp-
toms of intravascular and interstitial volume overload
and manifestations of inadequate tissue perfusion

ASSESSMENT
SUBJECTIVE DATA
Fatigue
Effort intolerance
Anorexia
Dyspnea
Nocturia

OBJECTIVE DATA
General
Cachexia
Nausea and/or vomiting
Tachypnea
Tachycardia
Pulsus alternans
Heart sounds: gallop rhythms (S_3, S_4)
Decreased peripheral perfusion: peripheral cyanosis,
  diminished pulses, cool skin, pale skin color
Anxiety
Restlessness
Lung sounds: crackles, rhonchi
Cheyne-Stokes respiration
Drug toxicity
  Digitalis toxicity
  Hypokalemia
Dysrhythmias

Left Ventricular Failure (LVF)
SOB
Restlessness
Fatigue
Dyspnea, exertional and/or at rest
PND
Orthopnea
Nocturia
Tachypnea
Dry, unproductive cough
Hemoptysis
Elevated BP
Tachycardia
Pulsus alternans
Left ventricular gallop: S_3, S_4
Auscultation: crackles, rhonchi
Cyanosis

Right Ventricular Failure (RVF)
Increased venous pressure (rise in "a" and "v" waves)
Distended neck veins
Firm, pitting edema
Peripheral edema
  Sacrum
  Genitalia
  Ascites
Right upper quadrant abdominal tenderness
Hepatosplenomegaly; hepatojugular reflex
Diaphoresis
Weight gain
Right ventricular gallop: S_3
Decreased urine output
Nausea, indigestion
Anorexia

DIAGNOSTIC TESTS
General
Serum
  Hct, Hgb
  BUN, creatinine
  Electrolytes
    Hyponatremia
    Hyperkalemia
    Hypokalemia
  Bilirubin: hyperbilirubinemia
  Enzymes: AST, ALT, LDH
  PT/INR
  Albumin
  Glucose
  TSH, T_4 (for patients >65 years or patients with atrial
    fibrillation)
Arterial blood gases: decreased Pao_2, Sao_2
Urine
  Specific gravity
  Protein
  Creatinine
  Sodium
ECG
Ambulatory electrocardiographic recording (Holter)
Chest x-ray examination

Echocardiogram
Radionuclide ventriculography (to measure ejection traction)
MUGA
Hemodynamic monitoring
Pulmonary function tests

Left Ventricular Failure
ECG: left ventricular hypertrophy (LVH), left atrial hypertrophy (LAH), dysrhythmias
Ejection fraction (EF)
LV systolic dysfunction: EF $< 35\%$ to 40%
Hemodynamic pressures:
Increased PCWP, SVR
Decreased CI, CO, MAP
Chest x-ray
Redistribution of pulmonary flow to upper lobes
Kerley B lines
Pleural effusion
Increased cardiac shadow
Pulmonary function test: decreased vital capacity (VC), residual volume, and total lung capacity

Right Ventricular Failure
ECG: Right ventricular hypertrophy (RVH), right atrial hypertrophy (RAH)
Elevated RA, RV pressure
Elevated CVP
Chest x-ray examination: generalized enlargement of cardiac shadow

POTENTIAL COMPLICATIONS
Pulmonary edema
Embolic phenomenon
Pulmonary infarction
Cardiogenic shock

MULTIDISCIPLINARY MANAGEMENT
THERAPEUTIC MANAGEMENT
Sodium-restricted diet (2 to 3 g/d)
Medications
ACE inhibitors
Diuretics
Vasodilators
Beta-blocking agents
Inotropic drugs
Morphine sulfate
Potassium
Oxygen therapy
Hemodynamic monitoring: CI, SVR, PVR, MAP, PAWP
SVO_2
Intraaortic balloon pump (IABP)
Ventricular assistive devices (VAD)
Surgical
Cardiac transplantation

PATIENT PROBLEMS—NURSING DIAGNOSES/INTERVENTIONS

▼ Decreased cardiac output related to increased/decreased preload, increased afterload, or decreased contractility

Assess and monitor BP, apical pulse, HR, and R q4h or as indicated *to detect signs of decreased CO*
Maintain bed rest as indicated to conserve energy; elevate head of bed 30 to 60 degrees *to facilitate ventilation;* lean patient forward on padded overbed table as needed
Assess: skin for warmth and color; distal pulses bilaterally for strength, regularity, capillary refill (<3 seconds)
Monitor and record hemodynamic pressures *to evaluate preload, afterload parameters, and contractility to assess response to therapy*
Administer medications as ordered, titrating to enhance contractility
Monitor for signs of drug toxicity; monitor drug levels
Restrict activities as indicated by condition
Provide bedside commode
Implement measures that *prevent fatigue*
Plan rest periods between procedures
Have patient rest before and after meals
Maintain planned rest periods
Provide emotional support, offer simple explanations

Expected Outcomes
Vital signs within acceptable limits for age
HR, CI, CO, PCWP SVR within acceptable limits
Urine output increased
Activity tolerance is increased

▼ Fluid volume excess related to fluid retention secondary to decreased renal perfusion

Assess and monitor for signs of fluid retention, increased congestion, and/or response to therapy
Check for increase or decrease in JVP
Auscultate chest for breath and heart sounds (S_3, S_4) q4h to 8h
Measure intake and output; record output qh; report output, <30 ml/hr
Monitor serial BUN and creatinine levels *to assess renal function* (BUN >20 and creatinine >1.5 suggest renal dysfunction)
Weigh patient daily (same time, scale, and clothing); report increase of 500 g/day or greater
Maintain parenteral fluids by microdrip when ordered; avoid rapid and excessive hydration; use concentrated IV infusion to *decrease volume administration* when possible
Administer diuretics and vasodilator therapy as ordered; observe for effect and toxicity
Estimate diaphoretic fluid loss
Monitor electrolytes to assess for signs of hypovolemia, hypokalemia, dehydration
Maintain sodium-restricted diet and maintain fluid *restrictions to control sodium resorption and fluid*

retention; assist patient with planning distribution of fluids over waking hours

Expected Outcomes

Exhibits no signs of fluid overload as evidenced by the following:

Absence of edema

Weight loss, return to baseline

PAWP, PAP within normal limits

Lung sounds clear; heart sounds normal (i.e., no S_3, S_4)

No signs of increased JVP

▼ Impaired gas exchange related to alveolar-capillary membrane changes caused by increased pulmonary capillary pressure

Assess and monitor for changes in respiratory function *to detect signs of impaired ventilation and perfusion*

Monitor serial arterial blood gases (ABGs) to *identify hypoxemia, hypercapnia*

Auscultate lung sounds q4h *to detect increases in congestion*

Monitor chest x-ray examinations for changes

Monitor hemodynamic parameters that are indicators of degree of pulmonary congestion: PAP, PCWP

Elevate head of bed; have patient lean forward on padded overbed table; reposition q2h to 4h as indicated *to optimize ventilation and gas exchange*

Administer oxygen therapy *to maintain arterial oxygen saturation by* Spo_2 *>90%;* prepare for intubation and assisted mechanical ventilation if required *to increase surface area for appropriate gas exchange*

Provide humidified inspired air *to liquefy secretions as ordered*

Instruct patient to cough and breathe deeply *to facilitate ventilation and remove secretions*

Administer medications as ordered

Morphine

Rapid-acting diuretics

Instruct patient to avoid using tobacco products

Provide brief explanations of all treatments and procedures *to prevent hyperventilation resulting from fear or anxiety*

Expected Outcomes

Demonstrates improved gas exchange as evidenced by the following:

Effortless breathing

Improved respirations

Absence of cyanosis

Lungs clear on auscultation

Po_2, Pco_2, and O_2 at (Sao_2) levels within normal limits

▼ Risk for impaired skin integrity related to impaired circulation and metabolic state

Assess skin integrity and bony prominence daily for signs of redness, scaling, breaks, or ulcerations

Initiate measures *to maintain skin integrity and enhance circulation*

If patient is on bed rest, turn and reposition q2h

Provide alternative preventive devices

Alternating pressure mattress

Air pressure bed (Clinitron)

Prevent and eliminate pressure and friction; position pillows or other supports between pressure areas *to avoid two skin areas touching*

Assist patient out of bed frequently or as ordered

Administer skin care q2h

Keep skin clean and dry

Massage bony prominence q2h to 4h using lanolin-based lotion

NOTE: To prevent skin excoriations, do not massage reddened area

Initiate pressure sore care at first signs of tissue breakdown or ulceration (p. 711)

Expected Outcomes

Demonstrates maintenance of skin integrity as evidenced by the following:

Skin intact

Warm and dry, normal color

Signs of healing over areas of breakdown

▼ Altered nutrition: less than body requirements related to impaired absorption of nutrients secondary to decreased cardiac output

Observe daily for signs of malnutrition and cardiac cachexia

Dry body weight 20% or more under the ideal for age, height, and frame

Decreased triceps skinfold (TSF) measurements

Stomatitis

Anorexia

Increasing fatigue and weakness

Decreased serum albumin, transferrin, iron-binding capacity, BUN

Lack of interest in food

Determine patient's baseline weight

Weigh patient daily (same time, scale, and clothing) *to determine accurate weight and caloric needs*

Administer oral hygiene q2h to 4h

Administer medications to relieve nausea and/or vomiting; arrange medication schedule so it does not interfere with mealtime

Maintain diet as ordered; consult with dietitian *to evaluate nutritional status and to assist in selection of foods*

Do not force patient to eat

Tempt appetite with food preferences compatible with diet restrictions and cultural values

Remove unsightly and odorous items from room during mealtime

Serve small, frequent meals

Supplement with high-calorie foods *to maintain minimum required caloric intake*

Initiate caloric count if nutritional status fails to improve

Initiate tube feedings or parenteral nutrition as indicated

Expected Outcomes

Demonstrates adequate nutritional status as evidenced by the following:

Dry body weight that is improved or normal for age and body build

Improved appetite

Good skin turgor, increased muscle mass

▼ Activity intolerance related to weakness secondary to decreased cardiac output

Assess and monitor for signs of activity intolerance

Check BP, HR, and R before and after activity *to detect orthostatic hypotension,* which can result from prolonged periods of bed rest and inactivity

Maintain patient on bed or chair rest with feet elevated as indicated

Identify factors known to cause fatigue; restrict and/or limit activities as indicated (e.g., number of visitors and their length of stay) *to promote energy conservation*

Space treatments and procedures *to allow for periods of uninterrupted rest;* provide periods of rest throughout day and evening to ensure periods of complete rest

Implement measures that will improve activity tolerance by minimizing fatigue (e.g., bathing in shower with chair rather than self-bathing); using bedside commode rather than bedpan to limit energy expenditure

Increase activity level as indicated; assess activity tolerance and activity progression *to evaluate improved myocardial performance*

Expected Outcomes

Demonstrates improved activity tolerance

Verbalizes improved energy to perform ADLs

ECG, BP, HR (<20 beats/min above baseline during activity, HR returns to baseline 5 minutes after activity), and R within acceptable limits during and after activity

Additional Nursing Diagnoses to Consider

Fatigue

Risk for ineffective coping; patient, family

Caregiver role strain

Noncompliance related to side effects of medications

PATIENT/FAMILY TEACHING

Assess level of understanding

Discuss nature and cause of disease process and underlying cause

Review symptoms of early heart failure to report to physician

Decreased exercise tolerance

SOB

DOE

PND

Persistent cough

Swelling of extremities

Sudden weight gain of >3 lb (6.6 kg) in a 24-hour period (1 kg approximates 1000 ml fluid)

Nocturia

Discuss need to avoid persons with infections, especially URIs

Explain importance of not using tobacco

Teach patient/family to monitor and record heart rate and report any changes

Discuss medications: name, dosage, time of administration, purpose, and side effects

Explain importance of avoiding extreme temperature changes

Explain importance of ongoing care

DISCHARGE/HOME CARE PLANNING

Discuss importance of daily weighing (same time, scale, and clothing) and reporting increases of >2 lb within 24 hours

Refer to home health agency for assistance with ADLs as necessary

Activities

Discuss importance of pacing activities to avoid overexertion and fatigue

Alternate exercise and other activities with rest periods

Use energy-saving techniques (e.g., sitting to brush hair and prepare foods)

Diet

Discuss importance of maintaining prescribed diet and fluid amounts; need to avoid food high in sodium

Instruct patient to limit sodium intake to 2 to 3 g/d; to limit alcohol to no more than one drink per day

Instruct patient to read labels for sodium content before buying

Provide information on alternative ways to season foods

Refer to dietitian for diet planning

■ SHOCK

A clinical syndrome in which blood flow to the tissues is insufficient to sustain normal cell metabolism, resulting in a generalized decrease in perfusion to vital body function (see Box 3-5 and Table 3-8)

hypovolemic shock ("cold" shock): Deficient return of venous blood to the heart caused by external losses of blood plasma or extracellular fluid or caused by internal sequestration of plasma (hemorrhagic shock)

vasogenic (warm shock): Shock syndrome that results in massive vasodilation from an increase in total vascular capacity; most common form is sepsis but may occur as a result of other factors, including anaphylactic reactions (septic shock)

cardiogenic shock: Shock caused by inadequate tissue perfusion that results from LV dysfunction

<table>
<tr><td>Box 3-5</td><td>**Shock Syndrome: Causes/Etiologies**</td></tr>
</table>

HYPOVOLEMIC SHOCK

Loss of blood volume (hemorrhage, gastrointestinal bleeding, wounds)

Loss of plasma volume (dehydration, burns, peritonitis)

CARDIOGENIC SHOCK

Acute myocardial infarction

Structural problems: septal rupture aneurysm, cardiomyopathies, valvular dysfunction

Other causes (pulmonary emboli, cardiac surgery, tamponade)

VASOGENIC SHOCK

Sepsis

Immune-mediated reactions (anaphylaxis)

Deep anesthesia effects

Table 3-8	Early and Late Signs of Shock Syndrome	
Signs	**Early**	**Late**
Blood pressure	↓ Pulse pressure ↑ Diastolic pressure	↓ Systolic pressure
Urine output	↓ Urine sodium concentration ↑ Urine osmolality	↓ Urine volume
Acid-base changes	↑ Respiratory alkalosis Metabolic alkalosis	Metabolic acidosis
Tissue perfusion	Occasionally warm, dry skin Slight restlessness	Cold, clammy skin Cloudy sensorium

From Shock *1976, The Upjohn Company. Reproduced with permission of The Upjohn Company.*

ASSESSMENT

SUBJECTIVE DATA

Restlessness

Anxiety

Irritability

Dizziness

Faintness when sitting up

OBJECTIVE DATA

Hypovolemic Shock

Decreased or falling BP: determined by patient's baseline pressure

Narrowed pulse pressure

Hemodynamics

    Interarterial pressure

        Early: normal

        Late: decreased

    Decreased RAP, PAP, PCWP

    Decreased CI, CO

    Decreased CVP (<3 cm H_2O pressure)

    Increased SVR

Low SVo_2

Flat neck veins

Collapsed peripheral veins

Tachycardia: weak, thready pulse

Tachypnea: shallow respirations

Extreme weakness

Altered levels in mental status

    Lethargy

    Semiconsciousness

    Coma

Circumoral pallor

Conjunctival pallor

Lip cyanosis

Skin

    Pale

    Cool

    Clammy

    Cyanotic

    Mottling of extremities

Subnormal temperature

Excessive thirst

Nausea, vomiting

Renal status

    Urinary output below 30 ml/hr

    Elevated serum creatinine

    Elevated serum urea nitrogen

    Low urine sodium (less than 20 mEq/L)

Internal or external circulating blood volume loss because of the following:

    Hemorrhage

        Postsurgical

        After trauma

    Plasma volume losses

        Burns

        Excessive diarrhea, vomiting

Vasogenic Shock

Early stage

    Normal or slightly decreased BP

    Decreased or normal SVR

    Hemodynamics

        Decreased or normal PCWP

        Greatly increased CO, CI

        Warm skin

        Tachycardia: bounding pulse

Late stage

    Decreased BP

    Increased peripheral vascular resistance

    Decreased CO, CI

    Decreased PCWP

    Increased SVR, SVRI

    Metabolic acidosis

    Tachycardia

    Decreasing SVo_2

Excessive thirst
Nausea, vomiting
Tachypnea
Temperature
  Subnormal
  Elevated
Altered LOC
  Lethargy
  Semiconsciousness
  Coma
Skin
  Pale
  Cool
  Clammy
  Cyanotic
Renal status
  Urinary output below 30 ml/hr
  Elevated serum creatinine
  Elevated serum urea nitrogen
Wounds
  Swelling, redness
  Abnormal secretions
  Generalized urticaria, pruritus

Cardiogenic Shock

Decreased or falling BP; determined by patient's baseline
  pressure
Hypotension: systolic pressures <90 mm Hg
LV pressures
  Increased left ventricular end-diastolic pressure
    (LVEDP)
  Increased LAP
  Increased PCWP >18 mm Hg
  Decreased CI, CO < 2 L/min
  Decreasing stroke index (SI)
  Decreased ejection fraction (EF)
Increased SVR (>1600 dyne/sec/cm^{-5}), and SVR index
  (SVRI)
Elevated RV filling pressures
  Presence of jugular vein distension
  Increased CVP: above 15 cm H_2O pressure
  Positive hepatojugular reflex
Tachycardia
Thready radial pulse
Diminished or absent peripheral pulses
Presence of S_3, S_4 gallops or murmurs
Increased SVo_2
Respiratory distress
  Tachypnea
  Orthopnea
  Hypoxia
Alteration in LOC
  Apathy
  Lethargy
  Semiconsciousness
  Coma
Skin
  Pale
  Cool

Clammy
Cyanosis
Temperature
  Subnormal
  Elevated
Excessive thirst
Nausea, vomiting
Renal status
  Urinary output below 20 ml/hr
  Elevated serum creatinine
  Elevated serum urea nitrogen
ECG changes
  Ischemic changes
  Dysrhythmias
  Ventricular fibrillation
Pain
  Chest
  Abdominal

DIAGNOSTIC TESTS
Hypovolemic Shock

Electrolytes
Chemistries: rising BUN, creatinine
ABGs: elevated Pao_2, low HCO_3^-, low Pao_2
Specific gravity

Vasogenic Shock

Cultures
Blood
Sputum
Urine
WBC
ESR
Chest x-ray examination
Clotting profile

Cardiogenic Shock

Serum studies
  Chemistries: BUN, creatinine
  Electrolytes
  Drug levels
  Cardiac enzymes
ABGs
ECG
Chest x-ray examination
MUGA
Echocardiogram
Radionuclide ventriculography

POTENTIAL COMPLICATIONS
Hypovolemic Shock

Heart failure

Vasogenic Shock

Lactic acidosis
Adult respiratory distress syndrome (ARDS)
Disseminated intravascular coagulation (DIC)
Multisystem failure/Multiple organ dysfunction (MOD)
  Renal, GI, hepanic failure

Cardiogenic Shock

Metabolic acidosis
    Increased serum lactate levels
    Decreased pH
Electrolyte imbalances
Myocardial ischemia: elevated enzymes
Heart failure
Pulmonary edema
Adult respiratory distress syndrome
    Diminished breath sounds
    Pulmonary congestion

MULTIDISCIPLINARY MANAGEMENT
THERAPEUTIC MANAGEMENT

Admission to intensive care unit
Cardiac monitor
Hemodynamic monitoring
Assisted mechanical ventilation
Oxygen therapy
Medications
    Vasodilator, sodium nitroprusside
    Sympathomimetic: dopamine, dobutamine
    Osmotic diuretics
For vasogenic shock: epinephrine, antihistamine,
    hydrocortisone
Parenteral therapy
    Blood replacement
    Plasma volume expanders
    Fluid challenges
Mechanical circulatory support devices
    Ventricular assist devices (VAD)
    Intraaortic balloon pump (IABP)
    Extracorporeal membrane oxygen (ECMO)

PATIENT PROBLEMS—NURSING DIAGNOSES/INTERVENTIONS

▼Altered tissue perfusion (cerebral, cardiopulmonary, peripheral) related to decreased cardiac output

Assess for signs and symptoms of impaired tissue perfusion *to avoid rapid deterioration of vital functions associated with progressive shock*
Maintain complete bed rest; place patient in flat supine position; keep patient warm and position extremities *to minimize metabolic needs and facilitate circulation*
Maintain parenteral therapy as ordered: whole blood, plasmanate, volume expanders *to maintain adequate circulating volume*
Measure intake and output qh to evaluate kidney function and body volume
Connect indwelling urethral catheter to closed gravity drainage system; notify physician if urinary output is <30 ml/hr
Measure all body fluid loss; estimate loss in dressings or perineal pads
Administer medications as ordered
Assess for effects of drug therapy and signs of toxicity

Maintain NPO or only clear liquid diet as ordered
Check respirations, apical pulse, and femoral pulse q15min and prn *to assess for signs of vasoconstriction and tissue perfusion*
Monitor hemodynamic parameters hourly or more *frequently to assess clinical status and/or response to therapy:* PAP, PCWP, CO/CI
Monitor intraarterial pressure (IAP) q1h to 2h (NOTE: mean arterial pressure <60 mg Hg adversely affects cerebral and renal perfusion); check peripheral arm BP q15min if arterial line is not in place
Monitor SVo_2, *decreasing trend indicates decreased CO*
Apply pressure to wounds *to control bleeding if necessary*
    Pressure dressing
    Direct pressure
        Gastric tube with balloon
Apply shock trousers as ordered; patient may arrive in trousers
Prepare medications to control bleeding if ordered
    Vitamin K
    Protamine sulfate
Prepare for surgery
    Resuturing of the bleeding site
    Removal of ruptured organ or resection of bleeding site
    See General preoperative care/teaching (p. 10)
Avoid routine nursing functions during acute phase

Expected Outcomes

Tissue perfusion is maintained:
    Blood pressure is within normal limits; MAP 70 to 105 mm Hg
    CI 2.5-4 L/min/m^2
    Urine output is ≥30 ml/hr
    Skin warm and dry
    Patient alert and oriented
    Peripheral pulses more than 2T

▼Decreased cardiac output related to mechanical factors (preload, afterload, and myocardial contractility)

Maintain complete bed rest; position *to promote optimal ventilation;* elevate head of bed 30 to 60 degrees and avoid routine nursing functions *to promote energy, increase venous return, and avoid drop in BP*
Check BP, R, apical pulse, and femoral pulse q15min and prn
Monitor LAP, PAP, and PCWP q1h to 2h as ordered
Measure and calculate CO, CI q4hr *to evaluate cardiac function*
Monitor intraarterial pressure q2h as ordered
Calculate systemic vascular resistance *to determine left ventricular afterload; a rise in SVR index (SVRI) reflects increased afterload and myocardial oxygen consumption*

$$\frac{\text{Mean aortic pressure} - \text{Mean right atrial pressure (mm Hg)}}{\text{Cardiac output (L/min)}}$$

Initiate IV line: maintain an open vein

Monitor ECG continuously *to detect dysrhythmias that may result from depressed myocardial contractility*

Measure intake and output qh *to assess for signs of decreased CO or presence of hypovolemia*

Maintain parenteral fluids as ordered

Connect indwelling urethral catheter to closed gravity drainage system; notify physician if urinary output is <30 ml/hr

Check axillary temperature qh *to assess for elevations,* which can increase myocardial oxygen demand

Administer oxygen as ordered and prn

Administer medications as ordered

To decrease afterload and O_2 consumption
    Vasodilator
    Corticosteroid
    Adjust flow rate according to BP response

To increase myocardial contractility and reduce peripheral vascular resistance (PVR)
    Sympathomimetic
    Vasodilator
    ACE inhibitors
    Adjust flow rate according to BP response

Administer plasma volume expanders as ordered; adjust flow rate according to PAP and PCWP readings

Keep patient warm and dry

Auscultate heart sounds q2h to 4h

Prepare for insertion of mechanical circulatory support devices: IABP, VAD, ECMO; assess cardiac response

Restrict and plan activities; provide rest periods between procedures

Avoid constipation, straining, or rectal stimulation; give stool softeners or laxatives as ordered

Expected Outcomes
Demonstrates improved cardiac output as evidenced by the following:
    Vital signs within normal limits: MAP >60 mm Hg, systolic SBP > 90 mm Hg
    CI >2.2 L/min/m^2
    PAP and PCWP within normal limits
    SVR >600 or <1400 dynes/sec/cm^{-5}
    Improved mentation

▼ Impaired gas exchange related to increased pulmonary capillary permeability associated with LV dysfunction

Assess respiratory pattern, noting rate and depth of respirations, *to assess adequacy of blood oxygenation and determine need for intubation*

Auscultate lungs q1h to 2h *to assess for pulmonary congestion*

Monitor serial ABGs *to assess for decreased oxygen lung perfusion*

Monitor SVo$_2$; report SVo$_2$, <60% because *this reflects decreased tissue perfusion*

Monitor PAP/PCWP as rises may *indicate increased pulmonary congestion*

Administer oxygen as ordered *to ensure oxygen delivery and gas exchange*

Monitor O_2 saturation and maintain at ≥95%

Review serial CSR to *evaluate clinical status*

Suction as ordered *to ensure patent airway, clear airway, and improve oxygen delivery*

Assist and teach patient to cough and breathe deeply q1h to 2h

Expected Outcome
Demonstrates improved ventilation as evidenced by the following:
    Alert and oriented
    Effortless breathing; respiratory rate: 12 to 20/minutes
    Clear lungs
    Po$_2$ 80 to 100 mm Hg; Pco$_2$ 35 to 45 mm Hg
    O$_2$ sat ≥95%
    PCWP 4 to 12 mm Hg

▼ Anxiety/fear related to actual or potential biologic threat

Determine patient's source of fear and anxiety *to understand patient's perception of situation*

Explain all procedures and treatments; offer brief explanations *to minimize feelings of uncertainty*

Remain with patient *to offer reassurance*

Anticipate needs *to minimize expenditure of energy*

Maintain quiet, nonstressful environment

Allow family or significant other to remain with patient as condition permits

Encourage verbalization of needs and fears of dying

Maintain calm and reassuring manner

Expected Outcome
Verbalizes decrease in anxiety level

Additional Nursing Diagnoses to Consider
Altered nutrition: less than body requirements related to depleted glycogen stores

Risk for infection related to sepsis and impaired immune response

Risk for impaired skin integrity related to mechanical and internal factors

■ CARDIAC SURGERY (OPEN-HEART PROCEDURE)*
Care depends on whether the operation is an open-heart procedure, requiring use of the cardiopulmonary bypass machine, or a closed-heart procedure that does not require use of the bypass machine

---

The standard for postoperative care of the patient with open-heart surgery can be used in either cases of open-heart or closed-heart procedures. The patient with closed-heart surgery will usually require less specialized equipment with decreased frequency of nursing functions; however, such a patient may have complications that would also be seen with open-heart surgery (e.g., atelectasis and hypertension).

CLASSIFICATION OF CARDIAC SURGERY

CLOSED-HEART SURGERY
Coarctation of aorta
Palliative pulmonary shunts
    Blalock-Taussig
    Potts' anastomosis
    Glenn's
Closed mitral commissurotomy

OPEN-HEART SURGERY
CONGENITAL DEFECTS
Atrial septal defect (ASD)
Ventricular septal defect (VSD)
Transposition of great vessels
Tetralogy of Fallot
Truncus arteriosus
Tricuspid atresia
Aortic stenosis

ACQUIRED DEFECTS, DISORDERS
Coronary artery disease
Valvular heart disease
Aneurysm, ventricular, aortic

PROCEDURES
Coronary artery bypass graft (CABG)
Minimally invasive open heart procedures for CABG and
    congenital defects
Aneurysm, repair, resection
Valve repair: commissurotomy, reconstruction,
    annuloplasty
Valve replacement
Procedures for congenital heart defects
Cardiac transplantation

PREOPERATIVE CARE

ASSESSMENT
SUBJECTIVE DATA
Emotions
    Anxiety: adaptive versus maladaptive
    Euphoria
    Depression
    Denial
    Anger
    Fear

OBJECTIVE DATA
LOC
BP, T, P, and R
Skin
    Color
    Turgor
    Temperature
Peripheral circulation
Heart sounds
    Murmurs
    Rubs
    Gallops

Breath sounds: abnormal
    Decreased breath sounds
    Rales
    Wheezes
Smoking history
Weight and height
Activity tolerance
Medications being taken
    Cardiac medications
    Anticoagulants/antiplatelets
    Antidysrhythmics
    Birth control pills

DIAGNOSTIC TESTS
ECG: acute changes, increase in dysrhythmias
    12-Lead
    Rhythm strip
Chest x-ray examination
    Cardiomegaly
    Pulmonary vascular congestion
Echocardiogram (ejection fraction)
Laboratory studies:
    CBC, Hgb, Hct
    Blood type and cross match
    Coagulation studies: PT, INR, APTT, and platelets
    Electrolytes
    BUN
    Creatinine
    Urinalysis
    Pulmonary function
        Vital capacity
        Tidal volume
        Minute ventilation

PREOPERATIVE TEACHING
Assess level of understanding
Involve family or significant other in care and
    instructions
Reinforce physician's explanation regarding operative
    procedure
    Location, type, and length of incision(s)
    Length of time anticipated for recovery
Explain preoperative procedures
    Skin preparation: shaving, antiseptic bath or shower
    Visits from anesthesiologist and respiratory
        therapist
Check whether dental clearance was given (dental
    checks should be done 10 to 14 days before
    operation)
Explain and review postoperative procedures and
    routines of CCU or ICU
    How special unit will differ from regular unit
    Types of noises to be experienced
    Visiting privileges
    Usual length of stay in unit
    Pain to be experienced and availability of medications
        as needed
    Method of communication while intubated
    Disorientation that may occur resulting from
        medications and/or lack of sleep

Assess patient's awareness, emotional status, and fears regarding
  Surgical procedure
  Heart-lung machine
  Short- and long-term outcomes
  Possible disabilities
  Previous surgical experiences
Report any *acute* changes in emotional status
  Anxiety
  Depression
  Fear of dying
Instruct patient on simple relaxation techniques such as guided imagery
Introduce patient to unit staff who will be providing care postoperatively
When possible, introduce patient and family to CCU or ICU, explaining equipment to be used
  Cardiac monitor
  Hemodynamic monitor
  Drainage tubes
  Pacing wires, pacemaker
  Respirator
  Nebulizer
  Oxygen administration
  IV therapy
    Blood transfusions
    Replacement fluids
Review postoperative medications, particularly those that will be long term, such as anticoagulants
Review procedures for and stress importance and purpose of the following:
  Turning
  Coughing
  Deep breathing
  Incentive spirometry
  Foot and leg exercises, use of support stocking
Instruct patient to practice these procedures 1 to 2 days before operation
Withhold medications as ordered (e.g., anticoagulants)
Refer to spiritual advisor or social service worker as indicated

▌ POSTOPERATIVE CARE

ASSESSMENT
OBSERVATIONS/FINDINGS
General
Neurologic: LOC
Pulmonary system
  Respirations
    Quality
    Rate
    Character
  Secretions
  Breath sounds: equal or decreased
    Dullness
    Crackles
    Rhonchi
  Chest drainage
    Amount

Quality
Color
Cardiovascular system
  Hemodynamic parameters
    Arterial BP
    HR, rhythms
    SVo_2 LAP, LVEDP, PCWP
    CVP
  Heart sounds
    S_1, S_2
    Rubs
    Murmurs
  Arterial pulses
    Quality
    Rate
    Rhythm
    Equality
Skin
  Color
  Turgor
  Temperature
ECG: check for presence of acute changes or dysrhythmias
Pacemaker: settings
Renal system
  Intake and output
  Urine output
    Amount
    Color
    Specific gravity
    Osmolality
  Electrolytes
  BUN, creatinine
Gastrointestinal system
  Nasogastric tube drainage
    Amount
    Color
  Absence or presence of bowel sounds
  Abdominal tone
    Flat
    Distended
    Tenderness
  Incision(s), location
    Midsternotomy
    Submammary
    Leg

Valve Replacement
Type of valve replaced
  Heterograft
  Mechanical
  Homograft
Valve sounds: normal
    Mechanical: opening, closing clicks
    Heterograft, homograft: produces no clicks
Valve dysfunction: occurrence of new regurgitant-type murmur
    Obstruction
    Perivalvular leak
    Rupture

Coronary Artery Graft

Graft site
  Saphenous vein
  Mammary artery

Congenital Heart Disease Repair

Type of repair: palliative, corrective
Use of conduits, grafts, baffles

DIAGNOSTIC TESTS

CBC, chemistries, electrolytes, platelet function, PT, INR, APTT
ABGs
Chest x-ray examination

POTENTIAL COMPLICATIONS
General

Cardiovascular system
  Dysrhythmias
    Premature ventricular contractions (PVCs)
    Ventricular tachycardia
    Atrial fibrillation
    Atrial flutter
    Asystole
    Complete heart block
  Fluid volume excess
    Dyspnea, orthopnea
    Increased JVD
    Lung sounds: crackles
    Heart sounds: S_3, S_4
    Elevated PAP, LAP, and PCWP
  Low CO syndrome
    Restlessness, lethargy
    Skin: cool, pale, peripheral cyanosis
  Tachycardia
  Decreased arterial pressure
  Decreased urine output
  Increased PCWP and LAP
  Increased SVR
  Hemorrhage
    Increased drainage through chest tubes
    Presence of bright red drainage
    Adults: blood loss >150 ml/hr
    Children: blood loss >5 ml/kg/hr
    Decreased Hct
    Hypotension
  Pericarditis
  Cardiac tamponade
  Shock
    Cardiogenic
    Hypovolemic
  Heart failure
  Postpericardiotomy syndrome
  Venous thrombosis
Pulmonary system
  Atelectasis
  Pleural effusion
  Diaphragmatic dysfunction
  Tension pneumothorax
  Respiratory failure

Neurologic system
  Altered LOC
    Postpump psychosis
      Restlessness
      Agitation
      Confusion
      Combativeness
      Visual and auditory disturbances
      Transient perceptual disorientation
  Cerebral embolism; CVA (p. 529)
Renal system
  Electrolyte imbalance
    Hyponatremia
    Hypokalemia
  Metabolic
    Acidosis
    Alkalosis
  Acute tubular necrosis (ATN)
Gastrointestinal system
  Stress ulcers
  Paralytic ileus
  Infection
    Sternal wound
    Leg wound

Valve Replacement

Disintegration of prosthesis
Vegetations from resected valve
Endocarditis

Mitral Valve Replacement

Brain embolism
Supraventricular tachydysrhythmias
  Atrial tachycardia
  Rapid atrial fibrillation
Low CO syndrome

Tricuspid Valve Replacement/Aortic Valve Replacement

Conduction defects
Subendocardial necrosis

Coronary Artery Bypass Graft

Acute myocardial infarction
Ventricular dysrhythmias
  PVCs
  Ventricular tachycardia
Low CO syndrome
Graft failure
  Angina
  Atrial fibrillation

Congenital Heart Disease Repair

Conduction defects
Atrial dysrhythmias
Conduit obstruction
Patch leaks

MULTIDISCIPLINARY MANAGEMENT
THERAPEUTIC MANAGEMENT
Admission to cardiac intensive care unit
Oxygen therapy with mechanically assisted ventilation
Cardiac monitor
Hemodynamic monitoring
SVo_2 monitoring
Medications
    Narcotics, analgesics
    Antihypertensives
    Antidysrhythmics
    Inotropic agents
        Dopamine
        Dobutamine
        Digoxin
    Vasodilators
    Anticoagulants
    Electrolytes
Parenteral therapy
    Blood replacement
    Plasma expanders
    Colloids
Pacemaker insertion
Intraaortic balloon pump (IABP)
Ventricular assist devices (VAD)

PATIENT PROBLEMS—NURSING DIAGNOSES/INTERVENTIONS (ADULTS)

▼ Impaired gas exchange related to hypoventilation and/or ventilation/perfusion abnormalities

Assess and monitor respiratory function while patient is on ventilator *to detect abnormal ventilation*/perfusion resulting from effects of anesthesia, hypoxia, acid-base abnormalities
Maintain patent airway
Administer oxygen and assisted ventilation as ordered
Elevate head of bed 45 degrees *to promote oxygenation*
Assess quality and rate of respiration
Monitor FIo_2 tidal volume to yield arterial Po_2 of about 100 mm Hg
Obtain and monitor ABGs as ordered; observe for and report signs of respiratory alkalosis or acidosis
Monitor SVo_2 as indicated
Auscultate lung sounds q1h to 2h *to assess resolving atelectasis and pulmonary congestion*
Suction q1h to 2h; hyperoxygenate 1 to 2 minutes before procedures; monitor and record any dysrhythmias
Assist and teach patient to turn; percuss chest and reposition q2h *to promote removal of secretions*
Encourage patient to turn, cough, and breathe deeply q1h to 2h in absence of endotracheal tube *to loosen secretions*
Have patient use high-humidity face mask after extubation *to avoid hypoxemia*
Obtain serial chest x-rays q4h to 6h as ordered *to detect signs of progressive pulmonary complications*

Expected Outcomes
Demonstrates adequate ventilation as evidenced by the following:
    Effortless breathing
    Absence of respiratory complications
    Clear, equal, and bilateral breath sounds
    Po_2 and Pco_2 within normal limits

▼ Decreased cardiac output related to mechanical factors (altered preload, afterload, contractility, heart rate) or electrical instability

Assess and monitor for signs of decreased CO *to detect early trends and changes*
Assess BP, apical pulse, and peripheral pulses q15min to 30min for 2 hours, then qh as ordered, reporting
    Systolic BP: drop of 20 mm Hg
    Systolic BP <85 or >160 mm Hg
    Diastolic BP >100 mm Hg
    Decreased amplitude in pulses
    Pulse rate <60 or >100 beats/min
Monitor PAP, arterial pressure, and SVo_2 q15min during immediate postoperative period, decreasing frequency as clinical status stabilizes
Calculate CO and SVR as ordered
Check temperature on admission once 2 hours × 24 hours, then q4h
Initiate rewarming procedures slowly; monitor for signs of shivering, which can *increase metabolic demand*
    Blankets
    Heat lamp
Auscultate heart sounds q2h to 4h
Monitor urine output qh; report outputs <30 ml/hr
Administer fluids, blood products *to maintain adequate tissue perfusion*
Perform laboratory studies q4h to 6h as ordered
    Cardiac enzymes, CPK-MB, SGOT, LDH *to detect ischemic changes*
    Electrolytes; potassium levels, magnesium q6h × 24 hours
    Hgb, Hct
Initiate IABP or VAD as ordered *to increase myocardial perfusion*
Avoid Valsalva's maneuver, such as caused by constipation
    Bedside commode
    Stool softeners
    Mild laxative
Monitor and record dysrhythmias *to avoid hemodynamic compromise*
    Record ECG rhythm strips q shift unless changes noted; measure rate plus P-R, QRS, and Q-T intervals
    Initiate temporary pacemaker *to maintain adequate CI;* check rate and milliamperes (MA)
    Administer antidysrhythmic agents as ordered
    Administer medications to increase myocardial contractility, decrease SVR, control dysrhythmias

Expected Outcomes

Demonstrates improved cardiac output as evidenced by the following:

Vital signs within normal limits

CO, LVEDP, and PCWP within acceptable limits

Increased activity tolerance

▼Risk for hemorrhage related to surgically induced fibrinolysis and/or inadequate reversal of heparin

Assess and monitor for clinical signs of excessive bleeding that may occur as result of the effects of heparin given intraoperatively (heparin rebound); platelet function is decreased

Perform blood studies q4h to 6h as ordered

Hgb, Hct

Coagulation: PT, INR, PTT, platelet count

Measure chest drainage qh; report drainage >150 to 200 ml/hr

Administer transfusions, platelets, and plasma expanders as ordered *to control bleeding and/or clotting disorders*

Administer drugs to correct coagulopathy

Protamine sulfate

6-Aminocaproic acid (Amicar)

Epsilon aminocaproic acid (EACA)

Vitamin K

Check dressings q1h to 2h

Note drainage: amount, color, and consistency

Change as indicated

Expected Outcomes

Demonstrates stable hemostasis as evidenced by the following:

Progressive decrease in chest tube drainage

Stable or improved Hct, Hgb

Normal bleeding times: PT, INR, PTT, platelet count

▼Ineffective breathing pattern related to decreased lung expansion

Assess rate and quality of respiration *to detect signs of decreased lung expansion or splinting*

Observe and maintain patency of chest tubes *to ensure proper drainage;* record drainage amount and color q1h to 2h and prn

Auscultate chest for diminished breath sounds q1h to 2h and later q4h to 6h *to detect and monitor signs of atelectasis*

Encourage patient to cough and breathe deeply q1h to 2h *to mobilize secretions*

Assist and encourage patient to use incentive spirometer q1h while awake

Administer oxygen therapy as ordered

Expected Outcomes

Demonstrates fully expanded lung

Bilateral equal excursion

Full and clear breath sounds

▼Risk for infection related to compromised host defense and environmental exposure

Monitor suture sites for local redness, drainage, and swelling *to detect developing infectious process*

Assess rectal, oral, or axillary temperature q2h as indicated *to detect infectious or inflammatory process*

Change incisional dressings daily

Administer antibiotics as ordered

Change IV and pressure lines and dressings according to protocol *to prevent nosocomial infections and cross contamination*

Remove urethral catheter when patient awakens or as soon as possible *to prevent urinary tract infection*

Obtain laboratory studies as indicated

CBC with differential

Blood and urine cultures

Expected Outcomes

Shows no signs of infection

Afebrile

Wounds: no signs of irritation or redness

▼Altered thought process related to biophysical changes (cerebral hypoxia, age, metabolic alterations, CNS depressants, sleep deprivation)

Assess LOC and neurologic signs q15min to 30min for 2 hours, then qh or as indicated

Deal with any personality or psychologic changes

Use reality orientation

Offer explanations of all procedures

Administer sedatives as ordered

Reorient patient to time of day and surroundings

Use simple, clear sentence structure

Anticipate needs

Maintain quiet environment; minimize external stimuli as much as possible

Remain with patient

Allow family to visit and participate in care when possible

Provide assurance of daily progress

Maintain patient safety; use soft restraints

Expected Outcomes

Regains baseline LOC

Arouses easily

Clear mentation

Oriented to time, place, situation

Additional Nursing Diagnoses to Consider

Fluid volume excess related to expanded extracellular fluid volume

Ineffective family and individual coping: family, individual related to situational disorganization

PATIENT/FAMILY TEACHING

Assess level of understanding

Review nature and type of operative procedure, emphasizing precautions and complications associated with surgery

Explain importance of wearing medical alert band if
  patient has (is taking)
  Prosthetic valve
  Pacemaker (p. 148)
  Anticoagulants (p. 157)
Explain need to avoid persons with infections, especially
  URIs
Discuss symptoms of wound infection to report to
  physician
  Chest discomfort
  Elevated temperature
  Rapid, irregular pulse
  Chills
  Anorexia
  Redness
  Pain
  Swelling
  Drainage
Explain care of incision
Discuss importance of ongoing care
Discuss importance of contacting spiritual advisor or
  social worker as necessary
Discuss medications: name, dosage, time of
  administration, purpose, and side effects
Explain need to avoid taking over-the-counter
  medications without physician approval
Discuss diet as ordered
  Refer to dietitian for specific diets
  Restrict salt intake
Discuss symptoms to report to physician
  SOB
  Swelling of hands and legs

DISCHARGE/HOME CARE PLANNING
Discuss activity limitations and allowances
  Ambulate to tolerance; avoid excessive physical
    exertion, lifting heavy objects or performing
    isometric exercises; restrict driving first 4 to 6
    weeks
  Instruct patient to increase activity gradually to avoid
    fatigue
  Avoid fatigue and sitting for long periods
  Explain that sexual activity may be contraindicated for
    2 to 4 weeks; need to check with physician for
    ability to resume
  Review ADLs
    Showers permitted, but no baths
    No driving for 6 weeks

VALVE REPLACEMENT
Provide instruction regarding anticoagulation therapy
  Mechanical valves: life-long therapy
  Heterografts: 3 to 6 months as ordered
Explain importance of reporting to physician signs and
  symptoms of endocarditis
  Elevated temperature
  Chills, diaphoresis
  Anorexia
Discuss importance of reporting to physician any event
  that may predispose to bacteremia

Dental and gum manipulation
Genitourinary procedures
Gynecologic procedures (D & C)
Childbirth
Skin boils, infective acne
Discuss importance of notifying all physicians, dentists,
  urologists, and obstetricians of valve replacement
  before any treatments
Encourage wearing medical alert bracelet or neck chain
Discuss need to maintain good oral hygiene
  Daily care
  Regular visits to dentist
  NOTE: Patient should wait 6 weeks after surgery before
    seeing a dentist
Explain significance of prophylactic antibiotic therapy
  before procedures that predispose to bacteremia

■ CARDIAC TRANSPLANTATION

ASSESSMENT
OBSERVATIONS/FINDINGS
Rejection
  Mild to moderate: usually no clinical symptoms
  Severe: weakness, fatigue, malaise, anorexia, nausea and
    vomiting, decreased urine output, weight gain,
    peripheral edema, distended neck veins, increased
    jugular pulsations, decreased perfusion, cool and
    pale skin, diminished pulses, diaphoresis, confusion,
    restlessness, pulmonary venous congestion, DOE,
    cough, tachycardia, dysrhythmias
  S_3, S_4
  Shock state
  Cardiac arrest

POTENTIAL COMPLICATIONS
Infection: cytomegalovirus (CMV)
Lymphoma
Obstructive coronary atheroscleroses

DIAGNOSTIC TESTS
ECG: atrial dysrhythmia (e.g., PAC, atrial fibrillation)
NOTE: With cyclosporine, these ECG changes may not be
  seen
Chest x-ray examination: increased C-T ratio (cardiomegaly)
Echocardiogram: thickening of LV, decreased LV function,
  contractility
Endomyocardial biopsy (EMB)
  Lymphocytes (findings vary with degree of rejection)
  Mild, occasional WBCs
  Moderate: myocyte necrosis
  Severe: perivascular infiltration of lymphocytes,
    interstitial edema, myocyte, necrosis
  Increased CPK-MB, SGOT, LDH

MULTIDISCIPLINARY MANAGEMENT
THERAPEUTIC MANAGEMENT
NOTE: Postoperative care is similar to that for any patient
  who has had cardiac surgery (p. 199)
Strict reverse isolation

EMB: once a week for 1 month, progressing to twice a week for 2 months

Diet: low saturated fat and cholesterol, sodium restriction (2 g)

Medications
　Cyclosporine (Sandimmune)
　Azathioprine (Imuran)
　Antithymocyte globulin (ATG)
　Orthoclone (OKT$_3$, Ortho)
　Corticosteroids
　　Prednisone
　　Methylprednisone (Medrol, Depo-Medrol, Solu-Medrol)
　Antihistamines
　Acetaminophen

PATIENT PROBLEMS—NURSING DIAGNOSES/INTERVENTIONS

▼Risk for injury (rejection) related to noncompliance with prescribed medical regimen

Assess and evaluate patient for understanding of prescribed lifelong therapy *to identify potential adherence problems*

Encourage discussion regarding anticipated changes in lifestyle that may have a positive or negative effect

Ensure that patient is aware that skipping cyclosporine will result in rejection

Review prescribed medical treatment and drug therapy

Anticipate and allow questions regarding prescribed therapy

Expected Outcomes
Demonstrates no signs of rejection
No new change(s) in EMB results
No clinical signs of rejection

▼Risk for infection related to immunosuppressive drug therapies

Assess and monitor for signs of infection *to begin medical therapy*
　Take temperature q4h
　Obtain cultures as indicated: sputum, throat, urine, any suspicious drainage in wounds
　Obtain and evaluate CBC; chest x-ray examination as indicated (NOTE: Laboratory values may be altered if steroids are taken)

Minimize or avoid use of invasive lines and/or procedures *to decrease risk of nosocomial or bacterial infections:* IVs, indwelling catheters

Change IV tubing, bags, and dressings every day using strict aseptic techniques

Do not place patient in room with another patient who is at risk for infection *to avoid potential cross contamination*

Institute reverse isolation for staff and visitors according to institutional protocol *to decrease potential new infections*

Minimize number of visitors; restrict visitors with signs of infections (e.g., colds, herpes simplex)

Expected Outcomes
Demonstrates no signs of infection
Baseline temperature maintained
CBC, urinalysis, cultures within normal limits

Additional Nursing Diagnosis To Consider
Risk for decreased cardiac output related to severe rejection

PATIENT/FAMILY TEACHING
Discuss and review signs and symptoms of rejection

Emphasize importance of keeping scheduled EMB appointments

Discuss lifelong need to take medications and need to take them exactly as prescribed; caution patient *never to stop* taking cyclosporine and to notify physician if dose is skipped

Review signs and symptoms of infection: elevation of baseline temperature, early signs of sore throat, cold, influenza

Discuss need to reduce risks of infection by avoiding individuals with infections or contagious diseases, avoiding large crowds

Discuss importance of lifelong follow-up: clinic visits, EMB appointments, and periodic stress test

Discuss activity allowances and limitations; instruct patient to check with physician before engaging in strenuous or competitive activities or sports

Discuss importance of daily weighing and reporting >2 lb weight gain in 24 hours

■ POSTCARDIAC INJURY SYNDROME
A group of signs and symptoms that occur after injury to the myocardium or pericardial cavity, which are thought to be a result of an immune response or hypersensitivity reaction to pericardial injury

　　postcardiotomy syndrome: After cardiac surgery (usually 7 to 10 days after surgery)

　　postmyocardial infarction syndrome (Dressler's syndrome): A late-appearing autoimmune response to myocardial necrosis; symptoms usually appear 3 to 6 weeks after MI

ASSESSMENT
SUBJECTIVE DATA
Chest pain or discomfort
Dyspnea
Anxiety

OBJECTIVE DATA
Elevated temperature
Diaphoresis
Pericardial friction rub
Malaise
Arthralgias

DIAGNOSTIC TESTS
Leukocytosis
Increased ESR
Chest x-ray examination: pleural effusions
Echocardiogram: pericardial effusion
ECG: Increased T wave

POTENTIAL COMPLICATIONS
Pericarditis
Cardiac tamponade

MULTIDISCIPLINARY MANAGEMENT
THERAPEUTIC MANAGEMENT
Medications
    Analgesics
    Antipyretics
    Antiinflammatory agents

PATIENT PROBLEMS—NURSING DIAGNOSES/INTERVENTIONS

▼Chest pain related to pericardial irritation

Assess quality of chest pain
Encourage bed rest; position patient for comfort
    Elevate head of bed 45 degrees
    Provide padded overbed table
Auscultate heart sounds q6h to 8h *to detect pericardial rub*
Administer medications as ordered
    Analgesics
    Antiinflammatory agents
    Antipyretics

Expected Outcomes
Verbalizes absence of chest pain
Activity level returns to normal

Additional Nursing Diagnosis to Consider
Anxiety related to perceived threat to health status

PATIENT/FAMILY TEACHING
Explain that syndrome commonly occurs after trauma or injury to heart and pericardial cavity and may clear up without specific treatment
Discuss symptoms to report to physician
    Elevated temperature
    Chest pain
    Chills, diaphoresis
    Difficult respirations
Explain need to avoid fatigue, alternate periods of activity with rest
Discuss name of medication, dosage, times of administration, purpose, and side effects

■ CARDIAC REHABILITATION
Comprehensive, long-term programs that include medical evaluation, prescribed exercise, cardiac risk factor modification, education, and counseling; designed to limit physiologic and psychologic effects of cardiac diseases and disorders

    indications: *MI, postcardiac bypass surgery, chronic stable angina*

    phases: *(1) Inpatient (2) supervised ambulatory outpatient program (3 to 6 months), (3) lifetime maintenance stage**

■ INPATIENT PROGRAM

ASSESSMENT
OBSERVATIONS/FINDINGS
Criteria for Terminating Exercise
Symptoms during activity and/or 30 minutes after activity or exercise session
    Severe dyspnea
    Chest pain
    Vertigo
    Diaphoresis
    Fatigue
    Leg claudication
    Disorientation or confusion
    Palpitations
Heart rate
    Increase >20 to 25 beats/min during activity or exercise
    Appearance of irregular rhythm
On telemetry: during exercise and rest periods
    ST elevation of 3 mm or more
    ST segment depression of 2 mm
    Multiple premature ventricular contractions (PVCs)

Activity Progression Program
Follow physician's orders for progressive activity program
Initiate program using a predeveloped in-hospital exercise program (Table 3-9)
Assess patient's progress on a daily basis and plan activity levels for the day (done by rehabilitation team and/or charge nurse and physician)
Increase activity levels gradually until discharge date
Avoid exercises
    After meals; allow 1 hour
    In the presence of dysrhythmias
    In the presence of CHF
Begin exercise program while patient is on telemetry
Record and report any signs or symptoms of SOB, fatigue, or nausea if they occur during or up to 24 hours after exercise
Obtain the following baseline information before activity
    On telemetry
        ECG rhythm strip, noting rate and rhythm
        Resting BP, P, and R, noting rate, rhythm, and quality
        Atrioventricular (AV) block
        Paroxysmal atrial tachycardia

---

*Definition from: Cardiac Rehabilitation: Clinical Practice Guideline *CHCPR, USDHHS, 1995.*

Table 3-9	**Cardiac Rehabilitation Program: Inpatient Activity (Myocardial Infarction)***				
Level	**Self-Care Activities**	**Position**	**Exercises**	**Repetitions**	**Education**
Level I (1 to 1.5 MET†)	1. Absolute bed rest, complete bed bath 2. Begin feeding self while sitting with head of bed elevated to 45 degrees and arms supported 3. Turn self	1. Supine *Advance to:* Supine 2. Supine	a. Passive ROM: all extremities (excluding shoulders in acute MI) b. Active exercises: all extremities except shoulders as tolerated Deep breathing exercises: all levels	5 times 3 times	
Level II (1.5 to 2.5 MET [except bedside commode])	4. Bed rest 5. Feed self, wash face and hands, brush teeth, and shave in bed 6. Bedside commode (3 MET) 7. Up in chair 20-30 min bid 8. Light recreational activity such as reading, writing	3. Supine	Active plantar and dorsiflexion ankle exercises qid		
Level III (1.5 to 3 MET)	9. In bed, patient assists with self-bath (not legs or back) 10. Patient stands and vital signs are taken 11. May walk to bathroom with help 12. Walk to chair and sit 15-30 min tid	4. Supine Sitting *Advance to:* 5. Supine Sitting Sitting	a. Advance active exercises to include neck rotation and shoulder flexion to 90 degrees as tolerated b. Active exercises: all limbs including shoulder flexion to 180 degrees c. Knee extension and hip flexion a. Active exercises: all extremities b. Knee extension and hip flexion c. Shoulder flexion to 90 degrees	5 times 5 times 3 times 7 times 7 times 7 times	Begin education a. Energy conservation b. Body mechanics c. Concepts of heart anatomy and physiology
Level IV (3 MET)	13. Same as 9 14. Begin dressing self (gown and pajamas) 15. If vital signs stable, see 10; walk to bathroom for toilet use only 16. Sit in chair 2 to 3 times a day 30-60 min with assistance	6. Supine Sitting 7. Supine	a. Exercise 5a b. Exercise 5b Instruct patient to perform independent exercise 3 times a day (patient to take own pulse)	7 times 7 times 5 times	d. Begin instruction in self heart rate measurement e. Discuss inpatient activity: importance of pacing, rest, relaxation f. Dietary assessment and referral if appropriate g. Begin discussion of: Signs and symptoms Risk factors

Modified from Guidelines for cardiac rehabilitation centers, *June 1985, copyright the American Heart Association Greater Los Angeles Affiliate.*
Recommended levels and times are for average patients and must be individualized.
†*MET: metabolic equivalent: the amount of oxygen consumed per kilogram of body weight per minute at rest. Approximately 3.5 cc kg/min.*

Table 3-9	**Cardiac Rehabilitation Program: Inpatient Activity (Myocardial Infarction)*—cont'd**				
Level	Self-Care Activities	Position	Exercises	Repetitions	Education
					Medication Warning signs Sexual counseling Activity progress
Level V	17. Sponge bathe self, sitting in bathroom (nurse bathes back) 18. Up in room and chair ad lib 19. Ambulate in hall 5-10 min with telemetry bid		Active exercises 5a, b, c; walk slow pace one half length of corridor (50 feet) with telemetry		
Level VI (3 to 4 MET)	20. Sit-down shower 21. Wash hair while seated 22. Shave, apply makeup in sitting position 23. Sit for meals 24. Full bathroom privileges 25. Up and about in room 26. Ambulate in hall 5-10 min bid with telemetry	8. Supine 9. Sitting 10. Walk 11. Ascend 12.	Active exercise 5a Active exercise 5b Increase distance walked, as tolerated, using moderate pace Three to six stair steps as tolerated May transport to cardiac rehabilitation center for low-level activity or test	5 to 7 times 7 times	Complete home instruction a. Diet b. Medications c. Activity allowances and limitations
Level VII (4 to 5 MET)	27. Same as level VI with addition of walking in hall 150 feet, advancing as tolerated 28. Evaluate any special requirements for home activities	13.	Continue stairs and ambulation as tolerated		
Level VIII	29. Same as levels VI and VII, advancing in frequency, distance, and time	14.	Establish progressive home activity program		

BP
  Drop of 15 to 20 mm Hg when patient stands
  Decrease in pulse pressure
  Increase in systolic-diastolic pressures:
    >20 mm Hg

MULTIDISCIPLINARY MANAGEMENT
THERAPEUTIC MANAGEMENT
Counseling referrals: nutrition, education, behavioral, and smoking cessation
Cardiac rehabilitation program
  Supervised structured group-based program
  Home-based exercise program with/without transtelephonic ECG monitoring
Prescription for inclusion to programs
Prescription for exercise program

PATIENT PROBLEMS—NURSING DIAGNOSES/INTERVENTIONS
MI
Maintain bed rest for initial 12 to 24 hours with use of bedside commode in hemodynamically stable patients

Progress to chair rest
Avoid prolonged bed rest
CABG
  Maintain bed rest for first 1 to 2 days postoperatively or as ordered by physician
  Start activity levels within 24 hours or as ordered by physician
  Off telemetry obtain resting BP, P, and R, noting rate, rhythm, and quality
Assist patient with performing activity
Obtain peak exercise heart rate
Obtain the following information during and 2 minutes after exercise
  On telemetry
    ECG rhythm strip toward end of activity, noting rate, rhythm, and ST segment changes or dysrhythmias
    Postexercise heart rate
  Off telemetry
    BP and HR at 1- and 2-minute intervals at end of exercise and at any signs of fatigue, pain, or SOB
Observe and report patient's tolerance

PATIENT/FAMILY TEACHING

Discuss and review the normal function of the heart, nature and causes of coronary heart disease

Discuss and stress the importance of identifying risk factors and need to modify or eliminate personal risk factors

Family history of heart disease

Patient history of heart disease

Diabetes

High BP

Overweight

High cholesterol and/or triglyceride levels

Smoking

Sedentary job and/or lifestyle

Stressful lifestyle

Dietary restrictions and limitations

Salt: limit to 2 to 3 g/d unless otherwise ordered

Lipids, cholesterol

Importance of controlling weight; provide target levels

Importance of verbalizing any questions and feelings regarding presence of heart disease

Importance of verbalizing any feelings of anxiety and fear regarding sexual impotency, return to work, and death

Review prescribed home exercise program; provide with names and number of referrals

Warning signs and symptoms of overexercising to report to physician

Excessive fatigue

Chest discomfort

Muscle pain

Dizziness

SOB

Palpitations

Discuss need to avoid isometric (static) activities and/or exercises (e.g., pushing heavy objects, doing pushups, or carrying heavy objects)

Importance of taking and recording HR before and after exercise, noting rate and rhythm

Importance of reporting heart rate increase >20 to 25 beats/min

Recommended limitations and allowances for first 2 weeks after discharge

Avoid heavy lifting and pushing

Refrain from extensive housework and gardening

Avoid sitting in same position for longer than 2 hours

Plan regular rest periods for at least twice a day

Avoid vigorous arm and shoulder exercises, especially those that require arms to be held above shoulders (e.g., washing windows or painting house)

Space activities, alternating activity with rest period

Avoid exercising at the following times

After meals; wait 1 hour

When feeling very tired

When suffering from a cold or other illness

Stop activity at onset of warning signs and rest

Importance of avoiding sexual activity for at least 2 weeks (check with physician when feasible to resume; once resumed, avoid after eating heavy meals, drinking alcoholic beverages in excess, or becoming emotionally stressed)

Need to avoid travel by car, bus, airplane, or train without first checking with physician

All walking and exercise activities must be preceded by warm-up exercises

INITIAL POSTDISCHARGE ACTIVITIES FOR CARDIOVASCULAR RECONDITIONING

Continue predischarge activities; actively exercise all extremities including shoulder flexion and knee extension

Distance walking

Week After Discharge	Total Distance (Mile)	Time (min)
1	0.25	8 to 10
2	0.25	5
3	0.5	15
4	1.0	30

Adjust speed and time to maintain HR at <100 beats/min

Record all exercise sessions, noting distance, time, and resting and peak heart rates (see chart below)

Exercise Record: Target Heart Rate: _____ beats/min

Date	Resting Heart Rate	Distance	Time	Peak Heart Rate	Comment
1-3-00	80	¼ mile	5 min	100	No complaints

Follow all exercise sessions with a cooling down period

CARDIOVASCULAR RECONDITIONING PROGRAM

Ordered approximately 6 to 8 weeks after discharge (done by physician)

Follow prescription for exercise determined by treadmill stress test before start of program

ELECTROCARDIOGRAM RHYTHMS

■ RHYTHMS OF SINUS ORIGIN

Rhythms originating in the sinus (sinoatrial [SA]) node (located in the right atrium near the opening of the superior vena cava, the sinus node functions as the normal pacemaker of the heart)

ASSESSMENT
SUBJECTIVE DATA
Palpitations
Dizziness
Lightheadedness
Chest pain
Syncope

OBJECTIVE DATA
Skin
   Pallor
   Diaphoresis
Heart rate
   Normal with ectopy
   Tachycardia
   Bradycardia
Heart rhythm
   Normal or irregular
Hypotension

DIAGNOSTIC TESTS
12-Lead ECG
24-Hour ambulatory ECG
Electrophysiologic (EP) studies
Signal average ECG

■ NORMAL SINUS RHYTHM (Figs. 3-13 to 3-15; Table 3-10)

ASSESSMENT
OBSERVATIONS/FINDINGS
Rhythm: regular
Rate: 60 to 100 beats/min

P wave: normal configuration, one before each QRS
P-R interval: 0.12 to 0.20 second
QRS complex: 0.06 to 0.10 second

MULTIDISCIPLINARY MANAGEMENT
None indicated

■ SINUS BRADYCARDIA (Fig. 3-16)

A sinus rhythm <60 beats/min; etiology—may be normal or occur in response to drugs or increased vagal tone

ASSESSMENT
OBSERVATIONS/FINDINGS
Faintness
Dizziness
Syncope
Rhythm: regular
Rate: below 60 beats/min
P wave: normal configuration, one before each QRS
P-R interval: 0.12 to 0.20 second
QRS complex: 0.06 to 0.10 second

MULTIDISCIPLINARY MANAGEMENT
None indicated unless patient is symptomatic
Medications
   Atropine
   Isoproterenol—use cautiously
Pacing: external, temporary, transvenous, permanent

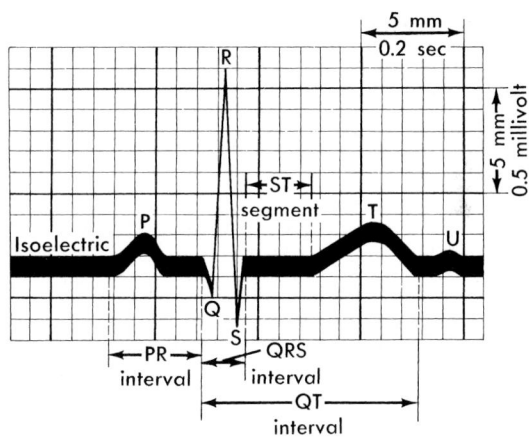

Fig. 3-13   Normal electrocardiogram complex.

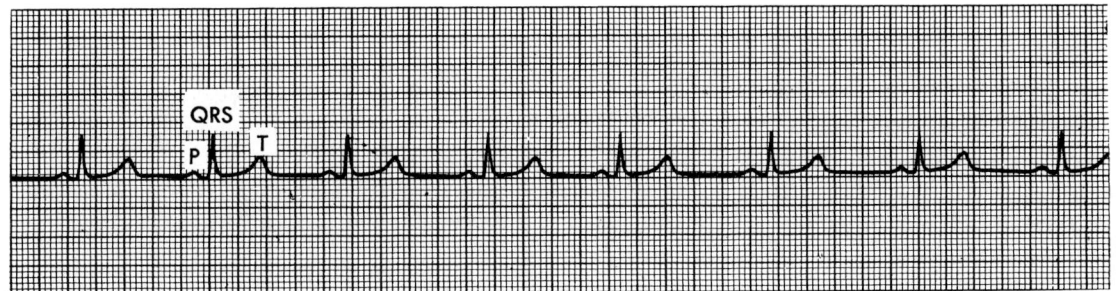

Fig. 3-14   Cardiac cycle. Basic cardiac cycle (P 5 QRS 5 T).
(From Goldberger AL: Clinical electrocardiography: a simplified approach, *ed 6, St Louis, 1999, Mosby.)*

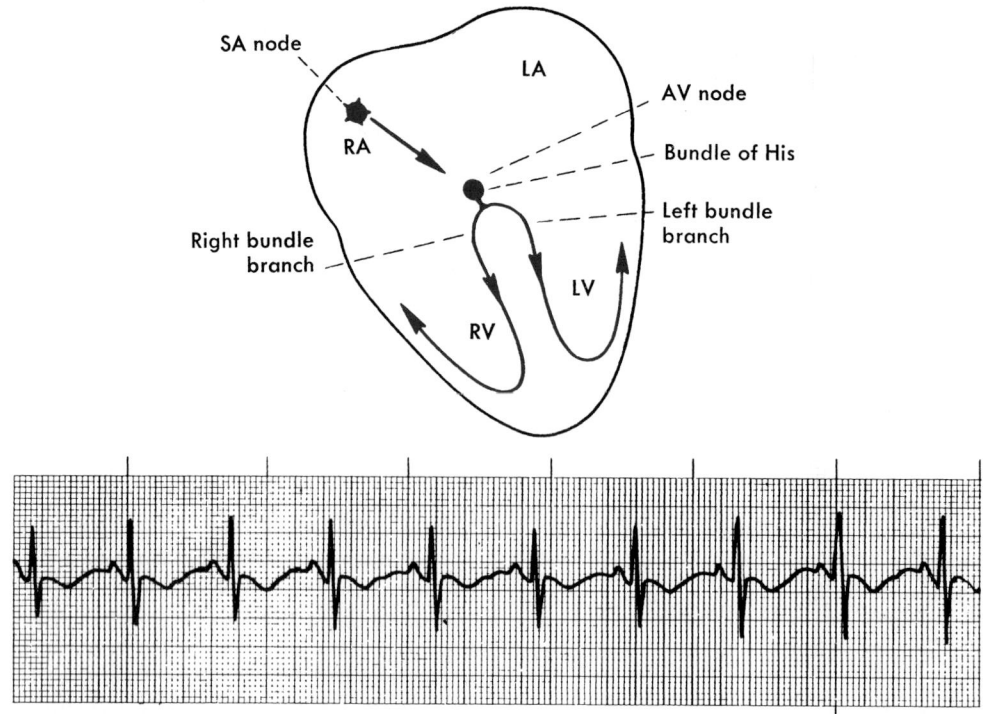

Fig. 3-15 Normal sinus rhythm.
(From Kinney M, Packa DR: Andreoli's comprehensive cardiac care, *ed 8, St Louis, 1996, Mosby.)*

Table 3-10	**Meaning and Significance of ECG Intervals***		
Description		**Duration (seconds)**	**Significance of Disturbance**
P-R interval: from beginning of P wave to beginning of QRS complex; represents time taken for impulse to spread through the atria, AV node, His bundle, bundle branches, and Purkinje fibers, to a point immediately preceding ventricular activation		0.12 to 0.20	Disturbance in conduction, usually in AV node, His bundle, or bundle branches, but can be in atria as well
QRS interval: from beginning to end of QRS complex; represents time taken for a depolarization of both ventricles		0.06 to 0.10	Disturbance in conduction in bundle branches and/or in ventricles
Q-T interval: from beginning of QRS to end of T wave; represents time taken for entire electrical depolarization and repolarization of the ventricles		0.36 to 0.44	Disturbances usually affecting repolarization more than depolarization such as drug effects, electrolyte disturbances, and rate changes.

From Kinney MR, Packa DR: Andreoli's comprehensive cardiac care, *ed 8, St Louis, 1996, Mosby.*
**Heart rate influences the duration of these intervals, especially that of PR and QT.*

INTERVENTIONS
Check BP and apical pulse q4h and prn
Monitor cardiac activity; check rhythm strips q6h to q8h and prn
Administer oxygen therapy as ordered
Inspect skin under external pacing electrodes *for burns*
Reposition electrodes as needed
Inspect insertion site of transvenous and permanent pacemaker *for signs of infection*

PATIENT/FAMILY TEACHING
Ensure that patient and/or significant other knows and understands
How to take radial pulse
Pacemaker insertion (p. 144), if indicated

SINUS TACHYCARDIA (Fig. 3-17)
A sinus rhythm >100 beats/min; causes—drugs, exercise, emotions, fever, increased sympathetic stimulation

II

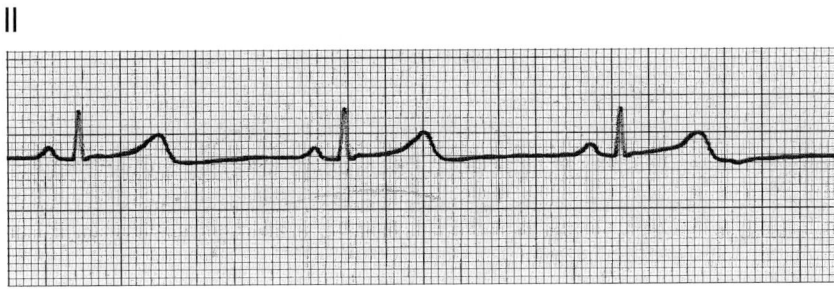

Fig. 3-16 Sinus bradycardia of 39 beats/min. The pacemaker is the sinus node, and conduction is normal.
(From Conover, MB: Understanding electrocardiography, ed 7, St Louis, 1996, Mosby.)

II

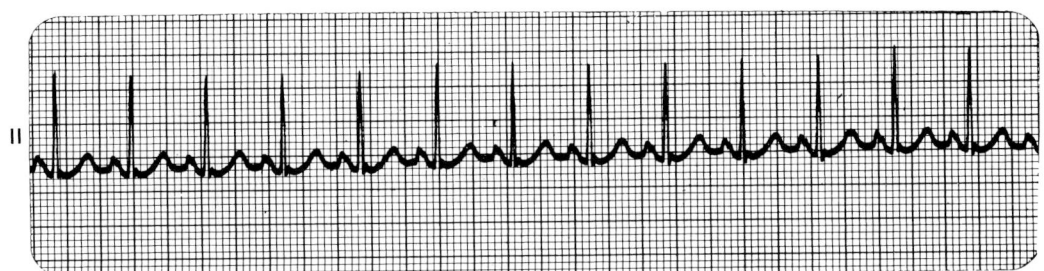

Fig. 3-17 Sinus tachycardia.
(From Goldberger AL: Clinical electrocardiography: a simplified approach, ed 6, St Louis, 1999, Mosby.)

Inspiration   Expiration   Inspiration

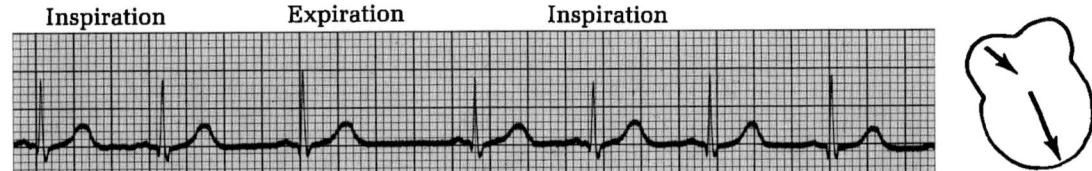

Fig. 3-18 Sinus dysrhythmia in a 4-year-old.
(From Conover MB: Understanding electrocardiography, ed 7, St Louis, 1996, Mosby.)

ASSESSMENT
OBSERVATIONS/FINDINGS
Fatigue
SOB
Rhythm: regular
Rate: 100 to 160 beats/min
P wave: normal configuration, one before each QRS
P-R interval: 0.12 to 0.20 second
QRS complex: 0.06 to 0.10 second

MULTIDISCIPLINARY MANAGEMENT
Treatment of underlying factors
Carotid sinus massage

INTERVENTIONS
Administer medications as ordered
Check BP, R, and apical pulse q4h to 6h and prn
Administer oxygen therapy as ordered
Initiate measures to decrease work of heart: rest,
    avoidance of caffeine intake and use of tobacco
    products

SINUS DYSRHYTHMIA (Fig. 3-18)

An irregular sinus rhythm; is normally found in children and young adults; causes—respiratory variation

ASSESSMENT
OBSERVATIONS/FINDINGS
Rhythm: irregular
Rate: 60 to 90 beats/min; may increase with inspiration
    and decrease with expiration
P wave: normal configuration, one before each QRS
    complex
PR interval: 0.12 to 0.20 second
QRS complex: 0.06 to 0.10 second

MULTIDISCIPLINARY MANAGEMENT
None indicated

SINUS ARREST (Fig. 3-19)

A rhythm in which a sinus impulse is not generated; causes—drugs, coronary artery disease, increased vagal tone, sinoatrial node disease

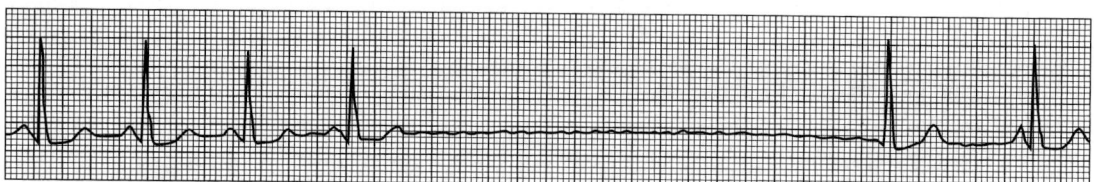

Fig. 3-19 Sinus arrest with asystole. Sinus arrest lasting 4 seconds and terminated with a junctional escape beat. *(From Kinney M, Packa DR:* Andreoli's comprehensive cardiac care, *ed 8, St Louis, 1996, Mosby.)*

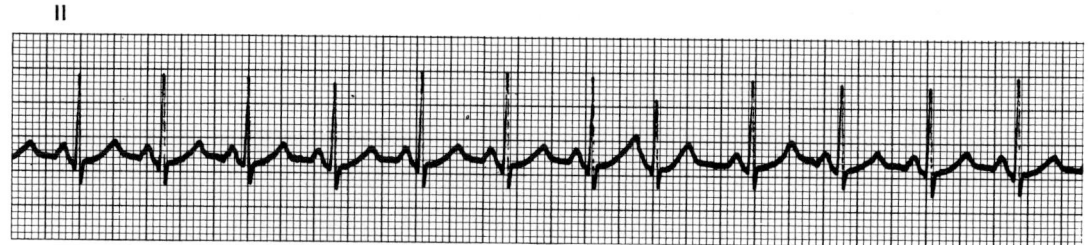

Fig. 3-20 Premature atrial contraction.
(From Conover MB: Exercises in diagnosing ECG tracings, *ed 3, St Louis, 1984, Mosby.)*

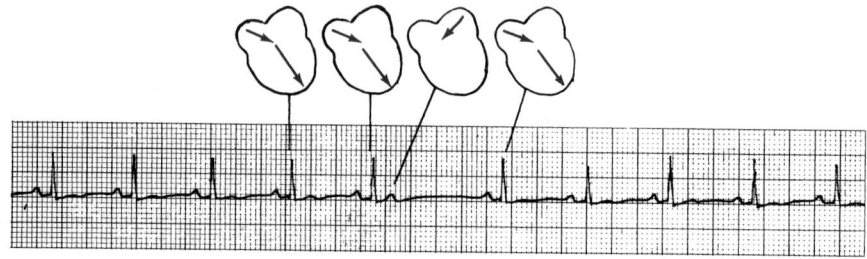

Fig. 3-21 Nonconducted premature atrial contraction (PAC).
(From Conover MB: Understanding electrocardiography, *ed 7, St Louis, 1996, Mosby.)*

ASSESSMENT
OBSERVATIONS/FINDINGS
Dizziness
Syncope
Rhythm: irregular during periods of arrest
Rate: variable
P wave: absent during periods of arrest
P-R interval: absent during periods of arrest
QRS complex: absent during periods of arrest

POTENTIAL COMPLICATION
Ventricular standstill

MULTIDISCIPLINARY MANAGEMENT
Medications: atropine
Cardiac pacing
Parenteral fluids
Cardiopulmonary resuscitation (CPR)

INTERVENTIONS
Monitor cardiac activity; check rhythm strips q4h to 6h and prn
Maintain bed rest as indicated
Check BP, R, and apical pulse q4h to 6h and prn
Administer oxygen therapy as indicated

■ RHYTHMS OF ATRIAL ORIGIN
Supraventricular or atrial rhythms that originate outside the sinoatrial node and above the bundle of His

▌PREMATURE ATRIAL CONTRACTIONS (PACS, APCS) (Figs. 3-20 and 3-21)

premature atrial contractions: Ectopic beats generated outside the sinoatrial node; causes—anxiety, ingestion of tobacco or caffeine, electrolyte imbalance, hypoxia, drug toxicity

ASSESSMENT
OBSERVATIONS/FINDINGS
Palpitations: skipped beats
Anxiety
Dizziness
Rhythm: irregular in presence of PACs
Rate: variable, may be normal or irregular in presence of ectopic beats
P wave: premature P wave is distorted; may be inverted or fused on preceding T wave
P-R interval: may be prolonged
QRS complex: may be normal or may show abnormal conduction in ectopic beat; no QRS will follow if P wave is blocked

II

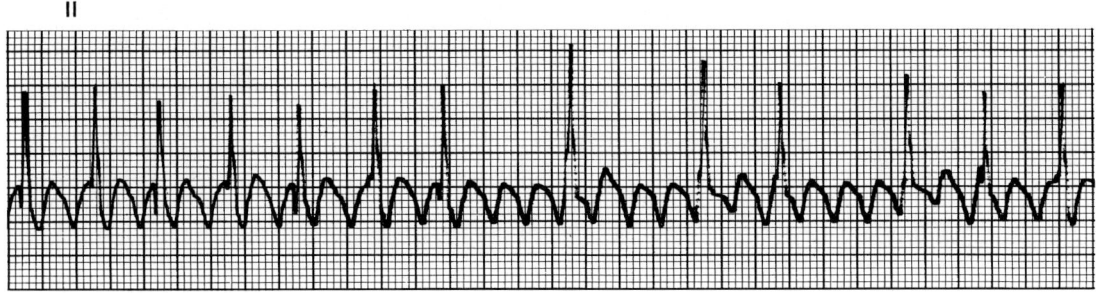

Fig. 3-22 Atrial flutter.
(From Conover MB: Understanding electrocardiography, *ed 7, St Louis, 1996, Mosby.)*

DIAGNOSTIC TEST
Holter monitor examination

POTENTIAL COMPLICATION
Atrial fibrillation

MULTIDISCIPLINARY MANAGEMENT
Treatment of underlying disease; none indicated for
    occasional PACs
Medications: antidysrhythmics

INTERVENTIONS
Monitor cardiac activity; check rhythm strips q4h to 6h
    and prn
Check BP, R, and apical pulse q6h to 8h
Restrict caffeine and nicotine as ordered
Correct electrolyte imbalance
Reduce anxiety

■ **ATRIAL FLUTTER** (Fig. 3-22)

*A rapid, regular ectopic atrial rhythm with character-
istic "flutter" waves; causes—most forms of cardiac disease*

ASSESSMENT
    OBSERVATIONS/FINDINGS
Tachycardia
Tachypnea
Palpitations
SOB
Rhythm
    Atrial: regular
    Ventricular: may be regular or irregular
    Emboli
Rate
    Atrial: 250 to 350 beats/min
    Ventricular: 100 to 150 beats/min
    P-R interval: unmeasurable
    P wave: absent; rhythm shows F waves in sawtooth
        shape
    QRS complex: usually normal

POTENTIAL COMPLICATIONS
Emboli
CHF
Shock

MULTIDISCIPLINARY MANAGEMENT
Treatment of underlying disease
Cardioversion
Carotid massage
Medications
    Antidysrhythmics
    Digitalis preparations
    Anticoagulation therapy
Atrial pacing
12-Lead ECG
Implanted antitachycardia pacemaker
AV Node radiofrequency ablation (RFA) with permanent
    pacemaker

INTERVENTIONS
Monitor cardiac activity; check rhythm strips q4h to 6h
    and prn
Check BP, R, and apical pulse q2h to 4h
Maintain bed rest as indicated
Administer oxygen therapy as ordered

■ **ATRIAL FIBRILLATION** (Fig. 3-23)

*A rapid, irregular, ectopic atrial rhythm with charac-
teristic "fibrillatory" activity; causes—coronary artery disease (CAD), valvular heart disease, hypertension, increased left atrial size in the elderly*

ASSESSMENT
    OBSERVATIONS/FINDINGS
Palpitations
Faintness
Syncope
Tachycardia
Irregular pulse
Pulse deficit (apical and radial pulses)
Chest discomfort
Nausea
Rhythm: irregular
Rate
    Atrial: 350 beats/min
    Ventricular: 90 to 100 beats/min
P-R interval: immeasurable
P wave: absent; rhythm shows "f" waves that are seen as
    undulations
QRS complex: usually normal

V_1

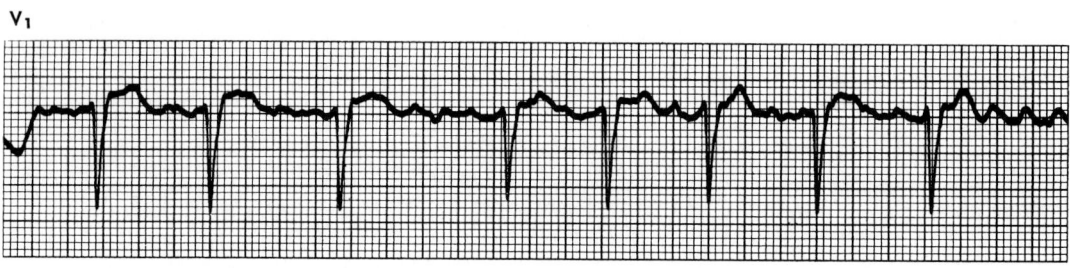

Fig. 3-23 Atrial fibrillation.
(From Conover MB: Exercises in diagnosing ECG tracings, ed 3, St Louis, 1984, Mosby.)

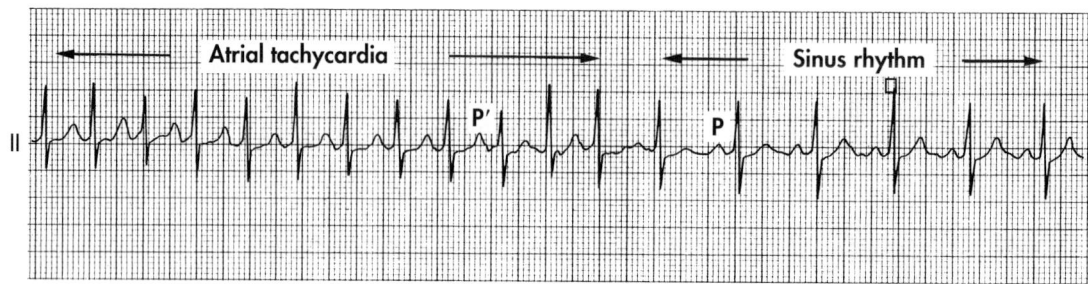

Fig. 3-24 Atrial tachycardia (a type of paroxysmal supraventricular tachycardia) terminating spontaneously with the abrupt resumption of sinus rhythm. The P waves of the tachycardia (rate: about 150 beats/min) are superimposed on the preceding T waves.
(From Goldberger AL: Clinical electrocardiography: a simplified approach, ed 6, St Louis, 1999, Mosby.)

POTENTIAL COMPLICATIONS
Mural thrombi
CHF
Shock

MULTIDISCIPLINARY MANAGEMENT
Medications: antidysrhythmics, anticoagulation therapy
Cardioversion
12-Lead ECG
AV node radiofrequency ablation (RFA) with permanent pacemaker insertion

INTERVENTIONS
Monitor cardiac activity; check rhythm strips q4h to 8h and prn
Check BP, R, and apical pulse q4h to 6h and prn
Administer oxygen therapy as ordered

■ SUPRAVENTRICULAR TACHYCARDIA (SVT) (Fig. 3-24)

An ectopic atrial rhythm that is regular and may start and stop abruptly, originating above AV node; causes— precipitated by sympathetic stimulation (e.g., emotion, caffeine, tobacco, fatigue, excessive alcohol intake); may also be associated with Wolff-Parkinson-White (WPW) syndrome

ASSESSMENT
OBSERVATIONS/FINDINGS
Palpitations
SOB
Lightheadedness
Syncope
"Frog sign"—rapid, regular venous pulsations in jugular veins during PSVT
Hypokalemia
Chest pain or discomfort
Abdominal discomfort
Polyuria
Tachycardia of short or prolonged duration
Rhythm: usually regular
Rate: 150 to 250 beats/min
P wave: normal or buried in QRS or T wave; may not be visible
P-R interval: usually normal
QRS complex: usually normal

DIAGNOSTIC TEST
Holter monitor examination
Electrophysiology study (EPS)

POTENTIAL COMPLICATIONS
CHF
Shock

MULTIDISCIPLINARY MANAGEMENT
Carotid massage (vagal stimulation)
Medications
    Antidysrhythmics
    Vagotonic preparations
Potassium replacement as indicated
Cardioversion

II

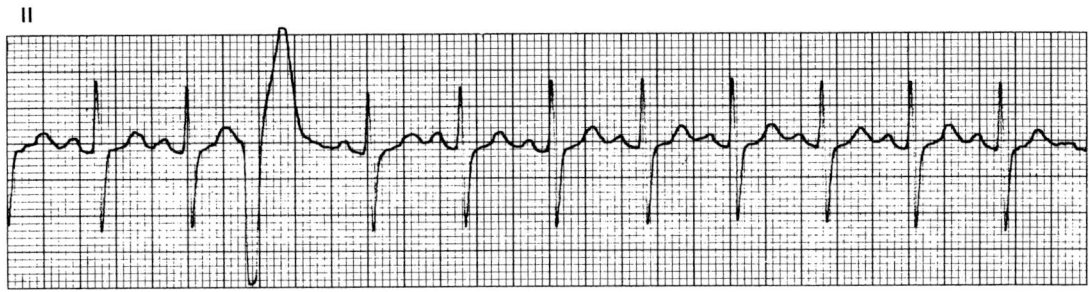

Fig. 3-25 Premature ventricular contraction (PVC).
(From Conover MB: Exercises in diagnosing ECG tracings, *ed 3, St Louis, 1984, Mosby.)*

V₁

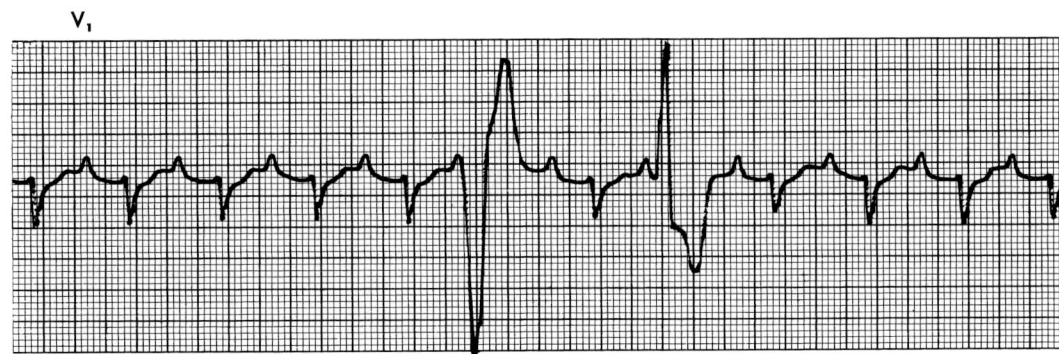

Fig. 3-26 Multifocal premature ventricular contractions (PVCs).
(From Conover MB: Exercises in diagnosing ECG tracings, *ed 3, St Louis, 1984, Mosby.)*

Atrial or ventricular pacing

12-Lead ECG

Treat underlying etiology

Radiofrequency catheter ablation for symptomatic dysrhythmias (e.g., Wolf-Parkinson-White syndrome [WPW])

INTERVENTIONS

Monitor cardiac activity; check rhythm strips q4h to 6h and prn

Administer oxygen therapy as ordered

Check BP, R, and apical pulse q2h to 4h

Maintain bed rest as indicated

Check serum potassium level if patient is taking digitalis preparations

Maintain quiet environment

■ RHYTHMS OF VENTRICULAR ORIGIN

Rhythms that occur as either escape or reentry (overdrive) rhythms arising within the ventricles

▌ PREMATURE VENTRICULAR CONTRACTIONS (PVCS)

(Figs. 3-25 and 3-26)

Premature beats arising in the ventricles below the bundle of His; may be a forerunner of ventricular tachycardia and ventricular fibrillation; causes—increased sympathetic stimulation (e.g., caffeine, to-bacco, emotion), most forms of heart disease, electrolyte imbalance

ASSESSMENT
OBSERVATIONS/FINDINGS

Palpitations

Precordial pain

Dizziness

Faintness

Momentary loss of consciousness

Rhythm: irregular

Rate

    Atrial: normal

    Ventricular: may be normal or rapid

P wave: does not precede premature beat; premature beat is usually followed by complete compensatory pause

P-R interval: immeasurable

QRS complex: premature beat is wide and bizarre in appearance, lasting longer than 0.12 second

DIAGNOSTIC TESTS

12-Lead ECG

Holter monitor examination

POTENTIAL COMPLICATIONS

Ventricular tachycardia

Ventricular fibrillation

MULTIDISCIPLINARY MANAGEMENT

Treatment of underlying disease
Medications: antidysrhythmics
12-Lead ECGs for
    Multifocal PVCs
    R on T phenomenon
    Coupling or paired PVCs
    Six or more PVCs/min

INTERVENTIONS

Monitor cardiac activity; check rhythm strips q4h to 6h
    and prn; report if more than 6 PVC/min or if they
    occur close to preceding T waves
Monitor BP, R, and apical pulse q4h to 6h and prn
Administer oxygen therapy
Restrict caffeine, nicotine, and hot and cold fluids

■ VENTRICULAR TACHYCARDIA (Fig. 3-27)

*Three or more consecutive PVCs; causes—ischemic
heart disease, significant chronic heart disease, drug
toxicity*

ASSESSMENT
OBSERVATIONS/FINDINGS

Anxiety
Palpitations
Dizziness
Precordial discomfort
Cyanosis
Confusion
Syncope
Altered LOC
Rhythm: usually regular
Rate: ventricular; 150 to 200 beats/min
P wave: absent; may be retrograde to atria
P-R interval: immeasurable
QRS complex: wide and bizarre in configuration, lasting
    >0.12 second

DIAGNOSTIC TESTS

Holter monitor
Signal average ECG
Electrophysiology study (EPS)

POTENTIAL COMPLICATIONS

Heart failure
Ventricular fibrillation

MULTIDISCIPLINARY MANAGEMENT

Treat underlying causes/diseases
Administer antidysrhythmics
Implantation of implantable cardioverter defibrillator (ICD)
    if patient's EPS shows polymorphic or sustained VT

INTERVENTIONS
IMMEDIATE CARE

Sedate patient as ordered
Apply direct current (DC) countershock
Administer antidysrhythmics medications as ordered:
    lidocaine bolus and drip
Initiate CPR; if patient has no pulse, treat as ventricular
    fibrillation (VF)
Initiate parenteral fluids as ordered
Take 12-lead ECG as ordered
Monitor BP, R, and apical pulse q15min to 30min as
    indicated
Administer oxygen as indicated

ONGOING CARE

Monitor cardiac activity; check rhythm strips q4h to 6h
    and prn
Monitor BP, R, and apical pulse q2h to 4h and prn,
    decreasing frequency as condition stabilizes
Administer medications as ordered
    Antidysrhythmics
    Sedatives
Maintain bed rest as indicated

■ VENTRICULAR FIBRILLATION (Fig. 3-28)

*Disorganized electrical activity of ventricles, which
leads to abrupt cessation of effective blood flow; causes—
severe heart disease, drug toxicity*

ASSESSMENT
OBSERVATIONS/FINDINGS

Anxiety
Palpitations

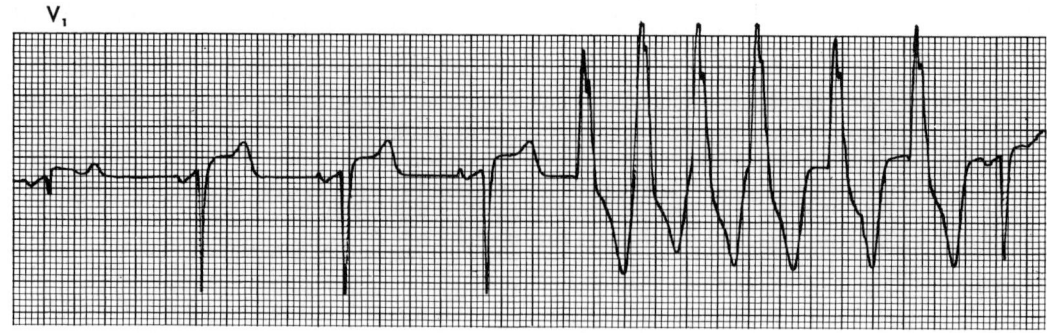

Fig. 3-27 Ventricular tachycardia.
(From Conover MB: Exercises in diagnosing ECG tracings, ed 3, St Louis, 1984, Mosby.)

Dizziness
Cyanosis
Precordial pain
Nausea, vomiting
SOB
Syncope
Absence of pulse
Rhythm: irregular
Rate: >210 beats/min; no beat-to-beat count
P wave: not seen; absent atrial activity
QRS complex: wide undulations; wandering, irregular
    baseline

DIAGNOSTIC TESTS

Holter monitor
Signal average ECG
Electrophysiology study (EPS)

MULTIDISCIPLINARY MANAGEMENT

Treat underlying causes
Implantation of implantable cardiodefibrillation (ICD)

INTERVENTIONS

IMMEDIATE CARE

Apply DC countershock
Administer CPR; usually indicated
Administer medications as ordered
Initiate parenteral fluids as ordered
Take 12-lead ECG as ordered
Administer oxygen with assisted ventilation as ordered
Monitor BP, R, and apical pulse q15min to 30min

ONGOING CARE

Monitor cardiac activity; check rhythm strips q1h to 2h,
    decreasing frequency as condition stabilizes
Monitor BP, R, and apical pulse q1h to 2h and prn
Maintain bed rest as indicated
Keep defibrillator and emergency cart at bedside until
    condition stabilizes

PATIENT/FAMILY TEACHING

Provide instruction for ICD as indicated (see p. 151)
Provide CPR instruction and training to family

TORSADES DE POINTE (POLYMORPHOUS VENTRICULAR TACHYCARDIA) (Fig. 3-29)

Atypical ventricular tachycardia occurring in the setting of delayed repolarization (prolonged Q-T interval); causes—drug toxicity such as quinidine; electrolyte imbalance

ASSESSMENT

OBSERVATIONS/FINDINGS

Palpitations
Faintness
Syncope
Rhythm: regular or irregular
Rate: ventricular, 150 to 300 beats/min
P-R interval: not measurable
QRS complex: wide and bizarre in configuration, lasting
    >0.12 second; amplitude and direction of QRS
    complex will vary
Q-T interval during baseline rhythm: >0.46 second or
    >33% of baseline
T wave during baseline: very broad and flat

POTENTIAL COMPLICATIONS

Ventricular fibrillation
Sudden death

MULTIDISCIPLINARY MANAGEMENT

Correction of underlying cause if identifiable (e.g., drug
    toxicity; quinidine, procainamide, amiodarone)
Correction of electrolyte imbalance: hypokalemia,
    hypomagnesemia
Medications (avoid drugs that prolong Q-T intervals, e.g.,
    quinidine, disopyramide [Norpace])
Overdrive pacing: rate set at 80 to 120 beats/min
Cardioversion
Left stellate ganglionectomy

INTERVENTIONS

Monitor cardiac activity; check rhythm strips q2h to 4h
    and prn, decreasing frequency as condition
    stabilizes
Monitor BP, P, and apical pulse q4h to 6h and prn

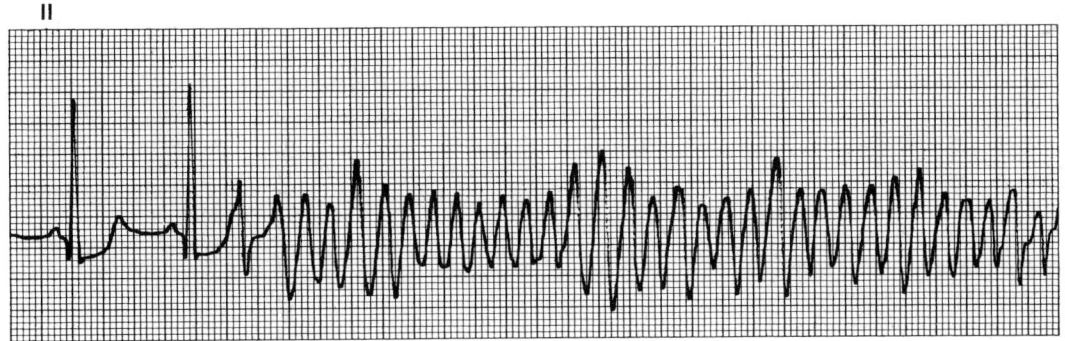

Fig. 3-28 Ventricular fibrillation.
(From Conover MB: Exercises in diagnosing ECG tracings, *ed 3, St Louis, 1984, Mosby.)*

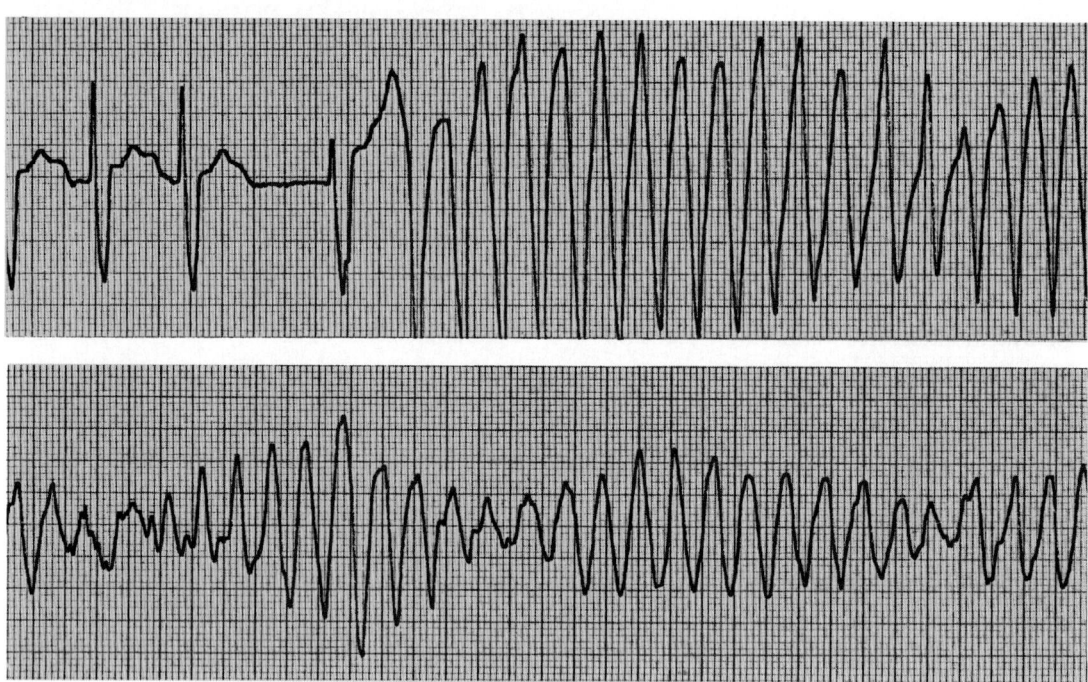

Fig. 3-29   Torsades de pointe.
(From the late Dr. Alan Lindsay collection, Salt Lake City, Utah. In Conover MB: Understanding electrocardiography, *ed 7, St Louis, 1996, Mosby.)*

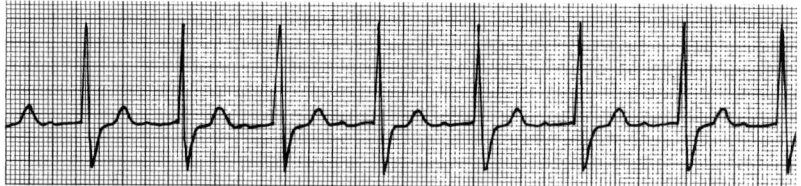

Fig. 3-30   First-degree AV block.
(From Conover MB: Understanding electrocardiography: arrhythmias and the 12-lead ECG, *ed 4, St Louis, 1984, Mosby.)*

■ ATRIOVENTRICULAR BLOCK

A conduction disturbance involving the AV junction, which normally functions as a bridge between the atria and ventricles

▌FIRST-DEGREE ATRIOVENTRICULAR BLOCK (Fig. 3-30)

A consistent delay in impulse conduction throughout the AV node; causes—digoxin toxicity, ischemic heart disease, hyperkalemia; congenital

ASSESSMENT
OBSERVATIONS/FINDINGS
Rhythm: regular
Rate: 60 to 90 beats/min
P wave: normal configuration; one before each QRS
P-R interval: prolonged, >0.20 second
QRS complex: 0.06 to 0.10 second

INTERVENTIONS
Monitor cardiac activity; check rhythm strips q4h to 6h and prn

Check BP, R, and apical pulse q4h to 6h and prn
Discontinue use of digitalis preparation or quinidine as ordered
Check serum levels of digitalis preparation and potassium as indicated
Observe for changes in P-R interval and measure

▌SECOND-DEGREE ATRIOVENTRICULAR BLOCK (Figs. 3-31 and 3-32)

An AV conduction disturbance characterized by non-conducted P waves and classified as type I or type II; causes—digoxin toxicity, ischemic heart disease

ASSESSMENT
OBSERVATIONS/FINDINGS
Rhythm: regular
Rate
  Atrial: regular
  Ventricular: irregular
P wave: may show one or more nonconducted P waves
  Type I: P-R interval progressively prolongs until one complex is completely blocked

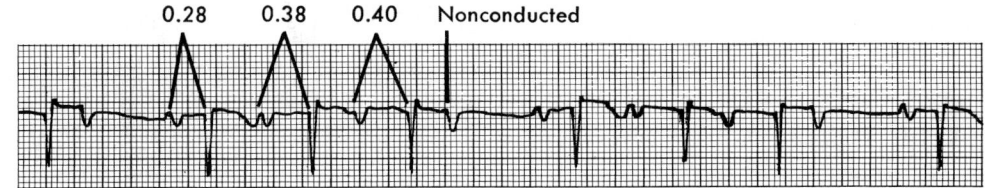

Fig. 3-31 Second-degree AV block: Mobitz type I (Wenckebach phenomenon) with narrow QRS complex. *(From Conover MB:* Understanding electrocardiography, *ed 7, St Louis, 1996, Mosby.)*

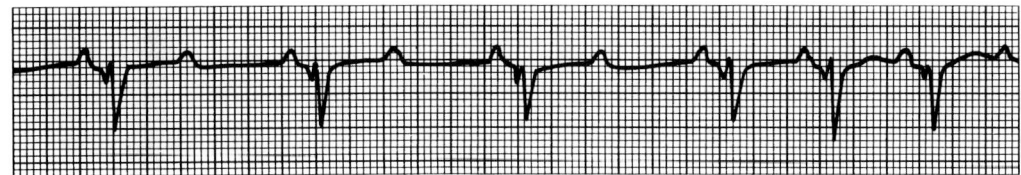

Fig. 3-32 Second-degree AV block: Mobitz type II. *(From Conover MB:* Exercises in diagnosing ECG tracings, *ed 3, St Louis, 1984, Mosby.)*

Type II: P-R interval remains constant with blocked impulses
QRS complex: 0.06 to 0.10 second

DIAGNOSTIC TESTS
Serum drug levels
His bundle recording

POTENTIAL COMPLICATIONS
Angina
Heart failure
Complete AV block
Asystole

MULTIDISCIPLINARY MANAGEMENT
Medications
    Atropine
    Isoproterenol
Temporary cardiac pacing

INTERVENTIONS
Monitor cardiac activity; check rhythm strips q2h to 4h
Monitor BP, R, and apical pulse q4h to 6h and prn
Observe for progression to higher degree of block

MOBITZ TYPE I (WENCKEBACH PHENOMENON) (Fig. 3-31)

Causes—digoxin toxicity, inferior wall myocardial infarction (MI), rheumatic fever

ASSESSMENT
OBSERVATIONS/FINDINGS
Rhythm
    Atrial: regular
    Ventricular: irregular
Rate: atrial > ventricular
P wave: may have multiple P waves before each QRS (characteristic "group beating")

P-R interval: becomes progressively prolonged (>0.28 second) until one P wave is blocked; cycle will then be repeated
QRS complex: 0.06 to 0.10 second; RR interval will shorten until QRS complex is dropped

MULTIDISCIPLINARY MANAGEMENT
Medications
    Atropine
External or transvenous pacing

INTERVENTIONS
Withdraw use of digitalis preparation as ordered
Check serum levels of digitalis preparation and potassium as indicated

MOBITZ TYPE II (Fig. 3-32)

Causes—digitalis toxicity, anterior MI

ASSESSMENT
OBSERVATIONS/FINDINGS
Dizziness
Weakness
Rhythm
    Atrial: regular
    Ventricular: irregular
Rate
    Atrial: 60 to 90 beats/min
    Ventricular: will vary according to degree of block
P wave: may have multiple P waves before each QRS
P-R interval: remains constant and may be greater than 0.20 second
QRS interval: usually normal or slightly prolonged

POTENTIAL COMPLICATIONS
Complete AV block
Asystole

MULTIDISCIPLINARY MANAGEMENT

Cardiac monitor

Medications

Atropine

External, temporary transvenous or permanent pacing

THIRD-DEGREE HEART BLOCK (COMPLETE) (Fig. 3-33)

Atria and ventricles are controlled by independent pacemakers

Causes—chronic conduction defect disease, digoxin toxicity, ischemic heart disease, congenital heart disease

ASSESSMENT

OBSERVATIONS/FINDINGS

Bradycardia

Syncope

Altered LOC

Angina

Seizure activity

Rhythm: regular; atrial and ventricular rhythms act independently of each other

Rate

Atrial: 60 to 90 beats/min

Ventricular: 25 to 45 beats/min

P wave: multiple P waves that occur independently of QRS

P-R interval: immeasurable

QRS complex

Normal if impulse originates above bifurcation of bundle of His (rate = 40 to 60 beats/min)

Greater than 0.12 second of impulse originates below bifurcation (rate = 15 to 40 beats/min)

POTENTIAL COMPLICATIONS

Heart failure

Shock

Ventricular fibrillation

Asystole

MULTIDISCIPLINARY MANAGEMENT

External, transvenous, or permanent pacing

Medications

Atropine

12-Lead ECG

INTERVENTIONS

Monitor cardiac activity; check rhythm strips q2h to 4h or prn

Monitor BP, R, and apical pulse q2h to 4h and prn

Administer oxygen therapy as ordered

Maintain bed rest as indicated

Administer IV fluids or vasopressor drips as ordered *to improve hypotension*

ATRIOVENTRICULAR JUNCTIONAL RHYTHMS

Dysrhythmias that originate at the AV junction; may include premature, escape, and accelerated junctional rhythm; causes—digitalis toxicity, MI, hypoxia, hyperkalemia, tricuspid valve surgery, rheumatic fever, SA node pathology

ATRIOVENTRICULAR JUNCTIONAL ESCAPE (Fig. 3-34)

ASSESSMENT

OBSERVATIONS/FINDINGS

Dizziness

Faintness

Heart block

Rhythm: regular

Rate: 40 to 60 beats/min

P wave: may precede or follow QRS; inverted in lead II

P-R interval: not measurable

QRS complex: 0.06 to 0.10 second; may be slightly abnormal

MULTIDISCIPLINARY MANAGEMENT

Treatment of underlying disease

Medications

Atropine

Ventricular pacing

12-Lead ECG as ordered

INTERVENTIONS

Monitor cardiac activity; check rhythm strips q4h to 6h

Check serum levels of digitalis preparation and potassium as indicated

WOLFF-PARKINSON-WHITE SYNDROME (VENTRICULAR PREEXCITATION) (Fig. 3-35)

Preexcitation of the ventricles over an accessory AV pathway: cause—congenital heart disease

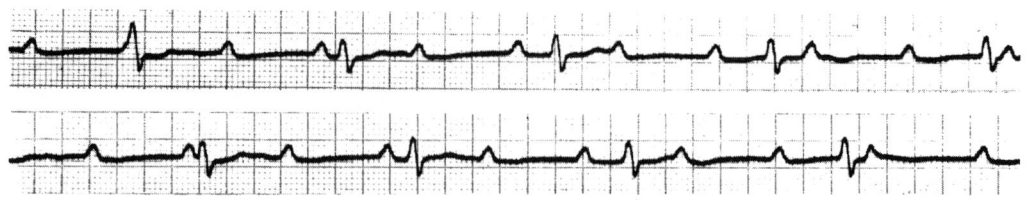

Fig. 3-33   Third-degree (complete) AV block.
(From Kinney MR, Packa DR: Andreoli's comprehensive cardiac care, *ed 6, St Louis, 1996, Mosby.)*

II

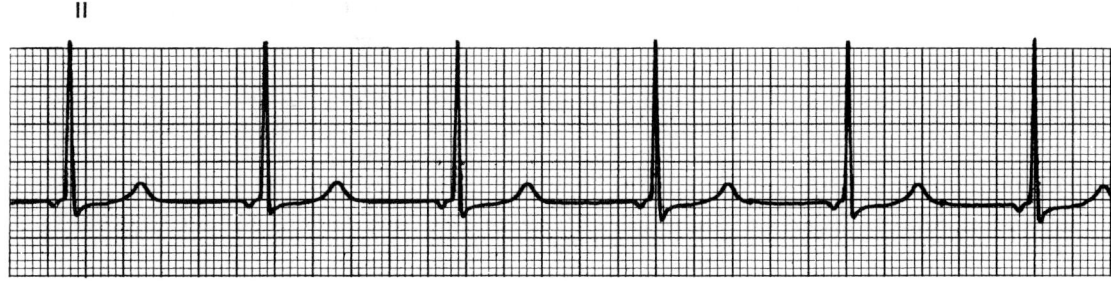

II

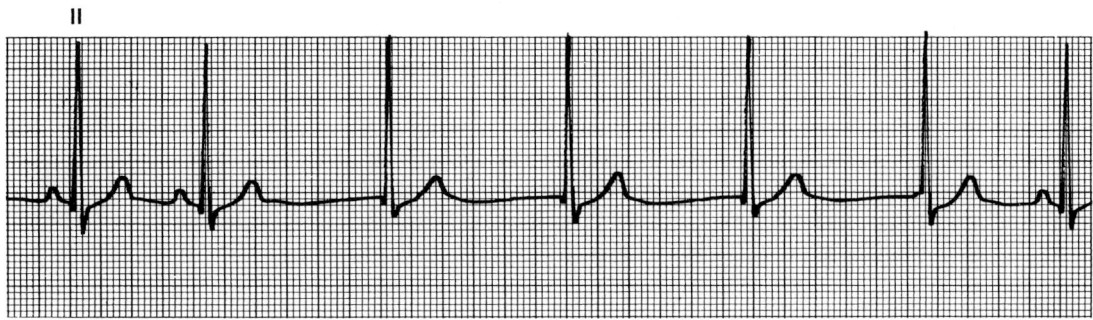

Fig. 3-34 Junctional escape rhythms.
(From Conover MB: Exercises in diagnosing ECG tracings, *ed 3, St Louis, 1984, Mosby.)*

ASSESSMENT
OBSERVATIONS/FINDINGS
Rhythm: regular
Rate: regular
P wave: normal configuration; one before each QRS
P-R interval: <0.12 second
QRS complex: when following shortened P-R interval, complex is widened and distorted, exhibiting delta waves

DIAGNOSTIC TESTS
Holter monitor examination
Electrophysiologic studies

POTENTIAL COMPLICATIONS
Atrial tachycardia
Atrial fibrillation
Paroxysmal supraventricular tachycardia (PSVT)
Ventricular fibrillation

MULTIDISCIPLINARY MANAGEMENT
Valsalva's maneuver; eyeball pressure
Medications as ordered
 Adenosine IV
 Calcium channel blocking agents
 Antidysrhythmics
Cardioversion
Radiofrequency ablation (RFA)

INTERVENTIONS
Monitor cardiac activity as indicated; check rhythm strips q4h to q6h; report any changes in rhythm to physician

PATIENT/FAMILY TEACHING
Discuss familial tendency for WPW

■ ELECTROCARDIOGRAM RHYTHMS
(Fig. 3-36)

MULTIDISCIPLINARY MANAGEMENT
PATIENT PROBLEM/NURSING DIAGNOSIS/INTERVENTIONS (GENERAL)

▼Anxiety related to altered heart action

Assess level of anxiety and degree of understanding *to identify source of anxiety and clarify any misconceptions*
Provide continuous explanation for various monitoring devices in use and procedures; *information alleviates anxiety*
Remain with patient during periods of heightened anxiety *to provide reassurance and comfort*
Promote physical rest *to decrease cardiac workload*
Administer sedation as ordered

Expected Outcomes
Anxiety level is reduced
Appears calm
Verbalizes fears and concerns, asks questions

Additional Nursing Diagnosis to Consider
Risk for decreased cardiac output related to electrical instability

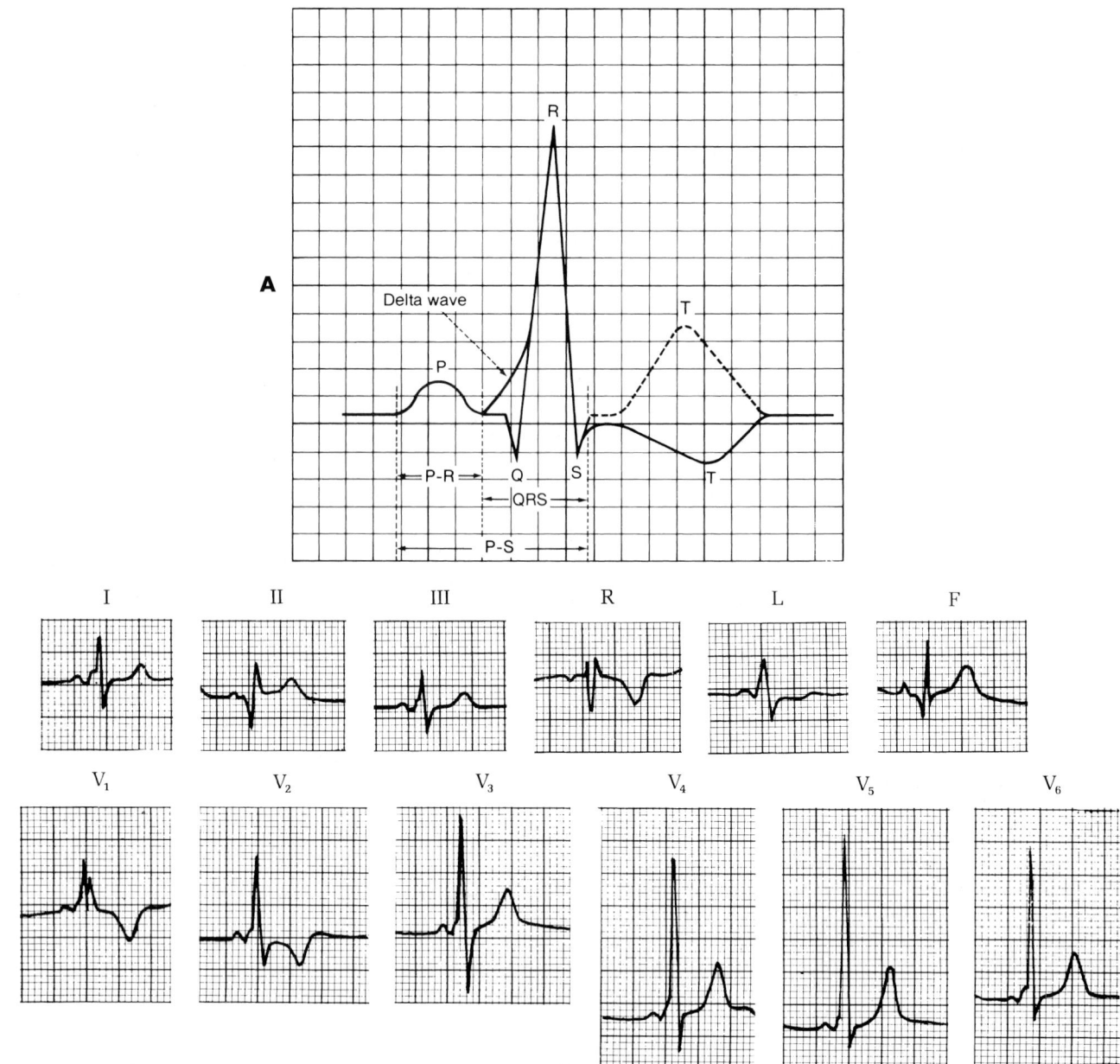

Fig. 3-35 Wolff-Parkinson-White syndrome. **A,** Contrast of the normal cardiac complex with a cardiac complex associated with preexcitation. Note the delta wave, widened QRS, and T wave inversion characteristic of preexcitation. **B,** Note that the ventricular complex is a fusion beat and that negative delta waves have produced Q waves in leads II and aV$_F$. The delta waves in leads I, III, and aV$_L$ and the precordial leads are nicely visualized.
(**A,** *from Kinney MR et al:* AACH's clinical reference for critical care nursing, *ed 4, St Louis, 1998, Mosby;* **B** *from Conover MB:* Understanding electrocardiography, *ed 7, St Louis, 1996, Mosby.)*

PATIENT/FAMILY TEACHING

Assess level of understanding

Explain purpose of treatment and equipment

Reinforce physician's explanation of rhythm disturbance and associated symptoms to report

Discuss need to exercise to tolerance and/or as ordered

Explain purpose and demonstrate method of taking pulse

Describe dietary restrictions as ordered; need to avoid caffeine and nicotine

Discuss medication: name, dosage, time of administration, purpose, and side effects

Need to avoid taking over-the-counter medications without checking with physician

Importance of ongoing patient care

Pacemaker care when indicated

■ PACEMAKER INSERTION

pacemaker: Electronic device used to electronically stimulate the myocardium to control or maintain the heart rate

Normal T wave

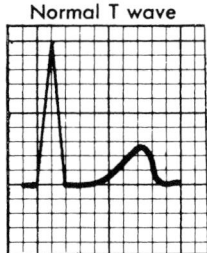

Nonspecific ST-T changes

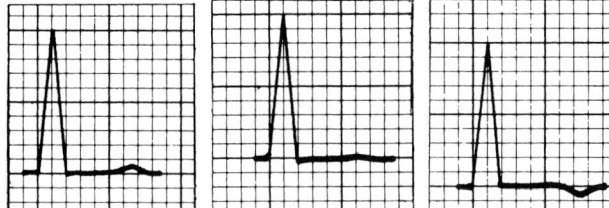

Fig. 3-36 Miscellaneous ECG changes. (Flattening of T wave or slight T wave inversion is abnormal but relatively nonspecific changes.) *(From Goldberger AL: Clinical electrocardiography: a simplified approach, ed 6, St Louis, 1999, Mosby.)*

PREPROCEDURE TEACHING

Reinforce physician's explanation of procedure
   How pacemaker functions
      To optimize cardiac function
      To restore and/or maintain AV synchronization
Indications
   To control bradydysrhythmias
   To control tachydysrhythmias
   To control ventricular fibrillation
Type or mode to be used
   Temporary
   Permanent
Method insertion
   Transvenous
   Transthoracic
   Epicardial
Ensure that patient and/or significant other knows and
   understands
      Procedure, duration of procedure, where it will be
         performed (operating room vs. procedure room),
         equipment that will be used (e.g., fluoroscopy), and
         type of anesthesia
Importance of restricting activities of affected arm to
   avoid lead dislodgement:
      First 24 to 48 hours use arm sling
      Avoid activities that raise arm over head (i.e., bowling,
         hunting, fishing) for 4 to 6 weeks
      Avoid lifting anything >10 lb for 4 to 6 weeks
Importance of being closely monitored postoperatively
Signs and symptoms of pacemaker malfunction
   Faintness
   Dizziness
   Dyspnea
   Twitching
      Pectoral muscles
      Abdominal muscles

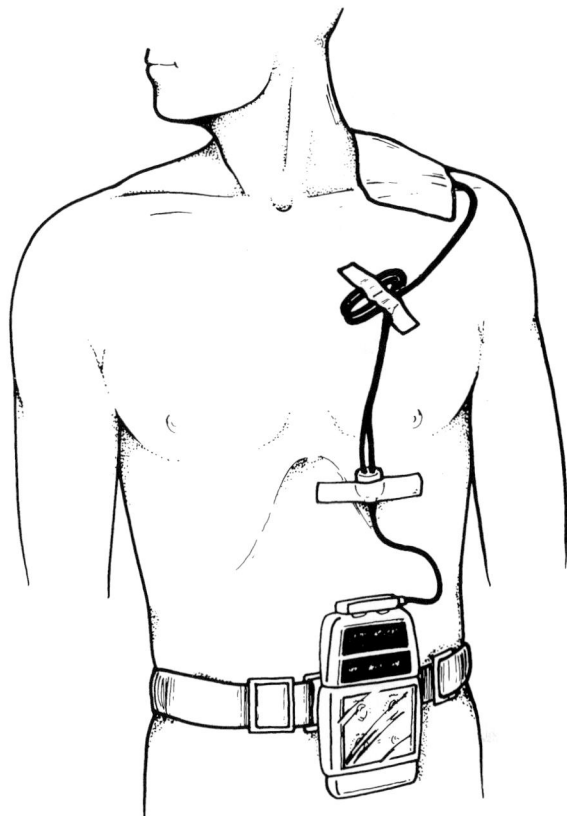

Fig. 3-37 Temporary external pacemaker.

Hiccups
Chest pain

POSTPROCEDURE ASSESSMENT
OBSERVATIONS/FINDINGS
Temporary Pacemaker (Fig. 3-37)
HR based on preset pacemaker setting
Pacemaker unit (Fig. 3-38)
   Firing at preset rate
   Output threshold (milliamperes)
   Sensing needle
   Terminal connections
Electrical grounding
ECG pattern (Fig. 3-39)
   Pacemaker artifact
   Capturing
   Patient's underlying rhythm
Battery failure
   Loss of capture
   Failure to sense
   Sensing needle: not moving

PERMANENT PACEMAKER
Pacemaker unit (Fig. 3-40)
   HR: based on preset pacer rate
   Location of pulse generator
   Mode (Box 3-6)
      Ventricular inhibited (demand): VVI
      AV sequential: DVI

Atrial triggered: AAT
Fully automatic: DDD
VVIR: Ventricular demand rate modulation
Programmable functions: rate modulation (see Box 3-6)
    Output (milliamperes)
    Sensitivity (to PQRS complex)

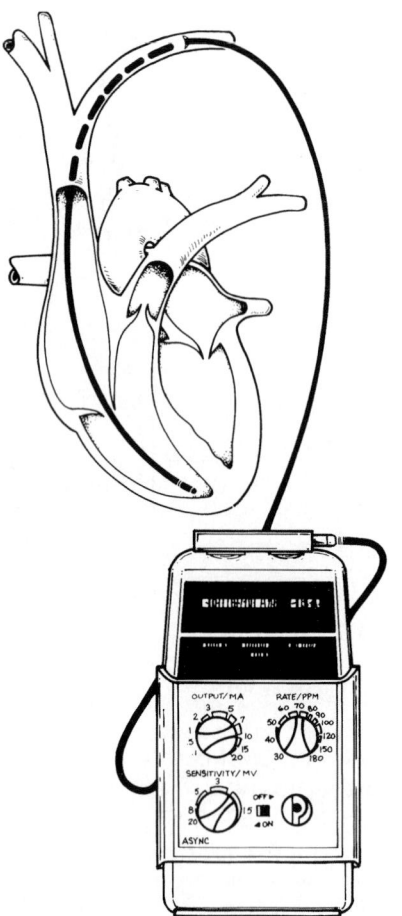

Fig. 3-38   Temporary pacemaker unit: transvenous approach.

POTENTIAL COMPLICATIONS

Pacemaker dysfunction
    Syncope
    Decreased BP
    Pallor or cyanosis
    Bradycardia
    Fatigue
    SOB
    ECG pattern changes
    Absent pacemaker artifact
    No ventricular response, absence of QRS complex
        after pacemaker artifact
    Competition; presence of pacemaker response
        complex and patient's own complex
    Runaway pacemaker; pacemaker artifact appears at
        several hundred per minute
Catheter dislodgment
    Change in QRS configuration
    Loss of artifact on ECG
    Failure to sense
    Hiccups
    Muscle twitching: chest, abdomen
Stokes-Adams syndrome
    Hypotension
    Vertigo
    Fainting
    Convulsions
    Coma
Cardiac dysrhythmias
    PVCs
    Ventricular tachycardia
Site of insertion
    Discoloration
    Pain
    Swelling
    Bleeding
Perforation
    Hiccup
Lead fracture
    Intermittent or loss of capture

Ventricular (VVI) Pacemaker

Lead II

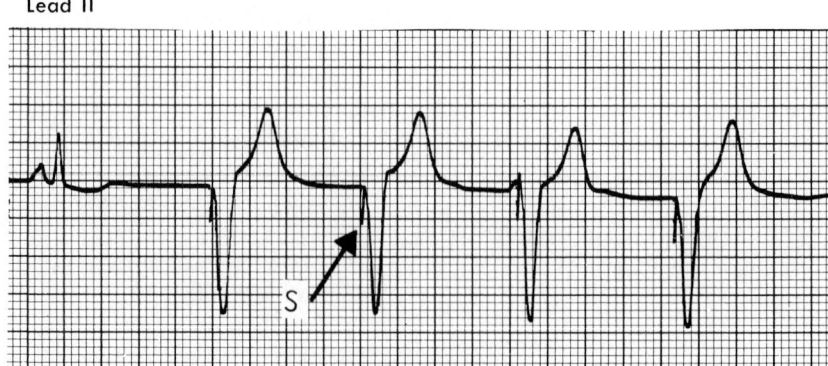

Fig. 3-39   Pacemaker beats. The first P-QRS cycle is from a normal sinus beat. It is followed by four pacemaker beats. Notice the pacemaker spike *(S)* preceding each paced beat. Pacemaker beats are wide and resemble bundle branch block beats. *(From Goldberger AL:* Clinical electrocardiography: a simplified approach, *ed 6, St Louis, 1999, Mosby.)*

Infection of incisional site
  Elevated temperature
  Redness
  Discoloration
  Pain, swelling
  Fluid collection, drainage
Cardiac tamponade

MULTIDISCIPLINARY MANAGEMENT
THERAPEUTIC MANAGEMENT
Cardiac monitor
Pacemaker
  Heart rate setting
  Threshold (milliamperes)
Medications
  Analgesics

PATIENT PROBLEM—NURSING DIAGNOSIS/INTERVENTIONS

▼ Risk for decreased cardiac output related to pacemaker dysfunction secondary to displacement or breakage of pacing catheter, infection, or bleeding

Assess patient and pacemaker unit *to detect signs of pacemaker failure*
Place patient on cardiac monitor *to evaluate pacemaker function*
Monitor BP, T, and R q4h; check apical pulse q1h to 2h for 7 hours then q4h *to detect signs of compromised cardiac function*

For temporary pacemaker
  Check settings: output, sensing, and rates
  Immobilize and secure extremity
Check rhythm strips on return to unit q4h and prn noting pacemaker function and rate
Examine site of insertion q2h to 4h; report any excessive bleeding to physician

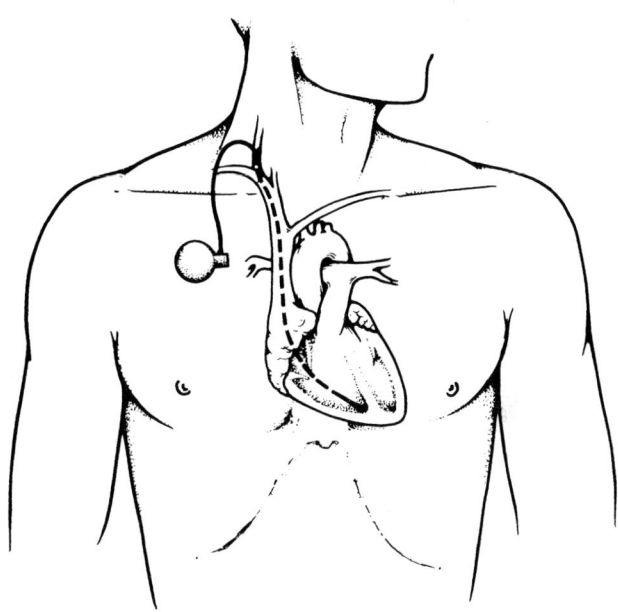

Fig. 3-40 Permanent pacemaker.

Box 3-6	**NBG Pacemaker Code (1987)**			
I	**II**	**III**	**IV** PROGRAMMABLE FUNCTIONS; RATE MODULATION	**V**
CHAMBER PACED	**CHAMBER SENSED**	**RESPONSE TO SENSING**		**ANTITACHYARRHYTHMIA FUNCTION(S)**
V-ventricle	V-ventricle	T-triggers pacing	P-programmable rate and/or output	P-pacing (antitachyarrhythmia)
A-atrium	A-atrium	I-inhibits pacing	M-multiprogrammability of rate, output, sensitivity, etc.	S-shock D-dual (P + S)
D-dual (A + V)	D-dual (A + V)	D-dual (T + I)	C-communicating functions (telemetry)	O-none
O-none S*-A or V	O-none S*-A or V	O-none	R-rate modulation O-none	

D D D R P

CHAMBER PACED	CHAMBER SENSED	RESPONSE TO SENSING	PROGRAMMABLE FUNCTIONS: RATE MODULATION	ANTITACHYARRHYTHMIA FUNCTION(S)
V = Ventricle	V = Ventricle	I = Inhibits pacing	R = Rate modulation	P = Pacing (Antitachyarrhythmia)

Modified with permission from Bernstein AD et al: NASPE/BPEG generic pacemaker code for antibradyarrhythmia and adaptive-rate and antitachyarrhythmia devices, PACE 10:794-799, 1987.
*Used by manufacturer.

Continue with immediate postoperative care and decrease frequency of nursing functions as patient's condition improves

Increase activity as tolerated and ordered

Change dressing daily as ordered, using aseptic technique *to prevent infection*

Expected Outcome
Demonstrates stable cardiac output; pacemaker unit functioning as programmed

Additional Nursing Diagnoses to Consider
Anxiety related to perceived and/or actual changes in health status

Pain related to incision and/or physical immobility of affected arm

PATIENT/FAMILY TEACHING
PERMANENT PACEMAKER
Assess level of understanding and degree of readiness to learn

Ensure that patient and/or significant other knows pacemaker model, date of insertion, location of pacer generator, and pacer rate

Demonstrate method of caring for pacemaker (Box 3-7)

Demonstrate changing of dressing

Demonstrate taking of pulse for 1 minute; give patient range of normal rates and instruct to report to physician if pulse is less than set range (i.e., <5 beats/min below set rate)

Deal with behavioral changes such as denial

Discuss living with pacemaker, assist patient to adjust to any limitations, and explain that pacemaker will eliminate feelings of faintness and fatigue

Discuss signs of pacemaker failure
  Pulse <60 beats/min or <5 beats/min below set rate
  Dizziness
  Faintness
  Palpitations

Box 3-7 Management of Pacemaker Equipment

TEMPORARY PACEMAKER
- Ground all equipment
- Secure all terminal connections
- Avoid use of electrical equipment such as shavers
- Insulate exposed pacemaker wires by enclosing pacemaker and connections with rubber glove
- Avoid wetting pacemaker
- Apply soft restraints as indicated

PERMANENT PACEMAKER
- Avoid exposure to electrical equipment that causes electromagnetic interference (EMI), such as diathermy and ungrounded equipment. Limit use of cellular phone; listen to phone with ear on opposite side of pacemaker site.
- Apply arm sling first 24 hours

Hiccups
Chest pain

Discuss method of reporting pacemaker failure
  Telephone monitoring
  Notifying physician

Discuss signs of infection around pacemaker generator
  Fever
  Heat
  Pain
  Swelling

Discuss medications: name, dosage, time of administration, purpose, and side effects

Explain need to avoid taking over-the-counter medications without checking with physician

Review prescribed diet

DISCHARGE/HOME CARE PLANNING
Explain importance of ongoing outpatient care: pacemaker clinic, use of transtelephonic system

Describe activity allowances and limitations
  Activity restrictions for 6 weeks after insertion:
    No lifting objects overhead
    No activity requiring swinging movement of arm on implant side (e.g., golfing, bowling, window washing)
  Avoid traveling for at least 3 months after insertion
  Discuss type of employment and make adjustments in work accordingly
  Resume sexual activity as tolerated
  Avoid engaging in body contact sports such as baseball, football, and basketball

Discuss need to wear nonrestrictive clothing over site of pacemaker

Discuss electrical safety
  Avoid working with radar or electrical equipment such as diathermy motors that may cause electromagnetic interference
  Ground home appliances so that they have little or no effect on permanent pacemakers
  Wear medical alert band
  Carry pacemaker card with information regarding type of pacemaker, set rate, date of implantation, and name of physician
  Inform dentist of pacemaker before any extensive dental work
  Limit use of cellular phone; listen to phone with ear opposite of pacemaker

■ CARDIAC CATHETERIZATION
An invasive cardiac procedure; assists in detection and localization of intracardiac problems, determines intracardiac measurements, and shows visualization of the cardiac chambers; performed with patient under local anesthesia

PREPROCEDURE TEACHING
Involve family or significant other in care and instruction

Assess level of understanding

Reinforce physician's explanation of purpose of procedure
Review routine preparation for procedure
    Clip hair from right and left groin area
    (NOTE: Shaving for skin prep is no longer appropriate based on 1985 CDC standards)
    Ensure that informed consent is obtained
    Review ordered labs tests and report any abnormal result to physician limits
        CBC and platelet count
        PT and PTT
        Electrolytes
        BUN and creatinine
        ECG—baseline
        Vital signs—baseline
    Medication for sedation may be ordered
    No food or water 6 to 12 hours before procedure
Review sensations to be experienced during procedure
    Palpitations
    Warm, flushed feeling during injection of dye
    Desire to cough
Review sensations to be expected after procedure
    Soreness at insertion site
    Possible backache from lying on table for 1 to 3 hours
    Fatigue
Stress importance of bed rest and immobility of extremity after procedure

POSTPROCEDURE ASSESSMENT
OBSERVATIONS/FINDINGS
Bleeding or hematoma at site of insertion
    Neck
    Antecubital fossa (brachial artery)
    Inguinal (femoral artery)
Vasospasm of affected extremity
    Numbness
    Tingling
    Cyanosis
    Loss of pulse
    Pain

POTENTIAL COMPLICATIONS
Dysrhythmias: atrial, ventricular, heart block
Vasovagal reaction
Contrast reaction/anaphylaxis/nephrotoxicity
Vascular injury
    Hemorrhage (local, retroperitoneal, pelvic)
    Pseudoaneurysm
    Thrombosis/embolus, air embolus
Cardiac perforation, tamponade
Myocardial ischemia, infarction
Local infection
CHF

POSTPROCEDURE CARE
Assess BP, T, R, apical pulse; and peripheral pulses, noting quality q15min × 4, then qh for 4 hours, then as ordered

Maintain bed rest for 6 to 8 hours after procedure or as ordered
    Elevate head of bed 20 to 30 degrees
    Keep extremity immobile for 6 to 8 hours after procedure as ordered
    Maintain sandbag over puncture site as ordered
Obtain 12-lead ECG as ordered
Monitor cardiac activity as ordered; check rhythm strips q4h and prn
Examine dressing at site of insertion q2h to 4h, noting amount and color of drainage; change daily and prn
Reinforce dressing as necessary
Inspect surrounding skin
    Redness or discoloration
    Swelling
    Irritation
Control pain as ordered
Ambulate as tolerated
Instruct patient to report any signs of pain, swelling, or discoloration of puncture site
Continue ongoing care for underlying disease process

PATIENT/FAMILY TEACHING
Reinforce physician's explanation of results of procedure and treatment plan

■ ELECTROPHYSIOLOGY STUDY (EPS)
An invasive cardiac procedure involving the placement of multipolar electrode catheter via the femoral vein into right atrium and ventricle and coronary sinus; indications: to determine the electrophysiologic properties of the conduction system, induce and analyze the mechanisms of dysrhythmias, and evaluate therapeutic interventions; performed under local anesthesia

PREPROCEDURE TEACHING
Involve family or significant other in care and instructions
Assess level of understanding
Reinforce physician's explanation of purpose of procedure
Review routine preparation for procedure
    Clip hair from right groin area and neck (coronary sinus catheter is usually inserted via the internal jugular vein)
    Administer sedation as ordered
    NPO for 6 to 12 hours
    Ensure that informed consent is obtained
    Review lab tests and report any abnormal results to physician
        CBC and platelet count
        PT and PTT
        Electrolytes
        Magnesium
        Drug levels
        EKG—baseline
        Vital signs—baseline
Review sensations to be expected during procedure
    Application of multiple electrodes, defibrillating gel pads, wires, and SpO_2 probe

Palpitations
Lightheadedness
Induced dysrhythmia—patient may need to be
   defibrillated to convert the dysrhythmia
Review sensations to be expected after the procedure
   Back discomfort from lying on procedure table for 1 to
      2 hours
   Anxiety from induced dysrhythmia
Stress importance of bedrest and immobility of extremity
   for 4 hours after procedure

POSTPROCEDURE ASSESSMENT
Admission to a monitored bed in a Cardiac Cath Recovery
   Unit or CCU (based on condition of patient)

OBSERVATIONS/FINDINGS
See Cardiac Catheterization, p. 118
Hematoma at insertion site

POTENTIAL COMPLICATIONS
Hemorrhage
Venous thrombroembolism
Phlebitis
Cardiac perforation and tamponade
Refractory ventricular fibrillation
Hemothorax and pneumothorax (internal jugular vein
   approach)

POSTPROCEDURE CARE
Assess vital signs, peripheral pulses, and insertion site
   q15min $\times$ 4, then q1h for 4 hours, then as ordered
Maintain bedrest for 4 hours after procedure or as
   ordered
Elevate the head of bed 20 to 30 degrees
Obtain 12-lead ECG as ordered
Inspect the insertion site q15min for 1 hour, then every 4
   hours for 24 hours
Assess skin integrity at site of defibrillator pads if used
Ambulate as ordered
Instruct patient to report any signs of swelling, pain, or
   discoloration of insertion site
Continue ongoing care for underlying disease process

PATIENT/FAMILY TEACHING
Reinforce the physician's explanation of the results of the
   EPS study
Provide medication instructions (if ordered) to patient
   and family
Provide ICD teaching (if indicated) (see p. 151)
Provide radiofrequency ablation (RFA) teaching if
   indicated

■ RADIOFREQUENCY ABLATION (RFA)
*An invasive cardiac procedure; involves the insertion
of an electrode catheter into the specific chamber in the
heart; the catheter is positioned close to the abnormal
electrical pathway; low-energy radiofrequency (RF) current is applied to permanently interrupt electrical conduction or activity in a region of arrhythmogenic cardiac
tissue*

PREPROCEDURE TEACHING
Involve family or significant other in care and
   instructions
Assess level of understanding
Reinforce physician's explanation of purpose of
   procedure
Review routine preparation for procedure
   Clip hair from right groin area and neck (coronary
      sinus catheter is usually inserted via the internal
      jugular vein)
   Administer sedation as ordered
   NPO for 6 to 12 hours
   Ensure that informed consent is obtained
   Review lab tests and report any abnormal results to
      physician
      CBC and platelet count
      PT and PTT
      Electrolytes
      Magnesium
      Drug levels
      ECG—baseline
      Vital signs—baseline
   Application of multiple electrodes, defibrillating gel
      pads, wires, and SpO$_2$ probe
Review sensations to be expected during procedure
   Palpitations
   Lightheadedness
   Chest discomfort
Review sensations to be expected after the procedure
   Back discomfort from lying on procedure table for
      several hours
   Anxiety from induced dysrhythmia
   May experience chest discomfort during application of
      RF energy
   Stress importance of bedrest and immobility of
      extremity for 4 hours after procedure

POTENTIAL COMPLICATIONS
Hypotension
Pneumothorax
Ventricular perforation with tamponade
Pericarditis
Stroke
Bleeding

POSTPROCEDURE ASSESSMENT
OBSERVATION/FINDINGS
See Cardiac Catheterization, p. 148
Successful ablation of dysrhythmia
Insertion site: bleeding, swelling
Hematoma at insertion site

POTENTIAL COMPLICATIONS
Hemorrhage
Venous thrombroembolism
Phlebitis

Cardiac perforation and tamponade
Refractory ventricular fibrillation
Hemothorax and pneumothorax (internal jugular vein
    approach)

POSTPROCEDURE CARE

Admission to a monitored bed in a Cardiac Cath Recovery
    Unit or CCU (based on condition of patient
Monitor vital signs q15min for 1 hour, then every 4 hours
    for 24 hours
Assess peripheral pulses, and insertion site q15min × 4,
    then q1h for 4 hours, then as ordered
Maintain bedrest for 4 hours after procedure or as
    ordered
Assess the integrity of skin at sites of the defibrillator and
    Bovie pads
Elevate the head of bed 20 to 30 degrees
Obtain 12-lead ECG as ordered
Obtain echocardiogram as ordered
Inspect insertion site q15min for 1 hour, then every 4
    hours for 24 hours
Ambulate as ordered
Instruct patient to report any signs of swelling, pain, or
    discoloration of insertion site
Continue ongoing care for underlying disease process

PATIENT/FAMILY TEACHING

Reinforce the physician's explanation of the results of the
    RFA

■ IMPLANTABLE CARDIOVERTER DEFIBRILLATOR (ICD)

A programmable electronic device capable of identi-
fying and treating life-threatening ventricular tachycar-
dia (VT) and ventricular fibrillation (VF); three different
types of tiered therapy can be delivered: antitachycardia
pacing and cardioversion for VT and defibrillation for
VT; VVI pacemaker is also available for slow (brady)
rhythms after electroshock therapy

FUNCTIONS OF ICD

To monitor the heart rhythm continuously
To detect any rapid (tachy) or irregular rhythm
To deliver electrical therapy to return the heart to normal
    rhythm (Fig. 3-41 and Box 3-8)
    Antitachycardiac pacing (ATP): rapid pacing delivered
        above the rate of VT
    Cardioversion (CV): if pacing is unsuccessful, low
        energy shocks can be delivered
    Defibrillation: high-energy shock delivered for fast VT
        and VF
To provide backup ventricular pacing after electroshock
    therapy
VVI pacing may be required after electroshock therapy
    until the electrical system of the heart recovers

INDICATIONS

Patients who have survived sudden cardiac arrest
Recurrent episodes of VT and VF despite antidysrhythmic
    therapy
Positive electrophysiology study (EPS)

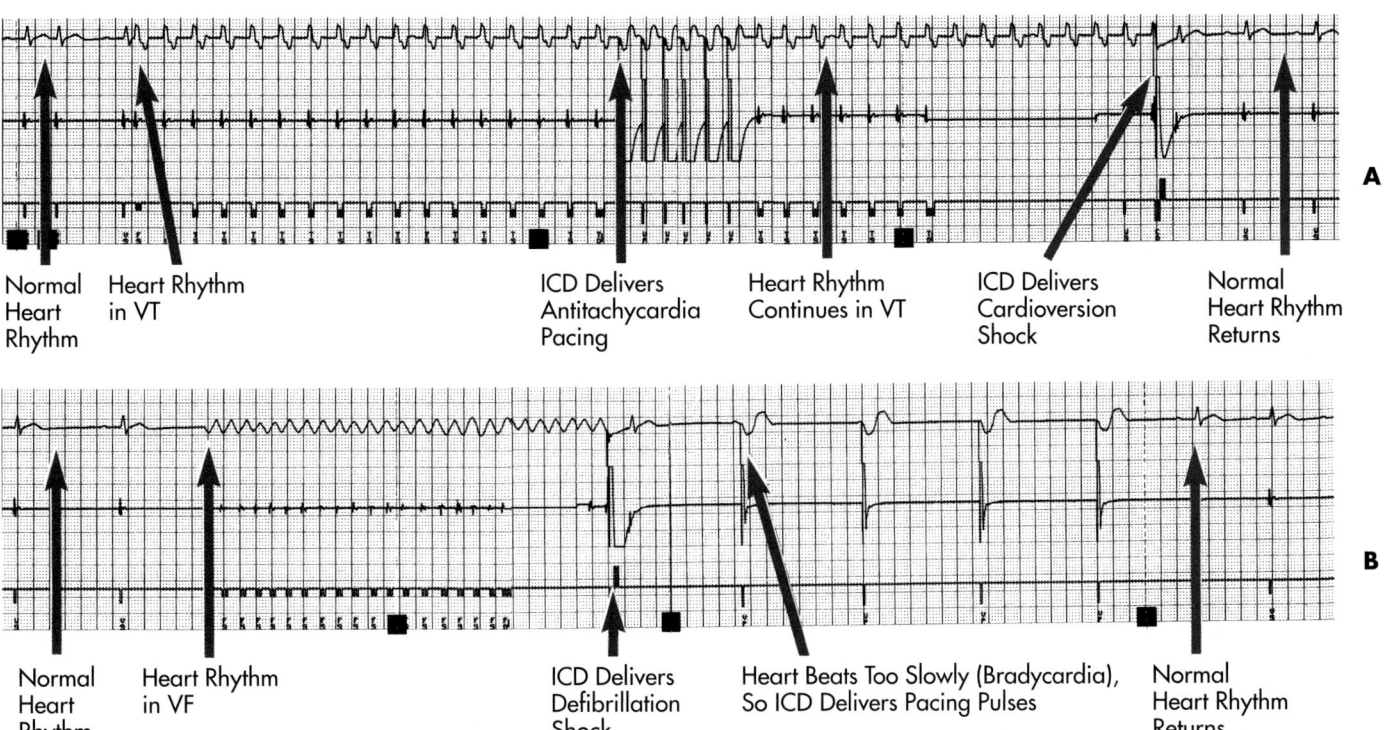

A

Normal | Heart Rhythm | ICD Delivers | Heart Rhythm | ICD Delivers | Normal
Heart | in VT | Antitachycardia | Continues in VT | Cardioversion | Heart Rhythm
Rhythm | | Pacing | | Shock | Returns

B

Normal | Heart Rhythm | ICD Delivers | Heart Beats Too Slowly (Bradycardia), | Normal
Heart | in VF | Defibrillation | So ICD Delivers Pacing Pulses | Heart Rhythm
Rhythm | | Shock | | Returns

Fig. 3-41 Delivery of cardioversion shock for ventricular tachycardia.
(*Restoring the rhythms of life, Minneapolis, 1996, pp 14-17, Medtronic, Inc.*)

Box 3-8	Types of Therapy Settings

The ICD can be programmed to deliver several types of therapies based on the patient's dysrhythmia. An ICD can deliver three types of therapy: **antitachycardia pacing (ATP), cardioversion (CV), and defibrillation.**

ANTITACHYCARDIA PACING (ATP)
If the patient's VT is relatively slow, the ICD can be programmed to detect the VT; deliver short, rapid pacing to over ride the VT; and restore normal rhythm. ICD devices can be programmed to perform multiple attempts of **ATP** to convert the VT. If **APT** fails to convert the patient out of the VT, additional programmed therapies will be delivered.

CARDIOVERSION (CV)
If the ATP fails to convert the VT, the ICD can be programmed to deliver low- to high-energy shocks to restore normal rhythm.

DEFIBRILLATION
The ICD can be programmed to detect ventricular fibrillation **(VF)** and deliver high-energy shocks to restore normal rhythm.

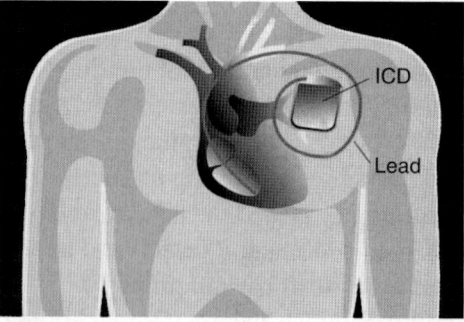
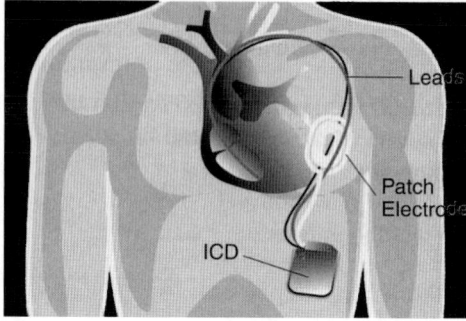

Fig. 3-42 ICD lead system placement. (Restoring the rhythms of life, *Minneapolis*, 1996, pp 14-17, *Medtronic, Inc.*)

Lead system (Fig. 3-42)
   One or two lead systems
   Transvenous or epicardial patches

INSERTION METHODS
ICD can be surgically implanted in operating room
   EP/Cath Lab
ICD is implanted either in the upper chest or abdominal area
Local anesthesia with IV conscious sedation is used for subcutaneous implantation of ICD device
Lead system usually inserted the via cephalic or subclavian vein—the most common approach
Epicardial patches requires general anesthesia and thoracotomy for insertion

PREPARATION
Withhold anticoagulation 1 to 2 days before procedure
Obtain informed consent
NPO 8 hours before procedure
Administer antibiotics if ordered
Obtain baseline data
   CBC and platelets
   PT and PTT
   ECG
   Chest x-ray
   Electrolytes
Skin prep
   Place monitoring electrodes on posterior shoulder areas
   Clip hair from neck to nipple line

PREPROCEDURAL TEACHING
Assess level of understanding and emotional status
Reinforce physician's explanation of procedure
Involve family or significant other in care and instruction
Explain and review postprocedure care
   Admission to CCU for first 24 hours for observation
Importance of restricting activities for first 24 to 48 hours to avoid lead dislodgment
Arm sling applied for first 24 to 48 hours

POTENTIAL COMPLICATIONS
Bleeding
Venous thrombosis
Cardiac perforation
Cardiac tamponade
Pneumothorax
Lead dislodgment or fracture
Malfunction of device
   Failure to sense and discharge
   Inappropriate discharges
Incision
   Infection
   Hematoma
Subclavian crush syndrome

POSTPROCEDURE TEACHING
Assess the level understanding and degree of readiness to learn
Discuss incisional care with family or significant other
Discuss predischarge device testing with patient and family
Discuss signs and symptoms of incisional infection
Encourage patient to discuss his or her emotional feelings concerning the ICD

DISCHARGE/HOME CARE PLANNING

ACTIVITIES

Keep incision clean and dry

Keep incisions dry—no showering until first
postprocedure visit with physician

Activity as ordered by physician

No lifting or swinging affected arm over head for 4 to 6
weeks—prevent lead dislodgment

Avoid tight clothing that may irritate skin over ICD

Avoid lifting more than 10 lb

Avoid excessive pushing, pulling, or twisting

Report any redness, swelling, or drainage

No driving until physician allows

INTERFERENCE WITH THE ICD

Avoid anything that has an electromagnetic field—
magnets or electrical items

Known as *EMI* (electromagnetic interference)

EMI can blind the ICD, preventing it from treating the
dysrhythmias or cause inappropriate therapy

Instruct patient to simply move away form the source
of EMI and the ICD will work normally

Teach patient and family which sources of EMI do/do
not affect the ICD

Household appliance, tools, and office equipment

Household appliances and tools that can be
operated safely (ICD have built-in feature to
protect it from most interference produced by
electrical appliances)

Microwave ovens

TVs, AM/FM radios, VCRs, and remote controls

Garage door openers

Tabletop appliances—toasters, blenders,
electric can openers, electric knives, etc.

Handheld appliances—hair dryers, shavers
(avoid holding against your implant side)

Washers and dryers, electric stoves,
refrigerator

Electric blankets and heating pads

Spark-ignited internal combustion engines,
lawn mowers, leaf blowers, automobiles, etc.

Personal computers, printers, electric
typewriter, fax machine, copying machine

Machine shop equipment—drills, table saws, etc.

Teach patient to keep tools 12 inches from ICD

Other sources of interference

Ask your physician about the following:

Industrial equipment

Arc and resistance welders

Induction furnaces

Large generators and power plants

Large magnets—such as the ones in stereo
speakers

Antennas for CB and ham radios

Large TV towers and power lines—maintain 25
feet between you and the lines or towers

Things to avoid

Maintenance or repair of any electrical or
gas-powered appliance or tool

Chain saws

Touching spark plugs or distributor on a running
lawn mower or car—turn engine off

MEDICAL PROCEDURES

Always inform any medial personnel that you have an ICD

The following medical equipment will not interfere
with the ICD

Diagnostic x-rays, CT scans, mammograms

Dental drill and ultrasonic probes

The following equipment may be used with ICD
providing the equipment is not placed directly over
the implant site

Therapeutic ultrasound, TENS, and electrolysis

Electrosurgery, diathermy, lithotripsy, and radiation
therapy produce high levels of interference—discuss
use with your physician

MRI is not recommended for ICD patients

SECURITY SYSTEMS

Instruct patient that he or she can walk through the
screening archways at airports, etc.

Do not stop in areas adjacent to the detection
equipment

ICD may set off the alarm

Show ICD ID card to personnel

Do not allow the personnel to use handheld wand (wand
can temporarily interfere with proper operation of the
ICD)

Ask to be hand searched

CELLULAR PHONES

Hold phone to ear opposite the side of ICD

Do not carry phone in breast pocket, or on belt or within
6 inches of ICD

IDENTIFICATION CARD

Instruct patient to carry a temporary ICD ID card until
the permanent card arrives in the mail

FOLLOW-UP VISITS

Discuss the importance of follow-up visits to ensure that
the ICD is functioning properly

Frequency of follow-up visits is every 3 months until
the battery status diminishes to replacement level

The ICD check is painless

Physician may reprogram the device at a follow-up
visit

Inform physician of any problems or change in
medications

REPLACEMENT

Discuss longevity of battery for ICD

Different for each manufacturer and how much the
device is used

ICD generator will be removed under local anesthesia
and replaced

Local anesthesia

Usually a same-day procedure

WHEN TO CALL THE PHYSICIAN

Instruct patient or family call the physician when the following occurs:

Receives a shock

Develops a rapid heart rhythm longer than 3 minutes

Has any questions about the ICD or medications

Plans to travel or move

Experiences any new or unusual symptoms

WHEN THE PATIENT RECEIVES A SHOCK

Ensure that the patient and family know what to do if the patient receives a shock

One shock—call physician's office

Two shocks—call physician's office and make arrangements for an ICD check

Three shocks—go to local emergency room

Stay calm and move to a place where the patient can sit or lie down

Have someone stay with the patient if possible

Have the family call an ambulance if the patient receives shocks and is unconscious for more than a minute

■ PERCUTANEOUS TRANSLUMINAL CORONARY ANGIOPLASTY (PTCA)

Invasive nonsurgical procedure using a balloon-tipped catheter to restore patency of coronary artery by compressing atheromatous plaques within the artery

directional coronary atherectomy (DCA): *Atherectomy is selective excision and removal of atheroma deposits from coronary vessel walls. Catheter contains a cylindrical cutter that shaves the plaque and deposits it into the nose cone of the catheter*

Percutaneous Transluminal Coronary Atherectomy (PTCRA)—Rotablator: *An elliptical steel burr coated with rough diamond chip attached to a flexible rotating shaft. The calcified plaque is pulverized as the burr spins at 200,000 rpms*

coronary stents: *A stainless steel scaffold that is inserted inside the lumen of the coronary artery to prevent abrupt closure of the vessel following PTCA, PTCRA, or DCA*

PREPROCEDURE TEACHING

Assess level of understanding and emotional status: fears of procedure and possible necessity of cardiac surgery

Involve family or significant other in care and instruction

Reinforce physician's explanation of purpose of procedure, desired outcome, and associated risks

Explain need to follow directions regarding administration and withholding of medications

Encourage verbalization and questions

Explain that procedure is similar to cardiac catheterization, identifying any previous negative experiences; procedure may last 45 min to 1½ hour

Review routine preparation for procedure

Medication for sedation may be ordered

No food or water for at least 8 hours before procedure

Explain sensations to be expected

During procedure

Palpitations

Warm, flushed feeling during injection of dye

Possible chest discomfort during balloon inflation

After procedure

Soreness at insertion site; arterial venous sheaths may remain in place until ACT/PTT has normalized

Possible backache from lying on table for 3 to 5 hours

Fatigue

Stress importance of bed rest and immobility of extremity after procedure

Stress importance of drinking fluids for first 6 to 8 hours to wash out contrast material

Explain and review postprocedure activities

Need to be admitted to CCU or Cardiac Cath Recovery unit for 24 to 36 hours for observation

Visiting privileges

Additional equipment to be used

Temporary pacing electrode

Cardiac monitor

Oxygen administration

Pulse oximetry (SpO_2)

Foley catheter

Knee immobilizer

IV therapy

NOTE: Cardiac surgical team should be available for emergent cardiac surgery procedure; see Cardiac surgery on p. 119 for brief explanation of differences in patient care after cardiac surgery

During procedure intraaortic balloon pump must be available on standby

PREPARATION

Obtain informed consent

Maintain NPO 8 hours before procedure

Withhold anticoagulation therapy 1 to 2 days before procedure

Administer medications as ordered

Salicylates and antiplatelet drugs may be ordered 2 days before procedure

Nitrates

Beta-blocking agents may be decreased

Calcium antagonists

Sedation

Obtain baseline data

CBC, platelet count

Electrolytes

BUN, creatinine

Blood type and cross match

Coagulation studies

ECG

Chest x-ray

POSTPROCEDURE ASSESSMENT
SUBJECTIVE DATA

Chest pain, pressure

SOB

Dizziness, lightheadedness
Anxiety

OBJECTIVE DATA
ECG changes
  ST elevations, depressions
  Ventricular dysrhythmias
Skin
  Pale
  Diaphoretic
Hypotension (systolic BP <90 mm Hg)
Bleeding or hematoma at site of insertion
Vasospasm of affected extremity
  Numbness
  Tingling
  Cyanosis
  Loss of pulse
  Pain
Dysrhythmias

DIAGNOSTIC TESTS
CBC, platelet count
Coagulation studies: APTT, activated clotting time (ACT)
Serum potassium and sodium
Cardiac enzymes: CPK
BUN, creatinine
12-Lead ECG

POTENTIAL COMPLICATIONS
Failure to dilate coronary artery
Abrupt coronary occlusion
MI
Bleeding
Rupture or dissection of coronary artery
  Cardiac tamponade
  MI
  Shock
  Cardiac arrest
  Death
Cannulated extremity
  Ischemia
  Vascular complication
    Hemorrhage
      Hematoma
      Retroperitoneal
      Pseudoaneurysm
      A-V fistula
  Thrombosis formation (clot or air)
  Aortic dissection
Renal hypersensitivity to contrast material

MULTIDISCIPLINARY MANAGEMENT
THERAPEUTIC MANAGEMENT
Admission to CCU or cardiac cath recovery unit for 24 to 48 hours
Bed rest
Cardiac monitor
Parenteral fluids
Medications
  Heparin infusion or antiplatelet infusion

Nitrates
Calcium channel blockers
  Aspirin
  Antiplatelet drugs

PATIENT PROBLEMS—NURSING DIAGNOSES/INTERVENTIONS

▼ Risk for altered tissue perfusion (peripheral) related to hematoma, thrombus formation, secondary to arterial cannulation

Assess pulses distal to site, noting quality, q15min × 4, decreasing frequency as ordered; note skin color, temperature
Observe for diminished pulses in extremity distal to cannulation site; report decreased or absent pulses immediately to physician
Maintain bed rest for 6 to 8 hours in supine position until arterial and venous sheaths are removed; when sheaths are removed maintain 5- to 10-lb sandbag over cannulation site
Inspect cannulation site for swelling, tenderness, discoloration, warmth, and drainage
Keep extremity immobile for 2 to 4 hours after procedure; log roll patient side to side; raise head of bed 15 degrees
Inspect dressing at site of insertion q2h to 4h, noting amount and color of drainage
Reinforce dressing as necessary
Inspect surrounding skin
  Redness or discoloration
  Swelling
  Irritation
Administer antiplatelets as ordered
Monitor coagulation studies, reporting prolonged PTT to physician

Expected Outcomes
Maintains adequate peripheral tissue perfusion
Pulse is full and bounding
Cannulation site: color is good, there are no signs of tenderness or swelling

▼ Risk for decreased cardiac output related to myocardial ischemia or dysrhythmias

Assess for signs of diminished CO
Monitor BP, R, and apical pulse q15min for 1 hour, then q30min for 1 hour, then qh for 6 hours, then as ordered
Monitor cardiac activity, check rhythm strips q4h and prn, observing for signs of ischemia or dysrhythmias
Obtain 12-lead ECG during episodes of chest pain; observe for and report any signs of ischemic change or dysrhythmias
Auscultate chest for heart and lung sounds q4h for 24 hours
Monitor intake and output; report output <30 ml/hr or inability to void within first 4 hours
Administer medications as ordered

Expected Outcomes

Maintains good CO
Vital signs are stable
Urine output is good
Mentation is clear

PATIENT/FAMILY TEACHING

NOTE: Refer to p. 90 for education for patients with angina
   pectoris
Assess level of understanding
Reinforce physician's explanation of postprocedure results
Review allowances and limitations of activity
   Avoid heavy lifting and pushing
   Ambulate at regular intervals
Explain importance of calling physician if chest pain
   occurs lasting longer than 20 minutes
Discuss medications: name, dosage, time of
   administration, purpose, and side effects
Explain importance of taking antiplatelet medications as
   ordered
Explain importance of ongoing outpatient care
Refer to standard for angina pectoris for patient teaching
   regarding
   Chest pain
   Risk factors
   Exercise, activities

Additional Nursing Diagnosis to Consider

Anxiety related to perceived biologic threat

■ THROMBOLYTIC THERAPY

*Infusion of thrombolytic agents to promote clot lysis, re-
store coronary blood flow, and limit myocardial ischemia*

PREPROCEDURE TEACHING

Assess level of understanding and anxiety level
Involve family or significant other in care and instruction
Reinforce physician's explanation of purpose of
   procedure, desired outcome, and associated risks
Describe procedure to be performed
   Intracoronary (IC) given
      Direct IC push via the guiding catheter over 15 to
         30 minutes.
   Intravenous: usually in emergency department or in
      CCU; infusion administered over 3-hour period
Explain and review intraprocedure and postprocedure
   routines
   Monitoring in CCU
   Visiting privileges
   Equipment to be used
      Cardiac monitor
      Oxygen administration
      Pulse oximetry (SpO$_2$)
      IV therapy
Explain need for bed rest during and after administration
   and need for frequent blood sampling to monitor
   clotting times
Instruct patient to inform nurse if chest pain develops

PREPARATION

Review past medical history to identify any
   contraindications (Box 3-9)
Obtain informed consents as required: thrombolytic therapy,
   cardiac catheterization, PTCA, and CABG surgery
Obtain baseline laboratory data
   To determine hemostatic status: CBC with platelets, PT,
      fibrinogen, fibrin split-product labels
   To determine degree of myocardial injury: CPK-MB
   Blood type and cross match, electrolytes, BUN,
      creatinine
Obtain diagnostic data
   12-Lead ECG/18-lead ECG
   Chest x-ray examination
Establish two to three patent IV lines
Administer medications as ordered

POSTPROCEDURE ASSESSMENT
OBSERVATIONS/FINDINGS

Successful myocardial reperfusion
   Abrupt cessation of chest pain
   ECG changes: return of ST elevations to baseline
   Dysrhythmias: sinus bradycardia, AV block with
      hypotension, ventricular tachycardia
   Isoenzyme: early peaking of CPK-MB (within 12 hours
      of onset of symptoms)
Bleeding/hemorrhage
   Surface bleeding: oozing from puncture or catheter
      insertion site, gingival bleeding, ecchymoses
   GI: hematemesis, tarry stools, positive occult blood
Coronary artery reocclusion
   Chest pain
   ECG: ST-T wave changes
   Dysrhythmias
Skin
   Pale
   Diaphoretic
   Clammy
Hypotension
Tachycardia
Anxiety
Shivering

Box 3-9	**Thrombolytic Contraindications**

CONTRAINDICATIONS
- Active internal bleeding
- Recent surgery or major trauma (within 2 months)
- Recent stroke (<6 months)
- CNS malignancy
- Bleeding diathesis (check PT, PTT, platelets, hematocrit)
- Severe uncontrolled hypertension (diastolic blood pres-
  sure >120 mm Hg, systolic blood pressure >200 mm
  Hg)
- Pregnancy

From Kern M: The cardiac catheterization handbook, *ed 3, St Louis,
1999, Mosby.*

Diagnostic Tests
CBC
Serum fibrinogen levels
APTT
CPK-MB

Potential Complications
Bleeding
Hemorrhage: GI, intracranial
Myocardial ischemia or infarction

Multidisciplinary Management
Therapeutic Management
Admission to CCU
Bed rest
Cardiac monitoring
Hemodynamic monitoring
Arterial pressure, PA, PWCP
PTCA
Medications
    During procedure
        Thrombolytic agents
            Streptokinase (SK)
            Urokinase (UK)
            Tissue plasminogen activator (t-PA)
            Anisoylated plasminogen-SK activator complex
                (APSAC)
        Diphenhydramine
        Heparin
    After procedure
        Heparin

Patient Problems—Nursing Diagnoses/Interventions

▼ Risk for fluid volume deficit related to bleeding/hemorrhage secondary to thrombolysis-induced coagulopathy

Assess for signs and symptoms of surface or internal bleeding
Monitor BP and HR according to unit protocol during first hour, decreasing frequency as condition stabilizes
Inspect puncture sites every 15 minutes; apply manual pressure when removing IV catheters
Initiate measures that prevent disruption of vascular integrity and/or keep venous or arterial puncture and injections to a minimum
Instruct patient to avoid vigorous tooth brushing
Avoid removing IV or arterial lines during first 24 to 48 hours or as indicated by specific agents
Use heparin lock for IV access or blood sampling
Monitor PTT valves

Expected Outcomes
Demonstrates no signs of bleeding
Hemostasis is reestablished
    Coagulation studies are within acceptable limits

No signs of surface or internal bleeding
Vital signs are within normal limits

▼ Risk for decreased cardiac output related to reperfusion dysrhythmias

Assess and record ECG changes during and after thrombolytic therapy
Assess and monitor BP, HR, R, and hemodynamic response to reperfusion dysrhythmias as they appear
Administer antidysrhythmic medications as ordered; keep medications and defibrillator at bedside

Expected Outcomes
Maintains good CO
ECG remains in stable or normal rhythm
Reperfusion dysrhythmias are controlled or absent
Vital signs remain stable

▼ Risk for chest pain related to decreased myocardial tissue perfusion secondary to reocclusion of coronary artery

Assess and monitor complaints of chest pain, noting patient's nonverbal expressions; compare with preprocedural chest pain complaints
Obtain 12-lead ECG during episode of chest pain, compare with baseline ECG taken after thrombolysis; report any changes
Maintain on bed rest
Monitor BP, HR, R
Administer analgesia: morphine sulfate
Prepare for possible catheterization, repeat thrombolysis, PTCA

Expected Outcome
Verbalizes absence of chest pain

■ Anticoagulant Therapy
anticoagulant: Medication administered to prevent or treat arterial or venous thrombosis; used in treatment of pulmonary embolism, cerebral embolism, and valvular heart disease, and with a heart valve prosthesis

Assessment
Observations/Findings
Therapeutic serum levels
    Warfarin: protime—1.5 to 2½ × control
    INR—2 to 3
        Heparin: PTT—
            2 to 3 × control
Hematuria
Pain
    Abdominal
    Flank
Tarry stools
Hematemesis
Epistaxis

Bleeding gums
Hemoptysis
Subcutaneous bleeding
Ecchymosis
Hematoma
Joints
   Pain
   Immobility
Site of incision
   Bleeding
   Immobility
Neurologic changes
Increased menstrual flow
Medications
   Potentiate anticoagulation
   Retard anticoagulation

INTERVENTIONS

Administer parenteral heparin as ordered
   Use heparin lock if ordered
   Give heparin at exact time ordered
   Give dosage over a period of 1 minute
   Never skip doses
   Do not remove heparin lock for 2 hours after last dose
   Maintain continuous heparin infusion if ordered; administer IV drip via infusion pump
   Administer subcutaneous heparin as ordered, rotating sites
   Coordinate all laboratory work; avoid multiple punctures
   Maintain manual pressure for at least 3 minutes after venous punctures
   Check puncture sites qh
   Monitor BP and P q4h to 8h
Avoid taking rectal temperature
Administer IM medications cautiously; apply manual pressure to injection sites until bleeding stops
Have protamine sulfate or phytonadione (Aqua-Mephyton) available
Administer routine medications cautiously; may potentiate or retard anticoagulation

◼ WARFARIN

PATIENT/FAMILY TEACHING

Ensure that patient and/or significant other knows and understands
   Name of medication, dosage, time of administration, purpose, and side effects
   Need to avoid taking over-the-counter medications without checking with physician; to read labels of all medications
      Cold prescriptions with aspirin
      Laxatives
      Vitamins
   Need to avoid aspirin (acetylsalicylic acid) without physician's order
   Importance of having laboratory work done as ordered and of contacting physician for possible dosage change

General side effects: anorexia, nausea, vomiting, abdominal cramps, dermatitis, and urticaria
Signs of bleeding to report to physician
   Hematuria
   Vomiting
   Elevated temperature
   Pain in joints, swelling
   Epistaxis
   Bleeding gums
   Easy bruisability
   Increased menstrual flow
Abdominal pain
Diet—moderate- to low-fat content without abundance of dark, leafy green vegetables; avoid excessive use of alcohol

DISCHARGE/HOME CARE PLANNING

Safety precautions to prevent injury
   Avoid vigorous nose-blowing and tooth brushing
   Avoid use of sharp-edged instruments such as razors
   Refrain from water-jet tooth cleaners; use soft-bristled toothbrush
   Refrain from engaging in dangerous hobbies or contact sports
   Wear shoes and slippers at all times
Importance of avoiding pregnancy while on medication; need to report to physician if pregnancy is suspected
Need to avoid use of intrauterine device (IUD) for birth control
Importance of ongoing outpatient care
Need to carry medical alert or identification card with name of medication
Need to inform physician when planning to travel in order to do the following:
   Obtain extra medications
   Arrange laboratory test
   Need to inform physician if a surgical procedure or cardiac catheterization is scheduled

◼ SUBCUTANEOUS HEPARIN INJECTION

ASSESSMENT

OBSERVATIONS/FINDINGS

Subcutaneous bleeding
   Hematoma
   Bruises
   Intraabdominal bleeding
   Pain
   Rigid, tender abdomen
Tarry stools
Bleeding gums
Epistaxis
Hematemesis
Hemoptysis
Hematuria
Injection sites
   Inflammation
   Bruises
   Tenderness
Increased menstrual flow

Allergic reactions
Itching
Urticaria
Redness
Joints
Pain
Immobility
Pain
Flank
Abdominal

PATIENT/FAMILY TEACHING
GENERAL GUIDELINES
Ensure that patient and/or significant other knows and
understands
Name of medication, dosage, time of administration,
purpose, and side effects
Importance of giving heparin injections at exact time
designated
Importance of not skipping any doses; keep record of
all missed doses
Need to avoid taking over-the-counter medications
without checking with physician
Aspirin
Salicylates
Need to avoid drinking alcoholic beverages while on
heparin therapy
Importance of having laboratory work done as ordered
Signs of bleeding to report to physician
Bleeding gums
Joint pain
Epistaxis
Hematuria
Tarry stools
Increased menstrual flow
Easy bruisability
Safety precautions to prevent injury
Avoid vigorous nose-blowing
Avoid vigorous tooth brushing
Avoid use of sharp-edged instruments such as razors
Refrain from engaging in dangerous hobbies or
contact sports
Importance of preventing pregnancy while on
medication; need to report to physician if
pregnancy is suspected
Need to avoid use of IUD for birth control
Importance of taking correct dosage at correct time
Demonstrate and explain purpose of each step of heparin
therapy
Preparation for injection
Rotation of injection sites
Action of heparin
Care of equipment
Have patient repeat steps verbally and then perform
procedure
Positively reinforce proper performance of procedure
and correct errors
Leave equipment at bedside for practice: syringe (1 to 2
ml with needle (25-gauge, ½ to ⅝ inch), vial of sterile
water, alcohol swabs, and flat sponge or orange

Arrange to have equipment that will be used at home
available
Have patient continue procedure with supervision while
in hospital

PREPARATION OF INJECTION
Ensure that patient and/or significant other demonstrates
Handwashing technique
Preparation of syringe and needle using sterile
technique
Withdrawal of exact heparin dosage
Ability to maintain sterile technique throughout
procedure

SITE OF INJECTION
Ensure that patient and/or significant other knows and
understands
Importance of using subcutaneous fatty tissue and
avoiding bruised areas, hematomas, incisions, or
scarred tissue and the area within 5 cm (2 inches)
of umbilicus
Importance of rotating site of injection with every
dose of heparin to prevent bleeding or tissue
damage
Importance of recording site of each injection

INJECTION
Ensure that patient and/or significant other demonstrates
injection technique
Select injection site (Fig. 3-43, A)
Prepare skin by cleaning with alcohol
Hold syringe filled with correct heparin dosage like a
pencil or a dart
Pinch up skin, forming a flat roll between fingers (Fig.
3-43, B)
Insert needle at 45-degree angle and quickly push it
into subcutaneous tissue up to hub of syringe; may
need to guide patient's hand at this point
(Fig. 3-43, C)
NOTE: Do not pull back on plunger
Inject medication slowly
Withdraw needle; gently release skin as needle is
removed
Press area gently; avoid rubbing or massaging area
Record date, time, site, and dosage of each injection on
home record (Table 3-11)

Table 3-11	**Heparin Home Record***		
Date	**Time**	**Site**	**Dosage**
1/1/00	6:30 AM	Right upper side	5000 U
	2:30 PM	Left upper side	5000 U
	10:30 PM	Right lower side	5000 U
1/1/00			
1/1/00			

Physician's order—5000 U heparin injected every 8 hours.

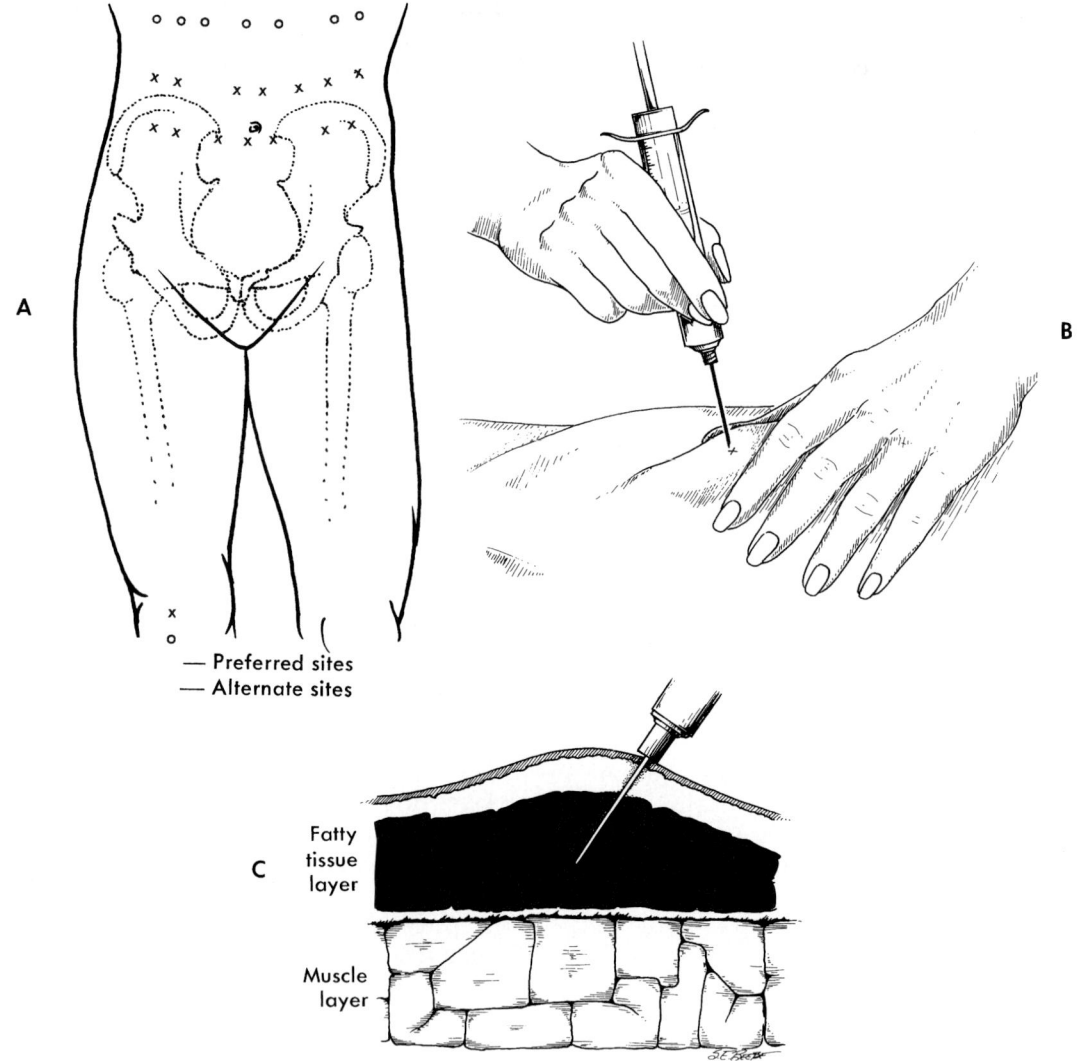

— Preferred sites
— Alternate sites

Fatty
tissue
layer

Muscle
layer

Fig. 3-43   Subcutaneous heparin injection. **A,** Sites to be used. **B,** Pinching skin to form a flat roll between fingers. **C,** Injection into fatty tissue layer.

BIBLIOGRAPHY

Agency for Health Care Policy and Research: *Clinical practice guidelines: "Cardiac rehabilitation,"* 1995; *"Heart failure: management of patients with left-ventricular systolic dysfunction,"* 1994; *"Unstable angina: diagnosis and management,"* 1994, National Heart, Lung and Blood Institute, U.S. Department of Health and Human Services, 1994.

American Heart Association: *Guidelines for cardiac rehabilitation,* ed 2, Los Angeles, 1982, The Association, Greater Los Angeles Affiliation.

Braunwald E, ed: *Heart disease: a textbook of cardiovascular medicine,* Philadelphia, 1988, WB Saunders.

Canobbio MM: *Cardiovascular disorders,* ed 3, St Louis, 1990, Mosby.

Canobbio MM: Cardiovascular system. In Thompson JM et al, eds: *Mosby's manual of clinical nursing,* ed 5, St Louis, 1998, Mosby.

Canobbio MM: Congenital heart disease in adults. In Clochesy JM et al, eds: *Critical care nursing,* ed 2, Philadelphia, 1995, WB Saunders.

Conn VS, Taylor SG, Casey B: Cardiac rehabilitation program participation and outcomes after myocardial infarction, *Rehabil Nurs* 17(2):58-62, 1992.

Conover MB: *Exercises in diagnosing ECG tracings,* ed 3, St Louis, 1984, Mosby.

Conover MB: *Pocket guide to electrocardiography,* ed 3, St Louis, 1994, Mosby.

Conover MB: *Understanding electrocardiography,* ed 7, St Louis, 1996, Mosby.

Ernst CB, Stanley JC, eds: *Current therapy in vascular surgery,* Philadelphia, 1991, BC Decker. *Mosby's Patient teaching guides,* St Louis, 1994, Mosby.

Pagana KD, Pagana TJ: *Mosby's diagnostic and laboratory test reference,* ed 3, St Louis, 1998, Mosby.

Ryan TJ, et al: Guidelines for percutaneous transluminal coronary angioplasty: a report of the ACC/AHA task force, *J Am Coll Cardiol* 22:2033, 1993.

Skidmore-Roth L: *Mosby's 1999 nursing drug reference,* St Louis, 1999, Mosby.

Smith S: AACN tissue and organ transplantation: implications for professional nursing practice, St Louis, 1990, Mosby.

Spillall JA: Office diagnosis of occlusive arterial disease, *J Cardiovasc Med*, 1984, p 107.

Swearingen PL et al: *Manual of critical care: applying nursing diagnosis to adult critical illness,* ed 3, St Louis, 1995, Mosby.

Teplitz L: Transcatheter ablation of tachyarrhythmias: an overview and case studies, *Prog Cardiovasc Nurs* 9:16-31, 1994.

Thelan L et al: *Critical care nursing: diagnosis and management,* ed 3, St Louis, 1998, Mosby.

Underhill S et al: *Cardiac nursing,* ed 3, Philadelphia, 1994, JB Lippincott.

Wright JM: Pharmacologic management of congestive heart failure, *CCQ* 18(1):32-44 1995.

Zelkovic M, Nichols GG: Carotid endathectomy in symptomatic patients, *Heart Dis Stroke* 2(4):313-316, 1993.

DIAGNOSIS ___ AORTIC PROCEDURES

SURGERY ___ AORTO-FEMORAL BYPASS/ANEURYSMS   DRG 111   ALOS 8.4

USC UNIVERSITY HOSPITAL
1500 San Pablo
Los Angeles, CA 90033 ©1991
SIDE 1   **MULTIDISCIPLINARY PLAN**

NAME ___
ALLERGIES ___
ADMIT DATE ___

DISCHARGE OUTCOMES

PHYSIOLOGICAL: Patient will maintain patent graft site(s) post-operatively. Patient will be hemodynamically stable, adequate nutrition maintained, and free from complications/infection.

COGNITIVE: Patient will verbalize acceptance of diagnosis and ask pertinent questions regarding future management of health care.

PSYCHOLOGICAL: Patient will verbalize acceptance of potential lifestyle changes, express concerns, and ask questions. Patient will exhibit appropriate coping mechanisms.

DISCIPLINE	PRE-OP/ PRE-ADMIT	DAY 1	DOS DAY 2	POD#1 DAY 3	POD#2 DAY 4	POD#3 DAY 5	POD#4 DAY 6
LOCATION		MED/SURG	SURGERY/PAR/SICU	SICU	SICU → DOU	DOU	DOU → MED/SURG
	DATE ___	DATE ___	DATE ___	DATE ___	DATE ___	DATE ___	DATE ___
LABS		Cell Saver T&C 6 units CBC Chem 20 UA PT PTT	Stat Hct on arrival to unit Spun Hct q 6° x 24° CBC Chem 7	CBC Chem 7	CBC Chem 7	DC daily labs p̄ eating Chem 7 qod	
CARDIO-PULMONARY		ECG Preop non-invasive vascular lab doppler study Pulse oximetry	Intubated → ventilator ABG Invasive monitoring Swan-ganz to monitor	Extubate ECG I.S. post-extubation	DC Swan Ganz & PA-line prior to transfer I.S. q1°	I.S. q1° W/A	I.S. q1° W/A
IMAGING/ NUCLEAR MEDICINE		CXR	Non-invasive intra-operative graft monitoring prior to closure.	CXR if pt remains intubated			
SOCIAL SERVICES D/C PLAN REHAB. SERVICES			Social worker consult Assess for potential home needs				
PHARMACY		Pre-op antibiotics Bowel prep c̄ phospha soda Ancef 1 gm IV	IV antibiotics x 24° Cardiac medication Pain medications Nipride drip for SBP>160 IV-D5LR 100-125cc/hr	If diabetic-pt will require Accu✓ c̄ insulin coverage	DC Nipride if not already done		Convert IV to S.L.
DIETARY/ NUTRITION		Clear liquids NPO p̄ midnight	NPO NG tube to LCS x 24°	DC NG tube Strict NPO		Clear liquids	Advance diet

Used by permission of USC University Hospital, Los Angeles, California.

PATIENT NAME: _____

MULTIDISCIPLINARY PLAN

DISCIPLINE	PRE-OP/ PRE-ADMIT	DAY 1	DOS DAY 2	POD#1 DAY 3	POD#2 DAY 4	POD#3 DAY 5	POD#4 DAY 6
		DATE __	DATE __	DATE __	DATE __	DATE __	DATE __
PATIENT ACTIVITY		Up as tolerated Betadine scrub to abdomen & lower extremities	Bedrest Turn q2° Compression boots	Dangle	OOB to chair Stand at bedside prior to transfer	Ambulate c̄ walker & assistance	Progressive ambulation DC compression boots when fully ambulatory
EDUCATION		Orientation to hospital Pre-op leg exercises I.S. C & DB Foley				Emphasize risk factors associated c̄ vascular disease including diet, smoking & pulse checks DC Foley	Pt to return demonstrate pulse checks Home expectations: • avoid heavy physical activity

COLLABORATIVE PROBLEMS

❶ Tissue perfusion, altered R/T graft, & hemodynamics.

❷ Alteration in comfort; pain R/T incisional site.

❸ Anxiety, fear R/T illness & hospitalization.

❹ Alteration in gas exchange/airway maintenance R/T intubation, mechanical ventilation, & general anesthesia.

❺ Potential for infection R/T surgical procedure & acute care stay.

❻ Knowledge deficit R/T discharge expectations, activity levels, & follow-up care.

OUTCOMES

❶ Pt will be free of tissue ischemia c̄ patent graft; adequate arterial blood flow; absence of thrombophlebitis.

❷ Pt will have absence or reduction of pain/discomfort.

❸ Pt will verbalize a reduction in anxiety c̄ provision of information & encouragement.

❹ Pt will display adequate respiratory function c̄ sats >92%.

❺ Pt will remain infection free & afebrile.

❹ Pt will demonstrate effective use of I.S. q1°

❶ Pt will be weaned off vasoactive drips & restarted or pre-op medications.

❷ Pt will exhibit a decreased requirement for pain medications; pain controlled on po medications.

❻ Pt will verbalize understanding of disease processes & risk factors. Able to verbalize expectations for follow-up care & ambulating independently.

KEY

❶ To initiate a problem or intervention, document under corresponding date.

❷ Document outcomes under appropriate date for achieving the goal.

❸ To discontinue an intervention or resolve a patient problem highlight, date, and initial.

Continued.

PLAN OF CARE DISCUSSED WITH		
DATE	INITIAL	S.O.	Pt.

Case Manager: _____

Consulting MD: _____

Social Service _____

Anointing of
The Sick
Date: _____

INTERVENTIONS

DAY 1	DOS DAY 2	POD#1 DAY 3	POD#2 DAY 4	POD#3 DAY 5	POD#4 DAY 6
DATE ___	DATE ___	DATE ___	DATE ___	DATE ___	DATE ___
—Explain disease process, expected outcomes, & provide information as needed	—Monitor all circulatory parameters distal to graft (designated by surgeon): • pulses • color • sensation • numbness • temperature • level of discomfort • immobility	—Check pulses by palpation or doppler q2° x 48°	—Nipride discontinued prior to transfer	—Check pulses by palpation or doppler q4° —Assist c̄ ambulation —Begin teaching in reference to risk factors associated c̄ disease	—Assess ambulation
—Encourage pt to verbalize fears	—Check pulses by palpation or doppler q1° x 24°	—Begin weaning off Nipride	—D/C O₂ sats if not on transfer orders	—Continue I & O —Assess pt ability to tolerate ordered diet	
	—Maintain hemodynamic lines; closely monitor hemodynamic profile & I & O				
	—Turn pt maintaining straight legs; support legs c̄ pillows				
	—Monitor for chest pain & ECG changes				
	—Avoid restriction of affected extremity				
	—Assess pt for nature of pain; note quality, site, & severity of pain				
	—Medicate c̄ analgesics as ordered. Assess for effectiveness				
	—Monitor for ↑ temperature, redness or drainage from surgical site, tachycardia & elevated WBC				
	—Maintain ventilator settings as ordered				
	—Monitor O₂ sats, assess breath sounds q4°; Nipride to keep SBP < 180 (or ordered parameter)				

MULTIDISCIPLINARY PLAN UPDATE

DATE	SIGNATURES	DATE	SIGNATURES	DATE	SIGNATURES

page 1 of 3

USC UNIVERSITY HOSPITAL
1500 San Pablo
Los Angeles, CA 90033 ©1991

SIDE 2   **MULTIDISCIPLINARY PLAN**

NAME _____
ALLERGIES _____
ADMIT DATE _____

DIAGNOSIS _____

SURGERY
AORTIC PROCEDURES
AORTO-FEMORAL BYPASS/ANEURYSMS   DRG _____ ALOS _____

DISCHARGE OUTCOMES	
PHYSIOLOGICAL	Patient will maintain adequate nutrition. Graft site will remain patent postoperatively. Patient will be hemodynamically stable & free from complications/infection.
COGNITIVE	Patient will verbalize acceptance of diagnosis & ask pertinent questions regarding future management of health care.
PSYCHOLOGICAL	Patient will verbalize acceptance of potential lifestyle changes, express concerns and ask questions. Patient will exhibit appropriate coping mechanisms.

DISCIPLINE	PRE-OP/ PRE-ADMIT	POD#5 DAY 7 DATE ___	POD#6 DAY 8 DATE ___	POD#7 DAY 9 DATE ___	POD#8 DAY 10 DATE ___	POD#9 DAY 11 DATE ___	POD#10 DAY 12 DATE ___
LOCATION		MED/SURG	MED/SURG→HOME				
LABS	Chem 7 CBC						
CARDIO-PULMONARY	I.S. q1°		Lower extremity ankle-brachial index prior to discharge				
IMAGING/ NUCLEAR MEDICINE							
SOCIAL SERVICES D/C PLAN REHAB. SERVICES	Discharge planner to re-evaluate home needs prior to discharge						
PHARMACY	DC S.L.		Discharge home c̄ po analgesics for pain control Patient will continue c̄ all pre-op prescribed medications				
DIETARY/ NUTRITION	Diet as tolerated						

Continued.

MULTIDISCIPLINARY PLAN

PATIENT NAME: _____

DISCIPLINE	PRE-OP/ PRE-ADMIT	POD#5 DAY 7 DATE ___	POD#6 DAY 8 DATE ___	POD#7 DAY 9 DATE ___	POD#8 DAY 10 DATE ___	POD#9 DAY 11 DATE ___	POD#10 DAY 12 DATE ___
PATIENT ACTIVITY		Progressive ambulation					
EDUCATION		Discharge teaching to include: • meds • s/sx to report to health care team	Review discharge teaching Discuss need to return to physician 10 days - 2 weeks post-discharge				

COLLABORATIVE PROBLEMS

DATE ___		COLLABORATIVE PROBLEMS	DATE ___		COLLABORATIVE PROBLEMS		DC DATE INIT
		❶ Tissue perfusion, altered R/T graft, & hemodynamics.					
		❷ Alteration in comfort; pain R/T incisional site.					
		❺ Potenial for infection R/T surgical procedure & acute care stay.					
		❻ Knowledge deficit R/T discharge expectations, activity levels, & follow-up care.					

OUTCOMES

					OUTCOMES		
		❶ Pt will have consistent quality of pulses by palpation or doppler.	❻ Pt will verbalize understanding of teaching provided, along c				
		❺ Pt will remain free from s/sx of infection.	understanding of required follow-up appointments.				
			❷ Pt will demonstrate pain control c prescribed po medications				

❶ To initiate a problem or intervention, document under corresponding date.

❷ Document outcomes under appropriate date for achieving the goal.

❸ To discontinue an intervention or resolve a patient problem highlight, date, and initial.

KEY _____

PLAN OF CARE DISCUSSED WITH			POD#5 DAY 7	POD# 6 DAY 8	POD#7 DAY 9	POD#8 DAY 10	POD#9 DAY 11	POD#10 DAY 12
DATE	INITIAL	S.O.	Pt.	DATE ____	DATE ____	DATE ____	DATE ____	DATE ____	DATE ____

INTERVENTIONS

—Review discharge teaching; assess pt understanding, & clarify any misunderstandings
—Assess ambulation & ability to perform ADLs
—Re-assess pt tolerance for prescribed diet

—Re-assess pt understanding of follow-up expectations

Case Manager: ____

Consulting MD: ____

Social Service ____

Anointing of The Sick
Date: ____

MULTIDISCIPLINARY PLAN UPDATE

DATE	SIGNATURES	DATE	SIGNATURES	DATE	SIGNATURES

BARNES

**CARE PATH® 207
23 HR.
CARDIAC CATHETERIZATION**

(1)

SERVICE		PHYSICIAN	
PRIMARY NURSE		PRIMARY NURSE	
DC DATE	ADM DATE	DATE OF SURGERY	**A-8**

Problem Number	PATIENT PROBLEMS/NURSING DIAGNOSES
#1	LACK OF KNOWLEDGE R/T POSSIBLE NEW DISEASE OR UNFAMILIARITY WITH PROCEDURE
#2	ACTIVITY INTOLERANCE R/T BEDREST IN SUPINE POSITION FOR 24 HRS.
#3	POTENTIAL ALTERATION IN NUTRITION R/T DECREASED INTAKE, NAUSEA, VOMITING
#4	POTENTIAL ALTERATION IN URINARY ELIMINATION R/T INABILITY TO VOID IN SUPINE POSITION
#5	POTENTIAL FOR INJURY R/T PROCEDURE
#6	ANXIETY R/T PROCEDURE AND COPING MECHANISM *** IF APPROPRIATE**

Problem Number		PRE-ADMISSION	PRE-CATH
#1 #2	ASSESSMENT / MONITORING	Clinical Coordinator calls pt. to evaluate: – hx of heart disease / symptoms – hx of CABG / PTCA – medication hx – allergy hx – previous CXR / ECG completion – advanced directive	Record height and weight in chart Complete pre-cath orders Complete pre-cath checklist for pts. coming to cath lab from floor **All labs and diagnostic data within acceptable parameters for cath completion** IV site condition, type Nutritional status Pedal pulses prior **VS WNL** and recorded
	CONSULTS	Social Work if Clinical Coordinator identifies need for emotional support, community resources, financial resources, advanced directive Dietary if risk factors identified Pastoral Care	
	PROCEDURE / TEST	Pre-cath labs completed SMA 6 SMA 12 PT / PTT CBC ECG CXR (PA-lateral) within past 6 months	**Pre-cath labs WNL** SMA 6 SMA 12 PT / PTT CBC ECG CXR (PA and lateral) completed within past 6 months
	TREATMENT		
#1 #2	ACTIVITY		Determine past pt. tolerance to maintaining bedrest and initiate plans to reduce discomfort post-cath

Used by permission of Barnes Hospital, St Louis, Missouri.

BARNES

**CARE PATH® 207
23 HR.
CARDIAC CATHETERIZATION**

(2)

CNS	DIETARY	RT
HOME HEALTH	OT	OTHER
PT	SW	OTHER

A-8

Problem Number	PATIENT PROBLEMS/NURSING DIAGNOSES
#7	POTENTIAL ALTERATION IN COMFORT R/T IMMOBILITY, INTERRUPTED SLEEP
#8	POTENTIAL ALTERATION IN BOWEL ELIMINATION R/T IMMOBILITY
#9	POTENTIAL ALTERATION IN SKIN R/T IMMOBILITY

POST-CATH	DC OUTCOMES	RESOURCE INFORMATION
1) VS with pulse check & groin check q 15 mins. x q 1 hr. x 4 and then q 4 hrs. if stable 2) Report the following to House Officer / Cath team / ASM MD immediately: Significant change in VS, diminution or loss of pulse, chest pain / angina equivalent hematoma, back pain, bleeding at groin 3) Notify House Officer / ASM MD if unable to void 4 hrs, post-cath **Pt. will be free of complications post-cardiac cath** I / O Pain / comfort Nutritional status	**Pt. will have no s/sx of impaired circulation R/T cardiac cath** **Groin site without hematoma** **Pedal pulse - normal** **Affected leg - color, temp sensation - normal**	**Cardiac Catheterization DC Instructions** The following information is intended to serve as a guide to assist with your care after DC following cardiac catheterization. 1. Resume your normal diet immediately, unless directed otherwise by your physician. 2. It is important to limit activity of the limb site used for the catheterization for 3 days. This includes, but is not limited to, activities such as aerobics, swimming, jogging, running, bicycling, bowling, dancing, rowing, or stair-stepping. If you are involved in activities not listed above, please ask your nurse or physician for specific instructions.
Contact intern / resident / ASM STAT on return of pt. from cath lab for immediate evaluation. Consult Cardiology Fellow or cath lab for significant changes in pt. condition. After hours contact **362-3796** for a cath lab team member. Pastoral Care	**Social Work consult completed** **Dietary completed or** **follow-up appointment arranged**	3. Avoid lifting for 2 days. 4. Gentle walking is permissible but only on level ground.
If hematoma occurs: - Consider Duplex scan and CBC VS **Cardiac cath completed**	**Pt. / signifcant other will verbalize understanding of diagnostic findings**	5. No driving for 2 days. 6. Restrict stair-climbing for 2 days, if possible. If stair-climbing is essential, climb with your non-catheterized leg, then bring the catheterized led up to the same step.
Keep 5 lb. sandbag to _____ groin for _____ hrs. post-cath		7. Customary sexual activity may be resumed after 2 days. Use postures that do not place a strain on the catheterized leg.
Maintain strict bedrest for _____ hrs. after cath. May raise HOB 30° at _____ if VS stable Use electric bed raiser Use orthopedic bedpan for female pts. Place bed in reverse Trendelenberg position to assist males in voiding Utilize appropriate comfort measures to relieve discomfort of bedrest: - pillow under knee of non-affected leg - rolled blanket under back	**Pt. will verbalize understanding of activity restriction the first 3 days post-cath**	8. Avoid straining for bowel movements for 7 days. If you tend to be constipated and/or regularly strain to pass stool, please inform your nurse of this so that a stool softening medication can be ordered. 9. It is common to have some bruising or purple discoloration of the skin near the puncture site.

Continued.

		PRE-ADMISSION	PRE-CATH
#1 #2	MEDS / IV	Clinical Coordinator will notify private MD of potential dye allergies to initiate pre-treatment med of Cimetidine, Prednisone and Benadryl	Administer pt. usual PO medications, unless otherwise ordered. Cardiac meds to be taken with sip of water If IDDM, evaluate need for AM insulin requirements and IV hydration. If Cr elevated, consider Mannitol Initiate and monitor IV fluid
#1	NUTRITION	NPO after midnight (except for medications). Limited water intake if specified in pre-cath orders	NPO except meds
#1	PATIENT / FAMILY EDUCATION	**Pt. / family verbalizes understanding of Care Path.** **Plan of care has been mutually set with pt. / family.** Clinical Coordinator completes pre-cath pt. teaching including: – Remind pt. to bring all current medications with them to hospital – Reminder to bring med records from private MD – NPO after midnight – Remain on bedrest after cath till following morning – No driving for 2 days after cath **Pt. / significant other verbalizes understanding of pre-cath preparation**	Instruct pt. they should wear dentures and may bring glasses to procedure. Remove jewelry and watches, tape rings. Ask pt. to empty bladder and bowel prior to procedure Instruct families that they may not accompany pt. to procedure. **Pt. followed pre-admission instructions** **Pt. / significant other verbalizes understanding of procedure**
#1	DISCHARGE PLANNING		
	PSYCHOSOCIAL / EMOTIONAL / SPIRITUAL NEEDS		Ensure pt. has transportation / accommodation arrangements completed for day of DC Provide opportunity to discuss implications / issues relating to procedure Pt. / significant other exhibits positive coping skills relating to procedure
	SIGNATURES		

3100-40 (Rev. 6/94)

POST-CATH	DC OUTCOMES	However, if any of the following occur, immediately contact your own physician.
IV fluids per orders. Resume previous medications when VS stable or as ordered by House Officer / ASM MD	**d/c IV if to be DC**	A. Bleeding from the catheterization puncture site, apply gentle pressure with a clean gauze or cloth (and call your physician or the Barnes Hospital Emergency Department immediately).
Encourage oral fluids, unless nausea / vomiting Withhold solid foods for _____ hrs. Resume previous diet after _____ . **Pt. will not have nausea or vomiting**	**If indicated, pt. verbalizes method to contact outpatient nutritional counseling office for follow-up appointment**	B. If a knot or lump under the skin increases in size, or C. If bruising appears to be worsening or tracking/moving down the leg rather than disappearing.
Pt. will demonstrate compliance with post-procedural instructions	Complete post-cath teaching and provide pt. with instruction sheet **Pt. will verbalize understanding of medication regime Pt. / significant other will verbalize understanding of invasive procedure, DC instructions and follow-up Pt. / significant other will verbalize s/sx to report to MD when at home**	D. If the leg used for catheterization appears pale in color and/or feels cooler to touch compared to the opposite leg. E. If the leg used for the catheterization appears reddened, swollen and/or feels warmer to touch compared to the opposite leg. 10. You may bathe or shower the day following the catheterization. Be careful to avoid slipping as your leg may feel stiff.
	For delays in DC contact cardiology nurse coordinator 24972	11. Resume the same medication you were taking before the catheterization unless otherwise ordered by your physician. 12. If you have any questions or concerns contact your private physician or call Barnes Hospital Emergency Department at **314 (362-9123).**
Provide opportunity to discuss implications / issues relating to procedure Pt. / significant other exhibits positive coping skills relating to procedure	**Pt. will have adequate transportation and accommodation arrangements for DC Pt. / significant other exhibits positive coping skills relating to procedure implications**	

3100-40 (Rev. 6/94)   Adapted from CareMap® System, The Center for Case Management

Continued.

BARNES

NURSE ADMISSION NOTE
C-2

5

Date _____ Time _____ Informant _____ *Age _____

T _____ P _____ R _____ B/P _____ Ht. _____ Wt. _____

Chief Complaint and History of Present Illness _____

_____

_____

_____

_____

ADDRESSOGRAPH

Medical / Surgical History	Date	Medical / Surgical History	Date	Medical / Surgical History	Date

Has received blood products in the past: ☐ Yes   ☐ No   If yes, list dates _____   Reactions: ☐ Yes   ☐ No

Allergies: _____   Advanced Directives: ☐ Yes   ☐ No

Medication / Dose / Freq.	Time of Last Dose	Patient Knows Med Rx	Medication / Dose / Freq.	Time of Last Dose	Patient Knows Med Rx	Medication / Dose / Freq.	Time of Last Dose	Patient Knows Med Rx

Patient Provided: ☐ Admission Kit   ☐ ID Band   ☐ Sensitivity / Allergy Band   ☐ Sensitivity / Allergy Sticker on Chart

Patient Instructed: ☐ Valuables Inventory ☐ Waiver Signed ☐ Smoking / Visitor Policy ☐ Nurse Call / Emergency / TV / Phone

☐ Patient's Rights / Responsibilities   SIGNATURE: _____

			Check if infusion device in use _____									
Amt.	Types of Fluid	Product # or Medication added	Date/Hr. Start	INT.	Date/Hr. Start	Int.	Amt. Rec'd	IV Site	Appearance	✓	IV Site Care Date/Hr.	Tubing Change Date/Hr.	Int.

GRAPHIC SHEET

TEMPERATURE

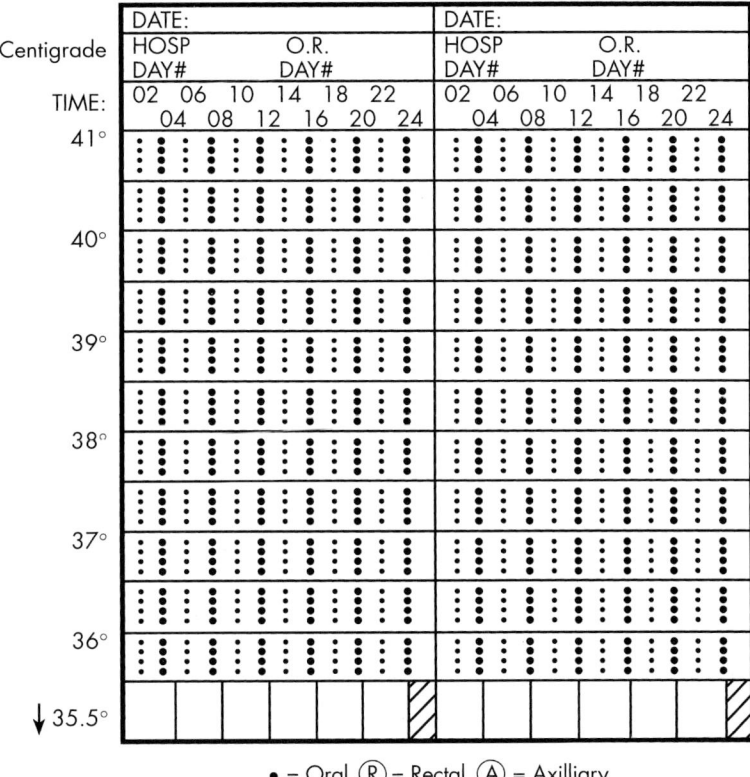

• = Oral Ⓡ = Rectal Ⓐ = Axilliary

BLOOD PRESSURE CHART

PULSE   X = Pulse a = Apical

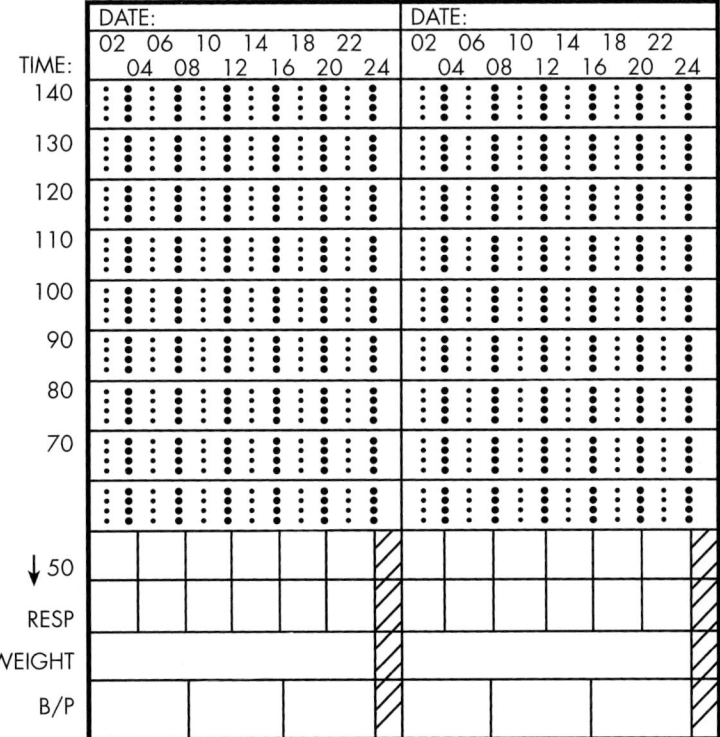

BARNES

C-10b

NURSING ASSESSMENT FLOWSHEET

DATE

INSTRUCTIONS: CIRCLE IF PRESENT.
WRITE IN ASSESSMENT.
INDICATE N/A NOT APPLICABLE OR NOT ASSESSED.

CODE: S - SELF,   A - ASSIST,   T - TOTAL,   I - INSTRUCTED,   C - COLLECTED

ADDRESSOGRAPH

NEURO / CEREBRAL	**NEURO / CEREBRAL**	ALERT CONFUSED MEMORY LOSS AGITATED ORIENTED X _____ _____	ALERT CONFUSED MEMORY LOSS AGITATED ORIENTED X _____ _____
COMFORT / SLEEP	**DISCOMFORT** INTERVENTION	_____ _____	_____ _____
	SLEEP STATUS	AWAKE SLEEP AT INTERVALS SLEPT	AWAKE SLEEP AT INTERVALS SLEPT
ACTIVITY / EXERCISE	**MOBILITY** LIMITATIONS / DEVICES **ACTIVITY**	INDEPENDENT ASSIST DEPENDENT _____ _____ _____	INDEPENDENT ASSIST DEPENDENT _____ _____ _____

SKIN / MUCOSA	**APPEARANCE**
	
	MATTRESS / EQUIPMENT
		WARM DRY TURGOR _____
		_____
		_____
		          HEEL AQUA K
		FOAM AIR PROTECTORS PAD TEDS
			WARM DRY TURGOR _____
			_____
			_____
			          HEEL AQUA K
			FOAM AIR PROTECTORS PAD TEDS

WOUND	**LOCATION** APPEARANCE **DRSG. CHANGE**	_____ _____ _____ X _____	_____ _____ _____ X _____
NUTRITION	**MEALS** TUBE-FEEDING INFUSION DEVICE	_____ CONTINUOUS BOLUS FLUSH X _____	% EATEN B: SATL: SAT CONTINUOUS BOLUS FLUSH X _____
ELIMINATION	**URINE** **BOWEL** BOWEL SOUNDS	CONTINENT INCONTINENT FOLEY _____ CONTINENT INCONTINENT GUAIAC _____ FREQ X: ABSENT PRESENT _____ ABDOMEN _____	CONTINENT INCONTINENT FOLEY _____ CONTINENT INCONTINENT GUAIAC _____ FREQ X: ABSENT PRESENT _____ ABDOMEN _____
RESPIRATORY	**AUSCULTATION**	_____ O$_2$ _____ COUGH / SECRETION _____	_____ O$_2$ _____ COUGH / SECRETION _____
CIRC	**CIRCULATION**	_____	_____
OTHER	**SPECIMEN**	I C TEST _____ _____	I C TEST _____ _____

SIGNATURE / STATUS	SIGNATURE / STATUS
HYGIENE: S A T	**HYGIENE:** S A T

HYGIENE	SAFETY	HYGIENE	SAFETY
BATH TUB SHOWER	ID BAND ON _____	BATH TUB SHOWER	ID BAND ON _____
SHAVE HAIR NAILS ORAL	SIDERAILS IN USE _____	SHAVE HAIR NAILS ORAL	SIDERAILS IN USE _____

Used by permission of Barnes Hospital, St Louis, Missouri.

page 1 of 3

USC UNIVERSITY HOSPITAL
1500 San Pablo
Los Angeles, CA 90033 ©1991

NAME _____
ALLERGIES _____
ADMIT DATE _____

SIDE 1   **MULTIDISCIPLINARY PLAN**

DIAGNOSIS **CAROTID ARTERY STENOSIS**

SURGERY **CAROTID ENDARTERECTOMY**   DRG _005_   ALOS _6.5_

DISCHARGE OUTCOMES	
PHYSIOLOGICAL	Patient will have improved carotid blood flow, be afebrile, healing incision, & VS stable. Patient will maintain baseline neurological status.
COGNITIVE	Patient will verbalize knowledge of risk factors & prevention of disease process as well as expected follow-up regimen.
PSYCHOLOGICAL	Patient will verbalize acceptance of potential lifestyle changes, express concerns, ask questions, & exhibit effective coping mechanisms.

DISCIPLINE	PRE-OP/ PRE-ADMIT	DOS DAY 1	POD#1 DAY 2	POD#2 DAY 3	POD#3 DAY 4	POD#4 DAY 5	POD#5 DAY 6
		DATE	DATE	DATE	DATE	DATE	DATE
LOCATION		SURGERY/PAR/SICU	SICU →DOU	DOU → MED/SURG	MED/SURG	MED/SURG → HOME	
LABS	CBC Chem 20 PT PTT UA Type & screen 4u	Hct stat post-op (Check Blood bank for autologous directed blood ⊤ or ⊤⊤ units)	CBC Chem 7				
CARDIO-PULMONARY	ECG	I.S. Pulse oximetry	D/C pulse oximetry on transfer				
IMAGING/ NUCLEAR MEDICINE	CXR Carotid duplex scan	Arteriogram during surgery Carotid duplex scan intra-op					
SOCIAL SERVICES D/C PLAN REHAB. SERVICES		Social worker support as needed Assess for potential home needs & discharge planning		Re-evaluate needs prior to discharge			
PHARMACY	ASA ⊤ prior to OR	Vasoactive drips for BP control (Nipride) Pain medication Start ASA post-op ⊤ qd	DC vasoactive drips Change IV to S.L. Change to po anti-hypertensives & pain medications	DC S.L.	Discharge medications: • po analgesics • ASA ⊤ tab qd • Continue pre-op prescribed medications		
DIETARY/ NUTRITION	NPO May have clear liquids when fully awake	Advance diet as tolerated					

Used by permission of USC University Hospital, Los Angeles, California.

Continued.

MULTIDISCIPLINARY PLAN

PATIENT NAME: _____

DISCIPLINE	PRE-OP/ PRE-ADMIT	DOS DAY 1	POD#1 DAY 2	POD#2 DAY 3	POD#3 DAY 4	POD#4 DAY 5	POD#5 DAY 6
		DATE ___	DATE ___	DATE ___	DATE ___	DATE ___	DATE ___
PATIENT ACTIVITY		HOB ↑30° Leg exercises compression boots	OOB to chair Ambulate c̄ assistance	Independent ambulation DC compression boots when fully ambulatory			
EDUCATION		Orient to environment Teach purpose/use of I.S., cough & deep breathe, foley, JP Acquaint pt c̄ equipment used for monitoring	Reinforce teaching Observe pt perform I.S. D/C foley	Discuss risk factors associated c̄ vascular diseases. Include diet, smoking, & pulse checks	Discuss home & follow-up expectations: • No driving x 1 week • Avoid heavy, physical activity • May resume usual ADLs • Walking is good exercise	Discuss need for surgeon's office appointment 10 days- 2 wks post-discharge Call office at any time for questions	

COLLABORATIVE PROBLEMS

DATE				DATE			

❶ Potential alteration in LOC, R/T stroke, nerve palsy, & swallowing difficulty.

❷ Alteration in tissue perfusion R/T hypertension (which may disrupt integrity of graft, sutures, newly manipulated vessel).

❸ Potential for alteration in gas exchange/airway clearance R/T airway occlusion from hematoma, bleeding, & post-anesthesia complications.

❹ Alteration in comfort, pain R/T incision site.

❺ Knowledge deficit R/T discharge expectations, activity levels, & follow-up care.

OUTCOMES

❶ Any S/SX of neurological damage postop will have immediate intervention & documentation.
   ❶ Pt will be able to swallow s̄ difficulty & is awake, alert, & oriented.

❷ Pt will be hemodynamically stable, including VS which are controlled on prescribed vasoactive medications.
   ❷ Pt will be weaned off vasoactive drips & restarted on pre-op medications.

❸ Pt will maintain patent airway c̄ respiratory distress & adequate gas exchange (refer to baseline ABG).

❹ Pt will have pain controlled/ relieved c̄ prescribed medications.
   ❹ Pt will demonstrate a decreased need for pain medications; po pain medications adequate for pain relief.

❺ Pt will verbalize understanding of disease process, risk factors, expectations for follow-up care, & ambulating independently.

---

❶ To initiate a problem or intervention, document under corresponding date.

❷ Document outcomes under appropriate date for achieving the goal.

❸ To discontinue an intervention or resolve a patient problem highlight, date, and initial.

KEY
△ = Change

	DOS DAY 1	POD# 1 DAY 2	POD#2 DAY 3	POD#3 DAY 4	POD#4 DAY 5	POD#5 DAY 6
PLAN OF CARE DISCUSSED WITH	DATE ____	DATE ____	DATE ____	DATE ____	DATE ____	DATE ____

INTERVENTIONS

	DOS DAY 1	POD#1 DAY 2	POD#2 DAY 3	POD#3 DAY 4	POD#4 DAY 5	POD#5 DAY 6
	—Neuro ✓'s q1° x 4, then q4°	—DC PA line p̄ Nipride no longer necessary		—Review teaching previously done —Assess pt understanding & clarify as needed	—Re-assess pt understanding of follow-up expectations	
	—Monitor for s/sx of bleeding: • hematoma • neck swelling • airway occlusion • stridor	—Assist OOB to chair —Assess activity tolerance	—Assist c̄ ambulation —DC compression boots when fully ambulatory	—Explain discharge instructions —Assess ambulation		
	—Maintain JP drain to bulb suction —Assess amount & consistency of drainage	—Assess breath sounds, respiratory status & airway q4° after transfer	—Neuro ✓'s q8° p̄ transfer	—Expect DC of JP drain		
Case Manager: _____	—Sequential compression boots until fully ambulatory	—I & O q8h				
	—Titrate Nipride to keep systolic BP within prescribed parameters					
Consulting MD: _____	—Monitor ECG for Δ's consist c̄ ischemia					
	—Assess breath sounds, respiratory status & airway q1° x 4, then q2°					
Social Service _____	—I & O q2° —Maintain integrity of hemodynamic lines					
Anointing of The Sick Date: _____	—Assess & document effectiveness of pain medications					
	—Assess for hoarseness; notify MD if this develops					

MULTIDISCIPLINARY PLAN UPDATE

DATE	SIGNATURES	DATE	SIGNATURES	DATE	SIGNATURES

Admission Date/Time: _____
Clinical Path Date/Time: _____
Discharge Date/Time: _____
Case Manager/Phone# _____

Rex Healthcare
Congestive Heart Failure (CHF)
Clinical Pathway
DRG 127
Expected LOS 5.0 Days

Addressograph

NOTE: DID YOU CONTACT YOUR M.D. PRIOR TO COMING TO THE ED? YES____ NO____
Advanced Directive? YES   NO
PATIENT/FAMILY TO CONTACT FOR FOLLOW-UP: PHONE: DATE:

Category	Preadmit/ED	Day 1/____ Unit	Day 2 ____	Day 3 ____	Day 4 ____	Day 5 ____
DIAGNOSTIC TESTING	EKG, CXR, CBC, M7, M12, Magnesium, Blood Gas or Pulse Ox, Coags*, Cardiac Enzymes*, Dig and other appropriate drug levels	Thyroid Profile (3) UA Echo (2) All admission lab and x-ray results on chart Copy of previous Echo report on chart	M7		M7* Dig and other appropriate drug levels*	
PATIENT CARE and TREATMENTS	Obtain previous Echo (US) Pulse Ox (RT)-------- Monitor Oxygen (RT) I&O (RN)----------- Baseline Weight (RN) Foley* (RN) Hep Lock---------- Cardiac Monitor------ Assessment: Neuro (RN)--------- VS (RN)----------- Breath Sounds (RN)---- Cardiac (RN)-------- Home Meds list (RN)---	Re-eval 02 (RT)-----> Daily Weight (RN) D/C Foley (RN) F/H Assessment (RN) Complete Survey–(RN) Nutrition/Medications/ Learning Needs Assessment (on back of path)	Spot Check (RT)- Re-Eval Cardiac Monitor		Repeat Learning Needs Assessment (on back of path)(RN)	■ ■ ■ ■ ■ ■ ■
MEDICATIONS	IV Diuretics (1) K supplements Nitrates or other Vasodilator Digoxin ACE Inhibitors------- Aerosolized Albuterol* Antianxiety medications Laxative of choice----- Morphine---------■		Change to Oral Medications (MD with RN or RP prompt)----------- --- Titrate ACE Inhibitors (MD)------			■ ■
DIET	Ice chips until respiratory status is stabilized (RN)	No added salt diet (RD, MD)---------- ___ml fluid restriction* (RD, MD)------				■ ■
ACTIVITY	Fowler's Positioning (RN) Bed rest (RN) Safety & Fall Precautions (RN)	BR with BRP/BR/BSC (RN) Safety & Fall Precautions (RN)	Advanced activity as tolerated (RN, PT)-			■
CONSULTS	Primary Care MD if D/C from Ed	PT, Cardiologist, Clinical Nurse Spec.	RT (4) Nutrition Screening (RD)			
DISCHARGE PLANNING	Preadmission Screening System (PFS or CM) Patient/Family Services or Case Management referral* (PFS or CM)-------- <------------	PFS/Case Management consult (PFS,CM)	PSF/Case Management assessment completed (PFS, CM) Confirm and communicate disposition with patient/family/MD [Rehab, SNF, HH](PFS) --Discharge Planning Rounds (all disciplines)----			■ ■
EDUCATION	Explain testing to patient (RN) Status report to patient/ family (RN) Explain safety measures to patient/family (RN) Discharge instructions if to home (RN) <----------	Orientation to floor, safety measures to patient/family (RN) ----Address specific learning needs (RN, RP, MD)----------	CHF video and pamphlet (RN)			■ Patient/Family education complete (RN) Patient/Family demonstrates knowledge of disease (RN) Medic-Alert bracelet, (RN, MD) wallet medication card, (RN) information given (RN, MD) Risk factor reduction (RN) Self-care (RN)

NOTE: * If individual patient's condition indicates appropriateness.

(1) Patient's potassium level to be monitored.
(2) If first time with CHF diagnosis or previous test is > one year. (3) If patient has atrial fibrillation or other evidence of thyroid disease, or if >65 and no obvious etiology for heart failure. (5) If inhaler is used.

KEY TO DISCIPLINES PERFORMING SERVICES

RN – Registered Nurse	MD – Physician
RT – Respiratory Therapist	RP – Registered Pharmacist
RD – Registered Dietitian	Lab – Laboratory
PFS – Patient & Family Services	US – Unit Secretary
CM – Case Manager	PT – Physical Therapist

Form Date: June 27, 1995
Form Revision Date: August 25, 1995

Used by permission of Rex Heathcare, Raleigh, North Carolina.

CHF Clinical Pathway						
Patient's NAME:						
Category	Preadmit/ED	Day 1	Day 2	Day 3	Day 4	Day 5
OUTCOMES	Actual weight obtained in ED Primary Care M.D. notified if patient D/C from ED Patient admitted to appropriate level of care Patient/Family demonstrates awareness of path Appropriate test/ treatments initiated based on patient severity of illness at presentation to ED	LV function defined within 24 hours O₂ Sat > 92% on oxygen therapy Negative fluid balance defined by: Output > Intake Weight loss Home meds list is obtained VS stable with increased activity — ■ (Day 4)	Electrolytes/lab values normalizing — ■ (Day 5) Weight loss — ■ No dyspnea at rest — ■ Patient voiding — ■ No symptomatic hypotension — — — — — — — — — — — — — — — — — — — ■ Patient/Family aware of confirmed D/C Plan		Patient/Family aware of need for med/ precautions — — — — — — — — — — — — — — — — ■ (Day 5) Compliance issues identified	

Nutrition — Medication Survey on Admission/Learning Needs Assessment

Nutrition

1. I am supposed to be on a special diet, but I am having trouble following it. yes no

2. I have gained or lost 10 lbs. or more without trying in the past 6 months. yes no

3. My appetite is poor and food does not taste good to me. yes no

4. I do not always have enough money to buy the food I need. yes no

5. (if over 65 years old) I eat alone most of the time. yes no

6. If "yes" to any question 1 – 5; go to # 15.

Medications

7. I do not know why I take each of my medications. yes no

8. I get my medications at different places. yes no

9. I do not always have enough of my medications. yes no

10. I have stopped taking my medicine. yes no

11. If "yes" to any question 7 – 10; go to # 15.

Learning Needs Assessment
(ASK QUESTIONS 12 – 13 – 14 AGAIN UPON DISCHARGE)

12. What is your understanding of your heart condition?
Admission response:_____
Discharge response:_____

13. Name some behaviors that will improve your health.
Admission response:_____
Discharge response:_____

14. Describe the importance of an accurate daily weight in assessing your heart condition and how you would do it.
Admission response:_____
Discharge response:_____

15. If any question(s) has a "yes" response, the nurse will order appropriate dietitian or pharmacist consult.

Pathway Daily Variance Tracking

Variance Type/Date Occurred	Initials	Reason/Comment	Initials	Action Taken/Date Resolved	Initials
1.					
2.					
3.					
4.					
5.					
6.					
7.					
8.					
9.					
10.					

Form Date: June 27, 1995
Form Revision Date: August 25, 1995

CHAPTER 4

Hematologic System

■ HEMATOLOGIC ASSESSMENT

▌ GENERAL OBSERVATIONS/FINDINGS

Age
Sex
Sociocultural factors
   Ethnicity
   Culture
   Economic status
   Occupation
   Family health history
   Physical environment
   Support systems
Appearance
   Stated age equals appearance
   Pallor
   Facial flushing
   Profuse perspiration
   Signs of pain
   Dehydration
   Abnormal body posture, movements, or gait
   Activity level
   Cachexia
Vital signs
   Blood pressure (BP), temperature (T), pulse (P), or
      respirations (R) changes
   Height and weight changes

▌ INTEGUMENTARY SYSTEM

Skin and mucous membranes
   Complaints of
      Pruritus
      Lesions, cuts, excoriations that do not heal
      Infections that recur or fail to resolve
Impaired skin integrity
   Skin tears
   Rashes
   Purpuric lesions
   Excessive ecchymosis
   Ulceration
   Erythema
Pallor
Cyanosis
Plethora
Jaundice

Petechiae
White patches
Telangiectasis
Subcutaneous nodules
Infiltrates
Vesicles
Uneven distribution of altered skin temperature,
   generalized or localized
Drainage
Turgor
Vascularity
Scars
Note distribution of abnormalities
   Pigmentary changes
Nails
   Color
   Brittle
   Ridges
   Flattened dorsal curvature
   Spoon shaped
   Clubbed
   Loosened
   Thickened
   Longitudinal striation
Hair
   Texture
   Growth patterns, loss or thinning
Eyes
   Edema
   Redness
   Inflammation
   Infection
   Enlarged/engorged vessels
   Vessel tortuosity
   Infiltration
   Hemorrhage
   Cataracts
   Conjunctival pallor
   Yellow sclera
   Position
   Alignment

▌ LYMPHATIC SYSTEM

Prominent lymph nodes
   Location

Size
Surface characteristics
Symmetry
Consistency
Fixation/mobility
Tenderness/pain
Heat
Vascularity
Erythema
Red streaks

GASTROINTESTINAL SYSTEM

Complaints of the following:
  Nausea
  Vomiting
  Dysphagia
  Anorexia
  Weight loss
Mouth
  Red mucous membranes
  Bleeding of gums and mucosa
  Stomatitis
  Purpura
  Telangiectasis
  Tonsillar hypertrophy
  Gingival hypertrophy
  Ulcers
  Tongue
    Complaints of pain
    Beefy or swollen appearance
    Texture
      Absence of papillae
      Furrows
  Color: red
Frank, occult bleeding in stool
  Hemorrhoids, anal/rectal fissures
Bowel habits
Abdomen
  Surface characteristics
    Contour
    Symmetry
    Masses
    Pulsations
Auscultation
  Bowel sounds
  High-pitched tinkling sound
  Friction rubs over liver or spleen
Percussion
  Decreased tympany
  Increased dullness
Palpation
  Hepatomegaly
  Splenomegaly
  Tenderness
  Rigidity
  Spasm
Anus
  Visual inspection

Inflammation
Breaks in mucosa

CARDIOVASCULAR SYSTEM

Complaints of the following:
  Palpitations
  Fatigue
    After exertion
    All the time
  Angina
Murmurs
Dysrhythmias
Tachycardia
Extremities
  Color
  Response to temperature changes
  Edema

RESPIRATORY SYSTEM

Percussion
  Compare anterior, lateral, posterior thorax
Auscultation
  Adventitious sounds
  Wheezing
  Crackles
Shortness of breath (SOB)
Orthopnea
Tachypnea
Dyspnea
Rhythm
Excursion
Rate
Effort and energy expenditure
Position required to ease respiratory effort
Hemoptysis

MUSCULOSKELETAL SYSTEM

Range of motion (ROM)
Joints/bones
  Swelling
  Pain
  Stiffness
  Tenderness
Soft tissue
  Edema
  Hematoma
  Abscess
Muscle loss/weakness
Posture
Flaccidity
Spasticity
Babinski sign

GENITOURINARY/RENAL SYSTEM

Hematuria
Incontinence
Impotence
Heavy menses

Retention
Difficult urination
Sexual maturity congruent with chronologic age
Scrotal masses
Kidneys
   Auscultation
      Systolic bruits in renal arteries
   Percussion
      Kidney tenderness/pain
      Dullness over bladder after urination
   Palpation
      Kidney tenderness
      Kidney lumps, masses
      Bladder tenderness
      Bladder lumps, masses

NEUROLOGIC SYSTEM

Headache
Numb, tingling extremities
Paresthesia
Weakness
Frequent napping
Sleeplessness
Behavior/mood changes
Changes in attention span and responses
Convulsions
Dyskinesia
Visual changes
Syncope
Tinnitus
Sudden or progressive changes in orientation
Sudden or progressive changes in level of
   arousal/wakefulness
Changes in motor and sensory capabilities
Changes in pupillary response

PERTINENT BACKGROUND INFORMATION

CONCURRENT DISEASES OR CONDITIONS
Frequent illness
Infectious processes
Blood transfusion/component therapy
Multiple allergies
Asthma
Bleeding tendency
Hemorrhage
Renal, cardiovascular, or liver disorders
Cancer
Gastric or duodenal ulcer
Diabetes mellitus, other endocrine disorders
Acquired immunodeficiency syndrome (AIDS)

PREVIOUS SURGERY OR ILLNESS
Gastric or duodenal ulcers
Gastric surgery
Hepatic surgery
Cardiac surgery
Renal surgery
Radioactive exposure and irradiation
Exposure to chemical agents
Recurrent infectious processes (e.g., frequent sore
   throats)
Splenectomy
Thyroidectomy

FAMILY HISTORY
Cancer
Blood dyscrasias, anemias
Immune disorders
Allergies

 Gerontologic Considerations

- The subjective symptoms of hematologic disorders (e.g., fatigue, weakness, dizziness, and dyspnea) may be mistaken for normal changes of aging or attributed to other disease processes commonly seen in the older adult.
- The most common blood disorders are forms of anemia.
- Decreased production of intrinsic factor in the aging gastric mucosa results in an increased incidence of pernicious anemia.
- Many older adults suffer from conditions such as colonic diverticuli, hiatal hernia, or ulcerations, which can cause occult bleeding. Older adults with these conditions should be observed for iron deficiency anemia.
- Age-related problems such as altered dentition, limited financial resources, difficulty in food preparation, and poor appetite resulting from emotional upset or depression can cause an increased incidence of iron deficiency anemia.

- Severe or persistent anemia can place additional stress on the aging or diseased heart.
- Administration of blood products should be done with caution, because the older adult is at increased risk of developing congestive heart failure. Careful assessment of cardiopulmonary function and intake and output is essential.
- Oral administration of iron preparations increases the risk of gastrointestinal irritation and constipation in the older adult.
- Ingestion of large amounts of aspirin and other antiinflammatory medications commonly taken by the older adult increases the risk of gastrointestinal bleeding and can lead to alteration in clotting.
- Chronic lymphocytic leukemia is the most common form seen with aging. This form of leukemia usually progresses slowly in the older adult and is rarely treated.

From Christensen BL, Kochrow EO: Foundations of nursing, *ed 3, St Louis, 1998, Mosby.*

Rh incompatibility
Cause of death of deceased family members

SOCIAL/CULTURAL HISTORY
Education level
Smoking
Alcohol use
Increased stress
Occupation; exposure to toxic substances
Radiation exposure
Environmental factors
Diet
   Recent changes
   Cultural or religious restrictions
   Decreased protein intake
   Fad diets
   Caffeine intake
   Low iron intake
   Supplements

MEDICATION HISTORY
Immunizations
Prescription medications

   Present medications
   Previously taken medications (e.g., chloramphenicol)
Over-the-counter medications
Home remedies
Use of other drugs (particularly quinidines and
   sulfonamides)

▮ DIAGNOSTIC TESTS

LABORATORY STUDIES (Figs. 4-1 and 4-2)
Complete blood cell count (CBC)
White blood cell count (WBC)/differential
Hematocrit (Hct)
Hemoglobin (Hgb)
T and B lymphocyte count
Reticulocyte count
Platelet count
Mean corpuscular volume (MCV)
Mean corpuscular hemoglobin concentration (MCHC)
Mean corpuscular hemoglobin (MCH)
Haptoglobin
Methemalbumin
Bleeding time

Red Blood Cells   **Platelets**

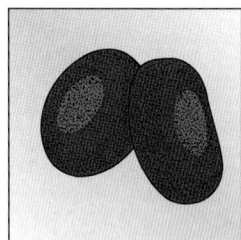   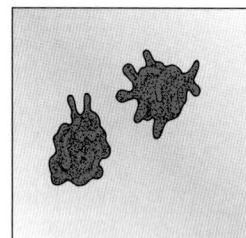

White Blood Cells (Leukocytes)

Granular leukocytes

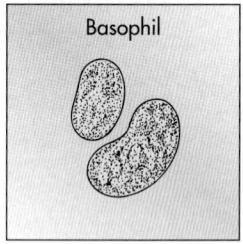 Basophil   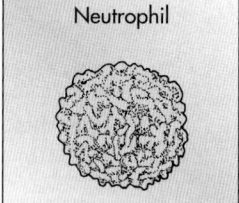 Neutrophil   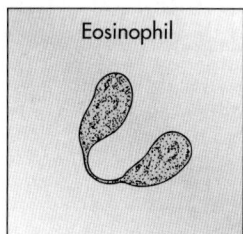 Eosinophil

Nongranular leukocytes

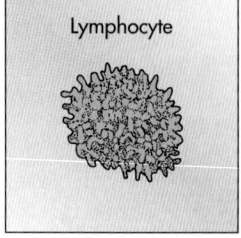 Lymphocyte   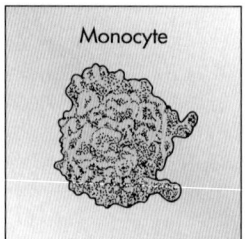 Monocyte

Fig. 4-1   Human blood cells.
(From Beare PG, Myers JL: Adult health nursing, ed 3, St Louis, 1998, Mosby)

Prothrombin time/International Normalized Ratio
(PT/INR)
Thrombin time
Activated partial thromboplastin time (APTT)
Sedimentation rate
Electrophoresis of serum proteins
Immunoelectrophoresis of serum proteins
Total protein
Fibrinogen
Electrolyte values
Bilirubin level
Direct/indirect Coombs' test
Factor assay
Total iron-binding capacity
Fibrin degradation products
Hemoccult/guaiac tests
Serum iron level
Ferritin titers
Sideroblasts
Gastric analysis
Schilling test
Human lymphocyte antigens (HLA)

Sickle cell test
ABO typing
Rh typing
Direct antiglobulin (direct Coombs')
Antibody screening test (indirect Coombs')

OTHER PROCEDURES

Biopsies
    Bone marrow
    Lymph nodes
    Spleen
    Liver
Chest and abdominal x-ray examinations
Magnetic resonance imaging (MRI)
Computed tomography (CT) scans
    Bone
    Liver
    Spleen
Intravenous pyelogram (IVP)
Uric acid
Urinary bilirubin
Urine culture

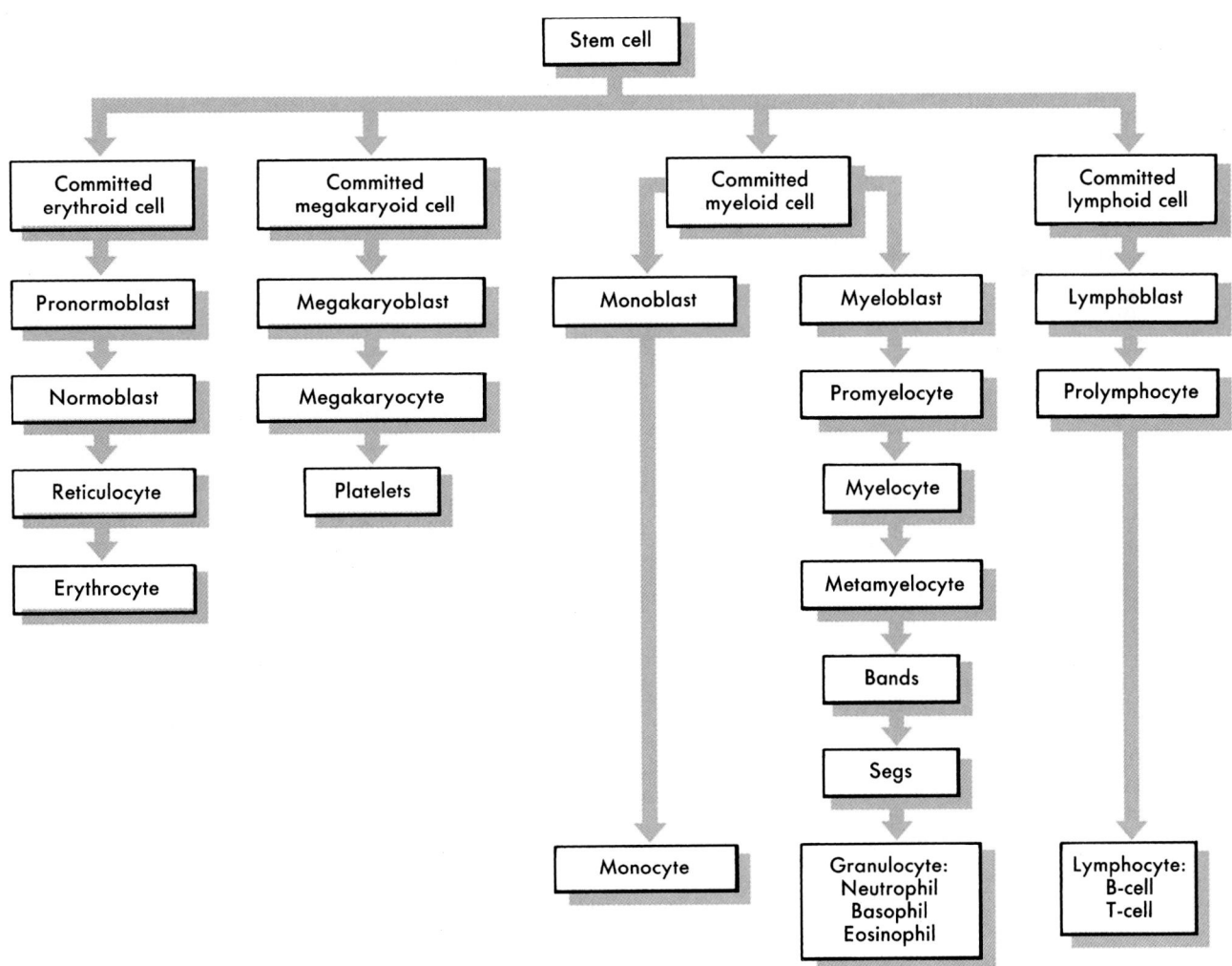

Fig. 4-2 Formation and Maturation of Blood Cells. All circulating blood cells originate from a common stem cell. *(From Beare PG, Myers JL:* Principles and practice of adult health nursing, *ed 2, St Louis, 1994, Mosby.)*

Lymphangiography
Renal ultrasound
Bence Jones protein
Intradermal skin tests

■ PERNICIOUS ANEMIA (CHRONIC, PROGRESSIVE, MACROCYTIC [MEGALOBLASTIC] ANEMIA)

Defective red blood cell (RBC) production caused by lack of intrinsic factor, which is essential for absorption of vitamin B_{12} (deficiency of vitamin B_{12} causes gastric, intestinal, and neurologic abnormalities)

ASSESSMENT
SUBJECTIVE DATA
Central nervous system (CNS)
  Weakness
  Fatigue
  Numbness and tingling in extremities
  Disturbances in taste, vision, hearing
  Poor memory
  Disturbances in coordination
  Irritability
  Depression
  Mood swings
Cardiovascular system
  Chest pain
  Shortness of breath (SOB)
  Difficulty breathing
  Palpitations
  Rapid heart beat
  Lightheadedness
Gastrointestinal system
  Loss of appetite
  Weight loss
  Abdominal pain
  Nausea
  Indigestion
  Sore mouth
  Sore tongue
  Bleeding gums
Integumentary system
  Itching
  Bruising easily
General
  Reports family history of disease

OBJECTIVE DATA
Central nervous system
  Impaired judgment
  Impaired fine finger movement
  Paresthesia of hands and feet
  Ataxia
  Disturbed coordination
  Positive Romberg's and Babinski signs
Cardiovascular system
  Tachycardia

Wide pulse pressure
  Palpitations
  Orthopnea
Gastrointestinal system
  Beefy, red, smooth, painful tongue
  Vomiting
  Flatulence
  Constipation or diarrhea
  Weight loss
  Pale lips, gums, tongue
Integumentary system
  Waxy pallor to lemon-yellow color
  Petechiae
  Purpura
  Jaundiced sclera
  Pale lips/gums
General
  Repeated infections
  Primarily Northern European background
  Usually between 50 to 60 years of age
  Previous history of gastrectomy

DIAGNOSTIC TESTS
Schilling test (<3% of radioactive B_{12} excreted in the first 24 hours after injection)
Erythrocyte count <3 million/dl
Hemoglobin reduced to 4 to 5 g/100 ml
Red blood cells (RBCs) decreased
MCH decreased
MCHC, MCV increased
WBC low
Platelet count low with large, malformed platelets
Bone marrow biopsy: increased megaloblasts
Bilirubin elevated: unconjugated forms
Serum vitamin B_{12} low
Serum folate normal or low
Gastric analysis: absence of free hydrochloric acid, decreased secretions, elevated pH
Therapeutic trial with parenteral vitamin B produces a large number of reticulocytes in the blood 4 to 5 days after injection
Upper gastrointestinal (GI) series: atrophy of gastric mucosa

POTENTIAL COMPLICATIONS
Permanent neurologic damage
Cardiomegaly
Congestive heart failure (CHF)
Gastritis
Paralysis
Paranoia
Hallucinations, delusions
Infection, usually genitourinary

MULTIDISCIPLINARY MANAGEMENT
THERAPEUTIC MANAGEMENT
Early parenteral vitamin B_{12} replacement
Lifelong vitamin B_{12} maintenance therapy
Digestants

Blood transfusions
Physical therapy
Respiratory therapy
Hematinic agents
Vitamin supplements
Antifungal, analgesic mouth rinse
Vital sign, pulse pressure monitoring
Diet high in vitamins, iron, and protein
Consultation with dietitian

PATIENT PROBLEMS—NURSING DIAGNOSES/INTERVENTIONS

▼ Activity intolerance related to weakness, fatigue, imbalance between oxygen supply and demand.

If patient on bed rest, maintain position of comfort *to promote ease of respiration and reduce energy expenditure*
Perform active or passive range of motion (ROM) exercises to patient tolerance *to maintain muscle strength and joint ROM*
 Assist with activities of daily living (ADLs) and ambulation *to conserve energy*
 Assist patient to identify causes of increased/decreased activity tolerance *to facilitate development of individualized, safe activity plan*
 Develop individualized activity regimen *to maintain cardiac performance and prevent muscle wasting*
 Plan and prioritize ADLs with patient *to reduce fatigue*
 Pace activity tolerance *to facilitate development of individualized, safe activity plan*
 Pace activities *to minimize demands on cardiac workload*
 Set goals with patient to increase activities as symptoms of intolerance decrease *to promote self-management of therapeutic regimen*
 Monitor physiologic responses to activities *to evaluate patient response to the ADL plan*
 Assess adverse responses to ADLs (e.g., tachycardia, dysrhythmias, dyspnea); refer to physician as needed
 Encourage use of coping strategies *to reduce fear and anxiety that may enhance activity intolerance*

Expected Outcomes
Participates in an activity plan within physiologic limitations without evidence of exertional dyspnea or tachycardia
Activity level progresses to preillness state
Monitors physiologic response to activity

▼ Altered nutrition: less than body requirements related to inadequate intake of iron and folic acid

Assess nutritional status and food preferences, including cultural, religious, or medical restrictions
Consult dietitian *for further assessment and nutritional support*

Provide small, frequent feedings *to avoid fatiguing patient with three large meals*
Provide dietary supplement as ordered *to ensure appropriate daily caloric intake*
Encourage family to bring patient's favorite foods from home if appropriate
 Avoid foods that are irritants, spicy, flatus-forming, or high in caffeine
Monitor intake and output every shift *to aid in early detection of inadequate intake*
Weigh patient daily (same time, scale, and clothing)
 Report 2% decrease in weight
Assist patient with meals as necessary *to conserve energy*
Encourage patient to perform oral hygiene before meals *to enhance taste*
Monitor and record character, amount, color, and frequency of stools; administer antidiarrheal medications as indicated

Expected Outcomes
Weight increases toward normal for height, age, sex, and body build
Taking balanced diet with fluids to 2000 ml, unless contraindicated
Intake and output are balanced

▼ Altered oral mucous membrane related to nutritional imbalance

Assess oral cavity every shift *to ensure early intervention and treatment*
Assist patient to perform oral hygiene every 2 hours when awake and before and after meals *to prevent buildup of plaque and bacteria*
Perform oral hygiene with dilute mouthwash or normal saline rinse and soft brush or sponge *to avoid irritation of mucous membranes*
Apply topical protective agents (water-based jelly, kaolin preparations) to lesions as ordered *to promote healing*
Apply topical analgesics 15 to 20 minutes before meals as ordered *to facilitate nutritional intake*
 Instruct patient to "swish and swallow" or "swish and spit"
Apply lubricating, water-based ointment to lips as ordered
Serve foods and fluids lukewarm or cold *to soothe inflamed oral mucosa*
Encourage patient to eat soft, easy-to-chew foods *to avoid tissue trauma and pain*
Encourage fluids, unless contraindicated; iced liquids or popsicles may be soothing
Instruct patient to avoid spicy/irritant foods *to decrease mucosal irritation*

Expected Outcomes
Oral mucosa, tongue, and lips are pink, moist, and intact
Verbalizes comfort in chewing, swallowing, and talking

▼ Risk for injury related to abnormal blood profile and hypoxemia

Provide safety measures when needed: side rails up, bed in low position when patient on bed rest, assist with ambulation as needed *to prevent falls*

Assess degree of cognitive impairment; monitor emotional state

Identify environmental risk factors *to promote safety*

Apply heat with caution; use extra blankets or layers of clothing instead of heating devices *to avoid burning the skin*

Assess skin twice a day for integrity, color, warmth, texture, and moisture *to detect peripheral and systemic changes*

Avoid use of restrictive clothing and shoes *to avoid impairment of skin integrity*

Have patient use support-type slippers or shoes and assistive devices as needed *to ensure safe ambulation*

Remind patient to call for assistance when needed

Expected Outcome
Avoids injury caused by cognitive impairment or abnormal blood profile

▼ Risk for infection related to compromised primary defenses: impaired skin integrity, inflamed mucosa; and compromised secondary defenses: impaired immune system, abnormal blood profile

Follow Standard Precautions *to minimize risk of nosocomial infection*

Assess for signs and symptoms of infection q8h to 12h

Administer antiinfective agents as ordered

Instruct patient/significant others in proper handwashing technique, including when to perform, *to reduce exposure to pathogens*

Assist patient to turn, cough, and deep breathe every 4 hours *to prevent stasis of secretions in lungs and airway*

Encourage fluid intake to 2500 ml per day, unless contraindicated, *to prevent stasis of urine, promote flushing of kidneys and bladder, and prevent urinary tract infection*

Encourage ambulation as tolerated *to prevent stasis of body fluids*

Provide for undisturbed rest and sleep periods *to promote healing*

Use soft toothbrush and stool softeners as ordered *to prevent injury to mucous membranes*

Expected Outcomes
Remains free of infection

Signs and symptoms of infection are recognized early and treated promptly

▼ Impaired gas exchange related to altered oxygen supply, altered blood flow, and altered oxygen-carrying capacity of blood

Maintain oxygen delivery as ordered *to prevent desaturation*

Monitor pulse oximetry *to assess changes in saturation*

Assess respirations for quality, rate, pattern, depth, dyspnea on exertion, guarding, use of accessory muscles

Assist patient to turn, cough, and deep breathe at least every 2 hours *to prevent stasis of secretions and body fluids*

Assess changes in mental status and behavior

Assist patient to maintain position of comfort for optimal respiratory effort *to promote lung expansion, increase air exchange, and maximize ventilatory effort*

Maintain bed rest with side rails up *to decrease cardiac workload*

Monitor P, BP, and R *to assess cardiac and respiratory function*

Assist patient with ADLs as needed *to conserve energy*

Increase patient's activity level as tolerated *to maintain cardiopulmonary fitness*

Provide reassurance as needed to reduce patient's anxiety *that may contribute to increased cardiopulmonary workload*

Instruct patient to report dyspnea and palpitations

Expected Outcomes
Hypoxemia is resolved or improved

Impairment of mental status and restlessness are absent or reduced

Vital signs are stable

Denies dyspnea

Demonstrates increasing activity tolerance

Additional Nursing Diagnoses to Consider
Altered family processes

Ineffective management of therapeutic regimen

Noncompliance

Altered protection

Altered role performance

PATIENT/FAMILY TEACHING
MEDICATION
Emphasize need to take medications as directed

Instruct patient in name of medication, dosage, time of administration, purpose, side effects, route of administration, and interactions

Instruct patient to avoid over-the-counter medications without checking with physician

DISEASE PROCESS
Discuss signs and symptoms of infection

Instruct patient/significant other in skin integrity maintenance

Instruct patient/significant other in oral hygiene techniques

Instruct patient to observe and report symptoms of recurrence to physician; explain that symptoms will recede with continuing therapy (check with physician for symptoms that may be irreversible)

Explain need to maintain planned rest periods and avoid fatigue

Arrange for visits by home health nurse as needed

Instruct patient to continue follow-up care with physician

NUTRITION
Explain need to maintain balanced diet and fluid intake
Review foods high in vitamin B_{12}, folic acid

ACTIVITY
Assist patient to practice physical therapy activities and general strengthening exercises
Explain need to increase activities gradually to desired level as tolerated
Instruct patient in measurement of pulse rate and rhythm during activity/exercise; instruct patient to stop if dysrhythmia is noted

DISCHARGE/HOME CARE PLANNING
Review history for presence of caregiver
Assess knowledge level of patient and caregiver about cause and correction of B_{12}/folic acid deficiency
Assess ability of patient/caregiver to learn home management techniques including daily weight, maintenance of nutrition log, selection of appropriate foods, oral hygiene, skin care

■ IRON DEFICIENCY ANEMIA (HYPOCHROMIC, MICROCYTIC ANEMIA)
Defective RBC production resulting from depletion of iron stores in the body needed to synthesize hemoglobin

ASSESSMENT
SUBJECTIVE DATA
Central nervous system
  Weakness
  Fatigue
  Numb, tingling extremities
  Headache
  Irritability
  Inability to concentrate
Gastrointestinal system
  Loss of appetite
  Indigestion
  Vague abdominal pains
  Sore mouth
  Difficulty swallowing
Cardiovascular system
  Palpitations
  Dizziness
  Rapid heart beat
  SOB with exertion
  Sensitivity to cold
General
  Reports history of taking anticoagulants, aspirin, steroids, or nonsteroidal antiinflammatory agents (NSAIDs)
  Mother reports history of unsupplemented breastfeeding, bottle-feeding of infant

OBJECTIVE DATA
Central nervous system
  Weakness

  Vertigo
  Paresthesia of extremities
  Listlessness
Gastrointestinal system
  Anorexia
  Pica
  Glossitis
  Angular stomatitis
  Dysphagia
  Weight loss
  Chronic diarrhea
  Flatulence
  Cachexia
Cardiovascular system
  Palpitations
  Tachycardia
  Tachypnea
  Dyspnea on exertion (DOE)
  Ankle edema
Integumentary system
  Pale ear lobes, palms, and conjunctivae
  Blue or pearl-white sclera
  Thin, brittle, spoon-shaped fingernails
  Brittle hair
General
  Chronic blood loss: GI bleeding, heavy menses
  Pregnancy
  Premenopausal woman
  Premature, low-birth-weight infant
Malabsorption syndrome: chronic diarrhea, partial or total gastrectomy, celiac disease

DIAGNOSTIC TESTS
Hgb reduced as low as 3.6 g/dl
Erythrocyte count rarely below 3 million/dl
MCH decreased
MCHC decreased
Hct reduced
Serum iron low with high binding capacity
Iron-binding capacity increased
Serum ferritin decreased
RBCs decreased with microcytic and hypochromic cells
Bone marrow studies: depleted or absent iron store; normoblastic hyperplasia

POTENTIAL COMPLICATIONS
Chest pain
Cardiomegaly
Hemoglobinuria

MULTIDISCIPLINARY MANAGEMENT
THERAPEUTIC MANAGEMENT
Iron therapy, orally or parenterally (Box 4-1)
Diet high in iron-rich foods to correct nutritional deficiency
Antifungal, anesthetic mouth rinse
Vital signs monitoring
Hematinic agents
Stool softeners, laxatives
Ascorbic acid

Box 4-1	**Precautions in Iron Therapy Administration**

ORAL ADMINISTRATION
Use straw to prevent staining teeth with liquid preparations

INTRAMUSCULAR (IM) ADMINISTRATION
Use second needle after withdrawing solution from ampule to avoid staining tissue
Use Z-tract method of injection
Inject 0.5 ml of air before removing needle from tissue

INTRAVENOUS (IV) ADMINISTRATION
Administer test dose
Remain with patient to assess for symptoms of nausea, headache, chest pain, dyspnea, rash, seizures, or shock
Use small-gauge needle
Cover solution with dark plastic

Consultation with dietitian
Physical therapy
Respiratory therapy

PATIENT PROBLEMS—NURSING DIAGNOSES/INTERVENTIONS

▼Altered nutrition: less than body requirements related to inadequate dietary iron intake, inability to absorb iron, and excessive chronic blood loss

Assess nutritional status and food preferences, including cultural, religious, or medical restrictions
Consult dietitian *for further assessment and nutritional support*
Provide small, frequent feedings *to avoid fatiguing patient with three large meals*
Provide dietary supplement as ordered *to ensure appropriate daily caloric intake*
Administer iron therapy as ordered *to supplement dietary intake*
Administer ascorbic acid as ordered *to supplement dietary intake*
Weigh patient daily (same time, scale, and clothing) *to monitor response to nutritional support*
Encourage family to bring patient's favorite foods from home if appropriate
  Avoid foods that are GI irritants, spicy, flatus-forming, or high in caffeine
Assist patient with meals as necessary *to conserve energy*
Monitor intake and output every shift *to aid in early detection of inadequate intake*
Review laboratory data *to monitor effectiveness of medication and nutritional support*

Expected Outcomes
Weight increases toward normal for height, age, sex, and body build

Taking balanced diet with fluids to 2000 ml, unless contraindicated
Consumes 100% RDA of iron and folic acid daily

▼Altered oral mucous membrane related to nutritional imbalance

Assess oral cavity every shift to ensure early intervention and treatment and monitor response to therapy
Assist patient to perform oral hygiene q2h when awake and before and after meals *to prevent buildup of plaque and bacteria*
Perform oral hygiene with dilute mouthwash or normal saline rinse and soft brush or sponge *to avoid irritation of mucous membranes*
Apply topical protective agents (water-based jelly, kaolin preparations) to lesions as ordered *to promote healing*
Apply topical analgesics 15 to 20 minutes before meals as ordered *to facilitate nutritional intake*
  Instruct patient to "swish and swallow" or "swish and spit"
Apply lubricating, water-based ointment to lips as ordered
Serve foods and fluids lukewarm or cold *to soothe inflamed oral mucosa*
Encourage patient to eat soft, easy-to-chew foods *to avoid tissue trauma and pain*

Expected Outcomes
Oral mucosa, tongue, and lips are pink, moist, and intact
Verbalizes comfort in chewing, swallowing, and talking

▼Risk for injury related to cognitive impairment, alteration in mental status, and abnormal blood profile

Provide a safe environment free of obstacles *to prevent injury to extremities*
Assess degree of cognitive impairment; monitor emotional state
Identify environmental risk factors *to promote safety*
Apply heat with caution; use extra blankets or layers of clothing instead of heating devices *to avoid burning the skin*
Assess skin bid for integrity, color, warmth, texture, and moisture *to detect peripheral and systemic changes*
Avoid use of restrictive clothing and shoes *to avoid impairment of skin integrity*
Have patient use support-type slippers or shoes and assistive devices as needed *to ensure safe ambulation*
Instruct patient to sit at side of bed and stand before walking *to prevent injury as a result of dizziness*
Remind patient to call for assistance when needed

Expected Outcomes
Avoids injury resulting from cognitive impairment or abnormal blood profile
Verbalizes precautions to prevent injury

▼Impaired skin integrity related to decreased tissue perfusion

Wash hair gently with conditioning shampoo *to prevent breakage and loss*

Assist patient with nail care as needed *to prevent damage*

Expected Outcomes

Hair is strong and shiny

Nails are strong and firm

▼ Sensory/perceptual alterations related to tissue hypoxia of the nervous system

Assess cognitive functioning every shift

Plan care with patient participation *to promote consistency and sense of calmness*

Maintain a warm environment

Maintain a safe environment *to prevent injury to extremities*

Assist patient with ambulation and positioning *to prevent injury resulting from a fall and increased dizziness*

Administer medications as prescribed *to manage headaches*

Anticipate patient needs, provide instructions and information, allow patient to verbalize concerns *to reduce irritability and manage altered concentration*

Assure patient that altered concentration will improve with therapy

Expected Outcomes

Exhibits increased concentration when performing ADLs and other activities

Signs of irritability decrease

Can change position and ambulate without dizziness or injury to limbs

Denies sensitivity to cold, headache

▼ Activity intolerance related to generalize weakness, fatigue, and imbalance between oxygen supply and demand

Maintain position of comfort

Perform active or passive ROM exercises

Assist with ADLs and ambulation *to conserve energy*

Assist patient to identify causes of increased/decreased activity tolerance *to facilitate development of individualized, safe activity plan*

Develop individualized activity regimen *to maintain cardiac performance and prevent muscle wasting*

Plan and prioritize ADLs with patient *to reduce fatigue*

Pace activities *to minimize demands on cardiac workload*

Set goals with patient to increase activities as symptoms of intolerance decrease

Monitor physiologic responses to activities *to evaluate patient response to ADL plan*

Assess adverse responses to ADLs (e.g., tachycardia, dysrhythmias, dypnea); refer to physician as needed

Provide uninterrupted rest periods *to maintain energy level*

Increase patient activity in small increments until tolerance level is reached

Expected Outcomes

Participates in an activity plan within physiologic limitations without evidence of exertional dyspnea or tachycardia

Activity level progresses to preillness state

Additional Nursing Diagnoses to Consider

Self-care deficit

Altered parenting

Impaired adjustment

PATIENT/FAMILY TEACHING

MEDICATIONS

Instruct patient in names of medications, dosage, time of administration, purpose, side effects, route of administration, and interactions

Inform patient that coffee, tea, eggs, and milk inhibit iron absorption; antacids decrease iron absorption; chloramphenicol delays erythropoiesis

Demonstrate method for parenteral administration of iron

Increase vitamin C/ascorbic acid intake to enhance iron absorption

Instruct patient to avoid over-the-counter medications without checking with health care provider

Explain need to continue iron therapy even when feeling better

Discuss color of stools expected and explain need and methods to avoid constipation

Emphasize need to take medications as directed

NUTRITION

Explain need to maintain balanced diet and fluid intake

Review dietary sources of iron

Explain importance of monitoring weight as instructed

DISEASE PROCESS

Discuss signs and symptoms of recurrence to report to health care provider (check with physician for symptoms that may be irreversible)

Instruct patient/significant other in maintenance of skin integrity

Instruct patient/significant other in oral hygiene techniques

Arrange for visits by home health nurse as needed

Instruct patient to continue follow-up care with physician and laboratory

Explain need to increase activities gradually to desired level as tolerated

Explain need to maintain planned rest periods and avoid fatigue

DISCHARGE/HOME CARE PLANNING

Review history for presence of caregiver

Assess patient's ability to provide balanced diet at home; initiate social services referral as needed

Assess knowledge level of patient and caregiver about cause and correction of iron deficiency

Assess ability of patient/caregiver to learn home management techniques including daily weight, maintenance of nutrition log, selection of appropriate foods, oral hygiene, ADL plan, medication administration

Assist patient/significant other to assess home environment for environmental safety hazards

■ HEMOLYTIC ANEMIA

Premature and accelerated destruction of erythrocytes in the presence of normal erythropoiesis; may be acquired or hereditary

ASSESSMENT

SUBJECTIVE DATA

Central nervous system
    Weakness
    Fatigue
    Headache
Gastrointestinal system
    Abdominal pain
    Loss of appetite
    Nausea
    Diarrhea
Genitourinary system
    Urinary changes
Cardiovascular system
    SOB
Integumentary system
    Pruritus
General
    Reports family history of disease
    Reports history of trauma, infection, systemic disease, exposure to drugs or toxins

OBJECTIVE DATA

Central nervous system
    Weakness
    Irritability
Gastrointestinal system
    Vomiting
    Abdominal tenderness
    Splenomegaly
    Diarrhea
Genitourinary system
    Nocturnal hemoglobinuria
    Urine changes
    Decreased urinary output
Cardiovascular system
    Chills
    Fever
    Venous thrombosis
Integumentary system
    Jaundice
    Pallor
Musculoskeletal system
    Bone deformities
    Edema

DIAGNOSTIC TESTS

Erythrocyte count low
Hgb low
Hct low
Reticulocyte count high
Erythrocyte fragility increased
Serum bilirubin increased
Urinary urobilinogen increased
Normocytic anemia
Bone marrow biopsy reveals erythroid hyperplasia

POTENTIAL COMPLICATIONS

Renal failure
Hemoglobinuria

MULTIDISCIPLINARY MANAGEMENT

THERAPEUTIC MANAGEMENT

Eliminate causative factors; treat underlying disorder
Management of primary condition
Maintenance of fluid and electrolyte balance
Consultation with dietitian
Transfusions as needed
Corticosteroids
Osmotic diuretics
Antidiarrheal medications
Antiemetic medications
Antipyretics as indicated
Splenectomy

PATIENT PROBLEMS—NURSING DIAGNOSES/INTERVENTIONS

▼ Fluid volume deficit related to active fluid loss and blood cell hemolysis

Monitor intake and output every shift *to assess fluid needs and prevent overload;* report imbalances

Weigh patient daily (same time, scale, clothing), report changes of 2% to 3% of original weight

Monitor vital signs and mental status every 4 hours

Assess skin turgor and peripheral pulses every shift *to determine adequacy of hydration*

Monitor character, amount, color, frequency of emesis, stools *to assess source, quality of active fluid loss*

Observe color, specific gravity, pH of urine *to ensure early detection of renal failure*

Provide oral fluid intake as tolerated *to maintain intravascular fluid volume*

Provide clear liquid diet *to reduce nausea;* progress to balanced diet as symptoms abate

Provide oral fluids in small, frequent amounts *to prevent abdominal distention*

Administer blood transfusions as ordered *to alleviate fluid deficit*

Force fluids to 2500 ml/day unless contraindicated

Administer intravenous fluids as ordered *to correct fluid deficit*

Administer urine alkalizers as ordered *to enhance renal function*

Arrange for quiet rest periods before and after meals *to alleviate nausea, vomiting, gastric distress*

Expected Outcomes

Skin turgor and color are normal

Intake and output are balanced

Renal function is adequate

Peripheral pulses are present

Extremities are warm with good color

▼Activity intolerance related to generalized weakness, fatigue, and imbalance between oxygen supply and demand

Develop an individualized activity regimen *to maintain cardiac performance and prevent muscle wasting*

Pace activities *to minimize demands on cardiac workload*

Assist patient with ADLs *to conserve energy*

Provide uninterrupted rest periods *to maintain energy level*

Set goals with patient to increase activities as symptoms of intolerance decrease

Monitor physiologic responses to activities *to evaluate patient response to the ADL plan*

Assess adverse responses to ADLs (e.g., tachycardia, dysrhythmias, dyspnea); refer to physician as needed

Expected Outcomes

Participates in an activity plan within physiologic limitations without evidence of exertional dyspnea or tachycardia

Activity level progresses to preillness state

▼Abdominal, back pain related to liver/splenic distention

Maintain position of comfort *to relieve pressure from enlarged liver/spleen*

Administer analgesics as ordered; provide pain-relief measures as needed *to relieve discomfort*

Offer antiemetics, oral care, other measures *to alleviate nausea and vomiting*

Encourage use of coping strategies *to reduce fear and anxiety that may exacerbate pain*

Assess pain for predisposing factors, intensity, frequency, duration, and effective methods of control *to facilitate development of a collaborative pain management program*

Expected Outcome

Verbalizes feelings of increased comfort on pain rating scale

▼Hyperthermia related to illness and increased metabolic rate

Administer antipyretics as ordered

Provide external sources of warmth *to warm when chilling occurs*

Expected Outcomes

Temperature is within normal limits

Does not experience chilling

▼Impaired skin integrity related to increased serum bilirubin, jaundice, or pruritus

Assess skin condition every shift

Monitor laboratory data daily *to assess liver function*

Provide frequent skin care *to promote comfort and decrease itching* (e.g., soothing baths: sodium bicarbonate, oatmeal)

Avoid skin dryness; apply lotions to slightly moist skin; cool sponge baths or tub soaks may be beneficial

Provide cool ambient temperature with adequate humidity

Avoid constrictive clothing *to prevent friction and impairment of skin integrity*

Elevate bedclothes with bed cradle; keep bed wrinkle-free *to prevent skin irritation*

Launder linen in nondetergent laundry products *to prevent skin irritation*

Advise patient to avoid scratching *to prevent irritation and injury*

Instruct patient to apply pressure or cool applications *to alleviate itching*

Expected Outcomes

Skin remains intact and moist without evidence of scratching

Skin is warm and dry with good turgor

▼Altered nutrition: less than body requirements related to liver dysfunction

Assess nutritional status and food preferences, including cultural, religious, or medical restrictions

Consult dietitian *for further assessment and nutritional support*

Provide small, frequent feedings *to avoid abdominal distention*

Provide balanced diet high in iron and protein *to promote erythropoiesis*

Provide dietary supplement as ordered *to ensure appropriate daily caloric intake*

Encourage family to bring patient's favorite foods from home if appropriate

Avoid high-fat foods *to minimize discomfort caused by stress on gallbladder*

Monitor intake and output every shift *to assess patient's appetite*

Weigh patient daily (same time, scale, and clothing) *to assess patient's response to nutritional therapy*

Assist patient as needed with meals *to conserve energy*

Review laboratory data, especially bilirubin, *to assess liver function*

Expected Outcomes
Eats a balanced diet
Weight increases toward normal for height, age, sex, and body build
Hepatosplenomegaly is absent

Additional Nursing Diagnoses to Consider
Social isolation
Altered parenting
Ineffective management of therapeutic regimen

PATIENT/FAMILY TEACHING
MEDICATION
Emphasize need to take medications as directed
Instruct patient in name of medications, dosage, time of administration, purpose, side effects, route of administration, and interactions
Instruct patient to avoid over-the-counter medications without checking with health care provider

DISEASE PROCESS
Instruct patient about type of hemolytic condition
   hereditary RBC deficiency: Patient is susceptible to hemolysis after ingestion of chemical oxidants; family members should be screened
   response to trauma or infectious disease: Explain that primary condition will be treated; discuss symptoms of recurrence to report
   acquired RBC deficiency: Explain that condition may be induced by infection, immunization, iron products, or plasma in whole blood transfusions
   Discuss symptoms of recurrence to report
Instruct patient/significant other to maintain skin hygiene and avoid scratching
Arrange for visits by home health nurse as needed
Instruct patient to continue follow-up care with health care provider

ACTIVITY
Explain need to increase activities gradually to desired level as tolerated
Explain need to maintain planned rest periods and avoid fatigue
Instruct patient in measurement of pulse rate and rhythm during activity/exercise; instruct patient to stop if dysrhythmia is noted
Instruct patient to seek assistance from others to conserve energy as needed

NUTRITION
Explain need to maintain balanced diet and fluid intake
Instruct patient to notify health care provider if intake or output decreases as indicated by change in weight

DISCHARGE/HOME CARE PLANNING
Review history for presence of caregiver
Assess patient's ability to provide balanced diet at home; initiate social services referral as needed
Assess knowledge level of patient/caregiver about cause and correction of iron deficiency
Assess ability of patient/caregiver to learn home management techniques, including daily weight, maintenance of nutrition log, selection of appropriate foods, oral hygiene, ADL plan, medication administration
Assist patient/significant other to identify environmental safety hazards in the home

■ SICKLE CELL ANEMIA AND CRISIS
A genetic disease that occurs in individuals with a defective hemoglobin molecule (HbS); this defect results in a major rearrangement, and rigid, elongated, crescent-shaped or sickle-shaped cells when oxygen tension is decreased; the microcirculation becomes slowed, and cells adhere to epithelium and clump, causing occlusion and infarction; crisis occurs when a critical point is reached and hemolysis occurs; sickle cell anemia is the most prevalent of the congenital hemolytic anemias and causes a shortened life span (Fig. 4-3)

ASSESSMENT
SUBJECTIVE DATA
Central nervous system
   Irritability
   Headaches
   Tiredness
Gastrointestinal systems
   Nausea
   Abdominal pain
Respiratory system
   Chest pain
   SOB
   Difficulty breathing
Cardiovascular system
   Chest pain
   Fatigue
   Rapid heart beat
   Palpitations
Musculoskeletal system
   Aching joints
General
   Reports family history of disease

OBJECTIVE DATA
Central nervous system
   Elevated temperature
   Irritability
   Lethargy
   Sleepiness
   Coma
Gastrointestinal system
   Vomiting
   Anorexia
   Hepatomegaly
   Splenomegaly
   Abdominal tenderness
   Pale tongue

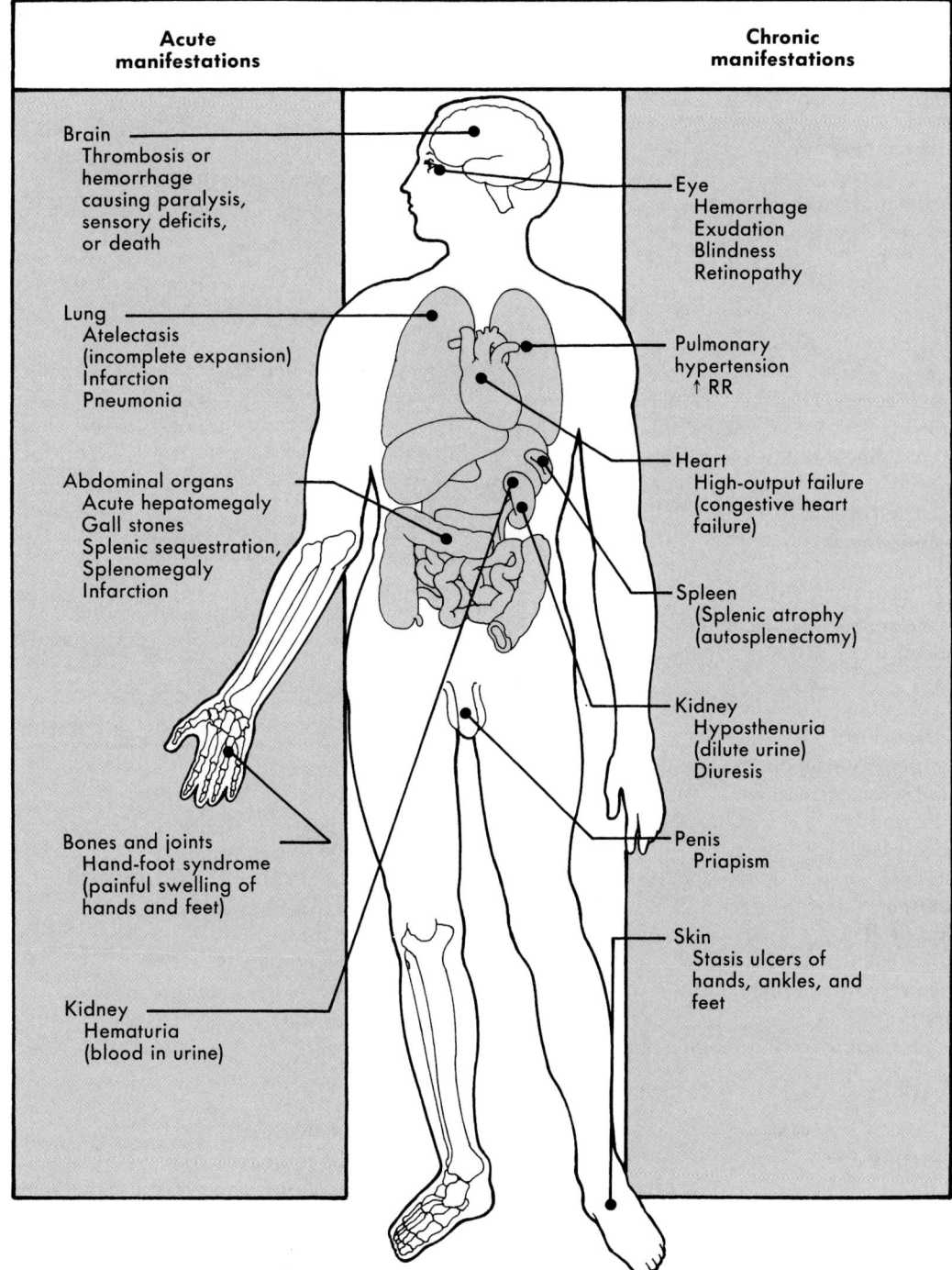

Acute manifestations

Brain
  Thrombosis or hemorrhage causing paralysis, sensory deficits, or death

Lung
  Atelectasis (incomplete expansion)
  Infarction
  Pneumonia

Abdominal organs
  Acute hepatomegaly
  Gall stones
  Splenic sequestration, Splenomegaly
  Infarction

Bones and joints
  Hand-foot syndrome (painful swelling of hands and feet)

Kidney
  Hematuria (blood in urine)

Chronic manifestations

Eye
  Hemorrhage
  Exudation
  Blindness
  Retinopathy

Pulmonary hypertension
  ↑ RR

Heart
  High-output failure (congestive heart failure)

Spleen
  (Splenic atrophy (autosplenectomy)

Kidney
  Hyposthenuria (dilute urine)
  Diuresis

Penis
  Priapism

Skin
  Stasis ulcers of hands, ankles, and feet

Fig. 4-3 Clinical manifestations of sickle cell disease.
(From Belcher A: Mosby's clinical nursing series: blood disorders, *St Louis, 1993, Mosby.)*

Musculoskeletal system
  Joint swelling
Integumentary system
  Pallor
  Leg ulcers above ankle
  Jaundice
  Pale lips, palms, nail beds
Genitourinary system
  Polyuria

Hematuria
Enuresis
Dark urine
General
  African descent
  Increased susceptibility to infection
  Infants and children: dacrylitis, failure to thrive, impaired growth and development with delayed puberty

Painful crisis
  Severe pain: abdomen, chest, back, joints, bones, muscles
  Increased jaundice
  Dark urine
  Low-grade temperature
Aplastic crisis
  Associated with infection, usually viral
  Temperature elevated to 100° F or 104° (37.7° C or 40°) for 2 days
  Pallor
  Lethargy
  Sleepiness, difficulty awakening
  Coma
  RBC hemolysis with bone marrow depression
Sequestration crisis
  Massive entrapment of RBCs in spleen and liver
  Pallor
  Progressive lethargy
  Hypovolemic shock

DIAGNOSTIC TESTS
Stained blood smear shows sickle cells
Hemoglobin electrophoresis shows HgbS
Low RBC
Elevated WBC
Elevated platelet count
Decreased erythrocyte sedimentation rate
Increased serum sedimentation rate
Increased serum iron
RBC survival decreased
Reticulocytosis
Low or normal Hgb
Increased bilirubin
Elliptocytosis
Sickle cell slide preparation of blood shows sickling after deoxygenation
Sickle solubility test shows turbid solution indicating presence of HgbS

POTENTIAL COMPLICATIONS
Sickle cell crisis (Box 4-2)
Autosplenectomy
Severe infections
Hypovolemic shock
Death
Hepatomegaly
Failure to thrive
Retinopathy
Neuropathy
Cerebrovascular accidents
Subarachnoid hemorrhage
Organ infarction
Renal failure
Respiratory problems
MI
CHF
Osteomyelitis
Priapism
Gallstones

Box 4-2   Sickle Cell Anemia—Crisis

Sickle cell anemia is a genetic disorder affecting black people. Sickle-shaped cells clump together, preventing oxygen and other products from reaching microcirculation, leading to more hypoxia and sickling. The causes are unknown, but factors thought to precipitate a crisis are hypoxia, infection, and dehydration. Tissue necrosis can result if prolonged.

ASSESSMENT
Pain in extremities, joints, abdomen
Weakness, pallor
Cardiac dysfunction: dysrhythmias, murmurs
Dyspnea, chest pain, cyanosis
Altered level of consciousness
Decreased urinary output
Signs of infection

INTERVENTIONS
Maintain airway, breathing, and circulation.
Administer high-flow oxygen (10-15 L) by mask.
Obtain IV access, hydration, lab studies.
Manage pain with medications, and positioning for comfort.
Provide rest environment for patient.
Monitor intake and output.

From Thompson, et al: Mosby's clinical nursing ed 4, *St Louis, 1997, Mosby.*

MULTIDISCIPLINARY MANAGEMENT
THERAPEUTIC MANAGEMENT
Rest
Heat application to joints
Hydration with IV fluids and electrolytes
Oxygen therapy
Analgesics
Sedation
Antipyretics
Antibiotics as indicated
Blood component transfusion
Exchange transfusions for aplastic, hyperhemolytic, and sequestration crises
Experimental use of antisickling agents: urea, cyanate, carbamoyl phosphate
Oral maintenance therapy with folic acid and/or iron
Consultation with respiratory therapist
Consultation with dietitian
Occupational therapy as indicated
Genetic counseling
Supportive care; social services

PATIENT PROBLEMS—NURSING DIAGNOSES/INTERVENTIONS

▼ Altered cardiopulmonary, cardiovascular, cerebral, renal, peripheral tissue perfusion related to increased blood viscosity, hypoxemia, impairment of microcirculation, and hypovolemia

Cardiopulmonary/cardiovascular system

Monitor BP q2h (or determine frequency based on condition) *to assess cardiac function and peripheral resistance to blood flow;* report changes immediately

Monitor respirations and auscultate chest for heart and breath sounds q2h (or determine frequency based on condition) *to assess pulmonary function and detect onset of respiratory failure;* report changes immediately

Maintain patient in semi-Fowler's position when in bed *to promote maximal respiratory excursion*

Encourage frequent rest periods and avoidance of strenuous activity *to decrease cardiac workload and minimize risk of sickling*

Maintain a stress-free environment *to minimize risk of sickling*

Assist with ADLs *to reduce oxygen demand*

Monitor administration of packed RBCs *to prevent circulatory overload and reaction*

Instruct patient to avoid caffeine, tobacco, and other stimulants *to prevent vasoconstriction*

Notify physician for complaints of chest pain, increased dyspnea, cyanosis, restlessness *to facilitate early intervention*

Administer oxygen therapy as ordered *to promote adequate tissue perfusion*

Administer anticoagulants as ordered *to promote tissue perfusion*

Initiate continuous pulse oximetry *to monitor oxygen saturation*

Administer sublingual nitroglycerin as ordered for angina

Review blood studies *to assess adequacy of tissue perfusion and blood flow;* report changes to health care provider

Cerebral system

Assess neurologic signs q2h *to detect increasing intracranial pressure (ICP)*

Maintain patient on complete bed rest with head of bed elevated *to conserve energy and lower ICP*

Provide quiet environment *to promote rest and reduce stress*

Instruct patient to avoid stimulants (caffeine, tobacco) *to prevent vasoconstriction*

Renal system

Provide oral/IV intake to 2500 ml/day unless contraindicated *to maintain fluid balance and promote renal perfusion*

Monitor intake and output every shift *to ensure balance is maintained*

Test urine for protein *to detect renal dysfunction*

Weigh patient daily (same time, scale, and clothes) *to monitor fluid retention*

Observe for presence of facial, extremity edema *to detect renal dysfunction, fluid retention*

Monitor vital signs q4h *to ensure adequacy of blood flow*

Expected Outcomes

Normal vital signs, pupillary responses, and reflexes

Alert and oriented

Denies having headaches

Intake and output are balanced

Skin is warm and dry with good turgor and color

Weight is stable

▼ Pain related to joint swelling, tissue hypoxia, stasis of RBCs, and sickling

Assess pain location, duration, intensity using pain rating scale *to facilitate development of pain management plan*

Collaborate with patient to develop pain management plan designed to prevent severe pain

Support affected joints with pillows in position of comfort *to minimize pain and discomfort*

Apply warm soaks to joints as ordered *to promote comfort*

Maintain anatomic alignment *to prevent deformity*

Perform back and pressure point care q2h *to prevent skin breakdown*

Move patient with slow, gentle movements *to minimize discomfort of repositioning*

Administer analgesics as ordered *to achieve goal of pain management plan*

Avoid restrictive clothing *to relieve pressure and promote comfort*

Position patient in semi-Fowler's position when in bed *to decrease abdominal pressure and increase intraabdominal space*

Provide small, frequent feedings *to prevent abdominal distention*

Auscultate bowel sounds *to detect obstruction*

Encourage use of alternative pain management techniques

Expected Outcomes

Demonstrates relaxed facial expression and posture

Verbalizes pain relief using pain scale

▼ Risk for impaired skin integrity related to altered tissue perfusion, tissue hypoxemia, and immobility

Inspect skin for redness, lesions, swelling, drainage q8h *to detect impairment of skin integrity*

Keep skin warm and dry *to prevent breakdown caused by environmental moisture*

Avoid use of constrictive clothing; maintain ambient and body warmth *to promote circulation and prevent possible sickling*

Assist patient with active and passive ROM exercises as tolerated *to maintain circulation*

Palpate peripheral pulses *to assess status of arterial circulation*

Review blood studies *to evaluate oxygen saturation, blood viscosity, and pH*

If ulceration occurs, maintain patient on bed rest in semi-Fowler's position *to prevent further injury and decrease peripheral vascular resistance*

Elevate affected limb *to promote venous return*

If ulceration occurs, implement wound care procedures as ordered *to remove drainage and necrosis, prevent infection, and promote healing*

Observe response of wound, lesions to therapy *to assess effectiveness of interventions*

Cleanse skin with mild soap, rinse well, dry thoroughly *to maintain integrity*

Apply protective cream after bathing and position change

Ensure that bed linens are wrinkle-free and nonconstrictive *to prevent mechanical injury*

Reposition patient q2h when on bed rest *to promote circulation and prevent stasis*

Expected Outcomes

Skin is warm and dry with good color

Skin is free of ulceration

▼ Risk for infection related to inadequate primary defenses, inadequate secondary defenses, and chronic disease

Follow Standard Precautions *to prevent transmission of pathogens*

Maintain aseptic technique for wound care

Limit visitors *to reduce exposure to pathogens*

Encourage high-calorie, high-protein diet as appropriate *to maintain optimal nutritional status*

Encourage fluid intake to 2500 ml/day, unless contraindicated, *to promote dilute urine and frequent emptying of bladder*

Encourage patient to turn, cough, deep breathe *to prevent stasis of secretions*

Administer antibiotics as ordered

Monitor vital signs and breath sounds q4h *to detect signs/symptoms of infection*

Administer antipyretics as ordered

Obtain cultures of infected areas as ordered *to determine causative agent*

Expected Outcomes

Remains free of infection

Vital signs are stable and within normal limits for patient

Infection is recognized and treated early

▼ Risk for injury related to alteration in mental status, abnormal blood profile, bone fragility, and joint swelling

Provide safety measures when needed: side rails up, bed in low position when patient on bed rest; assist with ambulation as needed *to prevent falls*

Assess degree of cognitive impairment; monitor emotional state

Identify environmental risk factors *to promote safety*

Have patient use support-type slippers or shoes and assistive devices as needed *to ensure safe ambulation*

Remind patient to call for assistance when needed

Reposition the patient frequently with joint support *to prevent trauma and injury*

Assist patient with active and passive ROM exercises *to promote circulation, joint movement, and maintenance of muscle strength*

Encourage consumption of diet high in calcium, protein, vitamins, as appropriate, *to prevent bone, tissue injury*

Expected Outcomes

Ambulates without assistance

Avoids injury

Denies joint or bone pain

Additional Nursing Diagnoses to Consider

Self-esteem disturbance related to physical, lifestyle, or role losses

Social isolation related to disease process

Sexual dysfunction related to disease process

Other self-perceptual, role, or coping diagnoses

PATIENT/FAMILY TEACHING

Discuss need to avoid conditions that precipitate crisis

Infections

Dehydration

Activities that may cause an increase in oxygen requirement: flying in unpressurized planes, high altitudes, cold weather, vasoconstrictive drugs

Explain nutrition requirements and importance of eating a well-balanced diet with fluids to 2000 ml/day; avoid iced drinks and foods

Instruct patient to avoid consumption of caffeine and other stimulants

Discuss importance of maintaining relationships with others and participating in meaningful activity and work

Teach that balancing exercise/activity with adequate rest is important

Use stress reduction methods daily

Instruct patient to maintain good hygiene

Teach signs and symptoms of infection to report to physician or nurse; need to avoid exposure to infectious persons, treat early symptoms, and have early childhood and yearly immunizations

Instruct about signs and symptoms of recurrence to report to physician

Pain

Persistent low-grade temperature

Decreased fluid intake

Decreased appetite

Increased lethargy or sleeping

Teach name of medication, purpose, side or toxic effects, time and frequency of administration

Explain that it is necessary to tell all health care providers about disease

Wear medical alert bracelet and keep follow-up
   appointments
Explain that childbearing may cause some risks to
   females and refer for gynecologic consultation
Refer family for genetic counseling and psychologic
   counseling when appropriate

DISCHARGE/HOME CARE PLANNING
Review history for presence of caregiver
Assess patient/significant other's knowledge level of
   disease process
Assess home environment for potential environmental
   hazards
Assess ability of patient/significant other to comply with
   instructions

■ APLASTIC ANEMIA
Anemia, aplastic or hypoplastic, resulting from destruction of or injury to the bone marrow stem cells or bone marrow matrix; exposure to toxins, specifically large doses of radiation, benzene, metabolites, alkylating agents, chloramphenicol, or sulfonamides, may cause pancytopenia (bone marrow failure with granulocytopenia, thrombocytopenia, and anemia)

ASSESSMENT
SUBJECTIVE DATA
Central nervous system
   Progressive fatigue
   Weakness
   Activity intolerance
   Headache
   Dizziness
   Confusion
Gastrointestinal system
   Nausea
   Indigestion
Cardiovascular system
   Nose bleeds
   Bleeding gums
   Heavy menses
   Bruising easily
Respiratory system
   Difficulty breathing
   Cold symptoms
   Cough
General
   Reports exposure to chemical toxin, radiation, or
      specific medications
   History of frequent infection

OBJECTIVE DATA
Central nervous system
   Irritability
   Slowed thought process
   Weakness
   Confusion

Gastrointestinal system
   Vomiting
   Bleeding gums
   Flulike symptoms
   Oral ulcers
   Rectal ulcers
   GI disturbances
   GI bleeding
Cardiovascular system
   Tachycardia
   Dyspnea on exertion (DOE)
Integumentary system
   Waxy pallor
   Ecchymosis
   Petechiae
General
   Elevated temperature
   Signs/symptoms of infection
   Cough
   Nonhealing cuts, lesions
   Burning on urination
Documented history of exposure to chemical toxin,
   radiation, or specific medications

DIAGNOSTIC TESTS
RBCs usually normochromic, normocytic potential
   macrocytosis, anisocytosis
Erythrocyte count usually <1 million/mm^3
Reticulocytes low
Serum iron elevated
Total iron-binding capacity normal or slightly reduced
WBC count decreased
Platelet count decreased
Coagulation tests abnormal
Bone marrow biopsy demonstrates fatty marrow,
   hypocellular or aplastic (Box 4-3)

Box 4-3	**Bone Marrow Study**

Bone marrow is obtained by aspiration or biopsy to examine types and numbers of cells, maturation level, and composition of supporting tissue; used for diagnosis and treatment response

INDICATIONS
Evaluation of the hematolymphatic systems for differential diagnosis of various anemias, neutropenia, leukemia, thrombocytopenia, immunoglobulin disorders, lymphoma, or granulomatous disease

CARE
Inform patient that pressure will be felt with insertion of needle and some pain with aspiration; position for good visualization; apply pressure and dressing at site; check BP, P, and R q30min × 2; maintain bed rest for 1 hour; assess site for bleeding, hematoma, infection

POTENTIAL COMPLICATIONS

Hemorrhage
Cirrhosis
Diabetes
Heart failure
Blood reactions
Overwhelming infections

MULTIDISCIPLINARY MANAGEMENT
  THERAPEUTIC MANAGEMENT

Removal of causative agent
Blood transfusion
Packed RBCs
Platelets
HLA-matched leukocyte
Bone marrow transplant
Respiratory support
Antibiotics in the presence of infection
Corticosteroids to stimulate erythroid production
Marrow-stimulating agents
Physical therapy
Nutritional support and consultation

  PATIENT PROBLEMS—NURSING
  DIAGNOSES/INTERVENTIONS

▼Activity intolerance related to imbalance between oxygen supply and demand, reduce number of RBCs, and generalized weakness/fatigue

Maintain position of comfort *to promote ease of respiration*
Perform active or passive ROM exercises *to maintain muscle and joint mobility*
Assist patient with ADLs and ambulation *to conserve energy*
Assist patient to identify causes of increased/decreased activity tolerance *to facilitate development of individualized, safe activity plan*
Develop individualized activity regimen *to maintain cardiac performance and prevent muscle wasting*
Plan and prioritize ADLs with patient *to reduce fatigue*
Pace activities *to minimize demands on cardiac workload*
Set goals with patient *to increase activities as symptoms of intolerance decrease*
Monitor physiologic responses to activities *to evaluate patient response to the ADL plan*
Teach patient to monitor physiologic response to activity *to facilitate self-management of activity plan consistent with physical status*
Assess adverse responses to ADLs (e.g., tachycardia, dysrhythmias, dyspnea); refer to physician as needed
Encourage use of coping strategies *to reduce fear and anxiety that may enhance activity intolerance*
Provide uninterrupted rest periods *to conserve energy*
Administer oxygen as ordered *to reduce dyspnea*

Expected Outcomes

Participates in an activity plan within physiologic limitations without evidence of exertional dyspnea or tachycardia
Activity level progresses to preillness state

▼Risk for injury, bleeding related to bone marrow malfunction, low platelet count, and impaired clotting

Avoid IM injections *to prevent interstitial bleeding*
Apply pressure to injection, venipuncture sites *to prevent extravasation*
Instruct patient to use an electric razor for shaving
Perform oral care with a soft toothbrush or foam stick *to prevent injury to oral mucosa*
Humidify oxygen *to minimize drying of mucous membranes*
Administer stool softener *to prevent constipation and prevent injury to intestinal mucosa*
Monitor and report changes in vital signs *to ensure early detection of signs of hemorrhage*
Check urine and stool for occult, frank blood
Assess skin for petechiae and ecchymosis
Monitor laboratory results *to ensure early detection of internal bleeding*
Administer blood components as ordered
Instruct patient to avoid scratching
Assist with ambulation and ADLs to prevent injury

Expected Outcomes

Vital signs are stable
Exhibits no signs/symptoms of bleeding
Skin and mucous membranes are warm, moist, with good turgor
Laboratory values are within normal limits

▼Altered nutrition: less than body requirements related to gastrointestinal disturbances

Assess nutritional status and food preferences, including cultural, religious, or medical restrictions
Consult dietitian *for further assessment and nutritional support*
Provide balanced diet high in proteins and vitamins unless contraindicated
Provide small, frequent feedings *to prevent abdominal distention and fatigue*
Provide dietary supplement as ordered *to ensure appropriate daily caloric intake*
Encourage family to bring patient's favorite foods from home if appropriate
Monitor intake and output every shift *to assess patient's appetite*
Weigh patient daily (same time, scale, and clothing) *to assess patient's response to nutritional therapy;* notify physician for decreases of 2% to 3%
Assist patient as needed with meals *to conserve energy*

Expected Outcomes

Eats a balanced diet with adequate fluid intake

Weight increases toward normal for height, age, sex, and body build

▼ Altered oral mucous membrane related to nutritional imbalance, bleeding, and infection

Teach and assist patient with routine oral care

Regularly inspect and palpate lips, gums, and buccal mucosa

Clean teeth and rinse mouth each morning, after meals, and at bedtime

Increase frequency of oral care to q2h if lesions are present

Choose dental equipment appropriate for state of oral cavity

Soft-bristled toothbrush if there are no breaks or lesions

Gauze or sponge-covered cleaners in the presence of breaks in skin or bleeding gums

Assess patient's denture fit

Avoid gumlike adhesives

Keep dentures scrupulously clean

Remove and clean dentures before using mouth rinse

Keep patient's mouth moist

Provide appealing, tepid liquids for sipping

Flavored ice pops may be soothing

Keep lips moist; use water-soluble gel

Expected Outcomes

Exhibits no oral lesions, or healing of lesions is progressing

Patient and/or caregiver demonstrates knowledge and practice of prescribed routine oral hygiene regimen

Reports oral comfort with swallowing and talking

▼ Risk for anxiety related to changes in health, poor prognosis, and uncertainty about tests and treatments

Assess patient/significant other's understanding of disease process, tests, and treatments *to collaboratively identify areas of knowledge deficit*

With patient/significant other, identify available support systems

Assess patient/significant other's coping strategies *to assist in development of effective stress-reducing and anxiety-reducing activities*

Engage patient/significant other in development of the plan of care *to ensure patient needs are met*

Provide care in a consistent and timely manner as agreed upon by staff and patient *to meet expectations and allay anxiety*

Provide instructions and information in a manner consistent with the patient's age, developmental level, and culture

Assess the patient/significant other's understanding of instructions and information

Provide referrals to social worker, clergy, other disciplines as indicated or requested *to assist with development of coping strategies*

Plan care to allow time for the patient/significant other to express fear, anxiety or ask questions

Expected Outcomes

Patient and significant other demonstrate knowledge of disease process, tests, and treatments

Expresses and discusses fears and anxiety about diagnosis

▼ Risk for infection related to suppressed immune system, bone marrow malfunction, replacement with factor, and altered blood profile

Prevent patient exposure to infected visitors and staff

Observe Standard Precautions *to minimize exposure to pathogens*

Wash hands before each contact with patient

Place patient in a private room for absolute neutrophil count <500 mm^3 *to minimize exposure to pathogens*

Monitor and report changes in T, P, and R q4h *to ensure early detection of signs of infection*

Monitor breath sounds daily; instruct patient to report sore throat, perirectal discomfort, vaginal itching, or burning on urination *to detect atypical signs of infection*

Observe body fluids for changes in color, odor, and consistency

Administer antibiotics, antifungals, and antivirals as ordered *to treat secondary or opportunistic infection*

Assist patient with daily hygiene and oral care

Assist patient with ambulation, turning, coughing, and deep breathing *to prevent stasis of body fluids*

Ensure fluid intake to 2500 ml/day, unless contraindicated, *to dilute urine and decrease risk of urinary tract infection (UTI) by promoting frequent emptying of the bladder*

Avoid invasive procedures; use strict aseptic technique when invasive procedures must be performed

Expected Outcome

Free of respiratory, urinary, GI, or other opportunistic infection

Additional Nursing Diagnoses to Consider

Ineffective coping

Ineffective thermoregulation

Self-care deficit

Altered parenting

Social isolation

PATIENT/FAMILY TEACHING
NUTRITION

Explain need to maintain balanced diet of preference and as tolerated; to use frequent, small feedings if preferred; and to avoid foods that irritate oral mucous membranes

Explain need to take fluids of preference—at least 2500 ml/day unless contraindicated

Explain need to perform mouth care routinely before and after meals and prn, to report early signs of mouth lesions or those that do not heal, and to use special mouth rinses as ordered

Demonstrate method of checking for and explain need to report signs and symptoms of mucositis

Explain need to weigh weekly (same time, scale, and clothing)

ACTIVITY

Instruct patient to alternate activities with rest periods to conserve energy

Explain need to gradually increase activity to tolerance

Instruct patient on placing personal items at hand and positioning furniture to prevent accidents

Demonstrate use of equipment to assist with ambulation when needed

Explain need to monitor activity tolerance (check pulse; if elevated or patient is feeling exhausted, rest, then continue)

Instruct patient to report symptoms of activity intolerance to physician if no relief occurs with rest

Demonstrate oxygen therapy administration
    Liters/minute ordered

Use of equipment: changing tank, cleansing or replacement of cannula

BLEEDING

Discuss signs and symptoms of bleeding to be reported to physician

Discuss emergency plan to follow if spontaneous hemorrhage occurs
    Have emergency numbers available
    Call paramedics
    Go to nearest emergency facility

Explain importance of telling dentist and other medical personnel about disease process and low platelet count

Explain importance of maintaining safe, clutter-free environment

Explain importance of avoiding over-the-counter medications, especially those containing acetylsalicylic acid (i.e., aspirin) without checking with physician

Instruct patient to avoid use of sharp objects whenever possible

Instruct patient to avoid harsh coughing and blowing of nose
    If cough persists, notify physician
    Take cough medication as ordered

Explain need to avoid activities and sports that may cause injury

Explain need to avoid constipation through diet, fluids, and stool softeners

Explain importance of ongoing outpatient care
    Routine laboratory appointments
    Return physician and nurse appointments

Ensure that patient and/or significant other demonstrates
    Method for applying pressure to bleeding site
        Apply dressing or clean material directly over site
        Apply pressure for 5 minutes
        Apply ice in covered plastic bag over site once bleeding stops
        Check site for further bleeding q15min for 1 hour
    Method for testing stool and urine for occult blood

INFECTION

Discuss signs and symptoms of infection to report to physician or nurse

Explain importance of avoiding persons who may be infectious or who have potentially contagious conditions, as well as persons who have been recently vaccinated and crowds

Explain need to avoid multiple sexual partners

Explain need to wash hands after using bathroom before eating or before performing any care procedures or food preparation

Discuss importance of preventing injury to skin
    Use electric razor
    Handle knives and sharp objects carefully
    Wear protective gloves when gardening and when using strong household cleaning solutions
    Wear broad-brimmed hat and sunscreen when in sun
    Avoid going barefoot
    Wear warm clothing and boots in cold weather
    Avoid cutting cuticles, corns, or calluses
    Wear padded gloves when using oven

Explain need to perform oral hygiene periodically throughout day and importance of daily hygiene, including perineal and rectal care

Explain importance of drinking up to 2500 ml of fluid each day unless contraindicated; need to avoid using common drinking fountain

Explain need to maintain clean home environment and handle food properly

Explain need to avoid contact with pets or other animals

Demonstrate method for taking and recording temperature

Demonstrate procedure for caring for very small cuts or breaks in skin

DISCHARGE/HOME CARE PLANNING

Review history for presence of caregiver

Assess patient/significant other's knowledge level of disease process

Assess home environment for potential environmental hazards

Assess ability of patient/significant other to comply with instructions

■ POLYCYTHEMIA

An increase in the number of circulating erythrocytes
polycythemia vera: *A chronic disorder in which over-production of myelocytes and thrombocytes, as well as*

erythrocytes, occurs with a resulting increase in blood viscosity, blood volume, and Hgb concentration.

secondary polycythemia: *A compensatory response to hypoxemia, which may result from chronic obstructive pulmonary disease (COPD), congenital heart disease, or prolonged exposure to low oxygen content (high altitude)*

relative polycythemia: *A result of decreased plasma volume; erythrocyte level is normal or decreased*

ASSESSMENT

SUBJECTIVE DATA

Central nervous system
  Headache
  Fullness in the head
  Dizziness
  Visual disturbances
  Fatigue
  Numbness of the fingers
  Double vision
Cardiovascular system
  Chest pain
  Calf pain with walking
  SOB with exercise
Gastrointestinal system
  Complaints of the following:
    Feeling full
    Constipation
    Weight loss
    Thirst
Integumentary system
  Pruritus
    Night sweats
Musculoskeletal system
  Joint pain

OBJECTIVE DATA

Central nervous system
  Paresthesia
  Engorged veins in the fundus and retina
  Congestion of the conjunctiva
  Altered mentation
Cardiovascular system
  Hypertension
  Intermittent claudication
  Thrombus
  Emboli
  Angina
  Hemorrhage
Gastrointestinal system
  Flatulence
  Constipation
  Hepatosplenomegaly in polycythemia vera
  GI bleeding
  Weight loss
  Gingival bleeding
Integumentary system
  Pruritus after hot bath
  Urticaria

Ruddy cyanosis
Ecchymosis

DIAGNOSTIC TESTS

Erythrocyte count up to 8 to 12 million/mm^3
Hgb 8 to 25 g/100 ml
Hct >60%
Mean corpuscular hemoglobin concentration (MCHC) decreased
Leukocytes increased
Thrombocytosis
Granulocytosis
Basophilia
Hyperuricemia
Total blood volume increased
Abnormal coagulation studies

POTENTIAL COMPLICATIONS

Hypervolemia
Thrombocytosis
MI
CVA
Gangrene of the digits
Hemorrhage
Splenic infarction
Renal calculi
Hypertension
CHF
Peptic ulcers
Leukemia (iatrogenic)

MULTIDISCIPLINARY MANAGEMENT

THERAPEUTIC MANAGEMENT

Phlebotomy
Pheresis transfusion
Myelosuppressive therapy (for control of symptoms related to myelocytosis, thrombocytosis, and hyperuricemia)
  Radioactive phosphorus PO or IV
  Antineoplastic agents
Smoking cessation
Rehydration
Stress management
Respiratory therapy support
Physical therapy
Nutritional support and consultation
Treatment of underlying disease, elimination of environmental causes (secondary polycythemia)

PATIENT PROBLEMS—NURSING DIAGNOSES/INTERVENTIONS

▼Altered cardiopulmonary tissue perfusion related to increased arterial pressure, increased total blood volume, and increased blood viscosity

Monitor BP *to assess cardiac function, peripheral resistance to blood flow, and effectiveness of therapy*

Monitor respirations and auscultate chest for heart and breath sounds *to assess pulmonary function and detect onset of congestive heart failure;* report changes immediately

Encourage frequent rest periods and avoidance of strenuous activity *to decrease cardiac workload*

Assist with ADLs *to reduce oxygen demand*

Apply antiembolic stockings *to enhance peripheral venous return*

Instruct patient to avoid caffeine, tobacco, and other stimulants *to prevent vasoconstriction*

Notify health care provider of complaints of chest pain, increased dyspnea, cyanosis, or restlessness *to facilitate early intervention*

Maintain a stress-free environment *to minimize risk of hypertension and maintain adequate cardiac output*

Administer oxygen therapy as ordered *to promote adequate tissue perfusion*

Initiate continuous pulse oximetry *to monitor oxygen saturation*

Administer sublingual nitroglycerin as ordered for angina

Administer medications as ordered *to promote vasodilation, diuresis, anticoagulation, pain relief, or treatment of other signs/symptoms and underlying causes*

Instruct the patient to avoid foods high in sodium *to reduce fluid retention*

Maintain the patient in semi-Fowler's position when in bed *to promote maximal respiratory excursion*

Assist the patient to turn, cough, and deep breathe *to ensure an open airway and prevent stasis of body fluids*

Assist the patient to ambulate as tolerated *to prevent stasis of body fluids, maintain cardiac function, and prevent injury caused by falls*

If phlebotomy is required, explain the procedure *to assure the patient that it will relieve distressing symptoms*

Monitor BP, P, and R *to assess patient response to the procedure*

Have the patient lie down during the procedure *to prevent vertigo and syncope*

Monitor the patient for tachycardia, clamminess, or complaints of vertigo; discontinue the procedure in the event these side effects occur

Check BP, P immediately after procedure

Instruct the patient to remain sitting for 5 minutes before ambulation *to prevent vasovagal attack or orthostatic hypotension*

Expected Outcomes
Vital signs are stable
Denies complaints of dyspnea, orthopnea, angina, dizziness, headache

▼ Altered cerebrovascular tissue perfusion related to increased intercranial pressure, intracranial bleeding, cerebral edema, and impairment of microcirculation

Assess neurologic signs *to detect increasing ICP*

Maintain the patient on complete bed rest with head of bed elevated *to conserve energy and lower ICP*

Promote a quiet environment *to promote rest and reduce stress*

Instruct the patient to avoid stimulants (caffeine, tobacco) *to prevent vasoconstriction*

Monitor vital signs and BP *to detect the presence of intracranial bleeding*

Assist the patient with ADLs and ambulation *to prevent injury*

Administer medications as ordered for vasodilation and anticoagulation

Expected Outcomes
Alert with normal and equal pupillary responses and reflexes
Denies visual disturbances, weakness in the extremities, or headache

▼ Altered peripheral tissue perfusion related to increased blood viscosity and vasoconstriction or microcirculation impairment

Observe color of the extremities, face, and mucous membranes *to assess disease status*

Perform passive, active ROM exercises *to prevent venous stasis*

Avoid excessive venipuncture; insert peripherally inserted central catheter (PICC), midline or Aquavene (Menlocare, Inc.) catheter for venous access, consolidate laboratory procedures

Monitor the patient's skin and mucous membranes *to detect lesions and impairment of skin integrity*

Monitor level of consciousness and pupillary responses *to detect cerebral insufficiency*

Expected Outcomes
Peripheral pulses are strong and equal
Skin is intact, warm, and dry

▼ Altered protection related to abnormal blood profile, drug therapies, and treatments

Assess patient for and report signs and symptoms of thrombus formation
  Changes in mental status
  Chest pain
  Sudden onset or increase in respiratory distress
  Abdominal pain
  Mottling or coolness of the extremities

Maintain position of comfort *to provide maximal respiratory excursion*

Avoid prolonged knee flexion *to prevent venous compromise*

Apply antiembolic stockings as ordered

Perform active/passive ROM exercises *to prevent venous stasis*

Avoid restrictive clothing and bed linens *to prevent injury to skin*

Keep the patient warm and dry *to prevent vasoconstriction*

Instruct patient to avoid sitting for long periods and avoid crossing legs when sitting *to prevent vasoconstriction*

Assist with ambulation *to prevent injury caused by falls*

Ensure that the environment is free of obstacles *to avoid injury caused by bumps and falls*

Instruct patient to call for assistance

Instruct patient to notify nurse for sudden onset of pain in the chest, head, extremities, or upon urination

Expected Outcomes

Verbalizes understanding of instructions to request assistance and notify nursing personnel of onset of pain

Exhibits no signs or symptoms of pulmonary, GI, GU, or neurologic involvement

Extremities are warm and dry with good color

▼Altered nutrition: less than body requirements related to inadequate intake of iron and folic acid

Assess nutritional status and food preferences, including cultural, religious, or medical restrictions

Consult dietitian *for further assessment and nutritional support*

Provide small, frequent feedings *to avoid fatiguing patient with three large meals*

Provide dietary supplement as ordered *to ensure appropriate daily caloric intake*

Encourage family to bring patient's favorite foods from home if appropriate

  Avoid foods that are GI irritants, spicy, flatus-forming, or high in caffeine

Monitor intake and output every shift *to aid in early detection of inadequate intake*

Weigh patient daily (same time, scale, and clothing)

  Report 2% decrease in weight

Assist patient with meals as necessary *to conserve energy*

Monitor and record character, amount, color, and frequency of stools; administer antidiarrheal medications as indicated

Expected Outcomes

Weight increases toward normal for height, age, sex, and body build

Taking balanced diet with fluids to 2000 ml/day, unless contraindicated

Intake and output are balanced

▼Risk for impaired skin integrity related to altered tissue perfusion, immobility, inadequate nutrition, mechanical forces, and itching

Inspect skin for redness, lesions, swelling, drainage q8h *to detect impairment of skin integrity*

Keep skin warm and dry *to prevent breakdown caused by environmental moisture*

Avoid use of constrictive clothing; maintain ambient and body warmth *to promote circulation*

Assist the patient with active and passive ROM exercises as tolerated *to maintain circulation*

Palpate peripheral pulses *to assess status of arterial circulation*

Review blood studies *to evaluate oxygen saturation and blood viscosity*

If skin impairment occurs, maintain patient on bed rest in semi-Fowler's position *to prevent further injury and decrease peripheral vascular resistance*

Cleanse skin with mild soap, rinse well, dry thoroughly *to maintain integrity*

Apply protective cream after bathing and position change

Ensure that bed linens are wrinkle free and nonconstrictive *to prevent mechanical injury*

Reposition patient q2h when on bed rest *to promote circulation and prevent stasis*

Inspect patient's feet frequently *to ensure early detection of gangrene*

Instruct patient to avoid scratching *to avoid injury to skin*

Expected Outcomes

Skin is warm, moist, and intact with normal color

Performs skin hygiene and does not scratch

Exhibits no signs or symptoms of gangrene

▼Pain related to musculoskeletal problems, impairment of microcirculation, disease process, abdominal distention, ulceration, and headache

Assess patient's pain for location, duration, and intensity using a pain rating scale *to facilitate development of a pain management plan*

Collaborate with patient, physician, and other health care team members to develop a pain management plan designed to prevent severe pain

Support painful joints with pillows in position of comfort *to minimize pain and discomfort*

Apply warmth to joints as ordered *to promote comfort*

Administer analgesics as ordered *to achieve goal of the pain management plan*

Use alternative pain management techniques *to achieve the goal of the pain management plan*

Auscultate bowel sounds *to determine presence of obstruction*

Monitor stool and emesis for presence of frank or occult blood *to detect GI bleeding*

Position the patient in semi-Fowler's position *to decrease abdominal pressure and increase intraabdominal space*

Administer antacids as ordered *to relieve epigastric distress*

Provide small, frequent feedings *to prevent abdominal distention*

Palpate the liver *to monitor size and location*

Maintain a quiet environment

Provide uninterrupted rest periods

Expected Outcomes
Verbalizes relief of pain using the pain management scale
Demonstrates a relaxed facial expression and posture
Denies headache, joint pain
Exhibits normal bowel sounds

Additional Nursing Diagnoses to Consider
Altered health maintenance
Altered parenting
Impaired adjustment
Activity intolerance related to immobility caused by joint pain or generalized weakness caused by anemia
Potential for injury related to risk of sensory dysfunction

PATIENT/FAMILY TEACHING
DISEASE PROCESS
Discuss symptoms of recurrence or progression of disease and complications to report to physician
Demonstrate how to check skin and peripheral pulses
Explain importance of regular follow-up care

COMPLICATIONS
Discuss trauma prevention
   Avoid restrictive clothing
   Wear comfortable shoes that fit well
   Keep home and work area free of clutter
   Use assistive devices when needed
   Use caution when performing oral hygiene
   Avoid sports and hobbies that may cause injury
   Handle equipment and sharp objects carefully
   Avoid extremes in environmental temperature

ACTIVITY
Instruct patient to balance rest and activity periods
Instruct patient not to cross legs when sitting or lock knees when standing; explain need to change position and exercise extremities frequently
Explain need to plan regular exercise program

NUTRITION
Explain importance of well-balanced diet; low-sodium or low-purine diet may be ordered
Instruct patient to take at least 2500 ml of fluid daily unless contraindicated
Discuss foods to avoid: gas-forming, acidic foods

MEDICATION
Teach name of medication, dosage, time of administration, purpose, and side effects
Instruct patient to avoid taking over-the-counter medications without checking with physician

Myelosuppressive treatment
Explain procedure to patient/significant other
Inform patient that risk of infection is increased
Instruct patient to avoid crowds
Instruct patient to notify physician for occurrence of signs and symptoms of infection

Inform patient of potential reactions to alkylating agents (nausea, vomiting, risk of infection); instruct patient to notify physician of side effects

Radioactive phosphorus
Explain procedure to patient/significant other
Inform patient that he or she may require repeated phlebotomies until the treatment takes effect
Instruct patient to lie down during IV administration to prevent extravasation and for 15 to 20 minutes after injection

DISCHARGE/HOME CARE PLANNING
Review history in presence of caregiver
Assess patient/significant other's knowledge level of disease process
Assess home environment for potential environmental hazards
Assess ability of patient/significant other to comply with instructions

■ THROMBOCYTOPENIA
A deficiency of circulating platelets. Idiopathic thrombocytopenic purpura (ITP) results from immunologic platelet destruction and is either acute (postviral) or chronic. Acute ITP generally occurs in children ages 2 to 6 years; chronic ITP affects adults under age 50. Secondary thrombocytopenia purpura results from viral infection, bone marrow failure, infectious mononucleosis, and drug hypersensitivity

ASSESSMENT
SUBJECTIVE DATA
Central nervous system
   Headache
   Confusion
   Weakness
   Fatigue
Gastrointestinal system
   Nausea
   Rectal pain
   Abdominal fullness
   Bleeding gums
   Vomiting blood
   Sore mouth
Cardiovascular system
   Rapid heart beat
   SOB
   Nose bleeds
   Bleeding gums
Genitourinary system
   Flank pain
   Blood in the urine
   Frequent, heavy menstrual periods
Integumentary system
   Bruising easily

General
    Reports family history of disease or recent exposure to NSAIDs, sulfonamides, histamine blockers, alkylating agents, or antibiotic chemotherapeutic agents
    Report of recent viral infection
    Report of recent excessive bleeding

OBJECTIVE DATA
Central nervous system
    Altered pupillary response
    Increased BP, P, and R
    Decreased LOC
    Sluggish reflexes
    Paresthesias of extremities
Gastrointestinal system
    Hematemesis
    Melena
    Guaiac-positive stool
    Abdominal distention
Cardiovascular system
    Tachycardia
    Tachypnea
    Epistaxis
    Oral blood-filled bullae
    Dyspnea
Genitourinary system
    Heavy menstrual flow
    Hematuria
Integumentary system
    Petechiae, purpura
    Ecchymosis
General
    Documented family history
    Documented recent use of specific medications
    Recent infection with Epstein-Barr virus or infectious mononucleosis

DIAGNOSTIC TESTS
Platelets <100,000/mm^3
Bleeding time prolonged
Normal coagulation time
Normal prothrombin International Normalized Ratio (INR) and activated partial thromboplastin time (APTT)
Increased capillary fragility
Bone marrow biopsy: increased megakaryocytes in the presence of increased platelet destruction

POTENTIAL COMPLICATIONS
Hemorrhage
Transfusion reaction
Death

MULTIDISCIPLINARY MANAGEMENT
THERAPEUTIC MANAGEMENT
Treatment of underlying cause, removal of causative agent
Plasmapheresis
Plasma transfusion
Platelet/blood component transfusion

Splenectomy
Corticosteroids
Respiratory support
Physical therapy
Nutritional support and consultation
Analgesics
Stress reduction

PATIENT PROBLEMS—NURSING DIAGNOSES/INTERVENTIONS

▼Altered protection related to abnormal blood profile

Maintain patient in a comfortable position; provide support with pillows
Avoid pressure to any area of body; use foam or gel pads, air mattress, and heel and elbow protection as needed *to prevent impairment of skin integrity*
Assist with hygiene *to maintain integrity of skin and mucous membranes*
Monitor vital signs and BP *to detect infection*
Assess skin and mucous membranes for bleeding tid
Check the stool and urine daily for presence of frank or occult blood
Monitor laboratory studies *to assess status of blood profile*
Avoid frequent venipuncture, IM injections *to maintain skin integrity and prevent bleeding*
    Consolidate necessary laboratory work
    Use fingersticks when possible
    Apply pressure at injection site for 5 to 10 minutes or until bleeding stops
    Observe injection sites for bleeding or hematoma every 15 minutes × 4 after injection
    Observe injection sites every shift for redness, pain, swelling, or infiltration
    Clean injection/venipuncture sites with povidone or other bacterial agent before procedure
Use sterile technique for dressing changes
Instruct the patient/significant other in the use of safety measures *to prevent trauma and bleeding*
Assist the patient with ADLs and ambulation *to prevent injury from falls*
Provide an environment free from obstructions *to prevent injury from bumps and falls*
Avoid use of constrictive clothing and linens *to prevent abrasion and impairment of skin integrity*
Pad side rails as needed
Use soft towels and cloths for hygiene; avoid vigorous skin care
Instruct patient to avoid straining at stool *to prevent increasing ICP and subsequent bleeding*
Administer stool softeners or laxatives as ordered
Assist patient to perform oral hygiene with soft toothbrush or foam stick *to prevent injury to oral mucosa*
Instruct patient to use an electric razor for shaving

Administer platelet transfusion as ordered *to treat complications of severe hemorrhage*

Administer platelets quickly *to prevent cell destruction*

Do not administer platelets in the presence of fever *to prevent cell destruction*

Monitor patient for signs and symptoms of febrile reaction during administration

Premedicate as ordered with acetaminophen and diphenhydramine

Administer corticosteroid and immunosuppressive therapy as ordered

Avoid use of antihistamines, phenothiazines, aspirin, and nonsteroidal antiinflammatory agents in patients with ITP *to avoid exposure to causative agents*

Instruct patient to avoid use of aspirin *to minimize risk of bleeding*

Prepare patient for splenectomy as ordered

Expected Outcomes

Vital signs are stable

Exhibits no signs or symptoms of bleeding

▼Altered oral mucous membrane related to altered blood profile

Assess oral cavity tid *to ensure early intervention and treatment*

Assist patient to perform oral hygiene when awake and before and after meals *to prevent buildup of plaque and bacteria*

Perform oral hygiene with dilute mouthwash or normal saline rinse and a soft brush or sponge *to avoid irritation of mucous membranes and disruption of bullae*

Apply topical protective agents (water-based jelly, kaolin preparations) to lesions as ordered *to promote healing*

Apply topical analgesics 15 to 20 minutes before meals as ordered *to facilitate nutritional intake*

Serve foods and fluids lukewarm or cold *to soothe inflamed oral mucosa*

Maintain diet of preference as ordered; avoid spicy/irritant food *to decrease pain from irritation of mucosa*

Encourage soft, easy-to-chew foods *to avoid tissue trauma and pain*

Encourage fluids, unless contraindicated; iced liquids or popsicles may be soothing

Measure intake and output every shift *to ensure adequacy of dietary intake*

Weigh the patient daily (same time, scale, and clothing) *to assess nutritional status*

Expected Outcomes

Oral mucosa, tongue, and lips are pink, moist, and intact with no bullae

Verbalizes comfort in chewing, swallowing, and talking

▼Pain related to altered sensations, paresthesias in joints and extremities caused by bleeding

Assess pain location, duration, intensity using a pain rating scale *to facilitate development of pain management plan*

Collaborate with patient, physician, and other health care team members to develop pain management plan designed to prevent severe pain

Support affected joints and extremities with pillows in position of comfort *to minimize pain and discomfort*

Administer analgesics as ordered *to achieve the goal of pain management plan*

Move patient with slow, gentle movements *to minimize discomfort of repositioning and promote relaxation*

Avoid restrictive clothing and linens *to relieve pressure on joints and extremities*

Encourage use of alternate pain management techniques *to enhance effects of analgesics*

Expected Outcomes

Demonstrates relaxed facial expression and posture

Verbalizes pain relief using a pain scale

▼Risk for impaired skin integrity related to altered tissue perfusion, mechanical forces, intradermal bleeding, immobility, and altered blood profile

Inspect skin for redness, lesions, swelling, drainage, petechiae, ecchymosis, hematomas tid *to detect impairment of skin integrity and evaluate need for further intervention;* notify physician of alterations

Keep skin warm and dry *to prevent breakdown caused by environmental moisture*

Avoid use of constrictive clothing and maintain ambient temperature and body warmth *to prevent trauma*

Assist the patient with active and passive ROM exercises as tolerated *to avoid injury and maintain circulation*

Avoid excessive venipuncture

Apply ice bag or manual pressure to any puncture site *to control local bleeding*

Gently assist patient with ambulation and repositioning *to avoid injury and tissue trauma*

Cleanse skin with mild soap, rinse well, dry thoroughly *to maintain integrity and avoid trauma*

Apply protective cream after bathing and position change

Ensure that bed linens are wrinkle free and nonconstrictive *to prevent mechanical injury*

Reposition patient every 2 hours when on bedrest *to avoid pressure injury*

Avoid invasive procedures

Expected Outcome

Skin is intact with no discoloration

▼Altered cerebral tissue perfusion related to impairment of microcirculation and intracranial bleeding

Assess neurologic signs q2 to 4h or as indicated by condition *to detect increasing intracranial pressure*

Maintain patient on complete bed rest with the head of bed elevated *to conserve energy and lower ICP*

Instruct patient to avoid coughing, straining at stool, or other Valsalva-type maneuvers *to minimize the risk of bleeding*

Provide a quiet environment *to promote rest and reduce stress*

Instruct patient to avoid stimulants (caffeine, tobacco)

Expected Outcome
Alert and oriented with normal reflexes

Additional Nursing Diagnoses to Consider
Ineffective coping
Self-care deficit
Altered parenting
Social isolation

PATIENT/FAMILY TEACHING
DISEASE PROCESS
Demonstrate method to assess for bleeding

Discuss signs and symptoms of recurrence to report to physician: continuous headache, coughing red-streaked sputum, persistent abdominal pain, vomiting frank blood or "coffee ground" material, increased areas of petechiae or ecchymosis, blood-filled bullae in oral cavity, blood in urine or stools

Demonstrate methods of checking for blood in stool and urine

Instruct patient to notify physician when contemplating pregnancy or when pregnancy is first suspected

Caution patient never to donate blood

Explain need to prevent trauma by

Avoiding constipation through diet, fluids, and use of stool softeners or laxatives if needed; avoiding vigorous nose-blowing or coughing; avoiding contact sports or other hazardous hobbies

Careful movements and careful handling of objects that may cause bleeding

Use of nonabrasive skin and mouth care products

Explain importance of notifying all health care providers of diagnosis and keeping follow-up appointments

NUTRITION
Explain importance of regular oral hygiene; discuss products to use or avoid; demonstrate method for daily inspection

Explain need to maintain balanced diet with adequate hydration; discuss foods to avoid to prevent trauma

ACTIVITY
Explain need to balance rest and activity periods; to increase activity as comfort increases; to use assistance when needed to prevent injury

MEDICATION
Teach name of medication, dosage, time of administration, purpose, and side effects

Teach how to read contents of over-the-counter medications, avoiding those that contain acetylsalicylic acid (antihistamines, phenothiazines, or nonsteroidal antiinflammatory agents in ITP)

DISCHARGE/HOME CARE PLANNING
Review history for presence of a caregiver

Assess the patient's ability to function independently

Assess the knowledge level of the patient and caregiver about the disease process, prevention of trauma, signs and symptoms of bleeding

Assess the patient/significant other's ability to perform necessary procedures and treatments

■ HEMOPHILIA
A bleeding disorder characterized by impaired coagulability of the blood and a tendency to bleed. Classic hemophilia (hemophilia A) and hemophilia B are hereditary X-linked recessive diseases. Hemophilia A, resulting from deficient or absent antihemophilic factor VIII activity, accounts for more than 80% of all hemophiliacs and is generally limited to males. Homozygous females with a hemophiliac father and a carrier mother are extremely rare. Christmas disease (hemophilia B) results from deficient or absent antihemophilic factor IX. Von Willebrand's disease is an autosomal dominant trait in both males and females manifested by deficiency of factor VIII and defective platelet adhesion

ASSESSMENT
SUBJECTIVE DATA
Central nervous system
  Confusion
  Fatigue
  Lightheadedness
  Headache
Gastrointestinal system
  Abdominal discomfort and fullness
  Bleeding gums, lips, tongue
  Rectal bleeding
Cardiovascular system
  Rapid heart beat
  Nose bleed
  Prolonged bleeding from wounds
Genitourinary system
  Blood in the urine
  Heavy menses
Integumentary system
  Bruising easily and excessively
  Clammy skin
Musculoskeletal system
  Joint pain and tenderness

OBJECTIVE DATA

Central nervous system
  Altered pupillary response
  Hyporeflexia
  Confusion
  Disorientation
  Seizures
Gastrointestinal system
  Melena
  Hematemesis
  Bleeding gums, tongue, lips
Genitourinary system
  Hematuria
  Menorrhagia
Cardiovascular system
  Hypotension
  Tachycardia
Respiratory system
  Hyperpnea
  Stridor
  SOB
Integumentary system
  Petechiae
  Purpura
  Ecchymosis
  Subcutaneous and intramuscular hematomas
Musculoskeletal system
  Hemarthrosis
  Joint swelling
  Joint deformity
  Impaired ROM

DIAGNOSTIC TESTS

Hemophilia A
  Factor VIII assay 0% to 30% of normal
  Prolonged APTT
  Platelet count normal
  Platelet function normal
  Bleeding time normal
  Prothrombin time normal
Hemophilia B
  Factor IX assay deficient
  Factor VIII normal
  Prolonged APTT
  Platelet count normal
  Platelet function normal
  Bleeding time normal
Severity of disease determined by percent of factor
  deficiency
  Mild = factor levels 5% to 40% of normal
  Moderate = 1% to 5% of normal
  Severe = less than 1% of normal
Von Willebrand's disease
  Bleeding time prolonged

POTENTIAL COMPLICATIONS

Hemorrhage
Respiratory distress
Hypovolemic shock

MULTIDISCIPLINARY MANAGEMENT
THERAPEUTIC MANAGEMENT

Replacement of deficient factor
Treatment for development of antibody inhibitors to
  specific factors
Packed RBC replacement for severe blood loss
Topical bleeding control
Analgesic, corticosteroids for joint pain
Desmopressin to stimulate release of stored factor VIII
Social Services
Occupational therapy as indicated

PATIENT PROBLEMS—NURSING DIAGNOSES/INTERVENTIONS

▼ Risk for fluid volume deficit related to hemorrhage

Monitor vital signs *for early detection of hemorrhage*
Monitor intake and output *to assess renal blood flow*
Monitor urine specific gravity *to assess degree of fluid
  deficit*
Encourage oral intake to 2500 ml/day unless
  contraindicated
Perform frequent physical assessment *to detect sites of
  bruising, bleeding*
Measure bruises, count and/or weigh dressings *to
  determine volume of blood loss*
Administer blood component therapy as ordered *to
  replace volume and deficient components*
  Monitor for transfusion reactions
Apply pressure to wounds if actively bleeding
Apply ice to affected joints, elevate and immobilize
  affected limb *to control bleeding*
Administer analgesics *to reduce joint pain*
Monitor laboratory values *to determine hemostatic
  status and efficacy of therapeutic regimen*
Avoid intramuscular injections
Assist patient with ambulation and ADLs
Monitor skin turgor, color, moisture
Monitor for circulatory overload during fluid replacement

Expected Outcomes

Vital signs are within normal limits
Intake and output is balanced, with urine output at least
  30 to 60 ml/hr
Urine specific gravity is within normal limits
Laboratory results are within normal limits
Reports relief of joint pain

▼ Risk for ineffective airway clearance related to
obstruction caused by tissue swelling and bleeding around the airway, nose, pharynx, and/or
esophagus

Assess the patient for head and neck trauma
Observe for bleeding from areas that may obstruct
  airway
Monitor vital signs, respiratory rate, and breath sounds *to
  facilitate early detection of respiratory compromise*

Instruct patient to report any respiratory distress

Apply pressure and packing *to control bleeding*

Perform gentle oral suction with a tonsil tip catheter *to clear the oropharynx*

Perform tracheal suction as ordered *to maintain a clear airway*

Assist patient to maintain position that promotes ease of respiration

Expected Outcomes

Reports ease of respiration

Airway is patent

Demonstrates respiratory rate, effort, excursion within normal limits

▼ Risk for sensory/perceptual alterations related to intracranial bleed

Monitor LOC, orientation, pupillary response, and reflexes *to facilitate early detection of neurologic changes*

Monitor vital signs *to assess for increased ICP*

Observe for and report altered pupillary responses, projectile vomiting, altered LOC

Encourage patient to avoid stimulants

Encourage patient to remain on bed rest with head elevated *to reduce ICP*

Use padded side rails if patient restless *to prevent injury*

Expected Outcome

Exhibits neurologic signs within normal limits

Additional Nursing Diagnoses to Consider

Ineffective coping

Knowledge deficit

Self-care deficit

PATIENT/FAMILY TEACHING
DISEASE PROCESS

Discuss information about disease severity

Discuss treatment plan with patient and caregiver

Inform patient of the need for prophylactic coagulation factor treatment before surgery and dental treatment

Discuss trauma prevention

Avoid restrictive, binding clothing

Avoid sports and hobbies that may cause injury

Handle equipment and sharp objects carefully

Use caution when performing oral hygiene

Encourage patient with hereditary forms of disease to seek genetic counseling

Instruct patient to report signs and symptoms of bleeding to a health care provider

MEDICATION

Avoid aspirin

Instruct patient/caregiver in self-administration of blood factors

DISCHARGE/HOME CARE PLANNING

Review history in presence of caregiver

Assess patient/significant other's knowledge level of disease process

Assess home environment for potential environmental hazards

Assess ability of patient/significant other to comply with instructions

■ DISSEMINATED INTRAVASCULAR COAGULATION (DIC)

Overstimulation of the normal coagulation process associated with underlying conditions such as snakebite, septicemia, severe hypotension, neoplasms, hemolysis, obstetric emergencies, acidosis, cancer chemotherapy, transplant rejection, and extensive burns, trauma, or surgery; the initial accelerated clotting process consumes large amounts of coagulation factors in the formation of fibrin clots; the fibrinolytic system is then activated to lyse fibrin clots into fibrin degradation products; the activity of these products and the depletion of plasma coagulation factors result in hemorrhage

ASSESSMENT
SUBJECTIVE DATA

Central nervous system
  Confusion
  Restlessness
  Visual changes
Cardiovascular system
  Chest pain
  Increasing heart rate
Gastrointestinal system
  Nausea
  Abdominal pain
Respiratory system
  Difficulty breathing
  Coughing up blood
Genitourinary system
  Vaginal bleeding
  Blood in the urine
Integumentary system
  Oozing of blood from the skin
  Slight blue discoloration of the hands and feet

OBJECTIVE DATA

Central nervous system
  Seizures
  Coma
  Altered LOC
  Restlessness
  Vasomotor instability
Cardiovascular system
  Increasing hypotension
  Postural hypotension
  Tachycardia
  Epistaxis

Shock
Acrocyanosis
Gastrointestinal system
  Nausea/vomiting
  Melena
  Hematemesis
  Increasing abdominal girth
Respiratory system
  Hemoptysis
  Dyspnea
  Tachypnea
Genitourinary system
  Hematuria
  Oligouria
Integumentary system
  Petechiae
  Eccymosis
  Hematoma
  Hemorrhagic bullae
  Diffuse oozing of blood or plasma
  Palpable purpura, initially on the chest and
    abdomen
General
  Presence of abnormal bleeding in the absence of
    history of a hemorrhagic disorder
  Severe muscle, joint, back pain
  Bleeding from surgical incisions, injection sites, IV
    insertion sites, around chest and nasogastric
    tubes
  Postpartum bleeding
  Bleeding into the fundus of the eye

DIAGNOSTIC TESTS

PT, prolonged >15 seconds
PTT, prolonged >60 to 80 seconds
Platelet count <100,000/mm^3
Fibrinogen level, decreased <150 mg/dl
Antithrombin III level decreased
Thrombin time prolonged
Fibrin degradation products elevated, >100 μg/ml
Plasminogen levels decreased
Levels of factors V and VIII decreased
Fragmentation of RBCs
Hgb decreased
Urine output, decreased <30 ml per hour
BUN elevated, >25 mg/100 ml
Serum creatinine elevated, >1.3 mg/100 ml
D-Dimer, present, >250 mg/L

POTENTIAL COMPLICATIONS

Shock
Acute tubular necrosis
Focal gangrene
Pulmonary edema
CHF
Convulsions
Coma
Failure of major organ systems

MULTIDISCIPLINARY MANAGEMENT
THERAPEUTIC MANAGEMENT

Elimination of causative agent
Correction of hypovolemia, hypotension, hypoxia,
  acidosis
Correction of homeostatic deficiencies
Management of septic shock
Administration of depleted blood components
Heparin (early stages and as a last resort for hemorrhage)
Antineoplastic agents
Antibiotics
Respiratory support

PATIENT PROBLEMS—NURSING DIAGNOSES/INTERVENTIONS

▼ Fluid volume deficit related to active fluid loss and bleeding (Table 4-1)

Monitor intake and output q8h to 12h *to assess fluid needs and prevent overload;* report imbalances
Weigh patient daily (same time, scale, and clothing); report changes of 2% to 3% of original weight
Monitor vital signs and mental status q4h
Assess skin turgor and peripheral pulses every shift *to determine adequacy of hydration*
Monitor character, amount, color, frequency of emesis, stools *to detect internal bleeding*

Table 4-1	Signs and Symptoms of Blood Loss		
Volume Lost			
ml	**% TBV**	**Clinical Signs**	
500	10	None; occasionally vasovagal syncope in blood donors	
1000	20	At rest there may be no clinical evidence of volume loss; a slight postural drop in blood pressure may be seen; tachycardia with exercise	
1500	30	Resting supine blood pressure and pulse may be normal; neck veins flat when supine; postural hypotension; exercise tachycardia	
2000	40	Central venous pressure, cardiac output, and systolic blood pressure below normal even when supine and at rest; air hunger, rapid thready pulse, cold clammy skin; tachycardia	
2500	50	Signs of shock, tachycardia, hypotension, oliguria, drowsiness, or coma	

From Lee GR et al: Wintrobe's clinical hematology, *ed 10, Baltimore, 1999, Williams & Wilkins.*
*Total blood volume.

Observe color, specific gravity, pH of urine *to ensure early detection of renal failure*

Provide oral fluid intake as tolerated *to maintain intravascular fluid volume*

Force fluids to 2500 ml/day unless contraindicated

Administer blood fractions as ordered *to alleviate fluid deficit*

Administer heparin as ordered *to control bleeding*

Review laboratory results *to assess degree of blood loss and patient response to therapy*

Apply ice packs and pressure to site of bleeding *to control blood loss*

Avoid injections, use of straight razors *to minimize risk of injury and bleeding*

Assist the patient with ADLs and ambulation *to minimize the risk of injury*

Use soft towels and cloths for hygiene; do not perform aggressive skin care *to prevent injury*

Expected Outcomes
Skin turgor and color are normal
Intake and output are balanced
Renal function is adequate
Peripheral pulses are present
Extremities are warm with good color

▼Pain related to tissue hypoxia

Assess location, quality, and intensity of pain; use pain rating scale

Place patient in position of comfort; provide support with pillows *to prevent stress on body parts*

Assist with care when patient is actively bleeding or experiencing discomfort

Maintain quiet environment

Provide adequate periods of rest; cluster activities and diagnostic studies, when possible, according to patient's tolerance

Assist patient with alternative comfort measures such as music therapy, imagery, or other distractions

Administer analgesics as ordered; assess effectiveness

Expected Outcomes
Verbalizes no discomfort
Body posture and face are relaxed

▼Anxiety related to threat of death and changes in health status

Assess level of patient's fear and current understanding of disease process, treatments, and interventions *to assist in development of an education plan*

Reassure patient as needed; remain with patient *to offer security during periods of anxiety*

Maintain a calm, tolerant attitude during interactions with patient

Provide continuity of care *to facilitate communication of anxieties and fears*

Orient or reorient patient to environment as needed *to promote a feeling of control and decrease anxiety, fear of the unknown*

Explain procedures simply and briefly; inform patient of what to expect and when to expect it

Maintain a quiet environment *to reduce stress-inducing stimuli*

Encourage patient to talk about anxiety and fear

Instruct patient to notify staff when he or she feels anxious or fearful *to promote a feeling of security*

Assist patient to develop coping strategies *to promote feeling of control*

Expected Outcomes
Appears calm and is able to verbalize fears and anxieties
Able to use coping measures independently

▼Impaired gas exchange related to altered oxygen supply, altered blood flow, and arterial hypotension

Maintain patient in semi-Fowler's position *to decrease diaphragmatic pressure and promote full respiratory excursion*

Encourage deep breathing *to prevent hyperventilation*

Maintain oxygen delivery as ordered *to prevent desaturation*

Monitor pulse oximetry *to assess changes in saturation*

Assess respirations for quality, rate, pattern, depth, dyspnea on exertion (DOE), guarding, use of accessory muscles

Assess changes in mental status and behavior *to evaluate patient's response to disease state and therapy*

Maintain bed rest with side rails up *to decrease cardiac workload*

Monitor BP, P, and R *to assess cardiac and respiratory function*

Assist patient with ADLs as needed *to conserve energy*

Increase patient's activity level as tolerated *to maintain cardiopulmonary fitness*

Provide reassurance as needed to reduce patient's anxiety, *which may contribute to increased cardiopulmonary workload*

Instruct patient to report dyspnea and palpitations

Assess skin color and temperature *to determine status of tissue oxygenation*

Expected Outcomes
Vital signs are stable
Denies dyspnea
Demonstrates increasing activity tolerance
Peripheral pulses are strong and regular

▼Decreased cardiac output related to decreased oxygenation

Maintain patient in semi-Fowler's to high-Fowler's position *to facilitate cardiac output and venous return*

Administer medications as ordered *to correct dysrhythmias*

Administer cardiotonic and vasoconstrictor medications as ordered *to increase cardiac tone*

Provide quiet, restful environment *to reduce stress that may increase cardiac workload*

Encourage patient to use relaxation techniques

Administer oxygen as ordered

Assess skin color and temperature *to determine status of tissue perfusion*

Monitor laboratory tests *to detect acidosis*

Monitor apical and all peripheral pulses *to determine status of tissue perfusion*

Expected Outcomes

Vital signs are within normal limits

Laboratory values are within normal limits

Able to participate in ADLs

Peripheral pulses are strong and regular

Skin is warm, dry, with good color

▼ Sensory/perceptual alterations (kinesthetic) related to altered sensory reception, hypotension, and hypoxia

Monitor vital signs and BP *to assess cerebral and peripheral blood flow*

Monitor neurologic signs *to assess cerebral blood flow*

Administer oxygen as ordered *to enhance cerebral blood flow*

Provide quiet, restful environment *to decrease stress on the CNS*

Instruct patient to avoid use of stimulants (caffeine, tobacco) *to minimize vasoconstriction leading to cerebral hypoxia*

Assist patient with ADLs and ambulation *to prevent injury resulting from falls*

Monitor ABGs *to detect impaired cerebral oxygenation*

Expected Outcome

Participates in ADLs and ambulates without difficulty

PATIENT/FAMILY TEACHING

Discuss signs and symptoms of DIC that should be reported immediately to physician

Instruct patient/significant other in heparin administration if ordered

Discuss medications prescribed including name, dose, route, time of administration, and side effects

Provide additional teaching applicable to underlying cause of DIC

Instruct patient in ways to prevent trauma and injury

Perform oral care with a soft toothbrush or foam stick

Perform skin care gently with a soft towel

DISCHARGE/HOME CARE PLANNING

Review history for presence of caregiver

Assess patient/significant other's knowledge level of disease process

Assess home environment for potential environmental hazards

Assess ability of patient/significant other to comply with instructions

■ SPLENECTOMY

Surgical removal of the spleen to treat traumatic injuries or blood dyscrasias in which hypersplenism occurs (the spleen produces leukocytes, lymphocytes, monocytes, and plasma cells; it also destroys nonfunctional red blood cells and platelets, stores blood, and assists in maintaining hemopoiesis; the spleen indiscriminantly sequesters normal RBCs and platelets, thereby removing them from the circulation when hypersplenism occurs)

POSTOPERATIVE ASSESSMENT
SUBJECTIVE DATA

Central nervous system
    Pain
    Fatigue
Cardiovascular system
    Rapid heart beat
Respiratory system
    Inability to take a deep breath
Gastrointestinal system
    Nausea
    Abdominal pain

OBJECTIVE DATA

Central nervous system
    Fatigue
    Weakness
Cardiovascular system
    Bleeding
    Tachycardia
    Thrombosis
Respiratory system
    Splinting with respiration, coughing
    Decreased breath sounds
    Tachypnea
    Atelectasis
    Subdiaphragmatic abscess
Gastrointestinal system
    Nausea/vomiting
    Dehydration
    Abdominal distension
General
    Signs and symptom of infection
    Dehiscence

DIAGNOSTIC TESTS

Thrombocyte level elevated

Normal bleeding, clotting times

Electrolytes

Hgb

Hct

POTENTIAL COMPLICATIONS
Hemorrhage
Infection
Paralytic ileus
Shock
Thrombophlebitis
Pulmonary embolus

MULTIDISCIPLINARY MANAGEMENT
THERAPEUTIC MANAGEMENT
Incentive spirometer
Nasogastric tube
Parenteral therapy
Pain management
Management of complications

PATIENT PROBLEMS—NURSING DIAGNOSES/INTERVENTIONS

▼Ineffective breathing pattern related to pain, anxiety, decreased energy, and decreased lung expansion

Assess respiratory effort, breath sounds, and rate
Position patient to optimize respiratory effort
Assist and teach patient to turn, cough, and breathe deeply q2h to 4h support incision
Teach patient to use incentive spirometer at least q4 hours
Assist with ambulation as soon as possible

Expected Outcome
Lungs are clear; respiratory excursion is adequate

Pain related to abdominal incision, drains, and tubes

Assess pain location, frequency, intensity, and duration; use pain rating scale
Assist patient with assuming position of comfort; support as necessary
Collaborate with physician to establish analgesic schedule and dosage to obtain maximum effectiveness; increased frequency usually required during immediate postoperative period
Teach alternative methods of pain relief (e.g., relaxation, imagery, music)
Administer pain medication before performing activities, thereby increasing compliance with the following:
Coughing and deep breathing
ROM exercises
Early periods of ambulation and self-care activities
If pain increases, assess for other factors (e.g., complications, exacerbation of primary condition)

Expected Outcomes
Verbalizes feelings of increased comfort
Performs activities without limitation
Body posture and face are relaxed

▼Risk for fluid volume deficit related to nasogastric tube, wound drains, blood loss in surgery, NPO status, and vomiting

Maintain NPO as ordered
Connect nasogastric sump tube to low, intermittent suction apparatus as ordered
Do not change position of tube
Maintain tube patency
Observe drainage q8h to 12h; report excessive bleeding
Assess skin turgor
Measure intake and output; report imbalance
Weigh patient daily (same time, clothing, and scale)
Replace fluids as ordered

Expected Outcomes
Intake equals output
Mucous membranes are moist
Skin turgor is good

▼Altered urinary elimination related to anesthesia, sensory motor impairment, neuromuscular impairment, and mechanical trauma

Observe voiding: frequency, amount, color, odor, discomfort, distention, q8h
Insert catheter when ordered for retention or overflow voiding; perform daily catheter care
Institute voiding measures as needed

Expected Outcome
Voids without difficulty and has no signs of infection

▼Constipation related to less than adequate dietary intake and bulk, medications, neuromuscular impairment, musculoskeletal impairment, pain on defecation, and emotional status

Auscultate abdomen for bowel sounds; report return of bowel sounds
Begin oral liquids, progressing to regular diet when ordered after return of bowel sounds; note tolerance
Encourage fluids to 2500 ml/day unless contraindicated
Monitor for first bowel movement after surgery; give stool softeners or enemas as ordered

Expected Outcomes
Takes regular diet and fluids to 2500 ml/day
Has had soft-formed bowel movement

▼Altered gastrointestinal and/or peripheral tissue perfusion related to interruption of flow, venous/arterial, hypovolemia, and hypervolemia

Monitor BP, T, P, R, and CVP q4h, decreasing frequency as indicated by condition
Assess for signs of bleeding or thrombosis
Check dressing for bleeding q2h to 4h for the first 48 postoperative hours

Reinforce as necessary
Report excessive bleeding to physician
Change dressing daily and prn; observe healing process; report early signs of infection when present
Position patient comfortably; assist with turning q2h; avoid knee hyperflexion or pillows under knees
Assist with and teach active or perform passive ROM exercises q4h
Provide correct-size antiembolic stockings when ordered *to promote venous return*
Plan uninterrupted rest and sleep periods *to prevent fatigue*
Assist with ambulation as necessary
Avoid sitting for long periods
Walk in place when standing

Expected Outcomes
Vital signs are within normal limits
Peripheral pulses are palpable
Color and temperature of extremities are normal
Incision is healing

PATIENT/FAMILY TEACHING
SELF-CARE
Instruct patient to shower daily, dry incision well
Teach patient to observe for and report increased pain, swelling, redness, or drainage
Emphasize importance of not applying creams, lotions, or powders to incision
Instruct patient to support incision, if needed, when deep breathing and coughing
Emphasize need for follow-up care

ACTIVITIES
Explain need to increase ambulation and activities each day and plan regular, uninterrupted rest periods
Explain need to exercise extremities routinely; demonstrate ROM and breathing exercises
Instruct patient to avoid sitting for long periods; explain importance of not crossing legs
Instruct patient to avoid heavy lifting and contact sports for 6 to 8 weeks or as directed by physician

NUTRITION
Instruct patient to maintain well-balanced diet, taking 2500 ml of liquids daily
Instruct patient to report inability to tolerate food or liquids, nausea, any vomiting, diarrhea, or constipation

■ APHERESIS THERAPY
Selective removal of blood or blood components for therapeutic goals; types of apheresis—procedures are named depending on the blood component to be removed (Table 4-2)

ASSESSMENT
Assess for appearance of complications during procedure (see Table 4-2)
Continue required assessment for primary condition

PREAPHERESIS CARE
Reinforce physician's explanation of procedure; include significant other
Obtain written consent after physician has explained procedure
Assess patient's existing condition and note routine and special nursing care requirements for primary condition
Check preapheresis laboratory values
Take and record vital signs and standing and lying BP
Assess patient's heart and lung sounds
Administer medications and fluids as ordered
NOTE: Wear protective gloves and gowns when handling blood components, needles, and centrifuge equipment

INTERVENTIONS
NOTE: Procedure is performed by a specifically qualified operator

DURING PROCEDURE
Assess vital signs, heart and breath sounds qh
Measure intake and output
Monitor infusions and rates qh
Administer routine medications
Continue care for primary condition

POSTAPHERESIS CARE
If antecubital veins are used for access
Never use for other venipunctures
Apply warm soaks qid
Teach arm-strengthening exercises
If arteriovenous fistula is used for access
Check patency daily
Never use for venipunctures
Never take BP in that extremity; no IM injections in same extremity
See standard of care for primary condition

PATIENT/FAMILY TEACHING
Ensure that patient and/or significant other demonstrates
Care of venous or arteriovenous fistula
Extremity exercises to perform daily
Ensure that patient and/or significant other knows and understands
Signs and symptoms of bleeding and infection to report to physician
To avoid exposure to persons with infections, especially upper respiratory tract infections (URIs)
See standard of care for primary condition

Table 4-2	Therapeutic Apheresis Procedures			
Considerations	**Plasmapheresis**	**Plateletpheresis**	**Leukapheresis**	**Erythrocytapheresis**
Indications	Hemolytic anemia (AIHA) acute idiopathic thrombocytopenic purpura (ITP), nonrelapsing thrombotic thrombocytopenic purpura (TTP), Guillain-Barré syndrome, myasthenia gravis, renal transplant rejection syndrome, Goodpasture's syndrome, systemic lupus erythematosus, rheumatoid arthritis, multiple myeloma, biliary cirrhosis, hyperlipidemia, hypercholesterolemia, cancer conditions in which plasma substances interfere with immune system	Thrombocytosis	Chronic lymphatic leukemia, rheumatoid arthritis, multiple sclerosis	Acute, severe sickle cell disease, polycythemia vera
Preapheresis laboratory/ diagnostic studies	Total albumin and protein, K, Mg, Ca, CBC, Hgb, Hct, platelet count, PT, activated PTT, hepatitis-associated antigen/VDRL, cold agglutinins, liver/renal function tests, HBsAg if history of hepatitis	Platelet count, CBC, Hgb, PT, activated PTT, cold agglutinins, liver and renal function tests, HBsAg if history of hepatitis	CBC, differential, Hgb, Hct, platelet count, PT, activated PTT, cold agglutinins, liver/renal function tests, HBsAg if history of hepatitis	CBC, Hgb, platelet count, PT, in activated PTT, cold agglutinins, liver/renal function tests, HBsAg if history of hepatitis
Complications	Electrolyte imbalance (hypocalcemia, hypokalemia), hypothermia, hypovolemia, fluid overload, vasovagal reaction, thrombus or air embolus, oliguria or anuria, shock	Air embolus, reaction from anticoagulation: (citrate) tingling, chills, seizures, hypotension, hemolysis, bleeding, fluid overload	Air embolus, reaction from anticoagulation: (citrate) tingling, chills, seizures, hypotension, hemolysis, bleeding, fluid overload	Hypovolemia, hemolytic transfusion reaction
Usual volume removed	2-4 L	1000 ml, depending on platelet count		
Replacement therapy	Volume removed replaced with normal saline and albumin or fresh frozen plasma (replaces Ig and coagulation factors but increases risk of hypersensitivity and hepatitis)	Albumin 5% add 0.9% NS or plasmanate	Albumin 5% add 0.9% NS or plasmanate	Amount removed replaced with washed, frozen, or WBC-poor RBCs
Usual length of each treatment	2-3 hr usually, depending on volume to be removed	2-4 hr	3-4 hr	Varies with condition being treated
Usual length of therapy	Six treatments	Varies with primary condition	18-20 treatments, depending on rate of cell proliferation	Varies with primary condition
Usual schedule of treatments	Every other day or every day to total required depending on antigen/complement levels	Varies with condition, continued until platelet count is at desired level	Three times week 1, two times week 2, then one time a week thereafter to total required	Varies with primary condition

■ BLOOD TRANSFUSIONS

ASSESSMENT
OBSERVATIONS/FINDINGS
Venipuncture site
  Pain
  Warmth
  Redness
  Swelling
  Leakage at insertion site
Position of extremity
Blood
  Type and Rh factor (Table 4-3)
  Flow rate
  Amount

POTENTIAL REACTIONS (Table 4-4)
Hemolysis
  Elevated temperature
  Decreased BP
  Hemoglobinuria
  Hematuria
  Chills
  Pain
Circulatory overload
  SOB
  Lung congestion: rales, rhonchi
  Frothy sputum
Pyogenic reaction
  Sudden chilling
  Elevated temperature
  Headache
Allergic reaction
  Urticaria
  Laryngeal edema
  Asthmatic wheezing
Blood-borne infections (e.g., hepatitis, cytomegalovirus
  [CMV], acquired immunodeficiency syndrome
  [AIDS])

PRETRANSFUSION CARE
Select equipment needed for venipuncture according to
  hospital policy, procedure, and physician's order
Prepare equipment and normal saline solution
Obtain blood no more than 30 minutes before
  administration; check blood according to hospital
  policy, ensuring that correct patient receives
  type-specific blood
Obtain baseline BP, T, P, and R
Prepare venipuncture site

CARE DURING TRANSFUSION
Flush blood tubing with normal saline solution before
  starting transfusion
Remain with patient for at least 15 minutes (or 50 ml)
  after starting blood; check vital signs and compare
  with baseline
Discontinue blood immediately if transfusion reaction
  occurs, call physician, change blood tubing, maintain
  patent IV line, and follow hospital procedure

POSTTRANSFUSION CARE
Apply pressure to venipuncture site
Apply adhesive bandage and/or dressing as indicated
Change blood tubing after transfusion
Observe for reaction 1 hour after infusion of blood
Record whether a reaction occurred

PATIENT/FAMILY TEACHING
Ensure that patient and/or significant other knows and
  understands the following:
    Importance of maintaining position of extremity
    Importance of reporting symptoms of reaction
    Rash
    Flushed feeling
    Chills
    SOB
    Chest pain
Importance of not regulating flow rate

Text continued on p. 224

Table 4-3	**Blood and Blood Components**			
Product	**Description**	**Indication(s)**	**Action**	**Administration**
Red blood cells, packed (PRC)	Concentrated red blood cells that remain after plasma is separated	To improve oxygen-carrying capacity of the blood (hemolytic anemia in aplastic crisis, chronic hypoplastic anemia, leukemia, lymphoma, and other malignant diseases with bone marrow failure); exchange transfusions; surgery; shock; conditions in which sudden changes in blood volume are not tolerated	Increases oxygen-carrying capacity; elevates Hct (3% if unit of PRC has Hct of 70%-80%) Increases Hgb 1 g/dl/unit in patients with no active bleeding	See blood administration standard; administer through a filter; regulate flow to 25 ml/hr for 15 min; remain with patient; observe for reaction; if no reaction, regulate flow to 100-200 ml/hr in adult with no cardiac failure or elevated central venous pressure (CVP) and in infants and children regulate flow to 2-6 ml/kg/hr; add sodium chloride to PRC before administration when ordered; *no other solution or medication may be added to red cells*
Red blood cells, leukocyte poor	Concentrated red cells with leukocytes removed, usually by continuous flow centrifuge or washing	See PRC; severe febrile transfusion reactions caused by antileukocyte or antiplatelet antibodies; candidates for transplantation	See PRC	See PRC
Red blood cells, frozen	Glycerol added to red cells to protect cell from hemolysis while suspended in hypertonic solution when frozen; glycerol is removed before administration	See PRC; hypersensitivity reactions to plasma components such as IgA	See PRC	See PRC
Whole blood	Plasma and RBCs; may or may not contain other cells and factors; dependent on length of time transpired after collection; unit usually contains 520 ± 45 ml of anticoagulated blood with Hct of about 40%	Restoration of decreased blood volume caused by hemorrhage or trauma in which more than 25% of volume is lost	Restores blood volume and increases oxygen-carrying capacity	Administer through a filter; remain with patient until 25-50 ml transfused, usually 15-30 min; observe for transfusion reactions; if no reaction, adjust flow rate to administer complete unit within 4hr; warm unit no higher than 37° C using special coils when refrigerated blood needs to be administered quickly
Whole blood, modified		Hypovolemic shock	Increases oxygen-carrying capacity and provides volume without adding platelets, which release serotonin (a vasoconstrictor)	See whole blood

Continued

Table 4-3	**Blood and Blood Components**—cont'd			
Product	**Description**	**Indication(s)**	**Action**	**Administration**
Whole blood with antihemophilic factor (factor VIII) removed	Prepared by removing factor VIII, using heparin in initial collection, or converting a previously collected unit of blood containing a citrate anticoagulant	Exchange transfusion in the adult	Provides volume without contributing to coagulation ability	See whole blood
Plasma	Plasma prepared from single donor unit of fresh blood	Burns; traumatic shock; replacement of certain coagulation factors	Provides plasma coagulation factors	Administer unit in less than 1 hr in hypovolemic patient; in normovolemic patient, administer at rate of 5-20 ml/kg
Plasma, fresh-frozen	Plasma prepared from single donor unit of fresh blood; it is frozen within 6 hr of collection	Source of fibrinogen and factors V and VIII	See plasma; 1 U usually contains approximately 400 mg fibrinogen, 200 U factors VIII and IX, and other stable and labile coagulation factors	Thaw frozen plasma in 37° C water bath with gentle agitation; *do not warm;* administer through a filter; *never add* medications or fluids
Plasma, liquid	Plasma prepared from single donor unit within 5 days after collection; stored frozen	Factor VII, IX, X, XI, and XIII deficiencies or abnormalities	Replacement of factors VII, IX, X, XI, or XIII	See plasma, fresh-frozen
Cryoprecipitated antihemophilic factor (factor VIII)	Preparation containing factor VIII is obtained from a single unit of blood; contains approximately 80 U factor VIII, and 200 mg fibrinogen in 15 ml of plasma	Hemophilia A; von Willebrand's disease (factor VIII deficiency)	Provides high concentrations of factor VIII and fibrinogen	Thaw in warm water bath at 37° C with gentle agitation; administer through filter rapidly within 6 hr after thawing if container not entered; 2 hr after thawing if container entered
Leukocyte concentrate	Leukocytes, platelets, and erythrocytes in varying amounts in 200-500 ml of plasma collected by apheresis; a compatible HLA donor is usually preferred (not identical donor whose use as a tissue donor is anticipated)	Bacterial sepsis not responsive to antibiotic therapy in presence of neutropenia; chronic granulomatous disease when bone marrow recovery is foreseen and temperature elevated for 24-48 hours	Provides granulocytes to more effectively control infection	Administer irradiated leukocytes to prevent engraphment and possible graft-versus-host disease (GVHD); regulate rate of flow to give 250-850 granulocytes/μl/M^2, usually 1 U/day is ordered; slow rate of transfusion at appearance of elevated T wave, chills, and urticaria; stop transfusion when symptoms of transient pulmonary infiltrate appear

Table 4-3	**Blood and Blood Components—cont'd**			
Product	**Description**	**Indication(s)**	**Action**	**Administration**
Platelet concentrate (random or single donor)	Platelets separated from whole blood suspended in plasma; collection from single donor preferred	Hemorrhage caused by thrombocytopenia; prevention of potential hemorrhage in bone marrow suppression caused by chemotherapy; abnormalities in platelet function	Corrects hemostatic deficit in thrombocytopenia and abnormally functioning platelets; 1 U usually increases platelet count 5000/ml in 70-kg adult	Administer through a filter (*never* a microaggregate filter); regulate flow rate to ensure administration of total unit in less than 20 min
Normal serum albumin, USP 25% solution hyperoncotic (NOTE: 5% solution is osmotically equal to plasma)	Derived from pooled venous plasma; contains 25 g normal serum albumin/100 ml	Hypoproteinemia; burns; shock caused by trauma, hemorrhage	Increases oncotic pressure; increases circulating volume by drawing 5 times the infused volume of albumin into circulation unless patient is dehydrated; reduces hemoconcentration and blood viscosity	Administer at flow rate <2-3 ml/min to prevent rapid rise in BP, circulatory overload, or pulmonary edema
Hespan, Hetastarch	A synthetic colloid derived from a waxy starch composed of amylopectin; it has a molecular weight suitable for use as a plasma expander; Hespan is 6% Hetastarch in 0.9% sodium chloride injection	An adjunct in treatment of hemorrhagic shock, burns, and septic shock Indicated in the treatment of hypovolemia when plasma volume expansion is required Not a substitute for blood or plasma	Volume expansion resulting from albumin-like properties Increases ESR when added to whole blood, thereby improving efficacy of granulocyte collection	Administer by IV infusion only. Total dose and rate depend upon amount of blood or plasma lost. Adults: usual dose 500-1000 ml at a rate of 20 ml/kg/hr for hemorrhagic shock, slower for other conditions. Contraindications: hypersensitivity to components, bleeding disorders, CHF, renal failure, elevated PT, PTT

Table 4-4	**Reactions to Transfusion of Blood and Blood Components**			
Product	**Type of Reaction**	**Onset**	**Observations**	**Nursing Actions**
Red blood cells (RBCs), all preparations	Febrile nonhemolytic	Initiation of transfusion to 24 hr post-transfusion	Chills, elevated temperature, headache, nausea, vomiting	Check and record baseline BP, T, P, and R; slow infusion; notify physician; administer antipyretic or antihistamines as ordered; check and record T, P, and R q15min; saline washed RBCs: frozen, thawed, washed RBCs or leukocyte filter may be ordered to decrease reaction
	Febrile hemolytic	Immediately to 30 min after initiation of transfusion or when 25-50 ml infused	Restlessness, anxiety, precordial oppression, elevated temperature to 105° F (40.6° C), tachycardia, tachypnea, flushed face, back and thigh pain, generalized tingling, chills, nausea, vomiting, shock, disseminated intravascular coagulation (DIC), renal failure, oliguria, hematuria, anuria	Stop transfusion immediately; change IV tubing; initiate normal saline at 4-6 ml/hr; cap blood tubing with sterile needle or cap; report symptoms to physician and blood bank; recheck identifying blood numbers with patient's numbers; monitor and record T, R, and cardiac rate and rhythm q10min-15min; measure and record urine output with each voiding or q½ hr; send first specimen to lab for testing; report output <15 ml/30 min or presence of bleeding; ensure that blood samples are drawn for testing; the following are usually ordered: Hgb, haptoglobin level, methemalbumin, bilirubin, differential agglutination, serologic studies, renal function tests, and aerobic and anaerobic cultures; complete transfusion record; send discontinued blood, tubing, and record to laboratory for testing; administer medications and fluids IV as ordered; diuretics, oxygen, electrolytes, and heparin may be ordered; prepare for dialysis
Whole blood	Allergic reaction to plasma proteins	Within 30 min after initiating transfusion	Mild reaction: chills, elevated temperature, backache, pain in legs	Check and record baseline BP, T, P, and R; stop infusion; initiate slow (4-6 ml/hr) infusion of saline using new sterile IV tubing; notify physician and blood bank; monitor T, P, R, and BP q10min-15min; ensure that blood specimen is drawn for testing; return remainder of blood product, tubing, and transfusion record to blood bank; indicate observations on transfusion record; usually red cells without IgA will be ordered for administration; oxygen, steroids, vasopressors, or epinephrine may be ordered for anaphylactic shock; prepare for resuscitation
		Immediately to 30 min after initiation of transfusion	Moderate-to-severe reaction: erythematous rash, urticaria, dyspnea, wheezing, hypotension, intestinal hyperperistalsis, anaphylactic shock	
		During transfusion to several days after	Urticaria, swelling of lymph nodes, sore throat	Slow transfusion rate; report observations to physician; administer antihistamines as ordered; blood obtained from a fasting donor may be ordered if reaction is severe

Table 4-4	**Reactions to Transfusion of Blood and Blood Components—cont'd**			
Product	**Type of Reaction**	**Onset**	**Observations**	**Nursing Actions**
	Circulatory over- load	During trans- fusion to 24	Sharp cough, precor- dial pain, back pain, dyspnea, cyanosis, increased venous pressure, distended neck veins, pro- ductive cough, frothy sputum, pleural rales	Slow transfusion rate; report observa- tions to physician; continue rate of flow as ordered; usually 2ml/kg/hr; monitor, BP, T, P, R, and CVP q15min-30min; see CHF (p. 112)
	Febrile (hemolytic)	*See* RBC	*See* RBC	*See* RBC
	Febrile (WBC and/ or platelet anti- bodies)	*See* Leukocyte concentrate	*See* Leukocyte con- centrate	*See* Leukocyte concentrate
Massive transfu- sions of RBCs or whole blood	Metabolic hyper- kalemia and citrate toxicity with acid citrate dextrose (ACD) anticoagulant	Citric acid eleva- tions of 100 mg/100 ml	Tremors, prolonged Q-T segment on ECG, hypocalcemia, acidosis then alkalosis, cardiac arrest if citric acid levels higher	When massive transfusions required, transfusion products with citrate- phosphate dextrose (CPD) antico- agulant usually ordered; monitor and record T, R, and cardiac func- tion q10min-15min; ensure that blood samples are drawn for elec- trolytes, calcium, pH, CO_2, bicar- bonate levels; administer calcium gluconate IV as ordered; adminis- ter oral or rectal cation exchange resins as ordered for hyperkalemia
	Pulmonary infiltrates	During transfusion	Chills, elevated temperature, tachycardia, nonproductive cough, dyspnea, respiratory distress syndrome (p. 270)	Stop blood immediately; change tub- ing; institute normal saline IV at 4-6 ml/hr; monitor and record BP, T, P, and R; auscultate chest for breath and heart sounds; report observations to physician; see Re- spiratory distress syndrome (p. 270)
	Bleeding tendency caused by dilu- tional effect	Transfusion volume equal to blood volume of patient	Bleeding in any body system, thrombo- cytopenia, coagu- lation abnormalities	Report observations to physician im- mediately; check and record BP, T, P, and R; q10min-15min; monitor cardiac function continuously; aus- cultate chest for heart and breath sounds q15min-30min; administer platelet concentrate, fluids, and medications as ordered; manage hemorrhage as indicated and or- dered
	Pulmonary air embolus	During transfusion	SOB, chest pain, cyanosis, syncope, hypo- tension, shock	Stop transfusion immediately; place patient on left side; administer oxygen as ordered; monitor vital signs, CVP q15min; see Pulmonary embolus (p. 256)
Leukocyte concen- trate	Acute reaction Transient pul- monary infiltrate	Immediately	Elevated temperature, chills Retrosternal constric- tion, pallor, cyano- sis, tachycardia, cough	Slow transfusion; monitor and record BP, T, P, and R q15min-30min; aus- cultate chest for breath and heart sounds q15min-30min; report observations to physician; see Respiratory distress syndrome (p. 270); medicate with Demerol when ordered

Continued

Table 4-4	**Reactions to Transfusion of Blood and Blood Components—cont'd**			
Product	**Type of Reaction**	**Onset**	**Observations**	**Nursing Actions**
	Graft-versus-host disease (GVHD)			Usually only irradiated leukocytes are administered for prevention of GVHD
	Graft-versus-host disease (GVHD)			Usually only irradiated leukocytes are administered for prevention of GVHD
Platelets	Febrile; usually caused by infusion of incompatible leukocytes contaminating platelet preparations	Immediately to 12-24 hr post-transfusion	Chills, hives, flushing	Check and record BP, T, P, and R q15min-30min; administer medications when ordered; reaction usually self-limiting; patient may develop antibodies and destroy platelets in subsequent transfusions; check platelet count 1 hr after transfusion
Plasma	Similar to whole blood	Similar to whole blood	Similar to whole blood	Similar to whole blood
Whole blood with factor VIII removed	Bleeding caused by heparin used as anticoagulant reactions as in whole blood	During and after transfusion when large volumes administered; see whole blood	Bleeding in any body system See Whole blood	Report observations to physician immediately, check and record BP, T, P, and R; monitor cardiac status continuously; administer protamine sulfate as ordered; measure and record urinary output See Whole blood
Normal serum albumin	Reactions are rare	During administration	Chills, elevated temperature, nausea	Slow transfusion rate; report observations to physician; check and record BP, T, P, and R q15min-30min
	Circulatory overload/bleeding during rapid infusion	During transfusion	Rising or elevated BP, circulatory overload, pulmonary edema; new areas of bleeding appear in hemorrhagic shock	Monitor rate of infusion carefully; slow rate of transfusion; report observations to physician; check and record T, P, R, and BP q10min-15min; monitor cardiac status continuously; auscultate chest for heart and breath sounds q15min-30min; observe closely for new sites of bleeding

BIBLIOGRAPHY

Beare PG, Myers JL: *Adult health nursing,* ed 3, St Louis, 1998, Mosby.

Belcher A: *Blood disorders,* St Louis, 1993, Mosby.

Fitzpatrick L et al: Blood transfusions: keeping your patient safe, *Nurs '97* 27(8):34-43, 1997.

Gulanick M et al: *Nursing care plans: nursing diagnosis and intervention,* ed 4, St Louis, 1998, Mosby.

Guyton AC: *Textbook of medical physiology,* ed 8, Philadelphia, 1990, WB Saunders.

Holms H et al, eds: *Illustrated handbook of nursing care,* Springhouse, Pa, 1998, Springhouse.

Jaffe M, Skidmore-Roth L: *Home health nursing assessment and care planning,* ed 3, St Louis, 1997, Mosby.

Kaiser Foundation Hospital/Health Plan, Northern California Region: *Nursing standards of practice manual, 1998: blood transfusion standard,* Oakland, Kaiser Foundation Hospitals.

Kim MJ, McFarland GK, McFarlane AM: *Pocket guide to nursing diagnoses,* ed 7, St Louis, 1998, Mosby.

Kinney MR et al, eds: *AACN clinical reference for critical care nursing,* ed 3, New York, 1993, McGraw-Hill.

Lee GR et al: *Wintrobe's clinical hematology,* ed 10, Baltimore, 1999, Williams and Wilkins.

Pagana KD, Pagana TJ: *Mosby's manual of diagnostic and laboratory tests,* St Louis, 1998, Mosby.

Phillips L: *Manual of IV therapeutics,* Philadelphia, 1993, FA Davis.

Thompson JM et al: *Mosby's clinical nursing,* ed 4, St Louis, 1997, Mosby.

Westphal RG, Kasprisim DO: *Current status of hemapheresis: indications, technology and complications,* Arlington, Va, 1987, American Association of Blood Banks.

MULTIDISCIPLINARY PLAN OF CARE

Diagnosis: **Sickle Cell Crisis**

Type of Surgery:_____   DRG #: <u>395</u>   Expected Length of Stay: <u>2 Days</u>

Resuscitation Status: ☐ No Code/DNR   Date: _____   Date of Admission: _____

    ☐ Other: _____   Date:_____   Date of Surgery: _____

Date/ Initials	Disci-pline	Patient Problem(s)	Patient Goal(s)	Date Resolved/ Initials
		Pain	Pain decreased and/or controlled	
		Potential for severe aplastic anemia, respiratory complications, infection	Stable blood pressure & CBC (based on patient's baseline), Hgb >5, Retic. Count >3, O2 SAT >90, afebrile	
		Knowledge deficit Re: disease process & treatment	Patient demonstrates knowledge of Sickle Cell Disease and Pain Management techniques	

This Plan of Care and guidelines do not purport to reflect all relevant medical considerations and are not intended to replace clinical judgment. REVISED 6/11/96, Approved by Pharmacy & Therapeutics Committee 8/96, Medical Records Committee 8/96, Executive Committee 9/96
DRG395.DOC
(Used by permission of Kaiser Permonente Medical Center Los Angeles Calif.)

MULTIDISCIPLINARY PLAN OF CARE

ASPECT OF CARE	Sickle Cell Crisis	
DISCHARGE OUTCOMES	**DATE:** Admission Day	
CONSULTS Consults completed	___ Social Medicine intervention per criteria	___
	___ Hematology consult, or list primary Hematology Physician:_____	___
		___
	___	___
DIAGNOSTIC STUDIES Results within acceptable limits	___ CBC, Reticulocytes, Lytes	___
	___ Chest X-ray	___
	___ Type & Hold/Type & Cross	___
	___	___
	___	___
TREATMENTS, PROCEDURES, & MONITORS Tolerating treatments & procedures well, VSS	___ V.S. q 4 hrs	___
	___ Record level of pain, level of consciousness with V.S.	___
	___ Reduce pain rating/severity to ≤5/10 utilizing Pain Control protocol	___
	___ Heat to affected area	___
	___ O$_2$	___
	___	___
	___	___
	___	___
MEDICATIONS/ LINES Routine oral meds, knowledge of pain control	___ IV fluids (D/C when taking 3-4 liters PO q d)	___
	___ Pain medications as ordered	___
	___	___
	___	___
	___	___
	___	___
NUTRITION Tolerating diet well	___ Diet as tolerated	___
	___ Encourage fluids	___
	___	___
ACTIVITY/ MOBILITY Ambulatory with independent ADLs	___ Bedrest with BRP	___
	___	___
	___	___
	___	___
PATIENT/FAMILY EDUCATION Knowledge of disease and self management skills	___ Determine knowledge of disease	___
	___ Discuss expected LOS with patient/family	___
	___ Review Advance Directives and incorporate into plan	___
	___	___
PSYCHO-SOCIAL Coping with illness and/or stressors	___ Psychosocial needs identified:	___
	___ specify _____	___
	_____	___
DISCHARGE PLANNING Adequate resources identified	___ Assess discharge needs PRN	___
	___ Home Health	___
	___	___
	___	___

MULTIDISCIPLINARY PLAN OF CARE

ASPECT OF CARE	Sickle Cell Crisis	
DISCHARGE OUTCOMES	**DATE:**	**Day 1**
CONSULTS Consults completed	___ ___ ___ ___	___ ___ ___ ___
DIAGNOSTIC STUDIES Results within acceptable limits	___ Lab per MD order ___ ___ ___ ___	___ ___ ___ ___ ___
TREATMENTS, PROCEDURES, & MONITORS Tolerating treatments & procedures well, VSS	___ V.S. q 4 hrs ___ Record level of pain, level of consciousness with V.S. ___ Reduce pain rating/severity (moderate 3-4/10) utilizing Pain Control protocol Heat to affected area ___ O₂ ___ ___ ___	___ ___ ___ ___ ___ ___
MEDICATIONS/ LINES Routine oral meds, knowledge of pain control	___ IV fluids (D/C when taking 3-4 liters PO q d) ___ Reevaluate pain medication, adjust as needed ___ ___ ___ ___ ___	___ ___ ___ ___ ___ ___ ___
NUTRITION Tolerating diet well	___ Diet as tolerated ___ Encourage fluids ___	___ ___ ___
ACTIVITY/ MOBILITY Ambulatory with independent ADLs	___ Bedrest with BRP ___ ___ ___	___ ___ ___ ___
PATIENT/FAMILY EDUCATION Knowledge of disease and self management skills	___ Reinforce teaching Sickle Cell Disease ___ Pain management ___ ___	___ ___ ___ ___
PSYCHO-SOCIAL Coping with illness and/or stressors	___ Follow-up needs: ___ specify:_____ ___ _____	___ ___ ___
DISCHARGE PLANNING Adequate resources identified	___ ___ ___ ___	___ ___ ___ ___

MULTIDISCIPLINARY PLAN OF CARE

ASPECT OF CARE	Sickle Cell Crisis	
DISCHARGE OUTCOMES	**DATE:**	
		Day 2
CONSULTS	___	___
	___	___
	___	___
	___	___
DIAGNOSTIC STUDIES	___ Labs per MD order	___
	___	___
	___	___
	___	___
	___	___
TREATMENTS, PROCEDURES, & MONITORS	___ V.S. q shift & PRN	___
	___ Record level of pain and level of consciousness with V.S. q shift	___
	___ Reduce pain rating/severity (mild 1-2/10) utilizing Pain Control protocol	___
	___ Heat to affected extremity	___
	___ O_2	___
	___	___
	___	___
	___	___
MEDICATIONS/ LINES	___ D/C IV	___
	___ Reevaluate pain medication, adjust as needed	___
	___	___
	___	___
	___	___
NUTRITION	___ Diet as tolerated	___
	___ Encourage fluids	___
	___	___
	___	___
ACTIVITY/ MOBILITY	___ Ambulatory and independent with ADLs	___
	___	___
	___	___
	___	___
	___	___
PATIENT/FAMILY EDUCATION	___ Continue reinforcement of teaching & evaluate understanding	___
	___	___
	___	___
	___	___
PSYCHO-SOCIAL	___ Follow-up needs:	___
	___ specify _____	___
	___ _____	___
DISCHARGE PLANNING	___ If pain mild or controlled for 8 hrs, may be discharged	___
	___	___
	___	___

Respiratory System

■ RESPIRATORY ASSESSMENT

▊ SUBJECTIVE DATA

Cough
Pain
    Chest
    Abdomen
Wheeze
Shortness of breath (SOB)
Number of pillows used
Amount of exercise tolerated
Fever
Chills
Rapid breathing
Tiring easily
Change in voice
Dizziness
Sweating
Swelling of feet and hands
Expectoration

▊ OBJECTIVE DATA

Anxious facies
Dyspnea
Dyspnea on exertion (DOE)
Flaring nostrils
Red, swollen nose
Nasal discharge
Color
    Cyanosis
        Lips
        Circumoral area
        Nail beds
        Gums
        Earlobes
        Soles of feet
        Palms of hands
    Pallor
    Ashen
    Gray
    Cherry red
    Red
    Reddish blue
Confusion, restlessness
Hallucinations

Cough
    Onset and duration
    Characteristics
    Dry hacking, barking, congested
    Severity
    Nonproductive
    Productive
    Sputum
        When produced
            Upon awakening (morning)
            Afternoon
            Continuously
        Characteristics: color, odor, consistency, amount
Hemoptysis
Stridor
Wheeze
Assuming upright position: orthopnea
Clubbing of extremities: nail beds
Use of accessory muscles of respiration
Telegraphic speech pattern: short, choppy sentences
Eyes
    Engorged veins
    Papilledema
Elevated temperature
Diaphoresis
Anorexia
Weight
    Obese
    Underweight
    Gain
    Loss
Ascites
Rash
Respirations (R) (Tables 5-1 and 5-2)
    Bradypnea
    Tachypnea
    Long expiratory phase
    Irregular
    Asymmetric
    Periods of apnea
    Cheyne-Stokes
    Shallow
    Pursed-lip breathing
    Biot's
    Kussmaul's

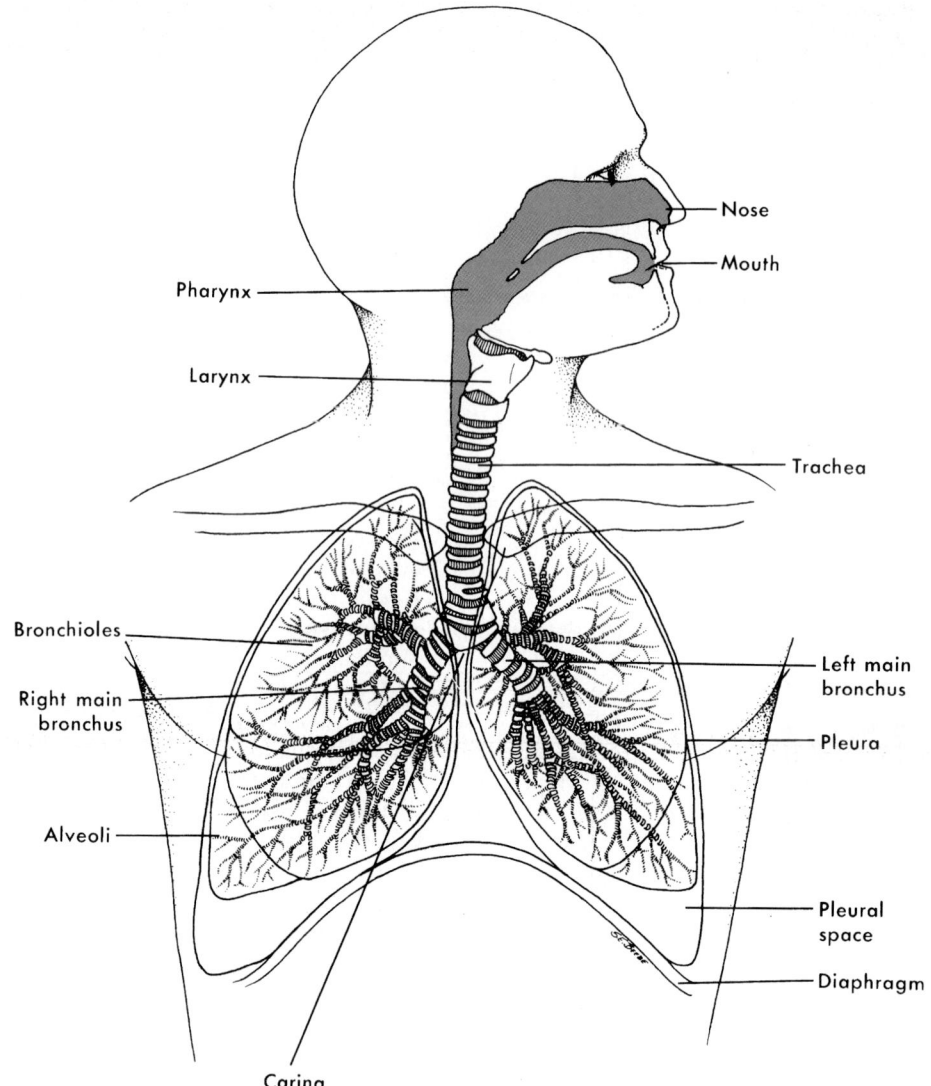

Fig. 5-1   Respiratory system.

Apneustic
   Hyperventilation
Retractions
   Suprasternal
   Supraclavicular
   Substernal
   Intercostal
Cardiac status
   Elevated BP
   Tachycardia
   Bradycardia
   Sinus dysrhythmia
Congestive heart failure (CHF)
   Crackles
   Rhonchi
   Jugular venous distention
   Edema
   Abdominal distention and pain
   Hepatosplenomegaly

Thoracic examination
   Scoliosis
   Kyphosis
   Kyphoscoliosis
   Pectus excavatum (funnel chest)
   Pectus carinatum (pigeon chest)
   Barrel chest
   Unequal shoulder height
Palpation
   Thoracic expansion
   Fremitus (vocal/tactile)
   Tracheal deviation
   Crepitus
Percussion
   Resonance
   Hyperresonance
   Tympany
   Dullness
   Flatness

Table 5-1	**Patterns of Respiration**	
Type		**Characteristics**
Normal respiration		Rate 14-20/min in normal adult Rhythm, regular
Cheyne-Stokes respiration		Periods of apnea alternating with series of respiratory cycles Rate and amplitude of successive respiratory cycles increase to a maximum and then decrease until terminated by period of apnea in a crescendo-decrescendo pattern
Biot's ataxic respiration		Variation of Cheyne-Stokes respiration in which periods of apnea alternate irregularly with periods of breaths of equal depth
Sighing respiration		Deep, audible sighs that interrupt normal respiratory rhythm
Painful respiration		Interruption of normal respiratory rhythm caused by pain; breathing frequently becomes shallow during interruption
Ataxic respiration		Gross irregularity in rate, rhythm, and depth of respiration; also referred to as meningitic respirations

Modified from Abels LF: Mosby's manual of critical care, *St Louis, 1979, Mosby.*

Table 5-2	**Normal Respiratory Findings**	
Area of Concern	**Normal Adult Findings**	**Variations in Older Adult**
General appearance	Appears relaxed Breathing is quiet and easy without apparent effort Facial expressions and limb movements are relaxed	
Breathing pattern	Diaphragmatic-thoracic pattern is smooth and regular May have occasional sighing respirations Breathing is quiet, and exhalation is passive	Pattern is same as for adults, but calcification at rib articulation points may decrease chest expansion
Respiratory rate	12-20 resp/min Ratio of pulse to respirations is 4:1	
Skin	Appears well oxygenated; no cyanosis or pallor present Palpation of skin and chest wall reveals smooth skin and a stable chest wall; there are no crepitations, bulging, or painful spots	
Nail bed, nail configuration	Minimal angulation between base of nail and finger No thickening of distal finger width	
Chest wall configuration	Symmetric, bilateral muscle development A:P to transverse ratio is 1:2 to 5:7; larger than these ratios is considered to be barrel chest Straight spinal processes Downward and equal slope of ribs; costal angle 90 degrees or less	Kyphosis is a common finding in older adults; there is dorsal scoliosis with slight tracheal deviation; this may also cause a slight increase in A:P to transverse ratio
Tracheal position	Midline and straight directly above the suprasternal notch	May be slightly deviated if kyphosis is present

Modified from Thompson JM et al: Mosby's clinical nursing, *ed 4, St Louis, 1997, Mosby.*

Auscultation (Table 5-3)
    Decreased or absent breath sounds
    Crackles
    Rhonchi
    Wheezing
    Friction rubs
    Whispered pectoriloquy
    Bronchophony
    Egophony

◼ PERTINENT BACKGROUND INFORMATION

CONCURRENT DISEASES OR CONDITIONS
Cancer
Heart disease
Renal disease
Liver disease
Ascites
Polycythemia
Obesity
Hypertension
Guillain-Barré syndrome
Myasthenia gravis or other neurologic disease affecting
    respiratory function

PSYCHOLOGIC RESPONSES
Response to stress
Methods of coping
Response to pain
Relationships with others

PREVIOUS RESPIRATORY CONDITION/MEDICAL HISTORY
Asthma
Bronchitis
Cystic fibrosis
Emphysema
Tuberculosis
Fibrocystic disease
Premature birth
Previous operations

FAMILY HISTORY
Heart disease
Hypertension
Diabetes
Cancers
Obesity
Pulmonary disorders

SOCIAL HISTORY
Smoking (past and present): packs per day × how many
    years
Alcohol use
Exercise and activity levels
Occupation: current and previous
Sleep patterns

Environmental factors: exposure to dust, fumes, asbestos,
    or chemicals
Recent exposure to infections
Travel out of country
Available family support
Age (see Gerontologic Considerations box)

MEDICATION HISTORY
Prescription medications
Over-the-counter medications

◼ DIAGNOSTIC TESTS

Chest x-ray examination
    Complete blood cell count (CBC)
    Arterial blood gases (ABGs): Pao_2, $Paco_2$, pH
    Lactic acid levels
Sputum evaluation
    Amount
    Color, odor, viscosity
    Cytologic study
    Gram stain
    Culture and sensitivity
Tracheal aspiration
Throat or nasopharyngeal culture
Blood cultures
Pulse oximetry (Spo_2)
Transcutaneous oxygen monitoring ($TcPO_2$)
End-tidal carbon dioxide monitoring ($PetCO_2$)
Alveolar-arterial oxygen gradient
Pulmonary function tests
    Tidal volume (V_T)
    Minute volume (V_E)
    Vital capacity (VC)
    Forced vital capacity (FVC)
    Forced expiratory volume (FEV); in 1 second
        (FEV_1)
    Inspiratory reserve volume (IRV)
    Maximal midexpiratory flow (MMEF)
    Peak expiratory flow rate (PEFR)
    Residual volume (RV)
    Functional residual capacity (FRC)
    Inspiratory capacity (IC)
    Expiratory reserve volume (ERV)
    Diffuse capacity carbon monoxide (DL_{CO})
    Total lung capacity (TLC)
Gastric lavage
Skin tests
Sweat test
Bronchoscopy
Bronchograms
Lung biopsy
Lung computed tomography (CT) scans
Ventilation/perfusion scanning
Thoracentesis
Direct laryngoscopy
Scalene node biopsy
Pulmonary angiography
Tomography

Table 5-3	Breath and Voice Sounds: Normal and Abnormal

Breath and Voice Sounds	Characteristics	Findings
NORMAL		
Vesicular	Heard over most of lung fields; low pitch; soft and short expirations	Low pitch, soft expirations
Bronchovesicular	Heard over main bronchus area and over upper right posterior lung field; medium pitch; expiration equals inspiration	Medium-pitch, medium expirations
Bronchial	Heard only over trachea; high pitch; loud and long expirations	High-pitch, loud expirations
ABNORMAL		
Bronchial when heard over peripheral lung fields	High pitch; loud and long expirations	
Bronchovesicular sounds when heard over peripheral lung fields	Medium pitch with inspirations equal to expirations	
Adventitious	Crackles: discrete, noncontinuous sounds	
	Fine crackles: high-pitched, discrete, noncontinuous crackling sounds heard during the end of inspiration (indicates inflammation or congestion)	
	Medium crackles: lower, more moist sound heard during the midstage of inspiration; not cleared by a cough	
	Coarse crackles: loud, bubbly noise heard during inspiration; not cleared by a cough	
	Wheezes: continuous musical sounds; if low pitched, may be called *rhonchi*	
	Sibilant wheeze: musical noise sounding like a squeak; may be heard during inspiration or expiration; usually louder during expiration	
	Sonorous wheeze (rhonchi): loud, low, coarse sound like a snore heard at any point of inspiration or expiration; coughing may clear sound (usually means mucus accumulation in trachea or large bronchi)	
	Pleural friction rub: dry, rubbing, or grating sound, usually caused by the inflammation of pleural surfaces; heard during inspiration or expiration; loudest over lower lateral anterior surface	
	Stridor: harsh, high-pitched sound; louder on inspiration than expiration (usually means partial upper airway obstruction)	
RESONANCE OF SPOKEN VOICE		
	Bronchophony: using diaphragm of stethoscope, listen to posterior chest as patient says "ninety-nine"	Negative response: muffled "nin-nin" sound heard Positive response: clear, loud "ninety-nine" response heard because the lung tissue is consolidated
	Whispered pectoriloquy: listen to posterior chest as patient whispers "one, two, three"	Negative response: muffled sounds heard Positive response: clear "one, two, three" is heard because of lung consolidation
	Egophony: listen to posterior chest as the patient says "e-e-e"	Negative response: muffled "e-e-e" sound heard Positive response: sound of sound *e* changes to an *a-a-a* because of consolidation

Modified from Thompson JM et al: Mosby's clinical nursing, ed 4, St Louis, 1997, Mosby.

Gerontologic Considerations

- The older person is generally able to maintain adequate ventilation and oxygenation, provided that there is no serious disease of the respiratory tract.
- However, changes of aging do have an impact on respiratory function:
  - Drier mucous membranes and decreased number of cilia affect the older individual's ability to humidify inhaled air and trap debris. These in turn increase the risk for inflammation and irritation of the upper respiratory tract.
  - Kyphosis and calcification of costal cartilage are common changes. These restrict expansion of the thoracic cavity and lead to a barrel-chested appearance.
  - Intercostal muscles and the diaphragm lose elasticity, resulting in a decreased ability to breathe deeply and cough, especially when lying down.
  - The elasticity of airways and alveoli decreases, alveoli thicken, and pulmonary blood flow decreases, resulting in increased risk for impaired gas exchange; vital capacity declines, and residual volume increases.
- Years of exposure to air pollution, smoke, and mechanical irritants increase the risk for respiratory disease in older adults, particularly those who have emphysema and chronic bronchitis.
- Inactivity and immobility increase the risk of stasis pooling of respiratory secretions, which then increases the risk of pneumonia.
- Signs and symptoms of pneumonia are often atypical in older adults. Fever, cough, and purulent sputum may be absent. Generalized signs and symptoms such as lethargy, disorientation, dyspnea, tachypnea, chills, chest pain, and vomiting, as well as an unexpected exacerbation of coexisting conditions, should be viewed with suspicion, because they may indicate pneumonia in the older adult.

- Adequate hydration is very important for the older person with pneumonia. It helps liquefy secretions and promotes expectoration.
- Many older adults have difficulty expectorating, which slows resolution of congestions and increases the difficulty of obtaining sputum specimens. Because deep breathing and coughing are difficult, the older person may require suctioning to remove respiratory secretions. This should be done with discretion, because too-frequent suctioning can stimulate increased production of secretions.
- Neurologic damage as a result of cerebrovascular accidents, Parkinson's disease, and other conditions is increasingly common in the older adult. Any neurologic disorder that decreases the gag or swallow reflexes increases the risk of aspiration of fluids and food, with resultant trauma to the respiratory tract.
- Cor pulmonale with right-side congestive heart failure, as well as left-side congestive heart failure with pulmonary congestion, are common complications of chronic obstructive pulmonary disease in the older adult.
- Older adults, particularly those living in institutions, should have routine skin tests for tuberculosis. Many older adults were exposed to tuberculosis during their childhood and have positive results on skin tests. These individuals should receive routine chest x-ray studies. Older adults who have histories of inactive tuberculosis should be watched for recurrence of active tuberculosis. Signs and symptoms are often vague and include loss of appetite and weight loss.
- Older immigrants and immunosuppressed older adults should be watched closely for drug-resistant strains of tuberculosis.

Modified from Christensen BL, Kockrow EO: Foundations of nursing, *ed 3, St Louis, 1998, Mosby.*

Barium swallow
Pulmonary echograms

■ FIBEROPTIC BRONCHOSCOPY

Direct visual examination of the trachea and tracheobronchial tree by means of a bronchoscope; the flexible fiberoptic bronchoscope is commonly used because it permits better visualization and identification of obstruction, tumor, or foreign body in tracheobronchial tree; indicated in diagnosis of pulmonary infection and disease, permits procurement of a specimen; therapeutically it is used to remove foreign bodies, treatment of atelectasis, drainage of abscess, and control of hemoptysis

PURPOSE/INDICATIONS
Collect secretions for laboratory examinations
Obtain tissue for biopsies
Locate and perform biopsy on tumors
Diagnose hemoptysis, lesions, or masses
Remove foreign bodies or mucous plug secretions
Treat lung abscesses, pneumonia, or aspiration

PREPARATION
Explain procedure to patient and the need to not talk during procedure; procedure may be done under local or general anesthetic
Maintain NPO for 6 hours before procedure
Manage pain with sedation as indicated; assess effectiveness of pain relief measures
Provide emotional support (patient may be fearful of discomfort and/or possible findings)
Remove dentures
Place patient in sitting or supine position as directed
Instruct patient to breathe in and out through nose with mouth open during procedure
    Fiberoptic bronchoscope is inserted through nose or mouth

POSTBRONCHOSCOPIC ASSESSMENT
OBSERVATIONS/FINDINGS
Difficulty in breathing
Stridor
Nasal flaring
Suprasternal and/or supraclavicular retractions
Hemoptysis
Hypotension
Tachycardia
Tachypnea
Hyperresonance
Wheezing
Cyanosis
Nausea, vomiting
Absence of gag and cough reflexes
Dysphagia
Hoarseness
Coughing
Throat or nasal pain
Chest pain

POTENTIAL COMPLICATIONS
Crepitus and/or subcutaneous emphysema
Absence of breath sounds
Decreased Sao_2
Pneumothorax
Hemoptysis

IMMEDIATE POSTBRONCHOSCOPIC CARE
Check blood pressure (BP), pulse (P), and R q15min for 1
    hour, then q2h to 4h and prn
Assist and teach patient to
    Not eat or drink until gag reflex returns, usually 3 to 4
        hours
    Maintain bed rest; elevate head of bed 45 degrees
    Dispose of tissue after coughing
    Understand importance of not using tobacco
    Report signs of crepitus to physician
    Manage pain as indicated; assess effectiveness of pain
        relief measure(s)
    Establish means of communication
        Call bell within reach
        Pad and pencil, Magic Slate*, or laptop computer
Auscultate chest for breath sounds q2h to 4h and prn
Report absent or diminished breath sounds to physician
Perform postural drainage as ordered
Perform oropharyngeal suctioning prn
Administer oxygen as ordered

CONVALESCENT CARE
Check BP, temperature (T), P, and R q8h and prn
Assist and teach patient to
    Gargle with warm saline solution q2h to 4h as
        indicated
    Maintain position of comfort

Western Publishing Co., Inc., Racine, Wis.

    Progress from liquids to diet as tolerated; avoid
        extremely hot foods

PATIENT/FAMILY TEACHING
Ensure that patient and significant other(s) know and
    understand
    Importance of not driving self home if procedure is
        done as outpatient
    Importance of maintaining liquid or soft diet as
        ordered until throat pain disappears
    Importance of forcing fluids to 3000 ml daily unless
        contraindicated by patient's condition
    Need to avoid extremely hot foods and liquids
    Need to avoid tobacco use
    Symptoms to report to physician
    Chest pain
    Difficulty in breathing
    Inability to swallow
    Increased hemoptysis
    Change in color and amount of sputum
Importance of ongoing outpatient care
Name of medication, dosage, time of administration,
    purpose, and side effects
Need to avoid taking over-the-counter medications
    without checking with physician
Importance of avoiding persons with upper respiratory
    infections (URIs)

■ THORACENTESIS
*Puncture of the chest wall with a large-gauge needle to
remove fluid from the pleural space*
Indications:
    *Diagnostic: collect fluid to examine for
      inflammation, infection, malignancy*
    Therapeutic: drain and relieve lung congestion

PREPARATION
Auscultate chest for breath sounds
Obtain chest x-ray examination as ordered by
    physician
Obtain baseline BP, T, P, and R
Prepare local anesthetic as ordered
Position patient on edge of bed with feet supported; head
    and arms should be resting on overbed table; if patient
    is unable to sit on edge of bed, have patient lie on
    unaffected side with head of bed elevated and arm
    raised over head
Provide emotional support
Obtain signed informed consent

PREPROCEDURE TEACHING
Ensure that patient and significant other(s) know and
    understand
Procedure to be performed
Importance of remaining immobile during procedure
Importance of not coughing during procedure; patient
    may be asked to exhale completely and hold or

breathe shallowly during procedure *to decrease risk of puncture*

That sensations of pain and pressure are to be expected

ASSESSMENT DURING AND AFTER THORACENTESIS
OBSERVATIONS/FINDINGS
During Procedure

Chest tightness
Difficulty in breathing
Tachypnea
Tachycardia
Vertigo
Hypotension
Cyanosis
Diaphoresis
Pallor
Anxiety

Postprocedure

Difficulty in breathing
Chest pain
Uncontrollable cough
Hemoptysis
Decreased BP
Tachycardia
Tachypnea
Absent or diminished breath sounds
Crepitus
Hyperresonance
Diminished chest wall movement on affected side
Distended neck veins
Cyanosis
Elevated temperature
Deviation of larynx and trachea

POTENTIAL COMPLICATIONS
Mediastinal shift
Pneumothorax
Hemothorax
Subcutaneous emphysema
Hypoxemia
Acute fluid shifts

IMMEDIATE POSTPROCEDURE CARE
Check BP, P, and R q15min for 1 hour, then q2h to 4h and prn
Check temperature q4h for 24 hours
Apply adhesive bandage or dressing to site of puncture
Check dressing q15min to 30 min
Turn patient on unaffected side for 1 hour, then to position of comfort
Manage pain as indicated; assess effectiveness of pain relief measure(s)
Administer oxygen as ordered
Measure and record total amount of fluid removed; note color and character
Auscultate breath sounds q2h × 2; then q4h for 24 hours; report diminished or absent breath sounds and audible crepitus to physician

Obtain chest x-ray examination to rule out pneumothorax as ordered

ONGOING CARE
Continue with immediate postprocedure care and decrease frequency of nursing functions as patient's condition improves
Change dressing prn
Assist and teach patient to
    Turn and deep breathe q2h to 4h
    Ambulate as tolerated
    Maintain diet as ordered

PATIENT/FAMILY TEACHING
Ensure that patient and significant other(s) know and understand
    Importance of deep breathing
    Importance of avoiding tobacco use
Care of puncture site
Symptoms to report to physician
    Difficulty in breathing
    Chest pain
    Vertigo
    Elevated temperature
    Diaphoresis
    Uncontrollable cough
    Continued drainage of fluid from puncture site
    Hemoptysis

■ ASPIRATION OF SECRETIONS (INDIRECT SUCTIONING)

PREPROCEDURE ASSESSMENT
OBSERVATIONS/FINDINGS
Restlessness
Wheezing
Inability to expectorate
Difficulty in breathing
Tachycardia
Diaphoresis
Crackles
Rhonchi over large airways
Decreased breath sounds
Cyanosis
Pulse oximetry saturation reading if indicated (use for ventilated patients)

PREPROCEDURE TEACHING
Explain procedure to patient
Discuss what is expected of patient during procedure
Demonstrate suction equipment
Assist and teach patient to cough and deep breathe before and after procedure

ASSESSMENT DURING PROCEDURE
OBSERVATIONS/FINDINGS
Tachycardia
Hypoxemia

Trauma to airway; bloody aspirate

Bronchospasm

Aspirate

Color

Consistency

Amount

Cyanosis

Tachypnea

Dyspnea

Nausea

POTENTIAL COMPLICATIONS

Hypotension

Sudden hypertension

Hypoxemia

Bradycardia

Cardiac dysrhythmias

Atrioventricular (AV) heart block

Premature ventricular contractions (PVCs)

Cardiac arrest

CARE DURING PROCEDURE

Auscultate breath sounds

Maintain sterile technique

Use closed ventilation suction system for ventilated patients or use vented catheter

Lubricate sterile catheter

Choose correct catheter to prevent airway occlusion and/or trauma; should be half diameter of airway (general guide)

Adult: 12 to 18 French

Infant: 5 to 6 French

Hyperoxygenate and hyperinflate lungs for four to five breaths × 1 minute

Avoid use of force when inserting catheter

Apply suction only while removing catheter; do not exceed 10 seconds

Rotate catheter while removing; avoid moving catheter up and down while suctioning

Suction pressure must not exceed

Adult: 80 to 120 mm Hg

Ventilate patient for four or five breaths or longer if necessary as soon as suction has been released

Use closed ventilation suction catheter for tracheal suctioning

Use Yankauer suction tip catheter for oral suctioning

Assess patient for the following:

Adequate chest expansion

Cyanosis: lips, earlobes, fingertips

Increased restlessness

Increased pulse rate

Cardiac dysrhythmias

Bronchospasm

Decrease in O_2 saturation

If bronchospasm, bradycardia, PVCs, or AV block occurs, stop suctioning immediately and ventilate and hyperoxygenate patient

Observe aspirate: if purulent or colored, obtain specimen for culture

NASOTRACHEAL SUCTION

Avoid nasotracheal suction if patient has a spinal fluid leak or epistaxis

Elevate head of bed 60 to 90 degrees

Hyperoxygenate and hyperinflate patient's lungs for four to five breaths before suctioning

Lubricate 6 to 8 cm of distal end of catheter with water-soluble lubricant or water and insert through nostril to pharynx

Have patient cough or deep breathe and advance catheter into trachea during inspiration

Suction no more than 10 seconds at a time

Hyperoxygenate and hyperinflate patient's lungs for four or five breaths after suctioning

ENDOTRACHEAL OR TRACHEOSTOMY SUCTION

Be aware that a coudé (curved-tip) catheter may be used in an attempt to suction left mainstem bronchus in certain disease states

Hyperoxygenate and hyperinflate patient's lungs for four or five breaths before suctioning

Suction oropharynx and discard catheter after each use

Suction endotracheal tube or tracheostomy tube with a sterile catheter

Suction no more than 10 seconds at a time

Hyperoxygenate and hyperinflate patient's lungs for four or five breaths after suctioning

POSTPROCEDURE ASSESSMENT
OBSERVATIONS/FINDINGS

Breath sounds

Crackles

Decreased

Increased

Rhonchi over large airways

Decreased

Increased

Arterial blood gases: decreased Pa_{O_2}, Sa_{O_2}

Bronchospasm

Tachycardia

Cyanosis

Increased work of breathing

IMMEDIATE POSTPROCEDURE CARE
GENERAL

Auscultate breath sounds; prepare to repeat suctioning procedure as indicated

Return oxygen concentration to setting as ordered

Check apical pulse and/or record ECG rhythm strip

Assist and teach patient to deep breathe after suctioning procedure

Monitor O_2 saturation via pulse oximetry tidal volume as ordered

■ OXYGEN THERAPY

Use of oxygen to relieve hypoxemia and avoid hypoxia; oxygen flow rate and concentration should be

regulated to maintain Pa_{O_2} between 60 mm Hg and 100 mm Hg

PREPROCEDURE ASSESSMENT
OBSERVATIONS/FINDINGS
Hypoxemia
  $Pa_{O_2} < 60$ mm Hg
  $Sa_{O_2} < 85\%$
Respiratory system
  Cyanosis
  Tachypnea
  Dyspnea
  Shallow respiration
Neurologic system
  Drowsiness
  Disorientation/confusion
  Restlessness
  Decreased attention span
  Impaired judgment
  Delirium
  Decreased long-term and short-term memory
Nausea
Nasal flaring
Muscle weakness
Retractions
Cardiovascular system
  Hypotension
  Sudden hypertension
  Bradycardia
  Tachycardia
  Cardiac dysrhythmias

PREPROCEDURE TEACHING
Explain procedure to patient
Demonstrate equipment to be used

ASSESSMENT DURING PROCEDURE
OBSERVATIONS/FINDINGS
Substernal pain with deep inspiration
Somnolence
Respiratory depression
ABGs
  Pa_{O_2}
  Pa_{CO_2}
  pH
  HCO_3
  Sa_{O_2}
Tidal volume (V_T)
Vital capacity (VC)
Elevated temperature
Tachycardia
Psychosocial problems
  Anxiety
  Depression
  Dependence

POTENTIAL COMPLICATIONS
Oxygen toxicity: time and dose related
  Decreased lung compliance
  Reduced VC

Sore throat
Nasal drying, bleeding
Cough
Diminished breath sounds
Crackles
CNS toxicity
  Nausea
  Anxiety
  Numbness
  Muscular twitching
Substernal pain with deep inspiration
Circulatory depression: falling pulmonary capillary
  wedge pressure (PCWP), central venous pressure
  (CVP)
Visual impairment
  Tearing eyes
  Papilledema

CARE DURING PROCEDURE
GENERAL
Assess patient for signs of hypoxemia
Maintain patent airway
Assist and teach patient to maintain position best suited
  for optimal lung expansion; head of bed usually
  elevated 45 to 90 degrees
Initiate and maintain oxygen flow rate and concentration
  with humidification as ordered; have portable oxygen
  tank or extension tubing available if oxygen is to be
  used continuously and patient is ambulatory or needs
  to be transported
Monitor BP, T, R, and apical pulse q15min for 1 hour, then
  q2h to 4h if stable
Assess level of consciousness (LOC) q15min for 1 hour,
  then q2h to 4h if no change
Auscultate breath sounds q2h to 4h; report diminished or
  absent breath sounds or audible crackles and rhonchi
  to physician
Administer oral and nasal hygiene q2h to 4h
Assist and teach patient to turn, cough, and deep breathe
  q2h to 4h
Provide emotional support; remain with patient if acutely
  anxious
Continue other nursing functions required for primary
  disease process
Avoid high concentrations of oxygen for patients who
  require some degree of hypoxemia to maintain
  respirations
Monitor ABGs as ordered
NOTE: Oxygen toxicity can occur with oxygen
  concentrations of 50% or higher administered for 24 to
  48 hours; symptoms include tachypnea, substernal
  pain, and dizziness; physiologic effects include
  atelectasis, ciliary dysfunction, and nitrogen washout;
  in carbon dioxide retainers, hypoventilation,
  somnolence, and apnea may occur with minimal
  elevations in Pa_{O_2}

GENERAL PRECAUTIONS
Provide humidification with oxygen administration
  especially for flow rate > 2 L/min

Always use sterile equipment when administering oxygen; change connecting tubing, humidification equipment, masks, and nasal cannulas every 24 to 48 hours

Do not allow tobacco use while oxygen is in use

Do not permit oil, grease, or other combustible material to come in contact with cylinders, regulators, gauges, valves, or fittings

Administer oxygen only with a safely functioning and properly fitting regulating device

Cylinders
    Secure safely to prevent falling
    Transport only in proper carrier
    Maintain valve in closed position when not in use
    Open valve slowly to full open position when using

CARE WITH USE OF VARIOUS DEVICES
Nasal Catheter
Check catheter patency before insertion

Lubricate catheter with water-soluble lubricant

Avoid kinking or twisting tubing

Position catheter so it cannot be seen when patient's tongue is depressed

Tape securely to nose

Remove catheter q6h to 8h

Reinsert new catheter in opposite nostril if possible

Assess patient for abdominal distention

Nasal Cannula (Prongs)
Useful for providing approximately 24% to 44% oxygen at flow rates of 1 to 6 L/min (flow > 6 L/min does not deliver more oxygen)

Approximate FIo$_2$ With Nasal Cannula	
1L 24%	4L 36%
2L 28%	5L 40%
3L 32%	6L 44%

Ensure proper positioning; avoid kinking or twisting, which impedes oxygen flow

Apply water-soluble lubricant to nares

Evaluate patient for pressure sores or nasopharyngeal irritation

Reposition q2h

Clean equipment daily

Simple Oxygen Mask
Can deliver 40% to 60% oxygen at flow rates of 8 to 10 L/min (rate < 5 L/min with face mask can lead to carbon dioxide retention in dead space of mask)

Choose correct size for patient

Remove mask q2h to 3h for a few seconds to do the following:
    Dry patient's face
    Observe for pressure areas
    Permit patient communication

Use face mask only with artificial airway in unconscious patient

Have nasal cannula available for patient to use while eating

Face Tent
Can deliver approximately 40% oxygen at flow rates of 8 to 10 L/min

Useful for patients who cannot tolerate a face mask

Remove periodically for a few seconds
    Dry patient's face
    Observe chin for pressure areas

Have nasal cannula available for patient to use while eating

Partial Rebreathing Mask With Reservoir Bag
Used for higher oxygen concentrations (40% to 60%) at flow rates of 8 to 12 L/min

Increases of 1 L/min increased FIo$_2$ by approximately 10%

Select correct size for patient

Ensure proper position of mask

Apply mask as patient exhales

Avoid twisting or kinking bag

Avoid letting bag totally deflate when patient is inhaling; increase oxygen flow rate if necessary

Remove mask periodically for a few seconds
    Dry patient's face
    Observe for pressure areas
    Apply water-soluble lubricant to lips

Provide means of communication

Have nasal cannula available for patient to use while eating

Monitor ABGs

Observe for signs of oxygen toxicity

Nonrebreathing Mask With Reservoir Bag
Provides 60% to 90% oxygen at flow rates of 6 to 15 L/min

Select correct size for patient

Ensure proper positioning of mask

Avoid letting bag totally deflate

Avoid twisting bag

Ensure that all rubber flaps stay in place

Remove mask periodically for a few seconds
    Dry patient's face
    Observe for pressure areas
    Apply water-soluble lubricant to lips

Observe patient for signs of oxygen toxicity; monitor ABGs as ordered

Have a nasal cannula available for patient to use while eating

Venturi Mask
Provides 24% to 50% oxygen at 4 to 8 L/min flow rate

Select correct size for patient

Ensure proper positioning; avoid kinking of tubing and blockage of oxygen intake parts, which alter FIo$_2$

Maintain oxygen flow rate as ordered by physician

Monitor ABGs

Remove mask periodically for a few seconds
    Dry patient's face
    Observe for pressure areas
    Apply water-soluble lubricant to lips

Rid tubing of excessive moisture as necessary

Have nasal cannula available for patient to use while eating

PATIENT/FAMILY TEACHING

Explain importance of not using tobacco or any open flames in the room with oxygen administration to avoid combustion and fire or explosion

Explain the necessity of checking all electrical equipment used in the same room with oxygen administration for frayed cords or potential for sparking to avoid combustion and fire or explosion

Instruct on proper removal and repositioning of the oxygen equipment because the patient may need to wipe off and dry his or her face, blow his or her nose, or eat

Teach the patient the proper oxygen concentration delivery ordered and the importance of maintaining the appropriate flow rate because high flow rates in CO_2 retainers can suppress the respiratory drive

Explain importance of humidification and adequate hydration because oxygen dries the mucous membranes

DISCHARGE/HOME CARE PLANNING

Explain that home oxygen is provided in one of three ways: compressed gas in a cylinder tank, liquid oxygen in a reservoir, or an oxygen concentrator

Provide referral for equipment and supplies
   To a home health agency for follow-up care at home;
   For patient and family support groups in the area

Demonstrate use, care, and cleaning of all equipment

Teach use of oxygen source, oxygen delivery device, and humidification source

Describe different home oxygen systems
   Liquid oxygen: a portable, relatively lightweight system that is easy to read but costly for continuous use or high flow rates
   Oxygen cylinders: small tanks that need to be changed frequently; least expensive if oxygen delivery is needed for ≤ 12 hr/day
   Oxygen concentrators: nonportable unit that delivers concentrated oxygen drawn out of room air; indicated for patient requiring oxygen 12 to 24 hr/day and only inside home
   Explain the importance of avoiding tobacco use, open flames, and frayed electrical equipment in area of oxygen equipment to prevent combustion, fires, or explosions
   Encourage walking and activities with portable oxygen as tolerated because continuous oxygen therapy can limit mobility
   Demonstrate care of skin and mucous membranes because oxygen devices can cause skin irritation and breakdown with prolonged wear and provide additional route for microorganisms

■ HUMIDITY AND AEROSOL THERAPY

Valuable in loosening thick secretions and in the delivery of medications; aerosol and humidity devices used to provide humidity when artificial airways are being used are as follows:

   jet nebulizers: Hand-held nebulizers commonly used to provide medicated aerosol treatment; these are large-reservoir nebulizers for continuous aerosol treatment with or without supplemental oxygen. Cool: delivers 40% to 50% humidity; heated: delivers 100% humidity

   ultrasonic nebulizers: Can be given to patients breathing on their own or installed into ventilator circuits; treatments generally last 20 to 30 minutes; deliver 100% humidity

   humidifiers: Used to prevent humidity deficit when artificial airways are in use; the most commonly used are the bubble humidifiers in conjunction with low-flow oxygen devices, cascade on ventilators

ASSESSMENT
OBSERVATIONS/FINDINGS
Patient
Respirations
   Quality
   Rate
   Depth
Breath sounds
   Crackles
   Diminished or absent
Secretions
   Amount
   Color
   Character
Fluid overload

Equipment
Oxygen concentration ordered
Oxygen concentration delivered
Heat control
Connecting tubing is patent, free from excess moisture

ONGOING CARE
PATIENT
Maintain patent airway
Monitor patient as frequently as indicated by disease or patient's condition during treatment
Suction as indicated
Auscultate breath sounds q2h to 4h; report absent or diminished breath sounds to physician
Position patient comfortably
Dry face of moisture as indicated
Assist and teach patient to turn, cough, and deep breathe q2h to 4h

EQUIPMENT
Use sterile distilled water in nebulizer; check water level in reservoir q4h—when adding water, empty reservoir, then refill to correct level
Free tubing of excess moisture q2h to 3h and prn
Check heat control q2h to 4h
Maintain temperature between 95° and 97.8° F (35° and 36.6° C) unless cool mist ordered

Change mask, adaptors, and tubing q24h

Secure and allow sufficient tubing for turning

PATIENT/FAMILY TEACHING

Teach the patient the importance of humidification and nebulization

Demonstrate use of equipment, how to fill humidifiers and nebulizers, and proper cleaning and disinfecting

Demonstrate administration of medication via handheld nebulizers

Teach use of medications, dosage, time of administration, purpose, and side effects

DISCHARGE/HOME CARE PLANNING

Teach use, care, and cleaning of equipment

Teach to inspect equipment for growth of mold and other organisms because water is a medium for growth of microorganisms

Check water in humidifiers and nebulizer q8h to maintain adequate level and refill as needed

Explain importance of maintaining temperature of humidifiers between 95° and 97.8° F

Ensure that humidifiers are placed in the room with the steam directed into room and set on a table at least 2 feet from walls and furniture

■ CHRONIC OBSTRUCTIVE PULMONARY DISEASE (COPD), CHRONIC OBSTRUCTIVE LUNG DISEASE (COLD)

Chronic condition associated with a history of emphysema (Fig. 5-2), asthma, chronic bronchitis (Box 5-1), bronchiectasis, cigarette smoking, or exposure to air pollution; there is persistent airway obstruction that progressively increases

ASSESSMENT
SUBJECTIVE DATA

Anxiety

Fear: suffocation, death

Fatigue

Malaise

SOB during exertions; ADLs

Decreased exercise tolerance

OBJECTIVE DATA

Audible expiratory wheeze

Prolonged expirations with considerable effort

Pursed-lip breathing

Use of accessory muscles of respiration

Increased A-P diameter of chest (barrel chest)

Breath sounds

    Diminished breath sounds

    Crackles

    Rhonchi

Bronchospasm

Restlessness

Anorexia

Weight loss

Cough

    Productive/unproductive

    Hacking, ineffective

Amount and character of sputum

Cardiac

    Hypotension

    Tachycardia

    Dysrhythmia

Pulsus paradoxus

Hypoxemia

Carbon dioxide retention

    Restlessness

    Confusion

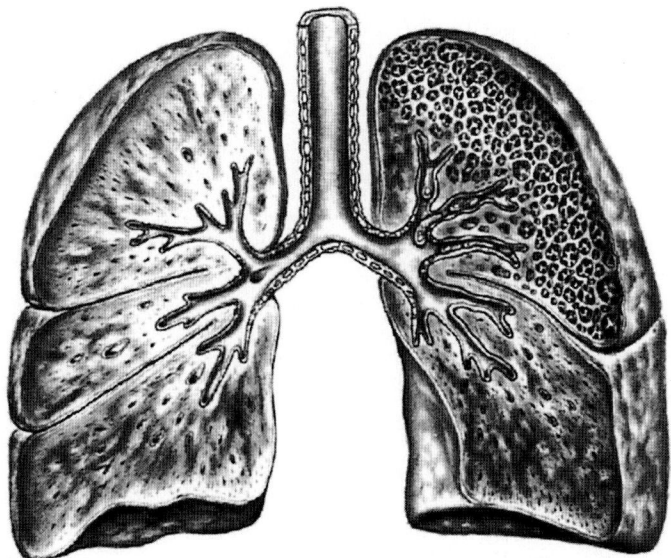

Fig. 5-2 Lobar emphysema.
(From Wilson SF, Thompson JM: Mosby's clinical nursing series: respiratory disorders, St Louis, 1990, Mosby.)

Box 5-1	**Diseases Contributing to Development of Chronic Obstructive Pulmonary Disease (COPD)**

CHRONIC BRONCHITIS

Mucosal swelling and inflammation of the bronchial mucous membrane with excessive mucous secretion in bronchial tree

ASSESSMENT
Observations/Findings
SOB
Cough
   Persistent
   Productive
Sputum (usually morning)
   Thick, tenacious, copious
   Mucopurulent
Breath sounds
   Scattered
   Moist crackles
   Rhonchi
Wheezing respirations
Bronchospasm
Cyanosis

Diagnostic Tests
Arterial blood gases
   Decreased Pao_2
   Increased $Paco_2$
   Increased HCO_3
   Respiratory acidosis
Sputum secretions
   Increased polymorphonuclear
      neutrophil leukocytes
Chest x-ray examination
   Increased peribronchial markings
      at both bases
   Increased cardiac size
Pulmonary function tests
   Decreased FEV_1/FVC ratio
   Increased residual volume
   FRC: may be normal in pure
      bronchitis
   FEV: decreased
   PEFR: decreased

EMPHYSEMA

Destruction of elastic tissues of the alveolar walls, causing a reduced expiratory flow rate and overinflated alveoli; a progressive disease that is irreversible

ASSESSMENT
Observations/Findings
SOB
Difficulty in breathing
Respirations
   Tachypnea
   Shallow
   Prolonged expiratory phase
Use of accessory muscles
   Intercostals
   Neck
   Shoulder
Cough: may be productive
Pursed-lip breathing
Orthopnea
Thoracic changes
   Barrel chest
   Unequal chest expansion
   Increased AP chest diameter
   Skin color: usually normal
Cachexia
Anorexia
Weight loss
Breath sounds
   Distant
   Expiratory wheezes
Hyperresonance
Weakness
Fatigue

Diagnostic Tests
ABGs
   Decreased Pao_2; normal or increased $Paco_2$
   pH within normal limits if compensation has occurred
Chest x-ray examination
   Hyperlucent lung fields; small, narrow heart; increased AP diameter; low, flat diaphragm; widened intercostals
   Apical bullae are common
   Decreased vascular markings
Pulmonary function tests
   Increased TLC
   Increased FRC
   Decreased PEFR, MMEF, FEV_1/FVC
Blood chemistry: α_1-antitrypsin

BRONCHIECTASIS

Chronic dilation of a bronchus or bronchi, secreting large amounts of purulent sputum

ASSESSMENT
Observations/Findings
Cough: paroxysms in early morning
Sputum
   Profuse (up to 200-300 ml/day)
   Purulent
   Foul odor
Wheezes
SOB
Prolonged expiration
Hemoptysis
Nasal stuffiness
Breath sounds
   Crackles
   Rhonchi
Recurrent infection, pneumonia
Elevated temperature
Chronic sinusitis

Diagnostic Tests
Chest x-ray examination
   Usually normal
   Air fluid levels and infiltrates
      may be seen in advanced diffuse
      disease
Bronchography
Sputum examination: staphylococci, streptococci, and pseudomonas commonly seen on sputum smears and cultures
Pulmonary function tests
   Normal or slightly decreased lung volumes
   Decreased flow rates
ABGs: mild decrease in Pao_2 and $Paco_2$ are common

Somnolence

Loss of memory

DIAGNOSTIC TESTS

ABG studies

Alveolar-arterial (A-a) oxygen gradient: widened

Decreased Pao_2, pH

Increased Pco_2

Chest x-ray examination

Flattened diaphragm

Increased AP diameter

Hyperinflation of lungs

Pulmonary function studies (see Box 5-1)

Sputum specimen analysis

CBC: polycythemia if chronically hypoxic

Serum electrolytes

ECG: atrial dysrhythmia low voltage, right axis deviation in advanced disease

POTENTIAL COMPLICATIONS

Dysrhythmias

Acute respiratory failure

Cardiac failure

Cor pulmonale

Peripheral edema

Hepatomegaly

Cyanosis

Distended neck veins

Loud P_2

Murmur of tricuspid regurgitation

Pulmonary hypertension

Blood gas abnormalities

Polycythemia

Peptic and esophageal reflux

MULTIDISCIPLINARY MANAGEMENT

THERAPEUTIC MANAGEMENT

Oxygen therapy

Artificial airway/mechanical ventilation as required

Chest physiotherapy

Pulse oximetry

Serial ABG assessment

Medications

Bronchodilators

Antibiotics

Corticosteroids

Diuretics

Vaccinations: influenza, pneumococcal

Alpha$_1$-antitrypsin therapy

Diet: high-protein, low-carbohydrate foods and fluids

Parenteral fluids

Restriction of tobacco use

Surgical: lung volume reduction

PATIENT PROBLEMS—NURSING DIAGNOSES/INTERVENTIONS

▼ Ineffective airway clearance related to retained tracheobronchial secretions or airway obstruction

Auscultate lungs q1h to 2h or as indicated: rhonchi, crackles, or wheezing *to determine progression of disease*

Assess secretions noting quantity, color, consistency, and odor *to identify symptoms of infection*

Assess hydration status: skin turgor, mucous membrane, q2h intake and output *to identify alterations in fluid status*

Increase fluid intake to 2000 ml/day unless contraindicated *to liquefy secretions*

Encourage incentive breathing with large tidal volumes *to open alveoli maximally*

Assist and teach patient to turn and cough q2h; position for optimal coughing: upright and flexed forward *to ensure maximum airway available*

Assist with and monitor chest physiotherapy: postural drainage, percussion *to assist with removal of secretions*

Provide periods of rest between treatments *to prevent fatigue*

Teach controlled cough techniques (Box 5-2)

Instruct patient in breathing retraining techniques: pursed-lip, diaphragmatic breathing (Box 5-3)

Provide humidification via mask, vaporizer

Suction nasopharyngeal airway or artificial airway as indicated *to remove secretions*

Administer medications as ordered

Bronchodilators: observe for therapeutic response; monitor theophylline level as appropriate

Antibiotics

Expected Outcome

Maintains a patent airway as evidenced by the following:

Improved breath sounds

Cough-produced thinned secretions

Box 5-2	**Controlled Cough Technique**

1. *Maximal inhalation*—an effective cough is contingent on filling the lungs and airways distal to the mucus so that the succeeding forced exhalation will propel the mucus up to the airways. Maximal inhalation also increases airway caliber; as a result, it is more likely that the air will pass distal to partially obstructing mucus or foreign matter.
2. *Hold breath 2 seconds*—this step permits the patient to prepare for exhalation and allows distribution of the inhaled air to the lung's periphery.
3. *Cough twice*—the first cough will loosen mucus; the second will propel the mucus. Further coughing may use excessive oxygen and energy at a time when the lung volume has already been expelled with the first two coughs, and the effort is thus wasted.
4. *Pause*—just long enough to regain control.
5. *Inhale by sniffing*—sniffing is recommended, because a deep inhalation through the mouth may drive loose mucus back down into the airways.
6. *Rest.*

Modified from Thelan LA et al: Critical care nursing: diagnosis and management, ed 3, St Louis, 1998, Mosby.

Box 5-3	**Breathing Retraining Techniques**

PURSED-LIP BREATHING

With mouth closed, inhale through nose.

Exhale through mouth with lips "pursed" (lips in a whistling or kissing position).

Make exhalation at least twice as long as inhalation (2 seconds in, 4 seconds out).

Rationale

Explain to the patient that this maneuver keeps airways open longer during exhalation and evacuates trapped air. The procedure for pursed-lip breathing can be used, along with diaphragmatic breathing, during episodes of SOB.

DIAPHRAGMATIC BREATHING

Have the patient place two fingers just below the xiphoid process and push in with his or her fingers while sniffing gently. Explain that the movement felt at the fingertips is the diaphragm moving as he or she sniffs and that this muscle requires exercise so that it can increase the efficiency of breathing.

Technique

Place one hand on chest, one hand on abdomen.

Inhale, pushing abdominal hand outward.

Exhale slowly (through pursed lips), allowing abdominal hand to fall inward.

Chest hand should remain still.

Rationale

Explain that this maneuver saves energy because the diaphragm uses oxygen more efficiently than the accessory muscles and that this technique retrains the diaphragm to assume the work of breathing. Diaphragmatic breathing is useful in terminating episodes of acute SOB but should also be incorporated into a regular routine of muscle retraining.

From Thelan LA et al: Critical care nursing: diagnosis and management, *ed 3, St Louis, 1998, Mosby.*

Normal rate and depth of respirations
Absence of dyspnea and cyanosis
Blood gases within acceptable levels

▼Impaired gas exchange related to alveolar capillary membrane changes

Assess respirations qh; note quality, rate, and use of accessory muscles: changes may indicate altered blood gas state

Auscultate breath sounds q1h to 2h or as indicated, noting area of abnormal sounds

Assess LOC, somnolence, and confusion, reporting any changes that *may indicate increase in impaired gas exchange*

Observe color, odor, and amount of secretions: *changes may indicate infective process*

Maintain bed rest in quiet environment during exacerbation of symptoms *to maximize energy*

Elevate head of bed 45 to 90 degrees
　Allow patient to assume position of comfort *to ease work of breathing*
　Padded overbed table may be helpful for patient's comfort and breathing

Administer humidified oxygen per nasal catheter or cannula at low flow as ordered *to maintain* Pao_2 *of no less than 55 mm Hg*

Observe for signs of cyanosis, which *indicates deoxygenation*

Monitor BP, T, and apical pulse q2h to 4h and prn *to assess for hemodynamic stability*

Monitor ABGs: report increase or decreases in $Paco_2$ and Pao_2 of > 10 mm Hg

Assist and teach patient to turn, cough, and deep breathe q2h; note type of cough and color and character of sputum *to maintain airway patency and detect infection*

Collect sputum for culture as ordered

Teach importance of absolutely no tobacco use

Monitor renal function, which may be altered secondary to chronic tissue hypoxia and alterations in metabolism

Administer medications as ordered
　Bronchodilators: observe for therapeutic response; monitor theophylline level as appropriate
　Antibiotics

Expected Outcome

Maintains adequate gas exchange as evidenced by the following:
　Improved mental status, skin color
　Blood gases within acceptable levels for patient
　Clear breath sounds

▼Altered nutrition: less than body requirements related to decreased oral intake and increased metabolic demand associated with dyspnea, anorexia, and fatigue

Assess nutritional status: weigh daily, monitor dietary intake *to detect signs and symptoms of malnutrition*

Record oral intake using calorie counts *to meet hypermetabolic requirements*

Monitor albumin and lymphocyte levels for indications of adequate protein

Place in high-Fowler's position at meals *to reduce dyspnea*

Encourage rest periods before meals *to reduce fatigue*

Provide liquid-to-soft, high-protein (which supports immune system), low-carbohydrate diet; avoid gas-producing foods, which can limit movement of diaphragm

Administer supplementary feedings

Provide attractive meals

Provide small, frequent meals *to decrease abdominal pressure on diaphragm*

Encourage significant other(s) to bring patient's favorite foods

Administer oral hygiene before meals *to enhance taste and appetite*

Administer medications *to relieve constipation* as indicated

Expected Outcomes

Nutritional status is maintained or improved as evidenced by weight remaining stable and within or moving toward normal range for patient's height, age, and build

Food intake is increased

Albumin and lymphocytes are within normal limits

▼ Anxiety related to threat of change in health status

Assess level of anxiety (mild, moderate, severe); identify any misperceptions of illness or treatment

Assess usual coping skills, which are previously used successful methods

Provide quiet, nonstressful environment *to increase relaxation*

Provide emotional support

Remain with patient during anxious periods

Encourage significant other(s) to participate in care

Be aware of patient's subjective statements

Encourage patient to ask questions and verbalize fears and concerns

Assess whether visitors are helpful during periods of heightened anxiety and limit visitation as indicated

Plan care to provide frequent rest periods

Avoid blaming attitude

Explain all procedures and treatment *to reduce fear*

Introduce support groups available to patient and family: Better Breathing Clubs of American Lung Association

Instruct on relaxation techniques such as guided imagery and use of autogenic techniques during periods of dyspnea

Expected Outcome

Experiences a decrease in fear and anxiety as evidenced by the following:

Relaxed facial expression

Verbalization of feeling less anxious

Verbalization of understanding hospital routines, procedures, and disease process

▼ Activity intolerance related to imbalance between oxygen supply and demand

Assess level of response to activities; monitor HR and respirations during and after activity

Plan care to provide optimal rest *to maximize energy*

Instruct patient on energy conservation measures

Perform activities such as bathing, shaving in sitting position; rest between activities

Encourage use of pursed-lip breathing during activities *to decrease the work of breathing*

Provide O_2 therapy as indicated; use portable O_2 to facilitate activities

Monitor for signs of extreme fatigue, chest pain, or diaphoresis during and after activity

Assist and teach patient progressive exercise conditioning *to increase strength and maintain muscle tone*

ROM exercises

Encourage participation in pulmonary rehabilitation program (see p. 249)

Determine methods of conserving energy while performing ADLs: stool in bathroom for shower

Expected Outcome

Demonstrates an increased tolerance for activity as evidenced by ability to resume ADLs without extremes of fatigue or dyspnea

Additional Nursing Diagnoses to Consider

Sleep pattern disturbance related to SOB and difficulty breathing

Infection, risk for, related to ineffective airway clearance

Altered sexual patterns related to chronic illness

PATIENT/FAMILY TEACHING

Disease process

Assess patient level of understanding regarding disease process and prescribed home health management

Encourage questions and discussion

Explain importance of maintaining optimal respiratory function by taking medications, eliminating tobacco use, and avoiding second-hand smoke

Explain need to avoid *respiratory irritants:* dust, fumes, smoke, perfume, aerosol sprays, cold temperatures

Explain need to avoid persons with infections, especially URIs

Explain importance of ongoing outpatient care

Discuss symptoms to report immediately

Elevated temperature

Sore throat

Increase in sputum production

Change in color and consistency of sputum

URI

Increased difficulty in breathing

Night sweats, chills

Decreased activity tolerance

Decreased appetite

Increased use of intermittent positive-pressure breathing (IPPB) and oxygen

Change in pulse or feelings of heart fluttering

Explain need to keep warm and prevent chilling

Explain importance of influenza immunization and pneumovax if ordered

Medications

Discuss name, dosage, time of administration, purpose, and side effects

Explain need to avoid taking over-the-counter medications without physician approval

Demonstrate use of bronchodilator nebulizers if ordered

Use tid or qid

Take one or two deep inhalations

Release medication only one or two times with each use

Watch for side effects such as tachycardia

Avoid overuse

Explain need to wear medical alert band identifying COPD

Discuss importance of avoiding emotional stress; teach stress reduction techniques

Diet

Explain need to maintain high-calorie diet as indicated; force fluids to 2000 to 3000 ml/day unless contraindicated

Explain need to avoid constipation and straining

Ensure that patient and significant other(s) demonstrate

Deep-breathing exercises, pursed-lip breathing

Positions for postural drainage if needed

Use of ventilator if applicable

Use of oxygen equipment if applicable

DISCHARGE/HOME CARE PLANNING

Initiate contact with Home Health Nursing or Visiting Nurses Association (VNA); determine need for home health care

Instruct patient and family on cleaning of all home respiratory equipment; refer to respiratory therapy as indicated

Assess home for presence of respiratory irritants; maintain environment free of irritants

Explain importance of environmental control, maintaining warm house 75° to 80° F (23.8° to 26.6° C)

Teach that some patients tolerate high humidity poorly and may need to have dehumidifier in the home

Provide detailed instruction on use of any oxygen or respiratory equipment to be used at home

Activity level: explain importance of alternating activity and rest periods

Exercise to tolerance

Need to limit activity on days of high air pollution

Plan rest periods during day

Rest before and after meals if SOB increases at mealtimes

Breathe deeply and slowly during periods of activity

Understand own lifestyle and avoid waste of energy

Need to space activities throughout day

Assess economic status and ability to purchase medications and supplies; refer to social services as indicated

■ ASTHMA

A reversible obstructive disease characterized by increased reactivity of the trachea and bronchi to stimuli, manifested by wheezing and dyspnea; narrowing is due to a combination of bronchospasm, mucosal swelling, and increased secretions

ASSESSMENT

SUBJECTIVE DATA

Dyspnea, labored breathing

Chest tightness, pain

Wheezes

Anxiety

Fear of suffocation, death

Decreased activity tolerance

History of allergies, cough

Nocturnal episode

OBJECTIVE DATA

Sudden onset of respiratory distress

Prolonged expiratory wheeze

Short inspiratory period

Intercostal and sternal retraction

Use of accessory muscles of respiration

Air hunger

Crackles

Breath sounds

Wheezes

Decreased

Absent

Assumes upright sitting position; leans forward

Diaphoresis

Tachycardia

Distended neck veins

Cyanosis

Circumoral area

Nail beds

Hard, dry cough; productive cough is difficult

Altered LOC

Hypoxemia

Hypotension

Pulsus paradoxus > 10 mm

Dehydration

DIAGNOSTIC TESTS

ABGs

Mild decrease in Pao_2 and $Paco_2$: normal ABGs common between attacks

Decreased Pao_2, increased $Paco_2$ with severe attacks

Chest x-ray examination
  Normal between attacks
  Hyperinflation with allergic attacks
Skin testing (extrinsic asthma)
Pulmonary function tests
  Normal or increased lung volumes
  Decreased FEV, PEFR, MMEF
  FEV_1; Improvement with bronchodilators by 12% or
    more
WBC and sputum examination
  Sputum and blood eosinophilia are common
  Serum IgE levels are elevated in extrinsic asthma

POTENTIAL COMPLICATIONS
Pulmonary edema
Respiratory failure
Status asthmaticus
Pneumonia

MULTIDISCIPLINARY MANAGEMENT
THERAPEUTIC MANAGEMENT
Oxygen therapy with humidification
Fluid and electrolyte management
Artificial airway and ventilatory support if necessary
Chest physiotherapy: percussion and vibration
Medications
  Bronchodilators (Table 5-4): parenteral, aerosols,
    oral
  Sympathomimetics
  Theophylline
  Corticosteroids: oral, parenteral inhalers
  Nonsteroidal antiinflammatory inhalers: cromolyn,
    nedocromil
  Antibiotics
Bronchoscopy
Saline lavage
Metered-dose inhalers
Peak flow meters

PATIENT PROBLEMS—NURSING DIAGNOSES/INTERVENTIONS

▼Anxiety related to threat of death secondary to
difficulty in breathing, fear of suffocation

Assess level of anxiety (mild, moderate, severe)
Assess usual coping skills, which are previously used
  successful methods
Provide emotional support *to increase relaxation and
  coping*
  Remain with patient during acute attack
  Anticipate patient's needs
  Provide quiet reassurance
  Maintain quiet environment
  Encourage significant other(s) to participate in care for
    support
Implement relaxation techniques: guided imagery, muscle
  relaxation *to relieve muscle tension*
Explain procedures; encourage questions *to reduce fear*

Maintain planned rest periods *to conserve energy and
  prevent recurrent attacks*
  Pace and plan ADLs
  Discourage talking if extremely dyspneic
  Limit visitors as necessary
  Encourage frequent rest periods

Expected Outcome
Demonstrates a reduction in fear and anxiety as
  evidenced by the following:
  Relaxed facial expression
  Verbalization of feeling less anxious
  Vital signs within normal parameters
  Verbalization of understanding procedures

▼Ineffective airway clearance related to retained
secretions and bronchospasm

Assess sputum for color, tenacity, and amount
Auscultate breath sounds q2h to 4h or as indicated for
  wheezes, crackles, or rhonchi
Assess respirations noting depth, ease, and rate *to
  determine adequate oxygenation*
Observe skin color and temperature q2h
Monitor ABGs
Monitor LOC; report changes to physician
Position to level of comfort *to optimize breathing*
  Elevate head of bed 60 to 90 degrees *to facilitate
    maximal air exchange*
  Support back with pillows for comfort
  Provide well-padded overbed table to lean over
  Place side rails up for safety and support
  Place humidifier or steam vaporizer at bedside as
    ordered *to aid in liquefying secretions*
  Administer low flow of oxygen by nasal catheter as
    ordered (avoid oxygen mask, which increases
    sensation of suffocation)
  Administer IPPB as ordered
  Encourage patient to cough effectively at frequent
    intervals *to clear secretion*
Initiate or assist with chest physiotherapy
Administer medications as ordered
  Sympathomimetic preparations
  Xanthine derivatives: aminophylline—monitor
    levels
  Antihistamines
  Expectorants
  Corticosteroids
  Nonsteroidal antiinflammatory inhalers
Force fluids as ordered to keep secretions thin
Collect sputum for culture as ordered
Suction prn: keep suction at bedside

Expected Outcome
Maintains a patent airway as evidenced by the
  following:
  Improved breath sounds
  Normal rate and depth of respirations
  Absence of dyspnea

Table 5-4	Bronchodilators		
Generic Name	**Brand Names**	**Availability**	**Adult Dosage Range**
SYMPATHOMIMETICS			
Albuterol	Proventil, Ventolin	Tablets: 2, 4 mg Aerosol: 90 µg Nebulizer: 0.5%-1%	PO: 2-4 mg 3-4 times daily Inhale: 2 inhalations every 4-6 hr
Ephedrine	Ephedrine	Tablets: 25 mg Capsules: 25, 50 mg Syrup: 11, 20 mg/5 ml Injection: 25, 50 mg/ml	PO: 25-50 mg every 3-4 hr SC, IM, IV: 25-50 mg
Epinephrine	Primatene, Vaponefrin, Bronkaid Mist	Nebulization: 1:100 Aerosol: 0.2, 0.25, 0.3 mg Injection: 1:200, 1:100	See manufacturer's recommendations
Ethylnorepinephrine	Bronkephrine	2 mg/ml	SC or IM: 0.5 ml
Isoetharine	Bronkosol, Beta-2, Bronkometer	Nebulization: 0.125, 0.2, 0.5, 1% Aerosol: 0.61%	See manufacturer's recommendations
Isoproterenol	Isuprel, Aerolone, Norisodrine	Nebulization: 0.25, 0.5, 1% Aerosol: 0.2, 0.25% Injection: 0.2 mg/ml SL: 10, 15 mg tabs	See manufacturer's recommendations
Metaproterenol	Alupent, Metaprel	Tablets: 10, 20 mg Syrup: 10 mg/5 ml Aerosol: 225 mg Nebulization: 5%	See manufacturer's recommendations
Terbutaline	Brethine, Bricanyl	Tablets: 2.5, 5 mg Injection: 1 mg/ml	PO: 5 mg q6h SC: 0.25 mg; repeat, if needed, in 30 min
XANTHINE DERIVATIVES			
Aminophylline		Tablets: 100, 200 mg Elixir: 250 mg/15 ml Liquid: 105 mg/5 ml Suppositories: 250, 500 mg Injection: 250, 500 ml Others	See manufacturer's recommendations
Dyphylline	Dilor, Dyflex, Lufyllin	Tablets: 200, 400 mg Liquid: 100 mg/5 ml Elixir: 100, 160 mg/15 ml Injection: 250 mg/ml	PO: 15 mg/kg, 5 times daily IM: 250-500 mg slowly
Oxtriphylline	Choledyl	Tablets: 100, 200 mg Elixir: 100 mg/5 ml Syrup: 50 mg/5 ml	200 mg 4 times daily
Theophylline	Bronkodyl, Elixophyllin, Theolair, others	Tablets: 125, 200, 225, 300 mg Capsules: 50, 100, 200, 250 mg Elixir: 80 mg/15 ml Liquid: 80 mg/15 ml Syrup: 80 mg/15 ml Suspension: 300 mg/15 ml Others	9-20 mg/kg/24 hr in four divided doses

Modified from Clayton BD, Stock YN: Basic pharmacology for nurses, *ed 11, St Louis, 1997, Mosby.*

Absence of cyanosis

Blood gases within normal range

Additional Nursing Diagnoses to Consider

Ineffective breathing pattern related to decreased lung expansion during acute attack

Risk for infection

Risk for activity intolerance

PATIENT/FAMILY TEACHING

Assess level of understanding regarding disease process and self-care management during severe attacks

Explain importance of preventing future attacks

Avoid known irritants and allergens

Avoid stressful situations

Express anxieties and fears

Encourage communication with significant other and/or family

Provide adequate humidity

Nonflowering plants can increase humidity 5% to 10%

Humidifiers are helpful (provide instructions on use of humidifiers and need to keep clean)

Avoid persons with infections, especially URIs

Do not use tobacco; avoid second-hand smoke

Explain importance of breathing exercises such as pursed-lip breathing

Explain how to avoid air trapping by slow, extended exhalation through pursed lips

Avoid gaining weight

Explain importance of ongoing outpatient care

Discuss symptoms to report to physician

URI

Influenza

Elevated temperature

Discuss medications: name, dosage, time of administration, purpose, and side effects

Demonstrate proper use of inhalers, peak flow meters and maintenance of containers

Explain need to wear medical alert band identifying asthma

Discuss importance of taking medications as ordered

DISCHARGE/HOME CARE PLANNING

Provide detailed instruction on any equipment to be used at home

Assess home for presence of respiratory irritants that may trigger asthma attacks

Instruct patient and family on cleaning of all home respiratory equipment

Determine need for home care and initiate contact with home health or visiting nurses

Assess economic status and ability to purchase medications and equipment; refer to social services or appropriate agencies

Activity level: discuss importance of exercising to tolerance

Avoid fatigue

Plan rest periods

Limit activities during temperature extremes (hot/cold) and on smoggy days

Diet: explain importance of diet and fluids

Eat balanced, nutritious meals

Force fluids to 2000 to 3000 ml/day unless contraindicated

Develop transportation plan to local health care facility if symptomatic and if peak flow meter approaches "red zone" as determined by physician

■ PULMONARY REHABILITATION

An inpatient or outpatient program designed to increase exercise tolerance in patients with lung diseases while educating them to understand and assist in the management of their disease; components generally include physical therapy, respiratory therapy, exercise conditioning, medications, and education

ADMISSION CRITERIA

Symptomatic pulmonary disease (Table 5-5)

Dyspnea

Cough

Wheezing

Sputum production

Chest pain

Patient motivation

Restricted ADLs

Table 5-5	COPD Disability Scale
Class	**Observations/Findings**
Class I	No significant restriction of normal activities, but dyspnea on strenuous exertion
Class II	No dyspnea with essential activities of daily living; dyspnea on climbing stairs and in other climbs but not on level walking; employability limited to sedentary occupations
Class III	Dyspnea with some activities of daily living (e.g., showering, dressing), but can perform all such activities without assistance; able to walk at own pace for a city block, but cannot keep up while walking with normal others of the same age
Class IV	Dependent on others in some activities of daily living; not dyspneic at rest, but dyspneic with minimal exertion
Class V	Dyspneic at rest; dependent on assistance from others for most activities of daily living

From Hodgkin J, Zorn E, Connors G, eds: Pulmonary rehabilitation: guidelines to success, *Stoneham, Mass, 1984, Butterworth. Modified from Moser KM et al: Results of a comprehensive rehabilitation program,* Arch Intern Med *140:1596, 1980.*

No underlying condition that would interfere with the program (psychosis, alcoholism, drug abuse)

Medically stable: no signs of CHF, uncontrolled dysrhythmias, or myocardial infarction (MI) in previous 6 months

Adequate financial/insurance status

Family support system

EXCLUSION CRITERIA

Terminal cancer

Heart failure

Stroke

Alcoholism, active

Drug abuse

Psychiatric disorder, active/uncontrolled

Organic brain disease

End-stage COPD

▌ INPATIENT PROGRAM (see Box 5-4)

ASSESSMENT

OBSERVATIONS/FINDINGS

Heart rate

    Increase of 30 beats/min more than resting rate with activity

    HR < 50 during activity

    Consistent drop in HR of > 10 beats/min during activity

ECG rhythm: presence of irregular rhythm

Blood pressure

    Increase of 20 mm Hg above normal

    Diastolic increase of > 10 to 15 mm Hg

    Systolic drop to < 90 at rest; diastolic < 40

SYMPTOMS DURING ACTIVITY

Dyspnea

Dizziness

Fatigue

Pain

Palpitations

Diaphoresis

INDICATORS OF ENERGY EXPENDITURE DURING ACTIVITY

Arterial oxygen saturation values

Pao_2

Oxygen consumption rate

INDICATORS OF VENTILATORY RESPONSE DURING ACTIVITY

Minute ventilation

Respiratory rate

Carbon dioxide production

ONGOING CARE

Activity progression program

    Follow physician's activity prescription

    Initiate exercise program

Evaluate daily progress and plan activity levels

Box 5-4 — Pulmonary Rehabilitation Program: Suggested Class Content

Orientation to rehabilitation program
Anatomy and physiology of pulmonary system
Nutrition
Effects of stress and emotions on lung disease
Coping with chronic lung disease
COPD, specific diseases
Medications
Effect of COPD on family and friends
Oxygen, IPPB treatments
Principles of exercise
Relaxation techniques
Breathing exercises: pursed-lip breathing and diaphragmatic breathing
Energy conservation techniques
Postural drainage
Prevention of infection
Stop-smoking sessions
Discussions on sexuality

Maintain progressive increase in activities until discharge

Monitor ECG and respiratory parameters

Record and report any signs or symptoms of SOB, fatigue, or nausea during or after exercise

Assist patient in performing ADLs and monitor HR, R, and BP 1 and 4 minutes after activity (response to activity should return to preactivity level within 5 minutes; if it does not, monitor every 2 minutes until pretest levels are reached)

Observe, record, and report patient's tolerance

DISCHARGE EVALUATION

Self-care, ADL skills

Equipment needs for the home

Weekly schedule of exercise and rest

Assessment of level of knowledge

Knowledge of agency referral sources

▌ BENEFITS OF PULMONARY REHABILITATION PROGRAM

Reduced symptoms

Decreased anxiety and depression

Improved ability to perform ADLs

Increased exercise tolerance

Reduced hospital admissions, days, cost of care

Improved quality of life

■ PNEUMONIA/PNEUMONITIS

Inflammation of the lung parenchyma caused by bacteria, viruses (Table 5-6), chemicals, smoke inhalation, dust, allergens, and aspiration of gastric contents; lung tissue is consolidated as alveoli fill with exudate (Fig. 5-3). Pneumonias also may be classified as community-acquired or nosocomial (hospital associated)

Table 5-6	**Bacterial and Nonbacterial Causes of Pneumonia/Pneumonitis**	
Pathogen	**Persons at Risk**	**Complications**
BACTERIAL		
Streptococcus pneumoniae (pneumonococcus) Gram-positive coccus Accounts for 80% to 90% of community acquired cases	Infants Older adults Alcoholics People with debilitating diseases (diabetes mellitus, sickle cell anemia)	Bacteremia meningitis Emphysema Pericarditis Impaired liver function Pleural effusions Higher mortality if more than one lobe involved
Klebsiella pneumoniae Gram-negative bacillus/rods	Alcoholics Patients with diabetes mellitus or COPD	Lung abscess Emphysema Necrotizing pneumonitis Respiratory failure 25% to 50% mortality
Staphylococcus aureus Gram-positive diplococcus Accounts for 10% of cases in hospitalized patients and 1% of cases in unhospitalized patients	Infants Older adults As complication of influenza As secondary infection after surgery	Necrotizing infections Lung abscess Pleural effusion 15% to 50% mortality Slow response to antibiotics Adult respiratory distress syndrome
Haemophilus influenzae (type B) Gram-negative bacillus Accounts for 1% of cases	Children under 10 years of age Persons with COPD or immune disease	Bronchiolitis
Legionella pneumophila (Legionnaires' disease) Gram-negative	Older adults Smokers Persons with lung diseases	Hypotension Respiratory failure Acute renal failure Shock 15% mortality
Pseudomonas aeruginosa Gram-negative bacillus	Hospitalized patients: endotracheal intubation, respiratory inhalation therapy Burns	70% mortality Rarely occurs in previously healthy adults
NONBACTERIAL		
Mycoplasma (Mycoplasma pneumoniae) Atypical ("walking pneumonia")	School-age children Young adults Spreads within family	Interstitial infections Pulse-temperature dissociation
Pneumocystis (*Pneumocystis carinii* pneumonia) Protozoan organism	Patients with AIDS, immunosuppressed patients	Respiratory failure
Viral influenza A	Elderly Symptoms may begin 1 wk after viral infection	Secondary bacterial infection Respiratory failure
Aspiration pneumonia	Patients with altered LOC, impaired gag or cough reflex	With aspirated material Atelectasis Pulmonary edema Hemorrhage Necrosis

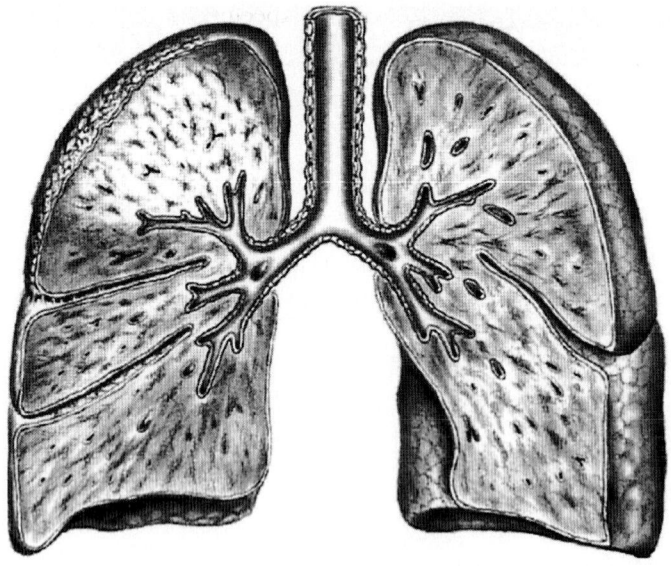

Fig. 5-3   Pneumococcal Pneumonia. Lobar pneumonia (right upper lobe).
(From Wilson SF, Thompson JM: Mosby's clinical nursing series: respiratory disorders, *St Louis, 1990, Mosby.)*

| Box 5-5 | **Observations/Findings of Viral and Bacterial Pneumonia** |

VIRAL

Symptoms
Usually mild at onset
Headache
Sudden onset of chills followed by fever
Cough (early, nonproductive)
Sputum (late)
    Mucopurulent
    Blood tinged
Myalgia
Photophobia
Anorexia
Nausea

Diagnostic Tests
Sputum examination: Gram stain and culture; influenza A, B, C, varicella, cytomegalovirus, adenovirus
Blood cultures
WBC normal or low; elevated lymphocytes
Elevated antibody titers
ABGs: hypoxemia
Chest x-ray examination
    Bronchopneumonic infiltrates

BACTERIAL

Symptoms
Sudden onset of high fever and shaking chills
Streptococcal pneumonia: afternoon, evening temperature; diaphoresis
Pleuritic chest pain
Cough
Sputum
    Rust colored, greenish, or yellow
    Purulent
Breath sounds
    Crackles
    Friction rub
Cyanosis

Diagnostic Tests
Sputum examination: Gram stain and culture streptococcal, pneumococcal, staphylococcal, *Haemophilus influenzae, Klebsiella pneumoniae*
Blood cultures
WBC leukocytes with shift to left
ABGs: hypoxemia
Chest x-ray examination
    Patchy areas of consolidation and infiltrates
    Pleural effusion

ASSESSMENT (SEE BOX 5-5)
    SUBJECTIVE DATA
Headache
Dyspnea
Cough
Myalgia
Chest tightness/discomfort

    OBJECTIVE DATA
Difficult and painful respirations
    Pleuritic pain
    SOB and grunting
    Tachypnea
Breath sounds over area of consolidation
    Diminished, progressing to absent

Crackles
Rhonchi
Egophony
Bronchial breath sounds
Asymmetric chest movements
Chills and fever (102° to 106° F [38.8° to 41.1° C]);
    delirium
Diaphoresis
Cough: productive, tenacious; unproductive, may be dry
    and hacking
    Incessant, painful
    Copious amounts of green-yellow sputum progressing
        to pink or rusty color
Restlessness, anxious
Cyanosis
    Circumoral area
    Nail beds
Tachycardia
Classic signs in elderly
    Increased respiratory rate
    Hypotension
    Change in mental status
    Loss of appetite
    Increase in frequency of falls
    Functional decline
    With/without fever

DIAGNOSTIC TESTS

Chest x-ray examination: patchy or diffuse infiltrates
    Pleural effusion
Sputum examination: Gram stain, culture, acid-fast stain
Serum studies (see Box 5-5): WBC, blood culture
Serologic studies: titers, cold agglutinins
ABGs
Transtracheal aspiration
Bronchoscopy

POTENTIAL COMPLICATIONS

Atelectasis
Empyema
Adult respiratory distress syndrome (ARDS)
Pleurisy
Pulmonary edema
Meningitis
Superinfection pericarditis
Lung abscess

MULTIDISCIPLINARY MANAGEMENT
THERAPEUTIC MANAGEMENT

Fluid management
Parenteral therapy
Oxygen therapy
Chest physiotherapy: postural drainage
Artificial airway or mechanical ventilation support
Medications
Electrolyte replacement
Antipyretics
Analgesics
Antimicrobials

Expectorants
Vaccines

PATIENT PROBLEMS—NURSING DIAGNOSES/INTERVENTIONS

▼ Impaired gas exchange related to lung consolidation with decrease in surface area available for gas exchange

Auscultate breath sounds q2h to 4h or as indicated
    monitoring *for adventitious sounds or decreased
    breath sounds*
Assess respiratory pattern, noting quality and rate
Monitor mental status and LOC *to assess for hypoxia/
    hypercapnia*
Observe color, odor, and amount of secretions *to assess
    for signs of infection*
Provide humidified oxygen by mask or nasal catheter as
    ordered *to avoid drying of upper airway;* maintain
    continuous vaporizer at bedside
Position patient *to optimize breathing*
Monitor oximetry readings; report O_2 saturation $\leq 92\%$
Administer oxygen therapy as ordered *to prevent
    hypoxia*
Assist and teach patient to turn, cough, and deep breathe
    q2h to 4h *to remove secretions*
Initiate or assist with chest physiotherapy *to mobilize
    secretions*
Assist with use of incentive spirometer *to open alveoli
    maximally*
Administer medications as ordered
    Antibiotics
    Expectorants
Pace activities to patient's tolerance *to decrease oxygen
    demand*
Monitor ABGs, CBC, and serum osmolality
Encourage fluid intake as tolerated *to liquefy secretions*
Assist with administration of mechanical ventilation as
    indicated

Expected Outcome
Maintains adequate gas exchange as evidenced by the
    following:
    Rate, rhythm, patterns of respiration within normal
        limits
    O_2 saturation $\geq 92\%$
    ABGs within acceptable range

▼ Ineffective airway clearance related to retained tracheobronchial secretions secondary to inflammatory process

Assess secretions noting quantity, color, and consistency
    to detect signs of infection or need to clear secretions
Assess hydration status: skin turgor, mucous membranes,
    24-hour intake
Auscultate breath sounds for crackles, rhonchi, and
    friction rubs q2h to 4h

Assist patient with use of incentive spirometer *to open alveoli maximally*

Perform nasopharyngeal or nasotracheal suctioning as needed

Force fluids as ordered *to help liquefy secretions*

Assist and teach patient to turn, cough, and deep breathe q2h to 4h *to maintain patent airway*

Monitor laboratory reports and serial chest x-ray examinations

Monitor response to antimicrobial therapy

Position patient *to optimize breathing and coughing*

Provide humidification as indicated

Expected Outcome

Maintains an effective breathing pattern as evidenced by the following:

Normal rate, rhythm, and depth of respirations

Clear lungs

Decreased dyspnea

Blood gases within normal range

Cough that has subsided

▼ Altered body temperature related to infectious process

Assess body temperature: measure temperature and pulse q4h; increase frequency during periods of chilling

Monitor skin color and temperature

Collect blood cultures and sputum cultures as ordered; monitor reports daily

Administer prescribed antipyretics as indicated

Encourage oral fluids as ordered *to ensure adequate hydration*

Administer cooling procedures as indicated: tepid sponge bath

Expected Outcome

Demonstrates no signs of elevated temperature as evidenced by the following:

Temperature within normal limits (96.4° to 99.1° F [35.8° to 37.3° C])

No signs of shivering, flushing

Pulse within normal limits

▼ Chest pain related to inflammation of lung parenchyma

Assess and monitor quality of pain, noting any changes; ask patients to rate on scale 1 to 10

Assist patient in chest splinting techniques during coughing episode *to reduce pain*

Administer medications *to suppress cough*

Administer analgesics as ordered

Be aware of potential for depression of respiratory function

Evaluate effectiveness

Provide additional comfort measures *to ease pain*

Plan rest periods

Bed rest

Quiet environment; soft or low light

Avoid unnecessary talking if necessary

Limit visitors as necessary

Expected Outcome

Experiences decreased pain as evidenced by the following:

Verbalization of pain relief

Relaxed facial expression and body movements

Improved breathing pattern

Effective cough

PATIENT/FAMILY TEACHING

Disease process

Assess level of understanding regarding disease process and underlying causes

Explain importance of avoiding transmission of disease

Turn head away when coughing and cover mouth with tissue

Use tissue once only

Dispose of tissue in waste container

Explain importance of gradual convalescence

Limit exercise and activity to tolerance

Plan two or three rest periods during day

Avoid fatigue

Explain importance of continuing postural drainage and deep-breathing exercises as ordered; continue deep-breathing exercises qid for 6 to 8 weeks

Diet: explain importance of maintaining diet as tolerated

Force liquids to 3000 ml/day unless contraindicated

Explain need to prevent recurrence of disease

Keep warm

Avoid chilling

Avoid persons with infections, especially URIs

Receive influenza vaccine and Pneumovax as ordered

Discuss symptoms to report to physician

Elevated temperature

Chill

Diaphoresis; night sweats

Difficulty in breathing

Persistent cough

Cold or influenza

Medications

Discuss medications: name, dosage, time of administration, purpose, and side effects

Explain need to avoid taking over-the-counter medications without physician approval

Ensure that patient and significant other(s) demonstrate methods of postural drainage

DISCHARGE/HOME CARE PLANNING

Explain need and use of vaporizer or humidifier at home

Explain importance of ongoing outpatient care

Assess home environment for any factors that would contribute to recurrence: adequate heat/cooling, absence of persons with infections

Assess economic status for ability to purchase medications and equipment; refer to social services or appropriate agency as indicated

Discuss importance of taking pneumococcal vaccine if at risk: all persons over 65 years, those with chronic disease, HIV infection, malignancy

■ PULMONARY EDEMA

Abnormal accumulation of fluid in the alveoli; causes an increase in pulmonary hydrostatic pressure, usually a result of cardiac disorders including acute myocardial infarction (AMI), mitral stenosis; noncardiogenic causes resulting from decreased colloid osmotic pressure

ASSESSMENT
SUBJECTIVE DATA
SOB, dyspnea
Anxiety, fear of suffocation

OBJECTIVE DATA
Respiratory distress
   Labored, noisy breathing
   Orthopnea
   Nasal flaring
   Tachypnea: shallow, moist respirations
Breath sounds—crackles: in dependent parts of lung initially, extending progressively upward
Cough: pink, frothy sputum
Bounding pulse
Hoarseness
Anxiety
Confusion
Restlessness, thrashing movement
Tachycardia: thready pulse
Diaphoresis
Pallor
Cyanosis
Heart failure (see p. 112)

DIAGNOSTIC TESTS
ABGs: variable
   Early: respiratory alkalosis
   Late: respiratory acidosis and hypoxemia
Chest x-ray examination
   Previous congestion
   Bilateral interstitial edema (Kerley B lines are common)
ECG
   Tachycardia
   Dysrhythmias
PCWP
   14 to 20 mm Hg: mild
   25 to 30 mm Hg: moderate to severe
Protein concentration of edema fluid
Cardiac catheterization
Echocardiogram
Thallium scan

POTENTIAL COMPLICATIONS
Respiratory failure
Respiratory/cardiac arrest

MULTIDISCIPLINARY MANAGEMENT
THERAPEUTIC MANAGEMENT
O_2 therapy: high flow by Venturi mask
Parenteral therapy
Intake and output
Hemodynamic monitoring
Cardiac monitor
Rotating tourniquets
Diet: low sodium
Medications
   Morphine
   Diuretics
   Cardiotonics
   Bronchodilators
   Vasodilators: nitroglycerin, nitroprusside
Mechanical ventilatory support
Intraaortic balloon pump (IABP)

PATIENT PROBLEMS—NURSING DIAGNOSES/INTERVENTIONS

▼Impaired gas exchange related to alveolar capillary membrane changes

Assess respirations, noting rate, depth, and use of accessory muscles
Assess LOC and mental status *to assess for hypoxia or hypercapnia*
Auscultate breath sounds qh
   Decreased breath sounds
   Crackles
Elevate head of bed 60 to 90 degrees with lower extremities dependent *to decrease venous return*
Monitor ABGs; intraarterial line may be required because of frequent need of samples
Monitor serial chest x-rays *to detect signs of improvement or exacerbation*
Administer bronchodilators *to relieve bronchospasm and respiratory effort;* vasodilators *to reduce systemic and venous pressure*
   Document response to diuretics or vasodilators
Administer oxygen therapy as ordered
Administer IPPB as ordered (p. 285)
Check BP, R, and apical pulse qh and prn
Assist and teach patient to cough and deep breathe qh and prn *to maximize air exchange*
Maintain bed rest during acute phase

Expected Outcomes
Adequate gas exchange as evidenced by demonstrated effortless breathing
Lungs clear to auscultation
Hemodynamic stability
Blood gases within normal range

▼Anxiety related to perceived biologic threat (fear of suffocation)

Assess degree of anxiety (mild, moderate, severe)

Provide emotional support

    Remain with patient

    Reassure that treatments will relieve symptoms

    Reduce environmental stimuli

    Explain procedures and treatments thoroughly

    Use short, simple sentences

    Use calm, reassuring voice

    Assess whether significant family member present would reduce anxiety

Position to level of comfort: high-Fowler's position with padded overbed table

Plan rest periods *to maximize relaxation and decrease oxygen demand*

Encourage patient to verbalize fears and concerns

Administer morphine sulfate or antianxiety medication *to calm patient*

Expected Outcome

Demonstrates decreased anxiety as evidenced by the following:

    Verbalization of reduced anxiety

    Demonstration that treatment is understood

    Decreased use of tranquilizers and pain medication

Additional Nursing Diagnoses to Consider

Fluid volume excess related to left ventricular dysfunction (see Heart failure, p. 112)

Ineffective breathing pattern related to tracheobronchial secretions and fluid overload

Activity intolerance related to imbalance between oxygen supply and demand

PATIENT/FAMILY TEACHING

Disease process

    Assess level of understanding regarding disease process and contributing factors

    Provide instruction regarding disease process

Explain need to exercise to tolerance

    Avoid strenuous exercise

    Plan frequent rest periods

Explain need to maintain a low-sodium diet as ordered

Explain importance of avoiding tobacco use

Discuss symptoms to report to physician

    Sudden weight increase of > 3 to 5 lb/wk

    Decreased urinary output

    Swollen feet and ankles

    Chest pain

    Difficulty in breathing

    Persistent cough

    Decreased activity intolerance

Discuss medications: name, dosage, time of administration, purpose, and side effects

DISCHARGE/HOME CARE PLANNING

Provide instruction regarding home management including respiratory therapy

Provide instruction on oxygen or respiratory equipment used at home

Teach the patient adaptive breathing techniques

Explain the importance of ongoing outpatient care

Explain the importance of avoiding contact with persons who have URIs

Assess economic status for ability to purchase medications and equipment; refer to social services or agency as indicated

■ PULMONARY EMBOLISM

Blockage of the pulmonary artery or one of its branches by thrombus; damage to the lung depends on the number of clots and the extent of obstruction to pulmonary circulation; most commonly associated with dislodged clot from systemic circulation such as deep veins of legs or pelvis, or atrial fibrillation

ASSESSMENT

SUBJECTIVE DATA

Sudden onset

    Dyspnea

    Pleuritic or nonpleuritic chest pain

    Cough

    SOB

    Restlessness

    Anxiety and feelings of impending doom

    Fear of suffocation/apprehension

History of symptoms of deep vein thrombosis (DVT)

    Unilateral swelling of thigh and/or lower leg

    Erythema

    Warmth

    Tenderness

OBJECTIVE DATA

Diaphoresis

Cyanosis, pallor

Tachypnea

Tachycardia

Hypotension

Hemoptysis (rare)

Cough (unproductive)

Breath sounds

    Decreased

    Crackles

    Pleural friction rub

    Wheezing

DIAGNOSTIC TESTS

Chest x-ray examination

    Wedge-shaped density

    Unilateral elevated diaphragms

    Atelectasis

    Hyperlucent lung fields

    Unilateral pleural effusion

    Area of consolidation (occasional)

ABGs

    Decreased Pao_2 (<80 mm Hg)

    Decreased $Paco_2$ (<40 mm Hg)

    Respiratory alkalosis

Elevated pH (>7.45)
Increased A-a gradient
ECG
Right ventricular strain (ST-T wave change in V_1-V_4)
Right axis deviation
Atrial fibrillation
Lung (ventilation/perfusion) scan
Pulmonary angiogram
Serum assays
Elevated lactate dehydrogenase (LDH), elevated
bilirubin
Fibrin split products (FSP)/fibrin degradation tests
Serum lipase
Pattern of abnormal perfusion in area of ventilation
Intraarterial filling defects
Pulmonary artery obstruction(s)
Spiral CT scans
Ultrasound of legs

POTENTIAL COMPLICATIONS
Extended/recurrent pulmonary embolism
Pulmonary infarction
Atelectasis
Pulmonary hypertension
Right ventricular (RV) failure
Cor pulmonale
Decreased CO
Shock
Cardiopulmonary arrest

MULTIDISCIPLINARY MANAGEMENT
THERAPEUTIC MANAGEMENT
Bed rest
Oxygen therapy
Cardiac monitor
Medication
Anticoagulants
Heparin
Warfarin
Thrombolytic therapy
Streptokinase
Urokinase
Parenteral fluids
Surgical therapy
Insertion of umbrella filter in the inferior vena cava for
multiple emboli
Embolectomy

PATIENT PROBLEMS—NURSING DIAGNOSES/INTERVENTIONS

▼ Impaired gas exchange related to ventilation/ perfusion abnormalities

Assess, monitor for, and report signs of restlessness, confusion, and irritability, *which may indicate hypoxia or respiratory distress*
Assess quality and respiratory rate q2h to 4h or as indicated

Administer oxygen as ordered; report O_2 saturation $\leq$ 92%; intubation and assisted ventilation may be indicated
Monitor BP, R, and apical pulse q1h to 2h and prn
Auscultate breath sounds q2h to 4h
Maintain bed rest during acute phase *to decrease metabolic demands;* instruct to turn and deep breathe q2h to 4h; avoid positions that bend knees, *which decreases venous return and can increase risk of pulmonary embolism (PE)*
Elevate head of bed 30 degrees *to improve ventilation*
Monitor serial ABGs: report changes in Pao_2 or $Paco_2$ > 10 mm Hg
Monitor ECG and cardiac status for dysrhythmias secondary to blood gas levels
Monitor for pulmonary hypertension, jugular venous distention, blood gas abnormalities, hepatomegaly, and cardiac compromise, which may indicate cor pulmonale

Expected Outcome
Experiences adequate O_2/CO_2 exchange as evidenced by the following:
ABGs within normal range
Reports exhibiting no signs of respiratory distress
Respiratory rate, rhythm within normal limits
Normal breath sounds

▼ Risk for injury related to increased bleeding from anticoagulant therapy

Observe for signs and symptoms of bleeding: stools— occult and frank bleeding, hematuria, sputum, bleeding gums, bruising skin
Monitor PTT/PT, INR, and clotting functions or coagulation factors daily as ordered
Administer anticoagulants as ordered
Do not administer aspirin-containing products
Provide antiembolic stockings as ordered *to prevent venous stasis*
Avoid constipation and straining; use stool softeners or mild laxatives
See Anticoagulant Therapy (p. 157) for further management

Expected Outcome
Experiences no bleeding or extension of embolism as evidenced by absence of blood in stool, urine, sputum, or other sites

▼ Anxiety related to fear of perceived threat (suffocation) or actual threat to biologic integrity

Assess verbal and nonverbal signs and symptoms of anxiety/fear; encourage questions
Provide emotional support; maintain quiet environment
Remain with patient during periods of heightened anxiety

Explain procedures and treatments; use simple
explanations

Assess whether significant family members present
decrease anxiety; assist them to provide care

Administer antianxiety medications as ordered

Expected Outcomes
Experiences a reduction in anxiety as evidenced by the
following:
Relaxed facial expression
Verbalization of feeling less anxious
Decreased use of sedatives and/or tranquilizers
Verbalization of an understanding of routines and
treatments

Additional Nursing Diagnosis to Consider
Altered tissue perfusion related to interruption of arterial
blood flow secondary to pulmonary embolism

PATIENT/FAMILY TEACHING
Discuss disease process
Assess level of understanding regarding disease
process and underlying cause
Provide information on prevention for patients at risk
for pulmonary embolism
Discuss symptoms of pulmonary embolism to report
Sudden, sharp chest pain
Bloody sputum
Difficulty breathing
Blood in stool
Medications
Discuss medications: name, dosage, time of
administration, purpose, and side effects
Explain need to avoid taking over-the-counter
medications without physician approval
Explain need to check for bleeding in urine, stools, and
sputum if sent home on anticoagulants (see
Anticoagulant therapy, p. 157)
Activity
Explain need to exercise to tolerance with planned
rest periods
Review strategies to prevent venous pooling
Avoid sitting or standing for long periods
Elevate legs while sitting
Do not cross legs
Use antiembolic stockings if ordered
Perform regular exercise such as walking
Explain importance of avoiding tobacco use
Explain need to wear medical alert band identifying use
of anticoagulants

DISCHARGE/HOME CARE PLANNING
Discuss any home management issues
Explain importance of ongoing outpatient care
Monitor exercise program
Assess economic status for ability to purchase
medications and equipment; refer to social services
and appropriate agency as indicated

■ PULMONARY HYPERTENSION
*An elevation of mean pulmonary artery pressure
(MPAP) > 20 mm Hg. Pulmonary hypertension may occur as a **primary** disorder or **secondary** to preexisting
diseases such as congenital heart disease or other pulmonary disease*

ASSESSMENT
SUBJECTIVE DATA
DOE and at rest
Fatigue
Syncope
Chest pain

OBJECTIVE DATA
Tachypnea
Breath sounds
Distant
Decreased at periphery
Crackles
Cyanosis
RV failure (Fig. 5-4)
Distended jugular veins
RV heave
Loud, accentuated P_2
RV diastolic gallop
Murmur of tricuspid insufficiency
Peripheral edema
Chest pain

DIAGNOSTIC TESTS
Chest x-ray examination
Enlarged pulmonary artery
RV dilation or hypertrophy
ECG
Right axis deviation
Right bundle branch block (RBBB)
Echocardiogram
Enlarged right atrium (RA), RV
Diminished wall motion
Pulmonary valve (PV) malfunction
Cardiac catheterization
Elevated pulmonary artery (PA) systolic and diastolic
pressure with normal PCWP
Decreased CO
ABGs
Pao_2 40 to 60 mm Hg
$Paco_2$ will vary depending on cause (40 to 70 mm Hg)

MULTIDISCIPLINARY MANAGEMENT
THERAPEUTIC MANAGEMENT
Oxygen therapy
Hemodynamic monitoring
Cardiac monitoring
Medications
Vasodilators
Prostacyclin
Hydralazine

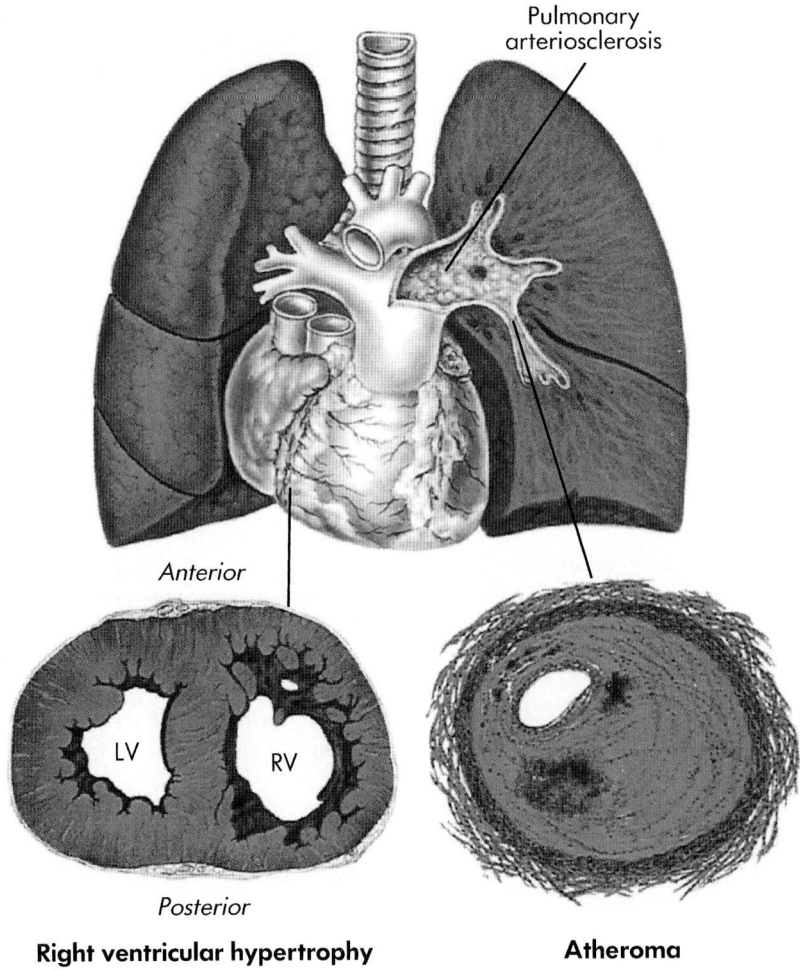

Pulmonary
arteriosclerosis

Anterior

LV   RV

Posterior

Right ventricular hypertrophy   **Atheroma**

Fig. 5-4   Right ventricular hypertrophy.
(From Wilson SF, Thompson JM: Mosby's clinical nursing series: respiratory disorders, *St Louis, 1990, Mosby.)*

Calcium channel blockers
ACE inhibitors
Diuretics
Digitalis (used for biventricular failure)
Lung transplantation (unilateral or bilateral)
Heart/lung transplantation

PATIENT PROBLEMS—NURSING DIAGNOSES/INTERVENTIONS

▼Impaired gas exchange related to alveolar-capillary membrane changes

Assess and monitor rate and depth of respirations, use of accessory muscles, air hunger, tachycardia

Assess skin color and capillary filling to determine circulatory adequacy

Auscultate breath sounds noting increase or decrease of rhonchi, crackles; report significant changes

Position patient in semi-Fowler's position *to optimize lung expansion*

Monitor serial ABGs and for signs of progressive hypoxemia and acidosis

Administer oxygen therapy as ordered *to optimize gas exchange*

Monitor chest x-ray examinations

Assist and instruct patient to cough and deep breathe; assess need to suction at regular intervals

Monitor for increasing signs of activity intolerance

Plan regular rest periods

Administer vasodilator as ordered

Expected Outcomes

Maintains adequate gas exchange
ABGs are within acceptable limits
Lung sounds are improved

▼Activity intolerance related to fatigue and dyspnea secondary to hypoxemia and decreased left ventricular function

Assess degree of reported activity intolerance; observe respiratory rate in response to activities

Assist and instruct patient to plan frequent rest periods, especially between activities

Monitor signs of progressive deterioration in performing ADLs; report to physician

Provide oxygen therapy as indicated *to prevent hypoxia:* report changes in Pao$_2$ and Paco$_2$ > 10 mm Hg

Assist patient to identify energy-saving methods while performing ADLs: shower chair, sitting while shaving

Instruct and encourage patient to use adaptive breathing techniques

Expected Outcome

Reports ability to perform ADLs and verbalizes a decrease in fatigue

Additional Nursing Diagnosis to Consider

Fluid volume excess related to RV failure (see p. 112)

PATIENT/FAMILY TEACHING

Disease process

Assess level of understanding regarding pulmonary hypertension, identifying any misconceptions

Provide patient and significant other(s) with information regarding disease process, signs and symptoms to report

Increasing SOB; noisy, wet breathing

Decreased activity tolerance

Changes in color, consistency of sputum

Increased cough

Swelling of legs, ankles, or abdomen

Discuss action to take during episodes of fatigue or dyspnea

Activity

Discuss importance of spacing heavy workloads and resting between activities

Teach energy-saving procedures: shower chair; sitting while shaving, combing hair, dressing, cooking

Discuss importance of taking prescribed medications: name, dosage, purpose, time of administration, and side effects

Discuss importance of avoiding tobacco or nicotine products

Provide instruction on adaptive breathing techniques

DISCHARGE/HOME CARE PLANNING

Assess home environment for energy-saving equipment: shower chair, grab bars

Monitor activity and exercise program: walking with rest periods

Teach use of home oxygen equipment

Assess economic status for ability to purchase medications and equipment; refer to social services and agencies as indicated

■ PULMONARY TUBERCULOSIS

A chronic acute or subacute infectious disease caused by the tubercle bacillus, Mycobacterium tuberculosis, *most commonly affecting the alveolar structure of the lung; clinical presentation varies from asymptomatic with*

Table 5-7	Diagnostic Classification for Tuberculosis Patients
Class 1	Exposed, not infected. Identified contact with contagious active TB patients. Negative PPD; may require close follow-up and empiric preventive therapy if exposure recent
Class 2	Latent TB (tuberculosis infection). PPD positive; no clinical radiologic or laboratory evidence of active TB
Class 3	Active TB. Positive for MTB or positive PPD with radiologic evidence of active TB
Class 4	Old disease, abnormal x-rays (fibronodular scarring), that have been stable over several months; negative cultures. Should be placed in class 5 while cultures and follow-up x-rays are pending
Class 5	Active TB suspected; diagnostic work-up recommended with in 3 months

From American Thoracic Society: Diagnostic standards and classification of tuberculosis, Am Rev Resp Dis *142:725-735, 1990.*

only a positive skin test to extensive pulmonary and systemic involvement (Table 5-7)

ASSESSMENT

SUBJECTIVE DATA

Fatigue, malaise

Headache

Anorexia

Chest pain

OBJECTIVE DATA

Low-grade fever, night sweats

Tachycardia

Weight loss

Cough: q2wk or greater duration nonproductive at first

Blood-streaked sputum

Mucoid or mucopurulent sputum

Lymph nodes

Inflamed

Painful

Crackles over apex of lung

Pleuritic chest pain

Irregular menses

DIAGNOSTIC TESTS

Skin testing

PPD: 5 units of purified protein derivative (PPD)

Mantoux test: PPD or OT—old tuberculin, injected intradermally with pressure gun

Tine test: OT pressed into skin with tine unit

Gastric washings

Sputum cultures: positive for *M. tuberculosis* within 2 to 3 weeks if active; positive acid-fast bacilli (AFB)

Chest x-ray examination (Box 5-6)

Calcification at original site, enlarged hilar lymph nodes, extensive infiltrates and large cavities

| Box 5-6 | **Tuberculosis: Chest X-ray Findings** |

PRIMARY
Appears as middle or lower lobe infiltrates/consolidation accompanied by hilar or mediastinal lymphadenopathy

REACTIVATED
Appears mostly in apical segment of the upper lobes and superior segment of the lower lobes

Pleural effusion or cavitation
CAUTION: Other lung abnormalities (pneumonia, tumors) can look like tuberculosis
Fiberoptic bronchoscopy
CT-guided needle biopsy of pleura
WBC: leukocytosis

POTENTIAL COMPLICATIONS
Atelectasis
Hemoptysis
Pneumothorax
Recurrence
Miliary tuberculosis
Tuberculosis pericarditis, peritonitis, meningitis, lymphadenitis

MULTIDISCIPLINARY MANAGEMENT
THERAPEUTIC MANAGEMENT
Antiinfective agents
  Primary drugs
    Isoniazid (INH)
    Ethambutol
    Rifampin
    Streptomycin
  Secondary drugs
    Paraaminosalicylic acid (PAS)
    Pyrazinamide (PZA)
    Ethambutol
    Capreomycin
    Cycloserine
Analgesics
AFB isolation until medication therapy initiated
High-protein, high-carbohydrate diet
Respiratory isolation as necessary (isolation room should have negative pressure)
Report to board of health for follow-up on family and contacts
Surgical therapy
  Drainage of lung abscess
  Lung resection

PATIENT PROBLEMS—NURSING DIAGNOSES/INTERVENTIONS

▼Ineffective breathing pattern related to muco-purulent secretions and poor cough effort

Assess quality and depth of respirations, use of accessory muscles; record any changes
Assess quality of sputum: color, odor, consistency
Auscultate breath sounds q4h for adventitious or decreased breath sounds
Position patient *to optimize breathing:* semi-Fowler's or high-Fowler's position
Assist and teach patient to turn, cough, and deep breathe q2h to 4h *to mobilize secretions and maximize lung expansion*
Instruct patient to splint chest *for more effective and productive cough*
Provide frequent rest periods, avoid fatigue, and exercise to tolerance
Monitor T, P, and R q4h
Administer medications as ordered
Encourage fluid intake *to liquefy secretions*

Expected Outcome
Maintains an effective breathing pattern
  Normal rate, rhythm, and depth of respirations
  Decreased dyspnea

▼Risk for infection, transmission related to insufficient knowledge of pathogen

Discuss importance of maintaining respiratory isolation; avoid direct contact with sputum until antibiotic therapy is initiated and necessary levels obtained
Teach patient to cough into tissues
  Turn head with coughing
  Dispose of tissues properly
  Use mask if unable to follow directions
Instruct patient how to collect and care for sputum cultures and use good handwashing techniques *to reduce risk of spreading infection*
Teach patient importance of not stopping antituberculosis medications until directed by physician

Expected Outcome
Decreased potential for transmission of disease as evidenced by failure of patient contacts to convert to positive skin test

▼Altered nutrition: less than body requirements related to fatigue, anorexia, or dyspnea

Obtain admission weight and monitor daily for changes
Assess nutritional status on a regular basis; consult with dietitian
Monitor percentage of meals eaten
Maintain high-protein, high-carbohydrate diet with small, frequent feedings
Assess for additional causes of malnutrition such as depression
Monitor albumin, prealbumin, and lymphocytes as *guide to nutritional status*

Place in high-Fowler's position at meals *to reduce dyspnea*

Encourage rest periods before meals *to reduce fatigue*

Encourage oral care before meals

Encourage significant other(s) to bring patient's favorite foods

Expected Outcome

Maintains an adequate nutritional status; weight remains stable and within normal range for patient's height, age, and build

PATIENT/FAMILY TEACHING

Disease process

Assess level of understanding regarding disease process; identify any fears or misconceptions

Explain nature of disease, mode of disease transmission, and purpose of treatment and procedures

Explain importance of good hygiene and handwashing (coughing into tissues, use of mask if unable to follow directions, how to dispose of tissues, to turn head if coughing, and to avoid direct contact with sputum)

Teach importance of maintaining respiratory isolation until necessary medication levels are obtained

Explain importance of exercise, frequent rest periods, and avoiding fatigue

Instruct on importance of avoiding close contact with others until advised by physician

Explain need to avoid crowds and persons with URIs

Discuss symptoms to report to physician

Hemoptysis

Chest pain

Difficulty in breathing

Hearing loss

Vertigo

Diet: explain importance of maintaining high-protein, high-carbohydrate diet; need to force fluids to 2000 to 3000 ml/day unless contraindicated

Discuss medications: name, dosage, time of administration, purpose, and side effects

Explain need to avoid taking over-the-counter medications without physician approval

Discuss importance of not stopping medication

DISCHARGE/HOME CARE PLANNING

Assess patient's ability to maintain isolation in home until necessary medication levels are obtained

Assess home for sanitary equipment for maintaining good hygiene: disposable trash bags, covered waste can for soiled tissues

Assess home for sleeping conditions, crowding, and persons with URIs; also children and others susceptible to infection

Evaluate economic status for ability to purchase medications and supplies; refer to social services and other agencies as indicated

Explain importance of ongoing outpatient care

Encourage PPD testing of family and contacts

■ PNEUMOTHORAX AND HEMOTHORAX

Collection of air or gas in the pleural space, causing the lung to collapse; may be partial or total collapse; open or communicating pneumothorax (sucking wound) occurs as result of an open chest wound that permits entry of air; spontaneous pneumothorax (closed) results from rupture of a bleb or bullae on the surface of the lung; may occur as a result of pulmonary disease (COPD, tuberculosis [TB]); or may be iatrogenically induced (thoracentesis)

tension pneumothorax: *An opening through the pleura that allows air to pass into the pleura on inspiration; however, the air cannot exit on expiration; this produces a shift in the affected lung and mediastinum toward the unaffected side (tension pneumothorax is a medical emergency) (Box 5-7 and Fig. 5-5)*

hemothorax: *Blood in the pleural space, causing the lung to partially or totally collapse; often appears as a complication of chest trauma and after chest surgery (see Box 5-7 and Fig. 5-6)*

NOTE: *Symptoms and treatment depend on size of pneumothorax:*

<15%: small

15% to 60%: moderate

>60%: large

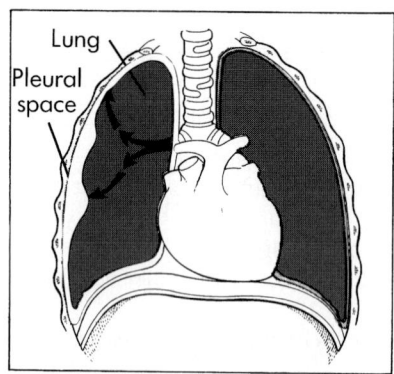

Spontaneous pneumothorax

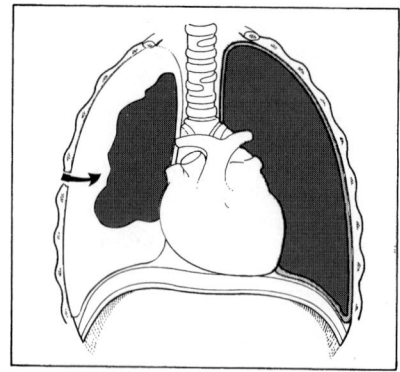

Traumatic pneumothorax

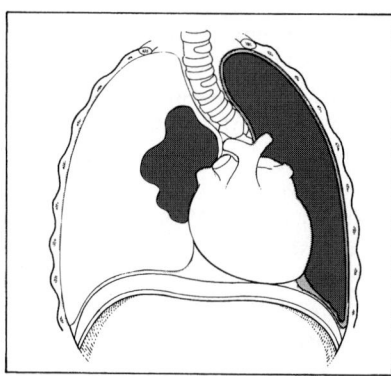

Tension pneumothorax

Fig. 5-5 Spontaneous, traumatic, and tension pneumothorax.

(From Wilson SF, Thompson JM: Mosby's clinical nursing series: respiratory disorders, *St Louis, 1990, Mosby.)*

ASSESSMENT

SUBJECTIVE DATA

Pain: pleural type, sudden, sharp pain radiating to
shoulder or arm of affected side
Anxiety
Dyspnea or SOB

OBJECTIVE DATA

Diaphoresis
Tachycardia
Cyanosis
Tachypnea
Absent or decreased breath sounds on affected side

BOX 5-7	**Assessment/Finding of Tension Pneumothorax and Hemothorax**

TENSION PNEUMOTHORAX DATA

Assessment

Subjective Data
Difficulty breathing
Anxiety, fear of death
Restlessness, agitation

Objective Data
Respiratory distress: sudden, severe
Use of accessory muscles of respiration
Tachycardia
Cyanosis
Tachypnea
Hypotension
Paradoxic chest movement
Hyperresonance over affected area on percussion
Tracheal and mediastinal shift: toward unaffected side
Breath sounds
   Absent (affected side)
   Diminished (unaffected side)
Distant heart sounds
Subcutaneous emphysema

Diagnostic Tests
Chest x-ray examination: complete lung collapse of affected
side, mediastinal or tracheal shift to unaffected side

HEMOTHORAX

Assessment

Subjective Data
Difficulty breathing
Pain
Anxiety, restlessness, fear of impending doom

Objective Data
Dullness on chest percussion
Distant to absent breath sounds on affected side
Asymmetric chest movements
Hypovolemic shock if blood loss is severe
   Tachypnea
   Tachycardia
   Hypotension
   Pallor

Diagnostic Tests
Chest x-ray examination
   Blunting of costophrenic angles
   Hazy appearance over lower chest
Hct decreased/Hgb

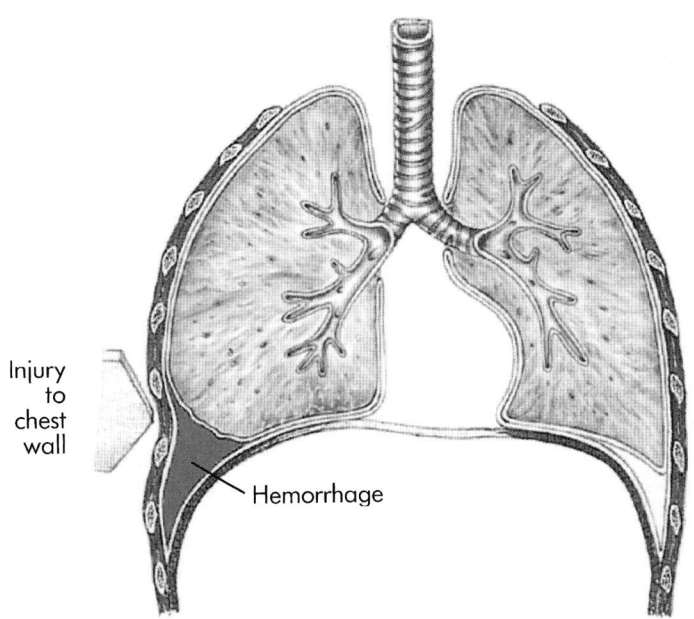

Fig. 5-6   Hemothorax.
(From Wilson SF, Thompson JM: Mosby's clinical nursing series: respiratory disorders, *St Louis, 1990, Mosby.)*

Hyperresonance to percussion over affected thoracic space

DIAGNOSTIC TESTS

Chest x-ray examination
  Unequal lung expansion
  Air in pleural space
  Mediastinal shift to unaffected side
ABGs
  Decreased Pao_2
  Decreased pH
  Increased $Paco_2$
Oxymetry: O_2 sat $\leq 92\%$
CBC

POTENTIAL COMPLICATIONS

Decreased cardiac output (CO)
Respiratory failure
ARDS
Infection
Cardiac arrest

MULTIDISCIPLINARY MANAGEMENT

THERAPEUTIC MANAGEMENT

Chest tube insertion (closed-tube thoracostomy)
Oxygen therapy
Parenteral therapy
Thoracentesis
Blood transfusion (hemothorax)
Thoracotomy

PATIENT PROBLEMS—NURSING DIAGNOSES/INTERVENTIONS

▼Ineffective breathing pattern related to inadequate chest expansion caused by air/fluid accumulation

Assess quality, rate, and depth of respirations, nasal flaring, retractions; report any changes
Note chest wall movement and position of trachea *to differentiate tension pneumothorax*
Auscultate breath sounds q2h to 4h *to detect absence of breath sounds*
Reassure and try to calm patient
Place patient in a position *to ensure optimal ventilation:* sitting position with head of bed elevated 60 to 90 degrees
Administer oxygen per nasal cannula at 2 to 6 L/min as ordered unless contraindicated *to treat hypoxia*
Assist with insertion of chest tube and provide chest tube care (see Chest tubes, p. 274)
Administer oxygen and IPPB as ordered
Monitor BP, T, R, and apical pulse q2h to 4h: *to detect changes in cardiac output, infective process, or oxygenation*
Assist and encourage patient to
  Turn and deep breathe q2h to 4h: diaphragmatic, segmental breathing; instruct patient to suppress cough

Avoid stretching, reaching, or sudden movements
Provide emotional support; remain with patient during periods of heightened anxiety
Continue with acute care and decrease frequency of nursing functions as patient's condition improves
Assess for tiring in relation to breathing attempts
Space activities *to provide periods of rest*

Expected Outcome

Maintains an effective breathing pattern as evidenced by the following:
  Normal rate, rhythm, and depth of respirations
  Chest x-ray examinations show full expansion
  Breath sounds are clear with full aeration

▼Impaired gas exchange related to decreased oxygen supply

Assess for signs and symptoms of hypoxemia: restlessness, confusion, irritability
Monitor ABG results: report changes in Po_2 or $Paco_2$ of >10 mm Hg
Observe for signs of respiratory distress: increased work of breathing, unequal lung expansion, complaints of increased dyspnea
Administer supplemental oxygen as ordered; assist with endotracheal intubation and mechanical ventilation as indicated
Monitor function and patency of chest tube
Provide periods of rest *to decrease oxygen demand*

Expected Outcome

Maintains adequate gas exchange as evidenced by the following:
  Usual mental status
  Usual skin color
  Blood gases within normal range

▼Chest pain related to pleural irritation/inflammation and physical factors (chest tube insertion)

Assess for presence of pain (verbal and nonverbal): rate pain on scale of 1 to 10
Administer analgesic as prescribed (30 minutes before initiating movement)
Assess effectiveness of pain relief measures
Medicate patient before breathing/coughing exercises
Instruct patient on splinting techniques; move as a unit *to enhance stability and comfort*
Secure chest tubes *to limit movement and resulting irritation*
Instruct patient to splint affected side when coughing or moving

Expected Outcome

Experiences decreased pain as evidenced by the following:
  Verbalizes pain relief
  Relaxed facial expression and body positioning

Improved breathing pattern
Increased activity

PATIENT/FAMILY TEACHING
Disease process
    Assess level of understanding regarding disease
       process and contributing factors
Explain importance of not smoking
Explain need to avoid persons with infections, especially
    URIs
Discuss symptoms to report: cold; sore throat; influenza;
    elevated temperature; cough; sudden, sharp chest pain;
    difficulty in breathing; any redness, pain, swelling, or
    tenderness of puncture wound
Diet
    Explain importance of maintaining diet as ordered;
       need to force fluids to 2000 to 3000 ml/day unless
       contraindicated to liquefy secretions and maintain
       hydration
Activity
    Explain need to exercise to tolerance, avoid fatigue,
       and plan rest periods
    Explain importance of avoiding strenuous activity or
       exercise, especially contact sports
Discuss medications: name, dosage, time of
    administration, purpose, and side effects

DISCHARGE/HOME CARE PLANNING
Explain importance of ongoing outpatient care for
    extended period following pneumothorax
Ensure that patient and significant other(s) demonstrate
    care of chest puncture wound (see Chest tubes p. 274)
Evaluate economic status for ability to purchase
    medications and supplies and refer to social services
    or agency as indicated
Teach patient adaptive breathing techniques to maximize
    lung reexpansion and prevent complications
Teach importance of avoiding persons with URIs or flu

■ ATELECTASIS
*Collapse of alveoli or airless condition of the lung
caused by mucous plugs, excessive secretions, compression of lung tissue by tumors, effusions, or pneumothorax, shallow breathing, or incomplete lung expansion at
birth*

ASSESSMENT
SUBJECTIVE DATA
Difficulty breathing
SOB
Localized pleuritic chest pain
Fatigue
Anxiety
Fear of air hunger

OBJECTIVE DATA
Elevated temperature
Breath sounds
    Absent or decreased over affected area

Crackles
Egophony and bronchophony
Tachypnea
Tachycardia
Labored breathing
Nasal flaring
Restlessness
Asymmetric chest movement on inspiration

DIAGNOSTIC TESTS
ABGs
    Decreased Pao_2: <80 mm Hg initially
    Normal or decreased $Paco_2$
    Significant atelectasis: increased $Paco_2$
Chest x-ray examination
    Elevated diaphragm on affected side
    Shift of trachea mediastinum toward affected side if
       large area is atelectatic
    Narrow rib spaces

POTENTIAL COMPLICATIONS
Pneumonia
Bronchiectasis

MULTIDISCIPLINARY MANAGEMENT
THERAPEUTIC MANAGEMENT
Oxygen therapy
Chest physiotherapy
Incentive spirometer
High tidal volume and/or PEEP for intubated patient
Bronchoscopy
Nutritional support
Fluid management
Medications
    Antipyretics
    Bronchodilators
    Antibiotics

PATIENT PROBLEM—NURSING DIAGNOSIS/INTERVENTIONS

▼Impaired gas exchange related to compressed
lung tissue

Assess for signs of hypoxemia: labored breathing,
    tachypnea, restlessness, pallor
Assess LOC for signs of hypoxia or hypercapnia
Auscultate breath sounds q2h to 4h
    Check quality and rate of respirations
    Note area of lung without breath sounds
Assist and instruct patient to turn, cough, and deep
    breathe q1h to 2h and prn *to enhance lung
    expansion and mobilize secretions*
Assist and instruct patient to perform postural drainage
    qid and prn; clapping may be ordered *to mobilize
    secretions*
Assist or initiate chest physiotherapy
Perform nasotracheal suction as indicated *to maintain
    patent airway*
Administer nebulization as ordered *to liquefy secretions*

Administer oxygen and IPPB as ordered

Instruct and encourage patient to use incentive spirometer as ordered

Encourage early ambulation as soon as possible *to facilitate lung expansion*

Monitor BP, T, and apical pulse q4h *to assess hemodynamics and infectious process*

Monitor ABGs as ordered

Administer medication as ordered: antipyretics

Expected Outcome

Gas exchange is improved

ABGs within acceptable limits

Lungs clear to auscultation

Normal rate and rhythm of respiration

PATIENT/FAMILY TEACHING

Assess level of understanding regarding disease process: identify fears and misconceptions

Instruct patient in coughing and deep breathing techniques; teach patient to splint chest when coughing

Instruct patient in use of incentive spirometer and how frequently to use if continued at home

Explain need to avoid persons with infections, especially URIs

Explain importance of avoiding tobacco use

Discuss symptoms to report to physician

URI

Influenza

Difficulty in breathing

Persistent cough

Elevated temperature

Explain importance of exercising to tolerance; need to avoid fatigue and plan rest periods

Discuss medications: name, dosage, time of administration, purpose, and side effects

Explain need to avoid taking over-the-counter medications without physician approval

DISCHARGE/HOME CARE PLANNING

Explain importance of ongoing outpatient care

Teach use of home oxygen therapy to patient and significant other(s)

Evaluate economic status for ability to purchase medications and supplies; refer to social services and other agencies as indicated

◼ PLEURAL EFFUSION

Excessive amount of nonpurulent fluid in the pleural space between the visceral and parietal layers; associated with primary diseases in which capillary fluid, lymphatic drainage membrane hydrostatic, and colloidal pressures of plurae are disturbed. Pleural effusion is rarely a primary disease

ASSESSMENT
SUBJECTIVE DATA

SOB

Localized pleuritic chest pain

Fatigue

Fear of suffocation

OBJECTIVE DATA

Related to underlying disease and may be asymptomatic if effusion is small

Breath sounds

Diminished or absent over affected area

Egophony over effusion area

Pleural friction rub

Asymmetric chest expansion

Elevated temperature

Cough

DIAGNOSTIC TESTS

Chest x-ray examination

Blunting of costophrenic angle

Partially obscured diaphragm

Complete "white out" (opaque densities) of involved area in large effusions

Mediastinal shift (large effusion)

Thoracentesis

Pleural biopsy

Cytologic examination of fluid

Gram stain, culture, and sensitivity of pleural fluid

POTENTIAL COMPLICATIONS

Pneumothorax

Pneumonia

Empyema

MULTIDISCIPLINARY MANAGEMENT
THERAPEUTIC MANAGEMENT

Bed rest

Chest tube insertion (see p. 274)

Thoracentesis

Sclerosing pleurodesis

Medications: antibiotics

Fluid management

Chest physiotherapy

Nitrogen mustard instillation or tetracycline via chest tube

Treatment of underlying disease process

PATIENT PROBLEM—NURSING DIAGNOSIS/INTERVENTIONS

▼Ineffective breathing pattern related to decreased lung expansion secondary to fluid accumulation in the pleural space

Assess rate, depth, and quality of respirations

Auscultate chest q2h to 4h for changes in breath sounds

Maintain bed rest; assist patient to assume position of comfort *to maximize breathing*

See Thoracentesis (p. 235) and Chest tubes (p. 274) if ordered

Monitor BP, T, P, and R q4h and prn to assess hemodynamics and detect any infective process

Administer medications as ordered

Assist and teach patient to

Turn, cough, and deep breathe q2h to 4h

Use incentive breathing *to maximize lung expansion*

Splint chest when coughing

Perform active ROM exercises to all extremities q2h to 4h

Incentive spirometer *to maximize lung expansion*

Increase activity as tolerated

Expected Outcome
Maintains an effective breathing pattern

Normal rate, rhythm, and depth of respirations

Decreased dyspnea

Chest x-ray examination clear

Additional Nursing Diagnoses to Consider
Impaired gas exchange related to alveolar-capillary membrane changes

Fear related to suffocation and dying

PATIENT/FAMILY TEACHING
Disease process

Assess level of understanding regarding disease process and allay fears and misconceptions

Discuss symptoms to report: difficulty in breathing, chest pain, elevated temperature, persistent cough

Instruct and encourage patient to cough, deep breathe to keep lungs well aerated

Explain importance of avoiding persons with URIs

Discuss symptoms of a cold or influenza to report

Explain importance of influenza vaccination as ordered

Medications

Discuss medications: name, dosage, time of administration, purpose, and side effects

Explain need to avoid taking over-the-counter medications without physician approval

Activity: explain need to exercise to tolerance

Plan rest periods

Avoid fatigue

DISCHARGE/HOME CARE PLANNING
Explain importance of ongoing outpatient care

Assess members living at home for possible URI or influenza; explain need for influenza vaccination

Evaluate economic status for ability to purchase medications and supplies and refer to social services or appropriate agency as indicated

◼ FLAIL CHEST
Chest cage abnormality usually resulting from crushing chest injury in which multiple fractures of ribs have occurred

ASSESSMENT
SUBJECTIVE DATA
Difficulty breathing

Pain: rib cage

Fear

OBJECTIVE DATA
Sharp chest pain

Respirations

Shallow

Paradoxic chest wall movement

Splinting

Tachypnea

Tachycardia

Cyanosis

Decreased breath sounds

Mediastinal and tracheal shift

Sputum

Copious

Blood tinged

DIAGNOSTIC TESTS
Chest x-ray examination

Atelectasis

Pneumothorax

Evidence of fractured ribs

ABGs

Decreased PaO_2

Increased $PaCO_2$

Pulmonary function tests: decreased lung volumes

POTENTIAL COMPLICATIONS
Tension pneumothorax

Hemothorax

Pulmonary edema

Cardiac tamponade

Respiratory arrest

Shock

MULTIDISCIPLINARY MANAGEMENT
THERAPEUTIC MANAGEMENT
O_2 therapy

Chest tube insertion

Intubation and mechanical ventilation with PEEP

Medications

Neuromuscular blockers

Sedatives

Antibiotics

Bronchodilators

Analgesics

PATIENT PROBLEMS—NURSING DIAGNOSES/INTERVENTIONS

▼Ineffective breathing pattern related to unstable chest wall movement

Maintain bed rest; assist patient in assuming position of comfort; do not turn patient onto flailed side

Understand that endotracheal tube (p. 276) or tracheostomy (p. 278) may be ordered

Place on continuous mechanical ventilation (p. 281) as ordered

　Positive-pressure ventilator

　Volume-cycled ventilator

　Respirations may be controlled by ventilator

Understand that chest tubes may be ordered (p. 274)

Monitor BP, P, and R q1h to 2h and prn for hemodynamic and respiratory changes

Auscultate breath sounds q1h to 2h and prn for adventitious or decreased sounds

Report decreased or absent breath sounds to physician

Perform oropharyngeal suctioning prn *to maintain patent airway and maximize lung expansion*

Monitor ABGs as ordered; report changes in Po_2 or $Paco_2$ of >10 mm Hg

Turn and reposition patient q2h to 4h and prn to provide comfort and skin care

Maintain body alignment

Assist and teach patient to deep breathe q2h to 4h and prn in absence of tracheostomy or endotracheal tube

Continue acute care management but decrease frequency of nursing functions as patient's condition improves

Administer IPPB with humidification as ordered

Assist and teach patient to use incentive spirometer as ordered

Expected Outcome

Maintains an effective breathing pattern

　Normal rate, rhythm, and depth of respirations

　Decreased dyspnea

　Blood gases within normal range

　Breath sounds clear

▼Chest pain, related to trauma

Assess for verbal and nonverbal signs of pain: rate pain on 1 to 10 scale

Manage pain as indicated; assess effectiveness of pain relief measure(s)

Prepare for possible intercostal nerve block

Establish means of communication of pain

　Call bell within reach

　Pad and pencil or Magic Slate

Explain all procedures thoroughly, using calm, reassuring voice

Expected Outcome

Experiences decreased pain as evidenced by the following:

　Verbalization of pain relief

　Relaxed facial expression and body positioning

　Improved breathing pattern

　Increased activity

PATIENT/FAMILY TEACHING

Disease process

　Assess level of understanding regarding disorder,

causes, treatment, and procedures; identify fears and misconceptions

Discuss symptoms to report to physician

　URI

　SOB

　Persistent cough

　Persistent chest pain

Activity: explain importance of exercising to tolerance; avoid overexertion, excessive sports and activities, and heavy lifting

Medication

　Discuss medications: name, dosage, time of administration, purpose, and side effects

　Explain need to avoid taking over-the-counter medications without physician approval

DISCHARGE/HOME CARE PLANNING

Explain importance of ongoing outpatient care

Monitor exercise and rest periods to increase strength

■ RESPIRATORY FAILURE

Inability of the respiratory system to maintain normal oxygenation of blood (hypoxia, Pao_2 < 60 mm Hg) or elimination of carbon dioxide ($Paco_2$ > 45 mm Hg) resulting from problems with ventilation, diffusion, or perfusion

Type I Hypoxemia without hypercapnia

Type II Hypoxemia and hypercapnia

Type III Hypoventilation causing hypercapnia

ASSESSMENT

SUBJECTIVE DATA

Difficulty breathing

Headache

Fear of suffocation, anxiety

Fatigue

OBJECTIVE DATA

Respiratory distress

　Nasal flaring

　Tachypnea or bradypnea

　Retractions—accessory and intercostal

　Use of accessory muscles of respiration

　Hyperventilation

　Dyspnea

Labored breathing

　Air hunger

　Diaphoresis

　Cyanosis

Breath sounds

　Crackles

　Rhonchi

　Wheeze

Skin

　Pallor

　Cyanosis

　Clammy

　Cool

　Plethora

Increased respiratory secretions
Altered LOC
    Early indicators
        Restlessness
        Headache
        Changes in mental status
    Intermediate indicators
        Confusion
        Lethargy
    Late indicator
        Coma
Impaired motor function; asterixis
Papilledema
Cardiovascular
    Tachycardia
    Hypertension
    Dysrhythmias
        Atrial
        Ventricular
        Tachycardia
Decreased urinary output

DIAGNOSTIC TESTS
ABGs
    Hypoxia
        Mild: Pao_2 < 80 mm Hg
        Moderate: Pao_2 < 60 mm Hg
        Severe: Pao_2 < 40 mm Hg
    Increased or decreased $Paco_2$, depending on stage of
        failure
Chest x-ray examination: documents underlying
    pathology or progressive disease process
Hemodynamic findings: type I—increased PCWP
ECG
    May show evidence of right-side heart strain
    Dysrhythmias

POTENTIAL COMPLICATIONS
ARDS
Dysrhythmia
Deterioration from type I to type II
Cardiac failure
Barotrauma

MULTIDISCIPLINARY MANAGEMENT
THERAPEUTIC MANAGEMENT
Oxygen therapy
    Low-flow oxygen delivery: nasal cannula, catheter,
        face mask, partial rebreathing mask with
        reservoir bag
    Mechanical ventilatory support with constant positive
        airway pressure (CPAP) or PEEP
    Nebulized inhalation
    Chest physiotherapy
    Hemodynamic/cardiac monitoring
    Parenteral therapy
    Medications
        Bronchodilators
        Steroids
    Nutritional support as needed

PATIENT PROBLEMS—NURSING DIAGNOSES/INTERVENTIONS

▼ Ineffective breathing pattern related to decreased lung expansion

Assess rate, depth, and quality of respirations, breathing pattern, and use of accessory muscles

Assess vital signs and LOC qh and prn: changes in LOC is one of first signs of acute respiratory failure (ARF)

Be aware that endotracheal tube may be inserted or tracheostomy done (see p. 276) if $Paco_2$ is > 50 mm Hg or Pao_2 is < 60 mm Hg

Administer oxygen with assisted ventilation and humidification as ordered *to correct hypoxia and liquefy secretions*

Monitor and record ABGs as indicated: assess for downward trend in Pao_2 or upward trend in $Paco_2$

Be aware that continuous mechanical ventilation (see p. 281) is indicated if $Paco_2$ is > 60 mm Hg, $Paco_2$ increases at a rate of 5 mm Hg or more per hour, Pao_2 cannot be maintained at 60 mm Hg or higher, patient manifests increased fatigue or mental depression, or secretions become difficult to control

Auscultate breath sounds qh for adventitious or decreased sounds

Maintain bed rest with head of bed elevated 30 to 45 degrees *to optimize breathing*

Encourage coughing and deep breathing; assist patient to splint chest during coughing *to optimize breathing and removal of secretions*

Instruct patient to use pursed-lip and diaphragmatic breathing *to reduce work of breathing*

Expected Outcome
Maintains an effective breathing pattern
    Normal rate, rhythm, and depth of respirations
    Decreased dyspnea
    Blood gases within normal range

▼ Ineffective airway clearance related to obstructed airway and poor ventilation secondary to retention of secretions

Assess rate and quality of respirations and use of accessory muscles

Auscultate breath sounds q2h for adventitious or decreased sounds

Assess, monitor, and record amount, consistency, and color of secretions: report changes to physician

Assist and teach patient to turn, cough, and deep breathe *to maximize breathing*

Encourage use of incentive spirometry (see p. 327)

Instruct patient in controlled coughing techniques

Position patient *to maximize breathing*

Assist and teach patient to perform postural drainage as ordered *to mobilize secretions*

Administer oxygen therapy as indicated *to correct hypoxia*

Provide airway humidification *to liquefy secretions*

Maintain adequate fluid intake *to liquefy secretions and prevent dehydration*

Suction secretions if necessary

   Use sterile technique

   Hyperoxygenate and/or hyperinflate patient's lungs for four or five breaths before and after procedure

Observe cardiac monitors for dysrhythmias during procedure

Administer medications as ordered

   Bronchodilators

   Mucolytic agents

Expected Outcome

Maintains a patent airway as evidenced by the following:

   Improved breath sounds

   Normal rate and depth of respirations

   Ability to expectorate secretions

   Blood gases within normal range

▼ Impaired gas exchange related to ventilation-perfusion abnormalities secondary to hypoventilation

Assess for signs and symptoms of hypoxia and hypercapnia

Assess BP, P, apical pulse, and LOC qh and prn; report changes in LOC

Monitor and record serial ABGs, *assessing for upward trend in Paco_2 or downward trend in Pao_2*

Assist with administration of mechanical ventilation as indicated; assess need for CPAP or PEEP

Auscultate for diminished breath sounds qh *for adventitious or decreased sounds*

Review serial chest x-ray examination, noting improvement or deterioration

Monitor cardiac rhythm for dysrhythmias

Administer parenteral fluids as ordered *to maintain hydration*

Administer drugs as ordered

   Bronchodilators

   Antibiotics

   Steroids

Evaluate ADLs in relation to decreased oxygen demands

Expected Outcome

Maintains adequate gas exchange

   Lungs clear

   Usual skin color

   Blood gases within normal range for predicted age

▼ Anxiety/fear related to perceived and actual biologic threat (inability to breathe)

Assess level of anxiety (mild, moderate, severe)

Encourage patient and family to verbalize fears and concerns and ask questions regarding procedures and condition

Explain procedures and treatments using simple sentences

Instruct patient on energy conservation techniques

   Pursed-lip breathing

   Diaphragmatic breathing

Use calm, reassuring manner

Monitor vital signs

Assess to determine whether significant other's participation in care relieves anxiety

Reassure patient that he or she will not be left alone

Describe and point out alarms to patient and significant other(s) and explain that these alarms will alert staff to any problems

Answer any alarms immediately

Expected Outcomes

Anxiety level is reduced

Appears calm and relaxed

Able to verbalize fear

Additional Nursing Diagnoses to Consider

Infection risk related to invasive procedures, inadequate primary defenses, chronic disease

Sleep pattern disturbance related to sensory alteration: illness, disrupted circadian rhythms

■ ADULT RESPIRATORY DISTRESS SYNDROME (ARDS)

Nonspecific result of acute injury to the lung, characterized by a group of symptoms that include decreased compliance of the lung, noncardiac pulmonary edema, and refractory hypoxemia (Fig. 5-7); etiology is diverse and includes shock, chest trauma, aspiration, fat embolism, and massive viral pneumonia; end result is a uniform hyaline membrane development that leads to gas exchange abnormalities; mortality is 50% to 60%

ASSESSMENT

SUBJECTIVE DATA

Difficulty breathing

Fear of suffocation or death

Anxiety

OBJECTIVE DATA

Early phase

   Dyspnea

   Tachypnea

   Color

      Pallor

      Cyanosis

   Diaphoresis

Breath sounds

   Crackles

   Wheezes

   Restlessness

   Cough

   Clear breath sounds

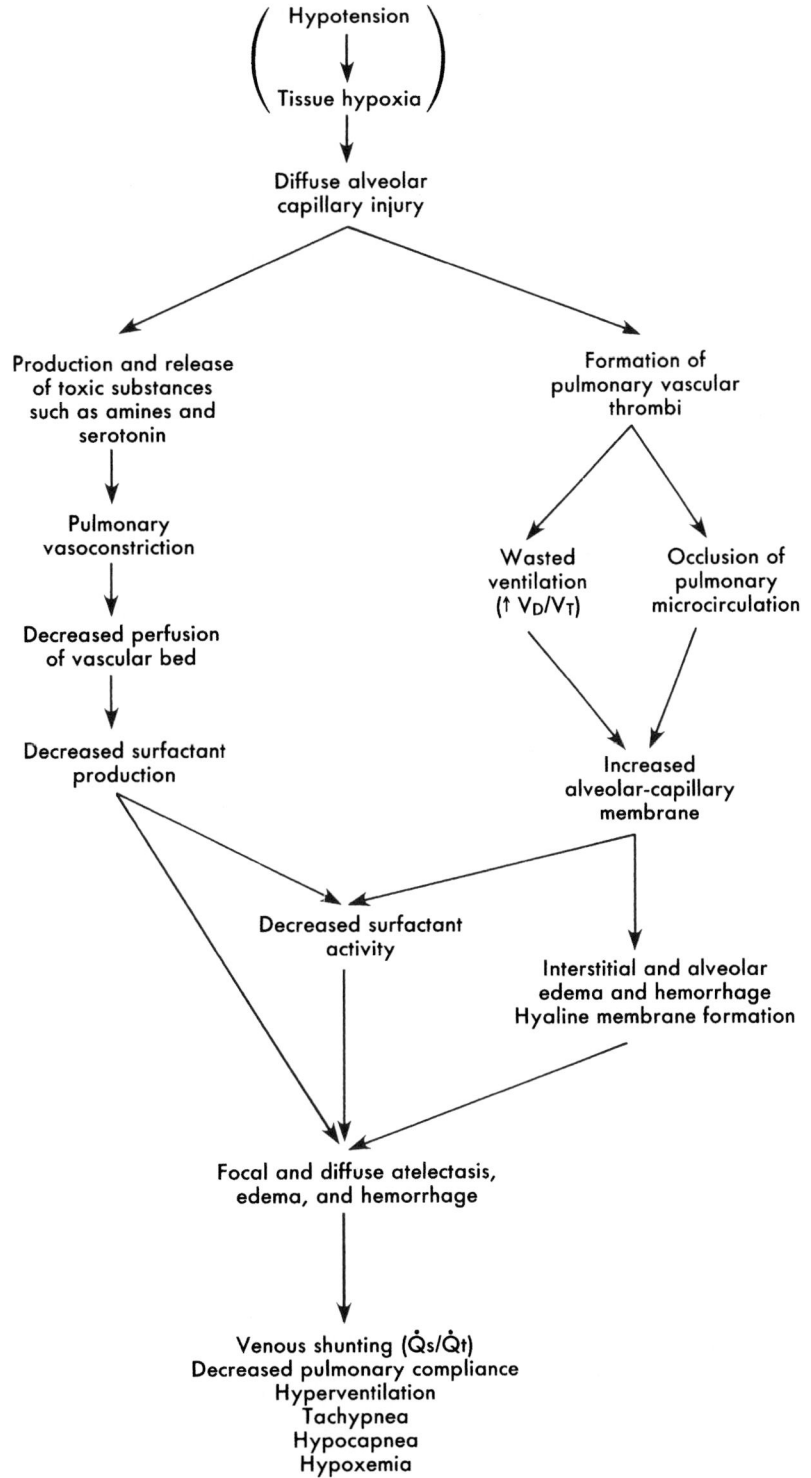

Fig. 5-7   Proposed pathogenesis for ARDS.
(From Thompson JM et al: Clinical nursing, *ed 3, St Louis, 1993, Mosby.)*

Late phase
    Grunting respirations
    Use of accessory muscles of respiration
    Severe dyspnea
    Rhonchi
Tachycardia
Confusion

DIAGNOSTIC TESTS
ABGs
    Decreased Pao_2 that is unresponsive to increasing FIo_2
    Decreased $Paco_2$ initially; then elevated $Paco_2$ in later
        stages
    pH initially > 7.45 mm Hg; as ARDS worsens,
        pH < 7.35 mm Hg

CBC
Chest x-ray examination
  Early: normal
  Late
    Diffuse bilateral pulmonary infiltrates
    "White out" on x-ray film, giving ground-glass appearance
Pulmonary artery pressures (PAP, PCWP)
  Early: normal
  Late: elevated ($\leq$18 mm Hg)
Pulmonary function tests
  Decreased VC, MV, FRC
  Decreased pulmonary compliance of $>$ 50 m/cm H_2O
Increased shunt fraction (Qs-Qt) $>$ 15% to 20% (normal 3% to 4%)
Increased lactic acid levels

POTENTIAL COMPLICATIONS
Dysrhythmias
Low CO
Renal failure
Infection/sepsis
Barotrauma
Disseminated intravascular coagulation (DIC)

MULTIDISCIPLINARY MANAGEMENT
THERAPEUTIC MANAGEMENT
Oxygen therapy
Intubation with ventilator support; use of CPAP, PEEP
Parenteral therapy
Nutritional support
Medications
  Sedation
  Steroids
  Heparin
  Diuretics
  Antibiotics
Cardiovascular support
  Cardiac monitor
  Hemodynamic monitoring
Nitric oxide
Kinetic therapy
  Kinetic treatment tables
  Air-fluidized turning beds

PATIENT PROBLEMS—NURSING DIAGNOSES/INTERVENTIONS

▼ Impaired gas exchange related to ventilation/perfusion abnormalities

See Respiratory failure (see p. 268)
See standard of care for primary condition
Assess and monitor rate, quality, and depth of respirations
Assess for signs of respiratory distress
Auscultate breath sounds for crackles and wheezes
Place patient on volume-cycled ventilator with PEEP or CPAP as ordered; PEEP is contraindicated in patients with COPD
Administer oxygen therapy, monitoring FIO_2

Assess ABGs; monitor for increases or decreases of Pao_2 and $Paco_2$
Monitor lactic acid levels
Administer parenteral fluids and electrolytes as ordered by physician
Monitor BP, P, and R qh; assess LOC qh and prn
Suction secretions if crackles or rhonchi are present
Administer corticosteroids and diuretics as ordered
Assess PAP and PCWP qh
Measure and record urinary output qh
Maintain bed rest with head of bed elevated 30 to 45 degrees *to maximize breathing*
Reposition from side to side q1h to 2h

Expected Outcome
Maintains adequate gas exchange as evidenced by the following:
  Return to baseline: LOC, skin color, respirations
  Blood gases within acceptable range

▼ Ineffective airway clearance related to excessive secretions secondary to interstitial edema

Assess and monitor rate and quality of respirations and use of accessory muscles
Assess characteristics of secretions; report changes to physician
Auscultate for breath sounds qh *to determine presence of adventitious or decreased sounds*
Review serial chest x-ray examinations to assess improvement
Assist and teach patient to turn, cough, and deep breathe if crackles or rhonchi are auscultated
Suction secretions as indicated to maintain patent airway
  If patient is intubated, hyperoxygenate and hyperinflate patient's lung for four or five breaths before and after procedure
  Observe cardiac monitor during suctioning procedure *for dysrhythmias caused by hypoxia*
Assist and teach patient to perform postural drainage as ordered *to mobilize secretions*
Administer bronchodilators and expectorants as ordered

Expected Outcome
Airway is patent
  Normal rate, rhythm, and depth of respirations
  Breath sounds clear
  Secretions are diminished/absent

Additional Nursing Diagnoses to Consider
Altered nutrition: less than body requirements related to insufficient intake versus increased metabolic demand
Activity intolerance related to fatigue of breathing
See standard of care for primary condition

DISCHARGE/HOME CARE PLANNING
Assess for lung damage as a sequela of ARDS to determine need for respiratory equipment including oxygen for home use

■ THORACOTOMY, LOBECTOMY, PNEUMONECTOMY

thoracotomy: Surgical incision of the chest wall
lobectomy: Removal of one or more lobes of the lung
pneumonectomy: Removal of an entire lung

PREOPERATIVE CARE
See general preoperative care/teaching

POSTOPERATIVE ASSESSMENT
SUBJECTIVE DATA
Difficulty breathing
Chest pain
Tenderness at chest tube insertion site

OBJECTIVE DATA
Patent airway
Respiratory distress
Labored breathing
Use of accessory muscles of respiration
Tachypnea
Shallow respirations
Dyspnea
Tachycardia
Breath sounds
   Present/absent
   Crackles, rhonchi
Elevated temperature
Hemoptysis
Crepitus
Cyanosis
Mediastinal shift
Incision
   Redness
   Pain
   Swelling
   Drainage
Arm contracture: operative side

DIAGNOSTIC TESTS
Chest x-ray examination
ABGs
ECG

POTENTIAL COMPLICATIONS
Pulmonary embolism
Pulmonary edema
Hemorrhage
Atelectasis
Tension pneumothorax
Infection
Bronchopleural fistula

MULTIDISCIPLINARY MANAGEMENT
THERAPEUTIC MANAGEMENT
O_2 therapy
Intubation and ventilator support
NPO until stable
Fluid and electrolyte therapy

Medications: analgesics
Chest tube insertion

PATIENT PROBLEMS—NURSING DIAGNOSES/INTERVENTIONS

▼ Ineffective breathing pattern related to pain secondary to surgical incision

Assess and monitor respiratory rate; note use of accessory muscles
Assess chest symmetry for mediastinal shift, paradoxic respirations, or splinting caused by pain
Assess severity and quality of pain: rate on a pain scale 1 to 10
Administer oxygen as ordered *to treat hypoxia*
Elevate head of bed 60 to 90 degrees *to facilitate maximal breathing*
Assist and teach patient to turn, cough, and deep breathe qh *to promote full lung expansion and promote drainage*
   Do not turn to unaffected side when pneumonectomy is done
   Pad area around chest tube when turned to operative side
   Splint chest to assist with coughing
   Administer IPPB as ordered
   Assist and teach patient to use incentive spirometer
Provide emotional support
Auscultate breath sounds q2h; report diminished or absent breath sounds on unaffected side to physician
Monitor ABGs
Check function of chest tube: note tidaling in the water-seal chamber, prevent dependent loops in tubing
Administer pain medications as indicated
Monitor for signs of gastric distension that may occur secondary to anesthesia or swallowing

Expected Outcomes
Maintains an effective breathing pattern: normal rate, rhythm, and depth of respirations
   Decreased dyspnea
   Blood gases within acceptable range
   Clear breath sounds

▼ Impaired physical mobility (arm on affected side) related to incisional pain and edema

Consult with physical therapy department to obtain ROM exercises *to prevent stiffness and ankylosis of shoulder on side of chest tube*
Assist and teach patient to exercise to tolerance
   Ambulate as ordered *to prevent thrombosis*
   Plan rest periods q1h to 2h
Begin ROM exercises, starting with passive and progressing to active
Encourage patient to rotate arm 360 degrees as ordered
Document progress
Medicate for pain as needed

Expected Outcome

Demonstrates full range of motion of affected side by discharge date; able to rotate arm in full 360-degree circles

PATIENT/FAMILY TEACHING

Disease process

Assess level of understanding regarding surgical procedure

Explain need to avoid tobacco use

Explain that some numbness, pain, or heaviness in operative area is expected; it is caused by interruption of intercostal nerves and is usually temporary

Explain need to avoid persons with URIs

Discuss symptoms to report to physician: persistent dyspnea, cough, elevated temperature, URI, redness, pain, swelling, drainage from incision

Activity

    Explain importance of exercising to tolerance

        Increase amount of exercise gradually

            Adjust activities according to degree of fatigue experienced

            Plan rest periods

Medications

    Discuss medications: name, dosage, time of administration, purpose, and side effects

    Explain need to avoid taking over-the-counter medications without physician approval

DISCHARGE/HOME CARE PLANNING

Explain need to continue coughing and deep breathing qid at home

Monitor gradual increase of exercise program and rest periods

Assess for URI or influenza in family members; encourage vaccinations

Explain importance of ongoing outpatient care

Ensure that patient and significant other(s) demonstrate care of incision

■ CHEST TUBES

Drainage tubes placed in the pleural space and attached to a water-seal drainage system and/or suction to remove air and/or fluid to allow expansion of the affected lung and reestablish negative pressure

Indications: pneumothorax/hemothorax, pleural effusion, empyema, postoperative thoracotomy

ASSESSMENT
OBSERVATIONS/FINDINGS
Patient

Chest drainage
    Amount
    Color
    Character
Dyspnea
Labored breathing
Tachypnea

Tachycardia

Nonsymmetric chest expansion

Breath sounds on affected side
    Diminished
    Absent
    Crackles
    Rhonchi
Crepitus

Equipment

Patency of tube(s) and water-seal drainage system

Continuous fluctuation of water or "tidaling" in water-seal drainage system

Water level in water-seal drainage system

Stability and security of water-seal drainage system

Amount of added suction applied to water-seal drainage system

Ensure all tubing connections are securely attached and taped

ONGOING CARE
Patient

Position patient on affected side with head of bed elevated 45 to 60 degrees after insertion of chest tube

Explain purpose of chest tube(s) to alleviate anxiety

Monitor and record BP, T, P, and R q4h and prn

Monitor and record amount, color, and character of drainage q2h to 4h; report drainage in excess of 100 ml/hr to physician

Manage pain as indicated; assess effectiveness of pain control measure(s)

Check chest tube site(s) and surrounding area q2h to 4h for crepitus and air leaks

Assist and teach patient to turn, cough, and deep breathe q2h *to facilitate lung reexpansion*

    Splint chest when coughing

    Pad area around chest tube(s) when patient is turned to operative side

Assist and teach patient to perform active or passive ROM exercises to extremities q2h to 4h *to prevent thrombus*

Ambulate patient as indicated

Auscultate breath sounds q2h to 4h; report diminished breath sounds in unaffected lung to physician

Change dressing as ordered

Equipment

Tape connecting tubing and secure chest tube to thorax securely

Maintain pressure if patient is on added suction as ordered

Inspect tubing for kinking and obstruction

Keep water-seal drainage system lower than patient's chest at all times

Secure connecting tubing and chest tube(s) to avoid tension and allow freedom of movement

Observe fluctuation of water in water-seal drainage system; if patient is breathing spontaneously, fluid level rises during inhalation and falls during exhalation

Change water-seal drainage system as indicated; never allow drainage to fill collection unit

Have petroleum jelly gauze at bedside for emergency use

Do not clamp the chest tube unless closed water-seal drainage system breaks and the lung is nearly expanded; it can result in a tension pneumothorax

If the system is broken, submerge the end of the tube in a cup of sterile water until another system is set up

PATIENT/FAMILY TEACHING

See standard of care for primary condition

Ensure that patient and significant other(s) know and understand

Purpose of chest tube(s), function, and care

Importance of turning, coughing, and deep breathing

Importance of keeping closed water-seal drainage system below level of patient's chest when sitting or ambulating

Importance of not placing tension on chest tube(s)

Need to report difficulty in breathing and chest pain to nurse and/or physician

Ensure that patient understands importance of and demonstrates coughing and deep breathing

▎REMOVAL OF CHEST TUBE

INTERVENTIONS

Place patient in a sitting position

Instruct patient to take a deep breath and hold it until chest tube is removed

Place pressure dressing with antibiotic ointment or petroleum jelly gauze over chest wall wound

Instruct patient to breathe normally

Chest x-ray after chest tube removal

Contact physician for pneumothorax

Auscultate chest for breath sounds q4h for 24 hours

Monitor respirations and drainage from pressure dressing

PATIENT/FAMILY TEACHING

See standard of care for primary condition

Ensure that patient and significant other(s) know and understand

Importance of reporting any sudden chest pain, difficulty breathing, redness, pain, swelling of puncture site

ARTIFICIAL AIRWAYS

▎PHARYNGEAL AIRWAYS

Pharyngeal airways can help restore and maintain an open airway. They are particularly useful when using a bag-valve-mask ventilation device. The airway separates the tongue from the posterior pharyngeal wall, restoring and maintaining an open airway. Two types of pharyngeal airways are used in clinical practice: the oropharyngeal and the nasopharyngeal airway

▎ORAL (OROPHARYNGEAL) AIRWAY

An artificial airway that extends from the lips to the pharynx, displacing the tongue anteriorly; oral airway is usually temporary, removed once patient regains consciousness or when more permanent airway is required for ventilation (Fig. 5-8, A)

▎NASAL (NASOPHARYNGEAL) AIRWAY

An artificial airway that extends from the nares to the pharynx (Fig. 5-8, B)

ASSESSMENT
SUBJECTIVE DATA
Difficulty in breathing

Anxiety

OBJECTIVE DATA
LOC

Airway obstruction

Restlessness

Stridor

Labored breathing

Retractions

Intercostal

Suprasternal

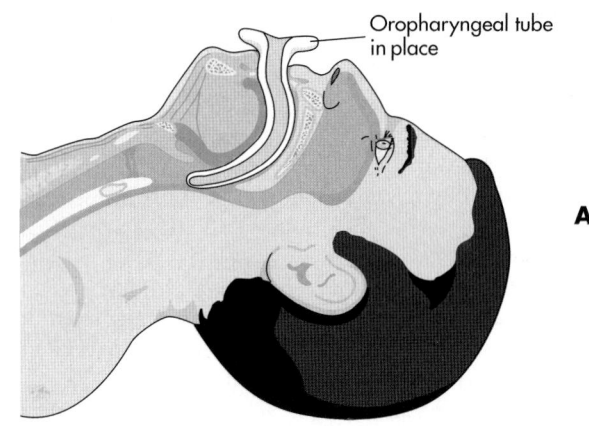

Oropharyngeal tube in place

A

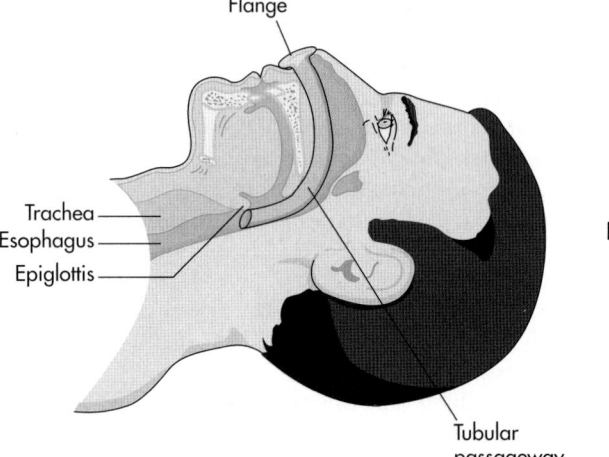

Flange

Trachea
Esophagus
Epiglottis

Tubular passageway

B

Fig. 5-8 **A,** Oropharyngeal airway. **B,** Nasopharyngeal airway. *(Beare PG, Myers JL:* Adult health nursing, *ed 3, St Louis, 1998, Mosby.)*

Supraclavicular
Nasal flaring
Cyanosis or pallor
Tachycardia
Breath sounds
Crackles
Rhonchi
Decreased
Secretion incrustations
Airway ports: patent or occluded
Oral airway
Gagging
Mouth infections
Oral lacerations or pressure sores
Position of tongue
Position of head and neck
Nasal airway
Mouth breathing
Pressure sores on nares
Position of head and neck
Complications: oral airways—airway obstruction,
aspiration

ONGOING CARE

GENERAL
Assess airway for patency and proper size of airway
Auscultate chest for breath sounds q2h and prn
Suction oropharynx or nasopharynx as indicated
Administer oxygen as ordered
Monitor pulse and respirations q4h and prn; note quality
of respirations
Administer oral hygiene q4h to 8h and prn

ORAL AIRWAY
Assess LOC
Choose correct oral airway size by measuring from the
angle of the jaw by the ear, following the natural curve
of the airway to the corner of the mouth
Inserting an oral airway can cause gagging, vomiting, or
laryngeal spasm; therefore oropharyngeal airways are
generally contraindicated in conscious and
semiconscious patients
Do not use if there is trauma to the oral cavity or
mandibular or maxillary areas of the skull
Do not use if a space-occupying legion or foreign object
obstructs the pharynx or oral cavity
If properly positioned, the tip of the oral airway will be
placed at the base of the tongue above the epiglottis
The flange of the airway must be positioned outside
the teeth
Incorrect placement can worsen the airway obstruction
Reposition airway q2h if flange contacts lips
Change airway every 24 hours
Apply water-soluble jelly to lips to prevent drying and
cracking

NASAL AIRWAYS
Choose correct oral airway size by measuring from the
earlobe to the tip of the nose

Generally the nasal airway is indicated in patients that
cannot tolerate an oropharyngeal airway, or when you
cannot separate the jaw
Do not use if there is trauma to the nasal region or if nasal
passages are obstructed by lesions or foreign objects
Lubricate the tip of the airway with water-soluble jelly
before insertion
Tilt head slightly back before insertion; insert *gently,* with
twisting motion if needed; do not use force
If resistance is met during insertion, try the other side
Once airway is inserted, ensure placement by listening to
breath sounds; try visualizing the tip of the airway
above the uvula using a tongue depressor
Change airway every 8 hours, alternating nares if possible
to prevent necrosis

REMOVAL OF AIRWAY
Assess LOC
Suction before removal
Remain with patient for 15 minutes after removal
Assess for any signs of respiratory distress
Monitor vital signs, noting any changes in rate and quality
of respirations
Auscultate chest for breath sounds q15 min to 30 min ×
3, then q2h to 4h as ordered

PATIENT/FAMILY TEACHING
Explain purpose of airway as indicated

■ ENDOTRACHEAL TUBE

*An artificial airway that extends from the nose or
mouth into the trachea (Fig. 5-9)*

*Endotracheal intubation is a preferred method of se-
curing the airway. In general, endotracheal tubes are required in cases of impending/actual airway compromise,
respiratory failure, or a need to maintain and protect the
airway. Endotracheal tubes maintain a patent airway, facilitate suctioning, ventilation, oxygenation, and provide
a route for administering drugs (see Fig. 5-9)*

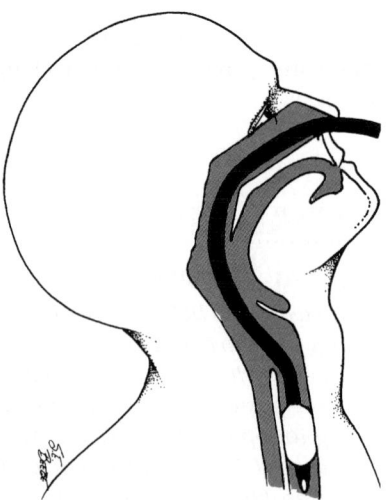

Fig. 5-9 Endotracheal tube.

INDICATIONS

Upper airway obstruction
Prevent aspiration
Remove airway secretions
Facilitate mechanical and spontaneous ventilation

INTUBATION CONSIDERATIONS

The airway must be inserted by a health care
    provider who has been trained and demonstrates
    proficiency in inserting, maintaining endotracheal
    tubes
Attempts to intubate must never interfere with providing
    adequate ventilation and oxygenation
Adequate ventilation and oxygenation must be provided
    between intubation attempts
Intubation attempts should never last longer than 20 to
    30 seconds
The airway cuff should be tested before intubation
Use of a water-soluble gel on the tip may ease tube
    advancement in the airway
Once the tube is place, the cuff should be inflated to a
    minimum occlusion volume. The pressure in the cuff
    should not exceed 20 to 25 mm Hg or 24 to 30 cm
    H_2O
Tube size (average adult) 7.5 to 9.0 mm

ASSESSMENT
OBJECTIVE DATA/FINDINGS
Patient
After insertion

Correct position of tube: assess for presence of bilateral
    breath sounds
Incorrect placement
    Right mainstem bronchus: unilateral (right) breath
        sounds; decreased breath sounds on left
    Carina: persistent coughing
    Esophagus: absent breath sounds
    Respiratory distress: cyanosis, tachypnea, restlessness,
        tachycardia, decreased Pao_2, increased $Paco_2$
Crackles
Rhonchi over large airways
LOC
Pressure sores/infection on nares, ears, lips
Anxiety
Equipment
    Tube placement should be assessed by chest x-ray
        showing the tip of the tube to be 2 to 3 cm above
        the carina
    Mode of ventilation and humidification per
        order

Potential Complications

Tracheal injury
    Tracheal ulceration
    Tracheal bronchial fistula
Aspiration
Dysrhythmias
Gag reflex
Pressure sores on nares, ears, lips
Airway obstruction

ONGOING CARE

Maintain patent airway
    Auscultate chest for breath sounds qh; report
        decreased or absent breath sounds to physician
    Suction secretions when crackles and/or rhonchi over
        large airways are heard
        Observe color of aspirate: if purulent or colored,
            obtain specimen for culture
        Irrigate with normal saline solution if ordered *to
            liquefy secretions*
    Check position of tube q½h to 1h *to prevent slippage
        into right or left mainstem bronchus;* average adult
        tube is placed at 25- to 26-mark at lips
    Obtain chest x-ray examination after insertion *to
        ascertain position of tube*
    Keep hand-held resuscitator with adaptor at bedside
Assess respirations for quality and rate qh
Be aware that respirations are usually maintained on a
    continuous mechanical ventilator
Use air or oxygen blow-by if indicated
Be certain cuff is inflated while patient is on ventilator
    Maintain inflated cuff with either a minimal leak or
        minimal occlusion volume technique
    Check cuff pressure: it should not exceed 20 mm Hg
Deflate cuff when patient is off ventilator for long
    periods; suction mouth and trachea before deflating
    cuff
Monitor ABGs as indicated
Assess LOC qh; establish means of communication if
    patient is conscious
    Call bell within reach
    Pad and pencil, Magic Slate, or communication board
        at bedside
Provide emotional support; explain all procedures
Administer oral hygiene q1h to 2h
Clean nares gently around endotracheal tube q8h and
    prn; use cotton-tipped applicator with saline solution;
    apply water-soluble lubricant to nares
Provide oropharyngeal airway or bite-block if patient
    bites on endotracheal tube
Apply soft restraints as necessary if patient is restless
Provide humidification to endotracheal tube when
    patient is off ventilator

◼ CARE DURING/AFTER EXTUBATION

ASSESSMENT
OBJECTIVE DATA/FINDINGS

LOC
Gag reflex
Respiratory distress
Laryngeal spasm
    Dyspnea
    Noisy breathing
    Use of abdominal or accessory muscles

ONGOING CARE

Assess whether patient is able to maintain spontaneous
    respirations at a rate sufficient to maintain normal
    ABGs

Auscultate chest for breath sounds: note adventitious or diminished sounds

Assess LOC: change in LOC is early sign of hypoxia

Elevate head of bed 45 to 90 degrees *to maximize breathing*

Preoxygenate and hyperinflate patient's lungs for four or five breaths

Suction oropharynx and/or nasopharynx *to maintain patency and remove secretions*

Suction endotracheal tube *to maintain patency and remove secretions*

Instruct patient to take a deep breath

Deflate cuff at peak of deep breath

Remove tube quickly as patient exhales, using a smooth, slightly downward motion

Administer humidified oxygen

Instruct patient to cough and deep breathe

Auscultate chest for breath sounds q15min × 4, then q1h to 2h; report absent or diminished breath sounds to physician

Monitor BP, R, and apical pulse q15min for × 4, then q1h to 2h

Monitor ABGs as ordered

Assess for signs of stridor and/or laryngospasm

Prepare for reinsertion of endotracheal tube if laryngospasm occurs or if patient is unable to maintain adequate respiratory rate

Administer oral hygiene

Provide emotional support

Remain with patient as much as possible

Explain that sore throat, hoarseness, and dysphagia are common after extubation and will resolve in a few days

Encourage patient to minimize talking for a few hours

Provide a pad and pencil, Magic Slate, or communication board

Have call light within reach

PATIENT/FAMILY TEACHING

Explain all procedures whether patient appears conscious or not; orient patient to date, time, and place

Explain why patient is unable to talk and that it is only a temporary condition

Establish means of communication

Call bell within reach

Pad and pencil, Magic Slate, or communication board at bedside

Emphasize importance of turning and coughing up secretions

■ TRACHEOSTOMY

Insertion of a tube into the trachea through a surgical incision (tracheotomy) (Fig. 5-10)

PREOPERATIVE CARE

See General preoperative care/teaching (p. 9)

Include as much of the following as possible:

Provide emotional support

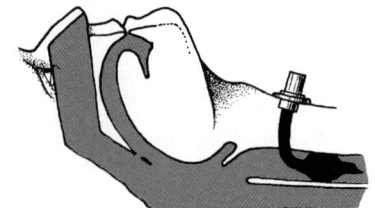

Fig. 5-10 Tracheostomy tube with cuff.

Explain purpose of tracheostomy

Remain with patient as much as possible

Speak calmly and act unhurried

Involve family or significant other(s) in care and instructions

Demonstrate: tracheostomy tube

Cleaning equipment

Suctioning equipment; explain suctioning procedure

Determine whether patient can read and write English or another language

Determine whether patient can hear

Explain that patient will not be able to talk postoperatively

Have pad and pencil, Magic Slate, or communication board at bedside

Have picture cards available if patient is unable to write

Explain that patient may be in critical care area after operation; tour critical care area with patient and family

Review means of contacting nurse

Call light

Tap bell

POSTOPERATIVE ASSESSMENT
OBJECTIVE DATA/FINDINGS
Patient

Position of tracheostomy

Cuff

Present

Inflated

Deflated

Bilateral expansion of chest

Sputum

Amount

Character

Stoma

Pain

Swelling

Drainage

Anxiety

Fear of suffocation

Helplessness

Hemorrhage

Airway obstruction
- Restlessness
- Tachycardia
- Tachypnea
- Noisy respirations
- Wheezing
- Stridor
- Pallor
- Cyanosis

Subcutaneous or mediastinal emphysema
Pneumothorax
Injury to thyroid, laryngeal nerve
Complications of tracheostomy
- Stomal infection
- Stomal hemorrhage
- Excessive cuff pressure

Infection
- Elevated temperature
- Purulent aspirate

Equipment

Tracheostomy tube
- Size
- Type: cuffed versus uncuffed
- Tubes used for weaning from mechanical ventilation
  - Fenestrate tube
  - Tracheostomy buttons

IMMEDIATE POSTOPERATIVE CARE

See Immediate general postoperative care (p. 10)
Maintain patent airway
- Administer humidification to tracheostomy *to liquefy secretions and prevent drying of trachea*
- Suction prn; need for suctioning is determined by auscultation of chest for breath sounds qh
  - Suction when crackles and rhonchi over large airways are heard
  - Use sterile technique when suctioning secretions
  - Hyperoxygenate and hyperinflate patient's lungs for four or five breaths before suctioning *to prevent hypoxia*
- Clean inner cannula (if present) q2h to 4h and prn
- Avoid occluding airway with bed linen or when turning patient
- Tape tracheostomy obturator to head of bed
- Have standby tracheostomy tube available: same size and type
- Have handheld resuscitator with adaptor at bedside

Elevate head of bed 45 to 60 degrees; prevent forward flexion of neck
- Remove pillow if necessary
- Place small towel under shoulder area

Administer oxygen or mechanical ventilation as ordered; see appropriate standard
If a cuffed tracheostomy tube is used
- Test pressure in inflated cuff q8h or as indicated; cuff pressure should remain <20 mm Hg
- Use a low-pressure, cuffed tube

Auscultate chest for breath sounds q2h to 4h; report diminished or absent breath sounds to physician

Monitor BP, P, R, and rectal temperature q4h for 48 hours, then qid
Maintain NPO
Assess stoma and neck q2h to 4h as indicated; report a constant ooze, subcutaneous emphysema, pulsation of tracheostomy tube
Assist and teach patient to turn, cough, and deep breathe q2h

ONGOING CARE

Continue with immediate postoperative care and decrease frequency of nursing functions as patient's condition improves
Maintain diet as ordered
- Assess swallowing ability
  - NOTE: Feedings may begin with nasogastric tube until swallowing ability returns
- Begin feedings with semisolid foods (e.g., gelatin)
- Inflate cuff before feedings and leave inflated for 30 minutes after each feeding
- Test swallowing reflex with gelatin; have suctioning equipment available
- Observe for signs of aspiration and tracheoesophageal fistula

Cleanse skin around stoma q4h and prn
- Wash with hydrogen peroxide
- Rinse with saline solution
- Pat dry
- Change and secure tracheostomy ties prn

Place 4 × 4 inch gauze under tracheostomy tube
Perform tracheostomy care
- Postintubation: q4h for 2 days
- Routine care: q8h and prn

Be aware that physician may change tracheostomy tube daily using progressively smaller sizes
If tracheostomy is permanent, begin to demonstrate tracheostomy care while patient watches in mirror
Establish means of communication
- Have pad and pencil, Magic Slate, or communication board available
- Avoid asking questions that require *yes* or *no* answers
- Wait for patient to write answer; do not anticipate end of sentence
- Read statements aloud
- Encourage patient to communicate feelings

Provide emotional support
- Encourage communication with significant other; help visitors and staff not to exclude patient from conversation or talk exclusively to one another
- Remain with patient as much as possible
- Answer call light promptly
- Deal with fear of suffocation and helplessness

Decannulate tracheostomy as ordered
- Be aware that a fenestrated tube may be used for decannulation process
- Partially plug tracheostomy tube
  - *Make sure cuff is deflated* throughout procedure
  - Observe patient for respiratory obstruction
- Progressively increase size of cork until tracheostomy is completely occluded; notify physician when

patient is able to tolerate complete occlusion of
tracheostomy for 24 hours
If tracheostomy is long term or permanent, provide
means of communication
Pad and pencil
Magic Slate or communication board
Laptop computer
Call light within reach
Tap bell
Initiate instruction on the following:
Care of tracheostomy and stoma; discuss and
demonstrate; provide mirror
Handwashing procedure
Suctioning procedure before tracheostomy care:
clean procedure, not sterile
Care of inner cannula: clean procedure, not sterile
Changing of tracheostomy ties
Cleansing skin around stoma bid
Use hydrogen peroxide
Rinse with water
Pat dry
Understand that patient may not be motivated to
participate initially
Have patient shower daily
Direct spray below neck
Cover tracheostomy with waterproof material

PATIENT/FAMILY TEACHING

Ensure the patient and significant other(s) know and
understand
Purpose of tracheostomy
Care of tracheostomy tube and stoma
Importance of clean not sterile technique; need to
wash hands before handling equipment: gloves not
necessary unless another person is cleaning
tracheostomy
Changing tracheostomy ties
Tracheostomy dressings are not recommended unless
excessive secretion occurs
Importance of reporting signs and symptoms of skin
irritation, infection, or changes in secretions
Humidification and infection control measures
Safety measures such as having an extra tracheostomy
tube and suction equipment available

DISCHARGE/HOME CARE PLANNING

Provide referral as necessary to the following:
Home health agency for follow-up care
Durable medical equipment company for required
equipment for home therapy: suction equipment,
humidifier, tracheostomy supplies
Diet
Maintain as ordered
Explain that tracheostomy tubes at home do not
usually have cuffs that need inflating during eating
Encourage patient to force fluids to 3000 ml/day
unless contraindicated *to help liquefy secretions*
ADLs
Explain need for daily shower; when showering use a

shower hose and direct spray below neck; avoid
getting soap into stoma
Instruct male patients to shave with electric razor or
safety razor; avoid getting lather into stoma
Encourage to exercise to tolerance; continue work,
hobbies, and activities except swimming; plan
regular rest periods as needed
Keep stoma covered at all times; wear clothing with high
necklines and scarves to protect against foreign
materials and warm air
Avoid areas with excessive dust, fumes, aerosols, smoke,
and powder
Avoid extremes in temperatures, which can irritate
tracheal mucosa
Wear medical alert identification indicating neck breather
for emergency situations
Avoid persons with URIs
Explain importance of ongoing outpatient care and
physician visits
Explain importance of covering stoma when coughing
and need to report persistent cough or change in color
of sputum to physician
Teach how to perform a *glottal stop* for secretion
removal: take a deep breath then momentarily occlude
tracheostomy tube opening; simultaneously cough and
move the finger from the opening; this substitutes for
the usual way intrathoracic pressure is increased to
move secretions into the trachea
Report any respiratory distress to physician
Discuss need to use commercial humidifier or pan of
water on stove to add comfort and prevent
encrustation; explain importance of changing water
daily to prevent growth of microorganisms
Explain the importance of not using tobacco and refer to
stop smoking groups as indicated
Teach name of medications, dosage, time of
administration, purpose, and side effects
Discuss the need to avoid taking over-the-counter
medications without physician approval
Demonstrate clean technique for tracheostomy care
Clean around stoma with mild soap and water as part
of hygiene
A pipe cleaner can be used to clean the inner cannula;
rinse with running tap water
For plastic tubes: use a clean bowl with half-strength
solution of hydrogen peroxide and tap water to
clean the tracheostomy tube
Demonstrate suctioning technique
Spontaneously breathing patient: three or four deep
breaths before and after suctioning is usually
sufficient for hyperoxygenation
Patients not immunocompromised may use clean
technique for suctioning
Describe care and cleaning of suction equipment
Rinse suction catheter and allow to dry thoroughly
between uses
Store in clean, self-sealing plastic bag
Catheters may be cleaned with hydrogen peroxide and
water and used for multiple days

After rinsing thoroughly in running water, soak in hydrogen peroxide 5 minutes, then rinse thoroughly

Place in boiling water 10 to 15 minutes and allow to air-dry on clean towel

Discard catheters when secretions cannot be completely removed

Assess body image, self-esteem, and sexuality and plan interventions as tolerated

■ PULSE OXIMETRY MONITORING

Pulse oximetry provides estimates of arterial oxyhemoglobin saturation (Sao$_2$) by utilizing wavelengths of light. It is a noninvasive monitor that provides trends and/or spot checks the oxygen saturation of functional hemoglobin (Fig. 5-11)

INDICATIONS

To monitor the adequacy of arterial oxyhemoglobin saturation

To monitor the response of arterial oxyhemoglobin saturation when administering therapeutic interventions

CONTRAINDICATIONS

If an ongoing need for the measurement of pH, Paco$_2$, total hemoglobin is present, this may be a relative contraindication to pulse oximetry

ASSESSMENT

OBJECTIVE DATA

Saturation of hemoglobin (Spo$_2$): normal 96% to 100%, however 95% is usually acceptable; an Sao$_2$ < 70% is life threatening

BP, P

Routine respiratory assessment (see Respiratory failure p. 268)

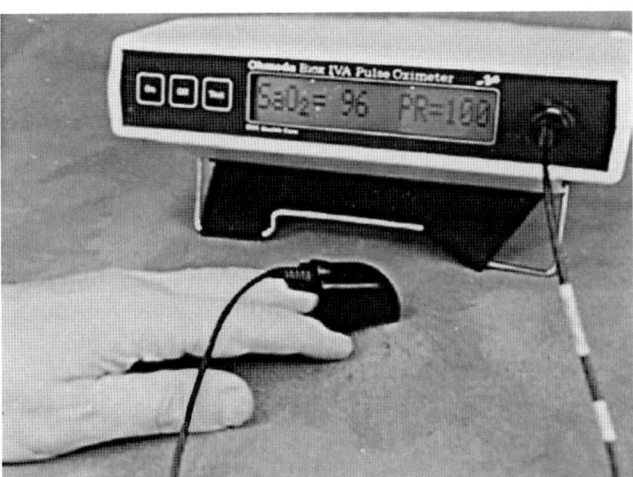

Fig. 5-11 Portable pulse oximeter displays oxygen saturation and pulse rate.
(Courtesy Ohmeda, Boulder, Colo.)

Activities that may positively or negatively affect oxygenation: suctioning, repositioning, changes in FIo$_2$, PEEP, medication, and clinical condition

ONGOING CARE

Identify type of probe/sensors (see Fig. 5-11) and select site by assessing area for warmth, capillary refill, and confirmation of arterial pulse; while finger is most commonly used, earlobe, toe, or external nares can be used as substitute

Place the window for the light source and the photodector directly opposite each other on each side of the arterial bed to ensure accuracy

Assess tissue at sensor site and rotate site q8h and prn to prevent tissue necrosis in hypoxemic patient

Set alarm limits and trouble-shoot according to specific patient needs

Shield the sensor from extreme light: heat lamps, procedure lights

Stress importance of not moving finger, because motion of finger may lead to false pulse rate and poor-quality wave forms

Remove nail polish or choose another site because it may interfere with light transmission

The pulse oximeter cannot distinguish if the hemoglobin is normal and thus can overestimate actual saturation

The pulse oximeter may not be accurate in people who are experiencing severe anemia

The pulse oximeter cannot determine accurate saturation when the pulse is weak or absent

PATIENT/FAMILY TEACHING

Discuss indications of pulse oximetry, use of equipment, and Spo$_2$ values expected

Explain alarms and problems or activities that can cause false alarming

■ CONTINUOUS MECHANICAL VENTILATION

A method of providing ventilatory support for those patients who are unable to spontaneously maintain adequate oxygenation of the blood, with or without carbon dioxide retention; two categories of ventilators are positive pressure (volume-cycled or pressure-cycled) and negative pressure (iron lung, cuirass), which is not commonly used; examples of time, volume-cycled, positive-pressure ventilators are Puritan-Bennett 7200, Siemann's Servo 300, Siemann's Servo 900C, Bear 1000, and Bird 8400ST. Volume-cycled ventilators include Bennett MA3 and the Bourns Bear 1 and 2. Pressure-cycled ventilators include the Bird Mark 7 and 8 and the Bennett PR2

INDICATION FOR VENTILATORY SUPPORT

Acute respiratory failure is the primary indication for the use of mechanical ventilation. There are six functional divisions of the respiratory system. If dysfunction occurs in any one division, it can cause respiratory failure. The divisions are:

1. Central nervous system
2. Peripheral nervous system
3. Chest wall
4. Muscles
5. Upper airway
6. Lung

MECHANICAL VENTILATION SHOULD BE CONSIDERED WHEN:

Pao_2 cannot be maintained above 50 torr by increasing the fraction of inspire oxygen (Fio_2)

$Paco_2$ rises above 50 torr and decreases the pH below 7.25

Effective spontaneous ventilation becomes ineffective and fatiguing to the patient (respiratory rate > 30/min or vital capacity < 20 ml/kg)

EXCEPTIONS

Patients with COPD may have compensated for $Pao_2 < 50$; use other indications for intubation

In cases of drug overdose, it may be necessary to intubate and ventilate early, based on suspicion of pending respiratory failure

MODES OF VENTILATORY SUPPORT

There are several modes of ventilatory support.
The health care provider determines which best meets the patient's needs. See Table 5-8 for modes of ventilatory support.

CARE OF PATIENT ON CONTINUOUS MECHANICAL VENTILATION

ASSESSMENT

SUBJECTIVE DATA

Apprehension
Anxiety
Dependence on ventilator
Difficulty in breathing

OBJECTIVE DATA

Position of airway
    Endotracheal tube
    Tracheostomy
Patency of airway
Hypoxemia
    Tachypnea
    Tachycardia
    Restlessness
    Anxiety (an early sign of hypoxemia)
    Diaphoresis
    Pallor
    Cyanosis
    Diminished, distant breath sounds
Breath sounds
    Crackles
    Rhonchi
Respiratory acidosis (acidemia)
    Decreased pH: <7.4 mm Hg
    Elevated $Paco_2$: >45 mm Hg
Respiratory alkalosis (alkalemia)
    Increased pH: >7.4 mm Hg

Table 5-8	Modes of Ventilatory Support	
Mode	**Description**
Continuous mandatory ventilation (CMV)	The application of positive pressure at the airway opening during *every* inspiration. Two major variations of CMV are based on whether the machine or patient initiates or triggers the breath
Control mode CMV (machine triggered)	Continuous mandatory ventilation in which the frequency of breathing is determined by the ventilator according to a preset cycling interval, *without* initiation by the patient
Assist/control mode CMV (machine- or patient-triggered)	Continuous mandatory ventilation in which the *minimum* frequency of breathing is predetermined by the ventilator controls, but the patient can trigger breaths at a faster rate
Intermittent mandatory ventilation (IMV)	Periodic ventilation with positive pressure, with the patient breathing spontaneously between breaths. As with CMV, these breaths may be machine-triggered only (control mode IMV) or machine or patient-triggered (synchronous IMV, SIMV)
Pressure support ventilation (PSV)	Patient-triggered, pressure-limited, flow-cycled ventilation designed to augment a spontaneously generated breath. The patient has primary control over the frequency of breathing, the inspiratory time, and the inspiratory flow
Continuous positive airway pressure (CPAP)	The maintenance of a pressure above atmospheric pressure at the airway opening throughout a spontaneous breathing cycle
High-frequency ventilation (HFV)	A form of positive-pressure ventilation provided at very rapid respiratory rates with a small tidal volume; usually used when high positive airway pressures aggravate lung injury

Modified from Scanlan CL, Wilkins RL, Stoller JK: Egan's fundamentals of respiratory care, ed 6, St Louis, 1994, Mosby.

Decreased Paco$_2$: <35 mm Hg
Pulse oximetry saturation $\leq$ 90%
Hypoxemia
Sputum
    Amount
    Color
    Consistency
  Atelectasis
Equipment
  Ventilation: mode (Boxes 5-8 and 5-9) and settings

POTENTIAL COMPLICATIONS

Disconnection from ventilator
Tracheal tube obstruction
Acid-base imbalance
Respiratory infection
Oxygen toxicity (time and dose related)
Fluid and electrolyte imbalance
Decreased CO
Pneumothorax
Barotrauma
GI bleeding

ACUTE CARE

Assess oxygenation status by monitoring and recording quality, rate, and depth of respirations; auscultate breath sounds q1h to 2 h
Assess for bilateral chest movement
Ensure that respirations are in phase with the ventilator
Maintain patent airway (see Care of Endotracheal Tube, p. 276; tracheostomy, p. 278)
  Suction prn; determine need for suctioning by auscultating chest for breath sounds qh; suction when crackles or rhonchi are present

Hyperoxygenate and hyperinflate lungs for four or five breaths before suctioning secretions
Suction patient with closed ventilation suction system
Monitor pulse oximetry saturation
Keep handheld resuscitator with adaptor and mask at bedside
Administer medications as ordered
  Sedatives
  Morphine sulfate
  Neuromuscular blocking agents
Monitor ABGs q shift or as indicated; allow 30 minutes after ventilation changes *to ensure equilibration*
Assess BP, R, and apical pulse q1h to 2h
Check rectal temperature q4h
Maintain position of optimal ventilation; elevate head of bed 45 to 90 degrees; turn q1h to 2h and prn, alternating postural drainage positions
Document ventilator settings q2 to q4h or as indicated; readjust as indicated
  FIO$_2$ (measure after suctioning): 60 mm Hg
  Sao$_2$ $\geq$ 90%
  Tidal volume (V$_T$): 8 to 10 ml/kg
  Airway cuff pressure
    Inspiratory flow: 40 to 60 L
    Sigh ventilation (if used): 1.5 to 2 $\times$ V$_T$
  Maintain temperature in inspiratory tubing between 89.6° and 95° F (32° and 35° C)
  Check ventilatory alarms
Obtain chest x-ray to confirm placement of tube
Administer parenteral fluids as ordered
Provide nutritional support
  Assess nutritional status daily
  Administer tube feedings, total parenteral nutrition (TPN) as ordered
Provide emotional support
  Answer call light promptly
  Establish means of communication: pad and pencil, Magic Slate, or communication board
  Allow patient sufficient time to communicate thoughts and feelings
  Maintain nonstressful environment

Box 5-8   Ventilation Equipment

CONTROL VARIABLES
Common parameters that can be manipulated by the ventilator are volume, flow, pressure, and time. Usually only one of the parameters is controlled during ventilation.
  For example, two common ventilators are:
1. Pressure-cycled positive-pressure ventilator: Delivers a flow of gas until a preset pressure is reached. The variable is volume of gas delivered.
2. Volume-cycled positive-pressure ventilator: Delivers a flow of gas until a predetermined volume is delivered. The variable is the pressure delivered.
  Modern technology has provided a means to manipulate mechanical ventilatory support by the control of the volume, flow, time, and/or pressure. The set parameters and documented data will depend on the type and mode of ventilation used.
  NOTE: Most ventilators deliver two types of breaths: spontaneous breaths (initiated and ended by the patient) and mandatory breath (can be initiated and/or terminated by the ventilator—also called a *machine breath*).

Box 5-9   Weaning Criteria

Discontinuing ventilatory support should be attempted with an agreed plan from a multidisciplinary approach.
  Common indicators include but are not limited to:
- Maximum inspiratory force (MIF) > 20-30 (−cm H$_2$O)
- Minute volume < 10 L/min
- Respiratory rate < 30 breaths/min
- Tidal volume > 5 mL/kg
- Vital capacity > 10-15 mL/kg
- Pao$_2$ (torr) > 60 on $\leq$ 0.40 oxygen
- Sao$_2$ (%) > 90% on $\leq$ 0.40 oxygen
- Paco$_2$ (torr) < 50
- pH > 7.35

Be calm, confident, and unhurried when caring for patient

Encourage communication with significant other(s)

ONGOING CARE: SUBACUTE

Continue with acute care and decrease frequency of nursing functions as patient's condition improves

Wean patient off respirator as ordered (see Box 5-9)

Explain weaning process thoroughly

Remain with patient during weaning process

Monitor respirations and apical pulse q5min to 15min after removal from ventilator

Place on ventilator immediately if respiratory distress occurs

Be prepared to repeat weaning process several times if necessary

CONVALESCENT CARE

See standard of care for primary condition

PATIENT/FAMILY TEACHING

Ensure that patient and significant other(s) know and understand

Purpose of ventilator

Importance of breathing with ventilator

Importance of coughing up secretions

Importance of artificial airway

Need to avoid placing any tension on airway; to never touch airway with hands

Need to communicate in writing

Technique for suctioning

Ventilator alarms and their implications

Use of manual resuscitator bag

ASSESSMENT AND CARE OF EQUIPMENT/DISCHARGE/HOME CARE PLANNING
GENERAL

Explain to patient/family that home ventilators are portable, easy to use, and small; home ventilation requires a great deal of commitment on the part of the family or significant other; refer to durable medical equipment company for equipment

Teach care of tracheostomy and suctioning; see Tracheostomy (p. 278)

Demonstrate ventilator connections, alarms, trouble-shooting, care, and cleaning

Teach how to drain and change tubing

Drain tubing to prevent fluid from entering lungs and partial obstruction of system

Properly draining and changing tubing is an infection-control measure

Demonstrate manual resuscitator bag and keep one at home in case of power failure

Activity

Teach and discuss importance of ROM exercises and chest mobility exercises if patient is unable to ambulate

Encourage patient to sit up in a chair as much as tolerated

Ambulation with assistance is possible with small, battery-powered ventilators placed on a small cart

Diet

Diet as ordered

Patient may be able to eat: check with physician for diet allowances; see Tracheostomy (p. 278)

If unable to eat, enteral or parenteral feedings are required

Assess body image, self-esteem, and sexuality and plan appropriate interventions

Refer to VNA or other home health agency for follow-up care

Refer family to support group for emotional support

Teach how to clean equipment and infection control techniques

EQUIPMENT

Ensure that patient/family understands care and management of equipment

Attached to gas source

Connecting tubing

Patent

Free of excess moisture

Air leaks

Cuff of endotracheal tube

Cuff of tracheostomy

Patent airway

Adequate humidification

Nebulizer

Heated humidification

Temperature of inspired gas

Settings as ordered

Total respiratory rate: should not be <12/min

Oxygen concentration: air-mix control

Inspiratory pressure control

Apnea control

Sensitivity control

ONGOING CARE

Maintain inspiratory rate and respiratory pressure as ordered

Patent airway

System free of leaks

Connective tubing patent and free of excessive moisture

Be aware that inspiratory, positive-pressure ventilators may not have alarm systems

Remain with patient as much as possible

Determine respiratory rate, oxygen concentration, and inspiratory pressure setting by ABGs

Establish flow sheet

Record ventilator settings

Record laboratory values

Maintain oxygen concentration as ordered; measure FIo_2 q8h and prn

Maintain respiratory rate as ordered

Measure tidal volume q8h and prn

Auscultate chest for breath sounds qh

Provide humidification

Make sure that equipment continues to cycle when cuff is deflated

Have patient sigh q15min or as ordered; use handheld resuscitator

Change connecting tubing, nebulizer, and humidification system q24h; replace with sterile equipment

VOLUME-CYCLED, POSITIVE-PRESSURE VENTILATOR

Delivers breathing gas at a predetermined volume; once the desired volume has been delivered, the ventilator will cycle and patient will passively exhale

ASSESSMENT AND CARE OF EQUIPMENT

Electrical system
  Plugged in
  Alarms on
Connecting tubing
  Patent
  Free of excess moisture
Air leaks
  Cuff of endotracheal tube
  Cuff of tracheostomy
Patent airway
Adequate humidification
  Heated humidification
  Nebulizer
Temperature of inspired gas
Settings as ordered
  Alarms
  Flow rate
  Inspiratory pressure
  Tidal volume (10 to 15 ml/kg body weight)
  PEEP
  CPAP
  Pressure support
  Ventilator rate: 10 to 16 breaths/min
  Oxygen concentration
  Sigh pressure
  Sigh volume
  Number of sighs per hour
  Ventilatory mode
    Control
    Assist
    Assist-controlled
    Synchronized intermittent mandatory ventilation (SIMV or IMV)
    Sensitivity
    Peak airway pressure (<40 cm H_2O)
    I : E ratio

ONGOING CARE

Maintain V_T as ordered
  Patent airway
  System free of leaks
  Connective tubing patent and free of excessive moisture
Determine ventilator settings by ABGs
Pulse oximetry and end tidal CO_2 monitors are excellent trending mechanisms

Establish flow sheet
  Record ventilator settings q2h
  Record laboratory values
Maintain oxygen concentration as ordered (determined by PaO_2); measure FIO_2 q8h and prn
Maintain respiratory rate as ordered
Provide heated humidification
Remove excessive water in tubing
Sigh pressure and volume if ordered
Avoid turning alarm system off
Measure V_T q8h and prn
Test alarm system q8h
Change connecting tubing, nebulizer, and humidification q48h; replace with sterile equipment

■ INTERMITTENT POSITIVE-PRESSURE BREATHING (IPPB)

intermittent positive-pressure ventilator: *A ventilator that delivers breathing gas until equilibrium is established between the patient's lungs and the ventilator; depends on pressure buildup in the patient's lungs rather than on time or volume; a valve mechanism shuts off the gas flow when the pressure has been reached and patient exhales passively; should be used only after less-expensive modalities have been tried*

PRETREATMENT ASSESSMENT
OBJECTIVE DATA/FINDINGS

Blood pressure
Pulse
Color
Respiratory effort
Breath sounds

PREPARATION

Observe BP and P before treatment
Auscultate chest for breath sounds
Place patient in sitting position
Prepare machine
  Secure all tubing connections
  Place medication or saline solution in nebulizer
  Set pressure and oxygen concentration as ordered
  Control nebulizer to produce fine mist

PREPROCEDURE TEACHING

Explain procedure and what is expected of patient
  Concentrate on using diaphragm
  Breathe at normal rate through mouth
  Allow machine to fill lungs to desired volume
  Prolong expiration
  Purse lips around mouthpiece

ASSESSMENT DURING TREATMENT
SUBJECTIVE DATA

Fatigue
Restlessness, nervousness
Chest pain

OBJECTIVE DATA
Respiratory rate
Chest expansion
Sudden respiratory distress
Hyperventilation
  Circumoral numbness
  Tingling of fingers
  Dizziness
Tachycardia
Function of equipment

ONGOING CARE
Take pulse one or two times during treatment
Remain with patient during initial treatment
Stop treatment if sudden respiratory distress or chest pain occurs
Have patient deep breathe slowly one or two times during treatment
Have patient cough one or two times during and after treatment
Check pressure gauge and adjust flow to avoid negative inspiratory pressure
Administer oral hygiene after treatment

PATIENT/FAMILY TEACHING
Ensure that patient and significant other know and understand
  Need to follow physician's instructions regarding use of IPPB
  Need to cough during and immediately after treatment
  Importance of using saline solution or medication in nebulizer
  Symptoms of respiratory distress to report to physician
  Need to stop treatment if dizziness, nervousness, chest pain, rapid pulse, or sudden respiratory distress occurs during treatment
  Symptoms of URI to report to physician
  Name of medication, dosage, time of administration, purpose, and side effects
  Need to avoid taking over-the-counter medications without physician approval

DISCHARGE/HOME CARE PLANNING
Ensure that patient and significant other(s) demonstrate
  Understanding of importance and purpose of treatments
  Preparation of machine for treatment
  Use of machine during treatment
  How to adjust pressure gauge and flow to avoid negative inspiratory pressure
  IPPB procedure
    Take pulse one or two times during treatment
    Deep breathing slowly one or two times during treatment
    Coughing techniques
    Stop treatment if sudden respiratory distress or chest pain occurs and contact physician
    Administer oral hygiene after treatment
    Care and cleaning of equipment

Explain importance of ongoing outpatient care and physician visits
Teach importance of avoiding persons with URIs
Refer to home health agency for follow-up care

■ INCENTIVE SPIROMETER
A mechanical device that assists patient in maintaining maximal inspiratory effort; effective when used by postoperative patients to prevent development of atelectasis and pneumonia; more physiologic and less hazardous than IPPB because it depends only on the patient's inspiratory effort (not on electricity, batteries, or gas)

ASSESSMENT
OBJECTIVE DATA/FINDINGS
Patient
Presence or absence of pain
Motivation
Weakness
Hyperventilation
  Dizziness
  Lightheadedness
  Numbness around mouth and nose
  Tingling in fingers and toes
Cough
  Productive
  Nonproductive
Breath sounds
  Diminished
  Absent
  Crackles
  Rhonchi over large airways

Equipment
Type of device
V_T

ONGOING CARE/DISCHARGE/HOME CARE PLANNING
Patient must be alert and cooperative
Assess degree of pain present
  Administer analgesics as ordered
  Assess effectiveness of pain relief measure(s)
Elevate head of bed 60 to 90 degrees or have patient sit in chair
Assist and teach patient to use incentive spirometer
  Exhale slowly
  Place mouthpiece in mouth between teeth
  Close lips tightly around mouthpiece
  Inhale through mouth only, taking a slow, deep breath
  Hold breath for 3 to 5 seconds
  Remove mouthpiece from mouth
  Exhale slowly
Repeat procedure 10 to 20 times qh
Caution patient not to breathe too rapidly
Observe for signs of hyperventilation; stop use of incentive spirometer if dizziness or lightheadedness occurs

Assist and teach patient to cough after using incentive spirometer

Auscultate chest for breath sounds q4h

Assist and teach patient to cough if crackles or rhonchi are heard

Report diminished or absent breath sounds to physician

Monitor patient's progress q4h

Increase V_T as patient tolerates it

PATIENT/FAMILY TEACHING

Ensure that patient and significant other(s) know and understand

Purpose of incentive spirometer

Importance of using it 10 to 20 times qh

Importance of holding breath for 3 to 5 seconds

Need to inhale through mouth

Importance of not exhaling into apparatus

Importance of reaching desired V_T

Importance of coughing after using apparatus

BIBLIOGRAPHY

Abels L: *Critical care nursing: a physiologic approach,* St Louis, 1986, Mosby.

Ahrens TS, Rutherford K: *Essentials of oxygenation,* Boston, 1993, Jones & Bartlett.

American Thoracic Society: Guidelines for the evaluation of impairment/disability in patients with Asthma, *Am Rev Resp Dis* 147:1056-1061, 1993.

Bates DV: *Respiratory function in disease,* Philadelphia, 1989, WB Saunders.

Boggs RL, Wooldridge-King M: *AACN procedure manual for critical care,* ed 3, Philadelphia, 1993, WB Saunders.

Burrell LO: *Adult nursing in hospital and community settings,* Norwalk, Conn, 1992, Appleton & Lange.

Clayton DB, Stock YN: *Basic pharmacology for nurses,* ed 11, St Louis, 1997, Mosby.

Corbett JV: *Laboratory tests and diagnostic procedure with nursing diagnoses,* Norwalk, Conn, 1992, Appleton & Lange.

Eflychou V: Clinical diagnosis & management of the patient with deep vein thrombosis and acute pulmonary embolism, *Nurs Pract* 21:365-371, 1996.

Fischback F: *A manual of laboratory and diagnostic tests,* Philadelphia, 1992, WB Saunders.

Guzzetta CE et al: *Critical care nursing: body-mind-spirit,* ed 3, Boston, 1991, Little, Brown.

Hopp L: Ineffective breathing related to decreased lung expansion, *Nurs Clin North Am* 22:193, 1987.

Hudak CM, Gallo BM: *Critical care nursing: a holistic approach,* ed 6, Philadelphia, 1994, JB Lippincott.

Kim MJ, McFarland GK, McLane AM: *Pocket guide to nursing diagnoses,* ed 7, St Louis, 1997, Mosby.

Kinney MR et al: *AACN's clinical reference for critical-care nursing,* ed 4, St Louis, 1998, Mosby.

Kozier B et al: *Techniques in clinical nursing,* ed 4, Redwood City, Ga, 1993, Addison-Wesley.

Laguatra I, Gerlach MO: *Nutrition in clinical nursing,* Albany, NY, 1990, Delmar.

Lehrer S: *Understanding lung sounds,* ed 2, Philadelphia, 1993, WB Saunders.

Luckmann J, Sorensen K: *Medical-surgical nursing,* ed 4, Philadelphia, 1993, WB Saunders.

McCance KL, Huether SE: *Pathophysiology: the biological basis for disease in adults and children,* ed 3, St Louis, 1998, Mosby.

Nakazaua H et al: Risk of aspiration pneumonia in the elderly, *Chest* 103:1636, 1996.

Scanlan CL, Wilkins RL, Stoller JK: *Egan's fundamental of respiratory care,* ed 7, St Louis, 1998, Mosby.

Schlichtig R, Ayers SM: *Nutritional support of critically ill,* St Louis, 1988, Mosby.

Swearingen PL: *Manual of critical care: applying nursing diagnosis to adult critical illness,* ed 3, St Louis, 1995, Mosby.

Thelan LA et al: *Critical care nursing: diagnosis and management,* ed 3, St Louis, 1998, Mosby.

Thompson JM et al: *Mosby's clinical nursing,* ed 4, St Louis, 1997, Mosby.

Tierney LM et al: *Current medical diagnosis and treatment,* Norwalk, Conn, 1994, Appleton & Lange.

Weilitz PB: *Pocket guide to respiratory care,* St Louis, 1991, Mosby.

Wilkins R, Shelden R, Krider S: *Clinical assessment in respiratory care,* ed 3, St Louis, 1995, Mosby.

Wilson S, Thompson JM: *Respiratory disorders,* St Louis, 1990, Mosby.

Wright JE, Shelton BK: *Desk reference for critical care nursing,* Boston, 1993, Jones & Bartlett.

ADULT PNEUMONIA CARE PATH

ADDRESSOGRAPH

PATIENT PROBLEM

1. Impaired gas exchange related to disease process.
2. Alteration in body temperature (hyperthermia) related to disease process.
3. Fluid volume deficit related to hyperthermia, excess insensible loss, and poor intake.
4. Knowledge deficit related to disease process

PATIENT OUTCOMES

1. Oxygen saturation > 94% and lung sounds clear before discharge.
2. Temperature will be 100° or below for 24 hours day before discharge.
3. Patient will be hydrated upon discharge as shown by intake and output within 100 cc and have a PO fluid intake of at least 2000 cc per day.
4. Patient will communicate discharge instruction.

DAY	DAY 1 — Emergency Department	DAY 1 — Inpatient	DAY 2	DAY 3	DAY 4	DISCHARGE DAY 5
DATE						
History / Physical	Prior history pneumonia, COPD, asthma, TB. Wheeze, rales, respiratory distress, shortness of breath, effusion					
Tests	☐ Chest x-ray, if significant effusion consider thoracentesis ☐ CBC, Lytes, Creat, Sputum gram stain STAT, Sputum C + S, Induce PRN ☐ Blood Cult x 2 if temp >101 ☐ Oxygen saturation-oximetry, ABG if indicated	☐ Pulse oximetry if on oxygen ☐ PPD, cocci, controls if indicated	☐ Pulse oximetry if on oxygen	☐ If oxygen saturation greater than or equal to 95% do room air oxygen saturation	☐ If oxygen saturation greater than or equal to 95% do room air oxygen saturation	None
Treatment	Assessment for following: ☐ Chest PT ☐ Cough, deep breath, q2h ☐ Incentive Spirometry q2h ☐ Deep suction PRN ☐ Suction if unable to cough		Assessment for following: ☐ Chest PT ☐ Cough, deep breath, q2h ☐ Incentive Spirometry q2h ☐ Deep suction PRN	☐ Continue treatments if indicated	☐ Continue treatments if indicated	None
Meds	☐ IVs ☐ Parenteral antibiotics ☐ oxygen if saturation <94% ☐ Nebulizer/metered dose inhaler with spacer (MDI) if indicated	☐ IVs ☐ Parenteral Antibiotics adjusted for gram stain ☐ Tylenol for temp >101 ☐ Med for pain ☐ Nebulizer/MDI	☐ DC IVs if PO intake tolerated ☐ Heparin lock ☐ Parenteral antibiotics ☐ Tylenol for temp >101 ☐ Med for pain ☐ Nebulizer/MDI	☐ DC Tylenol and pain meds ☐ Heparin lock ☐ Parenteral antibiotics ☐ DC oxygen if indicated ☐ Antibiotics adjusted for sputum/blood cultures if indicated	☐ Heparin lock ☐ Parenteral antibiotics	☐ DC Heparin lock ☐ DC parenteral antibiotics ☐ Discharge on PO antibiotics
Diet	☐ Diet & fluids as tolerated	☐ Regular diet ☐ Encourage fluids	☐ Regular diet ☐ Encourage fluids	☐ Regular diet ☐ Encourage fluids	☐ Regular diet ☐ Encourage fluids	☐ Regular diet

DAY	DATE — DAY 1 (Emergency Department)	DATE — DAY 1 (Inpatient)	DATE — DAY 2	DATE — DAY 3	DATE — DAY 4	DATE — DISCHARGE DAY 5
Activity or Treatment	□ Bed rest	□ BRP with assist and ad lib if tolerated	□ OOB in chair for 20 min. BID □ BRP □ Ambulate with assists × 1 or ad lib if tolerated	□ Ambulate × 3 in hall or ad lib if tolerated	□ Ambulate × 5 in hall or ad lib if tolerated	□ Ambulate ad lib
Assessment and Evaluation	□ Collect culture specimens □ Induce sputum if needed □ If sputum collection attempts are unsuccessful, notify physician □ Start antibiotics	□ Assess lung sounds □ Monitor temp. q4h □ I&O □ Assist with care due to shortness of breath □ Document sputum production and color □ Pulse oximetry daily if on oxygen	□ I&O □ Encourage fluids at least 2000 cc/day □ Assess lung sounds □ Monitor temp q shift □ Assist with care □ Document sputum production and color □ Pulse oximetry daily if on oxygen	□ Assess lung sounds □ Document sputum production & color □ Monitor temp q shift □ D/C I&O □ Encourage increased self-care □ Pulse oximetry daily if on oxygen	□ Monitor incentive spirometry □ Assess lung sounds □ Document any sputum □ Temp routine □ Increased self-care □ Ask patient to arrange transportation in preparation for discharge	□ Discharge instructions: Include incentive spirometry, fluid intake, MDI if needed □ Medication instructions
Teaching	□ Discuss initial plan of care with patient	□ Discuss plan of care with patient □ Inspirometer, cough, deep breathe	□ Discuss plan of care with patient □ Teaching continues from Day 1	□ Discuss plan of care with patient □ Patient demonstrates appropriate MDI, deep breathing and coughing technique	□ Discuss plan of care with patient □ Patient demonstrates appropriate MDI, deep breathing and coughing technique	□ Discuss plan of care with patient □ Discharge instructions □ Vaccinations □ Smoking cessation
Discharge Planning			□ Patient/family assessment	□ Post-hospital plans documented if needed. □ Discuss tentative discharge date with physician.		□ Arrangements made

DATE	SHIFT	SIGNATURE/TITLE	DATE	SHIFT	SIGNATURE/TITLE

5/93* THIS CARE PATH IS TO BE USED AS A GUIDELINE ONLY AND DOES NOT NECESSARILY IMPLY AS A STANDARD OF CARE

page 3 of 3

VARIANCE REPORT

Admission Date: _____

Discharge Date and Time: _____

Actual LOS: _____

Date Care Path Discontinued: _____

Implement Compromised Respiratory Status Standard

DATE	VARIATION	CAUSE	KEY	ACTION TAKEN	SIGNATURE	DATE RESOLVED	SIGNA

KEY:
1. PATIENT
2. SYSTEM

IF NOT, PLAN FOR RESOLUTION: _____

CHECK IF PATIENT OUTCOME WAS ATTAINED BEFORE DISCHARGE:

☐ Oxygen Saturation is above 94% and lung sounds are clear

☐ Temperature is 100° F or below during the last 24 hours

☐ The patient has taken oral fluids of 2000 ml/day. I and O is within 500 ml.

☐ The patient is able to communicate discharge instructions.

PATIENT LEARNING CHECKLIST   page 1 of 1

DIAGNOSIS PNEUMONIA

ADDRESSOGRAPH

INTERVENTION CODES	PATIENT/SIGNIFICANT OTHER CODES
A. QUESTIONS ANSWERED.	A. NEEDS INSTRUCTION/REINFORCEMENT.
B. INFORMATION PROVIDED. LIST WRITTEN MATERIALS.	B. DEMONSTRATES VERBAL UNDERSTANDING.
C. TASK DEMONSTRATED.	C. RETURNS DEMONSTRATION.
D. MULTIDISCIPLINARY REFERRALS. SPECIFY.	D. SEE FLOW RECORD.
E. REFER TO CLASS.	

TEACH/DEMONSTRATE	INTERVENTIONS				PATIENT/SIGNIFICANT OTHER RESPONSE				COMMENTS
	CODE	DATE	TIME	INITIAL	CODE	DATE	TIME	INITIAL	
A. Signs and symptoms of respiratory infection or bronchospasm: 1. elevated temperature 2. changes in character of sputum 3. increased respiratory rate 4. shortness of breath 5. wheeze or stridor									
B. Dietary regimen: 1. Nutritional Services Consultation									
C. Activity progression regimen: 1. Pace activities during day to avoid fatigue. 2. Arrange activities after respiratory treatment.									
D. Do not smoke or allow smoking in the home: 1. Refer to Health Education Stop Smoking Program (372-3357).									
E. Breathing techniques: 1. Respiratory Care Services consult 2. pursed-lip breathing 3. minineb/MDI 4. Refer to Health Education (372-3314).									
F. Adult Immunizations 1. Discuss pamphlet 2. Refer to physician									
G. Establish your care with a personal physician.									

INITIAL	SIGNATURE	TITLE	INITIAL	SIGNATURE	TITLE

Used by permission of Kaiser Permanente Medical Center, Kaiser Foundation Hospital, Martinez, California.

ADULT PNEUMONIA CARE PATH*
PATIENT COPY

	ADMISSION			DISCHARGE
TESTS	• Receive diagnostic examinations as ordered by your physician.	• Measurement of the oxygen level in your blood stream if you are receiving oxygen.	• Skin tests to rule out other causes of your illness if ordered by your physician.	
TREATMENT		• Discuss with your nurse the need to cough and deep breathe every 2 hours.	• You will be instructed on the use of incentive spirometry.	
MEDICATIONS	• Intravenous fluids and antibiotics if ordered. • Oxygen if needed. • Respiratory Therapy will instruct you in the use of a Metered Dose Inhaler if indicated.	• Tylenol for fever if needed. • Discuss pain medication needs with your nurse.	• Intravenous fluids will be discontinued if you are drinking adequate amounts of fluid. • IV entry port.	• Discuss need for continued pain medication with your nurse. • Discontinue oxygen if indicated.	• Discontinue the IV entry port. • Intravenous antibiotics discontinued. • Discharge on oral antibiotics if ordered.
DIET	• Diet and fluids as tolerated.	• Regular diet. • Discuss with nurse the need to drink an adequate amount of fluids.	• Regular diet. • Adequate fluid intake.	

Used by permission of Kaiser Permanente Medical Center, Kaiser Foundation Hospital, Martinez, California.
*Individual patient's course of therapy may vary from this guideline.

	ADMISSION		DISCHARGE
ACTIVITY	• Remain in bed. Activity increases your need for oxygen and may intensify any shortness of breath you are experiencing.	• Walk to the bathroom with help if you feel able.	• Up in a chair for 20 minutes twice a day if you are able. • Walk in the hall with help at least once a day or more if you are able.	• Walk in the hall three or more times a day if you are able.	• Up and about as you are able.
TEACHING		• Receive instruction in how to use incentive spirometer, cough, and deep breathe. • Please ask any questions you may have.	• Review instructions for use of Metered Dose Inhaler if you are using one. • Review incentive spirometry, coughing, and deep breathing.	• Receive discharge instructions. • Receive information about adult immunizations. • Receive information on nonsmoking.
DISCHARGE PLANNING			• Discuss discharge needs with your care provider. (For example: Is there someone at home to care for you?)	• Arrange for someone to drive you home. • Before discharge, establish or confirm the name of your personal physician.	• Discharge before 11:00 A.M.

page 1 of 2

Interdisciplinary Care Path:

ADULT COPD / Asthma

Expected Length of Stay: 4 days

This Plan of Care has been discussed with patient/significant other.

Date: _____

Signature: _____ ,RN

If discussed with someone other than the patient, specify.

Name: _____ Relationship: _____

If "NA," explain: _____

Addressograph

INTERVENTIONS

Patient Care Problems	Patient Outcomes	Emergency Dept. Date:	Admission Day Date:	Day 2 Date:	Day 3 Date:	Day 4 Date:
1. Impaired gas exchange related to the disease process.	1. The patient will communicate comfort in breathing. Date: _____ If not achieved, write a narrative note.	— Bed rest: positioned for optimal comfort and air exchange. — No caffeine — Chest x-ray — BUN,CBC,Lytes, Creatinine, Glucose — Peak Flow, Oximetry — Theophylline level — ABG — ECG for severe COPD — **IV/PO corticosteriods** — **IV/PO aminophylline** — Antibiotics if suspect infection — Oxygen — Nebulizer/MDI ☐ No Admission	— Bed rest: positioned for optimal comfort and air exchange. — No caffeine — Peak Flow — Oxygen — **Nebulizer/MDI**	— **BRP with assist and ad lib if tolerated. Provide portable oxygen.** — No caffeine — Oxygen — Peak Flow AM — Peak Flow PM — Oximetry — **Theophylline level** — Convert to PO meds	— **BRP ad lib if tolerated. Provide portable oxygen.** — No caffeine — Peak Flow AM — Peak Flow PM — Oximetry on room air if O$_2$ saturation is greater than 95% on oxygen. — DC oxygen if indicated — **Convert to PO meds**	— **Ambulate ad lib if tolerated. Provide portable oxygen.** — No caffeine — Peak Flow AM — Peak Flow PM — Oximetry on room air if O$_2$ saturation is greater than 95% on oxygen. — DC oxygen if indicated, or home on oxygen. — Convert to PO meds

INSTRUCTIONS FOR USE:

Initial if intervention *initiated*

Leave *blank* if intervention *not initiated*

Write NA if intervention *not applicable*

If the intervention is not initiated within 24 hours, document a narrative note. A narrative note is not required for "NA" (not applicable).

DAY SHIFT assures that the Care Path is reviewed and variances are documented.

Discharge to: Home ☐ SNF ☐ HH ☐ SOC ☐

Date: _____

Time: _____

SOC: _____

SSR:27Feb95

Used by permission of Kaiser Permanente Medical Center, Kaiser Foundation Hospital, Martinez, California.

INTERVENTIONS

Patient Care	Patient Outcomes	Emergency Dept.	Admission Day	Day 2	Day 3	Day 4
2. Knowledge deficit related to disease process and self-management.	2. The patient/ significant other will communicate understanding of disease process, treatments, and follow-up care. ___ Date: ___ *If not achieved, write a narrative note.*	___ Implement Emergency Department Teaching Guideline	___ Patient/family assessment ___ Implement Learning Checklist for Compromised Respiratory Status	___ Patient/family assessment ___ Continue Learning Checklist for Compromised Respiratory Status ___ Evaluate for MDI conversion and teaching: B-agonist, inhaled steroids. ___ Evaluate for DME, HH, SNF ___ Discuss discharge date with physician	___ Patient/family assessment ___ Continue Learning Checklist for Compromised Respiratory Status ___ Evaluate for MDI conversion and teaching: B-agonist, inhaled steroids. ___ Evaluate for DME, HH, SNF ___ Discuss discharge date with physician	___ Finalize arrangements ___ Complete Learning Checklist for Compromised Respiratory Status in preparation for discharge tomorrow
		GRASP: 8am - 4pm ___	GRASP: 8am - 4pm ___	GRASP: 8am - 4pm ___	GRASP: 8am - 4pm ___	GRASP: 8am - 4pm ___

Emergency Dept.			Admission Day			Day 2			Day 3			Day 4		
INIT	PRINT NAME	TITLE	INIT	PRINT NAME	TITLE	INIT	PRINT NAME	TITLE	INIT	PRINT NAME	TITLE	INIT	PRINT NAME	TITLE

All assigned registered nurses are responsible to update/review, and sign the patient care path each shift.

*6/94 This Care Path is to be used as a guideline only and does not necessarily imply a standard of care.

INSTRUCTIONS FOR USE: *Initial* if intervention *initiated* *Leave blank* if intervention *not initiated* *Write NA* if intervention *not applicable*	If the intervention is not initiated within 24 hours, document a narrative note. A narrative note is not required for "NA" (not applicable).	DAY SHIFT assures that the Care Path is reviewed and variances are documented.	Discharge to: Home ☐ SNF ☐ HH ☐ SOC ☐ Date: ___ Time: ___ SOC: ___

SSR:27Feb95

page 1 of 3

Admission Date/Time:	Rex Healthcare Clinical Pathway	
Critical Path Date/Time:	COPD, DRG 88	
Discharge Date/Time:		
Case Manager/Phone#:	LOS	Addressograph

MULTIDISCIPLINARY PATHWAY DOCUMENTATION

CATEGORY/DAY	Emergency Department	
ED/Patient Arrival	1. Does patient have an advanced directive? YES NO	2. Did patient contact physcian prior to coming to the ED? YES NO
ED/Presenting Assessment	Breath Sounds (RT) Cough (RT) Sputum produced (RT) Dyspnea (RT) Absent Moderate Severe **Recent infection? (RN)** describe_____	
ED/Diagnostic Testing	CBC M7 ABG CXR Sputum C&S Theo Level U/A ECG Pulse Ox	

ED/Outcomes for Discharge from ED	Patient/Family/Other aware of patient's
	  D/C instructions (RN)
	
	Appropriate Referrals made (PFS)
	
	Patient understands need to contact
	  MD/RN/RT when ill prior to ED visit?
	
	DISCHARGE CRITERIA: (MD)
	Lung sounds improved/clear
	Vital signs stable
	Peak Flow improved over baseline
	Pulse Ox improved
	Verbalized instructions
	Able to demonstrate proper use of MDI
	Aware of community resources
	Verbalizes self–care measures
	
	Discharge Criteria — Met Not Met	

ED/Outcomes for Admission	Results from all labs, ECG, test on chart (LAB) Sputum obtained and sent to lab (LAB) Sputum & other specimens collected by RN/RT Call abnormal results to MD (lab/x–rays) (US) Pulse Ox documented in progress notes (RT) Antibiotics started: Time administered_____ Recommended Antibiotics started PO / IV: TPM/SMX DS 1 tab BID or / Cefuroxime 750mg IV Q8H or Doxycycline 100mg BID or / Ceftriaxone 1mg IV Q24H Clarthromycin 500mg BID or Augmentin 500mg Q8H with food or Ceftin 500mg BID with food Pulse Ox/ABGs documented (RT) **Time of last respiratory treatment (RT)_____**	

NOTE: CLINICAL PATHWAYS ARE GUIDELINES FOR CONSIDERATION WHICH MAY BE MODIFIED ACCORDING TO INDIVIDUAL PATIENT NEEDS.

KEY TO DISCIPLINES PERFORMING SERVICES
RN — Registered Nurse	MD — Physician
RT — Respiratory Therapist	RP — Registered Pharmacist
RD — Registered Dietitian	Lab — Laboratory
PFS — Patient and Family Services	US — Unit Secretary
CM — Case Manager	PT — Physical Therapist

Form Date: June 14, 1995
Form Revision Date: August 16, 1995

Used by permission of Rex Healthcare, Raleigh, North Carolina.

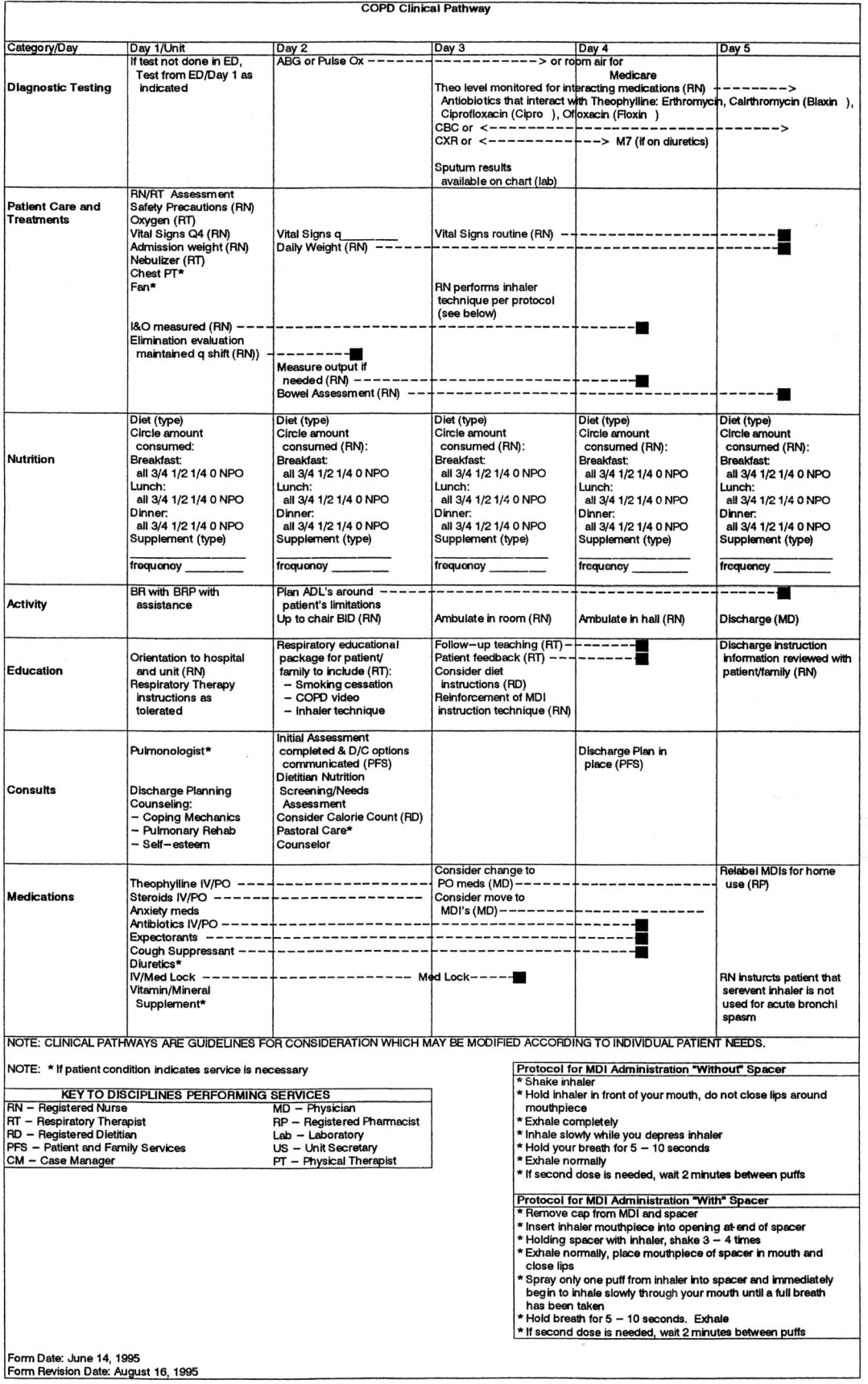

COPD Clinical Pathway

Category/Day	Day 1/Unit	Day 2	Day 3	Day 4	Day 5
Diagnostic Testing	If test not done in ED, Test from ED/Day 1 as indicated	ABG or Pulse Ox ----------------------> or room air for Medicare	Theo level monitored for interacting medications (RN) ------------> Antiobiotics that interact with Theophylline: Erthromycin, Calrthromycin (Blaxin), Ciprofloxacin (Cipro), Ofloxacin (Floxin) CBC or <------------------------------> CXR or <-----------------> M7 (if on diuretics) Sputum results available on chart (lab)		

Patient Care and Treatments	RN/RT Assessment
	 Safety Precautions (RN)
	 Oxygen (RT)
	 Vital Signs Q4 (RN)
	 Admission weight (RN)
	 Nebulizer (RT)
	 Chest PT*
	 Fan*
	
	 I&O measured (RN) ----
	 Elimination evaluation
	   maintained q shift (RN))
		Vital Signs q_____
		 Daily Weight (RN) ----
		
		--------------------- 	
		
		 ----------■
		 Measure output if
		   needed (RN) ---------
		 Bowel Assessment (RN) ---
			Vital Signs routine (RN) --------------------
			
			 RN performs inhaler technique per protocol (see below)
			
			 ---------------------- 	
			
			 --------------------- 	
			 -------------------- 	
				
				■
				
				■
					■
					 ■
					
					■

Nutrition	Diet (type)
	 Circle amount consumed:
	 Breakfast:
	  all 3/4 1/2 1/4 0 NPO
	 Lunch:
	  all 3/4 1/2 1/4 0 NPO
	 Dinner:
	  all 3/4 1/2 1/4 0 NPO
	 Supplement (type) _____
	
	 frequency _____
		Diet (type)
		 Circle amount consumed (RN):
		 Breakfast:
		  all 3/4 1/2 1/4 0 NPO
		 Lunch:
		  all 3/4 1/2 1/4 0 NPO
		 Dinner:
		  all 3/4 1/2 1/4 0 NPO
		 Supplement (type) _____
		
		 frequency _____
			Diet (type)
			 Circle amount consumed (RN):
			 Breakfast:
			  all 3/4 1/2 1/4 0 NPO
			 Lunch:
			  all 3/4 1/2 1/4 0 NPO
			 Dinner:
			  all 3/4 1/2 1/4 0 NPO
			 Supplement (type) _____
			
			 frequency _____
				Diet (type)
				 Circle amount consumed (RN):
				 Breakfast:
				  all 3/4 1/2 1/4 0 NPO
				 Lunch:
				  all 3/4 1/2 1/4 0 NPO
				 Dinner:
				  all 3/4 1/2 1/4 0 NPO
				 Supplement (type) _____
				
				 frequency _____
					Diet (type)
					 Circle amount consumed (RN):
					 Breakfast:
					  all 3/4 1/2 1/4 0 NPO
					 Lunch:
					  all 3/4 1/2 1/4 0 NPO
					 Dinner:
					  all 3/4 1/2 1/4 0 NPO
					 Supplement (type) _____
					
					 frequency _____

Activity	BR with BRP with assistance	Plan ADL's around -------- patient's limitations Up to chair BID (RN)	Ambulate in room (RN)	Ambulate in hall (RN)	---------■ Discharge (MD)
Education	Orientation to hospital and unit (RN) Respiratory Therapy instructions as tolerated	Respiratory educational package for patient/ family to include (RT): – Smoking cessation – COPD video – Inhaler technique	Follow-up teaching (RT) - --------■ Patient feedback (RT) -- --------■ Consider diet instructions (RD) Reinforcement of MDI instruction technique (RN)		Discharge instruction information reviewed with patient/family (RN)
Consults	Pulmonologist* Discharge Planning Counseling: – Coping Mechanics – Pulmonary Rehab – Self-esteem	Initial Assessment completed & D/C options communicated (PFS) Dietitian Nutrition Screening/Needs Assessment Consider Calorie Count (RD) Pastoral Care* Counselor		Discharge Plan in place (PFS)	
Medications	Theophylline IV/PO ---- Steroids IV/PO -------- Anxiety meds Antibiotics IV/PO ----- Expectorants --------- Cough Suppressant --- Diuretics* IV/Med Lock ---------- Vitamin/Mineral Supplement*	----------------------- ----------------------- ----------------------- ----------------------- ----------------------- Med Lock-----	Consider change to PO meds (MD)---------- Consider move to MDI's (MD)------------- ------------------ ------------------ ------------------ Med Lock-----■	 ■ ■ ■	Relabel MDIs for home use (RP) RN insturcts patient that serevent inhaler is not used for acute bronchi spasm

NOTE: CLINICAL PATHWAYS ARE GUIDELINES FOR CONSIDERATION WHICH MAY BE MODIFIED ACCORDING TO INDIVIDUAL PATIENT NEEDS.

NOTE: * If patient condition indicates service is necessary

KEY TO DISCIPLINES PERFORMING SERVICES	
RN – Registered Nurse	MD – Physician
RT – Respiratory Therapist	RP – Registered Pharmacist
RD – Registered Dietitian	Lab – Laboratory
PFS – Patient and Family Services	US – Unit Secretary
CM – Case Manager	PT – Physical Therapist

Protocol for MDI Administration "Without" Spacer
* Shake inhaler
* Hold inhaler in front of your mouth, do not close lips around mouthpiece
* Exhale completely
* Inhale slowly while you depress inhaler
* Hold your breath for 5 – 10 seconds
* Exhale normally
* If second dose is needed, wait 2 minutes between puffs

Protocol for MDI Administration "With" Spacer
* Remove cap from MDI and spacer
* Insert inhaler mouthpiece into opening at end of spacer
* Holding spacer with inhaler, shake 3 – 4 times
* Exhale normally, place mouthpiece of spacer in mouth and close lips
* Spray only one puff from inhaler into spacer and immediately begin to inhale slowly through your mouth until a full breath has been taken
* Hold breath for 5 – 10 seconds. Exhale
* If second dose is needed, wait 2 minutes between puffs

Form Date: June 14, 1995
Form Revision Date: August 16, 1995

Continued

COPD Clinical Pathway					
PATIENT'S NAME:					
OUTCOMES	Day 1/Unit	Day 2	Day 3	Day 4	Day 5
	Patient Age Appropriate Safety precautions taken		Patient lab values are returning to base line		
	Appropriate level of oxygen maintained		Patient exhibits no signs of Theophylline toxicity (1)		
			Patient is tolerating PO meds	Patient is independent on MDIs	Patient receives MDIs as relabeled for home use
		Patient activity level increased	Patient activity level increased	Patient activity level increased	Patient activity level increased
	Patient/Family aware of Clinical Path	Patient aware of educational material on disease management	Patient/Family education retained		Patient/Family aware of signs/symptoms that require patient to contact MD
	Patient/Family aware of activity expectations				Patient/Family understands instructions for medications
	Patient/Family aware Rex is smoke—free				
		Patient exhibits bowel function per patient's routine or Bowel Protocol initiated – – – –	– – – – – – – – – –	– – – – – – – – – –	– – – – – ■
		Patient/Family understands anticipated LOS and D/C options			
	Patient/Family understands importance of patient consuming adequate nutrition				Patient nutritional consumption is adequate

Daily Variance Tracing

Variance Type/Date Occured	Initials	Reason/Comment	Initials	Action Taken/Date Resolved
1.				
2.				
3.				
4.				
5.				
6.				
7.				
8.				
9.				
10.				

NOTE: * If patient condition indicates service is necessary.

(1) The following antiobiotics interact with Theophylline: Erythromycin, Clirthromycin (Biaxin), Ciprofloxacin (Cipro), Ofloxacin (Floxin), Norfloxacin (Noroxin)

Form Date: June 14, 1995
Form Revision Date: August 16, 1995

NOTE: CLINICAL PATHWAYS ARE GUIDELINES FOR CONSIDERATION WHICH MAY BE MODIFIED ACCORDING TO INDIVIDUAL PATIENT NEEDS

	Rex Healthcare Clinical Pathway Prevention of Noscomial Pneumonia for Ventilator ICU Patients	
Admission Date/Time:_____		
Clinical Path Date/Time:_____		
Discharge Date/Time:_____		
Case Manager/Phone:_____		
Patient/Family Contact/_____ Phone Number:		Addressograph

Category	Day 1/Placed on Ventilator	Day 2	Day 3	Day 1/Post Extubation	Day 2/Post Extubation	Day 3/Post Extubation
TESTING	M12 (1) ABG ------------------ CBC ------------------ M6 PT/PTT ---------------- EKG (1) CXR ------------------	M7------------	----- PRN ----- ----- PRN ----- ----- PRN ----- ----- PRN ----- PRN -----			■ ■ ■ ■ ■
MEDICATIONS	Sedation per Protocol (on back of path) Reassess to D/C antibiotic (2) Antacid: H2 Blocker until GI track function returns (5)	------------	------------	------------	------------	■
PATIENT CARE/ TREATMENTS	Assess for specialty bed Assess need for CPT Mouth Care Q4 and PRN per protocol (on back of path) Verify NG placement per protocol Verify NT or ET tube place- ment Q shift ---------- Suctioning PRN ---------- RN/RT document secretion PRN (based on assessment of patient) ---- Turning Q2H ------------ Skin integrity Q shift ----- I & O ------------------ Weight ---------------- Vent setting ------------ Nebulizer meds (2) if ordered/as ordered ---- Tube changing per Protocol Retaping ET tube (per Protocol to be developed) ---	PT assess OOB with RT/PT ------------ ------------ ------------ ------------ ------------ ----Daily Weight---- OOB ------------ ------------ ------------	------------ ------------ ------------ ------------ ------------	Incentive spirometry Swallowing Assessment post extubation or > 5 days intubated ■ ■ Assess for Ambulation ------ ■	 ------------ ------------ ------------ ------------	 ■ ■ ■ ■ ■ ■ ■
DIETITIAN		MD assess for enteral parenteral feeding Dietitian Screening				
CONSULTS	As directed: – Anesthesiology – Pulmonology – IM – Surgeon – Nephrology – Infectious Disease – Cardiology	Wound/Ostomy/Skin Care per Clinical Nurse Specialist				
DISCHARGE PLANNING	D/C Plan Consult	D/C Plan Assessment completed		D/C Plan in place or disposition determined		
EDUCATION	Use of Nebulizer Turning, coughing, deep breathing, splinting Trach Care education*			Incentive Spirometry Smoking Cessation (to be developed)		
PROCEDURES	A–Line IV: – CVP* – Swan* NG Dialysis*	MD assess for small bore feeding tube, Gastrostomey, Jejunostomy			MD assess for Small bore feeding tube	

NOTE: CLINICAL PATHWAYS ARE GUIDELINES FOR CONSIDERATION WHICH MAY BE MODIFIED ACCORDING TO INDIVIDUAL PATIENT NEEDS.

* As individual patient's condition indicates appropriateness.   (1) Required only if previously done >12 hours prior to intubation. (2) Prophylactic antibiotics discouraged. (3) Bed assessment guidelines/at reisk: (a) weight >250 lbs (b) age >60 (c) Neuro, abdominal and throacic surgery. (4) Recommended mertered dose inhaler as ordered. (5) Best oral antacid is Carafate (℞). Best IV antacids are Pepcid (℞), Tagamet (℞), or Zantac (℞).

KEY TO DISCIPLINES PERFORMING SERVICES	
RN — Registered Nurse	MD — Physician
RT — Respiratory Therapist	RP — Registered Pharmacist
RD — Registered Dietitian	Lab — Laboratory
PFS — Patient & Family Services	US — Unit Secretary
CM — Case Manager	PT — Physical Therapist

Form Date: July 5, 1995
Form Revision Date: August 23, 1995

Used by permission of Rex Healthcare, Raleigh, North Carolina.   *Continued*

**Prevention of Noscomial Pneumonia
for Ventilator ICU Patients**

Category	Day 1/Placed on Ventilator	Day 2	Day 3	Day 1/Post Extubation	Day2	Day 3
OUTCOMES	Lab WNL ------	------	------	------	------	■
	Chest x–ray clear ----	------	------	------	------	■
	Patient is comfortable and cooperative with treatment and tolerating vent status —	----------------	----------------	■		
	Patient will be free from signs of GI bleeding --	------	------	------	------	■
	Patient bed type is appropriate -------	------	------	------	------	■
	Patient has breath sounds WNL -----	------	------	------	------	■
	Patient exhibits mucosal intgrity -----	------	------	------	------	■
				Patient has normal gag reflex (immediatly post extubation)----	------	■
				Patient understands and independatly performs incentive spirometry (80%) of predictated value) --	------	■
	Patient has clear secretions ------	------	------	------	------	■
	Patient's skin integrity is is maintained ------	------	------	------	------	■
		Patient activity level increasing ------	------	------	------	■
		Patient is receiving adequate nutrition —	------	------	------	■
				Patient/Family verbilizes and understands D/C Plan		
				Patient demostrates understanding through performance of turning, coughing, deep breathing and splinting		

Pathway Daily Variance Tracking

Variance Type/Date Occured	Initials	Reason/Comment	Initials	Action Taken/Date Resolved	Initials
1.					
2.					
3.					
4.					
5.					
6.					
7.					
8.					
9.					
10.					

Protocol for Mouth Care and Assessment for Patient's with Endotracheal Tube

NOTE: The following information presents the standard of mouth care for patients who are intubated.

A. Comprehensive Mouth Care Performed q12h by RN and RT:
  1. RT loosens ties and manually holds the ET tube.
  2. RN brushes teeth using toothpaste and PlaqVac brush or removes dentures and soaks them in cleaning solution.
  3. Cleanse mouth by instilling diluted H_2O_2 (1 part H_2O_2 to 1 part NaC1) while maintaining continuous oral suction.
  4. Rinse mouth by instilling NaC1 (remove residual H_2O_2) while maintaining continuous oral suction.
  5. Apply moisturizer to mucosa (mouthcare kit) and lips.
  6. Inspect mouth for lesions, xerostomia, or stomatitis.
  7. Reposition ET tube and apply new ties PRN.

B. Routine Mouth Care performed q4h, with each ET suctioning and PRN.
  1. Suction mouth of all accumulated saliva.
  2. Rinse mouth by instilling diluted H_2O_2 while maintaining continuous oral suction.
  3. Rinse mouth by instilling NaC1 (remove residual H_2O_2) while maintaining continuous oral suction.
  4. Apply moisturizer to mucosa and lip balm to lips.

C. Minimize the following conditions by:
  1. Xerostomia (dry mouth)
    * Obtaining order for moisturizing spray and use per mouth care protocol and PRN.
    * Swabbing mouth with moist Toothette q4h and PRN.
    * Applying lip balm.
  2. Stomatitis:
    * Obraining order for magic mouthwash (MMW).
    * Using MMW with mouthcare q8h.
    * Obtaining Viscous Lidocaine order for placement on lesions PRN pain relief.

D. Post extubation, mouthcare should be performed at least qid by the patient or nurse. An oral assessment is done b.i.d.

E. For patients who are neutropenic and/or thrombocytopenic or on chemotherapy, see Nursing Division Protocol #242.

Form Date: July 5, 1995
Form Revision Date: August 23, 1995

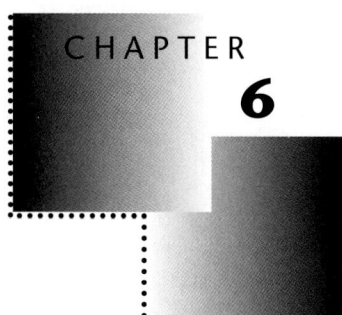

CHAPTER

6

Digestive System

■ GASTROINTESTINAL ASSESSMENT

▮ SUBJECTIVE DATA

Mouth, gums, tongue, lips
   Painful
   Tender
   Sores, lesions
Teeth
   Dentures, caps
   Loose teeth
Dysphagia
Eructation
Anorexia, change in appetite, weight loss/gain
Indigestion
Pyrosis (heartburn)
Fullness after eating
Pain, discomfort after eating certain foods
Nausea, vomiting; regurgitation without vomiting;
   hematemesis
Abdomen
   Pain (sharp, stabbing)
   Tender
   Cramping
Fatigue, malaise
Change in eating or bowel habits
Change in color, character, or frequency of stools
   or urine
Flatulence
Constipation
Diarrhea
Hemorrhoids, bleeding
Painful defecation
Use of laxatives or enemas
Change in skin color or texture; rash or itching
Edema of extremities

▮ OBJECTIVE DATA

General appearance, age (see Gerontologic
   Considerations box)
Vital signs
   Blood pressure (BP), pulse (P), and respiratory rate (R)
      Lying
      Sitting
      Standing

Temperature (T)
Weight
Urinary output, color, amount, specific gravity
Allergies
Mouth
   Stomatitis
   Condition and color of tongue, gums, mucous
      membranes, and teeth
   Halitosis
   Saliva production: increased or decreased
Abdomen
   Location of pain
   Rebound tenderness
   Distention, rigidity, ascites
   Increased abdominal girth
   Symmetry; asymmetry resulting from obesity,
      organomegaly, fluid or gas distention
   Hepatomegaly
   Keloid tissue, scars
   Visible peristalsis
   Bowel sounds
      Present
      Absent
   Visible palpable masses; hernia(s), lipomas
   Presence of ostomies
Perianal area
   Hemorrhoids, fissures
   Color and condition of area
   Odor
   Color, consistency, and frequency of stools
Sclera: jaundice
Skin
   Jaundice
   Turgor
   Pruritus
   Ecchymosis around the umbilicus (Cullen's sign)
   Spider angioma
   Purpura
   Moles
   Palmar erythema
   Peripheral edema
   Distended, tortous blood vessels
   Abdominal striae
   Scars

Gerontologic Considerations

- Loss of teeth and resultant use of dentures can interfere with chewing and lead to digestive complaints.
- Dysphagia is commonly seen in the older adult population and may be caused by changes in the esophageal musculature or by neurologic conditions.
- Hiatal hernias and esophageal diverticuli are significantly increased with aging because of changes in musculature of diaphragm and esophagus.
- There is decreased secretion of hydrochloric acid (hypochlorhydria and achlorhydria) from the parietal cells of the stomach. This results in an increased incidence of pernicious anemia and gastritis in the aged population.
- Peptic ulcers are common, but often the symptoms are vague and go unrecognized until there is a bleeding episode. Medications such as aspirin, nonsteroidal antiinflammatory drugs (NSAIDs), and steroids that are taken for the chronic degenerative joint conditions common with aging should be used with caution because they can contribute to ulcer formation.
- Frequency of diverticulosis and diverticulitis increases dramatically with aging and can contribute to malabsorption of nutrients.
- Constipation is a problem for many older persons. Inactivity, changes in diet and fluid intake, and medications can contribute to this problem. Bowel elimination should be monitored and a bowel regimen established to prevent impaction.
- Incidence of cholelithiasis increases with aging. Older individuals with histories of this problem should be observed closely for changes in the color of urine and stool or other signs and symptoms.
- The older adult may have increased amounts of subcutaneous fat on the lower abdomen and hips. Because of a thinner, softer abominal wall, the liver and kidneys are easier to palpate.
- Decline in absorption of vitamin B_{12} increases the incidence of pernicious anemia.

Modified from Christensen BL, Kockrow EO: Foundations of nursing, *ed 3, St Louis, 1998, Mosby.*

PERTINENT BACKGROUND INFORMATION

CONCURRENT DISEASES OR CONDITIONS

Carcinoma
Cardiovascular disease (hypertension)
Esophageal varices
Crohn's disease
Ulcers
Colitis
Alcoholism
Endocrine disorders
Severe burns
Psychologic problems
Chemical substance abuse
Neurologic conditions
Epistaxis

PREVIOUS SURGERY OR ILLNESS

Inflammatory bowel disease
Carcinoma
Gastrointestinal (GI) surgery
Cholecystectomy
  Gastric surgery
  Ostomies
  Other abdominal, pelvic, or rectal surgeries
Hepatitis
Cirrhosis
Pancreatitis
Diabetes mellitus
Hernia

FAMILY HISTORY

Obesity
Carcinoma
GI-related disease
Diabetes mellitus

SOCIAL HISTORY

Substance abuse
Personality type: tense, stressful
View of life's work
Cigarette use

NUTRITIONAL HISTORY

Eating patterns
Dieting attempts
Knowledge of food groups
Methods of meal planning
Types of food usually eaten
Cultural food preferences

MEDICATION HISTORY

Antacids
Laxatives, cathartics
Anticholinergics
Steroids
Antidiarrheals
Antiemetics
Tranquilizers
Sedatives
Antihypertensives
Barbiturates
Antibiotics
Acetylsalicylic acid
Hydrogen receptor antagonists (Tagamet, Zantac, Prilosec, Propulsid)

DIAGNOSTIC TESTS

Complete blood cell count (CBC), differential, platelet count
Alkaline phosphatase level

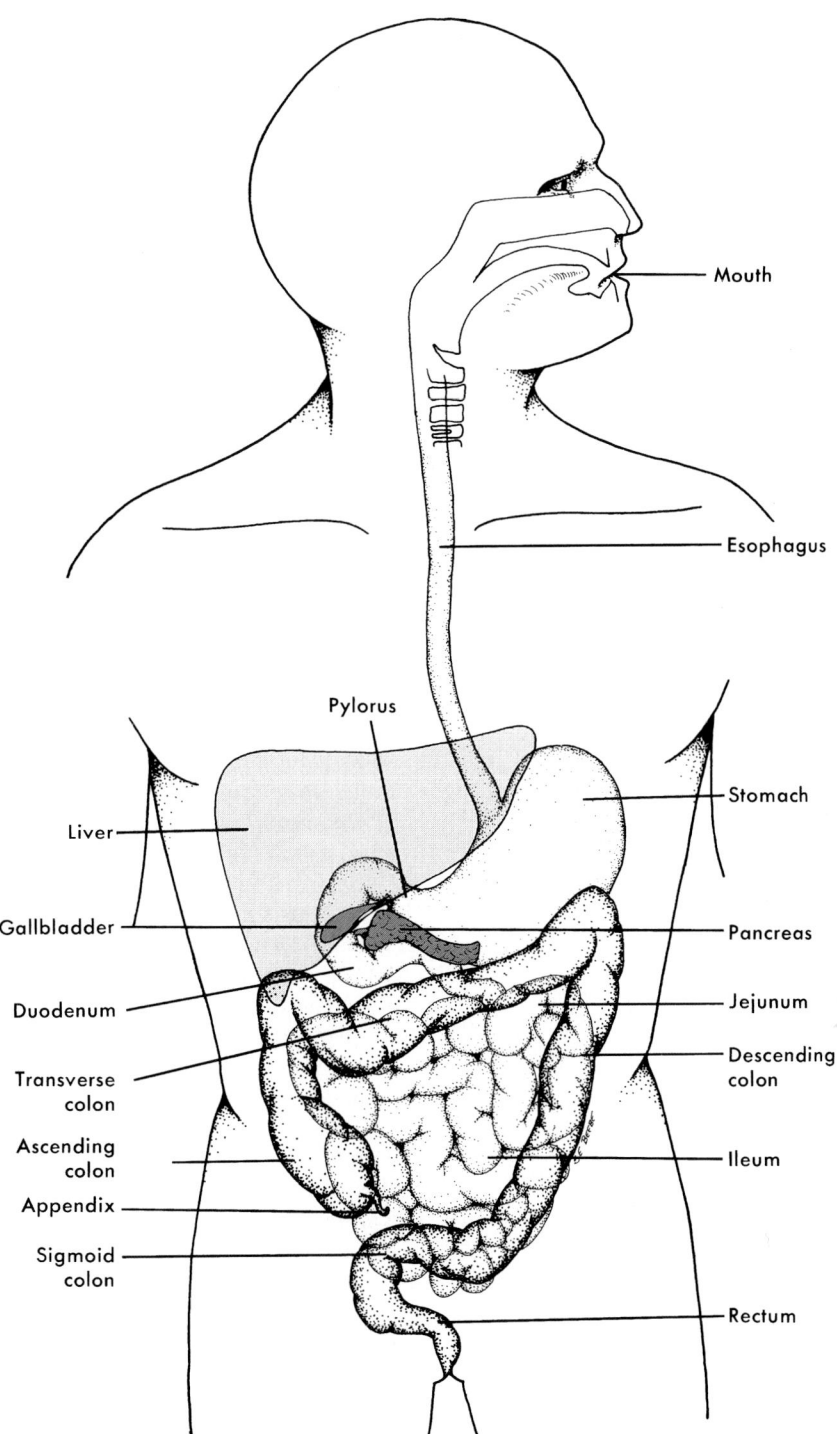

Fig. 6-1 Digestive system.

Bilirubin level
  Serum
  Urine
  Feces
Serum aspartate aminotransferase (AST)
Serum alanine aminotransferase (ALT)
5-Nucleotidase

Lactic acid dehydrogenase (LDH)
Prothrombin time/International Normalized Ratio
  (PT/INR)
Amylase level
  Serum
  Urine
Blood urea nitrogen (BUN)

Stool examination
   Occult blood, white blood cells (WBC)
   Fat
   Protein, pH
   Culture (parasite, ova)
Secretin stimulation test
Serum lipase, cholinesterase levels
Serum calcium level
Serum ammonia level
Serum gastrin level, parietal cell antibodies
Serum α-fetoprotein
Sulkowitch's urine test
Serum albumin level
Total protein level
Serum glucose level
Serum electrolyte profile
Serum carotene test
Xylose tolerance test
Lactose intolerance test
Schilling test
Albumin-globulin (A/G) ratio
Urobilinogen level, transferrin level
Galactose tolerance test
Insulin tolerance test
Carcinoembryonic antigen (CEA)

PROCEDURES
Esophagogastroduodenoscopy and biopsy
Water-soluble contrast studies; Gastrografin
Cine-esophagogram
Motility studies
Radioisotope scintiscan
Gastric acid stimulation test
Esophageal, anorectal manometry
Contrast radiography
Hypotonic duodenography
Radionuclide imaging
Computed tomography (CT) scan
Ultrasonography
Colonic transit study
Small bowel series
Barium enema or swallow gastrography
Barium air-contrast studies
Oral cholecystography
Intravenous (IV) cholangiography
T-tube cholangiography
Biopsy
   Liver
   Rectum
   Colon
   Small bowel
Digital rectal examination
Sigmoidoscopy
Colonoscopy
Proctoscopy
Rectal sensory function test
Complete abdominal x-ray examination
Hydrogen breath test
Gastric cytology

Percutaneous transhepatic cholangiography (PTC)
Celiac and mesenteric arteriography
Superior and inferior mesenteric angiogram
Splenoportography
Endoscopic retrograde cholangiopancreatography (ERCP)
Magnetic resonance imaging (MRI)

ESOPHAGUS

■ ESOPHAGEAL STRICTURE, ESOPHAGITIS, ACHALASIA, DIVERTICULOSIS

stricture: Narrowing of the wall of the esophagus (usually lower two thirds); most commonly resulting from gastroesophageal reflux, chemical ingestion, sliding hiatal hernia; neoplastic infiltration is a secondary cause

esophagitis: Acute or chronic inflammation caused by gastroesophageal reflux, trauma, bacteria, chemical ingestion, hiatal hernia, or overindulgence in alcohol and/or spices

achalasia: Disruption or absence of peristaltic action in the lower two thirds of the esophagus and failure of the cardiac sphincter to relax on swallowing

diverticulosis: Saclike protrusion in the esophageal wall, usually of a congenital nature

ASSESSMENT
SUBJECTIVE DATA
Midsternal or substernal pain; may radiate to back, neck, and arms; symptoms are similar to myocardial infarction (MI)
Discomfort after eating, when bending, or when in supine position
Sore throat
Nocturnal choking
Pyrosis (heartburn)
Nausea
Regurgitation without vomiting
Weight loss
Eructation
Dysphagia

OBJECTIVE DATA
Hematemesis

DIAGNOSTIC TESTS
Endoscopy with biopsy, cytology, and/or dilation
Barium swallow esophagogram
Splash-down time
Chest radiologic study
Manometry
CBC and electrolytes

POTENTIAL COMPLICATIONS
Aspiration pneumonia
Esophageal obstruction

Malnutrition
Esophageal stenosis
Esophageal perforation

MULTIDISCIPLINARY MANAGEMENT
THERAPEUTIC MANAGEMENT
High-calorie, low-fat diet according to tolerance
Antacids
Calcium-blocking agents, isosorbide dinitrate (Isordil), nifedipine (Procardia) (to reduce lower esophageal sphincter [LES] pressure)
H_2-Receptor antagonists, cholinergics
Topical liquid anesthetics
Stool softeners
Antibiotics
Dietary/nutritional consultation as indicated

PATIENT PROBLEMS—NURSING DIAGNOSES/INTERVENTIONS

▼Altered nutrition: less than body requirements related to dysphagia

Assess ability to swallow
Provide small, frequent meals *to ensure adequate intake* instead of large quantities at fewer meals; maintain caloric count
Teach patient to chew food well and eat slowly
Encourage patient to sit up during and after meals
Encourage fluids with meals *to assist patient in swallowing*
Avoid extremes in food temperatures
Measure intake and output *to ensure adequate hydration*
Administer liquid topical anesthetic before meals *to decrease dysphagia*
Encourage fluid intake to 2500 ml/day unless contraindicated
Provide high-fiber foods if tolerated *to assist in elimination*
Monitor CBC, electrolytes
Weigh patient daily (same time, scale, and clothing)
Maintain IV fluid, total parenteral nutrition (TPN) as ordered
Discourage tobacco use *because it increases LES pressure*

Expected Outcomes
Caloric and fluid intake is optimal
Electrolytes are within normal limits
Weight is maintained

▼Risk for aspiration related to impaired swallowing

Assist and teach patient to cough and deep breathe q4h
Monitor breath sounds q4h
Elevate head of bed 30 to 45 degrees after meals and at bedtime *to prevent regurgitation*

Avoid supine position *to aid digestion*
Provide planned rest periods
Assist with feeding as needed
Administer oral hygiene qid
Maintain suction, airway at bedside as indicated

Expected Outcomes
Demonstrates correct coughing and breathing techniques
Presents normal breath sounds

▼Pain related to esophageal inflammation and/or heartburn

Assess specific type of pain, duration, onset
Provide calm, nonstressful environment
Reinforce physician's explanation of disease process
Administer and monitor antacids for effectiveness, side effects
Administer cholinergics and H_2 receptors *to reduce LES pressure*
Provide soothing back rubs *to promote comfort*
Change patient's position in small ways *to promote comfort*
Encourage activities and self-care *to decrease discomfort*

Expected Outcomes
Reports a decrease in heartburn
Maintains activities at optimal level
Reports no pain or discomfort after eating

PATIENT/FAMILY TEACHING
Reinforce physician's explanation of disease and treatment goals
Provide patient/family with consultation from nutritional services/dietitian as indicated
Discuss with patient and/or significant other(s) the importance of diet and diet restrictions
 Explain need to avoid foods that cause dysphagia
 Provide and review high-calorie, high-protein diet instruction sheet if applicable
 Encourage increased fluid intake
 Advise patient to avoid tobacco, aspirin, phenylbutazone, and excessive intake of high-fat foods
 Advise elevating head while sleeping
Discuss methods of avoiding stress
Explain reasons why bending and stooping should be avoided
Discuss methods of avoiding constipation
 Recommend high-fiber foods if tolerated
 Encourage natural laxatives: bran, prunes, psyllium powder

DISCHARGE/HOME CARE PLANNING
Discuss need to avoid weight gain, straining, and/or wearing tight clothing such as belts, girdles
Increase patient's activities to tolerance
Discuss medications: name, dosage, time of administration, purpose, and side effects

Explain importance of follow-up care with physician
Discuss symptoms of recurrence or progression of
  disease to report to physician

■ BLEEDING ESOPHAGEAL VARICES

A condition usually associated with cirrhosis and portal hypertension in which the small esophageal veins become distended and rupture as a result of the increased pressure in the portal system; may be controlled medically, but surgery may be required

ASSESSMENT
SUBJECTIVE DATA
Restlessness
Confusion
Anxiety
Dizziness (vertigo)

OBJECTIVE DATA
Character, frequency, and amount of hematemesis
Respiratory distress
Altered vital signs
Aspiration of emesis
Disorientation
Dehydration
Electrolyte imbalance
Abdominal distention
Melena
Jaundice
Anemia

DIAGNOSTIC TESTS
Esophagoscopy
Mesenteric angiography
Sclerotherapy
CBC, platelets, PT, arterial blood gases (ABGs), electrolytes
Blood alcohol
AST, ALT, LDH, alkaline phosphatase
Liver function tests
Guaiac stools for blood

POTENTIAL COMPLICATIONS
Aspiration pneumonia
Hemorrhage
Shock
Hepatic coma
Death

MULTIDISCIPLINARY MANAGEMENT
THERAPEUTIC MANAGEMENT
NPO
Esophagogastric tamponade with suction and pressures
  to be maintained
Gastric lavages
Parenteral fluids with electrolytes
Fresh whole blood
Indwelling urinary catheter with hourly measurements
Orotracheal suctioning

Respiratory therapy consult as indicated
Oxygen therapy
Central venous pressure (CVP) line or Swan-Ganz catheter
Paracentesis
ABGs
Saline enemas
Vasopressin (Pitressin), neomycin, vitamin K, lactulose
Analgesics, usually phenobarbital
Histamine receptor antagonists (Tagamet, Zantac,
  Prilosec, Propulsid)
Esophageal sclerotherapy
Surgical intervention
Diet, activity
Social services

PATIENT PROBLEMS—NURSING DIAGNOSES/INTERVENTIONS

▼ Risk for aspiration related to esophagogastric tube, impaired swallowing

Maintain bed rest in quiet environment
  Position patient on side during vomiting episodes *to prevent aspiration*
  Elevate head of bed 30 degrees
Perform orotracheal suctioning prn
Auscultate chest for breath sounds q1h to 2h *to prevent respiratory compromise*
Administer oxygen therapy by mask or catheter
Assist and teach patient to turn and deep breathe qh; instruct patient not to cough *because it increases portal pressure*
Administer oral hygiene q1h to 2h; keep mouth and nares well lubricated with petroleum jelly *to promote comfort and skin integrity*
Maintain suction and airway at bedside

Expected Outcomes
Presents normal breath sounds
Manages secretions adequately
Demonstrates turning and deep breathing exercises accurately

▼ Altered tissue perfusion, cardiopulmonary, cerebral, gastrointestinal, renal, peripheral related to hypovolemia

GI system
Monitor bowel sounds; report changes to physician
Monitor stools for melena
Maintain esophagogastric tube
  Sengstaken-Blakemore tube (p. 311)
  Linton tube (p. 311)
  Monitor for signs of complications: aspiration, occlusion of airway, esophageal rupture
Monitor character and amount of gastric drainage q1h to 2h
Administer lavages via tube *to decrease bleeding*
Maintain NPO

Cardiopulmonary system

Assess for signs of hypovolemia: tachycardia; tachypnea; cold, clammy skin

Replace blood as needed; monitor for reaction: rash, fever, tachypnea

Monitor breath sounds

Provide oxygen prn

Maintain parenteral fluids with electrolytes, using large-bore catheter *to facilitate blood transfusion*

Monitor hemoglobin (Hgb), hematocrit (Hct), serum electrolytes, and PT/INR

Monitor CVP line or Swan-Ganz catheter

Monitor ABGs

Monitor BP, R, and apical pulse q15min to 30min

Take rectal temperature q2h while esophagogastric tube is in place

Renal system

Maintain urinary catheter to gravity drainage

Measure intake and output qh; if urine output is <50 ml/hr, report to physician

Monitor specific gravity of urine

Monitor serum pH, BUN, and creatinine

Cerebral system

Assess level of consciousness (LOC) and mental acuity

Establish baseline neurologic assessment

Orient to time, date, and place as needed *to prevent confusion*

Ensure safety with side rails and restraints as needed

Encourage family to sit with patient *to provide support/protection*

Administer lactulose *to prevent encephalopathy*

Peripheral system

Monitor pedal pulses

Encourage active/passive range of motion (ROM) exercises *to promote circulation*

Maintain warmth of extremities

Apply antiembolic stockings *to assist in venous flow*

Elevate legs *to increase venous flow*

Monitor medication administration; observe for effectiveness, side effects
    Antibiotics
    Vitamin K
    Vasopressin
    Antacids

Expected Outcomes

Gastric drainage is clear or clearing

Vital signs are normal

Electrolytes are within normal limits

Intake and output are balanced

Pedal pulses are palpable

Skin is warm and dry

Mental acuity is normal

▼Pain related to invasive procedures and therapeutic treatments

Assess specific type, onset, duration of pain

Maintain position of comfort within limits of ongoing treatments

Administer skin care and back rubs q2h to 4h *to promote comfort*

Keep patient warm and dry

Perform passive ROM exercises q4h

Assess pain intensity level
    Medicate according to pain scale
    Provide diversional activities where possible
    Provide alternative pain management techniques: imaging, deep breathing
    Assess effectiveness of pain relief measures

Increase activity as tolerated

Expected Outcomes

Reports reduction in pain/discomfort

Demonstrates relaxed affect

▼Anxiety related to uncertainty and threat to bodily health

Remain with patient at onset of bleeding as much as possible
    Use restraints if applicable: remove and reapply q4h
    Keep side rails up

Monitor mental acuity and for signs of ensuing coma (increased confusion, increased lethargy)

Plan care to provide rest periods *to prevent fatigue*

Orient patient to place, date, and time frequently

Explain each procedure

Reinforce physician's explanation of disease process

Maintain nonstressful environment
    Dim lights when possible
    Discourage loud talking and noises
    Encourage verbalization of fears and anxieties *to decrease stress*
    Promote relaxation techniques: deep breathing, imaging, relaxation techniques
    Discuss past successful coping behaviors to identify positive coping abilities
    Involve in self-care as much as possible
    Promote support by family/significant other(s)

Expected Outcomes

Expresses understanding of cause of anxiety

Demonstrates ability to cope independently with stress

Additional Nursing Diagnoses to Consider

Altered nutrition: less than body requirements related to anorexia, nausea, vomiting, diarrhea

Activity intolerance related to fatigue and anemia

PATIENT/FAMILY TEACHING AND DISCHARGE/HOME CARE PLANNING

Explain diet restrictions of carbohydrates, fats, and proteins

Consult nutritionist/registered dietitian for low-roughage diet plan

Discuss importance of avoiding alcohol

Explain about available counseling

    Alcoholics Anonymous

    Al-Anon, Al-Ateen

    Chemical dependency agencies

Instruct patient in a mild exercise-to-tolerance program with planned rest periods

Reinforce physician's explanation of effects of alcohol on disease process

Discuss medications: name, purpose, dosage, time of administration, and side effects; caution patient not to take over-the-counter medications (especially aspirin compounds) without checking with physician

Explain symptoms of recurrence or progression to report to physician

Discuss importance of follow-up care with physician

■ HIATAL HERNIA WITH ESOPHAGEAL REFLUX

A common condition in older adults, affecting females more than males; it is a protrusion of the stomach through the diaphragm at the normal esophageal hiatus; there are two types: in a sliding hernia the gastroesophageal junction and a portion of the stomach are above the diaphragm, and in a periesophageal hernia the gastroesophageal junction is normal, but a portion of the stomach is above the diaphragm and lies adjacent to it. A hiatal hernia becomes more significant if it is accompanied by gastroesophageal reflux disease (GERD), in which the gastric juices reflux into the esophagus and in turn cause irritation, scar tissue, and possible stricture (Fig. 6-2)

ASSESSMENT

SUBJECTIVE DATA

Gradual onset of symptoms

Burning sensation in throat after eating; increases in supine position

Regurgitation without vomiting

Dull substernal, epigastric pain; may radiate to shoulder

Dysphagia except for water

Nausea

Belching

Borborygmus

Pyrosis (heartburn)

Fear and anxiety: symptoms similar to MI and peptic ulcer

Decreased appetite

OBJECTIVE DATA

Abdominal distention

Tachypnea

Weight loss or gain

DIAGNOSTIC TESTS

CBC, urinalysis, electrolytes

Motility studies

Electrocardiogram (ECG) to rule out heart disease

Esophageal manometry

Esophagraphy (barium swallow)

Chest radiologic study

Endoscopy with biopsy and cytology

Stool for occult blood

POTENTIAL COMPLICATIONS

Esophageal stricture

Malnutrition

Electrolyte imbalance

Aspiration pneumonia

Hemorrhage

MULTIDISCIPLINARY MANAGEMENT

THERAPEUTIC MANAGEMENT

Antacids

Histamine receptor antagonists: cimetidine (Tagamet), ranitidine (Zantac), Prilosec, Propulsid

GI stimulants: metoclopramide (Reglan)

Cholinergics: bethanechol chloride (Urecholine)

Stool softeners

Diet, bland

Activity

Surgical intervention (fundoplication)

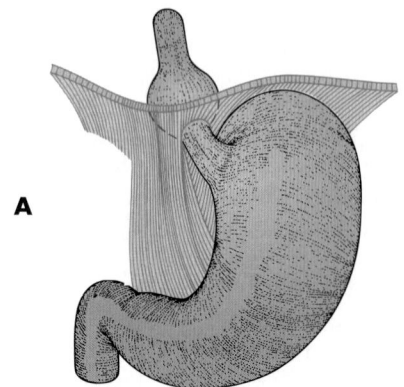 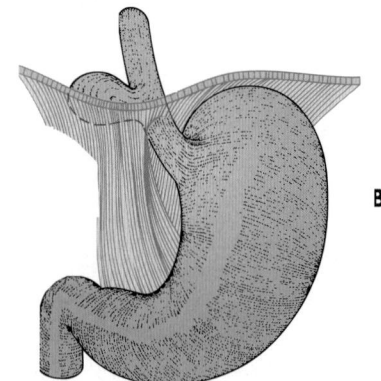

Fig. 6-2 Hiatal hernia. **A,** Sliding hernia. **B,** Rolling hernia.
(From Beare PG, Myers JL: Adult health nursing, *ed 3, St Louis, 1998, Mosby.)*

PATIENT PROBLEMS—NURSING DIAGNOSES/INTERVENTIONS

▼Altered nutrition: less than body requirements related to dysphagia and discomfort following meals

Maintain bed rest
  Place patient in sitting position *to facilitate swallowing*
  Avoid supine position *to prevent regurgitation*
Measure intake and output *to ensure balanced nutrition*
Administer GI stimulants *to increase gastroesophageal emptying* and cholinergics *to increase motility*
Assist with and teach patient to turn and deep breathe qid
Provide bland diet; small, frequent feedings *to prevent gastric distention*
Encourage water with meals *to cleanse esophagus and facilitate swallowing*
Maintain sitting position after meals for 1 to 2 hours *to aid digestion and prevent reflux*
Collaborate with nutritionist/registered dietitian for meal planning
Discourage smoking, alcohol, and spicy foods
Avoid constipation with stool softeners, natural laxatives *to prevent straining*
Encourage ambulation; caution against bending from waist
Discourage eating 1 to 2 hours before bedtime *to avoid heartburn/reflux*
Explain importance of weight loss if obese *to reduce pressure on gastroesophageal junction*

Expected Outcomes
Nutritional intake is adequate
Understanding of restrictions in diet and position are demonstrated

▼Pain related to reflux

Administer antacids after meals and hs *to decrease gastric acidity/discomfort*
Discuss importance of avoiding restrictive clothing: girdles, belts, longline bras
Provide diversional activities *to decrease attention on pain*
Explain association between food and discomfort
Provide list of foods that may cause pain

Expected Outcomes
Expresses increasing comfort with diet and position restrictions
Understands purpose and side effects of antacids

PATIENT/FAMILY TEACHING AND DISCHARGE/HOME CARE PLANNING

Instruct patient to elevate head of bed on 4-inch blocks and where to purchase needed supplies
Discuss patient's typical 24-hour diet

Discuss and provide dietary plan and the need to avoid fats, spicy foods, alcohol, chocolate, peppermint, caffeine, tobacco
Encourage patient to eat slowly; chew foods well; take small bites; and have small, frequent meals
Stress importance of exercise and weight reduction if applicable; some modification of activities may be needed
Explain disease process and symptoms to report to physician
Discuss stool softeners and natural laxatives as alternatives to cathartics/laxatives
Outline medication management as to name, dosage, purpose, time of administration, and side effects
Discuss importance of avoiding certain medications: anticholinergics, diazepam, nitrates, calcium blockers, beta-adrenergic antagonists
Stress importance of continuing follow-up care

■ ESOPHAGEAL SURGERY

fundoplication for hiatal hernia: Fundus of the stomach is wrapped around the lower 3 to 4 cm of the esophagus to produce an area of higher pressure; a thoracic approach may be used

perforated esophagus repair: Perforation is closed and the bleeding controlled

esophageal diverticulum: Outpouchings are repaired and the lumen of the lower esophagus reduced to normal size

ASSESSMENT
SUBJECTIVE DATA
Location and character of pain

OBJECTIVE DATA
Decreased breath sounds
Splinting with respirations
Tachypnea
Bradypnea
Function of chest tubes (thoracic approach)
Character and amount of gastric drainage and urine output

DIAGNOSTIC TESTS
CBC and electrolytes
Chest radiologic study

POTENTIAL COMPLICATIONS
Respiratory distress
Electrolyte imbalance
Gastroesophageal anastomosis leak
Hemorrhage
Shock
Tracheoesophageal fistula
Suture line infection
Pneumothorax (thoracic approach)
Pneumonia

MULTIDISCIPLINARY MANAGEMENT
THERAPEUTIC MANAGEMENT

Analgesics
NPO
Parenteral fluids with electrolytes
Whole blood if required
Nasogastric tube and urinary catheter
Respiratory therapy
Oxygen per mask or catheter as required
Incentive spirometer
Gastrostomy tube and type of feeding if appropriate
Diet, activity
Chest tubes

PATIENT PROBLEMS—NURSING DIAGNOSES/INTERVENTIONS

▼ Risk for aspiration related to anesthesia and naso-gastric tube

Assess ability to swallow
Auscultate chest for breath sounds q2h to 4h
Elevate head of bed 35 to 45 degrees *to promote coughing and prevent aspiration*
Teach and assist patient to turn, cough, and deep breathe q2h to 4h; splint chest as needed
Maintain oxygen and/or use incentive spirometer qh *to aerate the lungs and prevent atelectasis*
Place suction and airway at bedside

Expected Outcomes

Presents normal breath sounds
Performs turning, deep breathing adequately

▼ Risk for fluid volume deficit related to NPO state, and nasogastric tube

Maintain NPO; assess for signs of dehydration: poor skin turgor, fever
Maintain parenteral fluids with electrolytes *to replace volume loss*
Monitor serum electrolytes
Measure intake and output
Monitor vital signs q4h
Maintain nasogastric tube or gastrostomy tube to intermittent suction or gravity drainage *to promote patency/correct functioning*
Monitor placement of nasogastric tube; tape in place; if tube is dysfunctional, notify physician; *do not reposition because it may disrupt suture line*
Monitor character and amount of gastric drainage q8h
Monitor wound for excessive drainage/bleeding prn; report excess to physician
Encourage movement of legs, feet *to promote venous return*
After nasogastric tube removal
   Initiate oral fluids in small amounts *to assess tolerance and sphincter function*
   Progress to soft, bland diet as tolerated

Report pain, retching, or vomiting to physician because it may indicate dysfunctioning gastroesophageal sphincter
For gastrostomy tube: administer tube feedings (p. 20)

Expected Outcomes

Intake and output are balanced
Electrolytes are within normal limits
Vital signs are normal

▼ Pain related to surgical intervention

Assess type, location, and intensity of pain; use pain rating scale
Administer analgesics to maintain comfort; assess effectiveness of pain relief measures
Collaborate with physician to initiate patient-controlled analgesia (PCA)
Turn and change position q2h to 4h *to reduce fatigue, discomfort*
Provide back rubs and skin care *to promote comfort*
Maintain planned rest periods *to prevent fatigue*
Splint incision when coughing
Discuss alternative pain management techniques: deep breathing, imaging, relaxation techniques
Provide diversional activities *to decrease attention on pain*

Expected Outcomes

Reports reduction in or absence of pain
Demonstrates more relaxed affect

▼ Anxiety related to surgical procedure and possible changes in lifestyle

Reinforce physician's explanation of surgical procedure and expected outcome
Encourage and allow time for verbalization of concerns; involve significant others
Discuss stress management techniques: breathing, relaxation, imagery
Provide quiet, nonstressful environment
Explain nursing care plan and all procedures *to alleviate apprehension and increase awareness*
Assess present coping patterns; assist patient with identifying alternative and positive ways of coping
Explain needed changes in lifestyle in nonthreatening and positive manner *to assist patient in problem-solving techniques*

Expected Outcomes

Demonstrates progress in developing positive attitudes toward needed change in lifestyle
Uses family/significant other(s) for support group

PATIENT/FAMILY TEACHING

Discuss patient's typical 24-hour diet
Provide and discuss diet and dietary restrictions
   Eat small, frequent meals
   Chew foods well and eat slowly

Drink water with meals
  Elevate head of bed at night
Explain procedure for gastrostomy feedings (p. 20)
Discuss need to avoid smoking

DISCHARGE/HOME CARE PLANNING
Explain importance of balancing activity and rest
Discuss need to avoid constipation with natural laxatives
Demonstrate wound and dressing change care
Explain signs of wound infection: pain, redness, fever, drainage
Provide information on needed supplies and where to purchase them
Reinforce stress management techniques
Discuss importance of follow-up care with physician

■ ENDOSCOPY: ESOPHAGEAL, GASTRIC, DUODENAL
Insertion of a fiberoptic scope into the esophagus, stomach, or duodenum to determine pathologic conditions and/or obtain tissue specimens for diagnostic studies; also used to remove foreign bodies (Fig. 6-3)

PREENDOSCOPY CARE
Assess baseline vital signs
Encourage and allow time for verbalization of fears and concerns
Reinforce physician's explanation of procedure
Maintain NPO
Remove dentures and partial plates

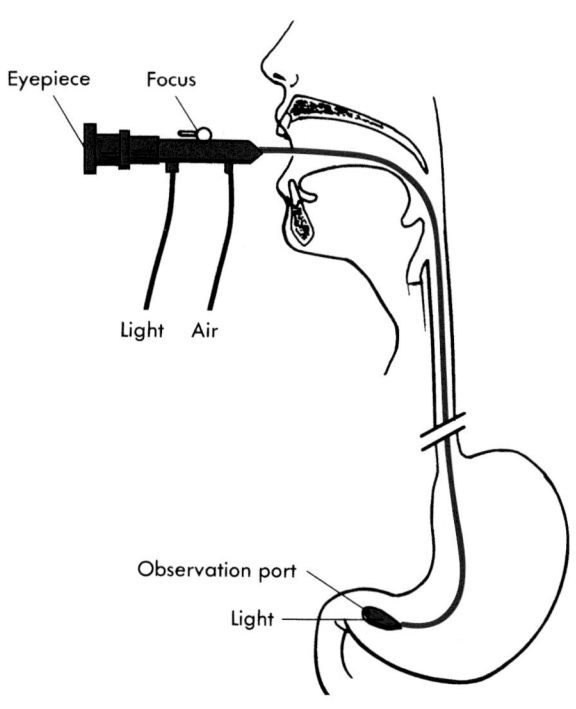

Fig. 6-3 Stomach may be visualized by means of a fiberscope. *(From Phipps WJ et al: Medical-surgical nursing: concepts and clinical practice, ed 6, St Louis, 1999, Mosby.)*

Labels in figure: Eyepiece, Focus, Light, Air, Observation port, Light

Administer oral hygiene
Administer premedications

POSTENDOSCOPY ASSESSMENT
SUBJECTIVE DATA
Sore throat

OBJECTIVE DATA
LOC and vital signs
Swallow and gag reflexes present
Respiratory rate and depth
Hoarseness

POTENTIAL COMPLICATIONS
Respiratory distress
Esophageal, gastric, or duodenal perforation
Dysphagia
  Subcutaneous crepitus in neck
  Extreme pain: increases with respirations or neck or shoulder movement
  Hematemesis

POSTENDOSCOPY INTERVENTIONS
Assist and teach patient to turn and deep breathe q2h *to maintain airway and aerate the lungs*
Administer warm saline gargles prn *to soothe sore throat*
Provide warm liquids until patient is able to swallow without discomfort, then increase diet as tolerated
Administer oral hygiene prn
Explain signs and symptoms to report to physician: increased pain, bleeding, difficulty breathing
Discuss deep-breathing exercises and oral hygiene
Encourage ongoing outpatient care
Keep suction and airway at bedside

■ SENGSTAKEN-BLAKEMORE TUBE OR LINTON TUBE
Sengstaken-Blakemore tube: *Nasoesophagogastric tube with three lumens and two pressure balloons: two lumens are used to inflate the balloons, and the third is for gastric drainage; used to control esophageal hemorrhage (Fig. 6-4, A)*
    Linton tube: *Three-lumen nasogastric tube for control of gastric hemorrhage: two lumens suction esophageal and gastric contents, and the third lumen inflates the gastric balloon (Fig. 6-4, B)*

PREINSERTION ASSESSMENT AND CARE
Baseline vital signs
Assess patient's ability to swallow and mouth breathe; maintain patent airway
Explain purpose of tube and procedure
Observe amount and color of emesis after stomach contents have been aspirated
Check tube for patency of each lumen and strength of balloon(s)

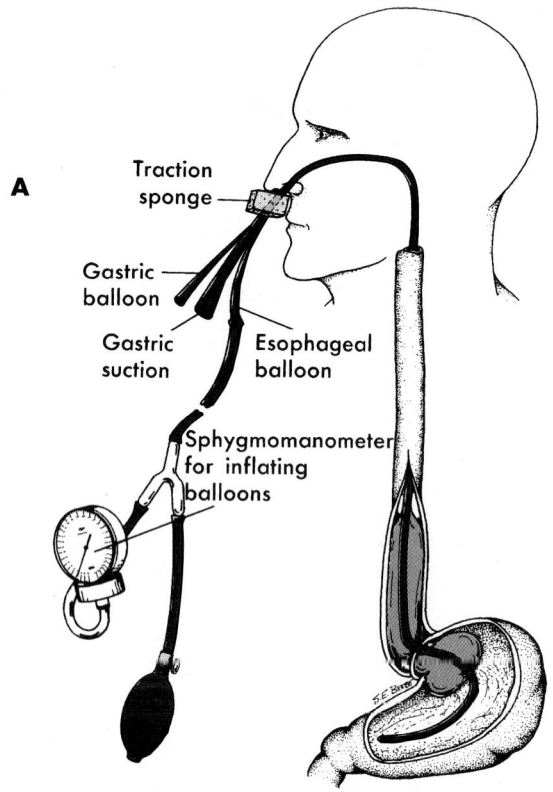

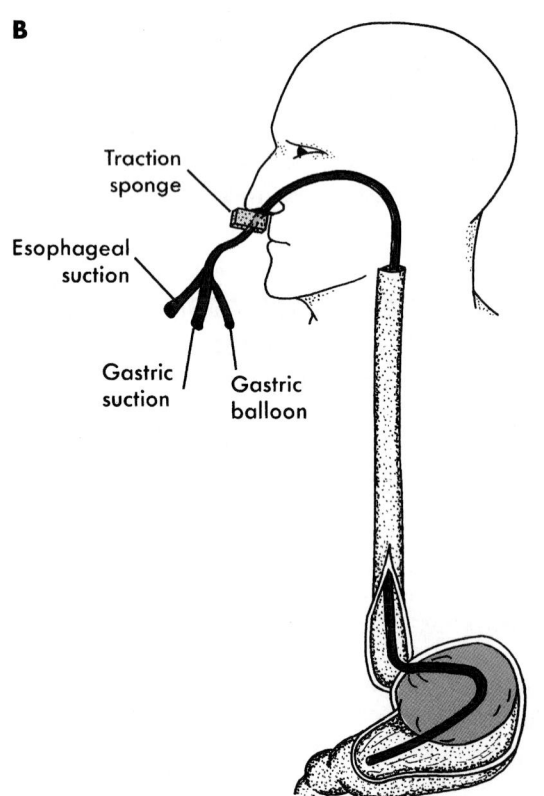

Fig. 6-4 **A,** Sengstaken-Blakemore tube. **B,** Linton tube.

Tube should be in good condition
　Use sphygmomanometer for balloon inflation of
　　Sengstaken-Blakemore tube
　Use 50-ml syringe for balloon inflation of Linton tube
　Lubricate and chill tube according to manufacturer's
　　instructions

POSTINSERTION CARE
Sengstaken-Blakemore Tube
Tube is inserted through nose into stomach
Balloons are inflated to 20 to 40 mm Hg each or as
　ordered (Fig. 6-3, *A*)
Lumens are securely clamped and labeled from each
　balloon
Gastric suction tube is labeled and attached to
　intermittent suction apparatus
Traction (¼ to 1 lb) is applied to gastric balloon as
　ordered
Tube is securely taped to nose or traction sponge

Linton Tube
Tube is inserted through nose into stomach
Gastric tube and esophageal tube are labeled and
　connected to separate intermittent suction
　apparatuses
Balloon is inflated with 100 to 200 ml of air or as ordered,
　and lumen is securely clamped and labeled (see
　Fig. 6-4, *B*)
Tube is taped to traction sponge and traction applied

POTENTIAL COMPLICATIONS
Respiratory distress
Aspiration pneumonia
Chest pain
Abdominal distention

INTERVENTIONS
Monitor vital signs
Maintain prescribed balloon pressure
Release traction, deflate balloon(s) q8h to 12h *to prevent
　necrosis of tissues*
Irrigate only gastric lumen of tubes
Tape tube comfortably and securely to cheek *to prevent
　pressure on oral/nasal tissues*

STOMACH

ANOREXIA NERVOSA/BULIMIA
　*anorexia nervosa: Disorder characterized by emaci-
ation occurring as a result of self-inflicted starvation; etiology appears to be primarily psychologic (severe body
image disturbance/morbid fear of obesity), but it may include underlying organic factors; subtypes include restricting type and binge-purging type*
　*bulimia: Eating disorder characterized by excessive
overeating and use of laxatives, diuretics, and/or self-*

induced vomiting to purge intestinal tract of food; sub-types include purging type and nonpurging type

bulimia nervosa: *A combination of anorexia nervosa and bulimia. Signs and symptoms, behaviors may overlap*

Persons with either of these disorders believe strongly that they can attain control of self and others, autonomy, and competence by dieting and losing weight; severe disorders manifest a multitude of physiologic changes: bradycardia, electrolyte imbalances, neurologic problems (seizures), amenorrhea, decreased testosterone and musculoskeletal maturation, hypotension, and death

Usual age: adolescence; predominantly females, but may affect males

Peak ages: 12 to 13 years; 19 to 20 years and into young adulthood

ASSESSMENT

Middle- to upper-class socioeconomic level
Conservative philosophy, high personal standards
Often dependent relationship with a passive father
Often dependent relationship with a dominant mother
Family members closely fused
Personal boundaries not respected
Mind reading prevalent
Sense of independence sabotaged
Expressions of anger, anxiety, or aggressiveness blocked
Arguments not allowed
Togetherness prized
Loyalty exaggerated
Excellence as the standard
Anorectic seeks love and approval, becomes
　perfectionistic, cannot achieve it, develops physical
　symptoms
Family attention focuses on and reinforces weight loss
　and poor eating

Prodromal Period

Increasing irritability
Eczema may develop
Abdominal discomfort
Headaches
Hyperactivity
Depression
Anxiety
Social withdrawal from friends
High level of investment in schoolwork and high-energy
　sports or high-stress employment

Organic Symptoms

Severe weight loss
Secondary amenorrhea
Bradycardia
Lowered body temperature
Decreased pH
Cold intolerance
Dry skin, poor turgor
Brittle nails
Lanugo hair

Decreased appetite
Feelings of satiety
Breasts atrophied
Axillary and pubic hair reduced
Sleep disturbances
Constipation
Increased susceptibility to infection

Affect/Behavior

Academically, professionally high achiever
Conforming behavior
Conscientious
Increased energy levels
Relentless pursuit of thinness and fear of fatness
Anorexia frequently precipitated by adolescent crisis
History of normal weight
Fear of developing feelings of sexuality
Disturbed body image of delusional proportions
　Defends emaciation as normal
　Feels rewarded by achieving and maintaining
　　emaciated state
　Is fearful of weight gain
　Interprets others' concerns as attempts to make
　　patient fat
　Admires emaciated self in mirror
Inaccurate and confused perception and interpretation of
　inner stimuli
　Does not recognize signs of nutritional need
　Is unable to assess amount of food taken
　Derives pleasure from refusal of food
　Hides food; may secretly flush it down toilet
　May induce vomiting after eating
　May use laxatives to speed passage of food
　Is preoccupied with food and related activities; may
　　plan and prepare meals for others, collect recipes,
　　count calories
　Increases activity to counteract weight gain
　May conceal weights on body before being weighed
　May hoard food, especially candy and nonnutritive
　　foods
Paralyzing sense of ineffectiveness
　Behaves with defiance and rebellion but is
　　overwhelmed by sense of ineffectiveness
　Feels he or she responds only to demands and wishes
　　of others
　Doubts ability of or right to self-assertion

DIAGNOSTIC TESTS

CBC with differential: leukopenia, lymphocytosis,
　anemia
Blood serum studies
　Hypoglycemia, hypocholesteremia, hypoproteinemia,
　　hypokalemia, hyponatremia
　Decreased estrogen/progestin levels, elevated BUN
　Fasting blood sugar; hypoglycemia
　Thyroid, pituitary studies
　ECG, T wave inversions
Urine studies: decreased urinary 17-ketosteroids, presence
　of ketones

POTENTIAL COMPLICATIONS
Lethal cardiac dysrhythmias

MULTIDISCIPLINARY MANAGEMENT
THERAPEUTIC MANAGEMENT
Dietary consultation
Determination of extent of nutritional deprivation
If severe, nasogastric feedings are ordered if food is refused by patient
Parenteral fluids with electrolytes/hyperalimentation for dehydration or life-threatening malnutrition
Medications: cypropheptadine (Periactin) to stimulate appetite, bicyclic antidepressant (fluoxetine [Prozac]); tricyclic antidepressants (Elavil), antianxiety agents: alprazolam (Xanax)
Daily weights when ordered
Referral to psychotherapist with family therapy approach to care, behavior modification therapy

PATIENT PROBLEMS—NURSING DIAGNOSES/INTERVENTIONS

▼Altered nutrition: less than body requirements related to anorexia, self-induced vomiting, laxative abuse, and/or distorted perception of body

Encourage patient's own selection of foods *to increase responsibility*
Limit mealtimes to 30 to 40 minutes *to prevent dawdling*
Six small meals may be required *to prevent gastric distention*
Diminish distractions during mealtimes
Encourage patient to eat slowly and relish the taste of food
Supervise patient following meals *to prevent vomiting*
Explain that food will not cause obesity at this time but will help patient maintain a normal weight
Avoid power struggles over food by minimizing attention paid to it
Be consistent in your own behavior *to increase patient confidence*
If tube feedings or TPN become necessary because oral intake is not adequate, explain the rationale in a calm, sensitive manner *to prevent patient from feeling a loss of control*
Monitor frequently to prevent patient from dislodging tube or needle
Involve nutritionist/registered dietitian in explaining meal planning, needed nutrients, and rationale for eating a variety of foods *to assist patient in feeling in control*
Monitor intake carefully *to ensure adequate nutrition*
Maintain strict calorie count after each meal
Provide at least 1200 to 1500 calories/day *to ensure balanced nutrition*
Obtain accurate weights *to ensure slow, steady weight gain*
Encourage feeling of responsibility for weight gain
Discourage patient from frequent self-weighing

Explain to patient that rehabilitation will be a long-term process

Expected Outcomes
Expresses understanding of nutritional needs
Ingests caloric intake adequate to maintain a slow, constant weight gain
Resumes eating pattern consistent with desired weight gain

▼Risk for fluid volume deficit related to dieting/purging

Monitor intake and output and maintain accurate records
Include patient in scheduling fluid intake times *to encourage compliance*
Explain and discuss methods to avoid use of laxatives/diuretics *to maintain fluid balance*
Monitor parenteral fluids with electrolytes/TPN as needed; accompany patient to bathroom to prevent emptying of IV fluids
Monitor vital signs q 1h *to evaluate adequate fluid volume*
Assess for hypotension, bradycardia

Expected Outcomes
Hydration is maintained adequately
Intake and output are balanced
Understanding of causative factors and behaviors is progressing

▼Body image disturbance related to inaccurate perception of self as fat; poor self-esteem

Assess patient's feelings about self, body
Give positive support and praise for things well done *to increase feelings of self-worth*
Foster successful experiences
Begin with tasks easily accomplished *to increase compliance and confidence*
Focus on positive traits *to assist patient to view body accurately*
Encourage patient to verbalize thoughts about self and body *to increase confidence*
Have patient draw picture of self and discuss perception of self
Encourage wearing loose clothing to avoid focusing on body, weight, appearance
Encourage good hygiene and grooming for feeling of well-being
Respond factually and consistently to patient's questions concerning diet and nutrition
Encourage and reinforce constructive physical activity (bed making, helping other patients) *to assist patient in viewing self as worthwhile*

Expected Outcomes
Begins to verbalize positive thoughts of self and self-worth

Begins to perceive self as thin and as an individual
Shows progress in accepting responsibility for actions

▼ Ineffective individual coping related to feelings of loss of control, fear of growing up, and/or personalized response to family dysfunction

Encourage ventilation of feelings; assist in identifying fears associated with bingeing, starving, and so on *to help patient deal with loss of control*
Observe and record responses to stress
Encourage speaking with staff when stressed *to promote patient's self-support*
Discourage (withdraw your attention from) rituals or emotional associations with meals, food, and so on
Support patient's attempts at self-determination, especially when with family, *to foster positive feelings about self and set realistic expectations*
Promote stress-reduction techniques: imaging, relaxation exercises, diversional activities
Encourage support by significant others
Discuss and teach problem-solving method *to promote positive communication skills*

Expected Outcomes
Begins to exhibit positive coping skills
Maintains weight during stressful periods
Seeks appropriate support and resources

▼ Ineffective family coping related to inability to communicate and inability to meet the needs of all family members

Assess patient/family on knowledge of eating disorder and altered communication skills *to facilitate the needed changes*
Encourage patient and family to verbalize thoughts, perceptions, and feelings
Point out areas where patient and family members disagree *to foster positive behaviors*
Determine each family member's perception of what another has said *to reinforce listening skills*
Emphasize with patient and family members importance of using "I" statements and taking responsibility only for self
With family members present, be patient's advocate and support attempts at self-determination and control
Redirect control conflicts between patient and parents/significant other(s) away from food and onto issues related to curfews, school activities, job satisfaction, and so on
Refer family to community resources for psychologic counseling as needed

Expected Outcomes
Begins to recognize needs of others
Identifies areas where needs and expectations are unmet

Responds positively to provided support
Seeks assistance as needed

Additional Nursing Diagnoses to Consider
Constipation related to laxative misuse
Powerlessness related to a feeling of loss of control over life
Impaired skin integrity, related to malnutrition
Sexual dysfunction related to decreased levels of estrogen, progestin, absence of menses

PATIENT/FAMILY TEACHING
Reinforce nutritional guidelines and how to manage diet
Weigh patient q week (same time, scale, and clothing)
Discuss with patient the need to reassess caloric requirements q2wk to 4wk
Reinforce use of stress-management techniques
Promote regular exercise program but discourage overexertion
Reinforce use of problem-solving and assertiveness skills to maintain sense of control over life
Discuss importance of socialization and other activities

DISCHARGE/HOME CARE PLANNING
Encourage patient to seek assistance in sexuality problems as needed
Refer to home health social worker as needed
Encourage patient to keep physician, nutritionist/ registered dietitian, and psychotherapist appointments
Refer to social services for local eating disorders association or to the national association:
American Anorexia Bulimia Association, Inc.
165 W 46th Street, Suite 1108
New York, NY 10036
Phone: (212)575-6200
www.aabainc.org

■ CHRONIC GASTRITIS
An inflammation of the mucosal lining of the stomach caused by Helicobacter pylori *bacteria, peptic ulcer, pernicious anemia, or stomach cancer. If* H. pylori *is the cause and is diagnosed and treated early, the risk of progression to peptic ulcer disease is greatly reduced; other etiologic factors implicated are long-term use of aspirin, NSAIDs, and alcohol (Fig. 6-5).*

ASSESSMENT
SUBJECTIVE DATA
Epigastric fullness, discomfort
Nausea
Abdominal tenderness
History of alcohol, aspirin ingestion
Anorexia, weight loss

OBJECTIVE DATA
Vomiting, eructation
Hematemesis
Melena

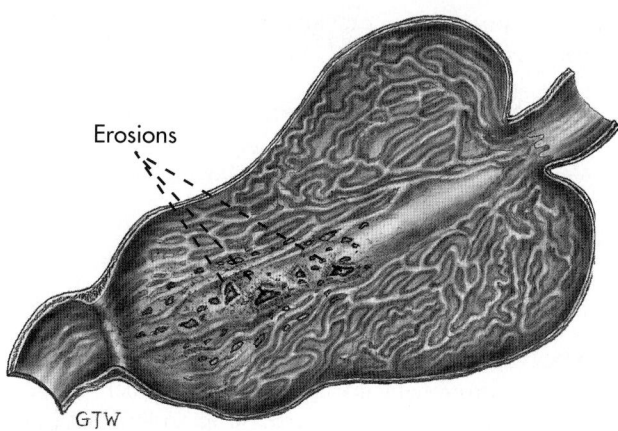

Fig. 6-5 Erosive gastritis (disruption of "tight cellular junctions" with back diffusion of H$^+$).
(From Doughty DB, Jackson DB: Mosby's clinical nursing series: gastrointestinal disorders, St Louis, 1993, Mosby.)

Diagnostic Tests

Enzyme-linked immunosorbent assays (ELISA)
Urease test with endoscopic biopsy
Serum gastrin, parietal cell antibodies, pepsinogen I level
Intrinsic factor antibodies
Antibodies to gastrin-producing cells
Breath tests to measure presence of bacteria
Biopsy
Endoscopy
Gastric analysis

Multidisciplinary Management
Therapeutic Management

For *Helicobacter pylori:*
　　Tetracycline (or amoxicillin) 500 mg qid for 14 days
　　Metronidazole (Flagyl) 250 mg qid for 14 days
　　Pink bismuth tablets (bismuth subsalicylate, Pepto-Bismol) two tablets qid for 14 days
H$_2$-Receptor antagonist (H$_2$RA) (Tagamet, Zantac) if being taken previously for hyperacidity
Diet restrictions
Iron products as indicated
Vitamin B$_{12}$ for pernicious anemia
Behavior modification for
　　Smoking
　　Alcohol consumption

Patient Problems—Nursing Diagnosis/Interventions

▼Pain related to epigastric distress and abdominal discomfort

Discuss importance of taking all medications as prescribed
For patients on tetracycline/metronidazole/bismuth regimen for *H. pylori*
　　Do not drink alcohol, beer, or wine or use tobacco products

Instruct patient to chew pink bismuth tablets thoroughly before swallowing
Take medications with a large glass of water *to promote absorption*
Do not take medications with milk *to avoid malabsorption*
Reassure patient that pink bismuth tablets may be taken with the tetracycline in this instance
Take antacids and or iron products, including vitamins with iron, 2 hours before or after the three prescribed medicines
Avoid long periods in the sun or under sun lamp during the 2-week period
Explain that symptoms may not improve immediately but will improve when treatment is finished

Expected Outcome
Reports reduction in or absence of pain

Patient/Family Teaching and Discharge/Home Care Planning
Review techniques to decrease stress (relaxation, deep breathing, etc.)
Avoid smoking and alcohol ingestion
Keep follow-up appointments
For patients on the *H. pylori* drug regimen
　　Explain that there may be some harmless side effects such as darkening of the tongue and/or urine/stool or metallic taste in the mouth; these are temporary
　　Notify physician if any of the following symptoms are present and bothersome:
　　　　Diarrhea, nausea, and abdominal pain
　　　　Vaginal discharge, itching
　　　　Skin rash
　　Take complete prescription as prescribed to ensure cure

■ Peptic Ulcer Disease (Gastric and Duodenal)

Peptic ulcer disease includes both gastric and duodenal ulceration of the gastric mucosa caused by an imbalance of acid and pepsin; however, the incidence, physiology, and some etiology are different for each

　　gastric ulcer: *Causative factors include medications (aspirin, antiinflammatories), chemicals (tobacco, alcohol); usually located in the distal portion of the stomach at the lesser curvature; the mucosa is normally protected by maintaining a neutral pH with release of mucus and bicarbonate; if this balance is altered, ulcer formation begins (Fig. 6-6)*

　　duodenal ulcer: *Causative factors include hypersecretion of gastric acid (40%) and decreased pepsin in gastric juices (60%); usually located at the pylorus end of the stomach and in the duodenum; ulceration occurs when acid secretion exceeds the protective ability of the mucosa, or when the pH of the duodenal juices is reduced and the pepsin damages the mucosa; genetic factors,*

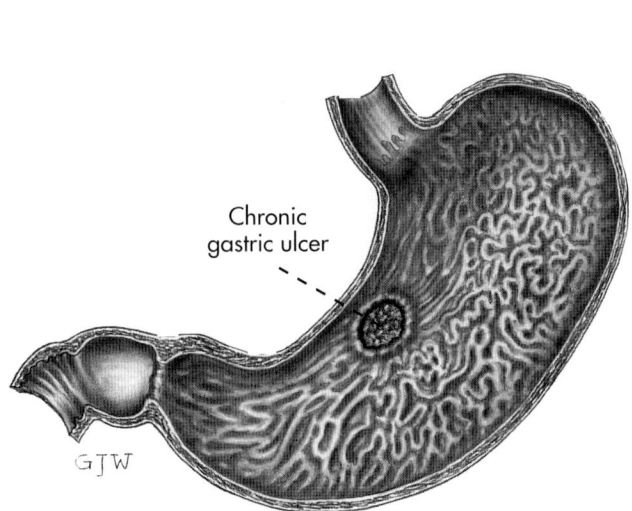

Fig. 6-6 Gastric peptic ulcer.
(From Doughty DB, Jackson DB: Mosby's clinical nursing series: gastrointestinal disorders, *St Louis, 1993, Mosby.)*

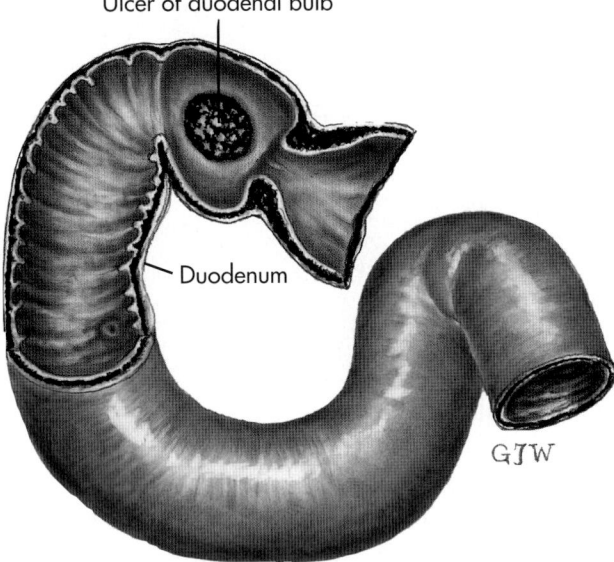

Fig. 6-7 Duodenal peptic ulcer.
(From Doughty DB, Jackson DB: Mosby's clinical nursing series: gastrointestinal disorders, *St Louis, 1993, Mosby.)*

stress, and medications may also be contributing causes (Fig. 6-7)

ASSESSMENT
SUBJECTIVE DATA
Gastric Ulcer
Left to midepigastric pain; may radiate to back, flank
Pain may or may not be relieved by antacids, food

Duodenal Ulcer
Right epigastric pain; may radiate to back or thorax; pain usually relieved by antacids, food

Common Data
Pyrosis (heartburn)
Fullness after eating
Eructation
Nausea
Vomiting
Bloating
Anorexia
Gnawing type of pain; not food related

OBJECTIVE DATA
Abdominal distention
Vomiting

DIAGNOSTIC TESTS
Endoscopy with biopsy and cytology
Barium studies
Abdominal radiologic studies
Gastric analysis
Hgb, Hct, blood pepsinogen, parietal cell antibodies, gastrin levels
Stool for melena

POTENTIAL COMPLICATIONS
Electrolyte imbalance
Gastric, duodenal hemorrhage
Perforation
Pyloric stenosis
Shock

MULTIDISCIPLINARY MANAGEMENT
THERAPEUTIC MANAGEMENT
Analgesics
Aluminum-magnesium antacids (Delcid, Mylanta-II)
H_2-Antagonists
    Cimetidine (Tagamet)
    Ranitidine (Zantac)
    Nizatidine (Axid)
    Famotidine (Pepcid)
Sucralfate (Carafate)
Cisapride (Propulsid)
Proton pump inhibitors (omeprazole, lansoprazole, pantoprazole)
Misoprostol (Cytotec)
Diet
Consultation with dietitian

PATIENT PROBLEMS—NURSING DIAGNOSES/INTERVENTIONS

▼ Altered nutrition: less than body requirements related to discomfort, anorexia

Assess patient's nutritional status: present diet, eating patterns, foods usually eaten, weight loss or gain
Assess patient's medication history: aspirin, steroids, vasopressors, antiinflammatories
Monitor vital signs q4h

Monitor intake and output q8h

Maintain nonstressful environment

Provide high-calorie, high-protein diet in small, frequent meals *to help neutralize the gastric acid*

Monitor effectiveness, side effects of antiemetics, antacids

Weigh as needed (same time, scale, and clothing) *to ensure maintenance of normal weight and assess loss or gain*

Expected Outcomes

Tolerates diet without discomfort

Intake and output are balanced

▼ Pain related to irritation, disruption of gastric mucosa

Assess pain: location, type, frequency, and duration; sudden severe pain may indicate gastric, duodenal perforation; use pain scale

Monitor effectiveness, side effects of analgesics/antacids

Provide diversional activities *to reduce attention on pain*

Administer back rubs, changes in position *to promote comfort*

Discuss and teach relaxation techniques: deep breathing, imaging

Expected Outcome

Reports reduction in or absence of pain

PATIENT/FAMILY TEACHING AND DISCHARGE/HOME CARE PLANNING

Discuss relationship of causative agents to peptic ulcer disease

Provide and review written instructions concerning medications, including name, purpose, dosage, time of administration, and side effects; instruct patient to take only antacids prescribed by physician and to avoid aspirin, steroids

Discuss dietary plan: importance of eating meals at regular times, necessity of not missing a meal, and benefits of small, frequent meals; avoid coffee, tobacco, and alcohol

Explain signs and symptoms of perforation: extreme epigastric pain and hematemesis

Avoid use of antiinflammatory agents

Describe importance of nonstressful environment, especially at mealtime

Discuss methods of stress management: relaxation, exercise, meditation

Encourage follow-up care with physician

■ GASTRIC HEMORRHAGE

Condition in which ulceration of the mucosa has progressed to the vasculature of the stomach or duodenum; may be insidious or acute

ASSESSMENT
SUBJECTIVE DATA

Nausea, vomiting

Abdominal tenderness, pain

Anxiety, fear

OBJECTIVE DATA

Decreased BP

Elevated pulse

Abdominal distention

Hematemesis

Melena

Hyperperistalsis

Increased bowel sounds

Dehydration

Chills, fever

DIAGNOSTIC TESTS

Endoscopy

GI series

Stools for occult blood

CBC, electrolytes, BUN

Blood type

POTENTIAL COMPLICATIONS

Electrolyte imbalance

Gastric perforation

Hemorrhage

Shock

MULTIDISCIPLINARY MANAGEMENT
THERAPEUTIC MANAGEMENT

Analgesics

NPO

Nasogastric tube or Linton tube, depending on bleeding site

Parenteral fluids with electrolytes and vitamins

Whole blood or packed red blood cells (PBCs)

Oxygen as indicated

CVP line, Swan-Ganz catheter

Urethral catheter

Cimetidine intravenously

Antacids via nasogastric tube

Gastric lavage (norepinephrine bitartrate [Levophed] may be added to produce vasoconstriction)

Endoscopy: endoscope electrocoagulation

Vasopressin arterially

Surgical intervention: repair or resection

Diet: nutritionist/registered dietitian consultation

Exercise, rest

PATIENT PROBLEMS—NURSING DIAGNOSES/INTERVENTIONS

▼ Altered tissue perfusion: cardiopulmonary, GI, peripheral, and renal related to blood loss

Cardiopulmonary system

O$_2$ prn

Auscultate chest for breath sounds q2h to 4h *to assess possible aspiration of emesis*

Maintain bed rest with head of bed elevated 30 degrees *to facilitate breathing*

Assess acuteness of bleeding and for signs of hypovolemia and shock: hypotension, tachycardia, tachypnea, decreased urine output

Monitor vital signs q15min to 30min until stable; take apical pulse

Maintain parenteral therapy: electrolytes, volume expanders, whole blood, packed cells *to prevent hypovolemia*

Monitor CVP line or Swan-Ganz catheter if appropriate

Balance treatments with rest periods *to prevent fatigue*

GI system

Auscultate abdomen for bowel sounds q4h

Monitor for abdominal distention

Monitor stools for melena

Maintain NPO

Monitor nasogastric tube and intermittent suction apparatus; measure gastric output q4h to 8h

Measure intake and output

Monitor electrolytes, Hgb, and Hct

Prepare for endoscopy; explain procedure *to reduce fear/anxiety*

Peripheral system

Monitor pedal pulses, capillary refill, and temperature of feet

Elevate legs *to increase venous flow*

Apply antiembolic stockings; remove at least twice daily

Maintain warmth of feet

Encourage active ROM of extremities *to promote circulation*

Renal system

Weigh patient daily (same time, scale, and clothing)

Maintain indwelling urethral catheter; monitor hourly output; if output is <30 ml/hr notify physician

Monitor urine pH and specific gravity

Monitor serum BUN, creatinine

Expected Outcomes

Vital signs within normal limits

Intake and output are balanced

Gastric drainage is clear or clearing

Pedal pulses, capillary refill are present

▼Altered nutrition: less than body requirements related to altered diet patterns, anorexia

When bleeding subsides and nasogastric tube is removed, initiate fluids in small amounts as tolerated

Progress to blended or soft foods in small, frequent meals

Collaborate with nutritionist/registered dietitian to provide high-calorie, high-protein diet; avoid increased calories if patient is overweight

Continue monitoring intake, output, and stools for melena

Monitor for complaints of fullness, nausea, vomiting *to avoid distention*

Administer saline enemas to clear bowel of old blood

Prevent constipation with natural laxatives: bran, prunes, psyllium powder

Assess effectiveness, side effects of antacids, vitamin K, cimetidine

Weight qod (same time, scale, and clothing)

Expected Outcomes

Tolerates diet well, and weight is stable

Tolerates medications

▼Pain related to disruption of gastric mucosa

Administer analgesics (e.g., morphine); meperidine is usually avoided because it can cause nausea and vomiting

Assess effectiveness of pain relief measures

Assist and teach patient to turn and deep breathe q2h to 4h

Use incentive spirometer as indicated

Administer back care and oral hygiene *to promote comfort*

Discuss and teach alternative pain relief measures: imaging, relaxation techniques

Change patient's position frequently *to provide comfort*

Keep patient warm and dry

Provide planned rest periods

Ambulate patient with assistance when tolerated *to decrease discomfort*

Provide diversional activities *to decrease attention on discomfort*

Expected Outcomes

Expresses reduction in or absence of pain

Appears relaxed and comfortable

▼Anxiety related to altered health status

Maintain quiet environment

Explain all procedures and treatments *to increase knowledge and reduce stress*

Encourage and allow time for verbalization of concerns

Assess level of anxiety, fear and current coping styles *to begin to help patient reduce anxiety* by using successful past coping behaviors

Discuss alternative coping behaviors and stress management techniques

Encourage communication with significant other(s) *to provide a support system*

Expected Outcomes

Demonstrates positive coping behaviors
Expresses a reduction in anxiety
Uses stress management techniques appropriately

PATIENT/FAMILY TEACHING AND DISCHARGE/HOME CARE PLANNING

Discuss nutritional plan, stressing importance of the following:
Small, frequent meals at regular intervals
Chewing food well and eating slowly
Avoiding caffeine, alcohol, tobacco, and aspirin
Reinforce physician's explanation of relationship of causative factors to disease process
Explain use of antiinflammatories and their relationship to ulcer formation
Always take with food
Take 1 hour after taking antacid *to avoid malabsorption of medication*
Reinforce stress management techniques
Provide medication instructions: name, dose, purpose, time of administration, and side effects; instruct patient to take only antacids prescribed by physician
Explain signs and symptoms of further bleeding: hematemesis, abdominal distention, tarry stools, fainting, dyspnea
Discuss importance of balancing exercise and rest periods
Check weight q week (same time, scale, and clothing)
Encourage follow-up visits with physician

■ GASTRIC SURGERY

gastric resection: *Removal of a gastric ulcer, leaving the stomach intact*

subtotal gastrectomy: *Removal of part of the stomach, usually the distal end, to prevent reformation of ulceration; the remaining part is anastomosed to the small bowel*

Billroth I: *Reshaping of the remaining stomach to reduce the curvature in order to merge it with the duodenum during the anastomosis*

Billroth II: *Following resection of part of the stomach and duodenum, the remaining stomach is anastomosed, side by side, to the remaining duodenum*

total gastrectomy: *Removal of the stomach, usually for cancer; the distal esophagus and proximal duodenum are also removed and an esophagojejunostomy is performed*

vagotomy: *Surgical interruption of the gastric vagal nerve to decrease gastric secretion and motility*

pyloroplasty: *Surgical procedure performed with a vagotomy to enlarge the gastric outlet and promote gastric emptying*

PREOPERATIVE ASSESSMENT AND CARE

Assess baseline vital signs
Assess respiratory status

Discuss and explain pain management
Reinforce physician's explanation of procedure
Teach patient to turn, deep breathe; methods of incisional splinting for coughing; use of incentive spirometer
Discuss placement of tubes, drains that may be present postoperatively
Insert nasogastric tube as ordered
Allow time for verbalization of concerns

POSTOPERATIVE ASSESSMENT
SUBJECTIVE DATA

Location, character of pain
Nausea

OBJECTIVE DATA

Vital signs
Splinting with respirations
Decreased breath sounds
Tachypnea
Bradypnea
Character and amount of gastric drainage
Vomiting
Urinary output
Abdominal distention
Pyrexia

DIAGNOSTIC TESTS

Hgb, Hct, electrolytes

POTENTIAL COMPLICATIONS

Dehydration, anemia
Electrolyte imbalance
Atelectasis
Anastomosis leak
Shock
Thrombophlebitis (p. 77)
Dumping syndrome (p. 322)
Paralytic ileus (p. 337)
Wound evisceration, infection
Postprandial hypoglycemia
Gastrojejunocolic fistula

MULTIDISCIPLINARY MANAGEMENT
THERAPEUTIC MANAGEMENT

NPO until bowel sounds return
Parenteral fluids with electrolytes until diet is allowed
Nasogastric suction
Analgesics
Antiembolic stockings
Dietary consultation
Respiratory therapy

PATIENT PROBLEMS—NURSING DIAGNOSES/INTERVENTIONS

▼ Fluid volume deficit related to altered digestive process, absorption, and nasogastric tube drainage

Maintain NPO; assess hydration status

Maintain nasogastric tube to intermittent suction apparatus

Monitor color and amount of gastric output q4h and include in total output

Monitor pH of gastric drainage 2 to 3 times qd

Do not reposition tube

Maintain patency of tube by irrigation with measured amounts of saline *only* if ordered

Note that after gastrectomy, drainage will be minimal

Report excessive bleeding to physician

Administer frequent oral hygiene with petroleum jelly; keep nares well lubricated *to prevent dryness from mouth breathing and irritation from tube*

Monitor electrolytes, Hgb, and Hct

Maintain parenteral fluids with electrolytes *to ensure adequate hydration*

Measure intake and output q4h to 8h

Weigh q2 days (same time, clothing, scale)

Expected Outcomes

Intake and output are balanced

Hydration is adequately maintained

Weight is maintained near normal

▼Altered nutrition: less than body requirements related to altered gastric functioning/absorption

Auscultate bowel sounds and passage of flatus q8h

When bowel sounds return, administer small amounts of water via nasogastric tube as ordered

Aspirate stomach 2 hours after last feeding of the day; contents should be <100 ml, and no pain, distention, or nausea should be present

Report to physician if amount is >100 ml and/or the above symptoms occur

Initiate oral fluids when nasogastric tube is removed

Offer 5 to 10 ml of warm water qh as ordered

Increase amounts until 90 to 120 ml is tolerated qh

Progress to small, frequent meals of soft foods; avoid milk *because it may cause dumping syndrome*

Discontinue feedings if pain, nausea, distention, or vomiting occur and notify physician

Continue measuring intake

Expected Outcomes

Tolerates increasing diet without discomfort

Ingests adequate calories to maintain normal weight

▼Ineffective breathing pattern related to discomfort of surgical incision

Assess respirations, observing for signs of distress

Maintain bed rest with head of bed elevated 30 degrees *to facilitate breathing*

Auscultate chest for breath sounds q4h

Assist and teach patient to turn, cough, and deep breathe q2h to 4h; provide support to incision *to reduce pain*

Administer incentive spirometer q4h *to a adequately*

Provide pain medication before deep brea to reduce discomfort*

Expected Outcomes

Demonstrates breathing techniques accurate

Exhibits normal respirations

▼Altered tissue perfusion: peripheral, cardiopulmonary, renal related to risk of hypovolemia

Peripheral system

Check extremities for temperature, color, and sensation

Monitor pedal pulses q4h

Do not hyperflex knees *because it may interrupt venous flow*

Apply antiembolic stockings and remove at least twice daily to inspect skin for redness, tenderness

Encourage ROM leg exercises qh *to promote venous return*

Cardiopulmonary system

Monitor vital signs q4h

Auscultate chest for breath sounds q4h

Monitor CVP/Swan-Ganz readings qh and prn

Monitor ABGs *to assess adequate arterial flow*

Renal system

Measure intake and output qh *to assess adequate kidney function;* if output is <30 ml/hr report to physician

Monitor urine specific gravity and serum BUN, creatinine

Expected Outcomes

Vital signs are normal

Intake and output are balanced

Laboratory values are within normal limits

▼Risk for infection related to surgical incision, inadequate primary defenses

Monitor dressings and incision for drainage and bleeding q4h

Change dressings prn and observe healing process

Observe for signs of wound infection: redness, drainage, pain, odor; report these to physician

Monitor and report elevated temperature to physician

Expected Outcomes

Incision is clean, dry, and intact

Wound is healing adequately

▼Pain related to surgical intervention

Assess location, type, and intensity of pain; use pain rating scale

ess effectiveness of analgesics; collaborate with
physician regarding patient-controlled analgesia
(p. 40)
Change position often and support with pillows *to
decrease discomfort*
Administer skin care and back rubs q4h *to promote
comfort*
Maintain quiet environment *to allow for adequate rest*
Schedule rest periods between treatments
Discuss alternative pain relief measures: imaging,
relaxation techniques, deep breathing
Provide diversional activities *to decrease attention on pain*
Encourage support from significant others

Expected Outcomes
Reports a tolerable level of pain/discomfort
Appears more relaxed

▼Anxiety related to change in health status

Explain all procedures and treatments
Reinforce physician's explanation of surgical procedure
and treatment
Encourage and allow time for verbalization of feelings
Assess present coping behaviors and support positive
responses
Teach stress management techniques
Encourage communication with significant other(s) *to
promote support*

Expected Outcomes
Expresses and identifies anxieties
Uses stress management techniques appropriately

Additional Nursing Diagnosis to Consider
Diarrhea related to malabsorption

PATIENT/FAMILY TEACHING
Discuss and explain dietary plan and restrictions
according to type of surgery performed
Eat small, frequent meals at regular intervals; avoid
excessive amounts of fiber foods, sugar, salt, caffeine,
alcohol, milk, and tobacco
Take fluids between meals, not with meals
Eat slowly and chew foods well
Measure weight q2h to 4h
Provide instructions and demonstrate wound care;
identify signs of wound infection
Reinforce importance of avoiding stressful situations,
especially at mealtimes
Reinforce stress management techniques
Explain symptoms of dumping syndrome: epigastric pain,
weakness, nausea, vomiting after eating
Discuss medications: name, dosage, time of
administration, purpose, and side effects; instruct
patient to avoid over-the-counter medications,
especially those containing aspirin
Discuss importance of adequate rest and exercise with
planned rest periods

Explain use of natural laxatives to avoid constipation
Encourage follow-up care with physician

DISCHARGE/HOME CARE PLANNING
Be certain that patient has names and phone numbers of
home health care team
Discuss where and what to purchase for dressing
changes
Provide information on community organizations for
meal delivery, home health care aides as needed

■ DUMPING SYNDROME
*Postgastrectomy, gastroduodenostomy, gastrojejunos-
tomy, or pyloroplasty syndrome caused by loss of the pyloric valve, allowing food and fluid to pass too rapidly
into the small bowel; this causes blood sugar level to rise
and increases insulin production, which in turn can
cause hypoglycemia; appears 1 to 3 weeks after surgery*

ASSESSMENT
SUBJECTIVE DATA
Time of onset of symptoms, usually after meals
Epigastric fullness
Nausea
Malaise
Palpitations
Vertigo
Urge to defecate
Sweating

OBJECTIVE DATA
Vomiting
Abdominal distention
Profuse diaphoresis
Tachypnea
Hypotension
Increased bowel sounds
Decreased blood sugar level (hypoglycemia)
Loss of weight

POTENTIAL COMPLICATIONS
Syndrome becomes chronic
ECG changes

MULTIDISCIPLINARY MANAGEMENT
THERAPEUTIC MANAGEMENT
Diet: high-protein, high-fat, low-carbohydrate plan
Anticholinergics, pectin powder
Surgery to alter dumping rate
Dietary consultation
Consult with Wound, Ostomy, Continence/ET Nurse as
indicated

**PATIENT PROBLEM—NURSING
DIAGNOSIS/INTERVENTIONS**

▼Altered nutrition: less than body requirements related to inability to absorb nutrients

Collaborate with physician and nutritionist/registered dietitian about diet

Provide six small meals a day

Do not give liquids with meals

Provide dry foods such as toast, crackers, and cereals

Provide diet low in carbohydrates and salt, moderate in fat, and high in protein

Avoid refined, concentrated carbohydrates *because they pass into intestines rapidly and cause increased insulin release*

Include foods containing pectin: citrus fruits, yellow vegetables, bananas, apples, apricots, cherries, beans

Avoid extreme temperatures in foods

Administer pectin powder; thoroughly mix with water: patient may experience a sense of oral dryness if mixture is not adequately liquefied

Provide liquids only between meals *to avoid increased dumping into intestine*

Administer anticholinergics 30 minutes before meals; assess for effectiveness

Monitor glucose levels *to assess for hypoglycemia*

Measure intake and output q8h

Weigh qod (same time, scale, and clothing)

Position patient in recumbent position after meals *to allow foods to pass more slowly into intestine*

Expected Outcomes

Tolerates diet without experiencing discomfort, distention, or nausea

Maintains weight and adequate nutritional status

PATIENT/FAMILY TEACHING

Discuss importance of dietary plan; stress small, frequent meals, foods to avoid, and foods to eat

Stress importance of eating slowly and chewing foods well

Explain that syndrome is usually only temporary, but its continuance after 2 to 3 weeks should be reported to the physician

Instruct patient to lie down on left side after meals and to avoid stressful situations, especially at mealtimes

Reinforce stress management techniques

Encourage follow-up visits with physician

DISCHARGE/HOME CARE PLANNING

Provide dietary plan with foods high in protein and fat and low in carbohydrates

Stress importance of not drinking liquids with meals

Provide names and phone numbers of home health care team members

Record weight weekly and notify physician of decreases

Refer to community agencies for assistance with meals as needed

Stress importance of maintaining normal weight

■ SURGICAL INTERVENTION FOR OBESITY

Insertion of two rows of staples across upper one tenth of the stomach to reduce capacity and ensure early satiety; performed for patients highly motivated to lose weight and for whom medical management of obesity has been unsuccessful; two types of surgery are performed:

gastric bypass: Anastomosis of jejunum to upper one tenth of the stomach, bypassing the remaining stomach (Fig. 6-8, A)

gastroplasty/vertical banding: Small opening left in rows of staples, allowing small amounts of food to pass into stomach (Fig. 6-8, B)

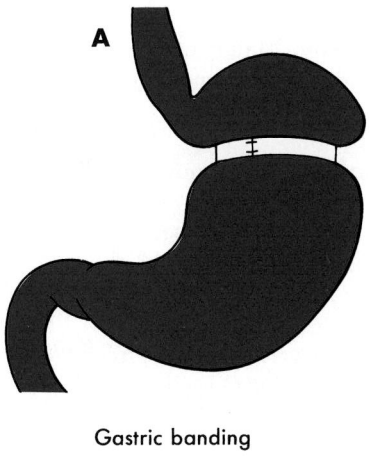

Gastric banding

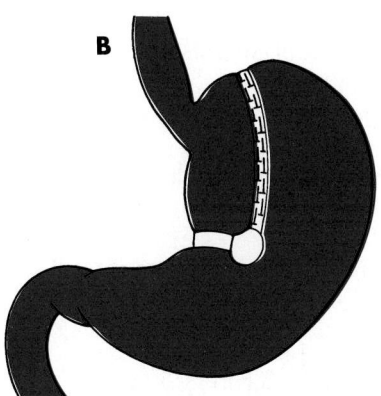

Vertical banded gastroplasty

Fig. 6-8 Examples of gastric-restriction procedures. **A,** Gastric banding. **B,** Vertical banded gastroplasty. *(From Beare PG, Myers JL:* Principles and practice of adult health nursing, *ed 2, St Louis, 1994, Mosby.)*

PREOPERATIVE ASSESSMENT
OBSERVATIONS/FINDINGS

Nutritional history
   Previous eating patterns and types of foods eaten
   Present weight >100 lb over ideal body weight
Medical history
   Absence of renal, cardiac, bowel, or liver disease
   No history of hypertension, diabetes, or arthritis
   No signs of upper respiratory infection or anemia
Psychologic adjustment to procedure
   Motivation to lose weight
   Weight loss minimal or absent after many attempts
   Presence of positive coping behaviors

DIAGNOSTIC TESTS

Renal and liver function studies
Abdominal and chest radiologic studies
Cholecystogram
Intravenous pyelogram (IVP)
Barium enema
Pulmonary function test
Serum glucose, insulin, cholesterol, triglycerides,
   creatinine, protein, iron, CBC, urinalysis, electrolytes
Baseline ABGs

MULTIDISCIPLINARY MANAGEMENT
THERAPEUTIC MANAGEMENT

Preoperative medication
Parenteral fluids with heparin
Nasogastric tube and indwelling urethral catheter
Consultation with dietitian
Respiratory therapy consult
PCA pump
Sequential compression device (SCD) on antiembolic
   stockings
Psychosocial support services

PATIENT PROBLEMS—NURSING DIAGNOSES/INTERVENTIONS

▼Anxiety related to hospitalization, procedures, surgery, and altered health status

Attempt to maintain nonstressful environment
Discuss stress management techniques
Orient patient to surroundings and provide comfortable
   armless chair
Encourage and allow time for verbalization of concerns
Assess coping skills and promote positive, successful past
   behaviors
Reinforce physician's explanation of preoperative and
   postoperative care and surgical procedure
Perform activities in an unhurried manner, explaining
   each as it occurs
Encourage verbalization with significant other(s)

Expected Outcomes

Expresses anxieties/concerns
Exhibits positive coping skills

▼Knowledge deficit related to lack of information about preoperative and postoperative care

Discuss with patient and teach
   Use of trapeze bar and how to get in and out of bed
   Method for turning, coughing, and deep breathing with
     incisional support
   Use of PCA pump
   Use of SCD or antiembolic stockings
   Use of incentive spirometer and diaphragmatic
     breathing procedure
   Procedure for sipping from a cup, 30 ml in 5 minutes
   Active ROM exercises, especially legs and feet
Explain that early ambulation (2 to 4 hours after
   surgery) will be required, and trapeze bars will be
   in place
Explain that preoperatively a nasogastric tube and
   indwelling urethral catheter will be inserted
Discuss postoperative dietary management: small
   sips of water increasing to 30 to 60 ml/hr as
   tolerated
Explain that IV line will be in place preoperatively, and an
   anticoagulant may be administered

POSTOPERATIVE ASSESSMENT
SUBJECTIVE DATA

Location and character of pain
Nausea

OBJECTIVE DATA

Splinting with respirations
Decreased breath sounds
Hypoventilation
Tachypnea
Character, color, and amount of the following:
   Gastric drainage
   Urine output
   Wound drainage
Placement and patency of nasogastric tube
Pressure delivered by suction machine
Vomiting
Abdominal distention

DIAGNOSTIC TESTS

Hgb, Hct, electrolytes
Chest radiologic study

POTENTIAL COMPLICATIONS

Dehydration
Electrolyte imbalance
Thrombophlebitis (p. 77)
Atelectasis
Anastomotic leakage
   Tachycardia
   Referred abdominal pain to left shoulder
Peritonitis (p. 332)
Hemorrhage
Shock
Wound infection

MULTIDISCIPLINARY MANAGEMENT
THERAPEUTIC MANAGEMENT
Analgesics, antidiarrheals
Anticoagulants as indicated
Ambulation q2h to 3h
Parenteral fluids with electrolytes
Nasogastric tube to intermittent suction; irrigation schedule
Indwelling urethral catheter to gravity drainage
Respiratory therapy
    Incentive spirometer
    ABGs, pulse oximetry
Diet, activity, rest
SCD or antiembolic stockings

PATIENT PROBLEMS—NURSING DIAGNOSES/INTERVENTIONS

▼Ineffective breathing pattern related to surgical incision, decreased lung expansion, anxiety fatigue

Maintain bed rest with head of bed elevated 30 degrees *to increase respiratory function and reduce thoracic pressure*
Monitor respirations q1h to 2h; observe for shallow breathing, splinting, hypoventilation, and respiratory distress
Auscultate chest for breath sounds q2h
Provide incentive spirometer qh
Place pads on side rails and encourage patient to use as arm rests *to aid in lung expansion*
Encourage diaphragmatic breathing *to reduce incisional pain*
Assist patient to turn, cough, and deep breathe q2h; support incision
Avoid abdominal binders *because they may hamper deep breathing and lung expansion*

Expected Outcomes
Exhibits normal respirations
Performs deep breathing exercises accurately

▼Altered tissue perfusion: cardiopulmonary, renal, and peripheral related to interruption of blood flow

Cardiopulmonary system
Monitor vital signs q4h; take rectal temperature while nasogastric tube is in place *because patient may mouth breathe because of nasogastric tube*
Monitor ABGs, CVP line or Swan-Ganz catheter, and pulse oximetry
Monitor Hgb and Hct
Assess heart and breath sounds

Peripheral system
Monitor pedal pulses q2h; assess color, temperature of feet
Avoid elevating knee hyperflexion

Check calves of legs for pain on dorsiflexion *because pain may indicate thrombophlebitis*
Discourage sitting with legs in dependent or crossed position *to prevent constricting venous flow*
Remove antiembolic stockings daily and inspect skin for pressure areas; remove and reapply at least twice daily
Encourage leg and foot movement qh
Ambulate with assistance and always have enough staff present to prevent injury
Administer heparin therapy *to prevent clot formation*

Renal system
Maintain indwelling urethral catheter to closed gravity drainage system
Monitor hourly urine output; if <50 ml/hr, notify physician
Measure intake and output
Administer catheter care and good perineal care *to prevent infection*

Expected Outcomes
Vital signs are stable
Urine output is normal
Lower extremities are warm and of normal color

▼Risk for fluid volume deficit related to gastric suction, electrolyte loss, and/or diarrhea

Maintain NPO; assess for signs of dehydration: reduced capillary refill, poor skin turgor, dry mucous membranes
Monitor parenteral fluids
Monitor serum electrolytes, magnesium, and calcium
Observe for muscle tone or strength loss and tremors caused by loss of magnesium, calcium
Measure intake and output; include gastric output, diarrhea in 24 hour total
Maintain nasogastric tube to intermittent suction apparatus
    Note color, consistency, and amount of drainage
    Label tube: *"Do not reposition"*
    Mark tube where it enters nose and avoid placing tension on tube
Irrigate gently with 20 to 30 ml of normal saline q2h to 4h *to maintain patency*
Auscultate abdomen for bowel sounds q4h
Weigh patient daily (same time, scale, and clothing)

Expected Outcomes
Gastric output is minimal
Electrolytes are within normal limits
Fluid volume is adequate for height and weight as evidenced by balanced intake and output

▼Risk for infection related to invasive surgical procedure and inadequate primary defenses

Maintain aseptic technique and proper handwashing procedure
Observe incision and dressings q2h to 4h; reinforce or change dressings prn; apply topical antibiotic creams as indicated
Monitor incision for signs of wound infection: redness, drainage, odor
Maintain dressings securely; avoid taping too tightly
Keep skin clean and dry
Monitor temperature q4h

Expected Outcomes
Exhibits clean, dry, and intact incision
Presents normal temperature
Exhibits no evidence of inflammation at or near the incision site

▼ Pain related to surgical intervention

Assess location, intensity, and character of pain; use pain rating scale
Administer analgesics and assess effectiveness of relief measure(s)
Collaborate with physician regarding PCA (p. 40)
Assess patency of nasogastric tube *because obstruction of tube may cause pain*
Medicate 20 to 30 minutes before procedures when possible *to reduce pain caused by activities*
Monitor type of pain closely and observe for abdominal distention, tenderness, and fever, *which may indicate infection/dumping syndrome*
Change position slightly at frequent intervals *to alleviate discomfort*
Encourage alternative pain management measures: imaging, deep breathing, relaxation exercises
Provide diversional activities *to decrease attention on pain*

Expected Outcomes
Expresses tolerable level of pain
Appears more relaxed

▼ Altered nutrition: less than body requirements related to decreased size of stomach

Remove nasogastric tube, usually third to fourth day postoperatively
Provide 1-oz medication cup and assist patient with sipping 30 ml/hr (adequate hydration demands almost constant fluid intake because of decreased stomach size)
Collaborate with nutritionist/registered dietitian regarding caloric intake and calorie counting
Progress to clear liquids, using 1-oz cup, until soft, high-protein, low-fat diet is tolerated
Assess tolerance of foods and fluids as they are introduced: *nausea may occur if stomach becomes overextended*

Instruct patient to heed feeling of satiety to avoid nausea or vomiting
Administer vitamin supplements including vitamin B_{12}, folate, and calcium *to prevent anemia from reduced oral intake*

Expected Outcomes
Tolerates frequent feedings adequately
Maintains desired weight loss

▼ Diarrhea related to induced malabsorption

Provide diet high in bulk with moderate fluid intake *because excess contributes to diarrhea*
Observe for signs of dumping syndrome (p. 322): nausea, distention, vertigo, palpitations
Provide perianal care after bowel movement; apply protective ointments as needed
Observe frequency, color, amount, and consistency of stools
Monitor electrolytes *because increased fluid loss may alter electrolyte balance*
Administer antidiarrheals

Expected Outcomes
Expresses understanding of rationale for diet regimen
Verbalizes factors causing diarrhea
Has bowel elimination that is returning to normal

▼ Risk for impaired skin integrity related to obesity, fluid deficit

Monitor incision for healing, drainage
Administer frequent skin care, especially in folds or on pressure points
Provide special air or foam mattress as indicated
Promote frequent position changes *to increase comfort;* support incision
Place clear skin barrier on heels and elbows *to prevent shearing*

Expected Outcomes
Incision is healing and surrounding skin is clean, dry, and intact
Skin integrity is maintained without evidence of any stage of dermal ulcer

PATIENT/FAMILY TEACHING
Discuss importance of following eating regimen
Eat and drink slowly and chew foods well
Always sit up while eating or drinking
Do not overeat: stomach will expand and void surgical procedure
Eat small amounts of all food and heed satiety feeling
Avoid drinking 30 minutes before and after meals
Eat with family, significant other(s)
Use small plate and glass to make portions appear larger

Do not snack between meals

Avoid carbonated beverages

Eat only two meals a day or as prescribed by physician

Explain importance of diet management

    Refer to nutritionist/registered dietitian as indicated; provide dietary list of foods to eat and avoid

    Have patient avoid high-calorie, high-carbohydrate foods and drinks, as well as gas-producing foods

    Maintain well-balanced, high-protein diet, 300 to 500 calories per day or as prescribed

    Discuss signs of hypokalemia: lower extremity muscle weakness, diarrhea, irregular pulse

Be accurate in measuring all food allowances

    Use 30-ml medication cup or 1½-tablespoon measuring scoop

    Maintain 1500 ml/day fluid intake or as prescribed

Add new foods to diet one at a time; intolerances can occur, especially with meat and poultry

    Discuss methods of processing foods with blender for gastroplasty patients

    Discuss availability of high-protein liquid supplements

Measure urine output daily

Keep accurate record of daily intake

Take chewable multivitamins daily

Weigh weekly because weight loss will be more noticeable

Instruct patient regarding rest and exercise

    Avoid heavy lifting and strenuous exercise

    Walk daily with goal of 1 to 2 miles per day within 4 weeks

    Maintain planned rest periods

Demonstrate incisional and perianal care

Explain symptoms to report to physician

    Elevated temperature

    Wound drainage

    Persistent nausea and/or vomiting

    Hematemesis

    Abdominal tenderness and/or pain

    Abdominal distention

    Urine output of <750 ml/day for 3 consecutive days

    Constipation or continuing diarrhea

Reinforce stress management techniques

Explain importance of avoiding over-the-counter medications without first consulting physician

Encourage follow-up visits with physician, nutritionist/registered dietitian, including laboratory testing as ordered

DISCHARGE/HOME CARE PLANNING

Provide information on what and where to purchase needed supplies: dressings, high-calorie supplements, blender

Explain signs of dumping syndrome: weakness, diaphoresis; may occur 2 to 3 weeks following surgery

Refer to community support groups to augment coping with altered lifestyle

Discuss maintaining a positive self-image by wearing attractive, comfortable clothing, and to avoid purchasing smaller-size clothing until ideal body weight is achieved

Encourage patient to dispose of large-size clothes so they are not available to convey the message that the weight loss will not be permanent

Discourage patient from seeking liposuction until ideal body weight is attained

■ NASOGASTRIC TUBES

nasogastric tube: *Tube used for gastric decompression, such as Levin or Salem sump (Fig. 6-9), or for administration of food, fluid, or medication; a Levin tube must always be connected to intermittent suction; a Salem sump tube is usually connected to low continuous suction (because it is air vented) but may also be connected to intermittent suction*

PREINSERTION ASSESSMENT AND CARE

Assess patient's ability to swallow and mouth breathe

Assess nasal patency; observe for deviated septum, fracture

Check tube for patency

Lubricate and chill tube according to manufacturer's instructions

Explain purpose of tube and procedure

POSTINSERTION ASSESSMENT

Character and consistency of gastric output

Patency of tube

Patency of sump if Salem tube is used

Placement for optimal drainage

Tube taped securely and comfortably to nose

Amount of pressure of suction apparatus

Nasal irritation

POTENTIAL COMPLICATIONS

Dehydration

Electrolyte imbalance

Aspiration pneumonia

INTERVENTIONS

Elevate head of bed 40 to 60 degrees *to reduce risk of aspiration or reflux*

Maintain NPO

Monitor character, amount, and consistency of gastric contents q4h; monitor gastric pH; if pH is <3.5, notify physician

Auscultate stomach for placement of tube prn by (1) inserting small amount of air in tube and listening for the air going into the stomach; use air vent on Salem tube and (2) aspirate tube and test liquid for pH (gastric fluid has pH <3)

Connect tube to low, intermittent suction apparatus as ordered; irrigate with measured amounts of normal saline solution as ordered; *do not use tap water because it can alter electrolyte balance of stomach*

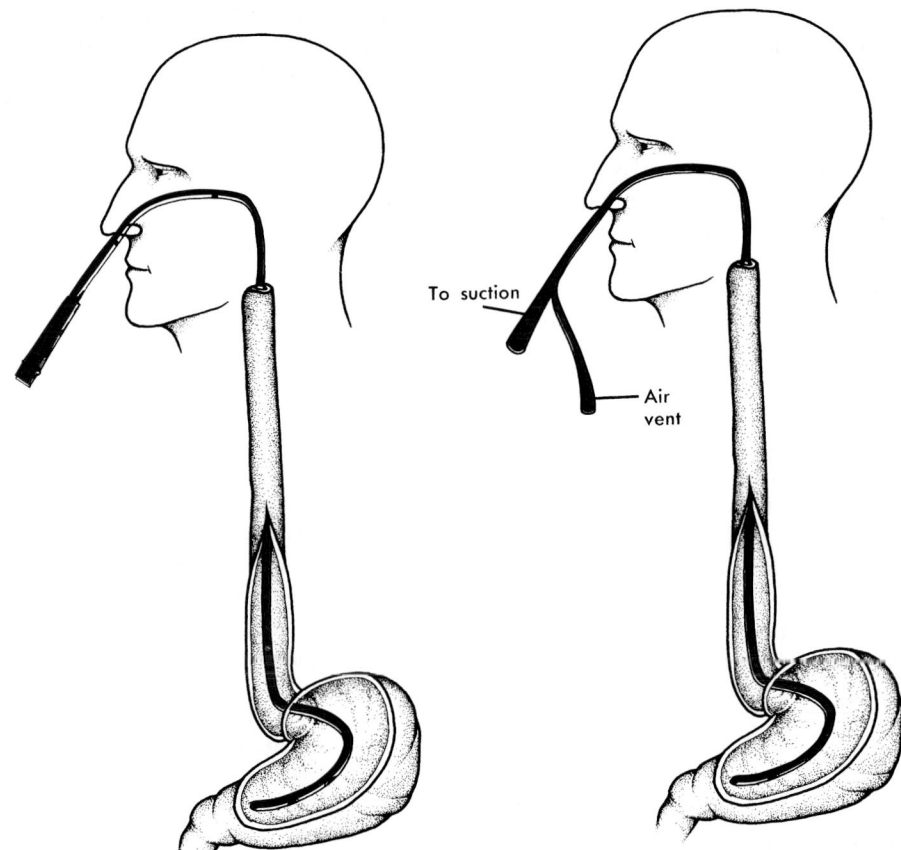

Fig. 6-9 **A,** Levin tube. **B,** Salem sump tube.

Salem sump tube
 Maintain patency of sump (air vent): keep opening higher than gastric tube and do not plug
 Sump tube may be irrigated, but instill 20 to 30 ml of air after irrigation to maintain patency
If nausea occurs, tube is usually obstructed and relief is obtained with irrigation
If vomiting occurs, turn patient on side to prevent aspiration; check for placement and obstruction
Avoid dislodgment: tape securely to nose and allow enough tube for freedom of movement
Apply lip balm or lubricant to nares and mouth prn
Check tape holding tube prn; observe for reddened area

■ ESOPHAGOSTOMY, GASTROSTOMY, DUODENOSTOMY-JEJUNOSTOMY MANAGEMENT

esophagostomy: Surgically constructed stoma used to drain saliva and other secretions in patients with esophageal carcinoma, stricture, dysphagia, or atresia; may be used to administer tube feedings for these conditions; this procedure is similar to gastrostomy except a longer catheter is used; the stoma may be permanent or temporary

gastrostomy: Surgically constructed stoma or opening for a catheter in patients with esophageal carcinoma,

stricture, trauma, atresia, and dysphagia; used for tube feedings or decompression and drainage; the ostomy is usually permanent, whereas the catheter is either temporary or permanent

percutaneous endoscopic gastrostomy: Feeding tube insertion using a gastroscope; the stomach is inflated with air and a cannula is inserted into the abdominal wall; a suture is threaded through and picked up by the scope and brought out through the mouth; the feeding tube is attached to the suture and drawn down into the stomach, out the abdominal wall, secured, and capped; this procedure is more cost effective and causes fewer complications

duodenostomy-jejunostomy: Surgical incision for placement of a catheter for the feedings or decompression and drainage in patients when oral intake is prohibited or after gastrointestinal-esophageal surgery; may be permanent or temporary

ASSESSMENT
SUBJECTIVE DATA
Tenderness or pain around ostomy site
Location, intensity of other pain

OBJECTIVE DATA
Type and patency of stoma or catheter
Placement of dressing or stoma appliances
Length of catheter from incision to distal end

Security of catheter placement
Pressure delivered by low, intermittent-suction
    apparatus
Placement of closed gravity drainage system, clamp, or
    other collecting device
Character, color, and amount of drainage
Skin integrity around catheter or stoma
Condition of lips and mouth
Weight
Urinary output and specific gravity
Abdominal distention
Diminished bowel sounds
Character and color of stool

LABORATORY/DIAGNOSTIC STUDIES
Electrolytes
Abdominal radiologic study for tube placement

POTENTIAL COMPLICATIONS
Dehydration
Nausea, vomiting
Electrolyte imbalance
Aspiration pneumonia
Wound infection
Hemorrhage, shock

MULTIDISCIPLINARY MANAGEMENT
THERAPEUTIC MANAGEMENT
Analgesics, antibiotics
Intermittent gastric suction or gravity drainage
Tube feedings, amount, and caloric content
Parenteral therapy with electrolytes and vitamins
Intake and output
PCA
Consultations
    Wound, Ostomy, Continence/ET Nurse
    Dietitian
    Respiratory therapy as indicated

PATIENT PROBLEMS—NURSING
DIAGNOSES/INTERVENTIONS

▼ Potential fluid volume deficit related to abnormal
loss of body fluids, electrolytes, or blood

Maintain NPO
Administer parenteral fluids with electrolytes and
    vitamins as ordered
Monitor vital signs
Measure intake and output q8h
For catheters (tubes)
    Check color and consistency of drainage q4h; measure
        amount q8h
    Connect catheter (tube) to suction apparatus or
        gravity drainage as ordered
    Measure length of catheter (tube) q8h
    Tape securely to abdomen or neck; allow sufficient
        tubing for freedom of movement

For prosthetic valve or ostomy
    Check dressings and place valve cap in safe place
    Place stoma appliance over ostomy
Auscultate abdomen for bowel sounds q8h; report return
    to physician
Check operative site *to assess bleeding q2h to 4h*
When bowel sounds return or drainage is less than 300 to
    500 ml/24 hr
    Clamp catheter, cap valve, or cover ostomy
        as ordered
    Instruct patient in signs of retention and bowel
        obstruction *to identify complications*
        Nausea
        Abdominal distention
        Abdominal pain
    If these symptoms occur, notify physician immediately
        and unclamp tube or uncap valve and connect to
        gravity drainage system
Initiate tube feedings as ordered; check residual
Weigh patient daily (same time, scale, and clothing)
Maintain fluid intake as ordered after parenteral therapy
    is discontinued: usually 2000 ml/24 hr unless
    contraindicated

Expected Outcomes
Hydration is adequate as evidenced by normal skin turgor
    and capillary refill
Intake and output are balanced
Fluid volume and electrolytes are within normal limits

▼ Ineffective airway clearance related to oral secretion management

Maintain bed rest with head elevated 30 to 45 degrees; do
    not maintain flexed knees
Assist and teach patient to turn, cough, and deep breathe
    q4h
Assist and teach patient to expectorate saliva rather than
    swallow it
Perform passive or assist with and teach active ROM
    exercises q4h

Expected Outcomes
Exhibits normal respiratory rate and rhythm
Breath sounds are clear

▼ Potential impairment of skin integrity related to
surgical procedure

Provide skin care around surgical site q4h to 8h
    Wash area gently with soap and water
    Rinse and pat dry
    Apply skin barrier as needed
    Reapply dressings and appliance prn
Provide skin care to lips and mouth as needed

Expected Outcomes
Wound heals without incident
Surrounding tissue is clean, dry, and intact

▼Alteration in comfort: pain related to surgical intervention

Administer analgesics as ordered; assess effectiveness of pain relief measures
Change position to position of comfort prn
Provide planned rest periods between procedures
Maintain clean, comfortable bed in safe environment

Expected Outcomes
Reports that pain is minimal to absent
Appears relaxed and comfortable

▼Ineffective coping by individual related to disease process, surgical procedure, and/or prognosis

Assess patient's present coping patterns and identify strengths
Encourage and allow time for verbalization; listen carefully
Assess past coping methods based on previous experiences
Involve patient in all care, explaining treatments and procedures
Encourage communication with significant other
Encourage diversional activities

Expected Outcome
Demonstrates adaptive coping behaviors

PATIENT/FAMILY TEACHING
Discuss with and demonstrate to patient procedure of tube feeding and tube feeding preparation, as well as amount and times of feeding
Discuss and demonstrate ostomy care (p. 350) and skin care around tube sites
Demonstrate dressing change procedure and care of prosthetic valve and cap
Explain importance of weighing q2d to 3d (same time, scale, and clothing)
Provide information on symptoms of bowel obstruction and wound infection
Demonstrate medication preparation via tube feeding; discuss name, dose, purpose, time of administration, and side effects
Encourage follow-up appointments with physician and Wound, Ostomy, Continence/ET Nurse

DISCHARGE/HOME CARE PLANNING
Provide information on vendors of needed equipment and supplies
Discuss signs and symptoms to report to physician
   Tenderness, drainage around ostomy
   Pain, eructation, or distention

INTESTINE

■ INFLAMMATORY BOWEL DISEASE: REGIONAL ENTERITIS (CROHN'S DISEASE, ILEOCOLITIS) AND ULCERATIVE COLITIS

regional enteritis: Chronic, recurrent nonspecific inflammation of unknown etiology affecting the entire intestine, usually the terminal ileum; it involves the mucosa and surrounding musculature and can lead to deep fissure formation

ulcerative colitis: Inflammatory intestinal disease of unknown cause, usually affecting the mucosal lining of the colon but may involve the entire large intestine; may be mild, chronic, or acute

ASSESSMENT
SUBJECTIVE DATA
Regional enteritis: cramplike abdominal pain; often in right lower quadrant with frequent diarrhea containing melena and/or steatorrhea
Ulcerative colitis: colicky abdominal cramps; pain is usually minimal; diarrheal stools are frequent and contain mucus, melena, and pus
Anorexia
Weight loss
Fever
Nausea
Generalized malaise

OBJECTIVE DATA
Vomiting
Hyperactive bowel sounds
Anxiety, depression
Decreased muscle tone, skin turgor
Dry mucous membranes
Dehydration
Malnutrition
Hypotension

DIAGNOSTIC TESTS
Barium studies of intestine
Sigmoidoscopy, colonoscopy
Biopsy, cytology
Radiologic study of abdomen
Serum iron, decreased
Serum electrolytes, decreased potassium and magnesium
Albumin, decreased
Liver function tests
Hematologic studies: anemia, leukocytosis
Complement fixation test
Stools for melena, fat
CBC
ESR, elevated indicating inflammation

POTENTIAL COMPLICATIONS

Electrolyte imbalance

Dehydration, malnutrition, anemia

Intestinal obstruction, perforation

Hemorrhage, shock

Fistula, peritonitis

Perianal abscess, fistula, fissure

Depression

MULTIDISCIPLINARY MANAGEMENT

THERAPEUTIC MANAGEMENT

Anticholinergics (Donnatal, Probanthine)

Immunosuppressants

Corticosteroids

Antimicrobial agents

Antidiarrheals

Sedative, analgesics

Diet high in calories, vitamins, protein; low-residue, milk-free

Monitor Hgb and Hct

Parenteral fluids, elemental diet, TPN (depending on severity of disease)

Nasogastric suction; NPO

Sitz bath

Dietitian consult

Surgical interventions: ileostomy, colostomy, resection

Wound, Ostomy, Continence/ET Nurse consultation for skin integrity problems or planned ostomy surgery

PATIENT PROBLEMS—NURSING DIAGNOSES/INTERVENTIONS

▼Risk for fluid volume deficit related to abnormal fluid loss (diarrhea)

Maintain NPO; assess hydration status

Maintain parenteral fluids with electrolytes and vitamins

Monitor for signs of circulatory overload

Measure intake and output including emesis q8h

Monitor electrolytes *to determine replacement needs*

Weigh patient daily (same time, scale, and clothing)

Monitor vital signs q4h; avoid taking temperature rectally; monitor for orthostatic changes

Administer antiemetics, antipyretics *to reduce fluid loss*

Expected Outcomes

Vital signs are stable

Hydration is adequate as evidenced by normal skin turgor and moist mucous membranes

Intake and output are balanced

▼Diarrhea related to inflammation of bowel

Maintain bed rest *to reduce intestinal motility and conserve energy*

Assess and monitor stools for amount, frequency, consistency, and color

Monitor stools for occult blood

Auscultate abdomen for bowel sounds q8h *to evaluate reduced peristalsis*

Monitor effectiveness and side effects of antidiarrheal, antibiotic, and steroid therapy

Balance rest with activity

Provide odor-free environment; keep covered bedpan within easy reach; empty, clean, and return promptly

Monitor for signs of bowel perforation: fever, tachycardia, lethargy, pain

Expected Outcomes

Expresses reduction in frequency of stools

States stool returning to normal consistency

▼Altered nutrition: less than body requirements related to diarrhea and altered absorption

Assess nutritional status and assist patient with identifying irritating foods such as raw fruits and vegetables, whole grains, carbonated beverages, whole milk

Provide diet high in calories, protein, and minerals; low in residue, fat, and fiber

Prepared elemental diets are available

TPN as indicated *to allow intestinal tract to rest*

Six small meals are beneficial

Encourage patient to participate in meal planning *to provide sense of control and increase intake*

Maintain intake record and avoid foods that cause cramping, diarrhea

Administer anticholinergics *to reduce motility and increase absorption*

Administer vitamin B_{12} *to correct malabsorption*

Encourage patient to eat slowly, chew well, and take small bites

Serve food attractively in a well-ventilated room

Administer oral hygiene *to increase desire to eat and enhance taste of foods*

Expected Outcomes

Maintains normal weight

Laboratory values are within normal limits

▼Risk for impaired skin integrity related to fluid/nutritional deficit and irritation from diarrhea

Assess perirectal area for inflammation, abscess, or fistula

Administer perirectal skin care after each bowel movement

Wash gently with soap and water

Pat dry and apply soothing protective ointments

Administer sitz baths *to reduce pain and irritated perianal tissue*

Provide skin care to bony prominences as needed *to reduce risk of skin breakdown*

Provide frequent position changes

Air mattress as indicated

Wound, Ostomy, Continence/ET Nurse consultation

Expected Outcomes
Perirectal tissue remains clean and intact
Skin turgor and color are normal

▼Pain related to bowel inflammation and irritation

Assess character, intensity, and location of pain using pain scale
Assess effectiveness, side effects of sedatives, analgesics, and rectal suppositories and ointments
Change patient's position frequently and administer back rubs *to relieve discomfort*
Provide diversional activities *to reduce attention on discomfort*
Ambulate patient with assistance as tolerated
Encourage and teach alternative pain management methods: imaging, deep breathing, relaxation techniques
Balance rest and activity

Expected Outcomes
Demonstrates a more relaxed affect
Verbalizes a tolerable level of pain

▼Ineffective individual coping related to multiple stressors and needed lifestyle changes

Assess present and past coping patterns *to increase ability in managing present problems*
Provide time for and encourage communication with significant other(s) *to provide a support system*
Establish a supportive relationship with patient and/or significant other(s)
  Explain all procedures and treatments
  Involve patient and/or significant other(s) in plan of care and realistically reinforce physician's explanation of disease process
  Maintain quiet, nonjudgmental, and nonstressful environment
  Encourage use of stress management techniques
  Provide undisturbed rest periods
  Accept patient's dependency and encourage independent activities as strength returns
Provide information about support groups such as the following:
  United Ostomy Association
  19772 MacArthur Blvd, Suite 200
  Irvine, CA 92612-2405
    1-800-826-0826
    (949) 660-8624
  FAX: (949) 660-9262

  Crohn's and Colitis Foundation of America, Inc.
  386 Park Avenue South
  New York, NY 10016-8804
    1-800-932-2423
    (212) 685-3440
  FAX: (212) 779-4098

Expected Outcomes
Expresses feelings/concerns more readily
Demonstrates understanding of needed lifestyle changes
Exhibits appropriate coping skills and behaviors

▼Sexual dysfunction related to altered body function, disease process, and lack of knowledge

Explore patient's knowledge of sexuality and current sexual practices and behaviors
Explain to patient and/or significant other that sexual activity needs to be curtailed only while perineal area is inflamed or fistulas or abscesses are present
Encourage patient and significant other to read about alternative sexual positions and techniques
Provide supportive and private environment

Expected Outcomes
Expresses understanding of needed changes in sexual practices
Verbalizes feelings and concerns

PATIENT/FAMILY TEACHING
Assess understanding of disease process and the cause/effect relationships of precipitating factors
Provide instructions in diet management, stressing foods to avoid: raw fruits and vegetables, alcohol, chocolate, and gas-producing foods
Discuss importance of introducing new foods one at a time
Discuss importance of avoiding stress during meals, need to chew food well and eat slowly
Explain causal relationship of stress to disease process and symptoms of recurrence or progression of disease to report to physician
Provide information about medications including name, dosage, purpose, time of administration, side effects, and interactions; explain need to avoid over-the-counter medications unless first discussed with physician
Encourage follow-up appointments with physician

DISCHARGE/HOME CARE PLANNING
Demonstrate procedure for perianal skin care
Stress importance of keeping area clean and dry
Discuss side effects of steroids: facial edema, ulcers, and reduced immune response to infection
Provide information about what and where to purchase needed supplies
Provide information on TPN if needed and discuss good aseptic technique
Discourage smoking
Provide names of community resources: Visiting Nurses Association (VNA), nutritionist/ registered dietitian, and social services

■ PERITONITIS (SECONDARY)
Inflammation of the peritoneal cavity caused by infiltration of intestinal contents from such conditions as a

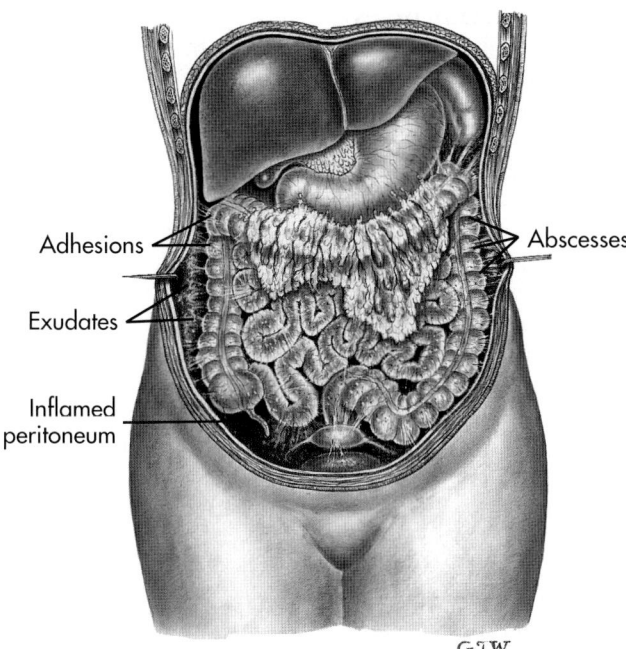

Fig. 6-10 Acute peritonitis.
(From Doughty DB, Jackson DB: Mosby's clinical nursing series: gastrointestinal disorders, *St Louis, 1993, Mosby.)*

ruptured appendix, gastric or intestinal perforation or trauma, and anastomotic leaks (Fig. 6-10)

Primary peritonitis is a bacterial infection of the peritoneal cavity not associated with bowel conditions; seen mostly in children with renal disorders and in patients with ascites

ASSESSMENT
SUBJECTIVE DATA
Abdominal pain and rigidity over area of inflammation
  Rebound tenderness
  May refer to shoulder, flank, back
Anorexia
Nausea

OBJECTIVE DATA
Vomiting
Abdominal distention
Decreased to absent bowel sounds
Failure to pass flatus or stool
Chills, fever
Tachycardia
Hypotension
Leukocytosis
Anxiety
Thoracic breathing: rapid, shallow
Fecal emesis

DIAGNOSTIC TESTS
CBC, electrolytes, WBC increased
Radiologic examination of abdomen

CT scan or ultrasound
Peritoneal aspiration of fluid and culture
Peritoneoscopy

POTENTIAL COMPLICATIONS
Electrolyte imbalance
Dehydration
Metabolic acidosis
Respiratory alkalosis
Hypovolemic shock

MULTIDISCIPLINARY MANAGEMENT
THERAPEUTIC MANAGEMENT
Parenteral fluids with electrolytes, antibiotics, and
  vitamins
Analgesics
Nasogastric suction, NPO
ABGs
CVP lines
Oxygen therapy, incentive spirometer
Peritoneal lavage with antibiotics
Surgical intervention

PATIENT PROBLEMS—NURSING DIAGNOSES/INTERVENTIONS

▼Fluid volume deficit related to increased blood flow to peritoneum, vomiting, and/or gastrointestinal perforation

Assess hydration status
Maintain NPO *to decrease intestinal motility*
Monitor vital signs and CVP qh or prn; observe for signs
  of shock
Maintain parenteral fluids with electrolytes, antibiotics,
  and vitamins
Weigh patient daily (same time, scale, and clothing)
Measure intake and output q1h to 2h; measure urine
  output hourly; if <30 ml/hr notify physician; *may
  indicate renal complications*
Assist with peritoneal aspiration/lavage, drainage
  Connect drain to gravity drainage as ordered
  Include drainage in output amount
  Send specimen for culture and sensitivity
Monitor electrolytes, blood gases, Hgb, and Hct
Perform passive or assist with and teach active ROM
  exercises q4h *to increase circulation*

Expected Outcomes
Hydration is adequate as evidenced by normal skin turgor
  and moist mucous membranes
Vital signs are stable
Intake and output are balanced

▼Ineffective breathing pattern, secondary to abdominal pain and distention

Assess respiratory status; monitor for shallow, rapid
  respirations

Maintain bed rest in quiet environment with head of bed elevated 35 to 45 degrees *to increase lung expansion*

Monitor oxygen therapy or incentive spirometer

Assist and teach patient to turn and cough q4h and deep breathe q1h to 2h

Auscultate chest for breath sounds q4h

Expected Outcomes

Exhibits normal respirations and breath sounds

Demonstrates ability to perform breathing exercises

▼Altered nutrition: less than body requirements related to vomiting and lack of intake

Monitor nasogastric tube or nasooral intestinal tube; connect to low, intermittent suction apparatus

Monitor character, amount, color, and odor of drainage

Provide frequent oral and nasal hygiene

Monitor for passing of flatus

Auscultate abdomen for bowel sounds q8h

Monitor TPN as indicated

When bowel sounds return and nasogastric-intestinal tube is removed, provide clear liquid diet as tolerated

If surgery is performed, see Intestinal surgery (p. 340)

Expected Outcomes

States absence of nausea/vomiting

Tolerates diet adequately

▼Pain related to inflammation and distention

Assess type, location, and severity of pain using a pain scale

Administer analgesics only after diagnosis has been made, *because they mask signs and symptoms*

Assess effectiveness of pain relief measures

Maintain position of comfort *to minimize stress on abdomen*

Change positions in small ways *to reduce discomfort*

Provide planned rest periods

Discuss and teach alternative pain management techniques: visualizing, imaging, deep breathing

Provide diversional activities *to reduce attention on pain*

Expected Outcomes

Verbalizes a tolerable level of pain

Exhibits improving ability to use alternative pain relief measures

▼Anxiety related to situational crisis

Assess anxiety level

Assess present coping skills

Encourage and allow time for verbalization of feelings

Explain all treatments and procedures

Reinforce physician's explanation of illness and treatment

Assist with and teach relaxation techniques

Provide periods of undisturbed rest

Encourage support of family/significant other(s)

Expected Outcomes

Expresses feelings and concerns and understands positive ways of coping

Appears more relaxed and comfortable

PATIENT/FAMILY TEACHING

Assess level of understanding of disease process

Discuss pain management and use of relaxation techniques

Stress importance of signs and symptoms to report to physician

Provide information about diet; increase to normal diet as tolerated; avoid irritating foods and introduce new foods one at a time

Discuss medications, side effects, and need to take all medications as prescribed

Encourage follow-up appointments with physician

DISCHARGE/HOME CARE PLANNING

Demonstrate wound care and importance of sterile technique

Provide information on what supplies are needed and where to purchase them

Provide names of community resources to assist with home care: visiting nurse, social services, home health aides

■ SHORT BOWEL SYNDROME

Malabsorption following small bowel resection; severity depends on the amount and portion of small bowel removed; the loss of >3 m of the small bowel will affect the body's ability to absorb nutrients and vitamins, especially if the ileocecal valve is removed

ASSESSMENT

SUBJECTIVE DATA

Diarrhea

Weight loss

Fatigue

Weakness

OBJECTIVE DATA

Frequent, watery diarrhea; may contain fat

Rapid dehydration resulting from malabsorption

Poor skin turgor

Purpura, generalized bleeding

Anemia

Malabsorption of fat and fat-soluble vitamins (A, D, E, K)

DIAGNOSTIC TESTS

Barium enema

Serum studies: reduced iron, vitamins B_{12} and A, calcium, folate, magnesium, electrolytes, CBC, carotene, cholesterol

PT/INR: increased

Stool for fat and culture

Lactose intolerance, elevated D-lactate level, decreased xylose tolerance

POTENTIAL COMPLICATIONS
Malnutrition
Electrolyte imbalance
Osteoporosis, osteomalacia
Night blindness
Tetany
Confusion, stupor

MULTIDISCIPLINARY MANAGEMENT
THERAPEUTIC MANAGEMENT
TPN, parenteral fluids (p. 24)
Antidiarrheals
Anticholinergics
Antibiotics
Antacids
Vitamin B_{12}, folate, multivitamins
Histamine-receptor antagonists (cimetidine)
Consult with dietitian
Elemental diet progressing to low-lactose, high-calorie diet
ECG as indicated

PATIENT PROBLEMS—NURSING DIAGNOSES/INTERVENTIONS

▼ Fluid volume deficit related to profuse diarrhea and fluid loss

Monitor parenteral fluids with electrolytes and vitamins
Assess for signs of dehydration and shock; check LOC q2h
Monitor vital signs q2h to 4h
Measure intake and output q8h
Weigh patient daily (same time, scale, and clothing)
Monitor serum electrolytes, Hgb, and Hct

Expected Outcomes
Vital signs are normal
Intake and output are balanced
Skin turgor is adequate
Electrolytes are within normal limits

▼ Diarrhea related to decreased intestinal absorption

Assess effectiveness, side effects of antidiarrheals, antacids, histamine-receptor antagonists
Monitor stools for color, consistency, amount, and frequency
Provide perineal care after each bowel movement; keep environment free of odor
Auscultate abdomen for bowel sounds q4h
Check stool for blood 3 times; report if positive

Expected Outcomes
Stools are less frequent
Stool consistency is more normal

▼ Altered nutrition: less than body requirements related to loss of absorptive surface of intestine

Maintain TPN as indicated
    Monitor urine for sugar and acetone qid
    Monitor blood glucose, report if <60 or >180 mg/dl
    Observe central IV line for infection, change dressing qod and prn
    Institute elemental diet (Vivonex, Precision LR), usually when weight gain is apparent and diarrhea is less frequent
    Administer diet through nasogastric tube or orally, depending on patient's appetite: 300 to 350 ml q2h
    When given orally, provide a straw because the taste may be unpalatable to some patients
    Discuss with and assist patient and significant other(s) with accepting revised nutritional plan, which may be necessary for a long period
    Collaborate with nutritionist/registered dietitian on diet and nourishments
    Assess effectiveness and monitor side effects of antacids and anticholinergics
    Measure intake after each meal; maintain calorie count

Expected Outcomes
Maintains weight at level normal for patient
Demonstrates understanding of changes needed in dietary regimen

PATIENT/FAMILY TEACHING
Discuss and provide written information about nutritional plan, usually low-lactose, high-calorie diet; introduce milk slowly and observe tolerance
Instruct patient and/or significant other(s) concerning signs and symptoms to report to physician: nausea, vomiting, diarrhea, or other intestinal problems
Discuss medication: name, dosage, purpose, time of administration, and side effects
Encourage follow-up visits with physician

DISCHARGE/HOME CARE PLANNING
Discuss and provide information on TPN if it is to be given at home
Involve nutritionist/registered dietitian and provide referral to home health services
Stress importance of signs of dehydration: poor skin turgor, dry mucous membranes, weakness
Provide names, phone numbers of home health team members
Monitor weight q week (same time, scale, and clothing)

■ INTESTINAL OBSTRUCTION
Blockage of the intestinal tract, which inhibits the passage of fluids, flatus, and food; may be mechanical or functional (neurogenic or vascular)

CAUSES
MECHANICAL
Adhesions
Strangulated hernia
Abscess

Tumor
Volvulus
Intussusception
Constipation

FUNCTIONAL
Paralytic ileus
Spinal cord lesions
Regional enteritis
Electrolyte imbalance
Uremia

ASSESSMENT
SUBJECTIVE DATA
Constipation
Anxiety
Anorexia and malaise
Small bowel
    Severe, cramplike abdominal pain, increasing with
      distention
    Mild distention
    Nausea
Large bowel
    Mild abdominal discomfort
    Severe distention

OBJECTIVE DATA
Fever
Tachycardia
Diaphoresis
Pallor
Abdominal rigidity
Failure to pass stool or flatus rectally or per
    ostomy
Increased bowel sounds (early obstruction)
Decreased bowel sounds (later)
Urinary retention
Small bowel
    Vomiting: early contains undigested food and chyme;
      later vomitus is watery and contains bile; finally,
      dark and fecal
    Rapid dehydration: acidosis
Large bowel
    Latent fecal vomiting
    Latent dehydration: rare acidosis

DIAGNOSTIC TESTS
Serum electrolytes, CBC, amylase
Barium enema
Radiologic studies of abdomen

POTENTIAL COMPLICATIONS
Dehydration
Electrolyte imbalance
Metabolic acidosis
Perforation
Shock

MULTIDISCIPLINARY MANAGEMENT
THERAPEUTIC MANAGEMENT
NPO
Nasointestinal suction
Surgical intervention: see Intestinal surgery
    (p. 340)
Parenteral fluids with electrolytes, antibiotics, and
    vitamins
Analgesics
Antiemetics
Oxygen therapy
Respiratory therapy consult as indicated

PATIENT PROBLEMS—NURSING DIAGNOSES/INTERVENTIONS

▼Fluid volume deficit secondary to nausea and
vomiting, fever, and/or diaphoresis

Monitor vital signs and observe LOC and for symptoms of
    hypovolemic shock
Maintain NPO; assess level of hydration
Measure intake and output
Monitor parenteral fluids with electrolytes, antibiotics,
    and vitamins
Insert and monitor nasointestinal tube and low,
    intermittent suction apparatus
    Measure drainage output q8h
      Observe contents for color, consistency; check for
        electrolyte loss or pH as prescribed
Position patient on right side, then left side *to
    facilitate passage into intestine;* do not tape
    nasointestinal tube to nose until tube is in correct
    position
Monitor tube for advancement qh
Indwelling urethral catheter may be inserted; report
    output of <30 ml/hr to physician
Monitor electrolytes, Hgb, and Hct
Prepare for surgery as indicated (p. 9)
If surgery is not performed, collaborate with physician
    and initiate oral fluids, either by clamping intestinal
    tube for 1 hour and giving measured amounts of water
    or tea or by giving these fluids after intestinal tube is
    removed
Open tube, if in place, at specified times as ordered *to
    estimate amount of absorption*
Observe abdomen for discomfort, distention, pain, or
    rigidity and report to physician
Measure abdominal girth q8h *to monitor distention*
Force fluids to 2500 ml/day unless contraindicated
Encourage ambulation *to stimulate peristalsis*
Observe initial stool for color, consistency, and amount;
    prevent constipation
Weigh patient qd (same time, scale, and clothing)

Expected Outcomes
Vital signs are normal
Intake and output are balanced

Patient is normovolemic with good skin turgor, stable weight, and absence of thirst

▼ Pain related to distention, rigidity

Maintain bed rest in position of comfort: do not hyperflex knees

Assess location, severity, and type of pain; use pain rating scale

Assess effectiveness and monitor for side effects of analgesics; avoid morphine *to prevent hypomotility*

Provide planned rest periods

Assist with and teach active or perform passive ROM exercises q4h *to prevent fatigue and promote peristalsis*

Change position frequently and administer back rubs and skin care *to promote comfort*

Provide oral care at frequent intervals

Auscultate bowel sounds; note increased rigidity or pain; give gentle enema if ordered

Report absence of bowel sounds to physician

Provide and teach alternative pain relief measures

Expected Outcomes

Verbalizes decreased discomfort; states pain is at tolerable level

Appears relaxed

▼ Ineffective breathing pattern related to abdominal distention and/or rigidity

Assess respiratory status; observe for shallow, rapid breathing

Elevate head of bed 40 to 60 degrees *to increase lung expansion*

Assist and teach patient to turn and cough q4h and deep breathe qh

Auscultate chest for breath sounds q4h

Monitor oxygen therapy

Support use of incentive spirometer q1h to 2h as indicated

Expected Outcomes

Demonstrates ability to perform breathing exercises

Exhibits respirations that are deep and slow

▼ Anxiety related to situational crisis and altered health status

Assess present coping behaviors and encourage use of past successful skills

Encourage and allow time for verbalization of anxieties and fears; provide quiet reassurance

Explain procedures and treatments and reinforce physician's explanation of illness, treatment, and prognosis

Maintain quiet, nonstressful environment; encourage support of family and significant other(s)

Expected Outcomes

Expresses understanding of present illness

Demonstrates positive coping skills in dealing with anxiety

PATIENT/FAMILY TEACHING

Discuss dietary management, stressing importance of eating slowly, chewing food well, and eating at regular intervals

Explain need to prevent constipation
    Use natural laxatives or stool softeners
    Maintain fluid intake of 2500 ml/day
    Increase activity as tolerated

Provide instructions on symptoms to report to physician: abdominal pain, cramps, distention, and/or nausea and vomiting

Encourage follow-up care with physician

If surgery was performed, see Intestinal surgery (p. 340)

DISCHARGE/HOME CARE PLANNING

Encourage patient to perform ROM exercises at home to increase strength

Promote increasing activity slowly but steadily to increase bowel function

Encourage short walks outdoors

Stress importance of adequate daily fluid intake

Monitor weight q week

■ PARALYTIC ILEUS

Temporary decrease in or absence of intestinal motility after intestinal or abdominal surgery or in connection with any severe metabolic disease; cause may be neuromuscular, resulting from lack of potassium, or gastrointestinal, resulting from gastric inactivity and air swallowing

ASSESSMENT
SUBJECTIVE DATA
Nausea

Feeling of fullness

Abdominal tenderness and distention

OBJECTIVE DATA
Absent or diminished bowel sounds

Vomiting

Lack of flatus

Decreased urinary output

Fever

DIAGNOSTIC TESTS
Electrolytes (decreased potassium)

Abdominal radiography series

POTENTIAL COMPLICATIONS
Dehydration

Electrolyte imbalance

Shock

Perforation of ileum

Peritonitis

Circulatory failure

Respiratory distress

MULTIDISCIPLINARY MANAGEMENT
THERAPEUTIC MANAGEMENT

NPO

Parenteral fluids with electrolytes

Nasointestinal, nasogastric aspiration

Oxygen therapy

Medications to promote peristalsis: dexpanthenol (Ilopan), bethanechol (Urecholine), neostigmine (Prostigmin), metoclopramide (Reglan)

Activity, diet

Enema, rectal tube

PATIENT PROBLEMS—NURSING DIAGNOSES/INTERVENTIONS

▼ Ineffective breathing pattern related to abdominal distention and rigidity

Maintain bed rest in position to facilitate respirations; do not hyperflex knees

Assess respiratory status

Auscultate chest for breath sounds q4h

Monitor oxygen therapy

Assist and teach patient to turn and cough q4h and deep breathe qh

Incentive spirometer q2h

Balance activity and rest

Monitor vital signs q4h

Expected Outcomes

Demonstrates ability to perform breathing exercises

Exhibits normal respirations and breath sounds

▼ Fluid volume deficit related to vomiting and distention

Maintain NPO; assess level of hydration

Maintain parenteral fluids with electrolytes

Maintain nasointestinal tube to low, intermittent suction apparatus

　Do not tape tube to nose; position patient to facilitate passage of tube into intestine

　Monitor advancement qh

Monitor character, amount, pH, and color of intestinal drainage q4h; report any change to physician

Nasogastric tube may be inserted in lieu of intestinal tube; connect to low, intermittent suction apparatus

　Tape securely to nose

　Irrigate with measured amounts of normal saline

　Monitor color and amount of drainage

Measure intake and output; report urine output of <30 ml/hr to physician

Monitor electrolytes

Collaborate with physician when intestinal or gastric output decreases and bowel sounds return to initiate feeding schedule

　Clamp tube

　Administer liquids (warm tea, carbonated beverages) in measured amounts (30 ml qh)

　　Monitor for pain, distention, nausea, and cramps; unclamp tube if these signs occur

　　Remove tube and progress to previous diet

Continue measuring intake and output until adequate for patient

Weigh patient qod (same time, scale, and clothing)

Expected Outcomes

Hydration is normal as evidenced by skin turgor

Intake and output are balanced

Bowel sounds are normal

Electrolytes are within normal limits

▼ Constipation related to decreased intake

Assess effectiveness of and monitor for side effects of medication used to increase peristalsis

Stool softeners as ordered

Auscultate abdomen for bowel sounds q4h; monitor for return of flatus and normal bowel elimination

Promote high-fiber diet and increased fluid intake as tolerated *to promote motility*

Encourage ambulation as tolerated *to increase peristalsis*

Expected Outcomes

Understands causative factors of constipation

Defecates soft, formed stool

PATIENT/FAMILY TEACHING

Reinforce physician's explanation of cause of paralytic ileus and that it is a temporary condition

Explain all procedures and treatments

Demonstrate technique for swallowing without ingesting air

DISCHARGE/HOME CARE PLANNING

Stress importance of increased fluid intake and activity to maintain peristaltic action

Maintain follow-up physician visits

◼ DIVERTICULAR DISEASE OF COLON

Herniation (pocket formation) along the mucosa of the large intestine caused by low-fiber diets and weakened intestinal wall (diverticulosis); an inflammatory process may occur when a diverticulum ruptures or feces become impacted in the diverticulum (diverticulitis); the incidence increases with age (60% of people older than 60 years of age have the condition) and is most commonly found in the sigmoid colon (Fig. 6-11)

◼ ACUTE DIVERTICULITIS

ASSESSMENT
SUBJECTIVE DATA

Cramplike pain and tenderness in left lower quadrant (LLQ), may radiate to flank and back

Anorexia

Nausea

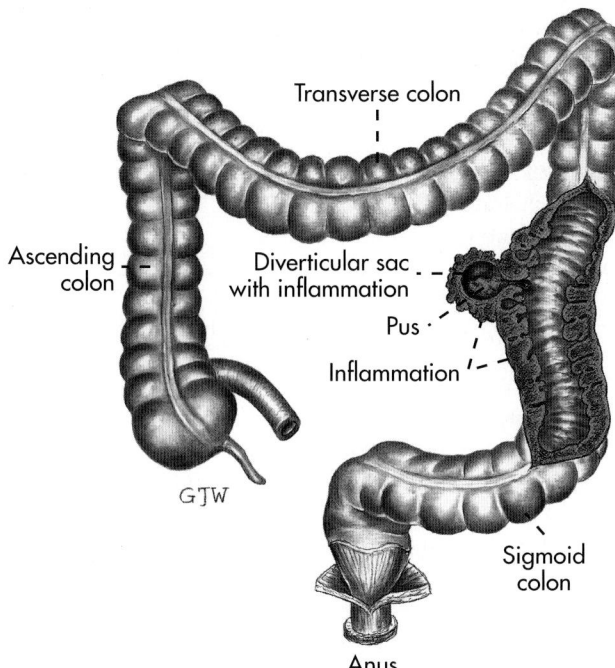

Fig. 6-11 Diverticulosis (diverticulitis).
(From Doughty DB, Jackson DB: Mosby's clinical nursing series: gastrointestinal disorders, *St Louis, 1993, Mosby.)*

OBJECTIVE DATA
Low-grade fever
Rebound abdominal tenderness
Irregular bowel function
    Constipation
    Diarrhea
    Mucus, blood in stool
    Increased flatulence
    Abdominal distention
    Decreased bowel sounds
Severe pain
    Tachycardia
    Hypotension
    Shallow respirations

DIAGNOSTIC TESTS
Water-soluble contrast enema
Sigmoidoscopy, colonoscopy with biopsy
Ultrasonography
CT scan
WBC, ESR: increased
Urinalysis, stool examination (including occult blood)
Examination of surrounding organs (kidney, bladder) for
    possible involvement

POTENTIAL COMPLICATIONS
Leukocytosis
Dehydration
Intestinal obstruction, perforation
Peritonitis
Fistula, abscess
Hemorrhage

MULTIDISCIPLINARY MANAGEMENT
THERAPEUTIC MANAGEMENT
Bed rest
Parenteral fluids with electrolytes and antibiotics
Nasogastric aspiration (severe vomiting, distention)
Analgesics, anticholinergics
Psyllium (Metamucil) laxative
NPO increasing to high-fiber diet
Surgical intervention (resection, colostomy)
Parenteral replacement of fluids as indicated
Consultation with dietitian

PATIENT PROBLEMS—NURSING DIAGNOSES/INTERVENTIONS

▼Risk for fluid volume deficit related to nausea, diarrhea, anorexia, risk of hypovolemia

Monitor vital signs q4h as needed
Maintain NPO; assess level of hydration
Maintain parenteral fluids with antibiotics and
    electrolytes
Monitor electrolytes
Collaborate with physician, nutritionist/registered
    dietitian; when pain and fever subside and/or
    nasogastric tube is removed, provide clear liquid diet
    and progress to soft diet until high-fiber diet can be
    tolerated
Force fluids to 2500 ml/day unless contraindicated
Assess and monitor amount of bleeding; check stools for
    occult or frank blood
Monitor Hct, Hgb as ordered
Monitor blood transfusions or PBCs
Assist with exercises of legs and feet q4h *to increase
    venous return*
Measure intake and output; report output of <30 ml/hr to
    physician
Weigh qod (same time, scale, and clothing)

Expected Outcomes
Hydration is adequate as evidenced by normal skin turgor
Intake and output are balanced
Vital signs are within normal limits

▼Constipation related to anorexia, low-fiber diet, and immobility

Monitor nasogastric tube and low, intermittent suction
    apparatus
    Maintain tube patency
    Irrigate with measured amounts of normal saline
    Measure gastric output q8h
Auscultate abdomen for bowel sounds q4h
Monitor stools for consistency, color, amount, and
    frequency; check for impaction
When nasogastric tube is removed, administer
    hydrophilic colloid laxative or psyllium (Metamucil) as
    tolerated *to promote defecation*
Ambulate as tolerated *to increase intestinal motility*

Expected Outcomes

Tolerates increasingly high-fiber diet

Defecates soft, formed stool

▼Pain related to inflammation, irritation of bowel

Maintain bed rest in position of comfort

Assess location, character, and severity of pain

Administer analgesics; avoid morphine; assess effectiveness of pain relief measures

Assist and teach patient to turn and deep breathe q2h; administer back rubs *to promote comfort*

Maintain planned rest periods

Change position frequently *to prevent pressure and fatigue*

Encourage and teach alternative pain management methods: relaxation techniques, imaging, deep breathing, warm baths

Expected Outcomes

Reports a tolerable level of pain

Appears relaxed

PATIENT/FAMILY TEACHING

Assess level of understanding of diverticular disease

Provide written dietary instructions and discuss relationship of diet to disease process

Include listing of high-fiber foods: bran, fruits, vegetables

Explain importance of regular meals, eating slowly, and chewing well

    Avoid large meals, extremely cold foods, caffeine and alcohol

    Increase fluid intake to eight glasses per day unless contraindicated

Discuss importance of elimination

    Establish regular bowel habits

    Avoid constipation, straining, enemas, and harsh laxatives

Use psyllium (Metamucil) or high-fiber wafers or powder

Encourage regular visits to physician

DISCHARGE/HOME CARE PLANNING

Discuss bowel training and establishing regular elimination habits

    Set aside a daily time for bowel movement

    Avoid anxiety and interruption

    Drink plenty of fluids and exercise regularly

    Maintain a high-fiber diet

Explain signs and symptoms of recurrence of condition to report to physician

    LLQ pain, cramps

    Diarrhea, constipation

    Blood in stool

■ INTESTINAL SURGERY WITH OR WITHOUT FECAL DIVERSION

Any surgery performed on the intestine from the jejunum to the colon for such conditions as carcinoma, obstruction, acute enteritis or colitis, benign tumors, trauma, appendicitis, incarcerated hernia, and diverticulitis; some of these conditions may require a fecal diversion, either an ileostomy or colostomy

PREOPERATIVE ASSESSMENT AND CARE

Assess respiratory status

Monitor potassium level

Prepare bowel

    Low-residue, clear liquid diet

    Magnesia preparations, oral antibiotics

    GoLytly bowel preparation

    Enemas until clear; avoid depleting debilitated or elderly patients with multiple enemas at one time

    Nasogastric/nasointestinal tube insertion

Provide patient with information regarding drains, tubes, and so on that may be present postoperatively (nasogastric tube, urinary catheter, or wound drains)

Teach patient to turn, cough, and deep breathe

Demonstrate methods for incisional support

Discuss importance of moving after surgery, especially feet and legs

Explain and discuss fecal diversion if appropriate, including purpose and placement of stoma

POSTOPERATIVE ASSESSMENT
SUBJECTIVE DATA

Location, type of pain

Nausea

OBJECTIVE DATA

Character and amount of gastric or intestinal drainage

    Urinary output

    Ostomy drainage, if applicable

    Wound drainage

Vomiting

Abdominal distention

Placement of nasogastric tube

Decreased, shallow respirations

Decreased breath sounds

DIAGNOSTIC TESTS

Electrolytes, Hgb, Hct

BUN, creatinine

Stool for guaiac

Urine culture after indwelling catheter is removed

Wound culture; suspected infection

POTENTIAL COMPLICATIONS

Dehydration

Electrolyte imbalance

Atelectasis

Hemorrhage

Shock

Peritonitis

Paralytic ileus

Pulmonary embolus

Thrombophlebitis

Wound evisceration

Wound infection

MULTIDISCIPLINARY MANAGEMENT
THERAPEUTIC MANAGEMENT
Parenteral fluids with electrolytes
Nasogastric aspiration
Indwelling urethral catheter
NPO progressing to prescribed diet
Analgesics, antibiotics, vitamins
Histamine inhibitors (cimetidine, ranitidine), antacids
Patient controlled analgesia
Oxygen therapy, incentive spirometer
Activity, antiembolic stockings; SCD
Jvac, Jackson-Pratt drains
Consultation with dietitian, social services, respiratory therapy
Wound, Ostomy, Continence/ET Nurse consultation

PATIENT PROBLEMS—NURSING DIAGNOSES/INTERVENTIONS

▼ Ineffective breathing pattern related to placement of incision and/or pain, anesthesia

Assess respiratory status: type, frequency, and character of respirations
Elevate head of bed 35 to 45 degrees *to promote lung expansion*
Auscultate lungs for breath sounds q2h
Assist and teach patient to turn and cough q2h and deep breathe qh; support incision
Provide incentive spirometer q1-2h
Administer pain medication before treatments as applicable *to reduce discomfort*

Expected Outcomes
Exhibits normal respiratory rate and rhythm
Presents breath sounds that are clear

▼ Risk for fluid volume deficit related to gastric suction, diarrhea

Maintain NPO, assess hydration status: skin turgor, moist mucous membranes, capillary refill
Maintain parenteral fluids with electrolytes, vitamins, and antibiotics
Monitor vital signs q2h to 4h
Monitor dressings for excessive drainage, hemorrhage
Place temporary appliance on ostomy if applicable; measure drainage q8h
Monitor nasogastric/intestinal tube and low, intermittent suction
  Measure output q8h
  Check color and consistency of drainage
  Irrigate with measured amounts of normal saline
Measure intake and output q8h and monitor for fluid shift: edema, weight gain, rales
Monitor serum electrolytes
Encourage position changes *to stimulate circulation*
Monitor indwelling urethral catheter and closed gravity drainage system; measure output q2h to 4h; if <30 ml/hr, report to physician

Perform guaiac test on stool for signs of intestinal bleeding
Observe for abdominal distention and monitor bowel sounds for 2 to 3 days postoperatively
Monitor peripheral pulses, signs of edema, capillary refill
Apply antiembolic stockings and remove daily for skin care
Encourage movement of legs and feet *to promote venous circulation*

Expected Outcomes
Vital signs are normal
Intake and output are balanced
Hydration is adequate as evidenced by normal skin turgor and capillary refill
Peripheral pulses are palpable

▼ Pain related to surgical intervention

Maintain bed rest in quiet environment
Monitor location, character, intensity of pain; use pain rating scale
Assess effectiveness of pain relief measures and observe for side effects
Initiate patient controlled analgesia (p. 40) if prescribed
Encourage patient to take pain medication as prescribed for 48 hours
Encourage ambulation *to reduce discomfort from intestinal gas*
Coordinate care to allow for planned rest periods
Change position frequently; administer back rubs *to promote comfort and ease fatigue*
Discuss and teach alternative pain relief techniques as needed: guided imagery, deep breathing

Expected Outcomes
Reports a tolerable level of discomfort
Appears more relaxed, comfortable

▼ Risk for impaired skin integrity related to increased wound drainage, altered circulation, nutrition

Administer nasal and oral hygiene frequently and keep nares and mouth moist
Change dressings as needed; use nonallergenic tape or Montgomery straps
  Assess healing process
  Monitor drainage for signs of infection; obtain culture prn
  Keep skin around incision clean and dry
Provide splinting of incision when coughing *to prevent dehiscence*
Maintain permanency of tubes and catheters by taping comfortably and securely
Initiate a wound pouching system if drainage is profuse
Assess color and condition of stoma and peristomal skin integrity if applicable (see Ostomy management p. 350)
Monitor perianal area if rectum was closed

Keep skin clean and dry
Change dressings as needed
Observe for increase in drainage
Encourage ambulation *to promote circulation and healing*

Expected Outcomes
Wound heals without incident
Surrounding tissue is clean, dry, and intact

▼ Bowel incontinence related to surgical manipulation, immobility, altered nutritional intake

Administer antiemetics *to prevent vomiting* and antacids or histamine inhibitors *to neutralize acids*
Assess preoperative bowel habits and nutritional intake; explain cause of alteration
Observe for passage of flatus
Auscultate abdomen for return of bowel sounds q8h; *indicates normal bowel function or possible paralytic ileus if sounds do not return*
Observe first postoperative bowel movement: assess color, consistency, amount, and frequency
Administer vitamin K if ordered, *because bowel preparation may inhibit absorption*
Administer stool softener *to promote peristaltic action*
Demonstrate and teach ostomy irrigation and appliance application if appropriate (p. 353)

Expected Outcomes
Understands causative factors of altered elimination
Defecates soft stool

▼ Altered nutrition: less than body requirements related to NPO status, nasogastric suction

Collaborate with physician, nutritionist/registered dietitian; after bowel sounds return and nasogastric/intestinal tube is removed or clamped, initiate clear liquids in measured amounts; observe for tolerance and discomfort or distention
Progress to soft or regular diet as tolerated
Assist patient in selection of high-protein, high-vitamin C foods *to promote healing*
Monitor for malabsorption syndrome after surgery of small intestine: steatorrhea, diarrhea, weight loss
Weigh patient daily (same time, scale, and clothing)
Monitor intake and output until adequate for age and weight

Expected Outcomes
Maintains normal weight
Tolerates diet without discomfort

PATIENT/FAMILY TEACHING
Provide written dietary instructions and restrictions
Demonstrate dressing changes, wound care, clean technique
Discuss signs of wound infection: pain, redness, swelling, odor, drainage
Reinforce ostomy care if applicable (p. 350)

Explain importance of preventing constipation and using natural laxatives or those prescribed
Discuss activities allowed and need for rest, mild exercise, and not lifting heavy objects (more than 5 to 10 lb) for 6 to 8 weeks
Reinforce physician's explanation of surgical procedure and outcome expected
Discuss medications: name, dosage, purpose, time of administration, and side effects
Encourage follow-up visits with physician

DISCHARGE/HOME CARE PLANNING
Discuss dietary plan to follow
Foods high in protein and vitamin C
Eat six small meals *to reduce feeling of fullness*
Drink plenty of fluids *to promote healing*
Eat slowly and chew foods well
Provide information on type of dressings needed and where to purchase them
Have patient return demonstrate clean technique, handwashing procedure, and dressing change
Discuss signs and symptoms of problems to report to physician
Tenderness, drainage, redness around incision
Increased pain, eructation, or distention
Bleeding from incision
Nausea, vomiting
Refer to community resources for assistance with food preparation, personal care, transportation

■ CONTINENT ILEOSTOMY (KOCK'S POUCH)
Surgical removal of the rectum and colon (proctocolectomy) with construction of an internal ileal reservoir, nipple valve, and stoma, allowing intermittent drainage of ileal contents; it is often performed in two stages, depending on age and physical condition of patient; performed for patients with ulcerative colitis, familial polyposis, or existing ileostomy diversion (Fig. 6-12); obesity is considered a contraindication to this procedure

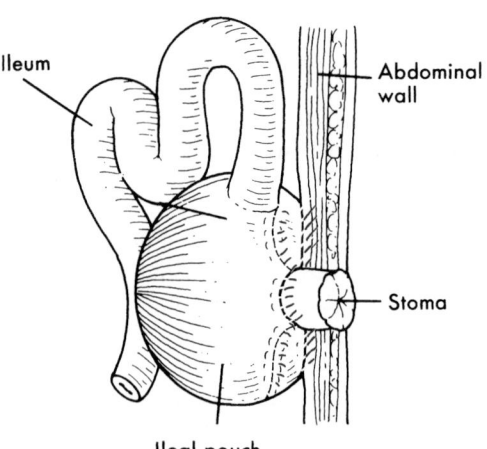

Fig. 6-12 Continent ileostomy (Kock's pouch).

PREOPERATIVE CARE

Administer prescribed bowel preparation
    Oral antibiotics
    Mild laxatives
    Colonic irrigations
Bowel preparation will depend on the following:
    Age and nutritional status
    Extent of disease process in colon
    Presence of existing ileostomy
    Stoma site selected
Insert nasogastric tube and indwelling urethral catheter
    as ordered
Involve enterostomal therapist in preoperative education;
    visit from a patient with a successful pouch is often
    beneficial
Reinforce physician's explanation of surgical procedure
    and postoperative care

POSTOPERATIVE ASSESSMENT
SUBJECTIVE DATA

Location and character of pain
Nausea
Abdominal cramps

OBJECTIVE DATA

Patency and placement of plastic ileal reservoir catheter
Patency of nasogastric tube
Placement of suture holding catheter in place or tube
    holding device with belt
Color and amount of the following:
    Ileal reservoir drainage
    Gastric drainage
    Urine output
    Wound drainage
Color of stoma
Vomiting
Abdominal distention
Diminished breath sounds

DIAGNOSTIC TESTS

Electrolytes, Hgb, Hct

POTENTIAL COMPLICATIONS

Electrolyte imbalance
Atelectasis
Intestinal obstruction, perforation
Peritonitis
Wound infection: stoma and rectum
"Pouchitis" (Box 6-1)
Bloody diarrhea, fever
Valve prolapse, leakage, blockage
Pouch perforation
Incisional dehiscence

MULTIDISCIPLINARY MANAGEMENT
THERAPEUTIC MANAGEMENT

Parenteral fluids with electrolytes
Nasogastric/ileal reservoir aspiration
Irrigating solution
Indwelling urethral catheter
PCA pump
Sitz baths
Analgesics, antibiotics, vitamins
Diet management; consult with dietitian
Consultation with Wound, Ostomy, Continence/ET Nurse

PATIENT PROBLEMS—NURSING DIAGNOSES/INTERVENTIONS

▼ Ineffective breathing pattern related to pain and risk of decreased lung expansion

Assess respiratory status and respiratory rate q2h to 4h
Assist and teach patient to turn and cough q2h to 4h and
    deep breathe qh; support incision
Auscultate chest for breath sounds q4h
Provide incentive spirometer q1h to 2h
Elevate head of bed 30 to 45 degrees *to increase lung
    expansion*

Expected Outcomes

Exhibits normal respiratory rate and rhythm
Presents clear breath sounds

▼ Risk for fluid volume deficit related to increased ileal output

Assess for dehydration: decreased skin turgor, dry mucous
    membranes, slow capillary refill
Maintain NPO *to allow intestine to rest*
Maintain parenteral fluids with electrolytes
Measure intake and output q8h
Monitor vital signs q4h
Monitor nasogastric tube and low, intermittent suction
    apparatus; irrigate gently with measured amounts of
    normal saline q2h to 4h
Monitor indwelling urethral catheter and closed gravity
    drainage system; report output of <30 ml/hr to
    physician; *may be indicative of hypovolemia*
Monitor serum electrolytes, Hgb, Hct, and urine specific
    gravity
Monitor for circulatory overload: tachycardia, neck vein
    distention, rales

Expected Outcomes

Vital signs are stable
Intake and output are balanced

Box 6-1 | **Pouchitis**

An inflammation of the reservoir caused by overgrowth of bacteria. Antibiotics such as metronidazole (Flagyl) or ciprofloxacin (Cipro) are used for treatment. Signs and symptoms of pouchitis are:
- Increased stool frequency, sudden or gradual
- Hematochezia
- Fever
- Malaise
- Pelvic discomfort

Hydration is adequate as evidenced by normal skin turgor, moist mucous membranes, and lack of thirst

▼Risk for impaired skin integrity related to acidity of ileostomy drainage and surgical procedure

Monitor dressings q1h to 2h for 24 hours; then q4h for 48 hours

Change dressings as needed; include rectal dressing

Place dressing around reservoir catheter *to prevent tension and absorb drainage from stoma*

Report excessive bleeding to physician

Monitor color of stoma (pink-red is normal); report any change to physician

Administer wound and stomal care prn

    Wash around stomal catheter and wound with clear water, pat dry, and allow to air-dry

    Apply skin sealant around stoma *to prevent irritation*

    Apply pouch if drainage is profuse or attach to bedside drainage bag

    Assess healing process

Administer sitz baths tid *to promote healing and comfort*

Expected Outcomes

Wounds are healing adequately

Surrounding skin is clean, dry, and intact

▼Altered bowel elimination related to ileostomy and ileal pouch reservoir

Monitor ileal reservoir catheter and closed gravity drainage system

Avoid placing tension on suture and catheter

Irrigate gently with 20 to 30 ml of normal saline q3h and prn, as determined through collaboration with physician, *to slowly increase pouch capacity*

Observe return flow: should equal amount instilled plus ileal contents

    Measure return; if less than amount instilled, include in intake

    Monitor color and consistency of drainage

Auscultate abdomen for bowel sounds q4h

Observe and monitor for signs of reservoir catheter obstruction

    Feeling of fullness in lower abdomen or around catheter

    Nausea, vomiting

    Increased pain or cramps

If symptoms of reservoir catheter obstruction occur, perform the following procedure, if ordered, after discussion with physician

    Gently irrigate catheter with 20 to 30 ml of normal saline

    If there is no outflow, carefully remove skin suture

    Retain suture around catheter because it marks length of insertion

    Gently irrigate with 20 ml of normal saline and rotate catheter clockwise until outflow begins

    If no results occur, notify physician immediately

Ileal catheter should remain in place 14 to 21 days to allow reservoir healing

Continue irrigations q2h to 3h with 30 to 40 ml of normal saline; contents will thicken as diet increases

Increase fluid intake to 3000 ml/day unless contraindicated

Provide grape and prune juice to keep ileal content thin

If plugging occurs, gentle milking of catheter and rotation clockwise while irrigating may help; having patient cough and applying light pressure to lower abdomen may also help

Catheter may be removed, rinsed, and reinserted if ordered

Expected Outcomes

Understanding of ileal pouch's function is clear

Pouch remains patent, and output becomes more normal

▼Altered nutrition: less than body requirements related to nasogastric aspiration and increased ileal output

Clamp or remove nasogastric tube as determined by physician when bowel sounds return or bubbles appear in ileal catheter

Provide water and clear liquids as tolerated; start with small sips and evaluate tolerance

Avoid carbonated beverages

Progress to soft, low-residue, low-fiber diet *to prevent catheter plugging*

Avoid gas-producing foods

Teach patient to chew foods well with mouth closed, eat slowly, and avoid talking while eating *to avoid swallowing air*

Have patient avoid drinking with straw *to prevent ingestion of air*

Consider patient's food preferences *to increase desire to maintain adequate diet*

Expected Outcomes

Demonstrates understanding of diet regimen

Tolerates diet, and weight remains stable

▼Pain related to surgical intervention

Maintain bed rest in quiet environment

Assess location, intensity, and character of pain; severe gas pains are usually present postoperatively

Administer analgesics and monitor effectiveness of pain relief measures; PCA may be beneficial for first 3 days

Assist with and teach active ROM exercises (especially for the feet and legs) q4h *to increase venous circulation*

Coordinate care to provide planned rest periods

Discuss and teach alternative pain relief measures

Change position frequently; administer back rubs *to promote comfort*

Provide diversional activities *to decrease attention on discomfort*

Ambulate with assistance *to increase peristaltic action and reduce gas discomfort*

Expected Outcomes
Reports a reduction of pain
Presents a more relaxed affect

▼ Body image disturbance related to altered bowel function (ileostomy)

Encourage and allow time for verbalization of feelings and concerns; provide privacy
Encourage patient communication with significant other(s)
Assess present coping behaviors and strengths
Offer praise for accomplishments in discussing, viewing, or exploring stoma
Introduce to Wound, Ostomy, Continence/ET Nurse and/or support group
Encourage patient to view stoma and catheter and discuss their positive aspects
Reinforce physician's explanation of procedure and treatment; clarify misconceptions

Expected Outcomes
Demonstrates understanding of fears/concerns
Begins to accept ileostomy as part of body
Uses positive coping skills to incorporate body changes into lifestyle

PATIENT/FAMILY TEACHING
Assist and teach patient to care for ileal reservoir catheter when patient is physically and psychologically able
Involve patient and significant other in plan of care
Set and explain daily goals, with ultimate goal being total patient management

PHASE I
Familiarize patient with anatomy and physiology of ileal reservoir
Explain that drainage will depend on food ingested and emphasize importance of high-liquid intake
Teach patient to irrigate catheter: use 50-ml syringe, normal saline, and 500-ml graduate
Instill 30 to 50 ml of normal saline
Measure outflow
Make certain all irrigating fluid is returned
Reconnect catheter to closed gravity drainage system

PHASE II
When ordered, clamp catheter for 1 hour, then release for 30 minutes and reclamp
Irrigate prn with normal saline if outflow is thick
Teach patient procedure in small segments until mastered
Explain that purpose of clamping procedure is to gradually increase reservoir capacity
Explain that clamping time will increase by 15 to 30 minutes daily until 3 to 4 hours is reached, usually in 5 to 6 days

Continue to connect catheter to closed gravity drainage system at night (Box 6-2)

PHASE III
When ordered, remove catheter and teach patient reinsertion procedure using the following equipment and guidelines
Equipment
No. 28 or No. 30 plastic catheter with insertion tube
50-ml graduate
50-ml syringe
Normal saline or tap water
Water-soluble lubricant
Tissues
4 × 4 dressing
Nonallergenic tape
Guidelines
Have patient sit on side of bed
Remove dressings and catheter; disconnect catheter from drainage system
Rinse catheter with water and lubricate tip; place other end into graduate
Place graduate below stoma
Gently intubate stoma until resistance of nipple valve is felt (2 inches or 5 cm)
Slide catheter through valve with gentle pressure to insertion line
If catheter meets resistance, do not force
Have patient lie down, relax, and take deep breaths
Insert catheter through valve during exhalation
Drainage time is about 5 to 10 minutes unless fecal material is thick; irrigating with 30 ml of normal saline or water will thin material

---

Box 6-2	**Method for Increasing Ileal Reservoir Capacity**

- Leave catheter in pouch with continuous drainage for first 3 weeks
- Week 4
  Intubate and irrigate catheter every 2 hours during day
  Connect to gravity drainage at night
  Irrigate once at night
- Week 5
  Intubate every 3 hours and irrigate bid
  Connect to gravity drainage at night
  Irrigate once at night
- Week 6
  Intubate every 4 hours and irrigate bid
  Intubate q5h at night
- Week 7 and thereafter
  Intubate pouch q6h
  Irrigate once daily until return is clear

Modified from Thompson JM et al: Mosby's clinical nursing, *ed 4, St Louis, 1997, Mosby.*

Air bubbles in catheter are normal

When drainage is complete, remove catheter and wash with soap and water; rinse well and dry; store in plastic bag

Cleanse stoma and skin with warm water; pat dry and apply 4 × 4 dressing; secure with tape

Discuss importance of maintaining drainage schedule

Time between drainage periods will increase as reservoir capacity increases

Provide and discuss written schedule (see Box 6-2)

Explain importance of diet regimen

Eat well-balanced, low-residue diet

Avoid gas-producing foods: cabbage, cauliflower, carbonated beverages

Avoid foods that can clog catheter: corn, nuts, mushrooms, lettuce, fruit peels

Eat at regular times, chew food well, eat slowly, and avoid straws

Maintain fluid intake of 2500 ml/day; drink prune and grape juices to help liquefy drainage

Discuss signs and symptoms of "pouchitis" to report to physician

Inability to intubate stoma

Abdominal distention

Nausea, vomiting

Increased abdominal pain

Elevated temperature

Incontinence of stool and/or flatus (nipple valve dysfunction)

Explain need to wear nonirritating clothing until wound heals

Demonstrate care of surgical incisions

Encourage follow-up visits with physician

DISCHARGE/HOME CARE PLANNING

Provide list of foods and fluids to eat and avoid

Observe and evaluate return demonstration of wound care, clean technique

Stress importance of handwashing

Provide information on what and where to purchase needed supplies

Teach patient procedure for sitz bath, if applicable; be certain water is not too hot

Reinforce signs and symptoms of "pouchitis"

Refer to community resources (VNA) for assistance with ADLs, personal care as needed

Provide medical alert identification

■ ILEOANAL RESERVOIR

A surgical procedure anastomosing the ileum to an ileal reservoir constructed at the anus, allowing normal bowel elimination without an ileostomy (Fig. 6-13); procedure may be performed in one, two, or three stages, depending on patient's age and physical condition

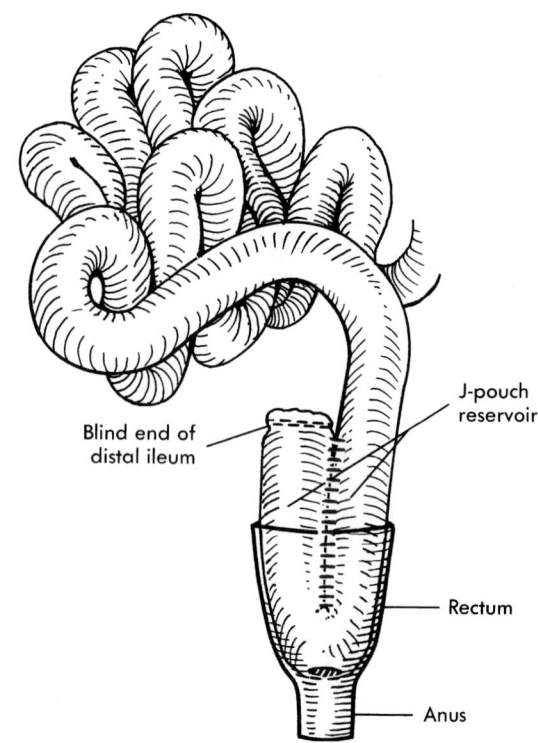

Fig. 6-13 Ileoanal anastomosis with a valveless ileal reservoir. Side-to-side anastomosis of a J-loop of terminal ileum is incised at apex and anastomosed to anal sphincter; remaining rectal mucosa provides support. Defecation occurs through anus. *(From Phipps WJ et al: Medical-surgical nursing: concepts and clinical practice, ed 6, St Louis, 1999, Mosby.)*

■ STAGE I: COLECTOMY, TEMPORARY ILEOSTOMY, AND CONSTRUCTION OF ILEAL RESERVOIR AT ANUS

PREOPERATIVE ASSESSMENT AND CARE

Reinforce physician's explanation of surgical procedure and expected outcome; clarify misconceptions

Contact Wound, Ostomy, Continence/ET Nurse for preoperative assessment and teaching

Monitor baseline vital signs

Prepare bowel as ordered: tap water enemas, oral antibiotics

Encourage and allow time for expression of concerns and feelings; promote positive aspects of surgical procedure

Explain possibility of nasogastric tube, indwelling urethral catheter, and presacral drainage tube exiting from abdomen postoperatively

POSTOPERATIVE ASSESSMENT
SUBJECTIVE DATA

Location, intensity, character of pain

OBJECTIVE DATA

Presence of nasogastric tube, urethral catheter

Respiratory function

Location of ileostomy and presacral drain
Presence of nasogastric tube, urethral catheter
Color, character, and amount of drainage
  Incisional (abdominal and rectal) drainage
  Gastric drainage
  Ileostomy drainage
  Presacral drainage
Skin integrity of ileostomy and rectal area
Urine output

DIAGNOSTIC TESTS
Electrolytes, CBC, urinalysis

POTENTIAL COMPLICATIONS
Skin erosion from ileostomy
Reservoir abscess, ischemia, fistula
Intestinal obstruction, adhesions
Wound infection
"Pouchitis" (inflammation of reservoir)
Cystitis, urinary retention
Phlebitis

MULTIDISCIPLINARY MANAGEMENT
THERAPEUTIC MANAGEMENT
Antidiarrheals, bulk-forming agents
Analgesics, antibiotics, dermatologic creams
Parenteral fluids with electrolytes and vitamins
Nasogastric suction, NPO
Irrigation of reservoir
Presacral catheter drainage apparatus
Indwelling urethral catheter
Sitz baths
Diet, rest, ambulation, exercise
Wound, Ostomy, Continence/ET Nurse

PATIENT PROBLEMS—NURSING DIAGNOSES/INTERVENTIONS

▼ Risk for fluid volume deficit related to risk of abnormal body fluid loss from ileostomy, gastric aspiration, and NPO status

Assess for signs of dehydration: poor skin turgor, dry mucous membranes, reduced capillary refill
Maintain NPO
Maintain parenteral fluids with electrolytes and vitamins
Monitor indwelling urethral catheter and closed drainage system; monitor output q2h to 4h for 12 hours; if <30 ml/hr, notify physician
Monitor nasogastric tube and low, intermittent suction apparatus; irrigate with measured amounts of normal saline to keep tube patent
Monitor ileostomy output; 800 to 1200 ml/day is not uncommon
Monitor presacral catheter, if applicable, and closed gravity drainage system; monitor output q2h for 12 hours, then q4h; include drainage in output

Calculate total intake and output q8h; assess for urinary retention
Monitor vital signs q2h until stable; then q4h
Weigh patient daily (same time, scale, and clothing)
Monitor electrolytes, Hgb, and Hct
Collaborate with physician and, when nasogastric tube is removed, initiate liquids and progress to well-balanced ileostomy diet as tolerated; monitor for tolerance of new foods as they are introduced

Expected Outcomes
Vital signs are stable
Intake and output are balanced
Ileostomy output is within normal limits
Electrolytes are within normal limits

▼ Risk for impaired skin integrity related to ileostomy and rectal/anal drainage

Monitor perianal area for drainage and mucus; may be copious and odorous
  Change dressings prn and clean area well; apply skin sealants and creams to promote healing, comfort, and skin integrity
  Cleanse skin around presacral drain and change dressing as needed
  Irrigate reservoir daily if ordered to remove mucus and other drainage and to prevent "pouchitis"
  Provide absorbent pads to wear while ambulating or at night
Assist with and teach patient ileostomy and skin care (p. 350) as soon as tolerated physically and emotionally
Apply suitable appliance as soon as possible

Expected Outcomes
Presents healing wounds, with surrounding skin clean, dry, and intact
Demonstrates increasing ability to manage ileostomy

PATIENT/FAMILY TEACHING
Reiterate ileostomy care and appliance change; observe return demonstration
Stress importance of and demonstrate skin care of perianal area and ileostomy site
Demonstrate prescribed daily reservoir irrigation
Discuss and teach patient Kegel exercises (squeezing and relaxing perineal muscles) to increase anal sphincter tone; begin exercises 6 weeks after surgery
Reinforce physician explanation of stage II procedure and answer questions
Explain that Gastrografin film of reservoir may be taken in about 6 to 12 weeks to assess reservoir capacity and anatomic location
Stress importance of well-balanced diet, rest, and exercise

Instruct patient about signs and symptoms to report to physician: increasing diarrhea, drainage, abdominal distention, absence of feces, foul odor from anus

Encourage follow-up visits with physician

STAGE II: ILEOSTOMY CLOSURE AND ANASTOMOSIS OF ILEUM TO ANAL RESERVOIR

PREOPERATIVE ASSESSMENT AND CARE
See Stage I (p. 346)
Irrigation of reservoir is sometimes ordered

POSTOPERATIVE ASSESSMENT
SUBJECTIVE DATA
Location, intensity, and character of pain

OBJECTIVE DATA
Respiratory function
Color, character, and amount of drainage
    Incisional drainage (abdominal)
    Gastric drainage
    Rectal drainage
Urine output
Skin integrity (perianal area)

DIAGNOSTIC TESTS
Electrolytes, CBC, urinalysis

POTENTIAL COMPLICATIONS
Reservoir abscess, ischemia, fistula
Skin erosion (perianal area)
Intestinal obstruction
Wound or reservoir infection
Cystitis, urinary retention
Phlebitis

MULTIDISCIPLINARY MANAGEMENT
THERAPEUTIC MANAGEMENT
Analgesics, antibiotics, antidiarrheals, dermatologic creams, ointments
Parenteral fluids with electrolytes and vitamins
Nasogastric suction, NPO
Ileal reservoir irrigation
Indwelling urethral catheter
Rest, ambulation, exercise
Sitz baths
Nutritionist/registered dietitian visits
Wound, Ostomy, Continence/ET Nurse visits

PATIENT PROBLEMS—NURSING DIAGNOSES/INTERVENTIONS

▼ Risk for fluid volume deficit related to abnormal body fluid loss from NPO status, nasogastric suction, and ileoanal reservoir

Maintain NPO; assess for signs of dehydration: decreased skin turgor, urinary output

Maintain parenteral fluids with electrolytes and vitamins
Monitor nasogastric tube and low, intermittent suction apparatus; irrigate with measured amounts of normal saline to keep tube patent
Monitor indwelling urethral catheter and closed gravity drainage system; monitor output q2h to 4h; if <30 ml/hr notify physician
Measure intake and output q8h
Monitor vital signs q4h
Weigh patient daily (same time, scale, and clothing)
Encourage patient to move feet and legs qh *to promote venous return*
Teach patient to turn, cough, and deep breathe qh *to increase cardiopulmonary function*
Monitor electrolytes, Hgb, Hct
Initiate voiding measures as needed after urethral catheter removal; observe for retention and signs of infection

Expected Outcomes
Vital signs are stable
Intake and output are balanced
Weight remains stable
Hydration is adequate as evidenced by normal skin turgor

▼ Risk for impaired skin integrity (perianal) related to diarrhea

Flush perianal area as needed with water and dry thoroughly with soft cloth or cotton balls; avoid toilet tissue
Cover with skin barrier after each defecation and use Tuck's pads *to reduce discomfort and pruritus and maintain skin integrity*
Administer sitz baths
Irrigate ileal reservoir daily if ordered and monitor return solution for blood, foul odor
Involve Wound, Ostomy, Continence/ET Nurse

Expected Outcomes
Perianal wound is healing
Surrounding skin is clean, dry, and intact

▼ Bowel incontinence related to ileal output and lack of sphincter control

Monitor bowel movements for frequency and consistency; will be frequent initially (10 to 20 per day)
Collaborate with physician and provide liquids progressing to ileoanal bland, low-residue diet after nasogastric tube removal; refer to nutritionist/registered dietitian
Monitor for effectiveness, side effects of psyllium (Metamucil), loperamide to control diarrhea
Promote Kegel exercises *to increase sphincter tone*

Expected Outcomes
Defecates fewer and more formed stools
Demonstrates ability to perform Kegel exercises

PATIENT/FAMILY TEACHING

Stress importance of protecting perineal area

After urinating or defecating flush area with water and dry thoroughly, using hair dryer when possible; take sitz baths prn

Apply skin sealants, lotions, and dermatologic creams after each bowel movement and prn

Avoid harsh, perfumed soaps and nylon underwear

Daily reservoir irrigation may be needed to prevent infection

Discuss bowel elimination; frequency will decrease (6 to 10/day) and eventually drop to 4 to 6/day

Some incontinence may be noted at night; pads may be worn as protection

Psyllium (Metamucil) and loperamide (Imodium) will help prevent diarrhea

Observe for abdominal distention

Avoid laxative use

Provide information about diet and foods that cause diarrhea (spices, fresh fruit, vegetables, and dairy products)

Instruct patient about signs and symptoms to report to physician: increasing diarrhea, drainage or foul odor from rectum, abdominal distention, absence of feces, pain, fever

Encourage follow-up visits with physician

DISCHARGE/HOME CARE PLANNING

Continue with sphincter exercises

Reemphasize importance of keeping perianal area clean and protected with skin barriers, sealants

Stress use of white, nonperfumed toilet paper and white cotton underwear

Wear absorbent pads between buttocks to reduce moisture and prevent friction

Stress importance of taking only medications ordered by physician

Avoid enteric-coated, large, and time-released medications because they may be incompletely digested

Avoid crushing pills without permission from physician

Encourage medical alert identification

■ MANAGEMENT OF NASO-ORAL INTESTINAL TUBE (CANTOR OR MILLER-ABBOTT TUBE)

Cantor or Miller-Abbott tube: *Intestinal tube, 6 to 10 ft (2 to 3.3 m) in length, that is passed through the nose or mouth into the stomach and intestine; a balloon for mercury is attached to the distal end; used for decompression and drainage in patients with bowel obstruction or paralytic ileus; tube is advanced manually, by peristaltic action, gravity, and weight of mercury (Fig. 6-14)*

PREINSERTION ASSESSMENT AND CARE

Reinforce physician's explanation of procedure and its purpose to patient and family

Assess patient's ability to swallow and willingness to cooperate

Assess abdomen for the following:

Size, shape, softness

Presence or absence of bowel sounds

Assess patient for presence of nausea, vomiting, and pain

Elevate head of bed 60 to 70 degrees; tilt head slightly forward to facilitate tube passage

Check tube for patency

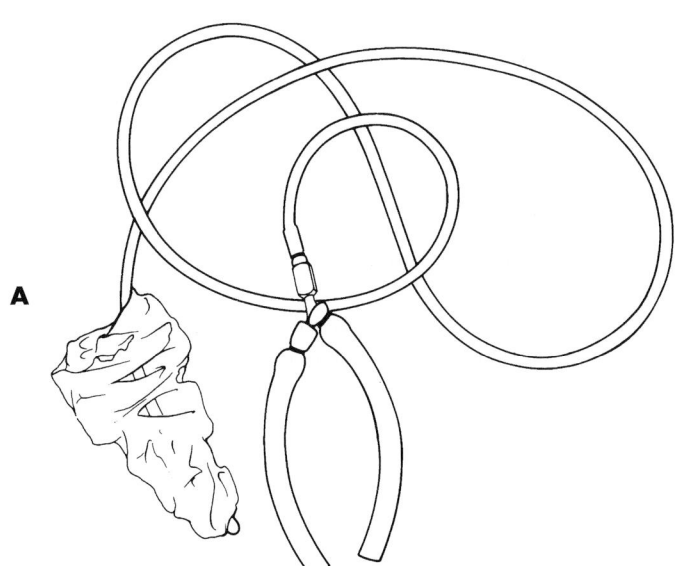 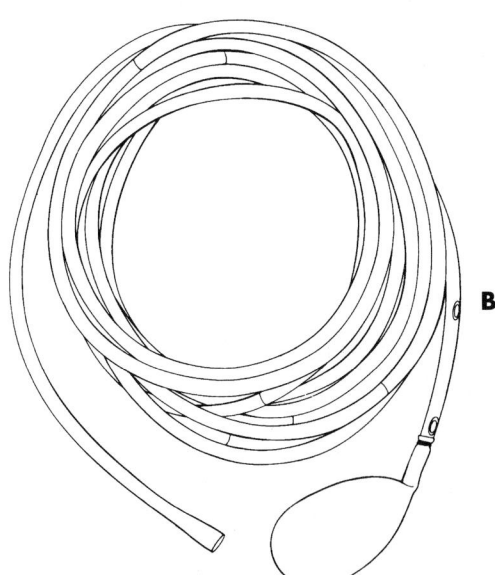

Fig. 6-14 Intestinal tubes.   **A,** Miller-Abbott tube. **B,** Cantor tube.
(From Phipps WJ et al: Medical-surgical nursing: concepts and clinical practice, ed 6, St Louis, 1999, Mosby.)

Check that balloon is securely attached and test for leakage by inserting water into balloon via correct lumen with syringe

Prepare syringe with correct amount of mercury

Cantor tube: mercury is injected into balloon via lumen before insertion

Miller-Abbott tube: mercury is injected into balloon via lumen after insertion

Ice tube according to procedure and lubricate with water-soluble jelly before insertion

INSERTION ASSESSMENT

Heart rate and rhythm: *dysrhythmias may occur as a result of vagal stimulation;* monitor with telemetry when ordered

Respiratory distress: *may occur if tube is inadvertently placed in trachea*

Vomiting

POSTINSERTION ASSESSMENT
SUBJECTIVE DATA

Nausea

Dysphagia

Sore throat

OBJECTIVE DATA

Vomiting

Character and amount of drainage

Accurate placement of tube in stomach

Pressure delivered by intermittent suction apparatus

Patency of tube

Position of patient and tube to facilitate passage of tube

Abdominal distention, pain, or cramps

Increasing bowel sounds

Erosion of nares

Condition of mouth

Blockage of eustachian tube on insertion side

POTENTIAL COMPLICATIONS

Dehydration

Electrolyte imbalance

Oliguria

Dysrhythmias

NURSING MANAGEMENT

Maintain NPO; assess for signs of dehydration

Insert prescribed amount of mercury into correct lumen of Miller-Abbott tube and label "mercury"

Connect nasointestinal tube to low, intermittent suction apparatus

Coil tube and pin to patient's gown; do not tape to nose; avoid placing tension on tube

Monitor color, pH, and consistency of intestinal drainage q4h

Irrigate tube gently with measured amounts of normal saline as ordered; if no return flow is obtained, include amount as intake

Auscultate abdomen for bowel sounds q4h; report increasing girth measurements

Turn patient to right side, to back, to left side until tube passes into intestine

Advance tube, usually 3 to 4 inches at specified times; lubricate intestinal tube thoroughly before advancing it

When bowel sounds return and/or flatus or stool is passed and after collaborating with physician

Clamp tube for 2 to 4 hours

Observe for signs of distention, cramps, or nausea

If these symptoms occur, unclamp tube and notify physician

If patient tolerates clamping procedure, administer small, frequent, measured amounts of water and observe tolerance

If patient tolerates fluids, tube is removed slowly, 2 to 3 inches at a time, or allowed to pass through rectum

Provide clear liquid diet and progress to regular diet as tolerated

Maintain bed rest in position of comfort: usually head of bed elevated 30 to 40 degrees

Administer oral hygiene q2h; provide lozenges or hard candy, if allowed, *to stimulate salivation*

Assess nares for irritation or dryness q2h; gently clean and apply lubricant as needed

PATIENT/FAMILY TEACHING

Discuss advancement of tube and how to avoid dislodgment

Discuss signs and symptoms to report to physician

Ear pain or fullness on side of insertion

Nausea or vomiting

Increased abdominal pain or cramps

Feeling of abdominal fullness or pressure

■ ILEOSTOMY, COLOSTOMY MANAGEMENT

ostomy: Surgical opening into the intestine to provide temporary or permanent passage of feces; necessitated by carcinoma, inflammation, trauma, fistula, or obstruction below the site of the ostomy; there are three types of colostomies:

end stoma: Bowel is cut and the distal end removed or sewn shut; the proximal end is pulled through the abdominal wall and a stoma made

double barrel: Bowel is cut and both ends pulled through the abdominal wall; proximal end will discharge effluent; distal end will drain mucus

loop: Bowel is not severed and a loop is pulled through the abdominal wall and supported with a rod until healing occurs; an opening is then made to discharge fecal material; this is usually temporary

ASSESSMENT
OBJECTIVE DATA

Type of ostomy

Ileostomy

Colostomy: ascending, transverse, descending; may be temporary or permanent

Removal and closure of rectum
Level of patient's understanding of surgical procedure
Emotional status
    Acceptance of ostomy
    Understanding of ostomy function
    Ability to verbalize feelings
    Acceptance of body image change
Character, frequency, and amount of feces
Size, location, and color of stoma
Condition of skin around stoma
Appropriateness of appliance and size
Placement of stoma
Hydration

DIAGNOSTIC TESTS
Electrolytes, Hgb, Hct

POTENTIAL COMPLICATIONS
Leakage under appliance
Signs of wound infection
Electrolyte imbalance
Malabsorption
Dehydration
Paralytic ileus
Intestinal obstruction
Hemorrhage
Stoma
    Prolapse
    Stricture
    Retraction
    Necrosis
    Mucocutaneous separation

MULTIDISCIPLINARY MANAGEMENT
THERAPEUTIC MANAGEMENT
Diet management
Nystatin powder
Odor-control preparation
Wound, Ostomy, Continence/ET Nurse

PATIENT PROBLEMS—NURSING DIAGNOSES/INTERVENTIONS

▼ Risk for impaired skin integrity (peristomal), secondary to ostomy drainage

Initiate peristomal care and apply ostomy appliance as soon as possible postoperatively
Measure stoma for correct appliance size at each appliance change; size should be ⅛ inch larger than stoma measurement
Change appliance prn and observe color, amount, and consistency of feces and color of stoma and surrounding skin; have extra appliances available at bedside
Maintain peristomal skin integrity
    Wash with water; start with a drainable pouch
    Pat skin dry with towel and apply effective skin barrier (Skin Prep, Stomahesive, Releaseal)

Instruct patient in caring for ostomy when physically and psychologically ready
Apply only clear appliance *to facilitate monitoring stoma*
Maintain a secure seal around stoma *to prevent leakage*
Involve Wound, Ostomy, Continence/ET Nurse if available
May control odor with deodorant drops or bismuth/chlorophyll preparations

Expected Outcomes
Presents a healing wound, and surrounding skin is clean, dry, and intact
Expresses understanding of ostomy function
Demonstrates understanding of ostomy appliance system

▼ Body image disturbance related to presence of ileostomy, colostomy

Assist patient and significant other in accepting ostomy
    Allow time for and encourage verbalization
    Answer all questions and explain treatments and procedures
    Provide care in a positive manner; avoid facial expressions connoting distaste
    Observe for signs of inappropriate denial, grief, or anger
    Provide privacy and a safe environment
Assess present coping patterns and explore strengths and resources
Encourage self-care and independence
Set goals with patient for the following:
    Viewing stoma
    Discussing self-care
    Taking steps in performing self-care
Give positive reinforcement for each step taken
Involve significant other(s) in training if desired by patient

Expected Outcomes
Expresses feelings and concerns
Demonstrates positive coping skills in dealing with presence of ostomy
Views stoma; discusses and performs some steps of care

▼ Sexual dysfunction related to ostomy and lack of knowledge

Assess stage of adaptation of patient to ostomy and explain its function
Encourage communication with significant other and explain the need to share feelings
Explain that normal sexual activity can be resumed when allowed
Discuss methods of controlling odor, general hygiene
Provide information about alternative sexual techniques and positions
Encourage counseling if patient is unable to discuss sexuality

Expected Outcomes

Verbalizes understanding of the information provided about sexual activity

Discusses feelings about sexuality with significant other

▼ Risk for fluid volume deficit related to increased fluid loss (ileostomy)

Assess for dehydration

Monitor intake and output and electrolytes q8h

Monitor stools for frequent, high-volume output, notifying physician if this occurs

Weigh patient daily (same time, scale, and clothing)

Monitor vital signs q8h

Expected Outcomes

Vital signs are stable

Intake and output are balanced

Weight remains stable

Hydration is adequate as evidenced by normal skin turgor

▼ Constipation (colostomy) or high output (ileostomy) secondary to shortened bowel

Assess patient's previous bowel habits and lifestyle

Reinforce physician's explanation of surgical procedure and anatomy and physiology of ostomy

Colostomy feces will be more solid; ileostomy feces will be liquid to pasty

Descending or sigmoid colostomy may be irrigated to establish near-normal elimination; ileostomy should never be irrigated

Involve significant other when appropriate

Demonstrate irrigation procedure and have patient return demonstration until patient can perform it alone (see Colostomy Irrigation, p. 353)

Provide information on where to purchase equipment and symptoms of intestinal obstruction or stomal prolapse to report to physician

Collaborate with physician and nutritionist/registered dietitian for diet instructions; each patient will differ in foods tolerated

Most ostomy patients are discharged on a general diet and given a list of foods that may cause gas or diarrhea

Follow these general rules

Patients with ileostomies should have foods high in sodium and potassium: bananas, bouillon, citrus juices, tea

Patients with ileostomies should initially avoid gas-producing, fried, rich, and highly seasoned foods; nuts; raisins; and all raw vegetables and raw fruits except bananas; fibrous foods such as celery, corn, and coconut may cause food blockage

Patients with colostomies should avoid gas-producing foods such as cabbage, beans, corn, broccoli, and cauliflower if gas is uncomfortable or embarrassing

Each patient will have to use a trial-and-error method to establish which foods can be tolerated

Introduce new foods one at a time

Stress adequate nutritional and fluid intake

Stress eating slowly, chewing food well, and eating regular meals

Advise avoiding carbonated beverages and extremes in temperature of foods

Involve patient and/or significant other(s) in meal planning

Auscultate abdomen for bowel sounds q8h; report absent sounds to physician

Discuss signs and symptoms of obstruction or stricture

Decreased drainage, constipation

Diarrhea

Cramps, abdominal distention

Nausea, vomiting

Expected Outcomes

Expresses understanding of ostomy function

Begins to care for stoma and ostomy

PATIENT/FAMILY TEACHING

Explain and demonstrate stomal care step by step and have patient and/or significant other(s) return demonstration

Discuss equipment used and where to purchase it; provide enough supplies to last a few days after discharge

Provide and explain written information on diet management

Provide information about outside support groups available and refer to home health care as needed

United Ostomy Association

19722 MacArthur Blvd.

Irvine, CA 92612-2405

(800) 826-0826

Web page: www.uoa.org

Discuss signs of wound infection, obstruction, prolapse to report to physician

Encourage follow-up visits with physician

DISCHARGE/HOME CARE PLANNING

Discuss and provide written information about the following:

Normal stoma color is pink-red, and any change must be reported to physician

Stoma will decrease in size and change shape during the first 6 to 8 weeks

Measure size frequently to maintain good appliance fit

Many appliances are available, but it is best to use one that needs changing only every 5 to 7 days

Change appliance when there is leakage or a burning sensation beneath or around appliance: *effluent can cause severe damage to skin*

Always use a skin barrier on the skin before applying pouch

Drink plenty of fluids to avoid dehydration because intake must compensate for output

Discuss changes in lifestyle that must be made: diet, gradual return to most activities

Avoid lifting for 6 weeks

Refer to ostomy support group

■ COLOSTOMY IRRIGATION

A procedure used by some patients with colostomies to clear the bowel of fecal matter and to help establish an evacuation schedule; may not be applicable for all patients; may be used occasionally to treat constipation

ASSESSMENT

OBJECTIVE DATA

Patient's emotional status

State of acceptance and desire for this optional procedure

　Knowledge and understanding of procedure

　Ability to comprehend

　Tolerance of procedure

Size and color of stoma

Location of stoma(s)

　Sigmoid colostomy

　Descending colostomy

Hydration of patient

Temperature and amount of irrigating solution

Retention of irrigating solution; dehydrated patients may retain some fluid and have poor return

Amount and character of return flow

Constipation

Diarrhea

Pain

Distention

POTENTIAL COMPLICATIONS

Stomal bleeding

Perforation

Obstruction

Prolapse

IRRIGATING PROCEDURE

Usually irrigations are ordered whenever patient is ready psychologically and physically

Explain procedure and equipment

　May be done every day or every other day

　Use equipment that will be used at home

　Demonstrate procedure step by step

　Assess patient's normal bowel habits

　Involve patient in assisting with procedure as soon as physically and emotionally able

　Use commode as soon as possible for irrigations *to provide a more normal environment*

　Provide diversional activities after instillation of irrigating solution

During procedure observe these precautions

　Have patient sit on commode when possible

　Prepare 500 to 1000 ml warm tap water

　　Remove all air in tubing

　　Hold bag at shoulder level or 12 to 18 inches above stoma

Apply irrigation sleeve over stoma; place end in commode

Insert lubricated cone tip gently into stoma; avoid using catheter, which may cause intestinal perforation

Allow solution to run into stoma slowly

Allow 45 minutes for return flow

　Position change and/or abdominal massage will help if return is slow

　Irrigation sleeve may be folded and clipped and patient encouraged to ambulate

Stoma dilation may be ordered but is generally not part of routine care

　Using glove, lubricate finger closest to size of stoma

　Insert finger gently into stoma, *never* force

　Rotate finger gently for 1 minute to dilate

　Involve significant other when appropriate

　Demonstrate procedure and have patient return demonstration until he or she can perform it unassisted

Provide information on where to purchase equipment and symptoms of obstruction or prolapse to report to physician

■ APPENDICITIS/APPENDECTOMY

appendicitis: *An inflammation of the appendix and the most common cause of an acute abdomen. Inflammation of the vermiform appendix may be classified as simple, gangrenous, or perforated (Fig. 6-15).*

appendectomy: *Surgical removal of the appendix via laparoscopic surgery or laparotomy*

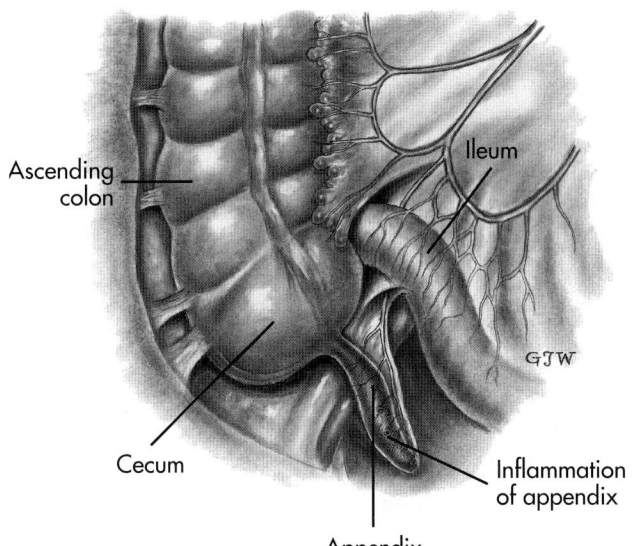

Fig. 6-15 Appendicitis (acute).
(From Doughty DB, Jackson DB: Mosby's clinical nursing series: gastrointestinal disorders, *St Louis, 1993, Mosby.)*

ASSESSMENT
SUBJECTIVE DATA
Mild to severe abdominal pain; usually in the right lower quadrant (RLQ); may radiate to other areas of abdomen and back; rebound tenderness; pain may increase with coughing
Anorexia
Nausea, vomiting
Constipation
Malaise

OBJECTIVE DATA
Fever
Positive rebound tenderness at McBurney's point; pain midway between iliac crest and umbilicus

DIAGNOSTIC TESTS
CBC with differential count
Ultrasound
CT scan

POTENTIAL COMPLICATIONS
Perforation
Peritonitis

MULTIDISCIPLINARY MANAGEMENT
THERAPEUTIC MANAGEMENT
Decreased activity, bedrest
NPO or clear liquid diet
Antibiotics
Surgical intervention (laparoscopic or open)

PATIENT PROBLEMS—NURSING DIAGNOSES/INTERVENTIONS

▼ Pain related to appendiceal inflammation and/or surgical intervention

Maintain position of comfort; bedrest
Administer skin care and back rubs to promote comfort
Keep patient warm and dry
Assess pain intensity level
Medicate according to pain scale
Provide diversional activities where possible
Provide alternative pain management techniques; imaging, deep breathing
Assess effectiveness of pain relief measures
Increase activities as tolerated

Expected Outcome
Subjective perception of pain decreases as documented by pain scale

▼ Risk for infection related to surgical incision

Monitor dressing and incision for signs of infection (increased pain, drainage, erythema, foul odor)
Monitor temperature q2h to 4h

Expected Outcomes
Incision is clean, dry, and intact
Wound is healing adequately
With laparoscopic procedure, incisions are without erythema or inflammation

▼ Anxiety related to surgical intervention and fear of unknown

Explain all procedures and treatments
Reinforce physician's explanation of surgical procedure and treatment
Encourage and allow time for verbalization of feelings
Assess present coping behaviors and support positive responses
Teach stress management techniques
Encourage communication with significant other(s) to promote support

Expected Outcome
Expresses and identifies anxieties

PATIENT/FAMILY TEACHING
Discuss and reinforce physician's instructions
Increase activity as tolerated; avoid lifting heavy objects for 4 to 6 weeks
Report difficulty in ambulation resulting from pain (may indicate retrocecal abscess)
Report fever, any increasing abdominal pain, chills, incisional pain, redness, swelling or discharge at site of incision
Provide wound or incisional care instructions
Avoid use of enemas in the postoperative period; may use stool softeners after third post-op day

DISCHARGE/HOME CARE PLANNING
Be certain that patient has names and phone numbers of physician
Discuss where and what to purchase for dressing changes

■ RECTAL SURGERY
Any surgery performed on the rectum necessitated by the following:
   anorectal abscess: *Localized infection of area with accumulation of pus in tissues of and around the rectum*
   anorectal fistula: *Abnormal opening between the rectum and perineal area*
   anal fissure: *Small tear in the lining of the anus*
   hemorrhoids (hemorrhoidectomy): *Collection of vascular tissue in the anus (internal) or prolapsed (external)*

ASSESSMENT
SUBJECTIVE DATA
Location, intensity, character of pain

OBJECTIVE DATA
Character and amount of rectal drainage
Placement of drain
Urinary output

DIAGNOSTIC TESTS
Anoscopy
CBC, urinalysis
Serum electrolytes
Digital rectal examination

POTENTIAL COMPLICATIONS
Abdominal distention
Urinary retention
Hemorrhage
Infection

MULTIDISCIPLINARY MANAGEMENT
THERAPEUTIC MANAGEMENT
Analgesic, topical anesthetic ointment
Ice packs, sitz baths, warm compresses
Stool softeners
Diet progression

PATIENT PROBLEMS—NURSING DIAGNOSES/INTERVENTIONS

▼ Pain related to surgical intervention

When on bed rest, turn patient side to side q2h
Administer analgesics as required; if ointments are ordered, test first for allergic reaction; assess effectiveness of pain relief measures
Have patient avoid supine position if possible; place pillows between knees while on side
Monitor effectiveness of warm, wet compresses or ice bag
Ambulate with assistance; provide Gelfoam or flotation pads for sitting; avoid rubber rings, *which tend to spread buttocks and cause further discomfort*
Provide planned rest periods; have patient avoid sitting in chair for long periods
Administer analgesic before removing packing
Monitor sitz baths for effectiveness

Expected Outcomes
Verbalizes increasing comfort level
Presents a more relaxed affect

▼ Risk for constipation related to NPO status and painful defecation

Maintain NPO until nausea subsides
Provide low-residue, soft diet as tolerated
Increase fluids to 2000 to 2500 ml/day unless contraindicated
Monitor for bowel sounds q4h

Administer stool softeners; encourage defecation as soon as urge occurs; provide privacy
Monitor effectiveness of stool softeners
Encourage activity and ambulation as soon as possible

Expected Outcomes
Bowel sounds are normal
Bowel movements are soft and formed

▼ Altered urinary elimination, related to proximity of surgical procedure to bladder

Measure intake and output for 24 hours; observe for signs of urinary retention
Use voiding measures if necessary: run water nearby, pour warm water over lower abdomen, place hands in water
Assist patient with voiding: assist males to stand and void; for females, elevate head of bed or use commode
Promote and assist with ambulation *to increase urge to void*

Expected Outcomes
Reports urine is clear and pale yellow and of adequate amount
Expresses ability to void without discomfort

▼ Risk for infection related to inadequate primary defenses

Monitor vital signs q4h, report increase in temperature
Observe dressings q2h to 4h: check for bleeding, drainage, odor, and packing
Change dressings prn; apply petroleum gauze
Cleanse perianal area after each bowel movement and keep area clean and dry
Assess for signs of healing
Shave area to prevent irritation, infection
Instruct patient in irrigating wound if applicable

Expected Outcomes
Wound is healing adequately
Surrounding tissue is clean, dry, and intact

PATIENT/FAMILY TEACHING
Discuss importance of diet management
    Maintain low-residue diet for 1 week
    Increase roughage as tolerated
    Include fresh fruits when appropriate
    Force fluids to 2500 ml/day unless contraindicated
    Monitor weight q week
Demonstrate care of incision and perirectal area
    Take sitz baths as ordered
    Use warm compresses
    Use petroleum gauze pads
    Cleanse perineal area well and dry thoroughly after each bowel movement
    Apply dressing

Discuss symptoms of wound infection and anal stricture
  to report to physician: redness, tenderness, swelling,
  drainage
Discuss maintaining soft bowel movements with use of
  stool softeners and natural laxatives
Explain importance of avoiding heavy lifting and straining
Encourage follow-up visits with physician

DISCHARGE/HOME CARE PLANNING

Demonstrate wound irrigation if applicable; may use
  Water Pik, shower massager
Explain how to use a mirror to inspect area
Provide information of types of and where to purchase
  needed supplies
Inform patient that mesh panties are available to hold
  dressings, as well as sanitary belt and pads; men will
  find jockey shorts more effective

GALLBLADDER

■ BILIARY OBSTRUCTION (STONES, INFECTION)

*Obstruction of the common and/or cystic bile ducts
caused by stones, which inhibit the drainage of bile and
cause an acute inflammatory process to occur*
  cholelithiasis: *Presence of stones in the gallbladder
(Fig. 6-16)*
  choledocholithiasis: *Presence of gallstones in the
common bile duct*
  cholecystitis: *An acute inflammatory process of the
gallbladder (Fig. 6-17)*

ASSESSMENT

SUBJECTIVE DATA

Nausea
Weight loss
Anorexia
Pain (biliary colic)

OBJECTIVE DATA

Midepigastric colicky pain
Pain may radiate to shoulder
Vomiting
Fever with chills
Dark, concentrated urine
Clay-colored feces
Tachycardia
Tachypnea
Abdominal distention

DIAGNOSTIC TESTS

WBC (elevated >12,000)
Serum bilirubin: elevated
Urobilinogen tests
Serum amylase: elevated
Ultrasound/radiologic abdominal series
Percutaneous transhepatic chiolangiography

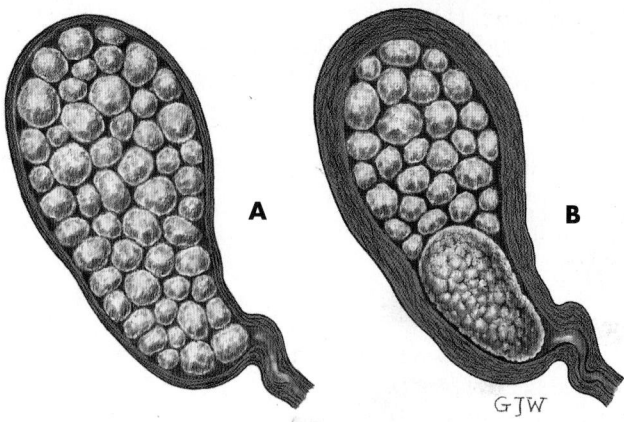

Fig. 6-16 Cholecystitis. **A,** Multiple-faced stones. **B,** Large and numerous small stones (in chronic cholecystitis). *(From Doughty DB, Jackson DB: Mosby's clinical nursing series: gastrointestinal disorders, St Louis, 1993, Mosby.)*

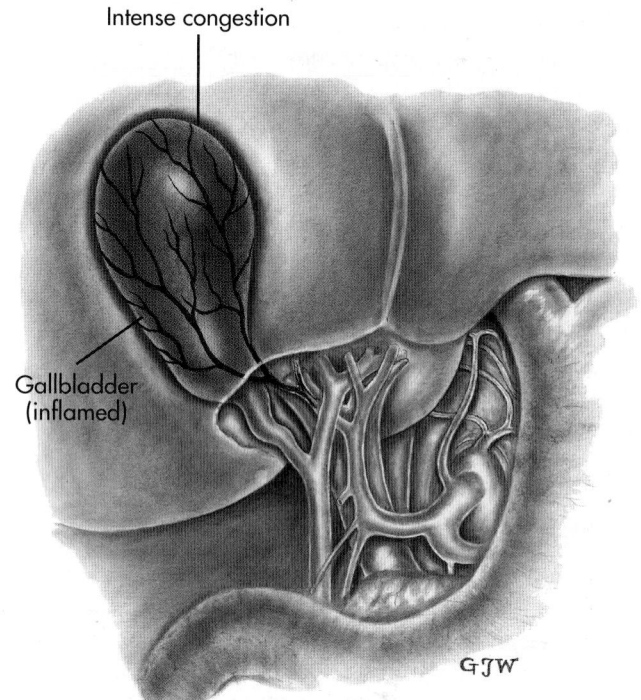

Fig. 6-17 Cholecystitis (acute). *(From Doughty DB, Jackson DB: Mosby's clinical nursing series: gastrointestinal disorders, St Louis, 1993, Mosby.)*

Radioisotope scan—HIDA (hepato-iminodiacetic acid
  [lidofenin] scan)
Endoscopic retrograde cholangiopancreatography (ERCP)
CT scan
Cholecystogram (for chronic cholecystitis only)
Chest radiographic study (to rule out pneumonitis)
Prothrombin time/International Normalized Ratio
  (PT/INR): decreased

POTENTIAL COMPLICATIONS

Jaundice
  Skin
  Sclera

Dehydration
Electrolyte imbalance
Bleeding tendencies (vitamin K deficiency)
Peritonitis if rupture occurs

MULTIDISCIPLINARY MANAGEMENT
THERAPEUTIC MANAGEMENT
Analgesics, antibiotics, antiemetics, anticholinergics, vitamin K
NPO
Nasogastric suction
Parenteral fluids with electrolytes
Diet and activity
ERCP with stone extraction
Surgical intervention: cholecystectomy with exploration of common bile duct or cholecystotomy (see p. 360)
Extracorporeal shock wave lithotripsy (ESWL)/biliary lithotripsy (see p. 359)

PATIENT PROBLEMS—NURSING DIAGNOSES/INTERVENTIONS

▼Risk for fluid volume deficit related to abnormal loss of body fluids from NPO status, gastric suction, vomiting

Maintain NPO, assess for signs of dehydration: poor skin turgor, dry mucous membranes, reduced capillary refill
Monitor vital signs q4h and prn
Maintain parenteral fluids with electrolytes, vitamin K, antibiotics
Monitor nasogastric tube and low, intermittent suction apparatus; irrigate with measured amounts of normal saline prn, monitor pH q4h
Auscultate abdomen for bowel sounds q4h
Administer oral hygiene prn *to reduce dryness of mucous membranes*
Assess for bleeding from gums, injection sites *(resulting from reduced PT)*, bile obstruction
Measure intake and output q8h; note color and consistency of urine, stools, and gastric contents
Monitor serum electrolytes to assess for depletion *caused by gastric suction, vomiting*
Observe for jaundice, pruritus, vitamin K deficiency and PT/INR results
Monitor stools for clay color or return of bile
Monitor skin turgor q8h
Administer antiemetics *to reduce nausea*

Expected Outcomes
Vital signs are stable
Intake and output are balanced
Electrolytes are within normal limits
Hydration is adequate as evidenced by normal skin turgor

▼Pain related to disease process, presence of stones, infection

Assess character, location, and intensity of pain; use pain rating scale
Administer analgesics and anticholinergics; assess effectiveness of pain relief measures
Avoid morphine, *which may cause sphincter of Oddi spasms and increase discomfort*
Maintain bed rest in position of comfort: usually head of bed elevated 30 to 45 degrees *to increase respiratory function*
Teach alternative pain relief measures: imaging, deep breathing, relaxation techniques
Change position frequently in small ways *to promote comfort*
Provide diversional activities *to decrease attention on discomfort*
Administer skin care *to reduce itching and discomfort as needed*

Expected Outcomes
Reports a reduction in pain intensity
Appears more relaxed

▼Altered nutrition: less than body requirements related to vomiting and decreased nutritional intake

After removal of nasogastric tube, collaborate with physician to initiate clear liquid diet and progress to low-fat, soft diet *to reduce stimulation of the gallbladder and consequent pain and possible recurrence*
Perform a calorie count after each meal *to assess nutritional deficiencies*
Monitor bowel sounds; observe for abdominal distention
Monitor serum BUN, albumin
Encourage fluids to 2500 ml/day unless contraindicated
Monitor for food intolerances
Discuss food preferences
Provide quiet, nonstressful environment at mealtimes
Encourage activity and ambulation *to stimulate gastric, intestinal motility*
Weigh patient daily (same time, scale, and clothing)

Expected Outcomes
Maintains desired weight
Tolerates prescribed diet

PATIENT/FAMILY TEACHING
Review and discuss disease process as outlined by physician; allow time for questions
Review signs and symptoms to report to physician: fever, nausea/vomiting, pain, jaundice, itching, dark urine, bleeding from mucous membranes, blood in stools/urine, clay-colored stools
Provide and discuss written dietary instructions on low-fat diet: avoid ice cream, butter, whole milk, gravies, fried foods
Avoid gas-producing foods: cabbage, cauliflower, beans, carbonated beverages, brussel sprouts

Avoid spicy foods, caffeine, citrus fruits that irritate gastric mucosa

Advise patient and/or significant other(s) to increase fat in diet slowly

Discuss need for weight loss if appropriate

Discuss importance of rest, especially after eating

Stress importance of activity as tolerated

Encourage follow-up visits with physician

DISCHARGE/HOME CARE PLANNING

Discuss importance of following dietary plan; involve nutritionist/registered dietitian to assist in explanation of reduced fat diet and weight loss program, if appropriate

Explain the need to rest in semi-Fowler's position following meals *because it increases bile flow*

Discuss importance of nonstressful environment at mealtimes

Encourage fluid intake of 2500 to 3000 ml/day unless contraindicated

Encourage walking and increasing level of exercise, *which stimulates digestion and improves gastric tone*

Refer to reputable weight loss clinic if needed

■ BILIARY SURGERY

Surgery of the gallbladder

cholecystectomy: *Removal of gallbladder*

choledocholithotomy: *Removal of stones in common bile duct*

choledochojejunostomy: *Anastomosis of the common bile duct to the jejunum*

ASSESSMENT
SUBJECTIVE DATA
Location, intensity, and character of pain

OBJECTIVE DATA
Respiratory distress

Diminished breath sounds

Splinting with respirations

Tachypnea

Bradypnea

Character and amount

Gastric drainage

Bile drainage (T tube)

Drainage from incision

Urinary output

DIAGNOSTIC TESTS
Electrolytes, Hgb, Hct

POTENTIAL COMPLICATIONS
Dehydration

Electrolyte imbalance

Hemorrhage

Shock

Peritonitis

Jaundice (3 to 4 days postoperatively)

Signs of wound infection

Thrombophlebitis

Atelectasis

Pulmonary embolus

MULTIDISCIPLINARY MANAGEMENT
THERAPEUTIC MANAGEMENT
Analgesics, antibiotics, vitamin K

Nasogastric suction, NPO

Parenteral fluids with electrolytes

Patient controlled analgesia (PCA)

Incentive spirometer

Oral replacement of bile salts: florantyrone (Sancho), dehydrocholic acid (Decholin)

T tube drainage and clamping

Respiratory therapy

PATIENT PROBLEMS—NURSING DIAGNOSES/INTERVENTIONS

▼ Ineffective breathing pattern related to decreased lung expansion and pain

Assess respiratory status; observe for splinting and shallow, rapid breathing *to prevent atelectasis*

Auscultate lungs for breath sounds q2h *to assess for congestion*

Administer incentive spirometer q2h to 4h

Administer pain medication to assist patient in moving and deep breathing

Assist and teach patient to turn and cough q2h and deep breathe qh; support incision *to reduce discomfort*

Elevate head of bed 20 to 30 degrees *to increase lung expansion*

Expected Outcomes
Demonstrates ability to turn, cough, and deep breathe

Uses incentive spirometer correctly

Exhibits normal respirations and breath sounds

▼ Risk for fluid volume deficit related to NPO status and increased body fluid loss from nasogastric suction

Maintain NPO; assess for signs of dehydration: poor skin turgor, dry mucous membranes, decreased capillary refill

Maintain parenteral fluids with electrolytes and vitamin K

Monitor vital signs q4h

Monitor nasogastric tube and low, intermittent suction apparatus; irrigate prn with measured amounts of normal saline *to maintain patency*

Monitor intake and output q8h; observe for urinary retention

Monitor T tube and closed gravity drainage system if applicable; observe color and amount of drainage q8h; report drainage >500 ml/day to physician; *may indicate obstruction*

Replace bile salts *to aid in fat digestion*

Monitor serum electrolytes, Hct, and Hgb; PT/INR

Monitor stools for clay-colored feces and assess urine for presence of bile

Monitor for vitamin K deficiency: bleeding mucous membranes, injection sites

Weigh patient prn with same clothes and scale

Encourage movement of feet and legs *to increase venous return*

Expected Outcomes

Intake and output are balanced

Vital signs are stable

Hydration is adequate as evidenced by normal skin turgor

▼ Risk for impaired skin/tissue integrity related to tube drainage, altered nutritional state, and invasive procedure

Monitor incision q2h for 8 hours, then q4h for increased drainage, bleeding

Reinforce and change dressing prn

Report excess drainage or bleeding to physician

Cover "stab wound" drain with ostomy appliance or sterile dressing *to facilitate measuring of output;* change prn

Administer injections with small-gauge needle and apply more pressure longer *to prevent bleeding from injection site*

Provide swabs for oral hygiene if bleeding gums are noted

Assess patency of T tube q2h; observe for kinks in tubing

Anchor tubing to allow for freedom of movement

Assess skin around T tube q2h to 4h; clean prn with soap and water; rinse and pat dry

Apply petroleum jelly gauze or Skin Prep as needed *to prevent irritation*

Apply Montgomery straps as indicated *to prevent adhesive burns*

Observe skin and sclera for jaundice or pruritus, *which may indicate obstruction of bile flow*

Provide distracting activities and remind patient not to scratch skin if pruritus is present

Collaborate with physician and clamp T tube after meals; observe for distention, cramps, and pain; if symptoms occur, unclamp T tube and notify physician

Ambulate with assistance as tolerated *to increase circulation and healing process*

Expected Outcomes

Wound is healing well

Surrounding tissue is clean, dry, and intact

▼ Pain related to surgical intervention

Assess location, type, and intensity of pain; use pain rating scale

Administer analgesics and assess effectiveness of pain relief measures

Collaborate with physician regarding PCA

Maintain bed rest in quiet environment

Change position frequently; administer back rubs *to promote comfort*

Discuss alternative pain management techniques: imaging, deep breathing, relaxation

Provide diversional activities *to reduce attention on discomfort*

Expected Outcomes

Reports a reduction of pain

Appears relaxed and comfortable

PATIENT/FAMILY TEACHING

Provide and review written diet instructions and restrictions; fats may be added as tolerated

Demonstrate care of incision and T tube (if applicable) T tube requires draining of collection bag at prescribed times

Discuss medications: name, dose, administration time, and side effects

Explain that florantyrone (Sancho), dehydrocholic acid (Decholin) may be required to assist in fat absorption

Explain signs and symptoms to report to physician: increased epigastric pain, dark urine, clay-colored stools, jaundice

Discuss importance of increasing activity as tolerated and planned rest periods

Explain that bowel movements may be loose for a while because of increased bile

Encourage follow-up visits with physician

DISCHARGE/HOME CARE PLANNING

Stress importance of aseptic technique for dressing changes, T tube management

Demonstrate handwashing technique and correct procedure for cleaning wound
   Cleanse area with mild soap and water
   Rinse well and pat dry
   Apply Skin Prep around incision to protect skin
   Maintain Montgomery straps as needed

Stress importance of draining T tube collection bag periodically *to reduce strain on tube*

Provide flow sheet for record keeping

Discuss importance of diet, eating slowly, and chewing foods well

Provide list of high-fat foods: whole milk, ice cream, butter, fried foods

Provide information on types of and where to purchase needed supplies

Refer to community resources for assistance with home care, ADLs as needed

■ BILIARY LITHOTRIPSY

extracorporeal shock wave lithotripsy: *Noninvasive procedure performed under analgesia, using high-energy shock waves to disintegrate gallstones, allowing them to pass through the common bile duct into the intestine*

ASSESSMENT
SUBJECTIVE DATA
Abdominal tenderness
Biliary colic; severe RUQ pain
Location and character of pain
Nausea

OBJECTIVE DATA
Condition of skin at treatment site: redness, bruising, hematoma
Hematuria
Vomiting

DIAGNOSTIC TESTS
Preprocedure: lipase, amylase, bilirubin, creatinine, PT/INR, activated partial thromboplastin time (APTT), Hgb, Hct, AST, ALT, electrolytes
Oral cholangiogram

POTENTIAL COMPLICATIONS
Retained fragments causing common duct obstruction
Jaundice, severe abdominal pain
Fever, nausea, vomiting
Acute cholangitis

MULTIDISCIPLINARY MANAGEMENT
THERAPEUTIC MANAGEMENT
Low-fat diet
Analgesics
Dicyclomine hydrochloride (Bentyl) for colic
Respiratory therapy as indicated

PATIENT PROBLEMS—NURSING DIAGNOSES/INTERVENTIONS

▼Ineffective breathing pattern related to decreased lung expansion

Monitor respirations for splinting and/or shallow, rapid breathing
Auscultate lungs for breath sounds q4h to 8h
Elevate head of bed 20 to 45 degrees *to increase lung expansion*
Assist and teach patient to deep breathe qh
Assess respiratory status q4h to 8h
Incentive spirometer if indicated

Expected Outcomes
Exhibits normal breath sounds
Demonstrates ability to perform breathing exercises correctly

▼Risk for fluid volume deficit related to abnormal fluid loss from NPO status

Assess for signs of dehydration: poor skin turgor, dry mucous membranes, reduced capillary refill
Maintain parenteral fluids until fully reacted
Monitor vital signs q4h

Monitor intake and output q4h; monitor for hematuria
Monitor for signs of jaundice
Encourage ambulation *to increase circulation*
Provide fluids to tolerance; 2500 to 3000 ml/day
Provide low-fat diet as tolerated

Expected Outcomes
Vital signs are stable
Intake and output are balanced
Tolerance for low-fat diet is without discomfort

▼Pain related to corrective procedure and treatment

Assess location, intensity, and character of pain
Evaluate effectiveness of pain relief measures
Provide diversional activities *to decrease attention on discomfort*
Change patient position frequently *to promote comfort*
Discuss alternative pain relief measures: imaging, deep breathing, relaxation techniques
Notify physician if pain is severe and long-lasting or does not respond to analgesics; *may indicate obstruction of bile*
Encourage ambulation *to increase circulation and healing*

Expected Outcomes
Reports a decrease in pain or no pain
Presents a more relaxed affect

PATIENT/FAMILY TEACHING
Encourage returning to normal activities
Provide and review written dietary instructions
    Low-fat to regular diet depending on tolerance
    High-fat foods may cause discomfort; dicyclomine hydrochloride (Bentyl) usually relieves the pain
Discuss signs and symptoms to report to physician
    Severe nausea, vomiting
    Fever above 101° F (38° C)
    Severe abdominal pain, jaundice
Encourage follow-up visits with physician for ultrasonography and laboratory tests

■ LAPAROSCOPIC, ENDOSCOPIC LASER CHOLECYSTECTOMY
Removal of the gallbladder without a surgical incision; four small punctures are made in the abdominal wall, and, with the use of a laparoscopic laser, the gallbladder is removed; 4.5 L of CO_2 is instilled in the abdominal cavity to allow freedom of movement (this is usually the main cause of postoperative pain and complications) (Table 6-1)

POSTOPERATIVE ASSESSMENT
SUBJECTIVE DATA
Nausea
Type, location, intensity of pain

Table 6-1	**Laparoscopic Procedures versus Open Surgical Procedures (Cholecystectomy, Appendectomy, and Bowel Resection)**	
	Laparoscopic	Open Procedure
Average length of stay	1-3 days	3-7 days
Typical post-op analgesic	PO medication (e.g., oxycodone)	Epidural or IV medication (e.g., morphine)
Post-op diet	Clear liquids to regular as tolerated	NPO (usually nasogastric tube) until return of bowel sounds
Incision care	"Bandaid" incisions; keep clean and dry	If open wound, may include packing, drains, referral to home health care prn
Activity	As tolerated; usually no restrictions	Slowly increase as tolerated; reinforce physician restrictions
Follow-up care	See physician in 1-2 wk; report fever, increase in drainage	See physician in 1-3 days; may include drain removal; report fever, increase in pain, erythema, drainage

OBJECTIVE DATA

Respiratory function
Location of puncture wounds
Amount of drainage, bleeding
Vomiting
Placement of nasogastric tube and attending suction apparatus
Placement of indwelling urethral catheter

DIAGNOSTIC TESTS

CBC
Electrolytes
Urinalysis

POTENTIAL COMPLICATIONS

Hemorrhage
Bile leakage into abdominal cavity

MULTIDISCIPLINARY MANAGEMENT

THERAPEUTIC MANAGEMENT

Amount of pressure on nasogastric tube suction apparatus; irrigating instructions
Analgesics
Diet
Activity and exercise
Respiratory therapy as indicated

PATIENT PROBLEMS—NURSING DIAGNOSES/INTERVENTIONS

▼ Ineffective breathing pattern related to decreased lung expansion and CO_2 inflation of the abdomen

Maintain bed rest until fully reactive
Place patient in Sims' position (left side with right knee and thigh flexed toward chest and right arm along thigh) *to facilitate absorption of CO_2*
Assess respiratory status including breath sounds q4h to 8h
Assist and teach patient to deep breathe qh

Incentive spirometer q2h
Ambulate with assistance within 3 to 4 hours postoperatively

Expected Outcomes

Exhibits normal breath sounds
Performs deep breathing qh

▼ Risk for fluid volume deficit related to risk of abnormal fluid loss from NPO status, nausea, and vomiting

Monitor vital signs q4h
Assess for signs of dehydration: poor skin turgor, dry mucous membranes, reduced capillary refill
Remove nasogastric tube when nausea decreases
Provide clear liquids as tolerated, avoiding carbonated beverages *to prevent distention*
Progress to regular or preprocedure diet as tolerated
Encourage fluids to tolerance unless contraindicated
Calculate intake and output q8h
Remove indwelling catheter when intake and output are balanced

Expected Outcomes

Vital signs are stable
Intake and output are balanced
Skin turgor is normal
Tolerance of diet and fluids is adequate

▼ Pain related to corrective procedure

Assess location, intensity, and character of pain using a pain scale
Assess effectiveness of analgesics
Notify physician if pain is unrelieved, severe, or long-lasting; *may indicate bleeding, obstruction*

Expected Outcomes

Reports decreasing or absent pain/discomfort
Presents a more relaxed affect

▼Altered protection related to abnormal blood profile caused by hemorrhage

Monitor dressings for bleeding or bile drainage; change prn
Assess abdomen for distention or severe pain
Monitor vital signs q4h; *tachypnea, hypotension may indicate abnormal bleeding*

Expected Outcomes
Dressing remains dry without evidence of bleeding
Vital signs are stable
Abdomen remains soft and nondistended

PATIENT/FAMILY TEACHING
Discuss care of puncture sites and signs and symptoms to report to physician
Wound drainage, redness, edema
Abdominal distention
Nausea, vomiting
Increased pain
Instruct regarding prescribed activities, usually not limited after 2 to 3 days (normally discharged in 24 to 48 hours)
Discuss importance of maintaining diet and fluid intake

DISCHARGE/HOME CARE PLANNING
Advise patient to remain on liquid diet on day of discharge and increase to light meals for 3 to 4 days
Stress importance of low-fat diet, avoiding ice cream, butter, whole milk, and fried foods
Explain that showering may begin on second day and dressings are to be removed at that time
Stress importance of not lifting heavy objects (>10 lb)

■ T TUBE MANAGEMENT
T tube: *Tube placed in the common bile duct to carry off excessive bile, decrease the amount of bile flowing into the intestine, and prevent backflow of bile into the liver when the common bile duct has been explored (Fig. 6-18)*

ASSESSMENT
OBJECTIVE DATA
Character, color, and amount of bile drainage; <500 ml/day is within normal limits
Patency of tube
Leakage around tube
Tube taped securely to skin
Skin integrity around tube
Color, consistency, and frequency of stools

POTENTIAL COMPLICATIONS
Jaundice: sclera, skin
Electrolyte imbalance

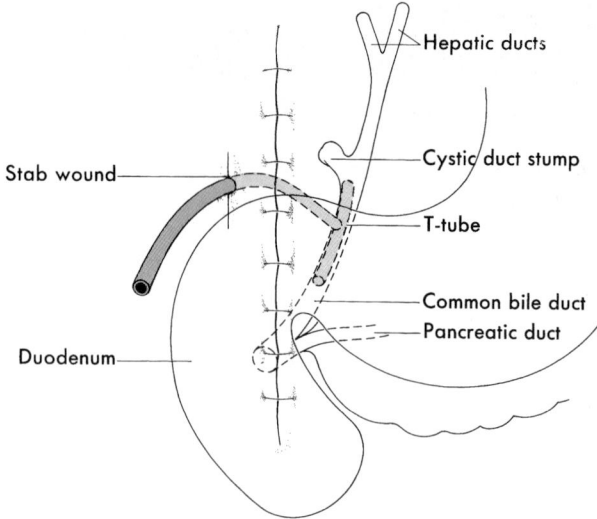

Fig. 6-18 T tube.
(From Beare PG, Myers JL: Adult health nursing, ed 3, St Louis, 1998, Mosby.)

Abdominal distention
Fat-soluble vitamin (A, D, E, K) deficiency

INTERVENTIONS
Connect T tube tubing to closed gravity drainage system placed well below incision
Secure connections with tape and allow enough tubing to allow for freedom of movement
Place rolled 4 × 4 pads under T tube at exit site and tape to skin to prevent tension
Monitor skin around T tube exit site; keep clean and dry; use Stomahesive wafer or Skin Prep to prevent irritation
Measure bile output q8h; report output >500 ml/day to physician
Auscultate abdomen for bowel sounds q8h; report return to physician
Observe first stool for color, consistency, and amount; should be dark (clay color may indicate bile duct blockage)
Collaborate with physician to clamp tube and observe for abdominal pain, distention, chills, fever, and nausea; if these occur, unclamp tube and notify physician
Increase time tube is clamped: usually before and after meals to facilitate digestion

PATIENT/FAMILY TEACHING
Explain T tube cholangiogram (7 to 10 days postoperatively); T tube is removed after 24 hours if bile duct is patent
Demonstrate care of skin, drainage system, and incision
Discuss measuring and clamping procedure of T tube
Discuss symptoms to report to physician: pain, increased drainage, distention, fever
Encourage follow-up visits with physician

■ TRANSHEPATIC BILIARY DECOMPRESSION CATHETER MANAGEMENT

A multivented catheter inserted through the abdominal wall, liver, and common bile duct and into the duodenum to allow bile to drain past the obstructed bile duct into the intestine; performed for hepatic dysfunction, biliary obstruction (jaundice), and inoperable malignancy of the biliary system

ASSESSMENT

OBJECTIVE DATA

Location of catheter, type of drainage system
Character, color, and amount of drainage
Presence of stabilizing device or sutures
Decreasing jaundice and serum bilirubin
Color, frequency, and amount of stool and urine

DIAGNOSTIC TESTS

Catheter usually inserted in radiology department
Postinsertion x-ray examination, cholangiography
Serum bilirubin, electrolytes
Stool for occult blood
Urine for bilirubin

POTENTIAL COMPLICATIONS

Biliary sepsis
Bleeding or increased retrograde flow of bile
Catheter obstruction
Hyponatremia, electrolyte imbalance

INTERVENTIONS

Maintain catheter with closed gravity drainage system; place stopcock between catheter and tubing; keep stopcock open
Monitor and measure amount of drainage q2h for 8 hours, then q4h; observe for increased amount of drainage; if >1500 ml/day, notify physician immediately
Monitor catheter site for drainage, type of sutures, and dressing q2h to 4h; change dressing prn and apply antibacterial ointment *to prevent infection*
Collaborate with physician to irrigate catheter through external port of stopcock, closing off drainage bag
Aspirate a few ml to ascertain patency
   Irrigate gently with prescribed amount of solution; this action may be painful for patient—explain before procedure
   Do not force irrigation if resistance is met; notify physician because catheter may be obstructed
   After instillation, open stopcock to allow irrigant to flow into drainage bag
   Assess patient's tolerance and observe for increasing, continuous pain, cramping, or abdominal distention (peritonitis, catheter slippage)
Collaborate with physician to clamp catheter and observe patient for decreasing jaundice

Monitor stools, urine, skin, and sclera
Monitor serum bilirubin
Tape catheter comfortably to abdomen; cover with sterile dressing
Monitor electrolytes, especially for hyponatremia; observe for lethargy or altered mental status

PATIENT/FAMILY TEACHING

Demonstrate and observe return demonstration for catheter irrigation and care
Provide and review written instructions for irrigating procedure
Discuss signs and symptoms of malfunction to report to physician
   Fever, chills, weakness
   Bleeding, increased bile output
   Increasing jaundice, abdominal pain, distention
   Dislodgment of catheter
   Food particles in catheter drainage
Explain need for prescribed visits to radiology department for evaluation of catheter position and function
Encourage follow-up visits with physician

DISCHARGE/HOME CARE PLANNING

Provide written information on what equipment and supplies to purchase and where to find them
Instruct patient and family or significant other(s) on aseptic technique and handwashing procedure
Evaluate caregiver/patient ability to care for catheter
Provide names, phone numbers of home health care team members

■ LIVER

■ CIRRHOSIS: PORTAL, POSTNECROTIC, BILIARY

Chronic liver disease characterized by the alteration and destruction of cells, progressive fibrosis, and eventual nodular formation that results from excessive alcohol intake (70% to 80% of patients), hepatitis, drug toxicity, biliary obstruction, metabolic disease, or congestive heart failure (CHF) (Fig. 6-19)

ASSESSMENT

SUBJECTIVE DATA

RUQ pain, may radiate
Generalized malaise/weakness
Anorexia
Nausea
Weight loss or gain
Diarrhea

OBJECTIVE DATA

Vomiting
Abdominal distention

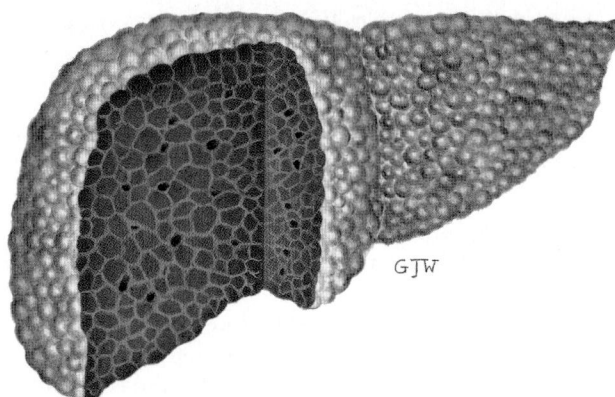

Fig. 6-19   Cirrhosis of the liver (septal cirrhosis). *(From Doughty DB, Jackson DB:* Mosby's clinical nursing series: gastrointestinal disorders, *St Louis, 1993, Mosby.)*

Hepatomegaly
Irregular bowel function
    Clay-colored stools
    Flatulence
    Melena
Ascites
Elevated temperature
Pruritus
Decreased urinary output; dark urine
Foul breath
Spider angiomas
Jaundice: sclera, skin
Edema of extremities
Gynecomastia
Dysrhythmias, CHF, jugular venous distention
Clubbing of fingers
Dehydration
Altered mental status
History of substance abuse
History of hepatitis or biliary obstruction

DIAGNOSTIC TESTS

Electrolytes
Serum bilirubin (elevated, jaundice)
AST, ALT, LDH, alkaline phosphatase (elevated)
Serum albumin (decreased), ammonia (elevated)
Glucose, BUN
CBC, PT/INR (prolonged), urinalysis
Stool for occult blood testing
ERCP (common bile duct obstruction)
Esophagoscopy (varices) with barium esophagography
Peritoneoscopy or laparoscopy
Liver biopsy, scans
Ultrasonography
Percutaneous transhepatic portography (visualizes portal venous system)
Paracentesis (ascites)
EEG
Psychometric testing

POTENTIAL COMPLICATIONS

Electrolyte imbalance
Malnutrition
Pneumonia
Ascites
Oliguria
GI bleeding
Portal hypertension, esophageal varices, *caput medusae* (umbilical venous distention)
Hepatomegaly, splenomegaly
Hepatic encephalopathy
Coma

MULTIDISCIPLINARY MANAGEMENT
THERAPEUTIC MANAGEMENT

Diuretics, analgesics, antibiotics, lactulose (ammonia detoxican)
Propanolol, vasopressin, hematinics, coagulants
Digestants (Cotazym, Kanulase), vitamins K and C, iron, thiamin, folic acid, antifibrinolytics
Cholestyramine for pruritus
Stool softeners
Parenteral fluids with electrolytes; TPN as indicated
Fresh whole blood, fresh frozen plasma, or platelets
Nasogastric suction
Dietitian consult
    Diet management according to disease process
Sodium and/or fluid restriction
Respiratory therapy
    Oxygen therapy, incentive spirometer
Social services

PATIENT PROBLEMS—NURSING DIAGNOSES/INTERVENTIONS

▼Altered nutrition: less than body requirements related to inadequate diet, vomiting, and/or anorexia

Maintain NPO if indicated *to reduce stress on liver*
Administer TPN as indicated *to maintain caloric intake*
Maintain bed rest in quiet environment
Provide small, frequent feedings of prescribed diet; amount of fat, carbohydrate, and protein will depend on patient's ability to metabolize these nutrients; salt may be restricted
Maintain calorie count
Provide salt substitute; avoid those containing ammonium *to reduce risk of encephalopathy*
Assist and encourage patient to eat; consider preferences in food choices
Provide oral hygiene prn, especially before meals
Weigh patient daily (same time, scale, and clothing)
Monitor for edema, ascites

Expected Outcomes

Tolerates prescribed diet
Demonstrates understanding of needed diet changes
Gains optimum weight

▼ Risk for fluid volume excess related to compromised regulatory mechanism (malnutrition), excess fluid, sodium intake

Assess for hydration status: good skin turgor, moist mucous membranes

Monitor for jugular vein distention; *may indicate vascular congestion*

Assess for dependent edema

Maintain parenteral fluids with electrolytes and vitamins; restrict fluid intake as ordered

Measure intake, output; assess for output less than intake

Note consistency, color, and frequency of stools and urine

Monitor serum and urine electrolytes; observe for signs of sodium and/or potassium imbalance

Auscultate lungs for breath sounds q4h *for signs of pulmonary edema*

Administer salt-poor albumin/plasma *to increase circulating volume and decrease edema*

Monitor vital signs q4h; observe for elevated temperature, dysrhythmias, and signs of CHF

Weigh patient daily (same time, scale, and clothing)

Assess for effectiveness/side effects of diuretics

Expected Outcomes

Vital signs are stable

Intake and output are balanced

Edema is decreasing; no jugular vein distention is present

Electrolytes are within normal limits

▼ Risk for impaired skin integrity related to edema, dehydration, and/or jaundice

Assess skin for breaks, reddened areas, pruritus, and jaundice

Provide sheepskin with alternating pressure mattress as indicated *to reduce tissue ischemia*

Administer skin care frequently; provide clean linen, use lotion, and clip nails as needed; administer cholestyramine for pruritus

Provide perineal care after urination and bowel movement; apply lotions *to prevent breakdown*

Turn patient q2h and administer back care; change position slightly prn *to promote comfort*

Perform passive or assist with active ROM exercises q4h *to increase circulation*

Expected Outcomes

Demonstrates understanding of needed techniques to prevent skin impairment

Participates in these activities

Maintains adequate skin integrity

▼ Ineffective breathing pattern related to debilitated state and ascites

Elevate head of bed 45 to 60 degrees or as needed *to maintain ventilation*

Assist and teach patient to turn and cough q4h; deep breathe q½h

Auscultate lungs for breath sounds q4h

Maintain O_2 as ordered

Assist and teach patient to use incentive spirometer q2h

Monitor blood gases, pulse oximetry for signs of atelectasis, pneumonia

Assess for signs of hypoxia (altered mentation)

Expected Outcomes

Blood gases are within normal limits

Respirations and mental acuity are normal

Breath sounds are clear

▼ Altered protection, hemorrhage related to risk of impaired blood coagulation or bleeding from portal hypertension

Monitor mucous membranes for signs of bleeding; avoid hard-bristled toothbrushes

Observe injection sites for prolonged bleeding; apply extra pressure and pressure bandage; use small-gauge needles

Monitor patient's use of razors and other sharp objects

Avoid straining during bowel movement and forceful nose blowing

Administer stool softeners

Monitor PT/INR and platelet count

Administer vitamin K and antifibrinolytic agents; assess for effectiveness/side effects

Observe for signs of bleeding: decreasing BP, increasing pulse, hematemesis, melena

Monitor vital signs, Hgb, Hct

Prepare for endoscopy if bleeding occurs

Monitor nasogastric tube and low, intermittent suction apparatus; measure gastric output qh and note color and consistency; irrigate, if ordered, with measured amounts of saline *to maintain patency*

Maintain parenteral fluids and/or transfusions

Administer vitamin K, vasopressin, and neomycin; avoid aspirin use

Expected Outcomes

Demonstrates understanding and ability to perform needed changes in activities

Exhibits absent or controlled bleeding

▼ Altered thought processes related to increased serum ammonia and hepatic coma

Monitor frequently for changes in mental status, lethargy, drowsiness, and confusion

Monitor neurologic status for decreased motor ability

Avoid use of sedatives, tranquilizers, and narcotics

Provide safe environment: side rails up and bed in low position

Monitor serum ammonia levels

Monitor for possible violent behavior

Reduce environmental stimulus

Provide rest periods

Acknowledge feelings of anger or fear

Assist patient to redirect aggressive behavior to an adaptive activity

Orient patient to time and place as appropriate with each interaction

Teach and assist with stress-reduction measures: imaging, deep breathing, relaxation techniques

Help to focus on accomplishing self-care activities; assist with ADLs only as necessary

Provide high-calorie, low-protein diet if mental deterioration occurs *because protein metabolism produces ammonia*

Expected Outcomes

Mental acuity is improving or normal

Orientation to name, time, place is accurate

Ability to focus on and accomplish ADLs increases

PATIENT/FAMILY TEACHING

Provide and discuss written dietary instructions from nutritionist/registered dietitian, listing amount of protein, carbohydrate, fat, and salt allowed

Discuss and teach stress management techniques

Discuss with patient importance of avoiding stress during meals and need to eat small, frequent meals

Reinforce physician's explanation of relationship between alcohol and cirrhosis if applicable

Provide information about medications, including name, purpose, dosage, time of administration, and side effects; caution against using any medicine not prescribed by physician

Explain importance of rest and exercise, avoiding exposure to infection

Discuss skin care if pruritus persists

Discuss signs of progression of disease to report to physician: hematuria, melena, abdominal distention, edema, fever, bleeding that does not subside, mental deterioration, personality changes

Encourage follow-up visits with physician

Ensure that significant other(s) know and understand symptoms of mental status change or behavior changes to report

Provide information about support groups in community

DISCHARGE/HOME CARE PLANNING

Reinforce information on use of items that may deter mucous membrane bleeding; soft toothbrush or Water Pik, electric razors

Discuss methods of reducing itching from pruritus

    Keep nails short

    Apply lotions to keep skin moist

    Wear soft clothing, undergarments

    Try to not scratch

Encourage counseling, Alcoholics Anonymous, substance abuse program

Provide information on where to purchase, rent alternating mattress, sheepskin

Stress importance of reducing salt/sodium intake, monitoring intake and output, and maintaining balance

■ VIRAL HEPATITIS

virus A (HAV): Rapid onset of symptoms and destruction of liver cells caused by contaminated water or food; usually affects young adults (Table 6-2)

    virus B (HBV): Slow onset of symptoms and destruction of liver cells caused by contaminated serum from needles and instruments; affects all age groups

    virus C (HCV): Causes liver destruction following blood transfusion (formerly non-A, non-B)

    virus D (HDV): Occurs in populations at risk for HBV infections

    virus E (HEV): Occurs mostly in young adults in developing countries

ASSESSMENT

SUBJECTIVE DATA

Nausea

Anorexia

Malaise

Headache

RUQ tenderness and pain

Arthritic pain (HBV)

OBJECTIVE DATA

Elevated temperature (HAV)

Jaundice

    Pruritus

    Urticaria

    Sclera

    Clay-colored stools

    Dark urine

Vomiting

Diarrhea

History of blood transfusions, foreign travel (Asia, Africa), clotting disorders, excessive alcohol ingestion

History of recent anesthetic (halothane)

History of IV drug use

History of accidental exposure to contaminated needles or instruments

History of exposure to hepatotoxic chemicals or medications

DIAGNOSTIC TESTS

Serum AST, ALT, bilirubin: elevated

Alkaline phosphatase, lactic dehydrogenase: elevated

PT/INR (prolonged in severe hepatitis)

Stool and serology for HAV

Serum antigen/antibody tests for HBV

CBC, urinalysis, electrolytes, fasting blood sugar (FBS)

Liver biopsy

Liver function tests: abnormal

Serum albumin: decreased

HbsRg (positive type B)

Anti-HAVIgM (positive type B)

Anti-HCV

Table 6-2	**Overview of Viral Hepatitis**				
	Hepatitis A	**Hepatitis B**	**Hepatitis C**	**Hepatitis D**	**Hepatitis E**
Occurrence	Worldwide; sporadic and epidemic, with a tendency toward cyclic recurrence; outbreaks in institutions	Worldwide; endemic; highest in young adults, homosexual men, heterosexuals with multiple sex partners, parenteral drug users, and health care and public safety workers	Worldwide; accounts for 90% of posttransfusion hepatitis in the United States	Worldwide; occurs epidemically and endemically in populations at risk for HBV infection	Epidemic and sporadic cases, particularly in developing countries; highest in young adults; rare in children or elderly
Etiologic agent	Hepatitis A virus (HAV)	Hepatitis B virus (HBV)	Hepatitis C virus (HCV)	A viruslike particle (HDV or the delta agent); coinfects with HBV	Viruslike particle (HEV)
Reservoir	Humans and captive primates	Humans and possibly captive primates	Humans, chimpanzees	Humans, chimpanzees	Unknown, possible nonhuman reservoirs
Transmission	Person to person by fecal-oral route; contaminated food, water, shellfish	Direct and indirect contact with blood, saliva, and semen; sexual contact; perinatal	Parenteral exposure to blood; person-to-person sexual and perinatal transmission have not been defined	Similar to HBV, including sexual contact	Contaminated water; person to person by fecal-oral route
Incubation period	15-50 days; average: 28-30 days	45-180 days; average: 60-90 days	2 wk to 6 mo; commonly 6-9 wk	2-10 wk	15-64 days; average: 26-42 days
Period of communicability	Latter half of incubation period to 1 wk after onset of jaundice	During incubation period and throughout clinical course of disease; carrier state may persist for years	From 1 or more wk before symptom onset, indefinitely during chronic and carrier states	Throughout acute and chronic disease	Not known; detected in stool 14 days after onset of jaundice
Susceptibility and resistance	Usually affects children and young adults; immunity after infection probably lasts for life	All age groups; disease is mild in children; lifetime immunity follows infection if antibody to HBsAg develops and HBsAg is negative	All age groups; degree of immunity following infection is unknown	All persons susceptible to HB, HBV carriers; disease is severe in children	Unknown; no explanation for epidemics among young adults; pregnant women in third trimester susceptible to fulminating disease
Report to local health authority	Mandatory case report	Mandatory case report	Mandatory case report	Mandatory case report	Mandatory case report

From Thompson JM et al: Mosby's clinical nursing, ed 4, St Louis, 1997, Mosby.

POTENTIAL COMPLICATIONS

Decreased urinary output

Dehydration and electrolyte imbalance

Altered mental status

Hyperglycemia or hypoglycemia

Hepatic coma

MULTIDISCIPLINARY MANAGEMENT
THERAPEUTIC MANAGEMENT

Activity, rest

Sedatives, antiemetics, antacids, vitamin K

Antivirals, antibiotics, corticosteroids

Consultation with dietitian

    Diet according to tolerance of protein, carbohydrates, and fat

Parenteral therapy with electrolytes and vitamins for vomiting or GI bleeding

Antihistamines and cholestyramine for pruritus

Immune globulin for patient's close personal contacts

Recombinant interferon as indicated

Social services

PATIENT PROBLEMS—NURSING DIAGNOSES/INTERVENTIONS

▼ Activity intolerance related to weakness or fatigue secondary to infection

Maintain bed rest in quiet environment *to conserve energy;* assist patient in assuming position of comfort; bathroom privileges may be allowed

Assist and teach patient to turn q2h and deep breathe q½h *to prevent skin breakdown and increase lung expansion*

Change position frequently *to promote comfort*

Administer sedatives *to provide restful sleep and build energy level;* assess for effectiveness, side effects

Provide diversional activities

Assist with and teach active or perform passive ROM exercises q4h while patient is in bed *to maintain muscle tone*

Coordinate care to provide planned rest periods

Ambulate with assistance when tolerated

Assess response to increased activity

Reinforce progress toward independence

Expected Outcomes

Expresses understanding of changes needed in activity levels

Increases activities as strength returns

▼ Altered nutrition: less than body requirements secondary to anorexia, vomiting, altered intestinal absorption

Collaborate with physician, nutritionist/registered dietitian and provide soft diet, monitoring intake of protein, fat, and carbohydrates

Offer small, frequent meals, attractively prepared

Encourage fluids to 2500 ml/day unless contraindicated; include fruit juices and carbonated beverages, which are easily digested

Assess for effectiveness, side effects of antacids and antiemetics; avoid prochlorperazine (Compazine) and chlorpromazine (Thorazine)

Weigh patient daily (same time, scale, and clothing)

Provide oral hygiene as needed, especially before meals *to increase desire for food*

Monitor blood glucose: hypoglycemia or hyperglycemia may be present, requiring adjustment in dietary intake

Expected Outcomes

Gains weight, progressing toward normal weight

Tolerates prescribed diet

▼ Risk for fluid volume deficit related to excessive loss of body fluids resulting from vomiting, fever, diarrhea

Maintain NPO if vomiting and/or anorexia are present

Maintain parenteral fluids with electrolytes and vitamin K

Assess for signs of dehydration: skin turgor, pedal pulses, dry mucous membranes

Measure intake and output q8h; include emesis/diarrhea in output

Monitor stool and urine for color, consistency, and frequency

Monitor for ascites, increasing jaundice, and mental deterioration

Monitor vital signs, electrolytes, Hgb, Hct

Monitor laboratory values for abnormal results

Expected Outcomes

Vital signs are stable

Intake and output are balanced

Skin turgor is normal

▼ Altered protection related to abnormal blood profile/coagulation

Assess for signs of bleeding: mucous membranes, injection sites, emesis, stool

Monitor coagulation studies *to identify risk for bleeding*

Use small-gauge needles for injections and apply increased pressure longer; rotate sites

Evaluate effectiveness of vitamin K administration

Expected Outcome

Free of bleeding as evidenced by clear skin, absence of bleeding at gums and injection sites, no occult blood in urine and feces, normal coagulation studies

▼ Risk for impaired skin integrity related to jaundice and ensuing pruritus

Administer frequent skin care; avoid soap or use superfatted soap

Provide shower or bath with baking soda or starch; apply
 lotions

Administer antihistamines *to control itching;*
 diphenhydramine (Benadryl)

Assess effectiveness of cholestyramine; *may cause
 nausea, constipation*

Offer frequent back rubs and changes in position *to
 promote comfort*

Encourage short fingernails or use of gloves

Provide diversional activities *to decrease attention on
 scratching*

Encourage patient not to scratch and to use knuckles if
 the urge is persistent

Expected Outcomes

Reports decreased pruritus/scratching

Participates in activities to maintain skin integrity

▼Risk for infection related to inadequate secondary defenses and malnutrition

Maintain isolation techniques according to hospital policy

Establish and explain blood and body fluid precautions *to
 prevent transmission to others*

Ensure that all contacts are protected against hepatitis

Maintain stringent handwashing technique

Assess temperature and breath sounds q4h to 8h

Restrict visitors with infections, especially URIs

Provide nutritious diet with fluids to 2000 ml/day *to
 promote cellular repair*

Administer antiviral medication: vidarabine (Vira-A),
 acyclovir (Zovirax)

Expected Outcomes

Demonstrates understanding of precautions by following
 guidelines

Maintains normal temperature; respirations are clear; no
 other evidence of infection

▼Disturbance in self-concept related to disease
process, hospitalization, and isolation

Encourage and allow time for communication of fears
 and concerns *to promote a trusting relationship*

Reinforce physician's explanation of disease process and
 treatment rationale

Explain purpose of isolation procedure to patient and/or
 significant other(s)

Assess present coping patterns and be supportive and
 understanding

Encourage communication with significant other(s)

Avoid making judgments about lifestyle *to promote
 self-esteem*

Encourage bright colors (red, blue) in clothing *to offset
 jaundice*

Expected Outcomes

Uses adaptive coping measures as evidenced by
 discussion of feelings

Uses diversional activities and maintains personal
 grooming habits

Patient/Family Teaching

Discuss techniques to prevent transmission

 HAV: perineal care, handwashing after toileting, and
 disinfection of soiled articles of clothing

 HAV and HCV: caution to not share razors or
 toothbrushes and to avoid serum or secretion
 contact with others

 Explain infectious nature of HAV, HBV, and HCV and
 the need to avoid infecting others (until laboratory
 values are normal); importance of not donating
 blood; need to avoid others with infections,
 especially URIs

 Provide information to family and close personal
 contacts regarding need for immune globulin as
 indicated

 Provide information about drug rehabilitation program
 if appropriate

 Stress importance of follow-up medical care for
 1 year

  Regular laboratory tests as ordered

  Routine follow-up care with physician

Encourage family members and friends to seek
 injection of gamma globulin, ISG, HBIG, hepatitis
 B vaccine

Discuss symptoms of recurrence to report to physician

Provide instructions about medication, including name,
 purpose, dosage, time of administration, and side
 effects; explain need to avoid medicines not
 prescribed by physician

Discharge/Home Care Planning

Reinforce physician's explanation of disease process so
 patient understands importance of the following:

 Diet instructions on amounts of protein, carbohydrate,
 and fat allowed

 No alcohol intake for at least 1 year

 Coordinating rest and exercise program to allow liver
 to regenerate

 Avoiding heavy lifting, contact sports

 Maintaining bowel function with adequate fluid intake,
 natural dietary bulk, stool softeners

Refer to community resources for assistance/counseling

Explain that it may require weeks to recuperate
 and to look for diversional activities to occupy
 the time

■ Hepatic Surgery

*Surgical removal or repair of portions of the liver re-
sulting from trauma or carcinoma*

Preoperative Assessment and Care

Assess cardiovascular, respiratory, cerebral, and
 renal status; obtain baseline vital signs; observe
 for jaundice

Prepare bowel as ordered: enemas, oral antibiotics, magnesium preparations; keep enemas to a minimum to prevent dehydration

Insert nasogastric tube and/or indwelling urethral catheter as ordered; monitor aspirate and/or urine for color and consistency

Administer vitamin K and/or blood transfusions

Reinforce physician's explanation of surgical procedure and postoperative care; explain that chest tubes may be present

Provide emotional support to patient and significant other(s)

POSTOPERATIVE ASSESSMENT
SUBJECTIVE DATA
Nausea

Location, character, type of pain

Dyspnea

OBJECTIVE DATA
Placement of chest tubes and drainage apparatus if applicable

Character and amount of the following:

Chest drainage if applicable

Gastric drainage

Urinary output

Wound drainage

Vomiting

Abdominal distention

Tachycardia

Tachypnea

Splinting of respirations

Decreased breath sounds

Elevated temperature

DIAGNOSTIC TESTS
Serum electrolytes

Albumin

Liver function studies

Electrolytes

CBC

Glucose

PT/INR

POTENTIAL COMPLICATIONS
Electrolyte imbalance

Decreased serum albumin levels

Hypoglycemia

Atelectasis

Pneumonia

Paralytic ileus

Hemorrhage

Shock

Subdiaphragmatic abscess

Jaundice

Ascites

Hepatic coma

Wound infection

MULTIDISCIPLINARY MANAGEMENT
THERAPEUTIC MANAGEMENT
Analgesics

Nasogastric suction, NPO

Parenteral fluids with electrolytes and vitamin K

Antibiotics, albumin, transfusions

Connection of chest tubes to underwater seal

Respiratory therapy

Oxygen therapy, incentive spirometer

Urethral catheter drainage

PATIENT PROBLEMS—NURSING DIAGNOSES/INTERVENTIONS

▼ Ineffective breathing pattern related to invasive procedure, chest tube placement, and/or pain

Elevate head of bed 30 to 45 degrees *to enhance lung expansion*

Assess placement of chest tubes and connect underwater seal to low, intermittent suction; monitor amount and color of aspirate q4h

Auscultate chest for breath sounds q2h; monitor respiratory rate and for signs of splinting

Assist and teach patient to turn and cough q2h and deep breathe q½h; support incision; medicate for pain before procedure when possible

Provide incentive spirometer q1h to 2h

Monitor pulse oximetry q8h, if applicable

Assist with ADLs *to conserve energy*

Expected Outcomes
Exhibits normal respirations

Verbalizes understanding of need for breathing exercises

Uses incentive spirometer routinely

▼ Risk for fluid volume deficit related to increased body fluid loss resulting from NPO status and/or nasogastric suction

Maintain NPO; assess hydration status: good skin turgor, moist mucous membranes, normal capillary refill

Maintain parenteral fluids with electrolytes and/or antibiotics

Monitor nasogastric tube and low, intermittent suction apparatus; irrigate gently with measured amounts of normal saline to maintain patency

Monitor urethral catheter and closed gravity drainage system; monitor output qh; report output of <30 ml/hr to physician

Measure intake and output q8h

Monitor vital signs qh until stable, then q4h

Encourage lower extremity movement *to increase venous return*

Apply antiembolic stockings; remove daily to inspect skin for redness, breakdown

Monitor serum electrolytes, albumin, and glucose

Monitor Hct to assess hydration status; *may be elevated in dehydration*

Auscultate abdomen for bowel sounds q8h
Monitor for peripheral edema; assess pedal pulses q8h
Monitor for signs of hypoglycemia: nausea, shakiness, lethargy
Monitor mental status q4h

Expected Outcomes
Vital signs are stable
Intake and output are balanced
Electrolytes are within normal limits
Skin turgor is normal

▼Altered protection related to abnormal blood profile, altered clotting factors resulting from hemorrhage

Monitor dressings and incision q2h for drainage or bleeding; reinforce and change dressings as needed
Monitor for signs of bleeding: tachycardia; hypotension; cold, clammy skin
Assess for bleeding tendencies resulting from reduced vitamin K: mucous membranes, injection sites
Use small-gauge needles; apply increased pressure longer to control bleeding
Monitor Hgb, Hct, and clotting times
Assess for effectiveness, side effects of vitamin K administration

Expected Outcomes
Blood profiles (Hgb, Hct, clotting time) are within normal limits
No evidence of bleeding at sites of injection or wound exists

▼Pain related to surgical intervention

Maintain bed rest in quiet environment in position of comfort; usually with head of bed elevated 35 to 45 degrees
Assess type, intensity, and location of pain; use pain rating scale
Administer analgesics and assess effectiveness of pain relief measures; medicate as prescribed for first few postoperative days
Consider patient controlled analgesia (p. 40)
Change position frequently; administer back rubs *to ease muscle soreness and promote comfort*
Discuss alternative pain relief measures: deep breathing, imaging, relaxation techniques
Provide diversional activities *to decrease attention on discomfort*
Encourage balanced activity/rest pattern

Expected Outcomes
Reports a decrease in pain
Appears relaxed and comfortable

▼Altered nutrition: less than body requirements related to NPO status, decreased energy

Collaborate with physician to remove or clamp nasogastric tube when bowel sounds return
Provide small amounts of water or clear liquids and monitor tolerance; *too much fluid may cause vomiting*
Progress to soft diet as tolerated; amounts of fat, carbohydrate, and protein will depend on ability of liver to metabolize these nutrients; involve nutritionist/registered dietitian
Measure intake and output *to assess for adequate balance*
Administer oral hygiene prn, especially before meals
Encourage fluids to 2500 ml/day unless contraindicated
Weigh patient daily (same time, scale, and clothing)

Expected Outcomes
Weight is maintained or returning to normal
Prescribed diet is tolerated without discomfort

PATIENT/FAMILY TEACHING
Provide and review written diet instructions with amounts of fat, carbohydrate, and protein allowed
Demonstrate care of incision and discuss signs of wound infection to report: tenderness, redness, drainage, fever
Provide information about signs and symptoms to report to physician
Decreased mental acuity, lethargy
Abdominal distention, pain
Jaundice, dyspnea, fever
Discuss medications: name, dosage, purpose, times of administration, side effects, and importance of taking only medicines prescribed by physician
Discuss need for balance between activity and rest
Encourage follow-up visits with physician

DISCHARGE/HOME CARE PLANNING
Provide information on what types of and where to purchase needed supplies: dressings, tape, disposable gloves
Review importance of handwashing technique
Explain necessity of taking all medications as prescribed
Discuss importance of weighing once a week and reporting loss to physician
Provide information on community resources for assistance at home with ADLs, meals, transportation

■ CONTINUOUS PERITONEAL–VENA CAVAL SHUNT FOR ASCITES
A subcutaneous shunt to remove ascitic fluid from the abdomen to the heart, and from there to reenter the systemic circulation and be excreted by the kidneys; there are two types used:
__La Veen shunt:__ Has a one-way, pressure-sensitive valve that remains open as long as the thoracic pressure is lower than the intraabdominal pressure
__Denver shunt:__ Has either a single or double valve; a fluid-filled pump is implanted close to the skin and allows

the patient to press and pump the device to keep the fluid moving and maintain patency

PREOPERATIVE CARE
Reinforce physician's explanation of surgical procedure
Monitor baseline vital signs
Monitor BUN, creatinine, Hgb, Hct readings
Administer antibiotics as prescribed
Prepare local anesthesia
Maintain IV line for IV analgesia

POSTPROCEDURE ASSESSMENT
Increased or decreased abdominal distention
Dyspnea
Diminished breath sounds
Tachypnea
Tachycardia, hypertension
Right upper quadrant pain
Jugular vein distention
Ankle edema
Increased or decreased urinary output
LOC
Leakage of fluid from incision site
Electrolyte imbalance; hypokalemia
Increased clotting time
Elevated bilirubin
Decreased Hgb, Hct, BUN
Disseminated intravascular coagulation
Wound infection

INTERVENTIONS
LAVEEN SHUNT
Maintain bed rest; elevate head of bed 60 to 90 degrees
Provide incentive spirometer *to increase intraabdominal pressure*
Apply abdominal binder *to increase pressure*

DENVER SHUNT
Maintain bed rest; must remain flat 30 minutes out of each hour for first 24 hours *to encourage abdominal fluid to flow toward the heart*
Teach patient to apply pressure to chamber slowly *to maintain patency of catheter*
Pump chamber about 10 times per hr or as ordered

COMMON INTERVENTIONS
Check vital signs q4h until stable, then q8h
Check neurologic signs q2h to 4h and report changes to physician
Check incision for excess bleeding or drainage and neck for edema q2h for 24 hours; then q4h for 24 hours; report presence of these signs to physician
Measure intake and output; report decrease in output to physician
Maintain NPO as ordered
Administer parenteral fluids with electrolytes and vitamins as ordered
Monitor serum electrolytes and blood clotting time; report significant changes to physician

Weigh patient daily (same time, scale, and clothing); if weight increases, notify physician
Auscultate chest for breath sounds q4h; report diminished breath sounds to physician
Manage pain as indicated; assess effectiveness of pain relief measure(s)
Assist and teach active or perform passive ROM exercises q4h *to increase venous flow*
Assist and teach patient to turn, cough, and deep breathe q2h to 4h *to maintain lung expansion*
Administer skin care and oral hygiene q2h to 4h
Evaluate incisions and report signs of wound infection: redness, tenderness, discharge, fever

PATIENT/FAMILY TEACHING AND DISCHARGE/HOME CARE PLANNING
Instruct patient on signs and symptoms of a clogged shunt: weight gain in excess of 2 lb, increased peripheral edema, and/or dyspnea
Stress importance of weekly weights
Provide rest and activity schedule *to maintain consistency and balance*
Encourage follow-up care with physician and laboratory tests

■ LIVER BIOPSY
Introduction of a special needle into the liver to obtain a specimen for pathologic examination; other noninvasive diagnostic procedures have replaced the biopsy, but it is still used when other procedures fail

PREBIOPSY CARE
Type and cross-match for possible transfusion
Monitor baseline vital signs
Assess mental alertness and ability to cooperate
Explain procedure and follow-up care
Administer analgesics or sedatives as ordered
Monitor for allergy to local anesthetic
Teach patient how to inhale and hold breath during needle insertion
Monitor bleeding, clotting, and PT results; report abnormal results to physician
Place on NPO 4 to 8 hours before biopsy
Have patient void immediately preprocedure

POSTBIOPSY ASSESSMENT
Intraperitoneal, intrahepatic hemorrhage
Pneumothorax

INTERVENTIONS
Monitor vital signs q15min × 4, then q30min × 4, then q4h or as ordered
Apply pressure to biopsy site for first 15 minutes after procedure *to prevent hemorrhage*
Maintain bed rest in supine position for 24 hours
Position patient on right side for first 6 hours *to keep pressure at site*

Observe biopsy site q30min × 4 for bleeding, swelling, or
increased pain

Monitor Hgb and Hct

Manage pain as indicated; epigastric pain or referred
shoulder pain may occur

Report increased respiratory rate, severe shoulder pain,
decreased breath sounds to physician; *indicators for
pneumothorax*

Administer vitamin K as ordered

Assist patient with eating and other activities as needed
for 24 hours

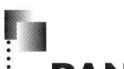

PANCREAS

ACUTE AND CHRONIC PANCREATITIS

*acute pancreatitis: Acute inflammatory disease in
which autodigestion of the organ occurs as a result of
obstruction of the pancreatic duct; exact cause is unknown, but various causative factors are thought to be
stones, tumors, trauma, and excessive use of alcohol
(Fig. 6-20)*

*chronic pancreatitis: Chronic, progressive disease
that may or may not follow acute pancreatitis; causative
factors include gallbladder disease, carcinoma, and excessive use of alcohol; pancreas becomes fibrotic and
necrotic, and enzyme action is markedly decreased or
nonexistent*

ASSESSMENT
SUBJECTIVE DATA
Acute pancreatitis
Sudden onset of severe pain in LUQ, often after a large
meal or alcohol intake

Increases in supine position; may radiate to shoulder and
thoracic vertebrae

Nausea

Chronic pancreatitis
Intermittent or constant epigastric pain: steady, dull, or
sharp
    Radiates to back
    Relieved when leaning forward
Nausea, anorexia
Weight loss

OBJECTIVE DATA
Acute pancreatitis
Fever, chills

Tachycardia, hypovolemia, hypotension

Respiratory impairment, tachypnea with or without
dyspnea, splinting; adult respiratory distress syndrome
(ARDS) may develop

Decreased urine output

Discoloration of abdomen and/or flanks

Mild abdominal distention

Diminished bowel sounds

Vomiting, diarrhea

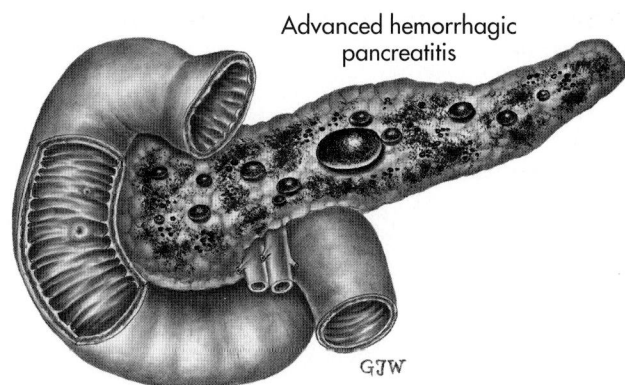

Fig. 6-20 Acute pancreatitis.
(From Doughty DB, Jackson DB: Mosby's clinical nursing series: gastrointestinal disorders, *St Louis, 1993, Mosby.)*

History of cholelithiasis, gastritis, gastric ulcers, trauma,
Crohn's disease

History of excessive use of alcohol, steroids, some
antihypertensives and antibiotics

Confusion, lethargy

Jaundice

Hyperglycemia

Chronic pancreatitis
Vomiting

Diarrhea, steatorrhea

Malnutrition

Minimal jaundice

Fat-soluble vitamin deficiencies

Symptoms of diabetes mellitus

DIAGNOSTIC TESTS
Acute pancreatitis
CBC, BUN, urinalysis, FBS

Arterial $P_{O_2} < 60$ mm Hg

Serum calcium, albumin (decreased)

Serum LDH, AST, ALT (increased)

Amylase: serum, urine, lipase (elevated)

Electrolytes: potassium decreased

Chronic pancreatitis
CBC, urinalysis

Alkaline phosphatase: elevated

Serum amylase, lipase: normal

ERCP

Acute and chronic pancreatitis
Endoscopy

Serum glucose: elevated

Radiologic abdominal films

Ultrasonography/CT scan

Upper GI series/cholangiography

Stool for fat and occult blood

POTENTIAL COMPLICATIONS
Electrolyte imbalance, hypocalcemia

Hyperglycemia

Respiratory, circulatory, renal failure
Paralytic ileus
Jaundice
Shock, hemorrhage

MULTIDISCIPLINARY MANAGEMENT
THERAPEUTIC MANAGEMENT

Analgesics, antacids, antiemetics, antibiotics, anticholinergics, H_2-receptor blockers (cimetidine, ranitidine, famotidine, nizatidine), oral enzyme supplements
Hemodynamic monitoring
Parenteral fluids with electrolytes, vitamins, serum albumin, and/or dextran
Nasogastric suction, NPO
TPN
Digestants (pancreatic enzymes) for chronic pancreatitis
Insulin for hyperglycemia
Paravertebral block for pain management
Respiratory therapy
Consultation with dietitian
Social services as indicated

PATIENT PROBLEMS—NURSING DIAGNOSES/INTERVENTIONS

▼ Risk for fluid volume deficit related to abnormal body fluid loss resulting from vomiting, fever, and/or gastric aspiration

Maintain NPO, assess hydration status: skin turgor, moist mucous membranes, normal capillary refill
Maintain parenteral fluids with electrolytes, vitamins, albumin, and antibiotics or TPN if indicated
Monitor nasogastric tube and low, intermittent suction apparatus; irrigate with measured amounts of normal saline; measure gastric output q4h and check pH
Auscultate abdomen for bowel sounds q4h
Observe for distention, vomiting, and decreased sounds after nasogastric tube is removed
Weigh as indicated to assess for loss (hypovolemia) or gain (edema, ascites)
Monitor vital signs q2h to 4h; *hypotension may occur as a result of pancreatic ischemia;* check apical pulse
Monitor CVP or Swan-Ganz catheter; monitor ABGs and pulse oximetry
Monitor urine output qh; report output <30 ml/hr to physician; *may indicate renal compromise*
Calculate intake and output q8h; report deficits; include gastric aspirate/emesis in output
Monitor mental acuity for decreased sensorium *as sign of hypovolemia, hypoxia*
Monitor for calcium imbalance: tremors, twitching
Monitor electrolytes, glucose, liver function studies, PT, and calcium
Monitor for peripheral/dependent edema
Assess pedal pulses

Encourage patient to move feet and legs qh *to increase circulation*
Antiembolic stockings, remove and reapply q shift

Expected Outcomes
Vital signs are stable
Electrolytes are within normal limits
Skin turgor is adequate
Intake and output are balanced

▼ Risk for infection related to inadequate primary defenses, nutrition imbalance

Monitor respiratory status: breath sounds, cough, sputum, shallow breathing, fluid collection
Change dressings promptly using aseptic technique; assess wound for signs of infection: redness, tenderness, increased drainage; obtain culture if present
Maintain aseptic technique when handling IV lines, catheters, tubes, drains
Promote good handwashing technique
Assist and teach patient to turn and cough q2h and deep breathe q½h, incentive spirometer q2h
Administer skin care and oral hygiene q2h to 4h; observe for reddened areas or breakdown
Observe for signs of jaundice: skin, sclera, urine
Monitor temperature for elevation; initiate cooling measures for temperature >101° F (38.2° C)
Monitor urine for infection
Administer antibiotics as indicated
Encourage small, frequent position changes *to enhance lung expansion*

Expected Outcomes
Patient is afebrile
Breath sounds are normal
Skin remains clean, dry, and intact
Urine is without infection

▼ Pain related to obstruction of pancreatic, biliary ducts

Maintain bed rest in quiet environment in position of comfort
Assess type, intensity, and location of pain; use pain rating scale
Assess effectiveness of pain relief measures
    Avoid morphine; small, frequent doses of meperidine are beneficial
    Medicate before pain becomes severe
    Teach alternative pain management techniques: deep breathing, relaxation, imaging
Change position frequently; administer back rubs *to promote comfort*
Perform passive or assist with and teach active ROM exercises q4h *to promote circulation and healing*
Coordinate care to provide for rest periods
Ambulate with assistance when allowed

Promote diversional activities *to decrease attention on discomfort*

Administer antacids *to neutralize gastric acid and reduce pancreatic enzyme production*

Administer cimetidine (Tagamet) *to decrease HCl and pancreas stimulation/pain*

Expected Outcomes

Verbalizes that pain is decreasing

Appears relaxed and comfortable

▼Altered nutrition: less than body requirements related to anorexia, vomiting, and/or decreased digestive enzymes

Monitor for presence of bowel sounds *to determine return of peristaltic action*

Collaborate with physician, nutritionist/registered dietitian and provide liquid to soft diet when tolerated

Provide high-protein, high-carbohydrate, low-fat, or diabetic diet in small, frequent meals

Administer bile pancreatic replacement if ordered; avoid taking with hot food/fluid, *which may inactivate enzymes*

Avoid coffee, tea, stimulants, and gas-producing foods

Monitor for food tolerances

Provide frequent oral hygiene, especially before meals *to increase appetite*

Administer antacids, insulin, and anticholinergics; assess for effectiveness, side effects

Weigh patient daily (same time, scale, and clothing)

Monitor stools for color, consistency, amount, frequency; test for presence of fat

Monitor urine for sugar/acetone *to assess for hyperglycemia/ketoacidosis*

Expected Outcomes

Demonstrates progressive weight gain/loss toward target weight

Tolerates balanced diet

Presents normal urine/stool

PATIENT/FAMILY TEACHING

Provide and review written dietary instructions

Reinforce causal relationship of alcohol use to pancreatitis; promote outside counseling with rehabilitation centers

Explain and teach about diabetes, blood testing, insulin therapy, and symptoms to report to physician

Discuss medications: name, schedule, dosage, purpose, and side effects; explain importance of taking only medicines prescribed by physician; promote discriminate use of narcotics

Encourage follow-up visits with physician

DISCHARGE/HOME CARE PLANNING

Discuss signs and symptoms to report to physician: fever, recurrence of pain, nausea/vomiting, abdominal distention

Explain importance of pancreatic enzyme replacement therapy, if applicable; do not take with hot liquids/food *because the heat destroys enzyme potency*

Reinforce signs of hyperglycemia: polyuria, polydipsia, weakness, weight loss

BIBLIOGRAPHY

Ambrose MS: Pancreatitis: managing a flare-up, *Nursing '96* 26(4):33, 1996.

Aronson B: Update on peptic ulcer drugs, *Am J Nurs* 98(1):41, 1998.

Beare PG, Myers JL: *Adult health nursing,* ed 3, St Louis, 1998, Mosby.

Bradley M, Pupiales M: Essential elements of ostomy care, *Am J Nurs* 97(7):38, 1997.

Butler RW: Managing the complications of cirrhosis, *Am J Nurs* 94(3):46, 1994.

Cason CL, Seidel SL, Bushmair M: Recovery from laparoscopic cholecystectomy procedures, *AORN J* 63(6):1099, 1996.

Cole-Arvin C et al: Identifying and managing dysphagia, *Nursing '94* 24(1):48, 1994.

Crecelius SA, Souen MC: Transjugular intrahepatic portosystemic shunts for portal hypertension, *Gastroenterol Clin North Am* 24(2):201, 1955.

Doherty MM, Carver DK: New relief for esophageal varices, *Am J Nurs* 93(4):58, 1993.

Doughty DB: What you need to know about inflammatory bowel disease, *Am J Nurs* 94(7):24, 1994.

Faller N, Lawrence KG: Comparing low-profile gastrostomy tubes, *Nursing '93* 23(12):46, 1993.

Greenberg L: Fast action for splenic rupture, *Am J Nurs* 94(2):51, 1994.

Huston CJ: Ruptured esophageal varices, *Am J Nurs* 96(4):43, 1966.

Inturri P, Graziotto A, Rossaro L: Treatment of ascites: old and new remedies, *Dig Dis* 14(3):145, 1966.

Jackson MM, Rymer TE: Viral hepatitis: anatomy of a diagnosis, *Am J Nurs* 94(1):43, 1994.

Johns JL: When the patient has an ulcer, *RN* 54(11):44, 1991.

Kim MJ et al: *Pocket guide to nursing diagnoses,* ed 7, St Louis, 1997, Mosby.

Krasner D: Six steps to successful stoma care, *RN* 56(7):32, 1993.

Lockhart JS, Hoelsken R: Abdominal hemorrhage, *Nursing '93* 23(3):33, 1993.

Marchiondo K: When the dx is diverticular disease, *RN* 57(2):42, 1994.

Martin FL: Ulcerative colitis, *Am J Nurs* 97(8):38, 1997.

McCance KL, Huether SE: *Pathophysiology: the biological basis for disease in adults and children,* ed 2, St Louis, 1994, Mosby.

McConnell EA: Loosening the grip of intestinal obstructions, *Nursing '94* 24(3):34, 1994.

McGinnis C, Matson SW: How to manage patients with a Roux-en-Y jejunostomy, *Am J Nurs* 94(2):43, 1994.

McManhon AJ, O'Dwyer PJ, Baxter JN: Laparoscopic interventions in the gut: yesterday, today and tomorrow, *Dig Dis* 14(1):14, 1996.

Meissner JE: Caring for patients with ulcerative colitis, *Nursing '94* 24(7):54, 1994.

Meissner JE: Caring for patients with cirrhosis, *Nursing '94* 24(9):44, 1994.

Murphy D, Berry D: Mechanical lithotripsy, *Gastroenterol Nurs* 16(5):204, 1994.

NANDA Nursing Diagnoses: *Definitions and Classification 1999-2000,* Philadelphia, 1998, North American Nursing Diagnosis Association.

O'Hanlon-Nichols T: Gastrointestinal system, *Am J Nurs* 98(4):48, 1998.

Pagana KD, Pagana TJ: *Manual of diagnostic and laboratory tests,* St Louis, 1998, Mosby.

Ross Laboratories: Caring for a gastrostomy, *Nursing '94* 24(8):48, 1994.

Ruth-Sahd LA: Acute pancreatitis, *Am J Nurs* 96(6):38, 1996.

Surratt S et al: Troubleshooting a sump tube, *Am J Nurs* 93(1):42, 1993.

Thompson JM et al: *Mosby's clinical nursing,* ed 4, St Louis, 1997, Mosby.

Wound, Ostomy, and Continence Nurses Society: *Standards of care: patient with ileostomy; patient with colostomy,* Costa Mesa, Calif, The Society, 1992.

page 1 of 3

DATE INITATED _____

BY _____

USC UNIVERSITY HOSPITAL
1500 San Pablo
Los Angeles, Ca 90033

MULTIDISCIPLINARY PLAN

DRG ___196___

ALOS _____

ALLERGIES: _____

DISCHARGE OUTCOMES		
PHYSIOLOGICAL	Absence of infection. Pain controlled c̄ p.o. analgesics. Tolerating reg. diet.	
COGNITIVE	Aware of signs and symptoms to report to M.D.	
PSYCHOLOGICAL	Express fears/concerns R/T hospitalization.	

LAPAROSCOPIC CHOLECYSTECTOMY

ADMISSION DATE _____ TIME _____ DISCHARGE DATE _____ TIME _____

PLAN OF CARE DISCUSSED WITH

	PATIENT	SIGNIFICANT OTHER
	DATE	INITIAL	DATE	INITIAL

DISCIPLINE	PRE-ADMIT	DOS DAY	PO #1 DAY	DAY	DAY	DAY	DAY
		DATE	DATE	DATE	DATE	DATE	DATE
LOCATION		OR/SURGICAL	SURGICAL				
LAB		CBC, Chem PT, PTT Liver panel serum amylase					
CARDIO-PULMONARY		ECG (over 40 or prev. history) Incentive Spirometer ⟶					
IMAGING/ NUCLEAR MEDICINE		CXR (if over 40)					
SOCIAL SERVICES D/C PLAN		Initiate Discharge planning assessment	Patient will need someone at home for 48°. Someone must drive for MD appt. on 1st, 2nd, 3rd, 7th day				
REHAB. SERVICES							
PHARMACY		Preop. Ancef ⊤ gm. Postop. Pain mgmt.	→ Δ to oral analgesic				

Continued

Used by permission of USC University Hospital, Los Angeles, California.

MULTIDISCIPLINARY PLAN

DISCIPLINE	PRE-ADMIT	DOS DAY ___ DATE ___	PO #1 DAY ___ DATE ___	DAY ___ DATE ___	DAY ___ DATE ___	DAY ___ DATE ___	DAY ___ DATE ___
NUTRITION		NPO Post-op: Liquids	Advance to full diet				
PATIENT ACTIVITY		Post-op Dangle ambulate c̄ assist.	Independent ambulation				
EDUCATION		Teach I.S. D.B. Benefits of early amb. Splinting Rationale for IV	Activity Restrictions Wound care s-sx to report to MD: (infection, bleeding, N/V, GI disturbance				
COLLABORATIVE PT. PROBLEMS							
1		Pain					
2		Potential for in-effective breathing pattern.					
3							
4		Potential for fluid volume deficit.					
5							
6							
OUTCOMES							
1		Verbalize hosp. routines	Verbalize concerns re: hospitalization				
2		Verbalize pain control →					
3		Demonstrate DB, IS, splinting	Returns to ADL				
4		Verbalize importance of early ambulation	Nutrition is adequate: No N/V				
5			Skin integrity maintained				
6							

NME 413-170 (4-91)

	DOS DAY	PO #1 DAY	DAY	DAY	DAY	DAY	DAY
	DATE	DATE	DATE	DATE	DATE	DATE	DATE
SERVICE	INTERVENTIONS: Pre-op Teach	Monitor pain management					
CASE MGR	NPO, consent	Abdomen and lung assessment					
PT/OT	Notify MD of abnormal labs	Assess incision for signs of infection					
DIETICIAN	Betadine scrub night before & morning of procedure						
SOCIAL SERVICE	INTRA & POST-OP						
ECF	Thromboguards Post-op I/O						
OTHER	Pain management						

MULTIDISCIPLINARY PLAN UPDATE

SIGNATURES	DATE	SIGNATURES	DATE	SIGNA

DATE

USC UNIVERSITY HOSPITAL
1500 San Pablo
Los Angeles, CA 90033

MULTIDISCIPLINARY PLAN

NAME _____
ALLERGIES _____
MR# _____

DIAGNOSIS Familial Polyposis/Ulcerative Colitis or Colon CA

SURGERY Colon Resection, Ileal Pouch Anal Anastomosis/Segmental/Laparoscopic Colectomy

DRG _____ ALOS _____ ADMIT DATE _____

DISCHARGE OUTCOMES	
PHYSIOLOGICAL	Bowel function returns. Fluids & electrolytes within normal limits. Able to eat regular diet with adequate caloric intake. Pain controlled by po analgesics. Skin intact, no breakdown. Wound healing by first intention.
COGNITIVE	Verbalizes medical follow-up plan & signs and symptoms to report. Demonstrates wound & ostomy care with minimal or no assistance.
PSYCHOLOGICAL	Anxiety/fear controlled as evidenced by active participation in ADLs and decisions with medical care. Verbalizes positive feelings with personal adjustment achieved by D/C.

DISCIPLINE	PRE-OP/ PRE-ADMIT	PRO-OP DAY 1 DATE	D.O.S. DAY 2 DATE	P.O.#1 DAY 3 DATE	P.O.#2 DAY 4 DATE	P.O.#8 DAY 5 DATE	P.O.#4 DAY 6 DATE
LOCATION		Med/Surg	Med/Sur→OR→DOU	DOU	DOU→Med/Surg	Med/Surg	Med/Surg (home if Laparoscopic)
LABS		CBC with diff Chem 20 UA Type & Cross PRBC	K+ level at 5 a.m. CBC in p.m. If clinically indicated, CBC in PAR		CBC Chem 7		
CARDIO-PULMONARY		ECG I.S. initial teach	I.S. q 2° W/A	Evaluate for self I.S.			
IMAGING/ NUCLEAR MEDICINE		CXR					
SOCIAL SERVICES D/C PLAN REHAB. SERVICES		D/C planning Home health evaluation E.T. consult Mark stoma ASAP			Re-eval for home health needs E.T. to evaluate & teach ostomy care	Oncology consult prn	
PHARMACY		Bowel prep K+ supplement prn IV to begin at 2400 Sleeper If on steriods within last 6 months, the steriods on call to OR	Epidural of PCA Antibiotics x 3 doses IV fluids	Epidural of PCA IV fluids	Epidural or PCA IV fluids until adequate po intake For Laparoscopic Colectomy: Convert to po analgesia		Convert to po analgesics
DIETARY/ NUTRITION		Clear liquids NPO after MN	NPO	Advance diet as tolerated when bowel function returns—passing flatus		Nutritional guidelines	

Used by permission of USC University Hospital, Los Angeles, California.

page 2 of 6

USC UNIVERSITY HOSPITAL

1500 San Pablo
Los Angeles, CA 90033

MULTIDISCIPLINARY PLAN

DIAGNOSIS Familial Polyposis/Ulcerative Colitis or Colon CA

SURGERY Colon Resection, Ileal Pouch Anal Anastomosis/Segmental/Laparoscopic Colectomy

NAME
ALLERGIES
MR#
ADMIT DATE

DRG___　ALOS___

DISCHARGE OUTCOMES	
PHYSIOLOGICAL	Bowel function returns. Fluids & electrolytes within normal limits. Able to eat regular diet with adequate caloric intake. Pain controlled by po analgesics. Skin intact, no breakdown. Wound healing by first intention.
COGNITIVE	Verbalizes medical follow-up plan & signs and symptoms to report. Demonstrates wound & ostomy care with minimal or no assistance.
PSYCHOLOGICAL	Anxiety/fear controlled as evidenced by active participation in ADLs and decisions with medical care. Verbalizes positive feelings with personal adjustment achieved by D/C.

DISCIPLINE	PRE-OP/ PRE-ADMIT	P.O.#5 DAY 7 DATE___	P.O.#6 DAY 8 DATE___	P.O.#7 DAY 9 DATE___	P.O.#8 DAY 10 DATE___	P.O.#9 DAY 11 DATE___	P.O.#10 DAY 12 DATE___
LOCATION		Med/Surg	Med/Surg	Med/Surg→Home			
LABS							
CARDIO-PULMONARY							
IMAGING/ NUCLEAR MEDICINE							
SOCIAL SERVICES D/C PLAN REHAB. SERVICES		Confirm all home health arrangements					
PHARMACY							
DIETARY/ NUTRITION		Regular diet					

Continued

PATIENT NAME: _____

MULTIDISCIPLINARY PLAN

MEDICAL RECORD # _____

DISCIPLINE	PRE-OP/ PRE-ADMIT	PRE-OP DATE	DAY 1	D.O.S. DATE	DAY 2	P.O.#1 DATE	DAY 3	P.O.#2 DATE	DAY 4	P.O.#3 DATE	DAY 5	P.O.#4 DATE	DAY 6
PATIENT ACTIVITY		Up ad lib		BR		OOB with assistance		Ambulate TID to QID		Progressive ambulation			
				Daily wt at 6 a.m.		Daily wt at 6 a.m.		Daily wt at 6 a.m.		Daily wt at 6 a.m.		Daily wt at 6 a.m.	
EDUCATION		**Pre Op Teach** Aggressive TCDB Presence/Purpose of tubes/drains. Pain management Kegel exercises Early ambulation to promote return of bowel function		**Ileostomy Teaching** Give ostomy handout		Return of bowel function Quality/Quantity of stool will vary Quality - loose/watery may have leakage at night. (Not permanent)		Perianal skin care		Teach S/Sx of small bowel obstruction If ostomy: • Encourage to look at stoma • Peristoma skin assessment • Clamp application/ removal		If Ostomy/passing flatus, teach: Appliance application Empty/wash bag Return demo-clamp Perianal skin care	

COLLABORATIVE PROBLEMS

	DATE		COLLABORATIVE PROBLEMS	DC DATE INIT
1.			Knowledge deficit R/T hospitalization, surgery.	
2.			Fear/anxiety R/T hospitalization, post-op course.	
3.			Fluid/electrolyte imbalance, potential R/T bowel preps & diversion.	
4.			Alteration in comfort, pain R/T surgery.	
5.			Potential for infection R/T surgery.	
6.			Potential for injury complication R/T surgery.	

	DATE		COLLABORATIVE PROBLEMS	DC DATE INIT
7.			Impaired skin integrity, perianal, ostomy R/T bowel diversion.	
8.			Altered bowel elimination R/T surgery.	
9.			Altered nutritional intake (less than body requirements) R/T surgery.	
10.			Body image, altered R/T ostomy.	
11.			Self-care deficit R/T ostomy.	

KEY

1. To initiate a problem or intervention, document under corresponding date.
2. Document outcomes under appropriate date for achieving the goal.
3. To discontinue an intervention or resolve a patient problem highlight, date, and initial.

OUTCOMES

1. Able to verbalize medical plan/hospital routine.	4. Verbalize pain controlled within 30 min of intervention.	7. Skin remains intact. Wounds heal by first intention.
2. Fears, anxiety controlled as evidenced by ability to participate in care/education.	5. No infection throughout hospitalization.	10. Verbalizes feelings R/T body image changes.
3. Electrolytes/fluids within normal limits.	6. No complication throughout hospitalization.	

4. **Laparoscopic Surgery:** Pain controlled by po analgesic.	8. Bowel output returns.	9. Caloric intake supports maintenance of wt/wound healing.
9. **Laparoscopic Surgery:** Caloric intake supports maintenance of wt/wound healing.	11. Participation in education.	4. Pain controlled by po analgesics.

PATIENT NAME: _____

page 4 of 6

MEDICAL RECORD # _____

MULTIDISCIPLINARY PLAN

DISCIPLINE	PRE-OP/ PRE-ADMIT	P.O.#5 DATE___	DAY 7 ___	P.O.#6 DATE___	DAY 8 ___	P.O.#7 DATE___	DAY 9 ___	P.O.#8 DATE___	DAY 10 ___	P.O.#9 DATE___	DAY 11 ___	P.O.#10 DAY 12 DATE___
PATIENT ACTIVITY		Progressive ambulation Weight at 6 am		Independent ambulation Weight at 6 am								
EDUCATION		D/C Instructions **If Ostomy:** Assessment care of stoma Return demo—emptying, washing Application of water, odor control		Medications/Weight control **If Ostomy:** Colostomy Irrigation Return demo—changing bag, application of water								

KEY

1. To initiate a problem or intervention, document under corresponding date.
2. Document outcomes under appropriate date for achieving the goal.
3. To discontinue an intervention or resolve a patient problem highlight, date, and initial.

COLLABORATIVE PROBLEMS

DATE	COLLABORATIVE PROBLEMS	DC DATE / INIT	DATE	COLLABORATIVE PROBLEMS	DC DATE / INIT
	4. Alteration in comfort, pain R/T surgery.			9. Impaired skin integrity (perianal, ostomy) R/T bowel diversion.	
	5. Potential for infection R/T surgery.			10. Body image, altered R/T surgery.	
	6. Potential for complication R/T surgery.			11. Self-care deficit R/T surgery.	

OUTCOMES

OUTCOMES		OUTCOMES	
4. Pain controlled within 30 min of intervention by po analgesics.		10. Verbalizes positive feelings with personal adjustment.	
5. No infection throughout hospitalization.		11. Pt will be able to care for self. Support for home care prepared.	
6. No complications throughout hospitalization.		11. Verbalizes s/sx to report to medical team.	
9. Skin remains intact.		11. Independent in ostomy care.	

Continued

PLAN OF CARE DISCUSSED WITH

DATE _____ INIT _____ SO/P _____

_____

_____

CASE MANAGER: _____

CONSULTING MD: _____

SOCIAL SERVICE: _____

ANOINTING OF THE SICK DATE: _____

INTERVENTIONS

	PRE-OP DAY 1 DATE___	DAY 2 DATE___	P.O. #1 DAY 3 DATE___	P.O. #2 DAY 4 DATE___	P.O. #3 DAY 5 DATE___	P.O. #4 DAY 6 DATE___
	– Orient to hospital environment/routine. – Review medical plan. – Bowel prep as ordered. – Provide time for verbalization of feelings/questions. – Monitor labs & report abnormals. – Pre-Op Teach • Respiratory care: – TCDB/I.S. q 2° W/A • Pain control – Presence of tubes/drains: foley – May have NG, abdominal drains. – Presence/purpose of compression boots. RN required to know daily wt. & I/O.	– Weight at 6 am. – Report abnormal lab K+. – Post Op. – Epidural PCA management. Assess respiratory function, TCDB. – I.S. q 2° W/A – Encourage leg exercises, compression boots. – NG tube management. – Foley cath – I & O – Record q 4° × 24° – Call MD if urine output <30cc/hr × 2 hr – Report N/V to surgery team – JP's to low intermittent suction or as ordered (Expected output ≤400cc) – Zinc oxide at bedside. Apply to anus for skin protection. – Chart each shift condition of wound, dressing drainage. – Keep wound clean, dry. Change dressing, cleansing old drainage from wound.	– Weight at 6 am. – Inspect wounds, skin & document Q.shift. – Consult ET/skin nurse prn. – Use skin barriers as ordered (& for all ileal-anal anastomosis) to prevent skin breakdown. – Assess abdomen, bowel sounds, passing flatus, distention, nausea & vomiting q shift & prn. – Assess for dehydration. Replace fluids/electrolytes prn. – Monitor & document stool output. – Pain management. – Continual assessment for S/Sx of infection. – Allow time for expression of feelings. – Provide support prn. – Refer to MSW prn. – Continue strict I & O. – Encourage OOB & early ambulation. – Assess/monitor perianal skin. – Remove dressings after 24". – Continue JP's to low intermittent suction. (Expected output ≤300cc.)	– Weight at 6 am. – Aggressive pain management. Offer pain meds at ordered intervals before ↑ activity. – Continued bowel assessment. – Continued foley care. If Laparoscopic, DE foley – Assess/monitor nutritional intake when diet resumed. – Instruct to eat foods slowly and chew well. – Increase foods gradually. Teach to eat at regular times. – Encourage adequate fluid intake. – Continue respiratory care. – Continue monitoring for s/sx of infection & post op complication. – Consult RN coordinator if coping difficulties. – Continued JP's to low intermittent suction. (Expected output ≤200cc.)	– Weight at 6 am. Ileal Anal/Segmental/Colon Surgeries: – Teach • Monitor how foods affect consistency of stool. – Prevent constipation, fluid intake. – Prevent diarrhea – eat foods that thicken stool. • Foods that are incompletely digested should be avoided – Continued J.P. management. (Expected output ≤100cc.) – Continued abdominal/wound assessment/care. Laparoscopic Colon Surgery: – Teach routine follow-up care. – Ambulate at regular intervals. – Rest frequently. – Increase activities slowly. – Report S/Sx of redness, pain, drainage. – Report N & V, cramping, inability to evacuate bowel. – Avoid heavy lifting 6-8 weeks.	– Weight at 6 am. – Continued abdominal/wound assessment/care. – Continued pain management. – Continued assessment for post-op complication. – Monitor caloric intake. – Daily perianal skin assessment. Laparoscopic Colon Surgery: – Reinforce D/C teaching. – Teach: Dr. Beart available from 2000-2100 for questions/concerns.

DATE	SIGNATURES	DATE	SIGNATURES	DATE	SIGNATURES

	P.O.#5 DAY 7	P.O.#6 DAY 8	P.O.#7 DAY 9	P.O.#8 DAY 10	P.O.#9 DAY 11	P.O.#10 DAY 12
PLAN OF CARE DISCUSSED WITH	DATE ___	DATE ___	DATE ___	DATE ___	DATE ___	DATE ___

DATE   INIT   SO/P

_____

INTERVENTIONS

Teach routine follow-up care:
– Ambulate at regular intervals.

– Rest frequently.
– Increase activities slowly.

– Keep incisions dry.
– Report S/Sx of redness, pain, drainage.
– Avoid heavy lifting 6-8 weeks.

– Splint abdomen, chest coughing/sneezing.

– Driving – consult MD.

– Routine exercises (i.e., walking/swimming).

– Time release meds will only be partially absorbed – consult MD.

– Contact MD for diarrhea >24° or food blockage >4–6°.

– Normal ileostomy output 500–1000 cc/day.

– Stress doing Kegel exercises. Hold stool & increase capacity of pouch.

Review/Reinforce:
– Ostomy care.

– Follow-up medical plan.
– S/Sx to report to healthcare team.

– Report N & V, cramping, inability to evaluate bowel.

Teach Patient:
– Dr. Beart available from 2000–2100 for questions/concerns.

J-Pouch Ileal anal with ileostomy coloanal with colostomy:

Pouch irrigation starting 2 wks post-op with increasing amounts of saline will increase pouch capacity.

CASE MANAGER: _____

CONSULTING MD: _____

SOCIAL SERVICE: _____

ANOINTING OF THE SICK DATE: _____

MULTIDISCIPLINARY PLAN UPDATE

DATE	SIGNATURES	DATE	SIGNATURES	DATE	SIGNA

HARTFORD HOSPITAL CRITICAL PATHWAY
BOWEL RESECTION

HARTFORD HOSPITAL ADMISSION DATE/TIME _____
PATH INITIATED DATE/TIME _____

ADMISSION UNIT _____

POST OP UNIT _____
PATHWAY COMPLETED DATE _____

PATHWAY DISCONTINUED DATE/TIME _____
*document reason

DISCHARGE DATE: _____
CP010201

----DAY OF SURGERY----

PRE-OP	A	V	OR (INTRA OP) PACU	A	V	POST OP DAY 0	A	V	POST OP DAY 1	A	V
OUTCOMES			**OUTCOMES**			**OUTCOMES**			**OUTCOMES**		
1 Patient verbalizes understanding of need for surgical procedure			45 Patient hemodynamically stable-OR			89 Patient hemodynamically stable			133 Patient hemodynamically stable		
2 Tentative discharge plans identified			46 Patient hemodynamically stable-PACU			90 Patient demonstrates effective CDB, IS use			134 Surgical wound: (circle open or closed) - if closed, incision intact - if open, appropriate care implemented		
3 Evidence pre-op education completed			47			91 Patient verbalizes effective pain management ≤ 3 per scale			135 Patient demonstrates effective CDB/IS		
4 Patient verbalizes plan for post op pain management			48			92 Surgical incision intact			136 Patient ambulating		
5 Patient verbalizes plan for post-op diet advancement			49			93			137 Patient verbalizes effective pain management < 3 per scale		
6 Patient admitted day of surgery			50			94			138 Ostomy education needs identified if applicable		
CONSULT			**CONSULT**			**CONSULT**			**CONSULT**		
7 Anesthesia			51			95 Pain team (if epidural analgesia)			139		
8 CNS (if applicable)			52			96			140 Ostomy CNS		
ASSESSMENT			**ASSESSMENT**			**ASSESSMENT**			**ASSESSMENT**		
9 Presence of completed: -H&P -Admission database -RN assessment -Fall/Risk assessment			53 Perioperative nursing assessment			97 Surgical wound/ostomy assessment			141 Surgical wound/ostomy assessment		
10			54 PACU flowsheet			98 Pain per scale			142 Pain per scale		
TESTS			**TESTS**			**TESTS**			**TESTS**		
11 HCT and HGB			55 Surgical Path specimen sent			99			143		
12 Electrolytes			56			100			144		
13 Additional tests required per anesthesia protocol			57			101			145		
MEDICATIONS			**MEDICATIONS**			**MEDICATIONS**			**MEDICATIONS**		
14 Completed Bowel prep-Mechanical			58 Epidural first dosing(PACU)			102 Heparin SQ			146 Heparin SQ		
15 Completed Bowel prep-Oral antibiotics			59			103 Epidural/PCA analgesia			147 Epidural/PCA analgesia		
16 IV antibiotics on call to OR			60			104 IM/SQ analgesia ≥ Q 4 hr.			148 IM/SQ analgesia ≥ Q 4 hr.		
17 Heparin SQ			61			105 Antiemetic ≤ 2 doses			149 Personal medications restarted		
18 Personal medications administered			62			106			150		
TREATMENT/INTERVENTION			**TREATMENT/INTERVENTION**			**TREATMENT/INTERVENTION**			**TREATMENT/INTERVENTION**		
19 Phone call 48 hr pre-op			63 NG/OG tube			107 Vital signs.			151 Vital signs.		
20 Initiate IV site			64 Foley catheter			108 Foley catheter			152 Foley catheter		
21 Vital signs.			65 Compression boots (OR)			109 Compression boots			153 Compression boots		
22			66 Compression boots (PACU)			110 I&O Q shift			154 I&O Q shift		
23			67			111 DSD to surgical wound			155 DSD to surgical wound		
24			68			112			156 Change ostomy appliance		

PRE-OP	A	V	OR (INTRA OP)/PACU	A	V	POST OP DAY 0	A	V	POST OP DAY 1	A	V
MOBILITY/ACTIVITY			MOBILITY/ACTIVITY			MOBILITY/ACTIVITY			MOBILITY/ACTIVITIES		
25 Activity at baseline			69 Bedrest			113 OOB to chair with assistance			157 Ambulating with assistance in room		
26			70			114			158 Complete assistance with hygiene		
27			71			115			159		
PSYCHOSOCIAL MANAGEMENT			PSYCHOSOCIAL MANAGEMENT			PSYCHOSOCIAL MANAGEMENT			PSYCHOSOCIAL MANAGEMENT		
28 Notify clergy/offer spiritual support			72			116 Reassure patient/significant other			160 Reassess needs		
29 Presence of completed Advance Directive Form			73			117			161		
30 Patient has received Bill of Rights			74			118			162		
NUTRITION			NUTRITION			NUTRITION			NUTRITION		
31 Clear liquids 24 hr pre-op			75 NPO			119 NPO			163 NPO		
32 IV fluids as ordered			76 IV fluids as ordered			120 IV fluids			164 IV fluids		
EDUCATION			EDUCATION			EDUCATION			EDUCATION		
33 Explanation of surgery			77 Post-op instructions (PACU)			121 Reinforce pain management			165 Pain management		
34 Pre-op instructions completed including: -Incentive spirometer/CDB -Ostomy/wound care -Pain management			78			122 Reinforce CDB/IS			166 Wound and/or drain care		
35 Patient has reviewed Diet progression/Low residue diet packet.			79			123			167 Ostomy education		
36			80			124			168 Diet advancement		
37 Overview of expected stay			81			125			169		
DISCHARGE MANAGEMENT			DISCHARGE MANAGEMENT			DISCHARGE MANAGEMENT			DISCHARGE MANAGEMENT		
38 Completed discharge planning assessment form.			82			126			170 Discuss projected discharge date		
39 Tentative plans identified			83			127			171 F/U referrals initiated		
40			84			128			172		
OTHER			OTHER			OTHER			OTHER		
41 Old records available on unit			85 PACU report to unit RN			129			173		
42 Chart complete including surgical consent evening before surgery.			86			130			174		
43			87			131			175		
44			88			132			176		

Continued

NAME: MEDICAL RECORD #:

POST OP DAY 2	A	V	POST OP DAY 3	A	V	POST OP DAY 4	A	V	POST OP DAY 5	A	V
OUTCOMES			**OUTCOMES**			**OUTCOMES**			**OUTCOMES**		
Discharge plans identified			Patient has voided			Temp < 101 degrees			Temp < 100 degrees		
Patient verbalizes effective pain management ≤ 3 per scale			Patient verbalizes effective pain management ≤ 3 per scale			Patient verbalizes effective pain management ≤ 3 per scale			Patient demonstrates ADL's per baseline		
Patient empties ostomy pouch with assistance						Patient empties ostomy pouch independently			Return evidence of bowel function		
PO intake initiated						Patient completes ostomy site care with assistance			Patient tolerating diet		
Patient nausea free			Patient nausea free			Patient voiding WNL			Patient/significant other verbalizes understanding of: - medication - Follow-up appointment/test - Diet - Reportable signs and symptoms		
									Patient verbalizes effective pain management ≤ 3 per scale		
CONSULT			**CONSULT**			**CONSULT**			**CONSULT**		
						Dietary					
ASSESSMENT			**ASSESSMENT**			**ASSESSMENT**			**ASSESSMENT**		
Surgical wound/ostomy assessed			Surgical wound/ostomy assessed			Surgical wound/ostomy assessed			Surgical wound/ostomy assessed		
Pain scale			Pain scale			Pain scale			Pain scale		
TESTS			**TESTS**			**TESTS**			**TESTS**		
HCT ≤ 1											
Electrolytes ≤ 1 set											
NUTRITION			**NUTRITION**			**NUTRITION**			**NUTRITION**		
Sips clear liquids			Clear liquids			General liquids to low residue			Low residue		
IV fluids						D/C IV					
MEDICATIONS			**MEDICATIONS**			**MEDICATIONS**			**MEDICATIONS**		
Heparin SQ			Heparin SQ			P.O. Analgesia			P.O. Analgesia		
Epidural/PCA Analgesia			P.O. Analgesia			Personal medications			Personal medications		
IM/SQ Analgesia			Personal medications						Prescription to patient		
Personal medications											
TREATMENT/INTERVENTION			**TREATMENT/INTERVENTION**			**TREATMENT/INTERVENTION**			**TREATMENT/INTERVENTION**		
Vital signs			Vital signs			Vital signs			Vital signs		
I + O Q shift.			I + O Q shift.			I + O Q shift.			Wound/ostomy care		
Foley catheter (Pelvic), D/C Foley (Abdominal)			D/C Foley catheter at 12mn (Pelvic)			Wound/ostomy care			D/C staples		
Wound/drain/ostomy care			D/C Epidural			D/C Ostomy bridge					
D/C surgical dressing			D/C Drain								
D/C Compression boots			Wound/ostomy care								
MOBILITY/ACTIVITIES			**MOBILITY/ACTIVITIES**			**MOBILITY/ACTIVITIES**			**MOBILITY/ACTIVITIES**		
Ambulating with assist.			Ambulating with assist in hall.			Ambulating with assist in hall			Ambulation per baseline		
Partial assist with hygiene.			Partial assist with hygiene.			Partial assist with hygiene.			Hygiene per baseline		
PSYCHOSOCIAL MANAGEMENT			**PSYCHOSOCIAL MANAGEMENT**			**PSYCHOSOCIAL MANAGEMENT**			**PSYCHOSOCIAL MANAGEMENT**		

NAME: _____   MEDICAL RECORD #: _____

POST OP DAY 2	A	V	POST OP DAY 3	A	V	POST OP DAY 4	A	V	POST OP DAY 5	A	V
NUTRITION			**NUTRITION**			**NUTRITION**			**NUTRITION**		
Sips clear liquids			Clear liquids			General liquids to low residue			Low residue diet.		
IV fluids						D/C IV					
EDUCATION			**EDUCATION**			**EDUCATION**			**EDUCATION**		
Pain management.			Pain management.			Pain management.			Review written diet instructions.		
Wound and/or drain care.			Wound care.			Wound care.			Review reportable signs and symptoms.		
Ostomy education.			Ostomy education.			Ostomy education.			Review medications.		
Diet advancement.			Diet advancement.			Diet advancement.					
DISCHARGE MANAGEMENT			**DISCHARGE MANAGEMENT**			**DISCHARGE MANAGEMENT**			**DISCHARGE MANAGEMENT**		
Confirm discharge plans.						W-10/DC summary complete.			Provide written Home care instructions.		
						Transportation arranged.			Patient is discharged		
OTHER			**OTHER**			**OTHER**			**OTHER**		

A=Accomplished: intervention/outcome reached

V=Variance: intervention/outcome not reached

NA=Non-applicable: intervention/outcome deemed not clinically applicable

X=indicates no intervention/outcome for that day

This critical path was developed through the consensus of a multidisciplinary group and depicts the sequence and timing of those critical events which drive the achievement of progressive patient outcomes during an episode of illness. This is not meant to represent the o[nly] acceptable way to design the care for a given patient nor would all patients' needs necessarily be met by such a path, therefore the content may be tailored to meet the needs of the individual patient

The contents of this document incorporate the Standards of Patient Care.
Used by permission of Hartford Hospital, Hartford, Conn.

BARNES

CARE PATH® 550
MAJOR SMALL & LARGE
BOWEL PROCEDURE

SERVICE	PHYSICIAN
PRIMARY NURSE	PRIMARY NURSE

DC DATE	ADM DATE	DATE OF SURGERY

A-8

1

Problem Number	PATIENT PROBLEMS/NURSING DIAGNOSES
#1	ALTERATION IN COMFORT RELATED TO ABDOMINAL SURGERY
#2	ALTERATION IN BOWEL ELIMINATION RELATED TO ABDOMINAL SURGERY
#3	ALTERATION IN SKIN INTEGRITY RELATED TO ABDOMINAL INCISION AND RECOVERY FROM SURGERY
#4	LACK OF KNOWLEDGE RELATED TO HOSPITALIZATION AND SURGICAL PROCEDURE
#5	ALTERATION IN BODY IMAGE RELATED TO ABDOMINAL SURGERY AND OSTOMY

* IF APPROPRIATE

#	1, 2, 3	3, 4, 5	4	4	1, 4
	ASSESSMENT / MONITORING	CONSULTS	PROCEDURES / TEST	TREATMENT	ACTIVITY
DAY 1 PRE OP	Assessment: Nursing Admission lab results Monitoring: VS routine O₂ saturation x1 I & O	Nurse specialist (if ostomy is a consideration).	CBC, 6, 12, PT, PTT T & C x2 units (admission labs) ECG ≥ 40 years old CXR ≥ 50 years old UA with micro *Mark ostomy site	Antithrombolytic stockings Mechanical bowel preparation	UAL
DAY 2 DOS	Assessment: Wound/dressing q 4 hrs. Bowel function q 4 hrs. Stoma appearance q 4 hrs. Pulmonary status q 2 hrs. Comfort level q 2 hrs. Braden score x1 Patency of tubes and characteristics of drainage q 8 hrs. IV patency & site appearance q 8 hrs. Fall risk factors Monitoring: VS q 1 hr. x 2 q 2 hrs. x 2 then q 4 hrs. I & O q 4 hrs. O₂ saturation x1 x 2	Respiratory Therapy for O₂		Antithrombolytic stockings O₂ to maintain O₂ saturation ≥ 92% Oral care q 4 hrs. Assist with Incentive Spirometer and TCDB q 2 hrs. Gastric decompression and tube irrigation	Bedrest
DAY 3 POD 1	Assessment: Wound/dressing q 4 hrs. Bowel function q 4 hrs. Stoma appearance q 4 hrs. Pulmonary status q 2 hrs. Comfort level q 2 hrs. Braden score x1 Patency of tubes and characteristics of drainage q 8 hrs. IV patency and site appearance q 8 hrs. Fall risk factors Lab results **O₂ saturation ≥ 92%** Monitoring: VS q 4 hrs. I & O q 8 hrs. Room air O₂ saturation x1 x2	Social Work Respiratory (if O₂ or tx needed) Nurse specialist (if ostomy placed).	CBC, 6	Antithrombolytic stockings Oral care q 4 hrs. Assist with Incentive Spirometer q 2 hrs. Gastric decompression and tube irrigation d/c foley d/c O₂	Up in chair with assist x1 x2 x3 Ambulate in room with assist x1 x2 Bed bath
DAY 4 POD 2	Assessment: Wound/dressing q 4 hrs. Bowel function q 4 hrs. Stoma appearance q 4 hrs. Pulmonary status q 2 hrs. Comfort level q 2 hrs. Braden score x1 Patency of tubes and characteristics of drainage q 8 hrs. IV patency and site appearance q 8 hrs. Fall risk factors Lab results **Voiding without difficulty (UO ≥ 240 cc q 8 hrs.)** Monitoring: VS q 4 hrs. I & O q 8 hrs.	Dietary screening		Antithrombolytic stockings Oral care q 4 hrs. Assist with Incentive Spirometer q 2 hrs. Gastric decompression and tube irrigation *Abdominal wound wet to dry dressing Change TID	Up in chair with assist x1 x2 x3 Ambulate in room with assist x1 x2 Bed bath
	SIGNATURE	INIT.	SIGNATURE	INIT.	SIGNATURE	INIT.

310-93 (New 8/93)

Copyright 1993, Barnes Hospital - All Rights Reserved

550

Used by permission of Barnes Hospital, St Louis, Missouri.

BARNES

CARE PATH® 550
MAJOR SMALL & LARGE
BOWEL PROCEDURE

2

CNS	DIETARY	RT
HOME HEALTH	OT	OTHER
PT	SW	OTHER

A-8

Problem Number	PATIENT PROBLEMS/NURSING DIAGNOSES

1, 4	4	2, 3, 4	2, 3, 4	1, 4, 5	INITIALS (SEE KEY AT BOTTOM)		
MEDS / IVS	**NUTRITION**	**PATIENT / FAMILY EDUCATION**	**DISCHARGE PLANNING**	**PSYCHOSOCIAL/ EMOTIONAL/ SPIRITUAL NEEDS**			
IVF Laxative Oral antibiotic Bowel preparation Prn medication for sleep	Clear liquids NPO after MN	Nursing: Disease process Surgical procedure Primary nursing Plan of care Pre-op booklet (gastric drain, Incentive Spirometer, IV, Foley, TCDB, O$_2$, freq. VS, abdomen incision/wound Antithrombolytic device post-op analgesia). *Ostomy teaching process	Pt./family verbalizes understanding of care path. Plan of care has been mutually set with pt./family.	Provide emotional support for pt./family. Provide privacy.			
SQ Heparin IVF IV Antibiotics IV H$_2$ Antagonist Analgesic (PCA, Epidural, IM)	NPO	Reinforce post-op teaching **Demonstrates/verbalizes appropriate use of analgesic** **Verbalizes understanding of post-op teaching.**		Provide emotional support for pt./family. Provide privacy.			
SQ Heparin IVF IV H$_2$ Antagonist Analgesic (PCA, Epidural, IM)	NPO	Reinforce Incentive Spirometer *Initiate ostomy teaching record		Provide emotional support for pt./family. Provide privacy.			
SQ Heparin IVF IV H$_2$ Antagonist Analgesic (PCA, Epidural, IM)	NPO	Reinforce importance of post-op activity *Ostomy teaching record	Nursing: Assess Home Health needs *Caregiver available	Provide emotional support for pt./family. Provide privacy.			

SIGNATURE	INIT.	SIGNATURE	INIT.	SIGNATURE	INIT.

Continued

#	1, 2, 3	3, 4, 5	4	4	1, 4
	ASSESSMENT / MONITORING	**CONSULTS**	**PROCEDURES / TEST**	**TREATMENT**	**ACTIVITY**
DAY 5 POD 3	Assessment: Wound/dressing q 4 hrs. Bowel function q 8 hrs. **Bowel sounds present** Stoma appearance q 8 hrs. Pulmonary status q 8 hrs. Comfort level q 4 hrs. **Low risk Braden score** Patency of tubes and characteristics of drainage q 8 hrs. IV patency and site appearance q 8 hrs. Fall risk factors Lab results Hemodynamically stable Monitoring: VS q 8 hrs. I & O q 8 hrs.	Physical Therapy (if not ambulating in halls.)	CBC, 6	Antithrombolytic stockings Oral care q 4 hrs. Encourage Incentive Spirometer q 2 hrs. NG or gastric drain to gravity. *Abdominal wound wet to dry dressing Change TID	Up in chair with assist x1 x2 x3 x4 Ambulate in halls with assist x1 x2 x3 Bath with assist
DAY 6 POD 4	Assessment: Wound/dressing q 8 hrs. Bowel function q 8 hrs. Stoma appearance q 8 hrs. Pulmonary status q 8 hrs. Comfort level q 4 hrs. **Lungs clear** **No atelectasis** IV patency and site appearance q 8 hrs. Fall risk factors Monitoring: VS q 8 hrs. I & O q 8 hrs. Patency of tubes and characteristics of drainage q 8 hrs.	Home Health (if need identified).		Antithrombolytic stockings Uses Incentive Spirometer independently d/c NG or G-tube clamped per MD order *Abdominal wound wet to dry dressing Change TID	Up in chair with assist x1 x2 x3 x4 Ambulate in halls with assist x1 x2 x3 x4 Bath with assist
DAY 7 POD 5	Assessment: Wound/dressing q 8 hrs. Bowel function q 8 hrs. Stoma appearance q 8 hrs. Comfort level q 8 hrs. IV patency and site appearance q 8 hrs. Fall risk factors Monitoring: VS q 8 hrs. I & O q 8 hrs.			Antithrombolytic stockings **Uses Incentive Spirometer independently** G-tube clamped *Abdominal wound wet to dry dressing Change TID	UAL with minimal assist Bath with assist
DAY 8 POD 6	Assessment: Wound/dressing q 8 hrs. Bowel function q 8 hrs. Stoma appearance q 8 hrs. Comfort level q 8 hrs. IV site appearance q 8 hrs. Fall risk factors Monitoring: VS q 8 hrs. I & O q 8 hrs.	**Consults completed**		d/c antithrombolytic stockings d/c Incentive Spirometer use *G-tube clamped *Abdominal wound wet to dry dressing Change TID	UAL with minimal assist Bath with assist
DAY 9 POD 7	Assessment: Wound/dressing q 8 hrs. **Abdominal incision/wound without signs of infection.** Bowel function q 8 hrs. Stoma appearance q 8 hrs. Stoma visible **No phlebitis** **Fluid balance adequate** **(PO fluid intake ≥ 1000 cc/day and UO ≥ 720 cc/day)** Monitoring: VS q 8 hrs. d/c I & O			*G-tube clamped *Abdominal wound wet to dry dressing Change TID	UAL Independent with bath
DAY 10 DISCHARGE	Assessment: Wound incision x1 Bowel function x1 Stoma appearance x1 **Abdominal incision/wound without signs of infection.** **Bowel function normal** **Stoma viable** **Pain controlled with PO analgesics** **No skin breakdown** **No IV phlebitis** **Fluid balance adequate** **No fall** **Afebrile VSS**	**Consults completed**	**Hemodynamically stable**	G-tube d/c by MD prior to DC **No pulmonary or circulatory complications.** **DC home with dressing or wound closed** **No gastric tube.**	**Ambulating independently**
	SIGNATURE	**INIT.**	**SIGNATURE**	**INIT.**	**SIGNATURE**	**INIT.**

1, 4	4	2, 3, 4	2, 3, 4	1, 4, 5	INITALS (SEE KEY AT BOTTOM)		
MEDS / IVS	NUTRITION	PATIENT / FAMILY EDUCATION	DISCHARGE PLANNING	PSYCHOSOCIAL EMOTIONAL/ SPIRTUAL NEEDS			
SQ Heparin IVF IV H$_2$ Antagonist Analgesic (PCA, Epidural, IM)	NPO	Reinforce importance of post–op activity and NPO *Ostomy teaching record	Social Work (High risk screening)	Provide emotional support for pt./family Provide privacy.			
SQ Heparin IV fluids IV H$_2$ Antagonist Analgesic (PCA, Epidural, IM)	NPO	Pt. to verbalize importance of post–op activity. Instruct dietary advances. *Ostomy teaching record.	*Home Health plans initiated	Provide emotional support for pt./family Provide privacy.			
SQ Heparin IVF IV H$_2$ Antagonist Analgesic (PCA, Epidural, IM)	Diet as prescribed by MD	Pt./family observe abdominal wet-dry dressing change if wound open. Reinforce dietary specifics. *Ostomy teaching record.		Provide emotional support for pt./family Provide privacy.			
SQ Heparin IVF to hep lock d/c H$_2$ Antagonist d/c PCA, Epidural or IM Analgesia PO Analgesic Assess need to resume pre-op meds.	Diet as prescribed by MD	Instruct pt./family in: Wound care (and dressing change procedure if indicated) s&sx infection and problems with bowel function. *Ostomy teaching record.	DC plans finalized **Pt./family able to verbalize DC plans.**	Provide emotional support for pt./family Provide privacy.			
d/c SQ Heparin d/c hep lock PO Analgesics **Pain controlled with PO analgesics**	Diet as prescribed by MD	Pt./family to demonstrate wet to dry dressing change (if indicated) MD: Instuctions for activity and follow-up. ***Ostomy teaching record completed.**		Provide emotional support for pt./family Provide privacy.			
No adverse drug reactions.	**Tolerating diet** **Tolerating prescribed diet**	DC instructions per MD, nursing and consults. **Pt./family able to identify support systems and resources if needed.** **Pt. able to verbalize activity restrictions, s&sx of infection, appropiate bowel function and MD follow-up.**	**Pt. discharged** **Home with appropriate level of care**	Pt./family verbalizes feelings R/T surgery and diagnosis.			
SIGNATURE	INIT.	SIGNATURE	INIT.	SIGNATURE			INIT.

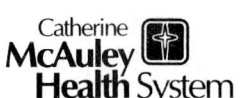

Nursing Service
5301 East Huron River Drive
P.O. Box 995
Ann Arbor, Michigan 48106

Nursing Care Plan Index

Diagnostic Conclusion Code:*
N - Nursing Diagnosis
C - Collaborative Problem

Primary Nurse _____   Associate Nurse _____

Primary Nurse _____   Associate Nurse _____

INDEX OF DIAGNOSTIC CONCLUSIONS

#	*DIAGNOSTIC CONCLUSION CODE	DATE IDENTIFIED	TITLE	SIGNATURE, TITLE	DATE RESOLVED
1	N		Knowledge Deficit R/T Preparation for Surgery and		
			Post-Op Recovery (N-K-077)		
			PER/OSTOMY		
2	N		Knowledge Deficit R/T Self Care Management of		
			New Ostomy (N-K-056)		
3	C		Post-Abdominal Surgical Procedure (C-A-091)		

SIGNIFICANT DATA	*(Safety level, cues needing followup, special considerations, patient assets/strengths, transfer dates)*	SIGNATURE, TITLE	DATE

PROJECTED DATE OF:

Transfer to _____ on _____

Discharge to _____ on _____

6102-001 N 2/93

REFERRALS MADE (Date, To Whom):

Dietary _____ Home Care _____ Other: _____

Social Service _____ Pharmacist _____ _____

Nursing _____ Pastoral Care _____ _____

St. Joseph Mercy Hospital
Ann Arbor, Michigan 48106
**NURSING CRITICAL PATH
OSTOMY 148/149**

To be used with NMP:
- Knowledge deficit R/T Prep of pre-abdominal/ostomy surgery
- Post-abdominal surgery
- Knowledge deficit - Self Care of Ostomy

page 2 of 4

	PPT/Admission	OR	POD 1 Date_____	POD 2 Date_____	POD 3 Date_____	POD 4 Date_____
PHYSICAL ASSESSMENTS	Weight - on admit Lung sounds - on admit VS & Temp - BID I & O including ostomy Skin assessment	Implement Post abdominal Surg Procedure NMP Assess: Dressing q 4 hr GI Status q 8 hr Stomal Integrity q 8 hr Lung sounds q shift VS & temp q 4 hr I & O q shift	Dressings q 4 hr GI Status q 8 hr Stomal integrity q 8 hr Daily Wt. q shift q 4 hr q 8 hr Braden Scale	Dressings/Incisions q s⌐ GI Status q shift Assess stoma and peristomal skin ⌐ VS & temp q shift	—— Continue —— BID/prn Lungs	—— Continue
DIAGNOSTICS MD ORDERS	UA ECG LTES CEA TS CXR CHEM PROF		CBC,LYTES	LYTES	LYTES,CBC	
TREATMENTS	Bowel Prep Protocol IV Diet: Cl Liq Maintain comfort	ABX IS, Cough, Deep Breathe IV Foley NG NPO Epidural/PCA	d.c ABX (if not ruptured) —— Continue ——	Soap and water wound care (ABX continue if ruptured) —— Continue ——	—— Continue —— d/c Epidural	
ACTIVITY	ad lib	Turn q 2 hr, leg exercises, up in chair	Chair	Hall BID Chair	Hall TID	Hall TID
CONSULTS/ REFERRALS	Barb Boylan-Lewis, ET APS Cardiology prn					
DISCHARGE PLANNING	Assess home situation/ D/C Plan Identify primary caregiver		HHC prn Social Work/Consult prn: ECF Psychosocial needs			
PATIENT EDUCATION	Implement KD R/T Preparation for Surgery and Postoperative Recovery N-K-077 PER/Ostomy	Implement KD: Self Care Management of New Ostomy N-K-056 PER/New Ostomy		Bag change with pt-S/O Give clamp to practice Y N Open and close clamp Y N Visualize stoma Y N	Teach soap and water wound care Y N Give closed wound care folder Y N Review Dietary Management - Flatus Blockage	Soap and water wound care per patient Y N Bag change - pt-S/O observed. pt-S/O prepare appliance Y N Teach emptying Y N Teach peristomal skin care T N
				Special considerations: Verbalize and/or demonstrate 1. Colostomy Irrigation 2. Drainage per rectum expected 3. Mucous fistula care 4. Interest in ostomy association visitor 5. Special concerns, i.e., hygiene occupation		
	RNSig_____ _____	RNSig_____ _____	RNSig_____ _____	RNSig_____ _____	RNSig_____ _____	RNSig_____ _____

Continued

St. Joseph Mercy Hospital
Ann Arbor, Michigan 48106
**NURSING CRITICAL PATH
OSTOMY 148/149**

To be used with NMP:
- Knowledge deficit R/T Prep of pre-abdominal/ostomy surgery
- Post-abdominal surgery
- Knowledge deficit - Self Care of Ostomy

POD 5 Date_____	POD 6 Date_____	POD 7 Date_____	POD 8 Date_____	POD 9 Date_____	POD 10 Date_____	Expected Outcomes
Incision q shift GI Status q 8 hr Stomal Assessment Peristomal skin Weight q day Lung Sounds prn VS & Temp q shift I & O q 8 hr	——Continue——	——Continue——	——Continue——	BID VS		Passing stool flatus Y N Stoma intact Y N Peristomal skin intact Y N Lungs at baseline Y N VS - afebrile Y N Voiding Y N
		Braden				
		Check Pathology if indicated				
Soap and water wound care IV Foley DD IS & cough Diet NPO/liquids PCA/PO pain meds	d/c IV d/c foley - ISC q 6 hr if no void Liquids PO Pain Meds prn	(d/c ABX *if ruptured) General				Wound healing without symptoms of infection Y N Tolerating pre-op diet Y N Pain Mgmt with PO Meds Y N
Hall TID up ad lib						Achieves baseline activity Y N
Dietary Refer prn		Oncology if indicated by Pathology				**Pt-S/O states/demonstrates** Resources: HHC/ET Nurse Ostomy Assoc. Ostomy Folder Y N
Follow up HHC Begin after ABD surgery D/C sheet		Order D/C supplies Give a patient Rx for supplies		Review D/C sheet		Rx for ostomy supplies Y N supplier Y N supply list Y N
						Incision care: Symptoms to report to physician Y N
		Reinforce Dietary Management				Bag preparation Y N

	Bag change by pt-S/O with RN assist/observe
	    Y N
			Bag change by pt-S/O
			    Y N
						Bag change Y N

						Emptying and cleaning Y N
Review emptying Review skin care	Pt emptying own bag Y N Skin care by pt-S/O					Symptoms of skin problems/treatment Y N Dietary Management Y N Thoughts R/T Ostomy: change in body Image, Incorporating ostomy into lifestyle Y N
RNSig_____	RNSig_____	RNSig_____	RNSig_____	RNSig_____	RNSig_____	RNSig_____

St. Joseph Mercy Hospital
Ann Arbor, Michigan 48106
**NURSING CRITICAL PATH
OSTOMY 148/149**

To be used with NMP:
• Knowledge deficit R/T Prep of pre-
  abdominal/ostomy surgery
• Post-abdominal surgery
• Knowledge deficit - Self Care of Ostomy

POD 11 Date____	POD 12 Date____	POD 13 Date____	POD 14 Date____	POD 15 Date____	Date____	
PHYSICAL ASSESSMENTS Dressing GI Status Stomal Integrity Weight Lung Sounds Temp & Vital Signs I & O Skin Assessment						
DIAGNOSTICS MD ORDERS						
TREATMENTS						
ACTIVITY						
CONSULTS REFERRALS						
DISCHARGE PLANNING						
PATIENT EDUCATION						
RNSig____	RNSig____	RNSig____	RNSig____	RNSig____	RNSig____	RNSig____

CHAPTER 7

Endocrine System

■ ENDOCRINE ASSESSMENT

▮ SUBJECTIVE DATA

Change in stamina and ability to perform activities of
    daily living (ADLs)
Excessive urination, thirst, or hunger
Fatigue
Numbness
Tingling
Paresthesia
Weakness
Bone pain
Change in mental status
Memory loss
Irritability
Anxiety
Nervousness
Depression
Headache
Syncope
Anorexia
Nausea
Abdominal pain
Change in body proportions
Palpitations
Shortness of breath (SOB)
Hoarseness
Anosmia
Decreased libido
Dysuria
Weight loss or gain

▮ OBJECTIVE DATA

General appearance: body development, proportion
    (Fig. 7-1, Table 7-1)
Vital signs: blood pressure (BP), pulse (P), respiratory rate
    (R), temperature (T)
Skin
    Temperature
    Turgor
    Hydration
        Dry, scaly
        Excessive perspiration
        Excessive oiliness

Texture
    Fine, smooth
    Coarse, leathery
    Acne
Color
    Increased pigmentation
        Gums
        Breasts
        Abdomen
        Scars/creases
    Bronze pigmentation
    Flushed/facial plethora
    Pale
    Cyanotic
    Ecchymosis
    Purple striae over areas of fat
    Vitiligo
Edema
    Face, eyelids
    Lower extremities
    Pitting/nonpitting
Lipodystrophy
Poor wound healing
Hair and nails
    Texture of nails
        Thick
        Brittle
        Thin
        Cracking
    Horizontal nail ridges
    Amount of hair
        Thin
        Increased
        Hirsutism
        Alopecia
    Distribution of hair
    Texture of hair
        Coarse, dry, brittle
        Fine, silky, soft
Musculoskeletal system
    Changes in height
    Changes in weight
    Fat distribution
        Central obesity
        Supraclavicular fat pads
        Dorsocervical fat pad (buffalo hump)

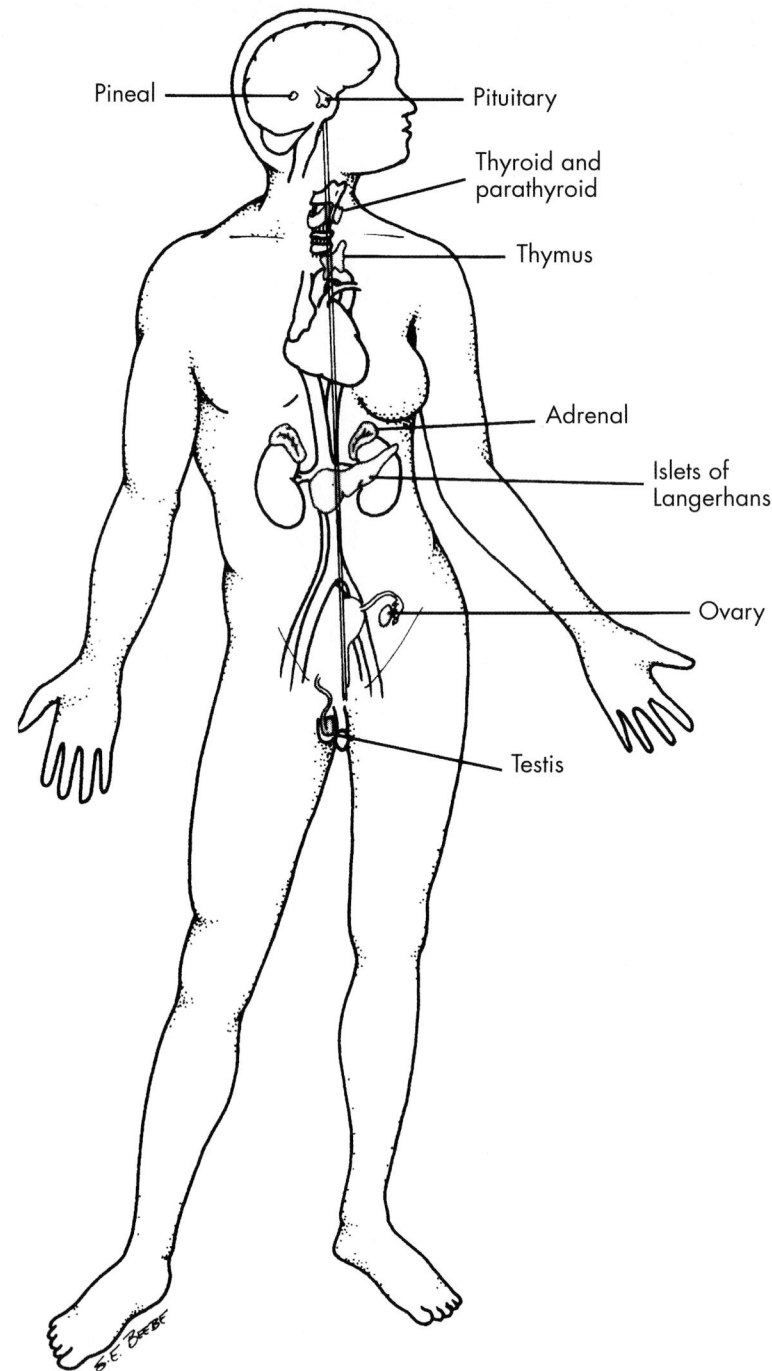

Fig. 7-1 Endocrine system (male and female).

Upper- to lower-body segment ratio
Muscle mass and function
    Atrophy
    Development
    Dystonia
    Tremors
    Spasms
    Wasting in extremities
    Tetany
    Ataxia
    Weakness
    Paralysis

Central nervous system (CNS)
    Personality changes
        Complacent
        Dull
        Lethargic
        Confused
        Mood swings
        Depressed
        Labile
            Euphoric to depressed
            Manic behavior
            Frank psychosis

Table 7-1	The Endocrine Glands

Endocrine Gland	Hormone	Function	Endocrine Disorders
Hypothalamus	CRH (Corticotropin-releasing hormone)	Stimulates anterior pituitary secretion of ACTH	Cushing's syndrome Adrenal insufficiency
	Dopamine	Inhibits secretion of PRL from the anterior pituitary	Galactorrhea
	GRH (Growth hormone–releasing hormone)	Stimulates anterior pituitary secretion of GH	Acromegaly Growth hormone deficiency
	GnRH (Gonadotropin-releasing hormone)	Stimulates anterior pituitary secretion of LH and FSH	Hypogonadism
	TRH (Thyrotropin-releasing hormone)	Stimulates anterior pituitary secretion of TSH	Thyrotoxicosis Hypothyroidism
	Somatostatin	Inhibits release of soma-totropin, thyrotropin, glucagon, insulin, cholecystokinin, adrenocor-ticotropic hormone	↑ Acromegaly, hypoglycemia ↓ Growth deficiency, pituitary insufficiency, hyperglycemia
Anterior Pituitary	GH	Promotes growth and retention of nitrogen for protein metabolism	↑ GH: acromegaly, gigantism ↓ GH: short stature
	TSH	Stimulates synthesis and secretion of thyroid hormones T_3 and T_4	↑ TSH: primary hypothyroidism ↓ TSH: secondary hypothyroidism, hyperthyroidism
	ACTH	Stimulates adrenal cortex to secrete cortisol, adrenal androgens, and mineralocorticoids	↑ ACTH: Cushing's disease ↓ ACTH: secondary adrenal insufficiency
	FSH	Women: promotes follicular growth and development and secretion of estrogen Men: stimulates Leydig cell of the testis to produce LH receptors; stimulates Sertoli cells to promote spermatogenesis	↑ LH, FSH: precocious puberty, menopause ↓ LH, FSH: delayed puberty, menstrual disorders, amenorrhea, infertility, impaired development of secondary sexual characteristics, Kallman's syndrome
	LH	Women: promotes ovarian maturation and ovulation; regulates gonadal steroid production (estrogens and progesterone) by the ovary; maintains corpus luteum Men: regulates gonadal steroid production (testosterone) by the Leydig cell of the testis	

Key: ACTH (adrenocorticotropin hormone or corticotropin)
CRH (corticotropin-releasing hormone)
GnRH (gonadotropin-releasing hormone)
GRH (growth hormone–releasing hormone)
GH (growth hormone)

FSH (follicle-stimulating hormone)
LH (luteinizing hormone)
PRL (prolactin)
TRH (thyrotropin-releasing hormone)
TSH (thyroid-stimulating hormone)

Continued

Table 7-1	**The Endocrine Glands—cont'd**		
Endocrine Gland	**Hormone**	**Function**	**Endocrine Disorders**
	PRL	Stimulates mammary glands of the breast to secrete milk	↑ PRL: hyperprolactinemia, galactorrhea, amenorrhea ↓ PRL: failure to lactate
Posterior Pituitary	ADH (Vasopressin)	Promotes reabsorption of water in the distal tubules of the kidney	↑ ADH: syndrome of inappropriate ADH (SIADH) ↓ ADH: Diabetes insipidus
	Oxytocin	Stimulates uterine contractions at parturition, stimulates mammary contractions during suckling, promotes maternal behaviors	None known
Adrenal Cortex	Glucocorticoids (cortisol)	Regulates metabolism of carbohydrates, fats, proteins; acts as antiinflammatory agent	↑ Cortisol: Cushing's syndrome ↓ Cortisol: primary adrenal insufficiency
	Adrenal androgens (androstenedione, DHA, DHEA, DHAS)	Masculinization of females	↑ DHA: hirsutism
	Mineralocorticoids (aldosterone)	Balances sodium, water, and potassium concentration	↑ Aldosterone: primary aldosteronism
Adrenal Medulla	Epinephrine Norepinephrine	Increases blood sugar; modulates vascular tone	↑ Catecholamines: pheochromocytoma
Pancreas Islets of Langerhans	Insulin (beta cells)	Promotes glucose entry into cells; initiates lipolysis	↑ Insulin: hypoglycemia, hyperinsulinism, insulin resistance ↓ Insulin: diabetes mellitus
	Glucagon (alpha cells)	Elevates blood glucose and stimulates lipolysis	↑ Insulin: glucagonoma
	C-Peptide	Indicates efficacy of beta cell secretory function	↑ Insulinoma, renal failure ↓ Factitious hypoglycemia, diabetes mellitus
Thyroid	Thyroxine (T_4) Triiodothyronine (T_3)	Regulates metabolic rate	↑ T_3, T_4: hyperthyroidism, Graves' disease ↓ T_3, T_4: hypothyroidism
	Calcitonin	Decreases serum calcium levels, bone remodeling	Marker for medullary carcinoma of the thyroid
Parathyroid	Parathyroid hormone (PTH)	Regulates serum calcium concentration	↑ PTH: hyperparathyroidism, hypercalcemia, osteoporosis, renal calculi ↓ PTH: hypoparathyroidism, hypocalcemia, tetany
Ovaries	Estrogens	Induces secondary sex characteristics, sexual functioning	↓ Estrogen (female): delayed or failed puberty, osteoporosis ↑ Estrogen (male): feminization
	Progesterone	Prepares and maintains endometrium for implantation	Infertility, menstrual cycle disorders
Testis	Testosterone	Induces secondary sex characteristics, sexual functioning	↓ Testosterone (male): primary hypogonadism; feminization, infertility ↑ Testosterone (female): hirsutism, virilization

Relationship Among Hypothalamic, Pituitary, and Target Gland Hormone Secretion

Hypothalamus	Pituitary	Target	Hormones
TRH	TSH	Thyroid	T_3, T_4
GHRH	GH	Liver	IGF-1
Dopamine	PRL	Breast	
CRH	ACTH	Adrenal	Cortisol
GnRH	LH	Ovary	E_2, progesterone
		Testis	Testosterone
	FSH	Ovary	E_2
		Testis	Inhibin, testosterone
GHRIH	GH	Liver	

The hypothalamus links the central nervous system with the endocrine system via the pituitary gland, which is stimulated to release hormones toward target cell membranes or organs. Hormones are released by some of the targets.

Key: ACTH, *Adrenocorticotropin hormone or corticotropin;* CRH, *corticotropin-releasing hormone;* GnRH, *gonadotropin-releasing hormone;* GHRH, *growth hormone–releasing hormone;* GHRIH, *growth hormone release–inhibiting hormone, somatostatin;* GH, *growth hormone;* FSH, *follicle-stimulating hormone;* IGF 1, *insulinlike growth factor;* LH, *luteinizing hormone;* PRL, *prolactin;* TRH, *thyrotropin-releasing hormone;* TSH, *thyroid-stimulating hormone;* T_3, *triiodothyronine;* T_4, *thyroxine.*

Alterations in consciousness
    Drowsy
    Slowing of cognitive ability
    Memory loss
    Inappropriate response to questions
    Somnolence
    Stupor
    Confusion
    Coma
  Small, reactive pupils
  Position sense
  Response to touch, vibration, and pain
Deafness
Speech
  Monotonous
  Slowed
  Weak
  Hoarse
Reflexes
  Hyperreflexia
  Hyporeflexia
  Trousseau's sign
  Chvostek's sign
Seizures
Head and neck
  Mouth: brown pigmentation
  Tongue
    Color
    Size: enlarged
    Tremors
  Face
    Coarse
    Protruding
    Moon face
    Erythema

Plethora
Edema
  Wide, puffy eyes
  Wrinkled eyelids
Broad, short, upturned nose
Enlarged lip
Enlarged nose
Anosmia
Eyes
  Visual acuity changes
  Visual field deficits
  Protruding eyeballs
  Drooping eyelids
  Cataracts
  Periorbital edema
  Ocular dysfunction
  Microaneurysms
  Hemorrhage
  Exudates
  Arteriolar narrowing
Thyroid
  Size
  Shape
  Symmetry
  Nodules
    Tenderness
    Systolic bruit
Gastrointestinal (GI) system
  Polyphagia
  Polydipsia
  Vomiting
  Diarrhea
  Steatorrhea
  Constipation
  Dehydration

Weight change
Increased abdominal girth
Obesity
Cardiovascular system
Easily bruised
Edema
Diaphoresis
Cold sweats
Tachycardia
Bradycardia
Hypotension: postural/orthostatic
Hypertension
Dysrhythmias
Cardiomegaly
Respiratory system
Hoarseness
Laryngeal stridor
Tachypnea
Kussmaul's respirations
Acetone breath
Stridorous respirations
Supraclavicular retractions
Renal system
Polyuria
Oliguria
Anuria
Enuresis
Dilute urine
Colic
Calculi
Reproductive system
Upper- to lower-body segment ratio
Precocious puberty
Menstrual cycle changes
Amenorrhea
Oligomenorrhea
Menorrhagia
Galactorrhea
Impotence
Female masculinization
Absent or minimal secondary sex characteristics
Changes in secondary sex characteristics
Genital atrophy
Breast atrophy

▌ PERTINENT BACKGROUND INFORMATION

CONCURRENT DISEASES OR CONDITIONS
Cardiovascular disease
Angina
Hypertension
Heart failure
Pericardial effusion
Myocardial infarction
Intestinal obstruction
Pulmonary edema
Psychologic problems/stress
Pathologic fracture
Obesity

PREVIOUS SURGERY OR ILLNESS
Cancer
Pancreatic disease
Burns
Renal disease
Cardiovascular disease
Transplant
Sarcoidosis
Diabetes mellitus
Diabetes insipidus
Trauma
Oophorectomy
Neck surgery
Adrenalectomy
Hypophysectomy
Gestational diabetes
Irradiation
Meningitis
Encephalitis

FAMILY HISTORY
Diabetes mellitus
Diabetes insipidus
Thyroid disease
Hypertension
Pheochromocytoma
Rheumatoid arthritis
Short stature
Hirsutism
Bone disease
Osteoporosis
Infertility
Renal calculi

SOCIAL HISTORY
Physical environment
Psychologic environment
Family structure/support
Occupation
Exposure to hazards
Shift work

MEDICATION HISTORY
Cardiovascular drugs
Respiratory drugs
Corticosteroids
Diuretics
Medication for sleep, nerves, and/or anxiety
Alcohol/chemical dependency
Insulin/oral antidiabetic drugs
Thyroid drugs

▌ DIAGNOSTIC TESTS
Blood
T_3 serum triiodothyronine; free T_3
T_4 serum thyroxine; free T_4
Thyroid stimulating hormone (TSH)
^{123}I or ^{125}I (radioactive iodine uptake)
Parathyroid hormone level (PTH)
Adrenocorticotropic hormone (ACTH)

Cortisol
Ketones
Testosterone or estrogen
Cholesterol
Triglyceride
Creatinine phosphokinase (CPK)
Catecholamine levels
Potassium
Sodium
Calcium
Phosphorus
pH
Carbon dioxide (CO_2)
Bicarbonate levels
Blood urea nitrogen (BUN)
Fasting blood sugar (FBS)
Glucose tolerance test (GTT)
Thyroid stimulation test
Metyrapone test
Insulin assay
Urine
    Calcium
    Glucose
    Urinary-free cortisol
    17-Hydroxycorticosteroids
    17-Ketosteroids
    Metanephrine
    Specific gravity
Imaging studies
    Bone x-rays
    Thyroid scan/ultrasound
    Computed tomography (CT) scans
        Thyroid
        Adrenal gland
        Parathyroid

Gerontologic Considerations

- Endocrine system normally functions well with the exception of the ovarian hormones, a lesser extent of the testicular hormones, and changes that occur in concentration of the parathyroid hormones.
- Glucose tolderance frequently decreases with aging, and blood glucose levels tend to increase.
- The classic signs and symptoms of diabetes may not be obvious in older adults.
- Dietary management may be complicated by a variety of social, economic, and financial factors.
- Hormone supplements must be administered with caution, because side effects are more likely to occur.
- Diabetes mellitus is the most common endocrine disorder seen in older adults.
- Older adult diabetics are at increased risk for infection and should be counseled to receive proper immunizations and seek regular medical attention for even minor symptoms.

From Christensen BL, Kockrow EO: Foundations of nursing, *ed 3, St Louis, 1998, Mosby.*

Adrenal angiography
Adrenal venography
Inferior petrosal sinus sampling
Endocrine tests
    Dexamethasone suppression test
    ACTH stimulation test
    Water deprivation test
    Thyroid stimulation test
    Thyroid suppression test

■ HYPOTHYROIDISM: MYXEDEMA

hypothyroidism: *A condition characterized by decreased activity of the thyroid gland; caused by surgical removal of all or part of the gland, overdosage with antithyroid medication, decreased effect of thyroid-releasing hormone secreted by the hypothalamus, decreased secretion of thyroid-stimulating hormone by the pituitary gland, or atrophy of the thyroid gland itself*

myxedema coma: *A severe form of hypothyroidism; develops after a prolonged period of untreated or uncontrolled hypothyroidism*

ASSESSMENT
SUBJECTIVE DATA
Poor memory
Difficulty thinking clearly
Difficulty seeing at night
Sore muscles, aches, and pains
Feel cold
SOB
Fatigue, tiredness
Poor appetite
Decreased libido
Paresthesia
Depression
Menstrual irregularities
Muscle cramps

OBJECTIVE DATA
Neurologic system
    Lethargy
    Slow, monotonous, slurred speech
    Memory impairment
    Slow cognition
    Personality changes: complacent, dull, apathetic
    Nystagmus
    Night blindness
    Perceptive hearing loss
    Intention tremor
    Slowed deep tendon reflexes
    Ataxia
    Somnolence
    Syncope
Musculoskeletal system
    Muscle stiffness or aching
    Myalgia
    Arthralgia
    Fatigue

Cardiovascular system
   Intolerance to cold
   Decreased sweating
   Low BP, P, and T
   Narrow pulse pressure
   Diminished heart sounds
   Precordial pain
Respiratory system
   Hoarseness or deepened voice
   SOB with mild exertion
Gastrointestinal/nutritional system
   Unexplained weight gain
   Anorexia
   Constipation
   Abdominal distention
   Ascites
   Enlarged tongue
Reproductive/sexual system
   Menorrhagia, metrorrhagia, amenorrhea
   Decreased libido
   Decreased fertility: spontaneous abortion
   Impotence
Integumentary system
   Skin: pale, cold, dry, coarse, scaling
   Nonpitting edema: hands, feet, periorbital area
   Upper eyelid droop
   Enlarged tongue and lips
   Coarse, thinning hair
   Nails: brittle, slow growing, thick

DIAGNOSTIC TESTS
Blood
   Decreased serum T_4 and T_3
   Decreased serum sodium
   TSH levels: decreased if secondary hypothyroidism;
      elevated if primary hypothyroidism
   Increased serum: cholesterol, triglycerides, CPK,
      alkaline phosphatase
   Arterial blood gases (ABGs): hypoxia, elevated CO_2
   Normocytic, normochromic anemia
Radioiodide uptake test (suppressed response)
Electrocardiogram (ECG): low-voltage, nonspecific ST
   segment changes, prolonged P-R interval, heart block,
   flat or inverted T wave
Thyrotropin-releasing hormone (TRH)

POTENTIAL COMPLICATIONS
Angina, dysrhythmias
Heart failure
Myocardial infarction
Intestinal obstruction
Pleural/pericardial effusions
Stupor
Coma

MULTIDISCIPLINARY MANAGEMENT
THERAPEUTIC MANAGEMENT
Synthetic thyroid hormone (levothyroxine sodium)
Glucocorticoids if adrenal insufficiency diagnosis
IV fluids, albumin

High-protein, high-fiber, low-calorie, low-sodium diet
Restrict fluids
Diuretics
Stool softeners
Monitor TSH

PATIENT PROBLEMS—NURSING DIAGNOSES/INTERVENTIONS

▼Fluid volume excess, extravascular, related to increased capillary permeability

Monitor intake and output q8h and prn
Monitor IV fluids, if administered, *to prevent overhydration*
Weigh patient daily and report significant gain to physician (significant gain is >0.5 kg daily)
Monitor for signs and symptoms *to identify excess extravascular volume*
   Periorbital edema
   Jugular vein distention
   Increasing abdominal girth
   Presence of abdominal fluid wave
   Dependent edema of extremities
   Pulmonary edema: dyspnea, orthopnea, and/or crackles in lungs; monitor chest x-ray results
Monitor serum albumin levels, electrolytes, creatinine
Maintain high-protein diet *to increase serum protein levels*
Restrict fluids as determined by collaboration with physician
Monitor vital signs q4h and observe for
   Increased pulse
   Labored respirations
   Development of S_3 gallop
Be cautious in administering sedatives, especially barbiturates, *because of increased sensitivity*
Notify physician of development or worsening of any of the previously mentioned signs or symptoms
Maintain patient on bed rest *to alleviate dyspnea and support edematous areas*

Expected Outcomes
Vital signs are stable; electrolytes are within normal range; intake and output are balanced; edema is resolving

▼Altered thought processes related to changed metabolic processes

Assess level of orientation q4h and reorient patient as necessary; explain procedures clearly and slowly; repeat as necessary; break down tasks into easy-to-accomplish segments
Help patient to focus on tasks and reach self-care goals
Provide a stable, calm, and nonstressful environment
   Be consistent in timing and performance of activities and procedures
   Restrict visitors as necessary
   Avoid frequent changing of personnel
   Prevent emotionally upsetting or confusing situations

Allow sufficient time for performance of procedures and activities

Plan care with patient *to engage patient as a partner in interventions designed to improve thought processes*

Allow sufficient time for patient to express needs and feelings

Assist patient to make choices and decisions

Provide diversional activities and materials

Assist significant other in acceptance of patient's slowness

Expected Outcomes

Oriented to time, person, and place

Accomplishes planned self-care activities

Makes choices known to others

Discusses feelings and responses with significant other(s)

▼ Risk for trauma related to potential for changes in sensory perception and coordination

Assess for development or worsening of perception/coordination defects q8h

Assess muscle strength and mobility daily

Explain necessary safety precautions *to prevent accident/trauma*

Assist patient with ambulation as necessary; provide aids to ambulation (walker, cane) as needed

Monitor pulse rate, complaints of dyspnea or chest pain during activity

Balance periods of activity and rest

Place articles patient may wish to use frequently within easy reach

Arrange environment simply; avoid unnecessary clutter

Remove potentially hazardous objects from patient's environment

Place bed in low position

Face patient when speaking *to obtain patient's attention*

Speak slowly and clearly

Serve foods at tepid temperature *to prevent thermal injury*

Assist with bathing, shaving, and toileting as necessary

Use safety measures (e.g., jacket restraint; avoid wrist restraints) as necessary

Instruct patient to call for assistance when getting out of bed *to prevent a fall*

Keep call light within easy reach at all times

Provide nighttime lighting

Keep side rails up at all times

Expected Outcome

Sustains no injuries

▼ Constipation related to decreased metabolic rate and/or decreased intestinal peristalsis and decreased dietary bulk and fluids

Maintain low-calorie diet that includes high-fiber foods

Administer fluids to tolerance; remind patient to drink fluids hourly if not restricted *to prevent constipation*

Monitor bowel pattern, consistency of color, odor of stool, and associated symptoms daily

Assess usual methods used *to prevent constipation*

Assess effectiveness of stool softener, laxatives administered

Provide privacy

Encourage exercise as tolerated

Teach patient to respond promptly to urge to defecate; avoid straining

Assist patient with recognizing activities that stimulate urge to defecate (drinking warm liquids)

Encourage patient to attempt defecation at same time each day *to establish a routine*

Expected Outcome

Stool is normal in color, consistency, odor, and frequency

▼ Impaired skin integrity related to edema; dry, scaly skin; and immobility

Assess for redness or breakdown q24h; if patient is on bed rest, assess q8h

Administer skin care to pressure points four times daily and as necessary *to retain skin integrity*

Use superfatted soap for bathing; apply lotion after each bath or handwashing *to prevent dryness*

Use elbow and heel protectors *to prevent friction rub*

Place patient on pressure ulcer–prevention mattress or bed

Elevate edematous extremities with pillows *to increase venous return*

Assist and encourage patient to make small position changes q½h to 1h; turn q2h

Encourage ambulation when able; avoid sitting for long periods *to prevent venous stasis*

Encourage patient to avoid crossing legs *to prevent venous stasis*

Maintain optimal nutritional status

Conserve body temperature by use of blankets, warm clothing

Expected Outcome

Skin turgor is good

Skin is intact

Patient uses preventive measures

PATIENT/FAMILY TEACHING

Explain basic concepts of the disease process and complications to report to physician

Explain reasons for physical and emotional changes

Teach name of medication, dosage, time and method of administration, purpose, side effects, and toxic effects

Emphasize that medication must not be discontinued without consulting physician

Emphasize importance of telling all health care personnel about disease and wearing medical alert band

Explain that condition is potentially reversible if treatment regimen is followed

DISCHARGE/HOME CARE PLANNING

Explain need to avoid taking over-the-counter medications without consulting physician

Prepare for home by providing information about
importance of
Ongoing outpatient follow-up
Understanding slowness and dullness
Increasing self-care
Avoiding very cold environments and stressful
situations
Adequate periods of rest alternating with increasing
activity/exercise
Maintaining balanced diet and adequate fluid intake
Preventing constipation
Discuss symptoms of infection to report to physician
Temperature above patient's normal
Cold or influenza symptoms
Redness or swelling around lesions
Frequency of or burning on urination

■ HYPERTHYROIDISM: THYROTOXICOSIS (THYROID CRISIS, STORM)

hyperthyroidism: Characterized by excessive amount of thyroid hormone; causes may be classified as autoimmune (Graves' disease), viral, hyperplastic, or neoplastic (thyroid adenomas); or secondary to an acute systemic illness and factitious (excessive thyroid hormone treatment results in increased sympathetic tone, which is responsible for many of the assessment findings that follow)

Graves' disease: Most prevalent form of hyperthyroidism; most commonly seen in women during the third and fourth decades of life

thyroid crisis: A medical emergency caused by acute exacerbation of the symptoms of hyperthyroidism; usually precipitated by a stressful event such as surgery, infection, trauma, acute cardiovascular disease, or an iodine load from contrast dye

ASSESSMENT
SUBJECTIVE DATA
Irritability/nervousness
Headache
Difficulty concentrating
Increased thirst and/or appetite
SOB
Palpitations
Weakness

OBJECTIVE DATA
Neurologic system
Hyperthyroidism
Tremors
Insomnia
Emotional lability
Diplopia
Brisk deep tendon reflexes
Muscle weakness or atrophy
Confusion
Memory loss
Easily distracted
Startled expression
Manic behavior
Thyroid crisis
Extreme restlessness
Confusion or disorientation
Psychosis
Apathy
Stupor or delirium
Coma
Eyes
Conjunctival irritation
Large, protruding eyes
Lid retraction
Periorbital edema
Tremor of eyelids
Weakness or paralysis of extraocular muscles
Cardiovascular system
Hyperthyroidism
Palpitations
Rapid, bounding pulses
Wide pulse pressure
Irregular pulse/dysrhythmias
Systolic cardiac murmur
Edema
Thyroid crisis
Profuse diaphoresis
Tachycardia disproportionate to change in BP
Atrial fibrillation
Weak pulse
Hypotension
Respiratory system
Hyperthyroidism
Dyspnea
Increased depth and rate of respirations
Thyroid crisis: pulmonary edema
Musculoskeletal system
Generalized muscle wasting
Gastrointestinal system
Hyperthyroidism
Weight loss/weight gain
Diarrhea
Hyperactive bowel sounds
Thyroid crisis
Anorexia
Metabolic system
Profuse sweating
Sensitivity to heat
Increased tolerance to cold
Enlarged thyroid gland
Bruit over neck
Integumentary system
Skin: soft, warm, moist, shiny
Reddened, hyperpigmented palms
Hair: thinning, fine, straight (silky)
Oily scalp
Separation of nails from nail beds
Reproductive/sexual system
Oligomenorrhea
Amenorrhea

Diminished libido
Decreased fertility
Gynecomastia in males

DIAGNOSTIC TESTS

Blood
  Elevated total and free T_3 and T_4
  Thyroid radioiodide uptake test (RAIU)
    Low uptake in thyroiditis or excess thyroid
      hormone medication (exogenous
      hyperthyroidism)
    High uptake in Graves' disease
Serum
  TSH
    May be increased with pituitary tumor
    Normal with thyroid hormone resistance
    Decreased with all other causes; toxic adenoma,
      Graves' disease, postpartum period, iodine
      induced

POTENTIAL COMPLICATIONS

Fever >106° F (41.11° C)
Marked elevation in BP and P
Dangerous dysrhythmias
Congestive heart failure (CHF)
Pulmonary edema
Widespread tremors
Circulatory collapse
Shock
Death

MULTIDISCIPLINARY MANAGEMENT

THERAPEUTIC MANAGEMENT

Medications
  Antithyroid medications
    Thioamides (PTU, ipodate agents, tapazole)
    β-Adrenergic blockers (propanolol), atenolol
    Glucocorticoids
  Palliative medications
    Acetaminophen
    Eye lubricants
Dietary changes
  High calorie
  High protein
  High carbohydrate
  High vitamin B
  3 to 4 L fluid per day (unless in CHF)
Comfort measures: cooling (hypothermia blanket)
Surgical intervention: subtotal thyroidectomy when
  euthyroid
Thyroid crisis
  Glucocorticoids
  Thioureas (propylthiouracil)
  β-Blockade
  Hyperthermia control (aspirin is contraindicated)
  Cooling measures
  Volume expanders and/or vasopressors for
    hypotension
  Digoxin and/or diuretics for CHF

PATIENT PROBLEMS—NURSING DIAGNOSES/INTERVENTIONS

▼ Altered thought processes related to increased stimulation of the sympathetic nervous system by high levels of thyroid hormone and sleep deprivation

Assess level of consciousness (LOC), orientation, affect, and perception q4h to 8h; report negative changes
Discuss feelings and responses to situations and people; reinforce those that are appropriate
Provide a stable, calm, nonstressful, and nonstimulating environment *to minimize confusion*
  Control extraneous noise *to facilitate clarity of thought processes*
  Be consistent in timing and performing of activities and procedures *to minimize confusion related to activities*
  Restrict visitors as necessary *to minimize stress*
  Avoid frequent changing of personnel
Plan care with patient; give clear, concise explanations *to facilitate concentration and understanding*
Anticipate needs *to prevent hyperactive reactions*
Inform patient that activities may be restricted *to minimize confusion*
Teach stress-reduction techniques and assess use by patient when patient is recovering from thyrotoxic episode
Provide diversional activities and materials that decrease stimulation; avoid those requiring fine motor manipulation
Reorient patient to environment as needed and provide orienting cues: clock, calendar, familiar pictures
Monitor for adverse reactions to medications

Expected Outcomes

Patient is oriented
Responds appropriately to situations and people

▼ Activity intolerance related to imbalance between oxygen supply and demand caused by increased resting metabolic rate and intolerance of heat

Assess baseline vital signs and prior activity level
Restrict activity to patient's level of tolerance by assessing physiologic response to activity (i.e., assess vital signs during activity and compare with baseline)
Allow patient to set priorities for care within limits
Space procedures *to allow adequate rest periods*
Provide needed equipment, supplies *to prevent expenditure of energy by patient before activity*
Discontinue activity at onset of signs of intolerance: dyspnea, tachycardia, fatigue
Assist patient with those activities patient is unable to perform because of weakness or tremors
Plan daily activity and rest pattern *to facilitate increasing tolerance for self-care*

Expected Outcomes

Completes planned activities without evidence of intolerance

Asks for assistance only when needed

▼ Sleep pattern disturbance related to an increased metabolic rate

NOTE: These measures are only useful when T_4 level decreases

Assess past and present sleep and activity patterns

Determine factors/techniques to induce sleep previously used by patient

Provide sleep aids requested by patient: warm drink, back rub, quiet music *to facilitate sleep and rest*

Discuss other sleep aids such as relaxation techniques

Discourage frequent daytime sleeping *to increase night sleeping;* provide nap times sufficient in length *to produce REM sleep*

Avoid intake of stimulants in diet *to avoid interference with sleep*

Assist patient with establishing a regular pattern of physical activity; reduce stimulating activities before sleep

Provide environment conducive to sleep: reduce lighting; close door to room; maintain quiet; maintain privacy

Avoid disturbing patient unnecessarily during the night for procedures *to allow uninterrupted periods of sleep and rest*

Schedule treatments and medications for daytime and evening hours when possible *to avoid interrupting sleep*

Assess effectiveness of sleep-promoting activities daily

Expected Outcomes

Sleep pattern is normal for patient

Expresses feeling rested, alert, with energy to accomplish daily tasks

▼ Altered nutrition: less than body requirements related to diarrhea, nausea, abdominal pain, and/or hypermetabolic state

Provide high-calorie, high-protein, high-carbohydrate, high-vitamin B diet *to compensate for loss of calories, protein, glucose, and vitamins from bowel hypermotility and increased metabolism*

Offer frequent, small meals and between-meal supplements

Consult patient as to food preferences

Avoid stimulants: coffee, tea, colas, or other beverages with caffeine or theobromine *to prevent peristaltic stimulation and fullness from empty calories*

Avoid foods with large amounts of fiber or highly seasoned foods *to prevent stimulating bowel motility*

Encourage fluid intake; avoid juices that may cause diarrhea

Provide environment with congenial visitors if patient desires

Weigh patient daily; same time, scale, clothing *to evaluate effectiveness of diet and health care plan*

Monitor intake and output q8h

Assess effectiveness of medication for nausea and abdominal pain

Expected Outcomes

Weight is increasing to that which is normal for patient

Takes prescribed diet without abdominal discomfort

Has no diarrhea

Intake and output are balanced

▼ Impaired tissue integrity (eyes) related to compromised protective mechanisms (inadequate tearing and lid closure in patients with Graves' disease)

Assess for eye changes: excessive tearing, feeling of foreign object, inability to close eyes, dryness, signs of infection, irritation, or abrasions q4h to 8h

Provide sunglasses during the day as necessary *to prevent injury from inadequate lid closure*

Administer artificial tears as ordered *to prevent injury to eyes from inadequate tearing*

Patch eyes during sleep *to protect exposed cornea*

Prevent foreign bodies from contact with eyes (dirt, dust)

Assist and teach patient to perform eye motion exercises

Discuss feelings and techniques related to improving appearance

Ensure that patient understands that surgical intervention may be needed

Expected Outcomes

Eyes remain moist without evidence of abrasions or infection

Uses methods to protect eyes and discusses feelings about appearance

▼ Hyperthermia related to hypermetabolic state

Maintain cool environment *to minimize discomfort related to hypersensitivity to heat*

Use light clothing and bed linens

Provide tepid sponge baths as necessary *to maintain normal body temperature*

Assess effectiveness of hypothermia blanket when in use; use measures to prevent skin breakdown

Administer acetaminophen as ordered (aspirin is contraindicated) *to control body temperature*

Increase fluid intake to 2500 ml/day *to cool body and prevent dehydration*

Monitor vital signs, LOC, urinary output q2h to 4h

Collaborate with physician in using additional cooling measures when condition indicates

Expected Outcomes

Alert and responsive

Vital signs and urinary output are normal

▼ Risk for trauma related to potential for altered mental status

Remove potentially hazardous objects from patient's environment and arrange furniture *to prevent bumps or falls (e.g., bed in low position)*

Provide fluids for drinking and bathing that will not burn patient if spilled or used immediately

Assess muscle strength, mobility, and mental status q4h to 8h

Provide information about need to follow safety precautions *to decrease risk for trauma*

Assist patient with ambulating as needed

Instruct patient to call for assistance when getting out of bed; keep side rails up

Keep call light within easy reach of patient

Keep personal articles patient may wish to use frequently within easy reach

Encourage use of nonskid slippers

Provide night light

Expected Outcomes

Patient is not physically injured

Understands safety precautions

Calls for assistance when needed

Patient/Family Teaching

Explain basic concepts of the disease process, signs and symptoms of recurrence, and complications to report to physician

Explain that symptoms of disease *may* be reversible if medical regimen is followed

Explain that nervous symptoms are part of the disease process and will decrease with treatment

Provide reasons for physical and emotional changes

Stress importance of discussing feelings about changes

Explain the need for a calm, stable environment

Provide patient and family with information about eye protection for patient with Graves' disease

Teach name of medication, dosage, time and method of administration, purpose, side effects, and toxic effects

Discharge/Home Care Planning

Discuss with patient and family the need for the following:

Family support to minimize the patient's potential for emotional upset

Planning daily activities and scheduling rest periods

Promoting an environment conducive to sleep

Diet to maintain weight and minimize bowel hypermotility

Regulation of environmental temperature

Emphasize importance of planned rest periods of adequate duration

Encourage high-calorie, high-protein, high-carbohydrate, and high-vitamin B diet with increased fluids until discontinued by physician

Explain need to avoid taking over-the-counter medications without physician approval

Emphasize importance of ongoing outpatient care

Instruct patient to inform health caregivers (physician, dentist) of presence of disease and wear medical alert bracelet

■ HYPOPARATHYROIDISM

A rare condition characterized by a deficiency of para-thyroid hormone (PTH); usually the result of damage to the parathyroid glands during thyroid or other neck surgery, radiation treatment, or parathyroidectomy; the cause also may be idiopathic. The parathyroid glands fail to produce an adequate amount of PTH to maintain serum calcium levels. The reduced action of PTH on bone and kidney leads to hypocalcemia and hypophosphatemia. Pseudohypoparathyroidism *refers to target organ resistance or unresponsiveness to PTH, not PTH deficiency*

Assessment
Subjective Data

Headache

Tingling

Irritability

Anxiety

Painful cramping

Stiffness

Fatigue

Palpitations

Depression

Numbness and tingling around mouth, fingertips, and feet

Objective Data

Neurologic system

 Emotional lability

 Changes in LOC

 Psychosis

 Papilledema

 Paresthesia: lips, tongue, fingers, feet

 Cataracts caused by calcification of lens

 Tremor

 Hyperreflexia

 Positive Chvostek's and/or Trousseau's signs

 Tetany

 Seizures

Musculoskeletal system

 Stiffness

 Twitching spasms

 Weakness

 Fatigue

 Dental abnormalities

Cardiovascular system

 Heart failure caused by hypocalcemia

 Cardiac dysrhythmias

 ECG changes: prolonged Q-T interval, peaked or inverted T waves, heart block

Respiratory system

 Hoarseness

 Laryngeal stridor

Laryngeal edema
Laryngeal spasm
Gastrointestinal system
  Nausea, vomiting
  Diarrhea
Integumentary system
  Dystrophic, dry, scaly skin and nails
  Cutaneous pigmentation
  Thinning hair
  Alopecia
  Horizontal ridges on nails
  Brittle nails

DIAGNOSTIC TESTS
Blood
  Serum calcium decreased
  Serum phosphorus increased
  Serum bicarbonate decreased
  Serum parathyroid hormone decreased or absent
Urine
  Hypocalciuria
  Hypophosphaturia

POTENTIAL COMPLICATION
Renal calculi

MULTIDISCIPLINARY MANAGEMENT
THERAPEUTIC MANAGEMENT
Calcium supplementation
Vitamin D supplementation
If acute tetany, IV calcium administration
Maintain serum calcium levels at 8 to 9 mg/dl to prevent
  hypercalciuria and nephrolithiasis
Respiratory therapy as indicated

PATIENT PROBLEMS—NURSING DIAGNOSES/INTERVENTIONS

▼ Risk for injury related to potential for seizures or tetany resulting from hypocalcemia

Monitor vital signs and reflexes
Monitor cardiac function if ECG abnormalities are present
Collaborate with physician *to manage early symptoms of tetany* by administering and monitoring effectiveness of parenteral fluids and calcium
Administer calcium cautiously *to prevent hypotensive thrombophlebitis*
Administer vitamin D and calcium supplements as ordered
Do not administer phosphate binders within 1 to 2 hours before or after calcium supplements or other medications
Monitor serum levels of calcium and phosphorus
When patient is on bed rest, pad rails and keep bed in low position *to prevent risk of injury if seizure occurs*
If seizure activity occurs when patient is out of bed
  Assist patient to floor
  Remove potentially harmful objects

Assess patient for injury after seizure
Inform patient of seizure and reorient if necessary

Expected Outcomes
Has no injuries
Reflexes are normal
Vital signs are stable
Takes diet and medications as prescribed

▼ Decreased cardiac output related to alterations in myocardial conduction

Assess vital signs
Monitor fluid balance, especially when nausea or vomiting occurs
Monitor cardiac function: Q-T interval changes, abnormal T and P waves reflect hypocalcemic interference with conduction

Expected Outcomes
Maintains adequate cardiac output
Vital signs remain stable

▼ Ineffective airway clearance related to laryngeal edema or seizure activity

Keep suction equipment and oral airway at bedside at all times
Have tracheostomy tray, oxygen, and manual resuscitation equipment readily available

Laryngeal edema
Assess respiratory efforts and voice quality
Auscultate for subtle laryngeal stridor
Report early symptoms to physician and collaborate *to maintain open airway*
Instruct patient to inform nurse or physician at first sign of tightness in throat or SOB
Position patient to optimize airway clearance: keep head in neutral position, midline

Seizure
If seizure occurs
  Maintain airway
  Clear immediate area *to avoid patient's self-injury during seizure*
  Monitor BP, P, R, and neurologic signs; check after seizure and prn
  Note frequency, time, LOC, body parts involved, and length of seizure activity
Be prepared to collaborate with physician in treating status epilepticus: intubation, medications
Monitor patient during postictal period
Continue preseizure care as indicated

Expected Outcomes
Respiratory rate, rhythm, and depth are normal for patient
Lungs are clear on auscultation

▼ Activity intolerance related to muscular weakness and/or fatigue

Assess past activity patterns

Assess for changes in musculoskeletal symptoms

Assess response to activity

Note changes in BP, P, R

Stop activity when changes occur

Increase participation in small increments as tolerance increases

Teach patient to monitor response to activity and alter, stop, or ask for assistance when changes occur

Plan care with patient *to determine activities patient desires to accomplish; schedule assistance from others*

Balance activity with rest *to prevent fatigue*

Keep articles and needed supplies within easy reach *to decrease energy expenditure*

Expected Outcome

Activity level is increasing daily without dyspnea, tachycardia, or elevated BP; performs ADLs without effort

Additional Nursing Diagnoses to Consider

Altered thought processes related to neurologic changes as evidenced by emotional lability

Risk for impaired skin integrity related to dry, scaly skin and immobility

PATIENT/FAMILY TEACHING

Explain basic concepts of the disease process

Discuss reasons for physical and emotional changes

Teach patient to check for and report early signs of tetany

Tingling sensations

Muscle twitching

Painful tonic muscle spasms

Facial spasms, grimacing

Positive Chvostek's and/or Trousseau's signs

Change in respiratory effort

Teach significant other(s) to recognize patient's seizure activity and determine course of action to take

Avoid restraining or interrupting behavior

Observe and record behaviors exhibited before and during seizure

Notify physician immediately

Remove hazardous objects; clear area around patient *to prevent injury*

Stress importance of daily activity and exercise to tolerance and reporting increasing muscle weakness or fatigue

DISCHARGE/HOME CARE PLANNING

Discuss importance of maintaining safe home environment

Teach name of medication, dosage, time and method of administration, purpose, side effects, and toxic effects and that medication needs to be taken for remainder of life

Explain need to avoid taking over-the-counter medications without consulting physician

Emphasize importance of ongoing follow-up care

Instruct patient to maintain high-calcium, high-vitamin D, low-phosphorus diet and increased fluid intake

The patient and significant other(s) should verbalize their understanding of disease process and principles of home and follow-up care and demonstrate method to check for Chvostek's and Trousseau's signs

■ HYPERPARATHYROIDISM

Hyperparathyroidism is the hypersecretion of parathyroid hormone (PTH) by one or more of the parathyroid glands, which leads to a state of hypercalcemia and hyperphosphatemia. Hyperparathyroidism may be due to primary or secondary causes; in primary hyperparathyroidism, hyperplasia of the gland is usually caused by a benign adenoma; secondary hyperparathyroidism is the result of excessive compensatory production of PTH that develops from conditions such as renal disease that cause a decrease in calcium levels

ASSESSMENT

SUBJECTIVE DATA

Fatigue

Slow mentation

Mood changes

Memory loss

Depression

Easy fatigability

Painful joints

Difficulty urinating

OBJECTIVE DATA

Neurologic system

Apathy

Decreased cognitive function

Drowsiness

Hyperactive reflexes

Musculoskeletal system

Muscular weakness (proximal)

Bone pain with weight bearing

Arthralgia

Bone deformities, shortened stature

Fractures

Painful joints

Hearing loss

Cardiovascular system

Hypertension

ECG changes: broad T wave, short or prolonged Q-T interval, bradycardia

Gastrointestinal system

Abdominal discomfort

Polydipsia

Anorexia

Nausea and vomiting

Weight loss

Constipation

Renal system
   Polyuria
   Dysuria; difficulty urinating
   Dehydration
   Renal colic
   Uremia
   Calculi

DIAGNOSTIC TESTS

Blood
   Elevated PTH
   Elevated serum calcium
   Low serum phosphate
   Elevated serum chloride
   Low serum HCO_3
   Anemia
Urine
   Increased urine phosphate and urine calcium
   cAMP (cyclic adenosine monophosphatase) reflects
      concentration of biologically active PTH
Imaging
   CT scan: neck
   X-ray examination: subperiosteal bone resorption
   Ultrasound: enlarged parathyroid gland
Endocrine tests: elevated parathyroid hormone (PTH)
   radioimmunoassay

POTENTIAL COMPLICATIONS

Renal failure
Pathologic bone fractures
Gastric ulcers
Pancreatitis
Stupor
Coma

MULTIDISCIPLINARY MANAGEMENT

THERAPEUTIC MANAGEMENT

Fluid replacement: 2000 to 3000 ml/day
Parenteral hydration: usually with normal saline
Avoidance of thiazide diuretics
Medications
   Glucocorticoids
   Calcitonin
Treatment of choice: surgical removal of the gland(s)

PATIENT PROBLEMS—NURSING DIAGNOSES/INTERVENTIONS

▼ Risk for fluid volume deficit related to hypercalcemia

Monitor IV and oral fluid intake *to promote adequate hydration:* 1000 ml/hr for short period may be given initially IV, then oral fluids to 3000 ml/day unless contraindicated
Monitor vital signs, central venous pressure (CVP), and breath sounds q4h as indicative of fluid volume imbalance
Monitor intake, output, and electrolyte values q4h *to assess hydration status*

Monitor cardiac rhythm for changes in T waves or Q-T intervals indicative of hypercalcemia
Assess muscle strength and mobility q4h *to evaluate effects of hypercalcemia*
Assess reflexes q4h *to evaluate for hyperreflexia*
Administer medications as ordered and observe for adverse reactions: hypotension with IV phosphates, extravasation with IV mithramycin
Weigh patient daily (same time, scale, and clothing)
Assess skin condition and turgor q8h *to evaluate hydration status*
Maintain low-calcium, high-phosphorus diet
Collaborate with physician if any changes in physical condition are detected

Expected Outcomes
Vital signs are stable
Intake and output are balanced
Electrolytes are within normal range
Skin is warm and moist with good turgor

▼ Risk for trauma related to potential for pathologic fracture

Assess for pain; may be indicative of fracture
Maintain correct body alignment as indicated *to prevent fractures*
Assist patient with ambulation as needed *to prevent falls*
Provide aids to ambulation: walker, cane
Place articles that patient may require frequently within easy reach *to prevent injury*
Arrange environment simply; avoid unnecessary clutter
Provide night light *to facilitate mobility at night*
Place call bell within easy reach at all times
Instruct patient to call for assistance before getting out of bed
Keep bed in low position with side rails up *to prevent falls*
Assist with personal hygiene as needed
Use safety measures (e.g., jacket restraint) as necessary if patient is confused
Remove potentially hazardous objects from patient's environment

Expected Outcomes
No physical injury occurs
Verbalizes no pain or increasing discomfort

▼ Altered thought processes related to slow mentation, depression, and/or drowsiness

Assess LOC and orientation q4h
Provide a stable, calm, and nonstressful environment *to prevent impaired cognitive operations*
   Be consistent in timing and performance of activities and procedures
   Restrict patient's visitors as necessary
   Avoid frequent changing of personnel
   Prevent emotionally upsetting or confusing situations if possible

Plan care with patient as appropriate *to promote cognitive mentation*
Anticipate patient's needs
Reorient patient to environment as necessary
Explain procedures slowly and clearly; repeat prn
Encourage patient to take active role in care
Avoid administration of narcotics or sedatives if possible

Expected Outcome
Alert, oriented, and accomplishes self-care as planned

PATIENT/FAMILY TEACHING
Instruct patient/family regarding low-calcium, high-phosphorus diet
Explain basic concepts of the disease
Discuss reasons for physical and emotional changes
Teach name of medication, dosage, time and method of administration, purpose, side effects, and toxic effects
Explain need to avoid taking over-the-counter medications without consulting physician
Instruct patient to maintain increased fluid intake
Emphasize importance of ongoing outpatient follow-up

DISCHARGE/HOME CARE PLANNING
Discuss potential alterations to patient's home environment to facilitate ADLs and minimize potential for trauma
Discuss importance of avoiding risks
Stress importance of maintaining a safe environment to reduce risk of injury, need to report signs of fractures to physician

■ ADRENOCORTICAL INSUFFICIENCY
Hypofunction of the adrenal cortex; primary adrenocortical insufficiency, Addison's disease, results in a deficiency of mineralocorticoids and glucocorticoids; secondary insufficiency results in a deficiency of only glucocorticoids. Primary insufficiency is usually caused by autoimmune atrophy of the cortex. Onset can be insidious with appearance of signs and symptoms after 90% of adrenocortical tissue has been destroyed. Secondary insufficiency is usually a result of suppression of pituitary function by exogenous glucocorticoid, pituitary tumor, radiation, or removal of pituitary

ASSESSMENT
SUBJECTIVE DATA
Fatigue
Headache
Depression
Dizziness
Apathy
Nausea; loss of appetite
Decreased libido

OBJECTIVE DATA
Musculoskeletal system
   Weakness
   Muscular atrophy
   Muscle and joint pain
Cardiovascular system
   Orthostatic hypotension
   Postural dizziness
   Decreased tolerance of cold or stress
   Hypopyrexia
   Hypovolemia
   Palpitations
   Diaphoresis
Gastrointestinal system
   Weight loss
   Anorexia
   Vomiting
   Abdominal pain
   Salt craving
   Diarrhea
Integumentary system
   Hyperpigmentation; bronze coloration
   Decreased body hair
   Vitiligo
Reproductive system
   Diminished secondary sex characteristics (especially females)
   Amenorrhea
   Premature menopause

DIAGNOSTIC TESTS
Blood
   Decreased plasma cortisol
   Increased serum adrenocorticotropin (ACTH) in primary; decreased or normal in secondary
   Hyponatremia
   Hyperkalemia (primary insufficiency)
   Normokalemia (secondary insufficiency)
   Metabolic acidosis
   Increased plasma renin levels (primary)
   Decreased plasma aldosterone (primary)
Imaging: x-ray examination—small heart, adrenal calcification
Endocrine studies: ACTH stimulation test
   Cortisol response in primary
   Normal/intermediate cortisol response in secondary

POTENTIAL COMPLICATIONS
Adrenal (Addisonian) crisis: medical emergency involving intensification of symptoms of adrenal insufficiency; usually precipitated by infection, trauma, surgery, or excessive loss of body salts
Observations/findings in adrenal crisis include
   Profound weakness, fatigue
   Severe hypotension
   Nausea, vomiting
   Dehydration
   Hyperpyrexia
   Hyponatremia
   Hyperkalemia
   Severe pain: back, abdomen, extremities
   Severe headache
   Fever in presence of infection

Shock
Cardiac arrest
Renal shutdown
Azotemia
Coma
Death

MULTIDISCIPLINARY MANAGEMENT
THERAPEUTIC MANAGEMENT
IV fluid and sodium replacement
Glucocorticoids: corticosteroid replacement
Mineralocorticoids: fludrocortisone replacement
In crisis: vasopressors, plasma expanders, supportive
   therapy (e.g., oxygen)

PATIENT PROBLEMS—NURSING DIAGNOSES/INTERVENTIONS

▼Risk for injury related to potential for adrenal
crisis

Assess vital signs q4h and prn; report abnormal findings
   and severe hypotension to physician immediately *to*
   prevent vascular collapse
Monitor cardiac rhythm continuously if dysrhythmias
   occur *to recognize and treat hyperkalemia*
   (initially), then hypokalemia
Monitor intake and output q4h and prn; report output
   greater than intake; also watch for decreased urine
   output and water intoxication
Monitor neurologic status q4h; report increasing
   headache and confusion
Position patient *to promote cardiovascular and*
   respiratory function
Collaborate with physician if adrenal crisis develops to
   administer IV fluids, vasopressors, corticosteroids, and
   oxygen

Expected Outcomes
Vital signs are stable and within normal limits
Alert and oriented
Intake and output are balanced

▼Risk for injury related to potential for inability to
tolerate environmental stresses

Select quiet, nonstimulating room with noninfectious
   roommate *to minimize stress and prevent infection*
   caused by reduced inflammatory responsiveness
Avoid exposure to cold: provide extra blankets; have
   patient wear bed socks and use warm robe when out
   of bed *to avoid stress from cold*
Administer steroid replacement therapy as ordered
   Consult physician in situations in which increased
      doses of steroids may be indicated during periods
      of stress: surgery, infection, trauma
   Always administer steroid therapy on time; do not
      discontinue or reduce dose abruptly
   Medicate for pain or nausea as required

Encourage regular rest periods alternating with activity
Anticipate stressful situations and defuse if possible
Avoid discussing stress-producing topics; inform
   visitors
Monitor and restrict visitors if patient desires
Plan daily schedule with patient and avoid unexpected
   events *to prevent unnecessary stress*

Expected Outcomes
Does not develop adrenal crisis
Begins to tolerate environmental stresses as evidenced by
   increased interest and participation in daily schedule
   and desire for visitors
Discusses disease process and asks questions

▼Risk for infection related to inability of adrenal cortex to produce steroids

Monitor for signs and symptoms of infection; report if
   detected (upper respiratory infection [URI], urinary
   tract infection [UTI], wounds, IV, or infection sites) *to*
   confirm and treat infection early
Have patient turn, cough, and deep breathe q2h while on
   bed rest *to prevent respiratory infection from stasis*
Avoid unnecessary invasive procedures (urinary
   catheterization) *to prevent opportunity for infection*
Maintain sterile technique when caring for any skin
   lesions, tubes, drains, or IV lines *to prevent infection*
   caused by contamination
Culture suspicious wounds or secretions
Maintain optimal nutritional and fluid status
Avoid placing patient in room with other potentially
   infectious patients
Avoid having nursing personnel with infections care for
   patient
Screen visitors and restrict those with potential infections
   or instruct to wear mask and wash hands before
   visiting

Expected Outcomes
Temperature is within normal range
No other signs of infection (respiratory, renal, or skin)
   present

▼Activity intolerance related to fatigue and weakness

Assess present activity level
Allow patient to ambulate and increase strength at own
   pace; *muscle weakness will diminish as hormonal*
   replacement is achieved
Assist with ambulation as needed
Assist with active or perform passive range-of-motion
   (ROM) exercises while patient is on bed rest *to*
   maintain muscle tone
Provide patient with assistive devices: walker, cane, over-
   the-bed trapeze, side rails *to prevent injury caused by*
   weakness and fatigue
Anticipate need for help with ADLs: grooming, feeding,
   toileting

Restrict patient's activities to level of tolerance

Discontinue activity at first signs of intolerance: tachycardia, fatigue, dyspnea, cardiac dysrhythmias, drop in BP, complaints of vertigo

Expected Outcomes

Performs ADLs without evidence of fatigue or weakness

Vital signs remain within normal limits during ROM exercises, ambulation, and ADLs

▼ Pain related to metabolic imbalance (headache, back, extremity, abdomen)

Provide hormonal replacement (hydrocortisone, fludrocortisone) as ordered

Identify with help of patient the location, severity of pain, and factors that increase or decrease pain

Assess need for and administer pain medication as ordered

Explore with patient available measures to reduce or relieve pain: positioning, use of pillows for support, warm or cold compresses, manipulation or massage of body part or area

Monitor effectiveness of interventions at routine intervals

Provide distraction (conversation, visitors, reading materials, quiet music) *to divert attention away from pain*

Assist patient with developing pain management techniques: progressive relaxation, guided imagery

Expected Outcomes

Recognizes and reports onset of pain as a sign of adrenal crisis

Reports relief of pain

Exhibits relaxed body position and facial expression

Begins using relaxation techniques

▼ Fluid volume deficit related to inability of renal tubules to retain sodium and water

Monitor serum sodium levels q8h *to recognize and treat hyponatremia*

Measure intake and output q8h and prn; be aware of risk for decreased urine volume and renal shutdown

Weigh patient daily (same time, scale, and clothing); observe for weight loss

Recognize presyncopal signs of lightheadedness, postural dizziness, and visual changes

Encourage patient *to minimize postural dizziness* by changing positions gradually

Encourage fluid intake to 2500 ml/day or as ordered

Administer IV fluids and sodium replacement as ordered *to prevent dehydration*

Assess for signs and symptoms of hypovolemia or dehydration: poor skin turgor, weak pulses, tachycardia, thirst, low BP, cool skin, increased body temperature, dry mucous membranes, change in mental status

Report occurrence of any of these signs or symptoms to physician immediately

Administer antiemetics as ordered

Provide diet high in sodium *to compensate for sodium lost in renal tubules*

Expected Outcomes

Intake and output are balanced

Skin is moist with good turgor

Mucous membranes and tongue are moist

Weight is stable within ideal range for body build and height

PATIENT/FAMILY TEACHING

Explain basic concepts of the disease process and symptoms of recurrence requiring medication dosage adjustment

Explain reasons for physical and emotional changes

Teach name of medication, dosage, time and method of administration, side effects, and toxic effects

Explain that hormone therapy must be continued throughout lifetime

Demonstrate to patient and significant other(s) method of administering intramuscular (IM) injections

Teach signs and symptoms of hypercortisolism that may result from overtreatment with glucocorticoids

Explain need to avoid persons with infectious diseases (especially URIs)

DISCHARGE/HOME CARE PLANNING

Provide patient with medical alert bracelet/identification and discuss its importance

Discuss plans to carry emergency medication

Discuss methods to incorporate diet, exercise, and rest periods into lifestyle

Remind patient of the need for lifelong hormonal replacement without interruption

Patient or family demonstrates ability to self-inject IM (hydrocortisone) before discharge if patient cannot take oral replacement therapy

Discuss stressful situations that may require additional steroid replacement

Infection

Fever, persistent cough, influenza, or cold

Wounds that are red and swollen

Injury (auto or other accident)

Surgery

Instruct patient to inform all health care providers of disease

Explain need for high-sodium, low-potassium diet with plenty of fluids

Instruct that emergency IM medication must be carried at all times for use in times of stress (trauma, illness)

Explain need to avoid taking over-the-counter medications without consulting physician

■ CUSHING'S SYNDROME (HYPERCORTISOLISM)

Results from the overproduction of cortisol by the adrenal cortex

Cushing's disease is caused by the overproduction of ACTH by a pituitary adenoma. There are two categories

of hypercortisolism: ACTH dependent (involving hyper-secretion of ACTH by the pituitary gland) and ACTH in-dependent (involving hypersecretion of cortisol by the adrenal glands)

ACTH-dependent *sources include Cushing's disease, ectopic ACTH (secretion of ACTH by nonpituitary tumor), ectopic corticotropin-releasing hormone (CRH) syn-drome (secretion of CRH by nonhypothalamic tumor)*

ACTH-independent *sources include adrenal ade-noma, adrenal carcinoma, micronodular adrenal hy-perplasia, and exogenous steroid abuse*

ASSESSMENT
SUBJECTIVE DATA
Anxiety
Paranoia
Irritability
Depression
Mood swings
Memory loss
Insomnia
Decreased energy
Decreased libido
Backache
Suicidal

OBJECTIVE DATA
Neurologic system
 Impaired cognitive function
 Lability of moods
 Panic attacks
 Agitated depression
 Increased intraocular pressure
Musculoskeletal system
 Weight gain and distribution
  Central obesity (face, neck, trunk, abdomen)
  Supraclavicular fat pads
  Dorsocervical fat pad (buffalo hump)
  Facial rounding (moon face)
  Proximal muscle wasting (thin extremities)
 Weakness: unable to rise from squat or chair without assistance
 Activity intolerance
 Osteoporosis
 Fractures
 Vertebral compression
Cardiovascular system
 Hypertension
 Fluid retention with pitting edema
 Dependent edema
 Vascular fragility
  Increased bruisability
  Venipuncture difficulty
  Facial plethora
 CHF
Gastrointestinal system
 Polydipsia
 Polyphagia

Renal system
 Polyuria
 Hypercalciuria
 Calculi
Integumentary system
 Hyperpigmentation
 Impaired wound healing
 Abdominal striae
 Thin/coarse hair
 Thin, transparent, fragile skin
 Bruises (caused by loss of connective tissue)
 Cutaneous fungal infections (nails, chest, oral)
 Acne
Reproductive/sexual system
 (Findings resulting from androgen excess)
 Hirsutism (mostly facial)
 Oily facial skin, acne
 Thinning scalp hair/temporal baldness
 Oligomenorrhea
 Decreased libido
 Impotence

DIAGNOSTIC TESTS
Blood
 Cortisol increased; loss of diurnal variation
 ACTH increased or decreased
 Sodium increased
 Potassium decreased
 Glucose increased
 White blood cell count (WBC) increased
 Eosinophils decreased
 Calcium and phosphorus normal
 Metabolic alkalosis
Urine
 24-Hour urinary-free cortisol increased
 24-Hour 17-hydroxycorticosteroids (17-OHCS) increased
 Calcium increased
Endocrine tests
 CRH test: administration of CRH to stimulate hypothalamic-pituitary-adrenal (HPA) axis
  Normal response: increased ACTH and cortisol
  Cushing's disease: highly increased ACTH and cortisol
 Dexamethasone suppression test: administration of dexamethasone to suppress HPA axis
  Normal response: decreased ACTH and cortisol
  Cushing's disease: no change in ACTH, cortisol
 Inferior petrosal sinus sampling (IPSS): to localize source of ACTH secretion by comparing *central* ACTH levels at the petrosal sinuses (pituitary gland) with *peripheral* levels of ACTH (arm); comparisons can be made before and after administration of CRH
Imaging
 CT scans
  Sella: pituitary macroadenoma or enlarged sella caused by adrenal hyperplasia
  Adrenal: enlargement or tumor

X-rays
>   Skull: sellar abnormalities
>   Chest: cardiomegaly
Bone densitometry: osteoporosis
Inferior petrosal sinus sampling (IPSS)

POTENTIAL COMPLICATIONS
Pathologic fractures
CHF
Peptic ulcers
UTI
Renal calculi
Steroid psychosis
Suicide

MULTIDISCIPLINARY MANAGEMENT
THERAPEUTIC MANAGEMENT
Transsphenoid hypophysectomy (p. 446) of pituitary
>   adenoma
Medications
>   Adrenocorticolytic agents (chemical adrenalectomy):
>   mitotane (glucocorticoid replacement essential)
>   Adrenal enzyme inhibitors
>   Ketaconazole
>   Trilostane
>   Etomidate
>   Metapyrone
Adrenalectomy (p. 444)

PATIENT PROBLEMS—NURSING DIAGNOSES/INTERVENTIONS

▼ Body image disturbance related to musculo-skeletal, integumentary, and sexual/reproductive changes

Encourage patient/family to provide old photographs *to assist health caregivers in assessment of physical changes related to onset of disease*
Provide information about reversibility of symptoms with treatment
Discuss feelings related to physical changes with patient
Assist patient with identifying and developing personal strengths and coping mechanisms *for dealing with physical changes*
Assist with grooming *to enhance appearance:* personal hygiene, hair removal measures, attractive clothing
Respect patient's wishes for privacy
Be sensitive to needs
Set aside time each shift for active listening *to provide emotional support*
Consult mental health nursing specialist

Expected Outcomes
Discusses feelings about changes in appearance
Verbalizes knowledge that reversal of symptoms will occur with treatment
Performs daily hygiene

Enhances appearance through judicious use of cosmetics and clothing if appropriate

▼ Risk for infection related to impaired immune responses

Monitor temperature and for other signs or symptoms of infection q4h *to enable early recognition and treatment of infections*
Have patient turn, cough, and deep breathe q2h while on bed rest *to prevent respiratory infection*
Avoid unnecessary invasive procedures (urinary catheterization)
Use sterile technique when caring for any skin lesions, tubes, drains, or IV sites *to prevent contamination and subsequent infection*
Obtain culture for suspicious wound sites or secretions
Maintain optimal nutritional status
Avoid placing patient in room with other potentially infectious patient *to prevent contagious infection*
Avoid having personnel with URIs or other infections care for patient; monitor visitors for signs of infection and restrict as needed or explain importance of handwashing and wearing mask before visit *to prevent transmission of infection*

Expected Outcomes
Temperature within normal limits
No evidence of infection in integumentary, respiratory, and renal systems

▼ Risk for impaired skin integrity related to fragile capillaries and/or thinning of skin

Exercise caution with venipuncture; apply pressure to venipuncture sites *to prevent hematoma formation*
Assess for redness or skin breakdown q8h; if patient is on bed rest, assess q4h
Instruct patient regarding good skin hygiene routine
>   Use oil or lotion in bathwater; rinse and dry well
>   Avoid use of harsh soaps or rough towels
Use elbow and heel protectors and pull sheets
Place patient on pressure ulcer–prevention mattress or bed
Assist and encourage patient to change positions frequently; teach and assist with ROM exercises; ambulate as soon as possible; have patient avoid sitting position for longer than 1 hour
Instruct patient to exercise caution in ADLs *to avoid minor trauma*
Keep environment clear of obstructions *to minimize potential for accidental trauma*
Instruct patient to wear protective clothing (socks and shoes) *to prevent trauma*
Maintain optimal nutritional status

Expected Outcomes
Interruptions in skin integrity are avoided
Skin is intact and without evidence of redness
Venipuncture does not produce hematoma

▼ Activity intolerance related to musculoskeletal weakness caused by increased protein catabolism

Allow patient to move at own pace; use side rails and overhead trapeze

Identify patient's priorities for energy expenditure

Alternate activity with rest periods *to aid in increasing tolerance*

Assist with and provide aids to ambulation (walker, cane, wheelchair) as necessary

Anticipate need for help with daily activities: grooming, toileting, feeding; provide needed supplies within reach *to reduce energy expenditure*

Restrict activities to patient's level of tolerance

Discontinue activity at first signs of intolerance: tachycardia, dyspnea, fatigue

Encourage patient to increase activity as tolerance increases but to seek assistance at appearance of symptoms of intolerance

Expected Outcomes

Increases participation in self-care and activities daily

Reports decreased feelings of weakness and fatigue

▼ Altered thought processes related to impaired cognitive functioning and memory loss from hypercortisolism

Explain to patient and family the effects of hypercortisolism on cognitive function, mood, and memory and reversibility of symptoms with treatment

Evaluate past and present coping methods

Encourage discussion of feelings of loss of control

Discuss reactions that are out of proportion to event and methods for future coping

Explain that mood swings will abate with treatment

Teach and assist with relaxation techniques

Provide a stable, calm, and nonstressful environment *to avoid impaired cognitive operations*

    Be consistent in timing and performance of activities and procedures

    Restrict visitors as necessary

    Avoid frequent changing of personnel

    Prevent emotionally upsetting situations

Plan care with patient and anticipate needs *to promote cognitive functioning*

Provide diversional activities and materials of preference

Reorient patient to environment as needed

Explain procedures slowly and clearly; repeat prn

Assist with problem solving

Be aware of suicide potential

Expected Outcomes

Alert, oriented, and not confused about activities or health care procedures

Discusses feelings easily

Acknowledges inappropriate responses to situations and discusses plan for managing response

Practices relaxation techniques

Family recognizes effect of disease on patient's thought processes

▼ Fluid volume excess related to excessive secretion of cortisol causing sodium and water retention

Monitor electrolyte values and report abnormal findings to physician *to confirm and treat early signs of fluid overload*

Monitor intake and output q8h

Weigh patient daily (same time, scale, and clothing); report increasing weight

Avoid excessive fluid intake when patient is hypernatremic

Monitor ECG for abnormalities associated with electrolyte imbalances, usually hypernatremia and hypokalemia, *to allow early recognition and treatment of imbalances*

Monitor BP, P, and breath sounds q4h and report significant changes from patient's baseline

Assess dependent areas for edema: provide support and skin care for edematous areas, turn and reposition q2h

Maintain high-protein, high-potassium, low-sodium, decreased-calorie diet

Expected Outcomes

Vital signs and electrolytes are within normal range for patient;

Intake and output are balanced;

Weight is stabilized and within patient's normal limits;

No evidence of edema present

Additional Nursing Diagnoses to Consider

Altered nutrition: less than body requirements related to charged carbohydrate metabolism and hyperglycemia (see Diabetes mellitus, p. 426)

Risk for trauma related to potential for pathologic fractures

Risk for injury related to potential for hypertension

Risk for injury related to suicidal tendencies

PATIENT/FAMILY TEACHING

Explain the basic concepts of hypercortisolism and signs and symptoms with emphasis on emotional and cognitive impairments

Emphasize importance of family role in recognizing emotional and cognitive impairments, appropriate interventions in decision-making process, and provision of emotional support

Discuss reversibility of signs and symptoms with treatment of disease

Explain the need for dietary restrictions related to glucose intolerance, low fat resulting from lipolysis, and additional protein to promote catabolism

If indicated, provide information on adrenalectomy and prepare patient as needed

If indicated, provide information on pituitary radiation therapy

If indicated, provide information on transsphenoidal hypophysectomy

DISCHARGE/HOME CARE PLANNING
Provide Medical Alert bracelet/identification and discuss its importance

Explain importance of maintaining a safe environment and balancing activity and rest

Teach name of medication, dosage, time and method of administration, purpose, side effects, and toxic effects

Explain that glucocorticoids must not be discontinued or reduced without consulting physician

If glucocorticoid replacement is indicated, discuss the importance of compliance and the potential need for doubling the dosage during times of stress; see Adrenal insufficiency (p. 415)

Patient/significant other should demonstrate ability to self-inject glucocorticoid IM

Avoid taking over-the-counter medications unless physician has been consulted

Emphasize importance of ongoing outpatient care

Explain importance of maintaining safe environment and balancing activity and rest during convalescence

Discuss the need for continued emotional support during convalescence and maintenance of reasonable expectations to avoid emotional crises

Discuss the potential for suicidal tendencies with depression

For other information, contact:
National Adrenal Diseases Foundation
505 Northern Blvd., Suite 200
Great Neck, NY 11021
516-487-4992
web page: www.medhelp.netusa.net

■ HYPERALDOSTERONISM: PRIMARY ALDOSTERONISM
Overproduction of mineralocorticoids (aldosterone) by the adrenal cortex caused by benign adenoma, hyperplasia of the adrenal cortex, or, less commonly, by carcinoma. Excess aldosterone leads to sodium reabsorption and hypovolemia causing hypertension; can be asymptomatic with spontaneous hypokalemia. Potassium depletion can lead to muscle weakness, fatigue, and alterations in cardiac conductivity, resulting in metabolic alkalosis; most common cause is adrenal adenoma

ASSESSMENT
SUBJECTIVE DATA
Frontal headaches
Fatigue
Muscle weakness
Paresthesia
Frequent urination
In presence of marked alkalosis
  Positive Chrostek's sign
  Positive Trousseau's sign
May be asymptomatic

OBJECTIVE DATA
Neurologic system
  Muscle weakness
  Paralysis of arms and legs
  Autonomic dysfunction
Cardiovascular system
  Hypertension
  Postural hypotension without reflex tachycardia
  Increased pulse when squatting
  Cardiomegaly
Renal system
  Polyuria, especially nocturnal
  Polydipsia

DIAGNOSTIC TESTS
Blood
  Potassium, decreased
  Sodium, increased
  Aldosterone, increased
  Renin, decreased
Urine: potassium, increased
  Hypervolemia
  Metabolic alkalosis
Imaging/procedures
  ECG
    Depressed ST segments and T waves; appearance of U waves
  Premature ventricular contractions
  CT scan of adrenal glands to localize an adenoma to differentiate hyperplasia from adenoma
  Adrenal venous catheterization with measurement of plasma cortisol and aldosterone to distinguish between unilateral and bilateral source of hyperaldosteronism
Endocrine tests
  Plasma renin activity
  Renin stimulation test
  Captopril test

POTENTIAL COMPLICATIONS
Renal failure
Heart failure

MULTIDISCIPLINARY MANAGEMENT
THERAPEUTIC MANAGEMENT
Unilateral adrenalectomy for adenoma
Aldactone (spironolactone) 200 to 400 mg qd
Antihypertensive therapy
Amiloride (potassium-sparing diuretic) may be indicated
ACE inhibitor; enalapril (Vasotec)
Low-sodium, high-potassium diet

PATIENT PROBLEMS—NURSING DIAGNOSES/INTERVENTIONS

▼Fluid volume excess related to hypernatremia

Weigh patient daily (same time, scale, and clothing); report to physician if gain >0.5 kg occurs

Measure intake and output q8h

Maintain low-sodium diet *to decrease fluid retention*

Monitor serum sodium levels q8h

Monitor for signs and symptoms of fluid overload: pulmonary edema (dyspnea, orthopnea, crackles in lung fields) *to allow early recognition and treatment of overload*

Monitor chest x-ray examination results

Monitor vital signs q4h and prn; observe for increased pulse, development of S_3 gallop, and labored respirations

Notify physician of development or worsening of any of the preceding signs or symptoms

Monitor pedal pulses q4h

Monitor effectiveness and side effects of diuretics

Expected Outcomes

Vital signs and breath sounds are within normal limits for patient

Intake and output are balanced

▼ Altered tissue perfusion: cardiopulmonary, related to dysrhythmias caused by hypokalemia

Maintain high-potassium diet: avocado, apricots, bananas, meat, poultry, potatoes, milk

Monitor serum potassium levels q8h and prn

Monitor for signs and symptoms of hypokalemia
     ECG changes (ectopic beats, decreased T wave amplitude, increased U wave amplitude)
     Muscular weakness
     Neurologic impairments

Administer potassium supplements as ordered *to correct electrolyte imbalance*

Collaborate with physician to alter development of any of the preceding signs or symptoms

Anticipate need for assistance with ADLs *to prevent injury and fatigue*

Expected Outcomes

Plasma potassium levels are within normal range

ECG exhibits normal sinus rhythm

Exhibits no signs of muscle weakness or paresthesia

▼ Activity intolerance and risk for injury related to muscle weakness, fatigue, paresthesia, autonomic dysfunction, and/or tetany

Assess neuromuscular function q4h to 8h; report changes indicative of potential tetany; increasing weakness or paresthesia

Allow patient to move at own pace; encourage use of side rails and trapeze for assistance

Assist with and encourage ambulation if patient is able; instruct patient to call before getting out of bed *to prevent injury*

Keep call bell within reach at all times

Provide aids to ambulation such as a walker or cane

Encourage changing positions gradually

Anticipate postural hypotension when patient gets out of bed or chair; if it occurs, have patient sit or lie down with head lower than heart *to promote circulation to head and prevent a fall caused by dizziness associated with postural hypotension*

Keep bed in low position and side rails up

Use safety measures (padded siderails for tetany; oral airway) as needed

Remove potentially hazardous materials and objects from patient's environment

Expected Outcome

Patient sustains no physical injury

PATIENT/FAMILY TEACHING

Explain basic concepts of the disease; signs and symptoms of hypokalemia, hypernatremia, and hypocalcemia to report to physician

Teach name of medication, dosage, time and method of administration, purpose, side effects, and toxic effects; if on spironolactone, teach signs of hyperkalemia to report

Discuss and prepare for adrenalectomy if planned

Emphasize importance of regular exercise alternating with rest periods

Discuss and provide information about therapeutic low-sodium, high-potassium diet

DISCHARGE/HOME CARE PLANNING

Discuss importance of continuing medication until physician indicates otherwise

Explain need to avoid taking over-the-counter medications without consulting physician

Emphasize importance of ongoing outpatient care

Emphasize importance of obtaining and wearing medical alert bracelet

■ PHEOCHROMOCYTOMA

A chromaffin cell tumor of the adrenal medulla that secretes an excess of the catecholamines: epinephrine and norepinephrine; the increased catecholamines cause severe hypertension, increased metabolism, and hyperglycemia

ASSESSMENT
SUBJECTIVE DATA

Neurologic system
     Anxiety/nervousness
     Feelings of impending doom
     Headache
     Nausea
     Sweating
     Flushing sensation
     Palpitations
     Abdominal or chest pain
     Tremors

OBJECTIVE DATA

Episodes are intermittent and frequency can vary from every 2 months to 25 times per day

Cardiovascular system

    Persistent or paroxysmal hypertension

    Tachycardia

    Palpitations

    Flushing

    Excessive diaphoresis

Respiratory system: tachypnea

Gastrointestinal/nutritional system

    Hyperglycemia

    Vomiting

Renal system: decreased urine output

Integumentary system: sweating (excessive and inappropriate)

Precipitating risk factors

    Postural change

    Exercise

    Laughing

    Smoking

    Urination

    Change in body or environmental temperature

    Vasovagal stimulus

    Any event that increases pressure on tumor (pregnancy)

DIAGNOSTIC TESTS

Blood

    Serum catecholamines elevated

    Hyperglycemia

Urine: elevated urine catecholamines, metanephrines, and vanillymandelic acid (VMA)

Imaging: abdominal CT scan or magnetic resonance image (MRI) showing tumor location; positron emission tomography (PET) scan; MIBG (metaiodobenzylguanidine) scan

Endocrine tests: clonidine supression test—failure of serum catecholamines to "suppress" after clonidine administration

Glucagon stimulation test

POTENTIAL COMPLICATIONS

Weight loss

Hypertensive encephalopathy

Myocardial infarction

Heart failure

Renal failure

Cerebrovascular accident (CVA)

Myocarditis

Dysrhythmias

Surgical morbidity or mortality

MULTIDISCIPLINARY MANAGEMENT
THERAPEUTIC MANAGEMENT

Surgical removal of the tumor(s)

Medications

    α- And β-adrenergic blockers

    α-Methylparatyrosine

    Catecholamine synthesis inhibitors

PATIENT PROBLEMS—NURSING DIAGNOSES/INTERVENTIONS

▼ Altered tissue perfusion: cardiopulmonary and renal related to hypertensive episodes caused by hypervolemia from excess catecholamines

Remain with patient during episodes of hypertension

    Monitor BP and pulse electronically q10min to 15min; use same arm consistently

    Be prepared to administer antihypertensive medications

    Position patient with head of bed elevated 30 degrees to minimize effects on intracranial pressure (ICP)

    Perform neurologic checks; auscultate chest for heart sounds, rate, and rhythm

    Monitor breath sounds; observe for dyspnea

    Measure urinary output qh; report if <30 ml/hr

    Provide a calm, low-stimulus atmosphere

Monitor orthostatic vital signs; report if difference >10 mm Hg

Monitor intake and output q8h

Review events occurring before episode *to determine etiology;* discuss methods of avoiding precipitating events, if present, with patient

Keep bed dry and wrinkle free if patient is diaphoretic

Provide quiet environment for adequate periods of rest

To minimize risk of hypertensive crisis:

    Do not palpate abdomen

    Avoid constrictive clothing

    Restrict activity

    Prohibit tobacco use

    Elevate head of bed

    Avoid Valsalva maneuver

    Identify and avoid factors that trigger hypertensive episodes

Expected Outcomes

Orthostatic vital signs are within normal limits

Intake and output are balanced with output >30 ml/hr

Verbalizes no palpitation, nervousness, or headache

▼ Sleep pattern disturbance related to increased levels of circulating catecholamines

Assess usual sleep pattern and use of any aids

Provide sleep aids requested by patient: quiet music, warm drink

Discourage frequent daytime sleeping *to support regular sleep pattern at night*

Avoid intake of stimulants in diet

Assist patient with establishing a regular pattern of activity

Provide environment conducive to sleep: reduce lighting; close door to room; maintain quiet and privacy; maintain comfortable ambient temperature

Avoid disturbing patient at night for unnecessary procedures

Schedule treatments, procedures, and medications for daytime and evening hours when possible *to support regular sleep periods*

Expected Outcomes

Reports feeling well rested after sleep

Maintains energy throughout day without need for naps

▼ Altered nutrition: less than body requirements related to increased metabolism and/or nausea

Assess nutritional status and food preferences

Assist patient to select daily menus and incorporate basic food groups *to promote appropriate dietary intake*

Provide several small meals if patient prefers

Ask patient's family to bring favorite foods from home, within limits of therapeutic diet

Assist patient with arranging meal tray and feeding if necessary

Provide dietary consultation *to reduce tyramine-containing foods in diet*

Monitor blood glucose; report if elevated

Monitor food intake daily

Weigh patient daily (same time, scale, and clothing)

Expected Outcome

Weight is increasing toward level required for body build and height

PATIENT/FAMILY TEACHING

Explain basic concepts of the disease process and potential risk factors

Discuss methods for avoiding hypertensive episodes

Provide written information about diet and reduction of tyramine-containing foods

Teach name of medication, dosage, time and method of administration, purpose, side effects, and toxic effects

Refer to Adrenalectomy (p. 444) for preoperative patient teaching if indicated

DISCHARGE/HOME CARE PLANNING

Explain need to avoid taking over-the-counter medications without consulting physician

Emphasize importance of ongoing outpatient care

Provide information for obtaining medical alert bracelet and card as indicated

■ HYPOPITUITARISM

Decreased or absent secretion of one or more of the anterior pituitary gland hormones; causes are varied and may include malignancies, other tumors, infection, vascular changes, physical injury such as head trauma, postoperative surgical removal of a pituitary tumor, or x-ray therapy to pituitary or surrounding tissue; hypopituitarism may be a disorder of the pituitary gland itself, may be caused by insufficient pituitary stimulation by the hypothalamus, or may result secondary to other conditions such as Sheehan syndrome

ASSESSMENT*
SUBJECTIVE DATA
Decreased libido

Weakness

Fatigue

Sensitivity to cold

Dry, scaly, pale skin

Decreased perspiration

Decreased energy

Constipation

OBJECTIVE DATA
General

    Wrinkled, waxy skin

    Hypothermia

    Low BP

    Low serum glucose

Gonadotropin deficiency

    Incomplete secondary sex characteristics

    Amenorrhea, menstrual irregularities

    Breast and uterine atrophy

    Loss of axillary and pubic hair

    Vaginal dryness, dyspareunia

    Small soft testicles

    Impotence, infertility

    Loss of muscle tone

Growth hormone (GH) deficiency

    Short stature

    Lack of development of secondary sex characteristics

    High-pitched voice

Thyroid-stimulating hormone (TSH) deficiency: see Hypothyroidism (p. 405); symptoms will be less severe

ACTH deficiency

    See Adrenocortical insufficiency (p. 415)

    No hyperpigmentation

    No sodium depletion

Prolactin deficiency: absence of lactation in postpartum women

DIAGNOSTIC TESTS
Urine 17-ketosteroids, 17-hydroxycorticosteroids and plasma cortisol: decreased

Deficiency of serum cortisol, thyroxine, testosterone, estrogen, and growth hormone

Lack of compensatory increased levels of serum ACTH, TSH, follicle-stimulating hormone (FSH), leutinizing hormone (LH), and growth hormone (GH)

Insulin tolerance test

Imaging

    X-rays: skull-sellar changes

    CT scan or MRI of head

---

*Assessment depends on which hormonal deficiencies are present.

Ophthalmologic examination
    Visual field deficit
    Decreased acuity
Endocrine studies: ACTH and TRH-stimulation tests

POTENTIAL COMPLICATIONS
Deficiencies are usually not severe (see specific disease
    entities)
Advanced cases may be associated with hypoglycemia,
    hypothyroidism, hypothermia, and hypotension

MULTIDISCIPLINARY MANAGEMENT
THERAPEUTIC MANAGEMENT
Microsurgical excision of tumor as indicated
Hormone replacement
    Glucocorticoids
    Thyroxine
    Gonadal steroids
    Growth hormone in children
    Gonadotropin or GnRH therapy to restore fertility

PATIENT PROBLEMS—NURSING DIAGNOSES/INTERVENTIONS

▼ Body image disturbance related to changes in physical characteristics and capabilities

Encourage verbalization by patient of feelings related to
    physical changes
Assist patient with developing coping mechanisms *to
    deal with changes*
Reinforce patient's qualities that have positive effect on
    self-image
Answer questions and clarify misunderstandings
    regarding diagnosis and permanence or regression
    of changes
Assist patient with developing a plan *to incorporate any
    permanent changes into lifestyle*
Demonstrate acceptance of patient and encourage others
    to do the same
Reinforce behaviors that demonstrate acceptance of
    changes

Expected Outcomes
Verbalizes feelings about physical changes to others
Discusses strengths and sets realistic goals

▼ Altered sexuality patterns related to hormonal deficiencies

Maintain privacy and confidentiality
Explore with patient and/or significant other usual
    patterns of sexuality and how current diagnosis
    may affect these patterns
Encourage patient and/or significant other to explore
    alternatives to usual patterns that consider limitations
    of the disease
Initiate referral to appropriate personnel if patient desires

Explore with patient and/or significant other alternatives
    to becoming parents if appropriate

Expected Outcomes
Begins to discuss feelings about sexuality with partner
Verbalizes understanding of effect of diagnosis on sexual
    patterns
Accepts referral for counseling

PATIENT/FAMILY TEACHING
Provide and discuss information*
    Basic concepts of the disease process
    Name of medication, dosage, time and method of
        administration, purpose, side effects, and toxic effects

DISCHARGE/HOME CARE PLANNING
Explain importance of the following:
    Regular outpatient follow-up
    Need to avoid taking over-the-counter medications
        without consulting physician
    Importance of discussing feelings regarding body
        changes with significant other
Provide referral for sexual counseling when appropriate
Discuss alternatives to usual sexual patterns

■ DIABETES INSIPIDUS (DI)
*Disorder of hypothalamus or posterior pituitary that
results in insufficient synthesis or secretion of vasopressin
(antidiuretic hormone); consequently, the renal mechanism for concentration of urine is impaired and large
amounts of dilute urine are excreted; causes may include
head injury, neurosurgery, and hypothalamic tumors*

ASSESSMENT
SUBJECTIVE DATA
Unquenchable thirst
Preference for ice water or cold beverages

OBJECTIVE DATA
Gastrointestinal system
    Polydipsia
    Weight loss
    Dehydration
    Constipation
Renal system
    Polyuria to 10 L daily
    Frequency
    Nocturia
Integumentary system
    Dry skin and mucous membranes
    Poor turgor

DIAGNOSTIC TESTS
Blood
    Serum osmolality >300 mmol/kg
    Increased sodium

For further interventions, refer to specific disease entity.

Urine
  Specific gravity $\leq$1.005
  Osmolality $\leq$200 mmol/kg
Endocrine tests
  Dehydration test: water deprivation with close
    observation, paired measurements of serum and
    urine osmolality, and body weight measurements
    Normal response: urine becomes concentrated
    Central DI: urine remains dilute
    Nephrogenic DI: urine remains dilute
  Psychogenic polydipsia: urine becomes concentrated
    (response may be slight if polydipsia is severe)
Dehydration followed by vasopressin administration:
  Normal response: slight increase in urine
    concentration
  Central DI: urine becomes concentrated
  Nephrogenic DI: no change
  Psychogenic polydipsia: urine becomes concentrated
Imaging/other tests
  CT scan of head: hypothalamic/pituitary lesions
  Visual field testing: defects related to
    hypothalamic/pituitary lesions

POTENTIAL COMPLICATIONS
Severe dehydration
Hypotension
Shock

MULTIDISCIPLINARY MANAGEMENT
THERAPEUTIC MANAGEMENT
Vasopressin: lysine vasopressin nasal spray
DDAVP (desmopressin acetate)

PATIENT PROBLEM—NURSING DIAGNOSIS/INTERVENTIONS

▼ Fluid volume deficit related to inability of renal tubules to concentrate urine in absence/or response to vasopressin

Provide sufficient fluid of patient's preference *to maintain equal intake and output for 24 hours*
Supplement oral intake with IV fluids as ordered
Monitor intake and output q2h; notify physician if output is >200 ml/hr and urine specific gravity is <1.005
Weigh patient daily *to assess fluid loss*
Check urine and plasma osmolality daily
Assess for signs and symptoms of dehydration: tachycardia, poor skin turgor, weak pulses, low BP, cool skin, increased body temperature, dry mucous membranes, changes in mental status, and weight loss
Report occurrence of any of preceding signs or symptoms to physician and initiate medical orders without delay
Administer vasopressin replacement therapy as ordered and monitor effectiveness
  Observe for side effects: hypertension, chest pain, uterine cramps, and increased peristalsis

Monitor for overhydration: headache, changes in LOC, confusion
  Report abnormal findings
Monitor for hypoglycemia if taking chlorpropamide; give rapid-acting carbohydrates if symptoms present; report to physician

Expected Outcomes
Intake and output are balanced
Intake is $\leq$2500 ml/day
Output is $\leq$100 ml/hr
Urine specific gravity is within normal limits
Skin is moist with good turgor
Weight is within patient's normal range
Vital signs are within normal limits

PATIENT/FAMILY TEACHING
Explain basic concepts of disease process
Teach name of medication, purpose, time and method of administration, dosage, side effects, and toxic effects
  Demonstrate how to administer vasopressin; discuss special considerations related to intranasal administration
  Explain need to monitor for side effects and report if present
  Demonstrate how to monitor urine specific gravity, color of urine, and measure intake and output
  Discuss parameters for as-needed administration based on urine output
  Instruct to weigh daily; report loss or gain (symptoms of recurrence or fluid retention) indicating change needed in medication dosage
  Demonstrate injection method if medication is to be taken IM
Emphasize importance of maintaining fluid intake equal to output
Explain need to avoid liquids that may cause a diuretic effect: coffee, alcohol, tea
Provide information to obtain medical alert bracelet and card

DISCHARGE/HOME CARE PLANNING
Emphasize importance of medical alert bracelet
Emphasize importance of monitoring output
Ensure understanding related to intranasal administration of DDAVP
Emphasize importance of regular outpatient follow-up
Explain need to avoid taking over-the-counter medications without consulting physician

■ DIABETES MELLITUS
Diabetes mellitus is a disorder of hyperglycemia caused by inadequate insulin; cases of extreme insulin deficiency can lead to diabetic ketoacidosis; diabetes is characterized by polyuria, polyphagia, polydipsia, and weight loss accompanied by an elevation in plasma glucose

insulin-dependent diabetes mellitus (IDDM), type 1 diabetes: Deficiency of insulin production requiring exogenous administration of insulin to prevent acidosis; results from autoimmune destruction of beta cells

non–insulin-dependent diabetes mellitus (NIDDM); type 2 diabetes: Caused by impaired insulin secretion, insulin resistance, and elevated glucose production by liver; may be managed by diet, oral hypoglycemic drugs, or supplemental insulin (Table 7-2)

ASSESSMENT
SUBJECTIVE DATA
Hunger
Thirst
Nausea
Headaches
Halos seen around lights

OBJECTIVE DATA
Gastrointestinal system
  Polyphagia
  Polydipsia
  Weight loss
  Obesity
Renal system
  Polyuria
  Glycosuria
  Frequency
  Nocturia
Neurologic system
  Numbness and tingling of lower extremities
  Decreased sensations of pain and temperature in distal extremities
  Blurred vision
  Cataracts
Cardiovascular system
  Cold extremities
  Weak pedal pulse
Integumentary system
  Shiny skin and atrophic
  Hair loss on feet/toes
  Infections/ulcerations
  Dermopathy
Reproductive/sexual system
  Impotence
  Vaginal discharge
  Susceptibility to vaginal infections

DIAGNOSTIC TESTS AND COMPLICATIONS
See Table 7-2

MULTIDISCIPLINARY MANAGEMENT
THERAPEUTIC MANAGEMENT
See Tables 7-3, 7-4, and 7-5
Consultation
  Dietitian
  Certified diabetic educator

PATIENT PROBLEMS—NURSING DIAGNOSES/INTERVENTIONS

▼ Fluid volume deficit related to absent or deficient insulin secretion

Assess vital signs q4h to 8h
Monitor intake and output q8h; check urine for ketones when blood glucose is >250 mg/dL
Assess skin turgor, moisture and condition of mucous membranes q4h to 8h
Assess mental status
Monitor blood glucose before or 1 to 2 hours after administration of insulin or oral diabetes medication and meals, and/or according to a predetermined schedule
Begin teaching self-blood glucose monitoring (p. 433) *to promote self-care*
Monitor effectiveness of administration of insulin: usually rapid acting ordered initially, then intermediate acting in split doses with or without addition of rapid acting (type 1); may need to use 70/30 insulin if patient has difficulty mixing the two different types of insulin
Monitor effectiveness of oral diabetes medications if ordered for type 2 diabetes
Assess for continuing signs of hyperglycemia (see Assessment, p. 428)
Assess for signs of hypoglycemia; blood glucose ≤60 mg/dl, dizziness, lightheadedness, tachycardia, sweating, shakiness, or altered LOC
Provide noncaloric fluids (as well as those allowed on ADA diet) to 2500 ml/day *to replace fluid loss from polyuria*
Monitor electrolyte and CO_2 laboratory values *for metabolic imbalance and acidosis*
Assess for disturbances in electrolytes and CO_2 (see Table 1-3, p. 26); be aware of potassium shift as fluid volume deficit improves
Assist with ADLs when patient is unable to complete because of weakness or malaise
Encourage self-care as condition improves

Expected Outcomes
Vital signs are stable and within normal limits for patient
Intake and output are balanced
Ketones are not present in urine; skin is moist with good turgor
Blood glucose, electrolytes, and CO_2 are within normal range
Patient completes ADLs without expression of fatigue or weakness

▼ Altered nutrition: less than body requirements related to diabetes mellitus, generally type 1 diabetes

Assess dietary intake pattern, preferences, and nutritional status

Table 7-2	**Two Major Classifications of Diabetes Mellitus**	
	Type 1 Insulin-Dependent Diabetes Mellitus (IDDM)	**Type 2 Non–Insulin-Dependent Diabetes Mellitus (NIDDM)**
DEFINITION		
Onset	<30 yr usually	>40 yr usually
Etiology	Beta cell destruction occurs resulting from autoimmune response in genetically disposed persons	Interaction between heredity and environmental factors such as obesity, diet, and lifestyle; impaired insulin secretion; insulin resistance and elevated glucose production
Insulin levels	Low to absent	Low, normal, or high
ASSESSMENT		
Observations/findings	Polyuria	May be asymptomatic in early stage
	Polydipsia	Fatigue
	Polyphagia	Polyuria
	Weakness	Polydipsia
	Fatigue	Vision changes
	Malaise	Tingling, numbness of extremeties
	Weight loss	Slow healing of cuts
	Irritability	Skin infections or pruritus
	See Diabetic ketoacidosis (DKA) (p. 436)	Drowsiness
		See Hyperosmolar hyperglycemic nonketotic syndrome (HHNS) (p. 438)
DIAGNOSTIC TESTS		
Fasting plasma glucose on at least two occasions	>140 mg/dl	>140 mg/dl
Oral glucose tolerance or random plasma glucose	>200 mg/dl	>200 mg/dl
Blood insulin level	Trace to absent	Normal to high
Serum osmolality	>300 mOsm/kg	>300 mOsm/kg
Plasma C-peptide	Absent	Low, normal, or high
Urine: ketonuria	Present in DKA	Usually absent, even in HHNS
COMPLICATIONS		
Acute	Diabetic ketoacidosis (DKA)	Hyperosmolar hyperglycemic nonketotic syndrome (HHNS)
Long-term	Microangiopathies	Microangiopathies
	Retinopathy	Retinopathy
	Nephropathy	Nephropathy
	Neuropathy	Neuropathy
	Macroangiopathies	Macroangiopathies
	Cardiovascular	Cardiovascular
	Cerebrovascular	Cerebrovascular
	Peripheral vascular	Peripheral vascular
THERAPEUTIC MANAGEMENT		
	Insulin preparations	Diet of 45%-55% carbohydrates, 30% fat, and 10%-20% protein
	Diet of 45%-55% carbohydrates, 30% fat, and 10%-20% protein	Oral diabetes drugs and/or insulin
	Regular exercise program	Regular exercise program
	Self-monitoring of blood glucose	Self-monitoring of blood glucose
	Treatment of existing complications	Treatment of existing complications

Table 7-3	Before Exercise Snacks	
Exercise*	**Blood Sugar Levels (mg/dL)**	**Snack**
SHORT WORKOUT		
Easy pace	Less than 100	1 fruit or
Examples: 15 min		1 bread or
Slow walk		4 oz milk
Easy swim		
Stretching	More than 100	No food needed
MODERATE WORKOUT		
Moderate pace	Less than 100	1 meat, 1 bread,
Examples: 25-40 min		and 1 fruit
Brisk walk		
Stationary bike	100-160	1 milk, 1 fruit,
Heavy housework		or 1 bread
Aerobics class	161-300	No food needed
LONG WORKOUT		
Hard pace	Less than 100	1 meat, 2 breads,
Examples: 1 hour		and 1 milk or
Shoveling snow		1 fruit
Skiing		
	100-160	1 meat, 1 bread, and 1 milk or 1 fruit
	161-225	1 milk and 1 bread
	226-300	1 milk or 1 bread

More food may need to be added than is given here if patient works out 2 to 4 hours after taking short-acting insulin. In 2 to 4 hours this type of insulin peaks, and blood sugar can drop very quickly. Always carry carbohydrate snacks during exercise.

Provide dietary consultation *to instruct patient and family on ADA diet*

Assist patient to select daily menu based on ADA program prescribed; reinforce correct choices

Monitor daily food intake; assist at mealtimes when necessary because of fatigue; provide exchanges for carbohydrate foods not taken at mealtimes

Provide relaxing environment and allow ample time for meals; visiting by support person may be helpful

Stress importance of regular meal and snack times, consistency of carbohydrate content of meals from day to day; remind not to save food for another meal

Collaborate with physician *to determine exercise program to meet patient's needs and lifestyle*
  Begin first phase of program
  Assist patient to check need for additional carbohydrates before exercise through use of self-blood glucose monitoring (see Table 7-3)

Weigh patient daily (same time, scale, and clothing)

Monitor blood glucose control

Monitor compliance with diabetes treatment regimen

Expected Outcomes

Maintains stable weight or increases weight to that predetermined for body build

Selects menus based on ordered ADA diet and eats meals and snacks as scheduled

Monitors blood glucose

Determines type of snack and takes extra snack if needed before exercise

▼ Altered nutrition: more than body requirements related to diabetes mellitus, usually type 2 diabetes

Assess baseline nutritional status: height, weight, activity level, eating patterns and preferences, psychosocial concerns related to overeating

Teach relationship of obesity to diabetes

Provide dietary consultation for calculation of caloric requirements and instruction of ordered ADA diet

Assist to select daily menu based on calorie-controlled, low-fat, ADA diet; reinforce correct choices; encourage patient to include foods high in complex carbohydrates (may assist in weight reduction)

Assess daily food intake; replace carbohydrate foods not eaten if taking insulin and sulfonylureas

Weigh patient daily (same time, scale, and clothing); give positive reinforcement for any weight reduction

Monitor blood glucose before meals or 2 hours after meals and at bedtime or before bedtime snack

Collaborate with physician to determine exercise program to meet patient's needs and lifestyle; begin first phase of program

Discuss need to monitor dietary intake and exercise level using a diary *to increase accuracy*

Explore with patient ways to increase activity in daily routine and add exercise program

Refer to diabetic and/or weight reduction support group *to provide additional support and guidance*

Expected Outcomes

Verbalizes understanding of relationship of obesity to insulin resistance

Verbalizes understanding of relationship between exercise, insulin resistance, and blood glucose levels

Selects meals and snacks based on prescribed mealplan

Monitors blood glucose as scheduled

Keeps diary of dietary intake and exercise level

Identifies persons or groups to use for support in making lifestyle changes

▼ Risk for impaired skin integrity related to reduced circulation and reduced sensation in distal extremities

Instruct patient on risks of injury and potential for poor wound healing

Encourage patient to not walk barefoot *to minimize trauma to feet*

Minimize environmental hazards

Table 7-4	**Insulins**						
Preparation	Brand	Mfr	Species	Onset (hrs)	Peak (hrs)	Effective Duration (hrs)	Route
Insulin analogue (lispro)	Humalog	Lilly	Human	<0.25	1	2.5-4	SC
Insulin injection regular (R)	Humulin R	Lilly	Human	0.5	2-4	6-8	SC,
	Novolin R	Novo-Nordisk	Human	0.5	2-4	6-8	IM, IV
Insulin isophane suspension (NPH) and regular insulin (R)	Humulin 70/30	Lilly	Human	See NPH and Regular	See NPH and Regular	See NPH and Regular	SC
	Humulin 50/50	Lilly	Human				
	Novolin 70/30	Novo-Nordisk	Human				
Insulin isophane suspension (NPH)	Humulin N	Lilly	Human	2-3	6-8	10-12	SC
	Novolin N	Novo-Nordisk	Human	2-3	6-8	10-12	
Insulin zinc suspension (L) (Lente)	Humulin L	Lilly	Human	2-4	6-10	12-16	SC
	Novolin L	Novo-Nordisk	Human	2-4	6-10	12-16	
Insulin extended zinc suspension (U) Ultralente	Humulin U	Lilly	Human	4-6	8-16	24-30	SC

NOTE: *All of above insulins are human insulins of recombinant DNA origin. Although animal-source insulins are still being manufactured, beef and beef-pork insulins were unavailable as of January, 1999; pork insulins are being phased out as well. Both Lilly and Novo-Nordisk manufacture purified pork insulins, which are more antigenic and may have slightly longer action times.*

Keep skin clean and dry; encourage patient to inspect skin regularly

Observe for early signs and symptoms of infection

Emphasize importance of foot care

Encourage measures to increase circulation to extremities

Expected Outcomes

Verbalizes understanding of risks and measures to avoid injury

Practices routine skin and foot care

Recognizes and reports early signs of skin lesions and infections

Additional Nursing Diagnoses to Consider

Altered tissue perfusion: peripheral, cardiopulmonary, cerebral, or renal related to microangiopathy or macroangiopathy

Sensory/perceptual alterations: visual related to retinopathy

Sexual dysfunction related to neuropathy

Risk for infection related to hyperglycemia

Noncompliance with therapeutic plan related to difficulty of integration of therapy into lifestyle

Altered urinary elimination related to nephropathy

PATIENT/FAMILY TEACHING

DISEASE PROCESS

Explain diabetes mellitus specific to patient's type

Discuss control of disease through managing interrelationship among diet, maintenance of ideal weight, exercise program, medication if ordered, and blood glucose changes

Refer to associations

American Diabetes Association

1701 North Beauregard St.

Alexandria, VA 22311

(800) ADA-DISC

web page: www.diabetes.org

Canadian Diabetes Association

15 Toronto Street, Suite 800

Toronto, Ontario M5C 2E3

(800) 226-8464

web page: www.diabetes.ca

PREVENTION OF COMPLICATIONS

Acute

Hypoglycemia (p. 440)

Diabetic ketoacidosis (DKA) (p. 436)

Long-term

Microangiopathies, macroangiopathies

Stress that maintaining control of blood glucose decreases the risk of or minimizes these complications

Discuss need to do the following:

Have regular medical follow-ups to check for early symptoms of complications: cardiovascular, peripheral, renal, neural, or visual

Visit ophthalmologist, dentist, and podiatrist regularly

Maintain control of BP and cholesterol

Stop smoking and tobacco use

Follow prescribed diet, exercise program; take medications; follow personal hygiene guidelines; and consult physician at first appearance of symptoms

Teach symptoms of long-term complications to report to physician

DIET THERAPY

Reinforce explanation of prescribed ADA and/or calorie-controlled diet

Assist with setting realistic goals for weight reduction

Have patient and/or significant other calculate dietary needs and choose a sample diet, cutting down on foods with high cholesterol, saturated fats, salt, sugar, and alcohol

Discuss need to eat meals and snacks at regularly scheduled times every day when taking insulin and sulfonylureas

Stress need to determine additional food requirements before exercise if taking insulin or sulfonylreas, by testing blood glucose before exercise

Stress that diet may be the only means of control for patients with type 2 diabetes, but that medications may be necessary during periods of acute stress or illness and as diabetes progresses

Provide written material, names of personnel, and telephone numbers for questions and assistance with meal planning

EXERCISE

Discuss need for exercise program: may decrease insulin resistance, assist with weight loss, improve blood glucose control

Collaborate with physician and patient to plan program of progressive exercise based on patient's interest and physical condition

Give details specifying exercise type, intensity, frequency, duration, warm-up and cool-down time

Teach pulse-taking to monitor target heart rate (HR) during exercise

Explain need to exercise 1 to 2 hours after meal and how to adjust dietary intake as required

Avoid exercise at peak insulin times

Check blood glucose before and 30 minutes after exercise

MEDICATIONS
Insulin

Provide information to patient and/or significant other about insulin

Action of the type(s) of insulin to be used

Time of day patient may expect to have reaction (peak action time; Table 7-4)

Factors that precipitate hypoglycemia reaction

Incorrect, increased dosage of insulin

Decreased food intake (especially carbohydrates) or delayed meals or snacks

Increased exercise or unusual exercise without increased food intake

Alcohol intake

Factors that may precipitate hyperglycemia:

Stress

Other disease processes

Cold

Influenza

Nausea, vomiting

Infection

Dosage may be adjusted according to blood test results as ordered by physician

Provide information about care of insulin and equipment

Keep opened insulin vial currently in use at room temperature and away from sunlight; keep no longer than 1 month or expiration date

Have at least one unopened vial stored in refrigerator, not in freezer

Observe expiration dates

Be sure units marked on syringe are understood; ½ ml or ³⁄₁₀ ml syringes are in increments of 1 unit/line; 1 ml syringes are in increments of 2 units per line for some brands

Handle syringe and needles carefully to avoid self-puncture

Maintain sterility of needle and syringe during procedure

Dispose of syringe and needle in safe container after use

Discuss use of special equipment for patients with vision problems or other handicaps

Provide instructions for preparing injection

Mix insulin by gently rolling bottle between hands; do not shake vigorously

Clean bottle top with alcohol

Read label and check expiration date

Insert air and withdraw exact dose

Withdraw rapid-acting insulin first if mixing two types of insulin (avoids contaminating rapid-acting with longer-acting insulin)

Read label again and check dosage

Discuss information about injection site with patient and significant other

Most rapid absorption occurs first in abdomen, then arms, and then thighs

Importance of rotating site of injection with each dose of insulin to prevent atrophy, fibrosis, lipodystrophy, and decreased insulin absorption

Rotation within one body area (e.g., abdomen) for a specific time of day is recommended to ensure same rate of absorption from day to day (Fig. 7-2)

Have patient and/or significant other demonstrate injection technique

Select site for injection

Hold syringe filled with correct insulin dosage as one would hold a pencil or a dart

Insert needle at 90-degree angle (45 degree if little subcutaneous tissue) and quickly push into tissue up to hub of needle

Inject medication

Withdraw needle; do not rub

Record any insulin dose changes, supplements, or decrements in diary

Table 7-5	**Oral Medications Used to Treat Type 2 Diabetes**			
Generic/Brand	Duration	Dosage Range	Side Effects	Metabolism
FIRST-GENERATION SULFONYLUREAS				
Tolbutamide (Orinase)	6-8 hr	1-2 g qd or bid	Dizziness, fatigue, hypoglycemia, malaise, headache	Dosing adjustment in hepatic impairment
Tolazamide (Tolinase)	10-24 hr	100-250 mg qd with breakfast	See above	
Chlorpropamide (Diabinese)	36-72 hr	100-500 mg qd	See above plus disulfiram reaction with alcohol, SIADH, prolonged hypoglycemia	Dosage adjustment in kidney and liver impairment
SECOND-GENERATION SULFONYLUREAS				
Glimepiride (Amaryl)	24 hr (t½ = 5-9 hr)	1-4 mg qd with meals (max = 8 mg)	Headache, nausea, dizziness, hematologic	Dosage adjustment in renal impairment; liver—no data
Glipizide (Glucotrol, Glucotrol XL)	24 hr (t½ = 2-4 hr)	2.5-20 mg qd 30 min before meals (20 mg bid or 40 mg/day max) (XL = 20 mg max)	Hypoglycemia, dermatologic effects	Dosage adjustment in liver impairment
Glyburide (DiaBeta, Micronase, Glynase)	24 hr (t½ = 5-16 hr)	1.25-20 mg qd or bid (Glynase 0.75-12 mg qd or bid)	See above	Dosage adjustment in liver and renal impairment
BIGUANIDES				
Metformin (Glucophage)	6 hr (t½ = 6 hr)	Initial 500 mg qd or bid with meals; (max = 2550 mg) titrate every 1-2 weeks	Nausea, diarrhea, rare lactic acidosis; discontinue if hypoxic (pneumonia, MI, surgery) or kidney dye studies	Dosage adjustment in renal failure; liver—can enhance toxicity

NOTE: First-generation sulfonylureas are rarely used today. Chlorpropamide should not be used in elderly patients. Acarbose: If taking a sulfonylurea, meglitinide, or insulin with acarbose, treat hypoglycemia only with glucose, fructose, or lactose (there will be delayed breakdown/absorption of sucrose and starches).

Oral Diabetes Medications

Provide information about medications when ordered: action and dosage (Table 7-5)

Monitor blood glucose level at specific times; times and frequency will vary according to type of medication, degree of diabetes control, and physician preference

Instruct patient to take sulfonylureas 30 minutes before meal(s)

Take meglitinides 0 to 30 minutes before meal(s)

Take metformin with meal(s)

Take alpha-glucosidase inhibitors with first bite of meal(s)

Take thiazalidinediones with meal unless otherwise indicated

Observe for hypoglycemic reactions (p. 438); if patient is taking sulfonylureas, meglitinides, or insulin; at first sign of reaction, test blood glucose if possible and treat if <60 mg/dL with 15 g simple carbohydrate; when blood glucose is >70 mg/dL, eat a small snack containing starch and protein if next meal or snack is more than 45 to 60 minutes away

Discuss other side or toxic effects to report to physician or nurse if they last longer than 24 to 48 hours

GI upset

Weakness

Paresthesia

Headache

Tinnitus

Skin rash

Jaundice

Photosensitivity

Intolerance to alcohol

Prolonged action of sedatives and hypnotics

Discuss planning for pregnancy with physician; notify immediately if pregnancy is suspected; oral agents need to be stopped before pregnancy occurs and

Table 7-5	**Oral Medications Used to Treat Type 2 Diabetes**—cont'd			
Generic/Brand	Duration	Dosage Range	Side Effects	Metabolism
ALPHA-GLUCOSIDASE INHIBITOR				
Acarbose (Precose)		Initial 25 mg qd to tid with first bite of meal; (≤60 kg max = 50 mg tid; >60 kg max—100 mg tid) titrate by 25 mg at a time each week	Flatulence, diarrhea, abdominal pain	Not recommended for GI problems, severe renal dysfunction
THIAZOLIDINEDIONES				
Troglitazone (Rezulin)	$t\frac{1}{2}$ = 16-34 hr; see effects in 2-8 wks	200-600 mg qd with breakfast; titrate every 2-4 wks	Nausea, vomiting, diarrhea, hepato-toxicity (check AST, ALT levels—d/c if 3× normal upper limit)	Do not use with liver impairment; may decrease effectiveness or oral contraceptives
Rosiglitazone maleate (Avandia)	$t\frac{1}{2}$ = 3-4 hrs	4-8 mg qd in single or divided dose with or without food	Mild anemia; slight weight gain	Resumption of ovulation in premenopausal women; monitor liver enzymes as a precaution; use with caution in patients with edema
MEGLITINIDES				
Repaglinide (Prandin)	$t\frac{1}{2}$ = 1 hr	0.25-4 mg 0-30 min before each meal (max = 16 mg/day)	Hypoglycemia, respiratory, GI, headache	Use cautiously in liver impairment; no adjustment required in kidney impairment unless hemodialysis

another regimen instituted in collaboration with physician

SELF-MONITORING OF BLOOD GLUCOSE (SMBG) AND URINE TESTING

Give reasons for testing blood glucose
  Maintain control of blood sugar
  Reduce risk of complications
Instruct about blood glucose test
  Frequency of testing: usually before meals or fasting and 2 hours after meals, before exercise, 30 minutes after exercise, and to monitor any symptoms of hypoglycemia or hyperglycemia
  Use only sides of fingertips; produces less discomfort (Fig. 7-3) (rotation of sites is unnecessary—patients will alter sites if discomfort occurs at a particular site)
  Advise that ring finger may have better blood flow

Methods to increase blood flow
  Wash hands with soap and warm water
  Hold hand below heart level and "milk" finger (Fig. 7-4)
Avoid using alcohol or povidone-iodine to clean finger because these products can interfere with test results
Dry hands well before beginning procedure
Procedure for using lancet and finger puncture device
Procedures to use glucose sensor meter (OneTouch by Life Scan, Accucheck by Boehringer Mannheim, etc.) or reagent strips
Care and storage of supplies and equipment
Disposal of lancets in safe container
Teach about urine testing
  Urine testing for sugar is an indirect method of assessing high *blood* glucose; positive urine glucose indicates serum glucose is above renal threshold for glucose (about 180 mg/dL in the average person)

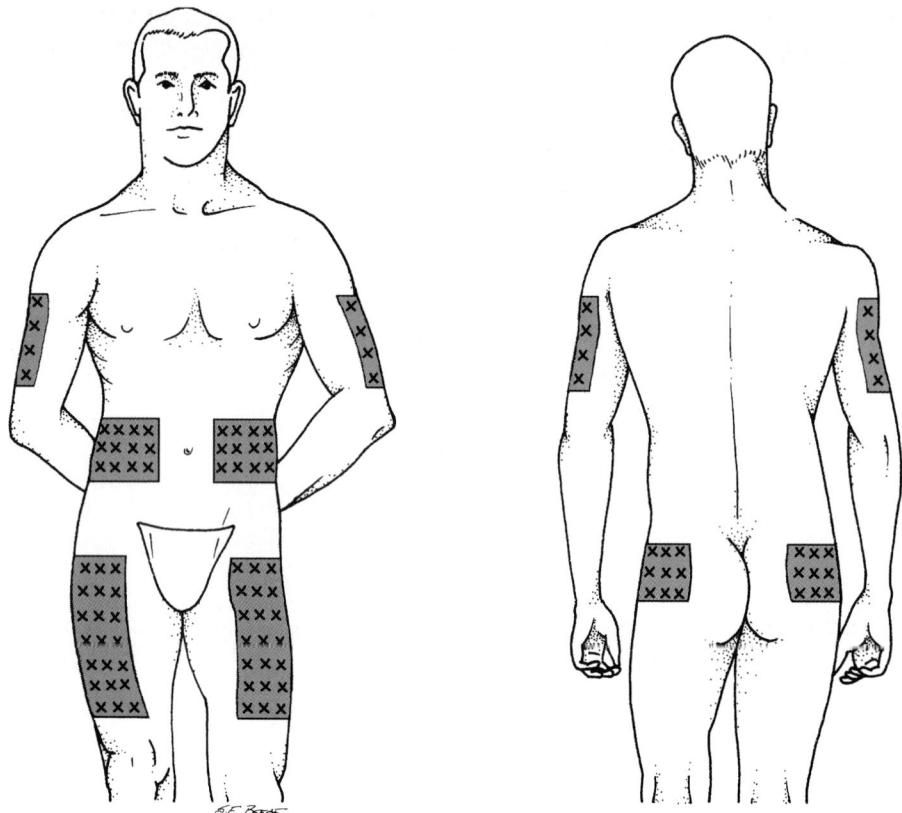

Fig. 7-2   Rotation of insulin injection sites.

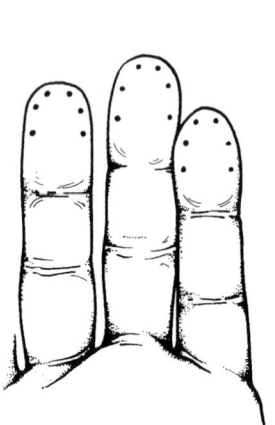

Fig. 7-3   Finger puncture sites.

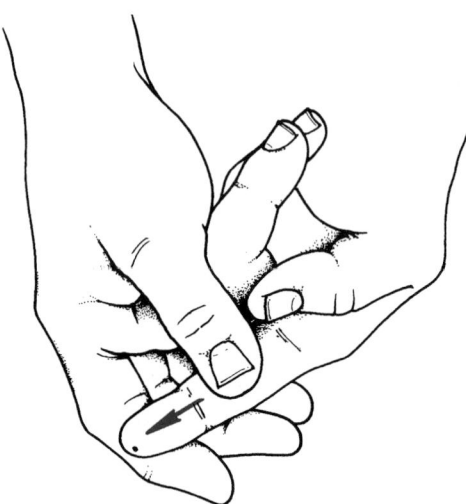

Fig. 7-4   Milking finger to obtain blood sample.

Test urine before meals and bedtime; follow directions
  on container

Test urine for ketones when experiencing symptoms
  of hyperglycemia or when blood glucose is >250 to
  300 mg/dL; urine ketones indicate high serum
  keytones. Ketones are a by-product of fat
  metabolism, which occurs in excess when
  inadequate insulin is available. Report presence of
  ketones to physician or follow predetermined plan

Store urine testing supplies in dry, cool, dark area away
  from oral medications and children

Record test results in diary; note that salicylates or
  ascorbic acid may give false-positive readings

Explain changes to make in diet, exercise, or medication
  as a result of blood glucose or urine test as determined
  through collaboration with physician

Discuss need to maintain diary to record
  Blood glucose/urine test
  Medication and dosage
  Exercise level
  Symptoms and interventions taken
  Missed meals or unusual situations

PERSONAL CARE AND HYGIENE
Skin, Foot, and Leg Care
Provide information about daily care
    Bathe or shower daily using tepid water; check standing water temperature with thermometer, especially when bathing feet
    Rinse and dry gently but thoroughly
    Apply lubricating lotion; do not leave skin wet; do not apply lotion between toes
    Inspect body, especially feet, legs, and groin area daily; use mirror if unable to see any body part (e.g., bottoms of feet)
    Check for cuts, cracks, blisters, corns, boils, calluses, or ingrown toenails; if found, wash with mild soap and water, dry well, and cover with dry, sterile dressing; notify physician if healing does not begin in 24 hours; avoid adhesive tape on feet
    Have podiatrist treat corns and calluses; do not use home remedies or devices (no "bathroom surgery")
    Keep feet dry; wear clean stockings (preferably cotton) daily
    Avoid tight-fitting stockings with elastic
    Wear well-fitting shoes; break in new shoes gradually; alternate two pairs of shoes; do not go barefoot
    Avoid one position for long periods; walk in place if standing, stand and walk if sitting
    Do not use hot water bottles or heating pads on extremities
    Wear protective clothing for warmth or sunshielding
    Use sunscreen, at least SPF 15, daily
    Use gloves when exposed to harsh soaps, gardening, using an oven, or handling heavy, rough objects
    Be cautious when using machinery, tools, and equipment

Care of Teeth
Teach patient about care of teeth
Brush teeth or clean dentures after sleep and meals and before bedtime
    Floss at least daily
    Examine mouth for irritated gums, bleeding, or ulcers; report those that do not begin to heal in 24 hours
    Schedule periodic dental examinations (usually every 6 months)
    Tell dentist about condition and check with primary physician before scheduling extensive dental care or surgery

Care of Eyes
Explain that eye changes (vision) may be temporary if blood sugar is high
Instruct patient to schedule yearly examinations with an optometrist or ophthalmologist to screen for eye changes related to diabetes
    Notify physician or ophthalmologist immediately if new onset of floaters, dramatic vision changes
Teach patient to maintain blood glucose in target range
Teach patient how to control hypertension

Urinary and Genital Care
Instruct patient in urinary and genital care
    Drink six to eight glasses of water/day (unless CHF, CRF, etc.)
    Be aware of symptoms of urinary tract and vaginal infections and immediately report to physician or provider so that treatment can be instituted
    Caffeine may elevate blood glucose, but small amounts generally have no significant effects
    Alcohol can be used in many patients using proper precautions and common sense; it should be avoided in patients with neuropathy
    Urinate as soon as urge is felt
    Wash and dry genital area daily
        Inspect for irritation and discharge
        Shower rather than take tub baths
            Wear underwear and/or pantyhose with cotton crotch
            Avoid douching except as ordered by physician
        Report to physician if following symptoms occur
            Urinary tract
                Difficulty in voiding
                Burning or pain on voiding
                Incontinence
            Vagina
                Heavy discharge
                Itching

SICK DAY RULES
Explain that any illness, injury, or change in body functioning causes a release of hormones that will increase the availability of glucose, elevating blood glucose levels
Advise that a change in medication and food is often required during these periods
Discuss signs and symptoms of illness, injury, or functional change that may require changes in medication or food
    Injuries
    Infections, including cold or influenza
    Nausea, vomiting
    Diarrhea
    Burns
    Dental care
    Surgery
    Pregnancy
    Emotional stress
    Unaccustomed physical activities: periodic jogging, swimming, tennis
Instruct to increase testing of blood glucose and urine ketones to every 4 hours or at least 4 times/day during this period
Explain importance of notifying physician when
    Blood glucose is 300 mg/dl and/or urine test results with ketones two successive times
    Experiencing an inability to take oral food/fluids
    Experiencing unusual thirst, increased urination, weakness, warm/flushed skin, blurred vision, or nausea and vomiting

Explain need to have blood glucose and urine ketone record sheet nearby to report to physician when experiencing symptoms of high blood glucose

Instruct about action to take

Drink a cup or more of broth, tea, nondiet carbonated drinks, gelatin, fluids with electrolytes, or water if able to eat. If unable eat, drink calorie-containing fluids, preferably caffeine-free, in amounts of about 15 g carbohydrate per hour or according to sick-day plan developed by dietitian, nurse educator, or physician

May need more insulin than normal during illness

Type 1 patients *always* need insulin, even when unable to eat. Less insulin than normal may be needed if vomiting or diarrhea occurs

Type 2 patients should generally take their medications unless nauseated and unable to tolerate; call physician if blood glucose >250 mg/dL two times in a row

Supplemental insulin may be needed; a predetermined sick day plan may be developed by physician or nurse educator; *or* patient should call provider for insulin doses during illness (NOTE: even more insulin is necessary if ketones are present)

TRAVEL TIPS

Discuss need to prepare for travel

Inform physician

Obtain immunizations well before trip when needed

Have generic prescriptions in duplicate for

Diabetic medications

Syringes and needles

Other medications needed

Carry letter describing condition and treatment (in language of country visiting if possible)

Buy and break in new shoes well in advance

Obtain medical identification bracelet or necklace if patient normally carries a card

Arrange for special meals while enroute

Importance of carrying supply of insulin and syringes in hand luggage to prevent exposure to extreme temperature and prevent loss

Need to take supply of emergency medication to prevent or treat possible travel complications

Importance of carrying emergency carbohydrates and a protein and carbohydrate snack or meal

Method to alter meal, medication, and activity needs when traveling to other time zones to maintain schedule

Where to obtain emergency assistance and how to express needs in language of country visited

International Association for Medical Assistance to Travellers: Directory of English Speaking Physicians Throughout the World

417 Center St.

Lewiston, NY 14092

(716) 754-4883

Importance of traveling with a companion when possible

■ DIABETIC KETOACIDOSIS

Acute complication of diabetes mellitus, characterized by marked hyperglycemia, metabolic acidosis, increased plasma ketones, and severe dehydration

ASSESSMENT

See Table 7-6

MULTIDISCIPLINARY MANAGEMENT
THERAPEUTIC MANAGEMENT

Regular insulin IV bolus or continuous drip (5 to 10 units/hr)

Rapid IV hydration: 1 L/hr (approximately 6 L); normal saline initially, then as serum glucose decreases to ≤250 to 300 mg/dL, glucose is added to hypotonic saline

IV potassium replacement unless potassium is >6.0 mEq/L or patient is anuric

ABG or total CO_2 content

Monitor ECG for signs of MI, hypokalemia, or hyperkalemia

Insulin subcutaneously after ketones have cleared

Treatment of infection if underlying cause

PATIENT PROBLEMS—NURSING DIAGNOSES/INTERVENTIONS

▼ Fluid volume deficit related to osmotic diuresis

Weigh on admission and every 6 to 12 hours

Monitor fluid intake and output every 1 to 2 hours

Monitor IV fluids; maintain large-bore IV *for rapid infusion*

Administer plasma expanders as ordered

Assess BP, P, R, mental status every 1 to 2 hours

Take temperature (rectal initially) every 8 hours

Test blood glucose (lab or finger stick) every 1 to 2 hours

Monitor urine ketones every voiding

Assess for signs and symptoms of hypovolemic shock, which include tachycardia; low BP; weak, thready pulses; cool skin; increased body temperature; change in LOC

Administer insulin; usually given IV initially

Rinse container and tubing with insulin per facility policy before adding prescribed dose *because insulin adheres to equipment and correct dosage may not be given*

Note that smaller doses are usually required for HHNS than for DKA

Assess effectiveness; report glucose level that continues to rise, falls too rapidly (>75 mg/dL per hour), or is 120 mg/dl or lower

Monitor plasma K^+, Na^+, Cl^-, HCO_3^-, serum ketones, arterial pH, Pco_2, Po_2, plasma phosphate, Mg^{2+}, Ca^{2+} as ordered

Assist with obtaining CBC, BUN, creatinine, urinalysis, cultures, chest x-ray to rule out infection

Do not stop insulin infusion unless subcutaneous insulin has been administered at least 30 to 60 minutes before

(IV insulin has a half-life of ~5 minutes; *stopping the infusion before a subcutaneous depot starts to absorb can precipitate a recurrence of DKA*)

Monitor ECG for changes; report signs of hyperkalemia or hypokalemia

Monitor electrolyte and ABG levels; report changes and collaborate with physician *to adjust fluids, electrolytes, and HCO₃*

Monitor CVP if inserted

Insert nasogastric tube as indicated; monitor gastric drainage

Insert indwelling urinary catheter to straight drainage *for exact assessment of output* if patient is incontinent or unable to void

    Monitor intake and output qh and report output <30 ml/hr

    Assess skin temperature, turgor, and capillary refill q2h

Expected Outcomes

Vital signs are stable

Intake and output are balanced

Skin turgor is good

Electrolytes are within normal range

Blood glucose is within patient's normal range

▼ Risk for injury related to confusion

Assess for presence of neurologic/sensory deficits and respiratory status q1h to 2h

Maintain oral airway at bedside

Keep bed in low position with padded side rails in up position when patient is on bed rest

Remove potentially hazardous materials from patient's immediate environment *to protect from injury*

Place articles frequently required within easy reach

Instruct patient to call for assistance before getting out of bed

Keep call light within patient's reach at all times

Be aware that patient's vision may be affected: assist with feeding, personal hygiene, and ambulation as needed

Maintain orientation to environment: assess LOC and orientation q4h and prn

Provide stimulation in the environment *that will assist in maintaining orientation:* pictures from home, calendar, clock, radio, television

Address patient by name; review day, date, time, and current events with patient as necessary

Expected Outcomes

Sustains no physical injuries

Remains alert and oriented to time, place, and person

▼ Risk for infection related to increased susceptibility caused by hyperglycemia and protein depletion

Monitor for signs of infection

    Sites of invasive lines

    Skin

    Respiratory and urinary systems

Maintain sterility of invasive sites (e.g., IV, catheters) *to avoid introducing infection;* provide meticulous, sterile daily care and rotate sites according to policy

Obtain culture for suspicious drainage *to identify source of infection and provide early treatment*

Teach and assist patient to turn, cough, and deep breathe q2h *to prevent respiratory infections*

Provide oral fluids to 2000 ml/day when allowed

Provide oral care q4h to 6h

Use aids *to promote circulation and prevent skin breakdown* when on bed rest

Expected Outcomes

Temperature is within normal range

Cultures show no evidence of infection

Lungs and urine are clear

Skin is dry and clear with good turgor

▼ Altered nutrition: less than body requirements related to deficiency of insulin

Assess diet and fluid intake before DKA

Provide ADA diet and fluids as prescribed

Weigh q12h initially, then daily

Administer insulin; assess effectiveness by monitoring blood glucose; collaborate with physician to adjust medication dosage as necessary

Determine possible factors leading to DKA episode

    Not taking insulin

    Not observing diet

    Reduction in level of exercise

    Infection, stress, injury

Expected Outcomes

Weight is stable or increasing toward predetermined level for patient's build

Blood glucose level is within normal limits

PATIENT/FAMILY TEACHING

Explain factors that predispose patient to ketoacidosis: omitted doses of insulin, failure to respond to increased need for insulin resulting from infectious process, stress, or pregnancy

Discuss early signs of DKA

    Blood glucose 300 mg/dl or more

    Ketones in urine

    Unusual thirst

    Increased urination

    Hot, dry, flushed skin

    Elevated temperature

    Drowsiness

    Nausea, vomiting, abdominal pain, diarrhea

    Deep-sighing respirations and "fruity" odor to breath

DISCHARGE/HOME CARE PLANNING

Teach action to take when early signs of DKA are noted

Continue diet and fluids; take calorie-containing liquid if unable to tolerate food

Table 7-6	**Comparison of Diabetic Ketoacidosis (DKA), Hyperosmolar Hyperglycemic Nonketotic Syndrome (HHNS), and Hypoglycemia**

Observations/Findings

Assessment	DKA	HHNS	Hypoglycemia
Diabetes type	Usually type 1	Usually type 2	Type 1 or type 2
Onset	Hours to days	Hours to days	Minutes to 1 hr
Renal	Polyuria; osmotic diuresis Dehydration	Polyuria; osmotic diuresis Dehydration	
Neurologic	Lethargy, drowsiness Paresthesia Slowed reflexes Confusion, disorientation Coma	Unconsciousness (50%) Drowsiness Confusion, disorientation Seizures Hemiplegia (reversible) coma	Inability to concentrate Headache Lack of coordination Numbness, tingling lips, tongue Weakness, anxiety Yawning, slurred speech Hyperreflexia, seizure activity Nighttime: nightmares, sleep-walking, restlessness
Respiratory	Tachypnea, Kussmaul's respiration Sweet, fruity breath	Tachypnea with shallow respiration	
Cardiovascular	Hypotension Tachycardia Weak pulses Warm to hot, dry, flushed skin Decreased turgor	Orthostatic hypotension Tachycardia Weak pulses Warm to hot, dry, flushed skin Decreased turgor Hypothermia or hyperthermia	Tachycardia Cool, clammy skin
GI	Polydipsia Nausea, vomiting Abdominal pain	Polydipsia Gastric distention Hematemesis	Hunger Nausea
Risk factors	Undiagnosed type 1 Insufficient insulin dosage	Undiagnosed type 2 Insufficient oral agent	Excessive insulin dosage, missed meal(s)

ARDS, *Adult respiratory distress syndrome;* DIC, *disseminated intravascular coagulation.*

Have patient take insulin as scheduled or change dosage as indicated by tests, with physician approval, using algorithms
Test urine for presence of ketones
Notify physician if signs of DKA persist
Increase frequency of blood glucose testing when glucose >250 mg/dl
Assess knowledge of diabetes mellitus and management through patient's maintenance of ADA diet, exercise program, diabetic medication schedule, and blood glucose monitoring
See Diabetes mellitus (p. 426)

■ HYPEROSMOLAR HYPERGLYCEMIC NONKETOTIC SYNDROME (HHNS)

Metabolic disorder in which the blood sugar level is extremely elevated, increasing the serum osmolality and resulting in hypertonic dehydration; serum ketosis is usually not present

ASSESSMENT
See Table 7-6

MULTIDISCIPLINARY MANAGEMENT
THERAPEUTIC MANAGEMENT
IV insulin administration
IV fluid administration, plasma expanders as needed
Electrolyte replacement as needed
    Electrolyte, blood glucose, and bicarbonate levels
    ABG or total CO_2 content
    Monitor ECG
    CVP monitoring as needed
    Insulin subcutaneously

PATIENT PROBLEM—NURSING DIAGNOSIS/INTERVENTIONS

▼ Altered tissue perfusion: peripheral, cerebral, cardiopulmonary related to risk of thromboembolism and DIC

Table 7-6	**Comparison of Diabetic Ketoacidosis (DKA), Hyperosmolar Hyperglycemic Nonketotic Syndrome (HHNS), and Hypoglycemia**—cont'd		
	Observations/Findings		
Assessment	**DKA**	**HHNS**	**Hypoglycemia**
Risk factors—cont'd	Stressors: surgery, injury, infection Pregnancy	Stressors: surgery, injury, infections Enteral or parenteral feedings Drugs such as cortico-steroids, diuretics Dialysis Nursing home resident	Unplanned increase in exercise without adequate food to compensate Vomiting or diarrhea Alcohol intake
DIAGNOSTIC TESTS **Blood**			
Serum glucose	<600 mg/dL	>800 mg/dL	<60 mg/dL
Serum osmolality	Usually <350 mOsm/Kg	Usually >350 mOsm/Kg	
Plasma ketones	>4+ in 1:1 dilution	<2+ in 1:1 dilution	
pH	Low	Normal	
Sodium	Normal or low	Normal or high	
Potassium	High, normal, or low	High, normal, or low	
bicarbonate	0-15 mEq/L	>16 mEq/L	
Urine			
Urine ketones	Strongly positive	Not present	Not present
POTENTIAL COMPLICATIONS			
	Shock Renal failure Cerebral edema Death occurs if untreated	DIC Acute renal failure ARDS Shock Seizures Coma Death occurs if untreated	Seizure Shock Delirium Unconsciousness Permanent brain damage is rare

Assess peripheral pulses q2h to 4h; report decreased amplitude or absence

Assess for thrombosis in extremities: vein—pain, swelling, tenderness, or Homan's sign; artery—mottling, cyanosis, coolness with delayed capillary refill

Teach active or assist with passive ROM exercises for extremities

Apply thromboembolic or pneumatic alternating-pressure stockings to lower extremities; remove daily, check condition of legs, then reapply

Assess vital signs, heart and breath sounds, and neurologic status q2h to 4h

　Assist patient to assume position *to enhance cardiopulmonary effort*

　Instruct patient to report sudden headache, chest pain, numbness in extremities

Expected Outcomes

Vital signs are stable and within normal limits

Reports no headache, chest pain, numbness, or pain in extremities

Alert and oriented

OTHER RELEVANT NURSING DIAGNOSIS

See Diabetic ketoacidosis for the following diagnoses (p. 436)

　Fluid volume deficit related to osmotic diuresis

　Risk for injury related to confusion and/or seizures

　Risk for infection related to increased susceptibility resulting from hyperglycemia and protein depletion

　Altered nutrition: less than body requirements related to deficiency of effective insulin

See Diabetes mellitus for altered nutrition: more than body requirements related to DM, usually type 2 (p. 429)

PATIENT/FAMILY TEACHING

Explain factors that predispose to HHNS

    Not taking oral hypoglycemic or insulin dosage

    Stressors: surgery, dental care, infections

    Pregnancy

Review symptoms of HHNS; see Assessment, see Table 7-6

DISCHARGE/HOME CARE PLANNING

Assess knowledge of diabetes mellitus management including patient maintenance of ADA diet, adherence to exercise program, monitoring blood glucose, and taking of medications; see Diabetes mellitus (p. 426)

Teach action to take when signs of HHNC are noticed

    Continue diet and fluids; take broth or tea if unable to tolerate food

    Increase frequency of blood glucose monitoring

    Take oral hypoglycemic as scheduled or change dosage as indicated by tests, with physician approval, using algorithm

    Explain that insulin may be required during these situations

    Notify physician if no improvement occurs

■ HYPOGLYCEMIA

In persons with diabetes treated with glucose-lowering agents such as insulin, sulfonylureas, or meglitinides, hypoglycemia is defined as blood glucose level <60 to 70 mg/dL

In persons without diabetes, hypoglycemia is generally defined as blood glucose <40 to 50 mg/dL. It may be caused by insulinoma, genetic or acquired conditions compromising hepatic glucose production (fasting hypoglycemia), or abnormal kinetics of glucose absorp-tion or insulin secretion in the fed state (reactive hypoglycemia)

ASSESSMENT

See Table 7-6

MULTIDISCIPLINARY MANAGEMENT

THERAPEUTIC MANAGEMENT

In persons with diabetes of insulinoma:

    15 g fast-acting oral carbohydrate

    If NPO or unable to swallow, IV glucose (15 to 25 g) or glucagon injection SQ or IM (0.5 mg if <age 5; 1 mg if >age 5)

In persons with reactive hypoglycemia:

    Treatment with starch/protein snack (not simple carbohydrate)

    Avoid by eating several small meals/day that contain protein and avoiding simple carbohydrate

Consultation with dietitian and Certified Diabetes Educator

PATIENT PROBLEMS—NURSING DIAGNOSES/INTERVENTIONS

▼ Risk for injury related to insufficient glucose to meet metabolic needs

Hypoglycemia requires immediate intervention

Obtain blood glucose stat and be prepared to administer 50% glucose IV if patient is a diabetic and is unable to swallow; then initiate IV of $D_{10}W$ if prescribed *or*

Obtain capillary blood glucose and give 15 g of fast-acting carbohydrate if patient is exhibiting early signs of hypoglycemia

Continue to monitor blood glucose q15min to 30min; slow-acting carbohydrate and protein may be needed *to prevent recurrence of symptoms;* give starch/protein snack when blood glucose >60 to 70 mg/dL if next meal or snack is more than 45 to 60 minutes away

Determine predisposing factor if possible

    Decreased food intake

    Increased exercise

    Wrong medication, dosage

Consult physician, if no predisposing factor determined, for adjustment of insulin or oral hypoglycemic dosage

Monitor neurologic and cardiovascular status q30min until fully reactive

Expected Outcomes

Blood glucose within normal limits after ingestion of carbohydrate or IV glucose

Vital signs are stable

Patient is alert and oriented

▼ Risk for trauma related to rapid onset of altered level of consciousness and seizure activity resulting from hypoglycemia

Keep oral airway and suction equipment at bedside

If indicated, pad side rails if patient is on bed rest *to prevent trauma* in the event of seizure activity

Assist to floor if patient is out of bed and remove hazardous objects *to reduce potential for trauma*

Note time, frequency, LOC, body parts involved, and length of seizure activity

Obtain stat blood glucose and administer IV glucose as ordered

Notify physician of seizure

Suction oropharynx as needed *to prevent aspiration*

Assess for injury

Check pulse and pupils

Reorient as necessary

Determine predisposing factor for hypoglycemia

Expected Outcome

Patient is free of injury

PATIENT/FAMILY TEACHING

Involve significant other and/or peers from work setting in teaching because patient may not be able to intervene

Teach factors that may precipitate hypoglycemia: too much insulin or oral hypoglycemic medication, increased length of time between meals, omission of a meal or snack, unplanned exercise, extremely stressful situation

DISCHARGE/HOME CARE PLANNING
Discuss symptoms of hypoglycemia
  Mild: shaky, sweaty, cool feeling, irritable, weak, headache, nervous, drowsy, or personality changes
  Moderate: nausea, faintness, disorientation, confusion
  Severe: coma, seizure
Explain that hypoglycemic reactions may be different for each person; any unusual feeling or symptom must be considered; each patient must become familiar with initial reactions
Identify the time reactions will most likely occur; relate to type of insulin prescribed (see Table 7-4)
Teach action to take immediately: take 15 g of quick-acting carbohydrate
Instruct patient that when driving or engaging in activities requiring clear thought processes and decision making, test blood glucose before and every 1 to 2 hours

The following foods contain 10 g of quick-acting carbohydrate:

Orange juice	4 oz
Apple juice	4 oz
Grape juice	3 oz
Coca-Cola	4 oz
Ginger ale	4 oz
7-Up	4 oz
Corn syrup	2 tsp
Honey	2 tsp
Granulated sugar	2½ tsp
Grape jam	2 tsp
Gumdrops	10 small
Jelly beans	6
Hard candy such as Life Savers	5 or 6
Dextrose tablets as labeled	
Glucose gel, amount indicated on label	

Emphasize importance of always carrying fast-acting sugar and keeping juice or other drink for easy, quick accessibility
Check blood glucose 15 minutes after taking quick-acting carbohydrates; retreat if BG <60 mg/dL. When blood glucose >60 to 70 mg/dL, take slowly digested carbohydrate such as milk, cottage cheese, bread, or peanut butter after response to fast-acting carbohydrate to offset a secondary reaction, if next meal or snack is more than 45 to 60 minutes away
Demonstrate method for glucagon administration to significant other; discuss action and dosage
Use if patient clamps mouth shut, is unable to swallow, or is unconscious; patient should respond in 15 minutes
Have patient eat a small meal after responding; may be nauseated; if so, drink carbohydrate-containing liquids until nausea subsides and able to tolerate solid food

Follow physician's orders if no response
  Telephone physician any time severe hypoglycemic episode has occurred
  Give another injection of glucagon if ordered
  Telephone for emergency help or take patient to emergency room of hospital
Explain need to observe closely for further reaction for the next few hours; avoid strenuous activity during this time
Determine predisposing factor after reaction is controlled
Emphasize importance of reporting frequent reactions to physician as directed
  Give time of onset and duration until response to care
  Discuss predisposing factor if known
Discuss prevention and early care
  Always carry some form of quick-acting carbohydrate (see list); take when first symptoms appear
  Eat correct diet regularly; remember between-meal nourishment when included in diet
  Test blood regularly for glucose; anticipate probable reactions
  Be aware of greater-than-normal activity or emotional stress; follow physician's directions to either notify physician, increase food intake, or decrease dosage of insulin
Discuss prevention of dosage errors
  Double check insulin dose before injecting
  Always wear medical alert band or chain and carry diabetic identification card
  Determine ability to manage diabetes mellitus

■ THYROIDECTOMY
Surgical removal of part (lobectomy, isthmusectomy, near total [95%] or total thyroidectomy) to treat hyperthyroidism (Graves' disease, toxic adenoma, nodules, carcinoma); usually reserved for patient who does not respond to medical treatment with antithyroid drugs; treatment of choice to remove very large goiters or those compressing surrounding structures; may also be performed for men and women of child-bearing age for whom radiation exposure is unwanted, patients allergic to antithyroid medications, and pregnant women

PREOPERATIVE ASSESSMENT
Assess baseline vital signs
Assess voice quality and ability to swallow

POSTOPERATIVE ASSESSMENT
SUBJECTIVE DATA
Hypocalcemia
  Numbness
  Tingling
Incisional pain
  Intensity
  Location
Choking sensation
Dysphagia

Complaints of heaviness or fullness in throat
Complaints of tight dressing

OBJECTIVE DATA
Increasing hoarseness
Change in tone or pitch of voice, vocal cord paralysis
Weak voice, inability to speak
Hypocalcemia
    Twitching
    Spasm, tetany
    Positive Chvostek's or Trousseau's sign
Incision site
    Color (redness)
    Pain: guarding of site
    Edema
    Drainage, bleeding
Airway
    Stridorous respirations
    Retraction of neck muscles
    Cyanosis

DIAGNOSTIC TESTS
Blood
    Serum: total and free T_3 and T_4
    Calcium levels

POTENTIAL COMPLICATIONS
Airway obstruction
Hemorrhage
Paralysis of recurrent laryngeal nerves
Hypothyroidism
Hypocalcemia; tetany

MULTIDISCIPLINARY MANAGEMENT
THERAPEUTIC MANAGEMENT
IV fluids progressing to regular diet
Treatment of complications
Pain management including throat spray or lozenges
Incentive spirometer

PATIENT PROBLEMS—NURSING DIAGNOSES/INTERVENTIONS

▼ Ineffective airway clearance related to bleeding and/or laryngeal edema

Monitor vital signs, LOC, orientation
Check dressing site for profuse bleeding (side of neck and back of head) every 15 minutes for 1 hour immediately after surgery *to identify signs of bleeding*
Keep dressing size minimized *to prevent impaired view of incision site*
Position patient on back with head of bed elevated 30 to 45 degrees *to promote ease in breathing*
Monitor for signs of respiratory distress or obstructed airway qh *to identify early signs of respiratory*

distress caused by tracheal edema: stridor, wheezing, coarse airway crackles, dyspnea, cyanosis, labored respirations
Teach and assist patient to turn, cough, and deep breathe q2h and prn *to prevent pulmonary complications*
If indicated, keep suction equipment at bedside; gently suction oropharynx only when necessary
Have tracheostomy tray and oxygen immediately available at bedside *to use if patient experiences severe respiratory distress*
Notify physician if dressing requires reinforcement more than one time

Expected Outcomes
Vital signs, respirations, and breath sounds are within patient's normal limits
No bleeding is present at surgical site

▼ Risk for injury (tetany) related to hypocalcemia caused by parathyroid suppression or removal

Evaluate reflexes q4h to 8h; report neuromuscular irritability *to aid in early recognition and treatment of hypocalcemia*
Monitor calcium levels *to watch for hypocalcemia*
Evaluate Chvostek's and Trousseau's signs with vital signs *to evaluate for hypocalcemia*
Collaborate with physician in treating symptoms of tetany: calcium and vitamin D supplementation

Expected Outcome
Exhibits normal reflexes

▼ Risk for infection related to invasive surgical procedure

Monitor vital signs and breath sounds q4h to 8h
Change dressing daily and prn when wet; observe for signs and symptoms of infection or impaired healing: redness, swelling, foul drainage, fever
Promote incision healing: prevent stress on incision line, cleanse site daily as ordered, and apply dry, sterile dressing
Use only necessary dressing and tape *to allow visibility of tissue around surgical sign* (edema, redness); remove tape toward incision *to prevent stress on suture line and possible interruption of wound healing*

Expected Outcomes
Incision is dry and clean
Vital signs are stable
Lungs are clear

▼ Impaired verbal communication related to damage and/or manipulation of laryngeal nerves

Monitor voice quality q2h *to evaluate damage to laryngeal nerves*

Monitor for edema at surgical incision and glottis

Reassure patient that voice should return to normal after a few days

If indicated provide alternative means of communication (e.g., pad and pencil)

Keep call bell within reach at all times

Report increasing hoarseness to physician

Anticipate patient's needs as indicated *to minimize patient's need to speak*

Expected Outcomes

Uses alternative communication methods for 48 hours postoperatively

Communicates verbally without voice change

Has no edema at incision

▼ Pain related to surgical incision

Assess patient for verbal and nonverbal signs of pain

Have patient use pain rating scale *to indicate intensity of pain*

Observe body language for evidence of pain *to ensure comfort despite impaired communication*

Discuss with patient factors that increase or relieve pain

Assist patient with finding physical position of comfort

Prevent flexion or extension of head and neck *to prevent tension on sutures*

Instruct patient to use hands to support head during movement

Assist patient with using distraction *to control pain:* guided imagery, progressive relaxation, soft music, reading, visitors

Monitor effectiveness of pain medications

Administer analgesic throat spray or lozenges as ordered and as patient desires *to minimize pain*

Expected Outcomes

Expresses feeling of well-being and comfort

Posture and face are relaxed

PATIENT/FAMILY TEACHING
PREOPERATIVE

Explain importance of not forcing speech postoperatively to prevent edema

Obtain pad and pencil for communicating postoperatively, if indicated

Teach patient to turn and deep breathe; include use of incentive spirometer

Explain that hoarseness will subside within 3 to 4 days

Discuss pain management, use of pain rating scale

Reinforce physician's explanation of procedure; clarify any misconceptions; allow time for questions

POSTOPERATIVE

Teach care of surgical incision

Discuss symptoms of recurrent hyperthyroidism, hypothyroidism, or hypocalcemia to report to physician

Discuss symptoms of wound infection to report to physician

Emphasize importance of rest and relaxation

DISCHARGE/HOME CARE PLANNING

Instruct patient to avoid driving vehicle for at least 1 week until neck is no longer stiff and can turn easily

Teach patient to massage incision tid for 2 weeks with lanolin-content lotions such as Keri, Lubriderm, or cocoa butter; use gentle circular motion

Instruct patient to perform neck circle exercises three times qid

Discuss with patient and family the importance of outpatient care and follow-up

Teach name of medication, purpose, time and method of administration, dosage, side effects, and toxic effects

Explain need to avoid taking over-the-counter medications without consulting physician

Teach patient to manage stressful situations and emotional outbursts with stress management techniques

Discuss proper nutrition and fluid intake

■ PARATHYROIDECTOMY

Surgical removal of the parathyroid glands; if surgery is performed for adenoma, total removal of all involved glands is necessary; if the cause of hyperparathyroidism is hyperplasia, three total glands are removed and three fourths of the fourth gland is removed, leaving sufficient gland to maintain normal calcium levels

POSTOPERATIVE ASSESSMENT
SUBJECTIVE DATA

Pain: location, intensity

Choking sensation

Heavy/full feeling in throat

Tingling

Paresthesia (numbness)

OBJECTIVE DATA

Signs and symptoms of hypocalcemia
  Stiffness
  Cramping
  Tremor
  Tetany

Respiratory system
  Hoarseness
  Laryngeal stridor
  Cyanosis

Incision site
  Redness
  Swelling

Drainage
Bleeding
Dysphagia

DIAGNOSTIC TESTS
Blood
   Serum calcium
   Serum phosphorus
   Electrolytes

POTENTIAL COMPLICATIONS
Hemorrhage
Hypocalcemia: seizures, tetany
Respiratory arrest

MULTIDISCIPLINARY MANAGEMENT
THERAPEUTIC MANAGEMENT
IV fluids, progressing to diet as tolerated
Treatment of complications
Pain management

PATIENT PROBLEM—NURSING DIAGNOSIS/INTERVENTIONS
See Thyroidectomy (p. 441)

▼ Altered nutrition: less than body requirements related to hypocalcemia

Assess Chvostek's and Trousseau's signs *to identify evidence of hypocalcemia*
Keep high-calcium snacks available to patient at all times *to treat symptoms of hypocalcemia*
Keep emergency calcium replacement available
Assess electrolytes *to monitor for fluctuations in calcium level*

Expected Outcome
Maintains adequate nutrition and appropriate calcium levels

PATIENT TEACHING AND DISCHARGE/HOME CARE PLANNING
Same as thyroidectomy (see p. 441)

■ ADRENALECTOMY
Surgical removal of the adrenal gland(s): unilateral removal is often indicated for treatment of benign adrenal adenomas, primary aldosteronism, or pheochromocytoma; bilateral adrenalectomy may be needed to treat ectopic ACTH-producing tumors, Cushing's disease (when other therapies have failed) or adrenal carcinoma

PREOPERATIVE ASSESSMENT AND CARE
Assess baseline vital signs to determine control of predisposing disease factors (e.g., hypertension in pheochromocytoma or primary aldosteronism)
If scheduled for bilateral removal, explain that patient must take glucocorticoid and mineralocorticoid preparations throughout life; if unilateral, for only 6 months to 2 years
Monitor blood glucose for control of hyperglycemia
Teach patient to turn, cough, and deep breathe
Encourage questions and discussion of fears and anxiety
Administer preoperative steroid

POSTOPERATIVE ASSESSMENT
SUBJECTIVE DATA
Headache
Pain
Restlessness
Confusion
Severe abdominal, leg, or back pain

OBJECTIVE DATA
Signs of adrenal crisis (p. 415)
   Falling BP
   Tachycardia; weak, thready pulses
   Hypopyrexia or hyperpyrexia
   Profound weakness
   Lethargy
   Hypoglycemia
   Electrolyte imbalance
   Seizures
Dehydration
Decreased urine output
Flatulence
Site of incision
   Redness
   Swelling
   Drainage, bleeding
   Impaired healing
Respiratory distress
   Decreased breath sounds
   Tachypnea, bradypnea

DIAGNOSTIC TESTS
Decreased serum cortisol levels
Decreased serum aldosterone levels
Hyperglycemia
Hyperkalemia
Hyponatremia

POTENTIAL COMPLICATIONS
Renal dysfunction
Atelectasis
Adrenal crisis
Coma
Cardiac arrest

MULTIDISCIPLINARY MANAGEMENT
THERAPEUTIC MANAGEMENT
IV fluids progressing to regular diet when bowel sounds return
Incentive spirometer
Treatment of complications
Pain management

PATIENT PROBLEMS—NURSING DIAGNOSES/INTERVENTIONS

▼Risk for injury related to potential for adrenal crisis

Administer IV fluids, vasopressors, and corticosteroids as ordered; assess effectiveness

Monitor cardiovascular, neurologic, respiratory, and renal function q4h

Assess vital signs q4h and prn; report abnormal findings to physician

Monitor neurologic status q4h; report increasing headache and confusion *to assess immediacy of risk for injury*

Monitor cardiac rhythm continuously if dysrhythmias occur *because of electrolyte imbalances*

Monitor intake and output q4h and prn; report output that is greater than intake

Position patient to promote cardiovascular and respiratory function

Expected Outcomes

Vital signs are stable and within patient's normal range
Intake and output are balanced
Alert and oriented when reactive

▼Pain related to surgery (surgical incision)

Assess for verbal and nonverbal signs of pain; use pain rating scale

Administer pain medications and assess effectiveness

Discuss with patient factors that increase or decrease pain to identify those that can be used to reduce perception of pain

Assist patient with finding position of comfort

Assist patient with using distraction *to control pain:* guided imagery, progressive relaxation, soft music, visitors

Maintain support of surgical incision during movement or ambulation *to minimize tension at incisional site*

Increase ambulation as tolerated

Expected Outcomes

Appears calm/relaxed
States pain is at tolerable level or absent
Uses learned pain control techniques

▼Risk for infection related to surgical incision and abnormal cortisol levels

Change dressing daily and when wet; observe for signs of infection, impaired healing, dehiscence, redness, swelling, foul drainage, fever

Culture suspicious drainage *to identify any source of infection*

Promote incisional healing/avoid infection
 Prevent stress on suture line
 Remove sutures/staples when ordered

Use dry, clean dressing when changing

Use only necessary amount of tape and remove in direction of incision

Cleanse site daily

Instruct patient to avoid touching incision site

Avoid unnecessary invasive procedures *to prevent potential for infection*

Assist patient to turn, cough, and deep breathe q2h

Monitor for signs of URI and UTI

Screen personnel and visitors for infections; restrict if present

Expected Outcomes

Temperature is within normal range
Breath sounds are clear
Incision is healing
Urine is clear

▼Risk for fluid volume deficit related to unstable levels of circulating steroids

Maintain IV fluids to 2500 ml/day

Monitor serum electrolytes q8h and prn

Calculate intake and output q4h to 8h; report intake less than output

Weigh patient daily; observe for weight loss

Administer sodium replacement as ordered in diet or IV fluids if NPO *to maintain fluid volume*

Assess for signs and symptoms of fluid/electrolyte imbalance: poor skin turgor, weak pulses, tachycardia, thirst, low BP, cool skin, cardiac dysrhythmias, increased body temperature, change in mental status

Report any of the preceding signs or symptoms to physician without delay and carry out medical orders received

Check blood sugar via fingerstick q8h

Expected Outcomes

Intake and output are balanced
Weight is stable
Skin is warm and moist with good turgor
Vital signs are stable
Blood glucose is within normal limits

PATIENT/FAMILY TEACHING

Discuss symptoms of adrenal crisis to report

Emphasize importance of reporting risk factors to physician immediately for medication adjustment (increase steroids)
 Infection: fever, cold, influenza, persistent cough, burning on urination, wounds that do not heal
 Injury, surgery, dental care
 Profuse sweating
 Strenuous, unusual activity
 Emotionally charged events
 Infections, no matter how minor

Explain need to avoid persons with infections, especially URIs *to avoid contracting contagious diseases while immunosuppressed*

Teach name of medications, dosage, time and method of administration, side effects, and toxic effects

Demonstrate IM injection method to patient and significant other

Explain that if bilateral adrenalectomy was performed, steroid therapy will be needed for remainder of life

Teach care of incision and to report signs of infection

Emphasize importance of the following:

Adequate rest

Moderate exercise

Good nutrition

Explain that if surgery was for Cushing's syndrome, symptoms of hypercortisolism will slowly recede

DISCHARGE/HOME CARE PLANNING

Patient/significant other demonstrates ability to give IM self-injection

Emphasize importance of carrying injectable cortisol for administration in emergency

Patient and family understand situations that can require administration of additional steroids (see Adrenal insufficiency, p. 415)

Discuss importance of ongoing outpatient care and informing all physicians, dentists, other health care providers of surgery and prescribed medications

Emphasize importance of wearing medical alert band or chain and carrying identification card

■ HYPOPHYSECTOMY

Surgical removal of pituitary gland to remove pituitary adenomas, craniopharyngiomas, and as palliative therapy in certain types of metastatic breast and prostate cancer; surgery is usually performed via transfrontal transsphenoidal approach; often the treatment of choice for Cushing's disease

PREOPERATIVE ASSESSMENT AND TEACHING

Assess for upper airway infection (colds, sinus infection), report if present (surgery will be delayed)

Discuss and teach postoperative care and rationale

Nasal packing

Graft site, usually thigh

Need for mouth breathing because of nasal packing

No toothbrushing (oral hygiene by rinsing)

Avoid coughing, sneezing, or noseblowing

Decreased senses of smell and taste

Encourage questions

Reinforce physician's explanation of procedure

Allow time for discussion of fears and anxiety

POSTOPERATIVE ASSESSMENT
SUBJECTIVE DATA

Pain

Location

Intensity

OBJECTIVE DATA

Signs and symptoms of increased intracranial pressure (ICP)

Increasing restlessness

Decreasing LOC

Unequal pupils

Visual changes

Widened pulse pressure

Bradycardia

Respiratory arrest

Gumline incision

Redness

Edema

Drainage or bleeding

Nasal packing

Intact

CSF drainage (may be postnasal drip): frequent swallowing, coughing

Bleeding

Patent airway

Thigh, graft site

Redness

Swelling

Drainage

DIAGNOSTIC TESTS

Hormone levels

Electrolyte levels

Glucose levels

Urine specific gravity

POTENTIAL COMPLICATIONS

Cerebrospinal rhinorrhea

Diabetes insipidus (p. 425)

Meningitis

Hemorrhage

Adrenal crisis (p. 415)

Severe hypoglycemia (p. 440)

Decreased levels of pituitary hormones (gonadotropins)

MULTIDISCIPLINARY MANAGEMENT
THERAPEUTIC MANAGEMENT

Indwelling catheter

Incentive spirometer

Monitor intake and output

IV fluids progressing to oral diet

Treatment of complications

Pain management

PATIENT PROBLEMS—NURSING DIAGNOSES/INTERVENTIONS

▼ Risk for injury, related to potential for intracranial pressure

Assess for signs and symptoms of increased ICP qh for first 24 hours, then q4h; check neurologic and vital signs

Notify physician at once if onset of restlessness or if pupillary or vital signs change

Maintain head of bed elevated 30 degrees *to promote circulation*

Avoid turning, extending, and flexing head for first 24 hours

Avoid having patient cough vigorously or use other Valsalva maneuvers for any reason *to prevent disruption of graft;* use stool softeners if needed

Maintain calm, dimly lit environment *to prevent stimulation*

Pace care *to avoid excessive stimulation;* allow adequate undisturbed rest periods

Expected Outcomes

Vital signs are within normal limits

Remains alert, oriented, with reactive pupils

Has no cough

▼Ineffective airway clearance related to nasal packing, postnasal drip, and/or dry oropharynx

Elevate head of bed 30 degrees *to avoid pressure at surgical site*

Assess for intactness of nasal packing q2h; determine whether packing is slipping posteriorly

Patient must maintain mouth breathing; maintain oral mucous membranes in moist condition

Provide oral care with saline solution or diluted mouthwash q2h and prn

Supply humidity to room or via face mask if necessary

Keep suction at bedside; gently suction oropharynx only when absolutely necessary

Remind patient to deep breathe and turn q2h, *to avoid forceful coughing*

Monitor for signs of respiratory distress: stridor, wheezing, labored respirations, cyanosis

Check dressing and oropharynx for bleeding or cerebrospinal fluid (CSF) leakage q2h to 4h prn

Expected Outcomes

Breath sounds, respiratory rate and rhythm are within normal limits

Nasal packing is intact without bleeding or postnasal drip

Mucous membranes are moist

Color is good

▼Risk for infection related to disruption in dura mater

Monitor incision *for signs and symptoms of infection* q4h

Evaluate drainage for CSF leakage (positive glucose reagent strip); report immediately

Assess for early signs of meningitis: chills, fever, malaise, headache, vomiting, nuchal rigidity; report immediately

Do not use toothbrush until incision is healed

Avoid foods that could irritate incision

Instruct patient not to touch dressing or packing; use sterile technique to change mustache pad each time it becomes damp

Expected Outcomes

Temperature is within normal limits

Nasal packing negative for CSF

Incision is clean without signs of infection

▼Risk for fluid volume deficit related to potential for surgically induced diabetes insipidus

Assess for signs of diabetes insipidus

Monitor intake and output q2h during first 24 hours postoperatively

Measure output qh; report if >200 ml/hr

Report intake >3000 to 4000 ml per 24 hours

Monitor urine specific gravity; report if <1.005

Collaborate with physician to correct condition if condition is present

Monitor vital signs, skin turgor, and mucous membranes q4h to 8h

Weigh patient daily (same time, scale, and clothing); monitor for weight loss *to identify/correct fluid volume loss*

Expected Outcomes

Vital signs are stable

Intake is <2500 ml/day

Urine output is <100 ml/hr, and specific gravity is within normal range

Weight is stable

Skin turgor is good

▼Pain at surgical site or headache

Assess patient for verbal and nonverbal signs of pain

Be aware that severe headache may be a sign of increased ICP

Discuss with patient factors that relieve pain; facilitate use of these measures if possible

Assist patient with finding position of comfort, maintaining neutral head position with head of bed elevated 30 degrees

Teach relaxation techniques *to reduce perception of pain*

Provide means of distraction from pain: guided imagery, soft music, visitors as tolerated

Administer pain medications as ordered; be aware that they may mask signs of increased ICP

Expected Outcomes

Verbalizes increasing comfort and no headache

Face and body are relaxed

Uses relaxation techniques

PATIENT/FAMILY TEACHING

Explain that decrease in senses of taste and smell and some numbness in upper gums is expected for several months

Explain need to avoid persons with infections, especially URIs

Discuss symptoms of incisional or systemic infection to report to physician

Emphasize importance of avoiding vigorous coughing, straining, and noseblowing

Emphasize importance of ongoing patient care

Discuss signs and symptoms of hormonal imbalances to report to physician (see specific disease relating to hormone deficiency)

Teach name of medication(s), dosage, time and method of administration, side effects, and toxic effects

DISCHARGE/HOME CARE PLANNING

Emphasize that hormone therapy may need to continue throughout lifetime

Explain need to notify caregiver about unusual stress so medication dosages can be changed if needed

Provide information for obtaining medical alert bracelet and card

BIBLIOGRAPHY

American Diabetes Association: Position statement: insulin administration, *Diabetes Care* 14(2):34-35, 1991.

Clayton LH, Dilley KB: Cushing's syndrome, *Am J Nurs* 98(7):40, 1998.

Dress JA, Peterson A: Type 2 diabetes, *Am J Nurs* 96(11):45, 1996.

Freeland BS: Diabetic ketoacidosis, *Am J Nurs* 98(8):52, 1998.

Hernandez D: Microvascular complications of diabetes, *Am J Nurs* 98(6):27, 1998.

Kim MJ et al: *Pocket guide to nursing diagnoses,* St Louis, ed 6, 1995, Mosby.

Kinney M, Packa D, Dunbar S: *AACN's clinical reference for critical care nursing,* ed 3, 1994, Bookmakers.

Kreisberg R: Diabetic ketoacidosis. In Rifkin H, Porte D, eds: *Ellenberg and Rifkin's diabetes mellitus theory and practice,* ed 4, New York, 1990, Elsevier.

Maffeo R: Helping families cope with type 1 diabetes, *Am J Nurs* 97(6):36, 1997.

Thompson JM et al: *Mosby's clinical nursing,* ed 4, St Louis, 1997, Mosby.

Wilson JD, Foster DW: *Williams textbook of endocrinology,* ed 8, Philadelphia, 1992, WB Saunders.

Wyngaarden JB, Smith LH: *Cecil textbook of medicine,* ed 18, Philadelphia, 1988, WB Saunders.

MULTIDISCIPLINARY PLAN OF CARE

Diagnosis: **Diabetic Ketoacidosis**_____

Type of Surgery:_____   DRG #: _294_   Length of Stay: **2 days**

Resuscitation Status: ☐ No Code/DNR   Date:_____   Date of Admission:_____

    ☐ Other: _____   Date:_____   Date of Surgery:_____

Date/ Initials	Disci-pline	Patient Problem(s)	Patient Goal(s) Met by Discharge	Date Resolved/ Initials
		Altered tissue perfusion related to decreased neurovascular function	VS within normal limits, blood glucose within acceptable limits	
		Non-compliance with prescribed treatment plan	Patient/caregiver acknowledges or agrees to treatment plan and accepts responsibility for self-care management of diabetes	

This Plan of Care and guidelines do not purport to reflect all relevant medical considerations and are not intended to replace clinical judgment. **REVISED 6/27/96**, Approved by Pharmacy & Therapeutics Committee 8/96, Medical Records Committee 8/96, Executive Committee 9/96.

DRG294.DOC

Used by permission of Kaiser Permanente Medical Center, Los Angeles, California.

Continued

MULTIDISCIPLINARY PLAN OF CARE

ASPECT OF CARE	Diabetic Ketoacidosis	
DISCHARGE OUTCOMES	**DATE:** **Admission Day**	
CONSULTS Consults completed	___ Endocrinologist ___ Diabetes Clinical Educator	___ Social Medicine intervention per criteria ___
DIAGNOSTIC STUDIES Serum HCO3 >18, resolution of ketoneuria	___ Lytes STAT and q 2 hrs ___ BUN CBC, RBS, Creatinine STAT and q 2 hrs ___ UA and C & S STAT ___ Serum ketones STAT ___ Ca (if phosphate administered) STAT & q 6 hrs ___ Blood glucose monitoring 30 minutes ac and HS at each meal	___ CXR ___ EKG ___ ABG ___ ___ ___
TREATMENTS, PROCEDURES, & MONITORS Tolerating treatments & procedures well, VSS	___ Strict I & O , straight cath if no urine output (UOP) in 2 hrs ___ Avoid Foley if posible ___ Weight on admission and q 6-12 hrs ___ VS q 1 hr x4, q 2 hrs x4, then q 4 hrs & PRN ___ Oxygen if needed ___ Cardiac monitor ___ NG (for vomiting) ___ Capillary blood sugar q 1-2 hrs ___ Initiate Sliding Scale with Regular insulin	___ ___ ___ ___ ___ ___ ___ ___
MEDICATIONS/ LINES Maintaining fluid & electrolyte balance	___ IV NS 2-3 L over 1st 3 hrs ___ 1/2 NS at 150-300 cc/hr, add D5 when glucose reaches 250 ___ If pH<7 Sodium bicarbonate 50mEq ___ Regular insulin 10 units IV push ___ Insulin 8 units/hr, double rate of infusion if no response in 2 hrs	___ Begin SQ Insulin when glucose <250 ___ D/C IV insulin one hr after first SQ dose ___ Potassium 10mEq/hr IV when K<6, and urine flow documented (supplement with PO KCl PRN) IV to Hep-Lock ___
NUTRITION Tolerating diabetic diet	___ NPO 	___
ACTIVITY/ MOBILITY Maintaining ADLs	___ Bedrest ___ ___ ___	___ ___ ___ ___
PATIENT/FAMILY EDUCATION Able to demonstrate survival skills	___ Discuss expected LOS with patient/family ___ Review plan of care ___ Introduction to Diabetes information (newly diagnosed) ___ Initiate Diabetic MPEPs with patient/family	___ ___ ___ ___ ___
PSYCHO-SOCIAL Coping with illness and/or stressors	___ Psychosoial needs identified: ___ Specify: _____ _____	___ ___
DISCHARGE PLANNING Adequate support identified	___ Assess discharge needs PRN ___ Refer to Home Health as indicated ___ ___	___ ___ ___ ___

This Plan of Care and guidelines do not purport to reflect all relevant medical considerations and are not intended to replace clinical judgment. **REVISED 6/27/96,** Approved by Pharmacy & Therapeutics Committee 8/96, Medical Records Committee 8/96, Executive Committee 9/96. DRG294.DOC

MULTIDISCIPLINARY PLAN OF CARE

ASPECT OF CARE	Diabetic Ketoacidosis	
DISCHARGE OUTCOMES	DATE: Day 1	
CONSULTS	___ Nutritionist ___ Diabetes Clinical Educator	___ ___
DIAGNOSTIC STUDIES	___ Blood glucose monitoring 30 minutes ac and HS at each meal ___ ___ ___ ___	___ ___ ___ ___ ___ ___
TREATMENTS, PROCEDURES, & MONITORS	___ Strict I & O (Straight cath if no UOP in 2 hrs) ___ VS q 4 hrs & PRN ___ Continued Sliding Scale insulin coverage ___ ___ ___ ___ ___ ___	___ ___ ___ ___ ___ ___ ___ ___ ___
MEDICATIONS/ LINES	___ Hep-Lock ___ Begin NPH insulin BID when patient taking PO intake ___ ___ ___ ___ ___	___ ___ ___ ___ ___ ___ ___
NUTRITION	___ Diet as tolerated ___ ___	___ ___ ___
ACTIVITY/ MOBILITY	___ As tolerated ___ ___ ___	___ ___ ___ ___
PATIENT/FAMILY EDUCATION	___ Review Diabetic MPEPs with patient/family and evaluate understanding ___ ___	___ ___ ___ ___
PSYCHO-SOCIAL	___ Follow-up needs: ___ specify _____	___ ___
DISCHARGE PLANNING	___ Assess discharge needs PRN ___ Nutritial referral ___ Diabetes Clinic referral ___	___ ___ ___ ___

This Plan of Care and guidelines do not purport to reflect all relevant medical considerations and are not intended to replace clinical judgment. **REVISED 6/27/96.** Approved by Pharmacy & Therapeutics Committee 8/96, Medical Records Committee 8/96, Executive Committee 9/96.

DRG294.DOC

Continued

MULTIDISCIPLINARY PLAN OF CARE

ASPECT OF CARE	Diabetic Ketoacidosis	
DISCHARGE OUTCOMES	DATE: Day 2	
CONSULTS	___ Nutritionist ___ Diabetes Clinical Educator	___
DIAGNOSTIC STUDIES	___ Blood glucose monitoring 30 minutes ac and HS at each meal ___ ___ ___ ___	___ ___ ___ ___ ___
TREATMENTS, PROCEDURES, & MONITORS	___ Strict I & O (Straight cath if no UOP in 2 hrs) ___ VS q 4 hrs & PRN ___ ___ ___ ___ ___ ___ ___ ___	___ ___ ___ ___ ___ ___ ___ ___ ___ ___
MEDICATIONS/ LINES	___ Hep-Lock ___ Discharge patient on combination NPH and regular insulin BID ___ ___ ___ ___	___ ___ ___ ___ ___ ___
NUTRITION	___ Diet as tolerated ___ ___	___ ___ ___
ACTIVITY/ MOBILITY	___ As tolerated ___ ___ ___	___ ___ ___ ___
PATIENT/FAMILY EDUCATION	___ Give copy of MPEPs to patient/family and evaluate understanding ___ ___	___ ___ ___
PSYCHO-SOCIAL	___ Follow-up needs: ___ specify _____	___ ___
DISCHARGE PLANNING	___ Assess discharge needs PRN ___ Nutritial referral ___ Diabetes Clinic referral ___ Refer to outpatient member health education	___ ___ ___ ___

This Plan of Care and guidelines do not purport to reflect all relevant medical considerations and are not intended to replace clinical judgment. **REVISED 6/27/96,** Approved by Pharmacy & Therapeutics Committee 8/96, Medical Records Committee 8/96, Executive Committee 9/96.
DRG294.DOC

CHAPTER

8

Musculoskeletal System

■ MUSCULOSKELETAL ASSESSMENT

■ SUBJECTIVE DATA

Pain and/or edema in muscles, joints, or bones with or
 without movement
Weakness in extremities
Limited activity and movement
Sensory changes
Anorexia; weight loss
Insomnia
Tires easily, fatigue
Unsteady gait or stance
Frustration, anger at self

■ OBJECTIVE DATA

General appearance
Age (see Gerontologic considerations box, p. 455)
Vital signs: blood pressure (BP), temperature (T), pulse
 (P), and respiratory rate (R)
Weight
Joint(s) inflamed, edematous, and/or warm to touch
Impaired neurovascular status of each extremity
Deformities
Paralysis
Contractures
Posture
Abnormal body alignment
Limited ability or inability to move in bed
Abnormal gait; needs assistance
Decreased handgrip and range of motion (ROM)
Internal and external rotation of extremities
Ability to perform ROM exercises
Contusions, lacerations, scars
Wounds: amount and type of drainage
Facial and body gestures indicating pain
Loss of extremity
Pressure ulcers
Skin rashes
Allergies
Tenseness
Presence of casts, braces, prostheses, crutches, traction,
 cane, or walker
Nutritional history
Ability to use trapeze in bed, sit up, and turn

Ability to perform activities of daily living (ADLs)
Constipation
Dependence, independence, and interdependence

■ PERTINENT BACKGROUND INFORMATION

CONCURRENT DISEASES AND/OR CONDITIONS
Diabetes
Spinal cord injury, nerve impairment
Cerebrovascular accident (CVA)
Rheumatoid arthritis
Arthritis
Bursitis
Polyneuritis
Multiple sclerosis
Muscular dystrophy
Myasthenia gravis
Fracture
Ruptured disc
Ménière's disease
Labyrinthitis
Osteoporosis
Congenital conditions
Low back pain
Lupus erythematosus
Gout
Blood dyscrasias
Older adult (see Gerontologic Considerations box)

PREVIOUS SURGERY AND/OR ILLNESS
Orthopedic surgery
Spinal surgery
Poliomyelitis
Hemiplegia, paraplegia
Cerebral palsy
Parkinson's disease
Ataxia
Alcoholism
Syphilis
Impaired vision and/or hearing
CVA
Hyperparathyroidism
Osteoporosis

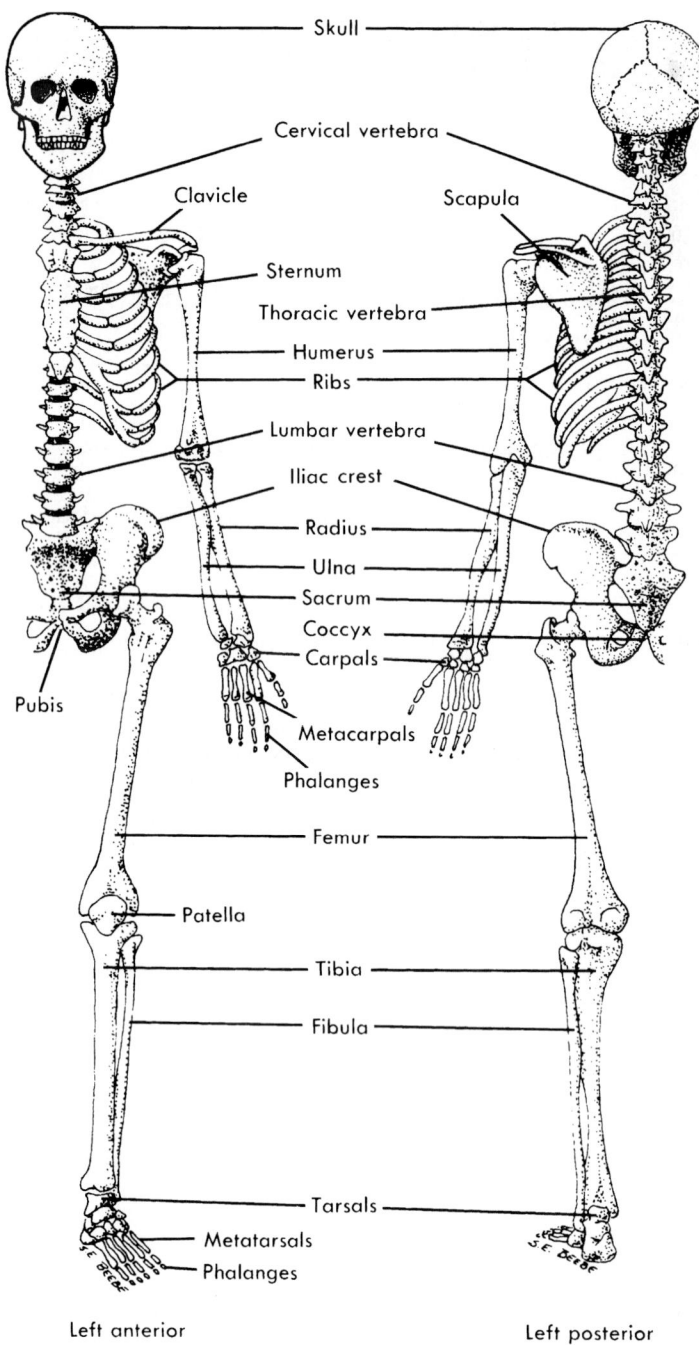

Skull

Cervical vertebra

Clavicle

Scapula

Sternum

Thoracic vertebra

Humerus

Ribs

Lumbar vertebra

Iliac crest

Radius

Ulna

Sacrum

Coccyx

Carpals

Pubis

Metacarpals

Phalanges

Femur

Patella

Tibia

Fibula

Tarsals

Metatarsals

Phalanges

Left anterior   Left posterior

Fig. 8-1 Musculoskeletal system.

Rickets, osteomalacia
Tuberculosis

FAMILY HISTORY
Carcinoma
Diabetes
Tuberculosis

SOCIAL HISTORY
Hazardous job or recreation (e.g., construction work or
    contact sports)
Safety measures used
Accident proneness
Alcohol, substance abuse, tobacco use

MEDICATION HISTORY
Antiinflammatory agents: steroid and
    nonsteroid
Sedatives
Tranquilizers
Analgesics
Acetylsalicylic acid
Antimalarials
Antiemetics
Anticoagulants
Antidepressants
Insulin
Oral hypoglycemics
Psychotherapeutic agents

Gerontologic Considerations

- Physiologic changes of aging result in decreased joint flexibility and muscular strength.
- Changes in bone mass, particularly in older women, increase the risk of fractures. Hip fractures and compression fractures of the spine are most common.
- Degenerative joint disease related to "wear and tear" on joints is common. Joint replacement is increasingly common and has done much to improve mobility and the quality of life.
- Changes in the foot can occur from a lifetime of use, poorly fitted shoes, or heredity. Bunions and hammer toe are commonly seen in older adults. These may cause pain and lead to decreased mobility. Older adults should be encouraged to wear properly fitted shoes to reduce discomfort. If discomfort is severe, surgical correction may be necessary.
- The older adult's home should be checked for safety hazards such as rugs that could cause falls.
- Climbing unsteady or uneven surfaces should be avoided, because coordination and balance change with aging and falls may result.
- Older persons should be instructed in the correct use of assistive devices such as canes or walkers. They should be encouraged to use these measures regularly to prevent injury.
- Older persons should be instructed to include regular podiatry care with trimming of toenails and treatment of fungus.

Modified from Christensen BL, Kockrow EO: Foundations of nursing, ed 3, St Louis, 1998, Mosby.

Antibiotics
Antihypertensive agents

DIAGNOSTIC TESTS

Serum
  Calcium
  Phosphorus
  Alkaline phosphatase
  Erythrocyte sedimentation rate (ESR)
  Creatinine clearance
  Blood urea nitrogen (BUN)
  Uric acid
  Aspartate aminotransferase (AST), alanine aminotransferase (ALT), creatinine phosphokinase (CPK)
  Coagulation studies
  Albumin
Urine
  Calcium
  Phosphorus
  Creatinine, uric acid

PROCEDURES

X-ray examination of bones
Arthrogram
Arthroscopy
Myelogram
Fluoroscopy
Arteriogram
Venogram
Bone marrow aspiration
Bone, synovial fluid, or muscle biopsy
Incision and drainage of joint
Aspiration of joint
Electromyogram (EMG): muscle and nerve conduction studies
Bone scintigraphy (scan)
Computed tomography (CT) scan
Thermography
Magnetic resonance imaging (MRI)
Lumbar puncture
Discogram

■ OSTEOPOROSIS

Overall reduction in bone mass and density, as a result of bone formation being less than bone resorption, causing increased porosity and brittleness; risk factors: prolonged immobilization, decreased blood estrogen, increased ratio of blood estrogen, increased ratio of blood calcium to phosphorus, excessive steroid therapy, and people with red-blond hair and freckles; disease predisposes patients to fractures and/or deformities

ASSESSMENT
SUBJECTIVE DATA
Acute/chronic neck or back pain
History of steroid therapy or smoking
Decrease in height

OBJECTIVE DATA
Age and sex of patient (usually more than 50 years of age and female)
History: inactivity, immobilization, previous fracture, vertebrae/hip/forearm, thoracic kyphosis
Nutritional history
  Lack of vitamins C and D and calcium
  Diets high in protein, salt, alcohol, and caffeine
  Excessive smoking
History of endocrine disease
  Diabetes
  Hyperthyroidism
  Hyperparathyroidism
  Cushing's syndrome
  Acromegaly
  Hypogonadism
Females: menopause, history of hysterectomy
Anorexia nervosa
Hematologic malignancies
Alteration in self-concept
Decreased mobility

DIAGNOSTIC TESTS
Bone densitometry with dual energy x-ray absorptiometry (DEXA),

Quantitative computed tomography (QCT), quantitative ultrasound
Radiologic studies
Bone biopsy
Serum studies: chemistries, complete blood count (CBC), ESR, parathyroid hormone (PTH), thyroid-stimulating hormone (TSH)

POTENTIAL COMPLICATIONS
Chronic pain
Respiratory compromise
Fractures: lower distal radius, femoral neck, vertebrae
Decreased mobility and dependence in activities of daily living (ADLs)

MULTIDISCIPLINARY MANAGEMENT
THERAPEUTIC MANAGEMENT
Diet: High protein; calcium, vitamin D supplements
Medications
    Calcitonin
    Biphosphonates (etidronate, alendronate [Fosamax])
    For postmenopausal women:
        Estrogen replacement
        Selective estrogen receptor modulator (SERM)
    Analgesics (nonsteroidal antiinflammatory drugs [NSAIDs], narcotics)
Increased activity, weight-bearing hyperextension and resistance exercises, orthopedic supports: back braces, corsets
Physical therapy consultation as indicated

PATIENT PROBLEMS—NURSING DIAGNOSES/INTERVENTIONS

▼ Impaired physical mobility related to decreased bone mass and pain

Assess degree of immobility and pain
Encourage ambulation with assistance; use walker or cane if indicated
Assist with and teach active ROM exercises q4h
Monitor and maintain body alignment; fractures can occur without patient's knowledge
Handle patient carefully and assist with and teach correct body mechanics *to prevent fractures*
Apply and teach patient the application of braces or corset *to prevent stress fractures*
Administer medications as prescribed and monitor response
Perform active and passive ROM *to maintain muscle and joint strength*

Expected Outcomes
Mobility is improved
Able to perform ROM exercises to tolerance
Uses walker, cane correctly
Demonstrates application of brace, corset correctly

▼ Body image disturbance related to actual/perceived physical changes secondary to increased kyphosis

Assess degree of bone deformity and limitation imposed by disease
Encourage and allow time for verbalization of feelings
Clarify any misconceptions about disease process and treatment
Discuss ways of altering clothes to ensure a better fit and the use of scarves, color schemes *to enhance self-concept*
Assist patient in identifying strengths that were successful in the past
Identify present coping behaviors and praise for tasks accomplished
Encourage communication with significant other(s)

Expected Outcomes
Appears more comfortable with limitations
Expresses desire to discuss clothing and ways to enhance self-image

Additional Nursing Diagnoses to Consider
Impaired gas exchange related to kyphosis
Risk for injury: falls, fractures related to progressive bone loss
Pain related to stress fractures

PATIENT/FAMILY TEACHING AND DISCHARGE/HOME CARE PLANNING
Discuss disease process and preventive measures to take
Review signs and symptoms to report: bone pain, deformity, decreased mobility
Stress importance of diet, activity, and rest
Encourage participation in regular (minimum 3 days/week) exercises: weight bearing, extension, resistant, and aerobic
Provide medication schedule including name, dosage, purpose, and side effects; discuss alendromate (Fosamax) therapy for bone replacement; discuss calcitonin—inhalant form of calcium
Discuss importance of safe environment and fall prevention
    Use ambulatory devices as needed; avoid slippery areas, loose rugs
    Maintain awareness of possible falls or fractures; avoid small rugs; use hand rails
    Avoid activity after taking analgesics or muscle relaxants
    Avoid quick movements that may cause fractures
    Provide information for personal emergency response system
Teach energy conservation techniques: use long-handled equipment
Encourage reduction of caffeine, alcohol intake, and smoking
Discuss importance of medical follow-up

■ ACUTE OSTEOMYELITIS
Infection of the long bones and knee joint caused by acute local infection or bone trauma, usually caused by Escherichia coli, Staphylococcus aureus, *or* Streptococcus pyogenes; *this condition may be asymptomatic for months, but once diagnosed, aggressive treatment is re-*

quired with a long rehabilitation to prevent recurrence of the infection; surgical intervention may be required to drain infected areas

ASSESSMENT
SUBJECTIVE DATA
Bone pain, muscle spasms in affected joint
History of trauma or newly acquired prosthetic device
Headache
Weakness
Restricted joint mobility

OBJECTIVE DATA
Redness, tenderness and swelling in affected joint; increases with motion
Chills, fever, leukocytosis
Diaphoresis
Tachycardia
Restlessness, Irritability
Pain with movement; reluctance to bear weight

DIAGNOSTIC TESTS
Serum studies: white blood cell (WBC) count, blood cultures (aerobic and anaerobic), ESR, C-reactive protein (CRP), CBC
Bone and joint radiologic study, CT scan, radionuclide scan, MRI
Culture of joint aspirate, bone, tissue, or pus
Radionuclide bone scan

POTENTIAL COMPLICATIONS
Limited motion, contractures, bone deformity, loss of function
Ankylosing of joint
Degenerative joint changes
Recurrence of infection
Chronic osteomyelitis
Amputation of affected joint, limb

MULTIDISCIPLINARY MANAGEMENT
THERAPEUTIC MANAGEMENT
Parenteral fluids with antibiotics
Antibiotics, analgesics
Irrigant solution
Immobilization of joint
Compresses: warm, moist, or alternate warm and cold
Dietary consultation as needed
Surgical management
    Excision, aspiration, drainage, irrigation of joint
    Placement of antibiotic-impregnated beads
Physical medicine
    Physical therapy
    Occupational therapy
Consultation with Wound, Ostomy, Continence/ET Nurse

PATIENT PROBLEMS—NURSING DIAGNOSES/INTERVENTIONS

▼ Impaired physical mobility related to pain and swelling

Maintain bed rest; handle affected extremity gently
Immobilize joint/extremity with use of cast, splint, and/or pillows to maintain alignment; elevate *to reduce edema*
Assist with and teach active or perform passive ROM exercises to unaffected extremities
Encourage self-care
Encourage diversional activities for pain and mood management
Increase activity after fever and swelling subside or drainage decreases
Initiate ROM exercise of affected joint/extremity when tolerated
Provide resistive exercises
Protect affected joint/extremity from trauma
Assist patient to chair; elevate affected extremity
Ambulate with crutches; advance to walker or cane as tolerated; involve physical therapy department
Provide a safe environment
Instruct patient in weight bearing
Provide encouragement and support for each accomplishment

Expected Outcomes
Mobility and joint use are improving with less discomfort
Participation in own care is increasing
Edema is diminishing

▼ Risk for altered body temperature related to bone and soft tissue infection

Assess and monitor vital signs q4h; institute cooling measures as needed
Draw blood cultures as ordered; monitor results
Administer parenteral fluids with prescribed antibiotics
Administer antipyretics as ordered *to reduce fever*
Encourage fluid intake *to prevent dehydration*
Monitor for chills and diaphoresis; if present check temperature
Keep patient comfortable and dry following episodes of diaphoresis
Maintain comfortable room temperature and light bedding *to promote comfort*

Expected Outcomes
Vital signs are stable
Temperature is approaching normal or is normal

▼ Pain related to inflammation and increased pressure at affected side

Assess location, intensity, and type of pain
Provide analgesics as indicated; assess effectiveness of pain relief measure
Administer intravenous (IV) antibiotics as ordered and monitor response
Assist patient with changing position frequently; support affected extremity; administer back rubs *to promote comfort*

Handle joint distal to site gently, because it may also be painful when extended

Immobilize affected extremity with splint or traction *to alleviate spasm and pain*

Provide diversional activities *to decrease attention on pain*

Expected Outcomes

Reports that level of pain is tolerable

Appears more relaxed, comfortable

Balances periods of activity with rest

▼ Impaired skin integrity related to incision and surgical intervention

Assess and monitor wound edges for adequate closure and condition

Change dressing as ordered to lessen odor and skin maceration

Collaborate with physician and prepare patient for excision and drainage as indicated

Take cultures of aspirated fluid

Consultation with Wound, Ostomy, Continence/ET Nurse specialist

Observe for skin breakdown

Monitor incision for bleeding; change dressing as needed; maintain rigid aseptic technique

Provide high-calorie, high-protein diet as tolerated *to promote healing;* assist with meals as needed

Encourage fluids to upper limits for age and weight

Remove splints daily if ordered and monitor skin condition

Reposition patient q2h *to increase circulation to affected site*

Expected Outcomes

Skin is clean, dry, and intact

Wound is closed with no signs of infection

WBC count is within normal limits

Verbalizes understanding of wound care regimen

Additional Nursing Diagnoses to Consider

Altered tissue perfusion: peripheral related to site edema/infection

Body image disturbance related to prognosis

Anxiety related to prolonged treatment

PATIENT/FAMILY TEACHING

Provide and discuss information on prescribed rehabilitation program: physical therapy and home instructions

Demonstrate incision care

Provide information about disease process and complications

Demonstrate administration of IV medication through intermittent infusion catheter

Initiate referral to social services for financial support to purchase medications if needed

Discuss signs and symptoms to report to physician

Tenderness, pain, discomfort

Fever, malaise

Drainage from incision

Provide medication schedule, including name, dosage, purpose, and side effects; instruct patient to take all prescribed medications

Stress importance of nourishing diet and increased fluid intake; avoid weight gain

Stress importance of good handwashing, especially after toileting and contact with wound drainage

Promote regular visits with physician

DISCHARGE/HOME CARE PLANNING

Assess home care needs and continue with patient/family teaching and monitor the following:

Environmental/safety status

Caregivers' ability to perform needed tasks (e.g., infusion therapy, wound care)

Accessible telephone and emergency numbers: physician, pharmacy, home health care team

Emergency call device to summon outside help

Absence of scatter rugs, unbacked carpets

Presence of stairs with hand rails

Grab bars at tub and toilet

Nonskid strips in tub

Adequate lighting for safe movement

Wide doorways to accommodate wheelchairs/walkers

Height of chair and bed for easy transfer on and off of each

Flashlights near bed and chair

Medications accessible and labeled

Availability of transportation to needed appointments

Needed supplies: what and where to purchase

Mobility status

Ability and desire to follow prescribed rehabilitation plan and exercises

Correct transfer techniques

Amount of weight bearing; reinforce wearing low-heeled, comfortable shoes

Correct use of walkers, canes, crutches

Status of immobilizing device

Neurovascular status of each affected extremity

Condition of device: wet, loose, clean, soiled

Condition of skin under device: clear, red, tender

Nutritional status

Understanding of basic food groups and what to eat to provide optimal nutrition with no weight gain

Signs of weight loss, dehydration

Ability to prepare meals; refer to social agency to provide meals

Elimination status

Presence of elevated toilet seat

Use of stool softeners, natural laxatives, bulk in diet

Ability to be physically active

Amount of fluids taken per day: increase to upper limits for age and weight

Use of fracture pan/urinal/female urinal

■ GOUTY ARTHRITIS

Acute and/or chronic arthritis of the joints caused by either overproduction or underexcretion of uric acid; uric acid crystals are deposited in the joint space, causing an acute inflammatory reaction; disease is thought to involve a hereditary renal defect in uric acid excretion leading to chronic hyperuricemia; commonly affects males in the fourth or fifth decade

ASSESSMENT
SUBJECTIVE DATA
Joint pain, tenderness
Increased heat at site
Anorexia
Headache
Constipation

OBJECTIVE DATA
Affected joint (usually metatarsophalangeal joint of great toe); other joints commonly affected by gout are the intertarsals, ankle, knee, wrist, finger, and elbow
Redness
Asymmetric swelling
Shiny
Vein distention
Deformity
Elevated temperature
Chills
Subcutaneous tophi: proximal ulnar surface of the forearm, the olecranon process, Achilles tendon, pinna of the ear

DIAGNOSTIC TESTS
Serum and uric acid elevated, WBC, ESR
Microscopic examination of joint aspirate
X-ray examination of affected area
Arthrocentesis

POTENTIAL COMPLICATIONS
Decreased urine output
Hypertension
Renal calculi
Joint deformities

MULTIDISCIPLINARY MANAGEMENT
THERAPEUTIC MANAGEMENT
Medications
NSAIDs: (e.g., indomethacin [Indocin], naproxen [Naprosyn], sulindac [Clinoril], phenylbutazone [Butazolidin])
Corticosteroids (intraarticular, oral, intramuscular)
Adrenocorticotropin hormone (ACTH)
Colchicine
Analgesics
For chronic management
Urate-lowering agents (e.g., allopurinol, probenecid, sulfinpyrazone)
Supportive Care
Cold compresses
Joint immobilization and decreased weight bearing

Dietary
Low-calorie diet with gradual weight reduction if overweight
Reduction in alcohol consumption
Reduction in intake of high-purine foods (organ meats, sweetbreads, sardines)
Consultation with dietition

PATIENT PROBLEMS—NURSING DIAGNOSES/INTERVENTIONS

▼Pain related to inflammation and edema

Assess intensity, location, and type of pain; use pain rating scale
Immobilize affected joint or extremity
Maintain patient in position of comfort with affected joint (initially foot) supported and in alignment; place cradle over foot/affected joint; no weight bearing
Apply hot or cold packs, ice bag to affected joint; avoid placing excess pressure on joint
Elevate affected area *to reduce edema and promote venous return*
Administer analgesics and antigout and antiinflammatory agents; observe for side effects
Colchicine: nausea, vomiting, bloody diarrhea, oliguria, hematuria
Phenylbutazone: nausea, vomiting, diarrhea, rash, edema, hypertension, leukopenia
Encourage fluids to 2500 ml/day *to increase elimination of urate salts*
Monitor serum uric acid levels

Expected Outcomes
Reports pain is at a tolerable level
Appears calm and relaxed
Exhibits lessening or absent edema

▼Impaired physical mobility related to joint pain and inflammation

Maintain bed rest with affected extremity elevated until edema and pain have lessened
Increase activity as pain and swelling subside
Ambulate with assistance; use walker or cane
Perform ROM exercise carefully to affected joint
Promote return to normal activities

Expected Outcomes
Performs ROM adequately in affected joint
Ambulates with walker or cane without discomfort

PATIENT/FAMILY TEACHING AND DISCHARGE/HOME CARE PLANNING
Discuss pain management
Take pain medication as needed; monitor for side effects of drugs
Apply ice/hot packs as ordered
Immobilize extremity as needed

Encourage bed rest and use cradle to keep sheets off
extremity
Review need to
Inspect skin for tophi formation
Apply lotions for dryness
Discuss importance of not sitting, lying in one position
for extended periods
Discuss preventive measures
Avoid high-purine diet if indicated
Avoid excessive use of alcohol
Encourage fluid intake up to 3 L/day if adequate
kidney function
Provide medication schedule including name, dosage,
purpose, and side effects and explain necessity of
taking colchicine hourly at onset of acute attacks
Report side effects of medications immediately; avoid
salicylates if taking probenecid
Discuss importance of diet, exercise, and rest program
Provide list of high-purine foods (liver, kidneys, sardines,
consommé, herring, anchovies); discuss foods to
substitute (chicken, fish, vegetables, cheese, eggs, milk)
Emphasize importance of maintaining normal weight
Explain importance of high fluid intake (2500 ml/day), if
not contraindicated
Encourage medical follow-up visits and laboratory tests to
monitor serum uric acid

■ FRACTURE

A break in bone continuity; types of fractures and their causes are listed in Box 8-1

ASSESSMENT
SUBJECTIVE DATA
Fracture site
Pain, tenderness, muscle spasm
Decreased sensation, numbness, tingling
Loss of function

OBJECTIVE DATA
Fracture site
Edema
Deformity
Crepitation
Skin open or intact
Color and temperature of surrounding tissues
Presence/absence of pulse distal from break
Bleeding, hematoma, soft tissue damage
Restricted, limited mobility
Abnormal position of extremity
Signs of shock: hypotension, tachycardia, pallor,
diaphoresis
Signs of fat embolism: chest pain, dyspnea, changes in
respiratory rate, decreased mental acuity

DIAGNOSTIC TESTS
Radiologic films of fracture, CT, MRI
CBC, electrolytes, prothrombin time/International
Normalized Ratio (PT/INR)

POTENTIAL COMPLICATIONS
Malunion, delayed union, or nonunion of fracture
Thrombophlebitis
Fat embolism
Compartment syndrome (knee, elbow)
Infection
Nerve compression

MULTIDISCIPLINARY MANAGEMENT
THERAPEUTIC MANAGEMENT
Surgery
Open or closed reduction of fracture
Joint arthroplasty or total replacement
Medications
Analgesics, narcotics, sedatives, antibiotics, muscle
relaxants, anticoagulants
Application of cast, traction, splint, sling, external fixation
device
Ice application
Antiembolic stockings and/or antithrombic pump
Diet, activity, rest, mobility restrictions
Physical therapy
Rehabilitation exercises
Crutch walking

PATIENT PROBLEMS—NURSING DIAGNOSES/INTERVENTIONS

▼Impaired bed mobility related to pain and limitations of fracture and injury

Assess extent of injury surrounding fracture site
Maintain bed rest in prescribed position *to facilitate
healing and rest*
Evaluate pressure points, change position q2h
Elevate affected extremity and apply ice bags as
indicated *to reduce edema and improve venous
return*
Support affected extremity above and below fracture
when moving, turning, and lifting
Monitor cast, traction, and sling qh initially, then q4h;
observe for cast integrity and position of traction
weights and sling
Assist with and teach use of trapeze and other methods
of moving and turning
Perform passive or assist with and teach active ROM
exercises to unaffected joints *to maintain joint
mobility*
Explain restrictions and limitations in activity
Assist with and teach patient use of urinal or bedpan for
elimination; administer perineal care as needed

Expected Outcomes
Moves from one bed position to another
Verbalizes understanding of progression from dependent
to independent repositioning in bed

▼Impaired physical mobility related to musculoskeletal impairment

| Box 8-1 | **Types and Causes of Fractures** |

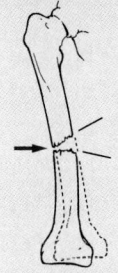

Angulated: Fracture with fragments at angles to each other
Cause: Direct or lateral force, causing break and loss of anatomic positions

Angulated

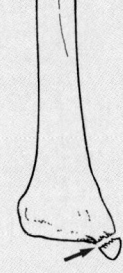

Avulsed: Fracture that pulls bone and other tissues from usual attachments
Cause: Direct energy or force, with resisted extension of bone and joint

Avulsed

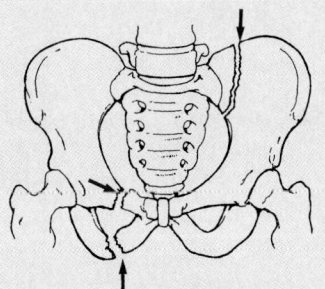

Bucket handle: Double vertical fractures of pelvis on same side, resulting in pelvic dislocation
Cause: Direct blow or anterior compression force, with or without sacral torsion

Bucket-handle

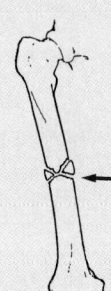

Butterfly: Butterfly-shaped piece of fractured bone, usually accompanying comminuted fracture
Cause: Direct, indirect, or rotational force to bone

Butterfly

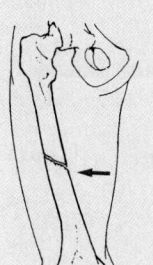
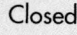

Closed: Skin intact over fracture
Cause: Minor force or energy

Closed

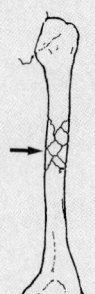

Comminuted: Fracture with more than two pieces; may have significant associated soft tissue trauma
Cause: Direct crushing injury or force to tissues and bone

Comminuted

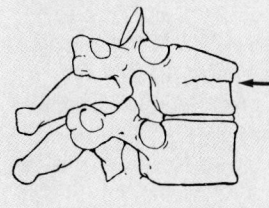

Compression: Fracture is squeezed or wedged together at one side
Cause: Compressive, axial energy or force applied directly from above fracture site

Compression

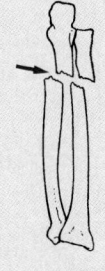
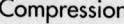

Displaced: Fracture with one, both, or all fragments out of normal alignment
Cause: Direct energy or force to site

Displaced

From Mourad LA: Mosby's clinical nursing series: orthopedic disorders, *St Louis, 1991, Mosby.*

Continued

Box 8-1	**Types and Causes of Fractures**—cont'd

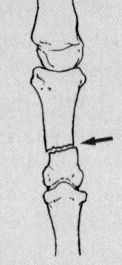

Extraarticular: Fracture near but outside a joint
Cause: Direct energy above or below a joint

Extraarticular

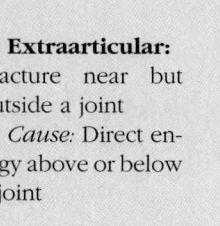

Greenstick: Break in only one cortex of bone
Cause: Minor direct or indirect energy

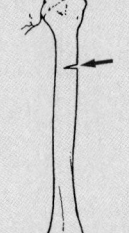

Greenstick

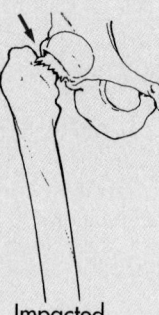

Impacted: Fracture with one end wedged into opposite end or inside fractured fragment
Cause: Compressive axial energy or force directly to distal fragment

Impacted

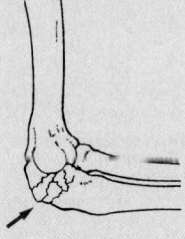

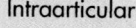

Intraarticular: Fracture involving bones inside a joint
Cause: Direct or indirect energy or force to joint

Intraarticular

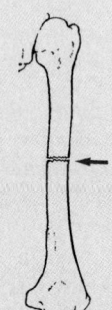

Linear: As a line, so can be transverse or oblique
Cause: Minor or moderate energy or force directly to bone

Linear

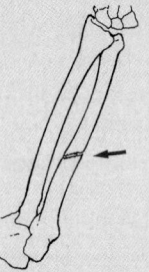

Nightstick: Fracture of ulna caused by blow to forearm elevated in defensive position
Cause: Direct force or blow to forearm

Nightstick

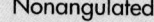

Nonangulated: Fracture with fragments in anatomic relationship to each other
Cause: Minor force or energy

Nonangulated

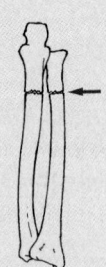

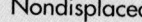

Nondisplaced: Fracture fragments in close approximation and anatomic position to each other
Cause: Minor-to-moderate force or energy

Nondisplaced

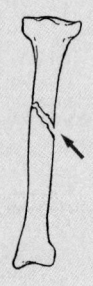

Oblique: Fracture at oblique angle across both cortices
Cause: Direct or indirect energy, with angulation and some compression

Oblique

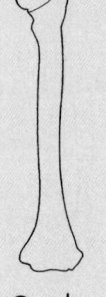

Occult: Fracture that is hidden or not readily discernible
Cause: Minor force or energy

Occult

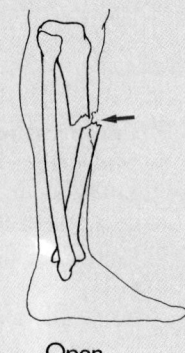

Open: Skin broken over fracture; possible soft tissue trauma
Cause: Moderate-to-severe energy that is continuous and exceeds tissue tolerances

Open

| Box 8-1 | **Types and Causes of Fractures** |

Pathologic: Transverse, oblique, or spiral fracture of bone weakened by tumor pressure or presence
Cause: Minor energy or force, which may be direct or indirect

Pathologic

Segmented: Fracture with two or more pieces or segments
Cause: Direct or indirect moderate-to-severe force

Segmented

Spiral: Fracture that curves around cortices and may become displaced by twist
Cause: Direct or indirect twisting energy or force with distal part held or unable to move

Spiral

Stellate: Central fracture point from which fissures radiate
Cause: Direct blow or force of moderate energy

Stellate

Straddle: Bilateral fractures of pelvic and pubic rami
Cause: Fall that causes or results in straddling of hard object

Straddle

Stress: Crack in one cortex of bone
Cause: Repetitive direct energy or force, as from jogging, running, or striking a lever, or from osteoporosis

Stress

Torus: Fracture of one cortex of shafts of radius and ulna (one cortex of each bone), shown as wrinkle or buckle
Cause: Direct blow to forearm or indirect compressive force, as from fall

Torus

Transverse: Horizontal break through bone
Cause: Direct or indirect energy toward bone

Transverse

Encourage patient to perform ADLs within scope of limitations; provide supplies; assist as necessary

Provide information about task simplification

Teach exercises to maintain strength: quadriceps, buttocks, sitting exercises q4h

Manage pain *to optimize physical mobility*

Ambulate as ordered; involve physical therapy department in use of crutches, walker, cane

Teach appropriate use of assistive devices *to ensure safety while improving mobility*

Expected Outcomes

Regains mobility to optimal level

Participates actively in treatment plan

Seeks assistance as needed

Verbalizes needed restrictions and understands rationale

▼Risk for altered peripheral tissue perfusion related to location of fracture and risk of arteriovenous flow alteration

Assess and monitor pulses distal from fracture q1h and observe for color, temperature, and sensation q2h

Monitor vital signs q2h to 4h

Assess capillary refill; report abnormal findings; compare with opposite extremity

Maintain body alignment and prescribed position *to ensure adequate circulation*

Observe for signs of compartment syndrome (p. 490)
Apply antiembolic stockings: remove daily *to inspect for pressure, pain, and redness*
Encourage small movements of affected digits *to maintain venous flow*

Expected Outcomes
Pulses distal to fracture are present
Skin is warm
Capillary refill is normal (2 to 4 seconds)

▼Risk for altered tissue perfusion: cerebral and/or cardiopulmonary related to fat embolus; *this dangerous complication requires immediate action; these emboli can occlude coronary arteries, pulmonary circulation, and cerebral flow; death may ensue if not treated promptly*

Assess cardiopulmonary status
  Monitor vital signs q2h to 4h; take apical pulse
  Monitor cardiac output, ABGs
  Observe for tachycardia, angina; instruct patient to report chest pain immediately
  Auscultate chest for breath sounds q4h; observe for diminished sounds
  Monitor respirations for tachypnea, dyspnea
  Assist with chest x-rays
  Assist and teach patient to turn and cough q2h and deep breathe qh
Assess cerebral status
  Monitor LOC, mental status orientation as to name, time, place q4h to 8h
  Assess pupils for size, equality, and reaction to light
  Instruct patient to report headache, dizziness, numbness/tingling of extremities immediately

Expected Outcomes
Presents normal vital signs
Exhibits clear breath sounds
Presents laboratory values within normal limits
Remains alert, oriented
Reports no headache or chest pain

▼Impaired tissue integrity related to surgical reduction, puncture wounds

Assess wound integrity and observe for signs of infection or drainage, especially at pin sites
  Administer antibiotics and assess effectiveness, side effects
  Monitor and change dressings prn using aseptic technique
  Monitor temperature
Monitor traction/casts for pressure points
  Provide frequent skin care to bony prominences and around cast/traction openings
  Turn patient frequently; maintain body alignment
  Maintain dry, wrinkle-free bed linen

Provide foam, air, or water mattress as needed; use bed cradle to prevent pressure

Expected Outcomes
Tissue integrity is maintained
Temperature is normal

▼Pain related to fracture and/or trauma

Assess location, intensity, and type of pain; use pain rating scale
Administer narcotics, analgesics, and muscle relaxants; avoid allowing pain to become severe; assess effectiveness of pain relief measures
Collaborate with physician regarding patient controlled analgesia (PCA)
Provide quiet environment initially and encourage diversional activities *to decrease awareness of discomfort*
Assist with and teach alternative pain management methods
Change position frequently and administer back rubs and massages *to promote comfort*
Encourage ambulation with assistance when tolerated

Expected Outcomes
Verbalizes relief or a reduction in pain
Appears comfortable; a relaxed manner

▼Anxiety related to altered health/situational crisis

Monitor patient's level of anxiety (p. 56)
Reinforce physician's explanation of treatment and expected outcome; clarify misconceptions
Encourage and allow time for verbalization of feelings
Teach and assist with stress management techniques
Assess present coping behaviors and encourage use of behaviors that were successful in managing past experiences
Encourage interaction with significant other and friends, relatives
Explain all procedures and treatments; involve patient in plan of care; provide options; encourage safe decision making

Expected Outcomes
Demonstrates relaxation techniques correctly
Verbalizes a feeling of less tension, apprehension
Appears calm and relaxed
Participates in activities appropriately

Additional Nursing Diagnosis to Consider
Impaired: transfer and/or wheelchair mobility

PATIENT/FAMILY TEACHING
Stress importance of prescribed rehabilitation plan of activity, rest, and exercise

Provide and review diet instructions regarding type and amount; need to avoid weight gain if applicable

Discuss medications: name, purpose, schedule, dosage, and side effects

Discuss signs and symptoms to report to physician: severe pain, changes in temperature, color, or sensation in extremity, foul odor or drainage from wound

Explain cast, splint, sling care as indicated (see Cast care p. 494)

Encourage follow-up visits with physician

DISCHARGE/HOME CARE PLANNING

Assess level of understanding of injury and continue with patient/family teaching and monitor the following:

Environmental/safety status

Caregivers' ability to perform needed tasks

Accessible telephone and emergency numbers: physician, pharmacy, home health care team

Emergency call device to summon outside help

Absence of scatter rugs, unbacked carpets

Presence of stairs with hand rails

Grab bars at tub and toilet

Nonskid strips in tub

Adequate lighting for safe movement

Wide doorways to accommodate wheelchairs/walkers

Height of chair and bed for easy transfer on and off of each

Flashlights near bed and chair

Medications accessible and labeled

Availability of transportation to needed appointments

Needed supplies: what and where to purchase

Mobility status

Ability and desire to follow prescribed rehabilitation plan and exercises

Correct transfer techniques

Amount of weight bearing; reinforce wearing low-heeled, comfortable shoes

Correct use of walkers, canes, crutches

Ability to apply brace, corset, removable cast

Status of immobilizing device

Neurovascular status of each affected extremity

Condition of device: wet, loose, clean, soiled

Condition of skin under device: clear, red, tender

Status of wound

Incision for healing, infection

Signs of infection: redness, pain, swelling, fever, drainage

Ability to care for wound; correct supplies and handwashing technique

Knowledge of where and what supplies to purchase

Nutritional status

Understanding of basic food groups and what to eat to provide nutrition with no weight gain

Signs of weight loss, dehydration

Ability to prepare meals; refer to social agency to provide meals

Elimination status

Presence of elevated toilet seat

Use of stool softeners, natural laxatives, bulk in diet

Ability to be active

Amount of fluids taken per day; increase to upper limits for age and weight

Use of fracture pan/urinal/female urinal

◼ MAXILLOMANDIBULAR FIXATION

Surgical procedure to reduce and repair jaw fractures or deformities, using wires and/or plate and additional fixation

PREOPERATIVE ASSESSMENT AND CARE

Assess respiratory status; observe for signs of upper respiratory infection

Explain purpose of wires after surgery and provide method of communication: pad and pencil, Magic Slate*

Assist with and teach patient method for pushing secretions through clamped jaw (if possible) and demonstrate use of oral suction catheter

Discuss importance of oral hygiene and oral suctioning and teach procedure

Demonstrate feeding procedure using straw or syringe

Explain possibility of nasopharyngeal airway and/or nasogastric tube and aspiration postoperatively

Perform facial scrub and oral hygiene preoperatively

Administer prescribed antibiotics

Answer all questions and allow time for verbalization of fears and anxieties

POSTOPERATIVE ASSESSMENT

SUBJECTIVE DATA

Location, character of pain

Nausea

Dyspnea

Apprehension

OBJECTIVE DATA

Edema of the following:

Face

Base of tongue

Front of neck

Nose

Vomiting; aspiration of emesis

Elevated temperature

Drainage from mouth

Location of wire cutters or scissors

DIAGNOSTIC TESTS

CBC, electrolytes

Radiologic examinations for alignment of fracture

Western Publishing Co, Inc, Racine, Wis.

POTENTIAL COMPLICATIONS

Upper respiratory infection with nasal congestion; respiratory distress

Aspiration pneumonia

Hemorrhage, shock

MULTIDISCIPLINARY MANAGEMENT
THERAPEUTIC MANAGEMENT

Medications

Analgesics, sedatives, antibiotics, antiemetics

Parenteral fluids

Nasogastric aspiration or nothing by mouth (NPO) if applicable

O$_2$ therapy

Consultation with respiratory therapist

Surgery

Wire and band cutting procedure

Activity, rest

Dietary

Diet (liquid) high in calories, protein, vitamins

Nutritious supplements: Ensure, Ensure Plus, milkshakes, and other dietary supplements

PATIENT PROBLEMS—NURSING DIAGNOSES/INTERVENTIONS

▼Risk for aspiration related to presence of wired jaws

Tape wire cutters or scissors to head of bed; if aspiration is imminent, cut wires as needed

Maintain bed rest with head elevated when reactive *to prevent aspiration*

Assess patient's ability to swallow *to prevent aspiration*

Perform oral suctioning prn; assist and teach patient to clear airway and perform suctioning

Provide and maintain suction apparatus at all times; observe for edema, drainage, and bleeding

Teach patient techniques to prevent vomiting: deep breathing, swallowing

Control with antiemetics prn

Monitor nasogastric tube and low, intermittent suction apparatus if applicable; maintain patency with normal saline irrigations prn

Apply ice bags *to reduce swelling*

Monitor vital signs, respiratory status q4h to 8h

Auscultate chest for breath sounds q4h to 8h *to monitor for possible aspiration*

Instruct patient to report immediately inability to manage self-suctioning or feeling of nausea

Maintain parenteral fluids and decrease amount as fluid intake increases

Provide clear liquid to full high-calorie liquid diet as tolerated after nasogastric tube has been removed

Assist and teach patient to use straw or feed with syringe; give small amount and wait for swallowing before continuing

Follow each feeding with water and mouth care

Provide small, frequent meals

Consult nutritionist/registered dietitian regarding alternatives in food selections (i.e., commercially prepared formulas)

Measure intake and output q8h

Expected Outcomes

Patient is able to:

Perform self-suctioning to remove secretions

Ingest liquid diet without nausea

Breath sounds are clear to auscultation

Vital signs are stable and within normal limits

▼Pain related to surgical procedure, edema

Assess type, intensity, and location of pain; administer prescribed analgesics; use pain rating scale; assess effectiveness of pain relief measures

Assist patient with changing position frequently while in bed *to promote comfort*

Maintain quiet environment *to provide adequate rest/sleep*

Administer back rubs *to promote comfort*

Offer diversional activities *to decrease attention on pain*

Administer frequent oral hygiene; use water jet, if available, or mouth swabs; keep lips well lubricated *to soothe irritated membranes*

Ambulate patient with assistance as needed *to change surroundings*

Assist with and teach alternative pain management techniques

Apply ice bags *to reduce edema/discomfort*

Expected Outcomes

Reports a tolerable level of pain

Appears calm, relaxed

Adequately balances sleep with activities

▼Impaired verbal communication related to jaw wiring

Maintain call light within easy reach

Provide means of communication: pad and pencil, Magic Slate, laptop computer

Allow time for patient to write out thoughts and questions

Encourage patient to express fears and anxieties

Maintain equipment for communication and place within easy reach

Expected Outcomes

Demonstrates ability to use alternative methods of communication

Appears comfortable with method selected

Additional Nursing Diagnoses to Consider

Altered nutrition: less than body requirements related to anorexia

Impaired tissue integrity related to trauma from injury

PATIENT/FAMILY TEACHING

Provide and review diet instruction for full liquid diet and foods allowed: blended junior foods, eggnogs, and milkshakes; demonstrate use of straw or syringe; introduce spicy foods slowly

Discuss importance and purpose of small, frequent meals

Stress and teach oral hygiene and demonstrate use of Water Pik and dental wax *to keep lips moist*

Demonstrate method for cutting wires and under what circumstances to cut (wires will remain for 6 to 8 weeks)

Discuss limiting strenuous activities/sports until wire removal

Explain signs and symptoms to report to physician: fever, increased pain, edema, foul odor from mouth

Discuss obtaining all medications in liquid form

Promote follow-up visits with physician

DISCHARGE/HOME CARE PLANNING

Assess and continue with patient/family teaching and monitor the following:
  Environmental/safety status
    Caregivers' ability to perform needed tasks
    Accessible telephone and emergency numbers: physician, pharmacy, home health care team
    Medications accessible and labeled
  Status of mouth/wires
    Correct oral hygiene procedures
    Wire-cutting procedure
    Condition of device: wet, loose, clean, soiled
    Condition of skin under device: clear, red, tender
  Nutritional status
    Ability to prepare nourishing liquid diet
    Signs of weight loss or dehydration

■ SPINAL SURGERY

Surgery performed to relieve pressure on the spinal nerves and/or cord caused by a herniated disk, trauma, displaced fracture, incomplete vertebral dislocation from rheumatoid arthritis, osteoporosis; incision may be anterior or posterior in cervical, thoracic, or lumbar areas

  laminectomy (hemilaminectomy): *Removal of part of the disk lamina*

  microdiscectomy: *Removal of part of the disk*

  microsurgical dorsal root rhizotomy: *Severing of the sensory nerve root to the painful area; provides symptomatic relief and causes loss of sensation and possible motor damage; performed when other treatments have been unsuccessful*

  facet joint rhizotomy: *Needle insertion into the facet joint with destruction of the nerve by microwave current; provides symptomatic relief*

  laser therapy: *Percutaneous incision and insertion of laser to remove bulging disks; the laser destroys the disk*

  chemonucleolysis: *Enzyme chymopapain is instilled into the disk to dissolve it; this procedure is not favored, because of anaphylactic reactions*

PREOPERATIVE ASSESSMENT AND TEACHING

Assess patient's neurovascular and respiratory status and location, intensity, and duration of pain

Discuss with and teach patient postoperative care and rationale
  Definition and importance of prescribed postoperative position and body alignment
  Methods for turning/log rolling, coughing, and deep breathing
  Use of trapeze and method for getting in and out of bed
  Necessary movement limitations and activities allowed ROM and isometric exercises
    Gluteal contractions, quadriceps setting

Explain that antiembolic stockings and sequential compression sleeves may be applied to lower extremities *to promote venous return*

Discuss and practice turning on side to eat and using a fracture bed pan

Discuss pain management and possible use of PCA; explain that discomfort may not be relieved at once following surgery because the nerves take time to heal

Encourage patient to ask questions; provide emotional support
  Reinforce physician's explanation of surgical procedure
  Allow time for and discuss patient's fears and anxieties

POSTOPERATIVE ASSESSMENT
SUBJECTIVE DATA
Location and character of pain

OBJECTIVE DATA
Neurovascular status of extremities
  Decreased sensation and motor activity
  Change in color, temperature, or pulse
Respiratory status (especially in cervical surgery)
  Difficulty in breathing
  Cyanosis
  Tachypnea
  Diminished cough
Body alignment: presence of immobilization devices
Character and amount of
  Wound drainage
  Urinary output

DIAGNOSTIC TESTS
CBC, electrolytes, clotting time
Spinal radiologic examinations
Urine for culture/sensitivity

POTENTIAL COMPLICATIONS
Neurovascular damage, leaking spinal fluid
Hemorrhage
Shock
Urinary retention, infection
Abdominal distention
Constipation
Paralytic ileus
Atelectasis, hypostatic pneumonia

Pulmonary embolus
Wound infection
Nonunion

MULTIDISCIPLINARY MANAGEMENT
THERAPEUTIC MANAGEMENT
Medications
Analgesics, antibiotics, antiemetics, stool softeners
Parenteral fluids with electrolytes
Urinary drainage catheter
Respiratory therapy consultation
O$_2$ therapy, incentive spirometer
Transcutaneous electrical nerve stimulation (TENS) unit (p. 42), PCA (p. 40)
Immobilization devices: brace, cast, corset
Diet, activity, rest
Antiembolic stockings
Physical therapy
Rehabilitation evaluation and planning
Ambulatory devices
Strengthening exercises

PATIENT PROBLEMS—NURSING DIAGNOSES/INTERVENTIONS

▼Risk for ineffective breathing pattern related to anesthesia, pain, or cervical spinal cord compression

Assess respiratory status q2h: monitor for signs of aspiration
Assist and teach patient to deep breathe qh
For cervical surgery
Check respirations q½h for rate, rhythm, quality, and distress signs
Maintain bed rest with head of bed elevated 30 to 45 degrees
Observe for diminished cough reflex
Assess face and neck for edema qh
Maintain comfort with analgesics *to improve respiration*
Auscultate chest for breath sounds q2h
Monitor vital signs
Provide incentive spirometer qh to 2h
Encourage ambulation as soon as prescribed

Expected Outcomes
Breath sounds are normal
Respiratory rate and rhythm are regular
Face and neck edema is absent

▼Altered peripheral tissue perfusion related to surgical procedure and interruption of arterial flow

Monitor vital signs q2h to 4h
Assess neurovascular status of both legs; report changes in color, temperature, pulse, sensation, or motor activity to physician
For cervical surgery: assess upper extremities for color, pulse, temperature, motor activity, and sensation q2h; report changes to physician

Monitor for peripheral edema q4h
Apply antiembolic stockings *to increase venous return;* remove daily and inspect skin for pressure areas
Apply sequential compression sleeves as ordered
Monitor capillary refill on both feet q2h to 4h
Avoid heavy blankets over feet and extreme cold exposure
Encourage moving toes and feet *to promote venous flow*

Expected Outcomes
Vital signs are stable
Capillary refill is within normal limits
Extremities are warm, of normal color, and pedal pulses are present
Motor activity and sensation are within normal limits

▼Risk for infection related to invasive procedure and reduced primary defenses

Monitor temperature q4h; report elevation immediately
Monitor hemoglobin (Hgb), hematocrit (Hct), WBC
Monitor dressing(s) for drainage q2h for 24 hours, then q4h; evaluate type of drainage; a clear or pink ring may indicate cerebrospinal fluid leakage; report to physician at once
Change dressings prn; physician may wish to do initial dressing; drainage is usually minimal
Report excess drainage, bleeding to physician
Obtain culture for suspicious drainage
Encourage adequate food and fluid intake *to promote wound healing*

Expected Outcomes
Incision remains clean, dry, and intact
Temperature is normal
Laboratory values are within normal limits

▼Altered urinary elimination related to anesthesia and/or bed rest

Measure intake and output q4h to 8h
If unable to urinate after 8 hours, catheterize per physician's order prn until voiding qs
Encourage fluids to 2500 ml/day if not contraindicated *to promote elimination*
Assist with ambulation when allowed

Expected Outcomes
Urinary output is normal for age and weight
Fluid intake is adequate

▼Impaired bed mobility related to postsurgical musculoskeletal limitations

Maintain bed rest, usually in supine or prone position with slight flexion of knees
Maintain immobilization of spine
Maintain body alignment throughout all procedures
For cervical surgery, a soft cervical collar may be ordered if no immobilization device is present

Do not flex head forward

Elevate head of bed 40 to 60 degrees

Turn patient only as prescribed

    Administer pain medication 30 minutes before turning when possible

    Use log-rolling method

    Turn q2h from back to side to side

    While turning

        Support patient's legs with pillow between knees

        Support head with small pillow

        Roll in one continuous motion

        Support back with pillows

        Administer skin care with each turn; assess pressure points

Balance rest periods with activity

Increase activity as prescribed

    Initiate quadriceps setting and gluteal contractions

    Assist with and teach active or perform passive ROM exercises q4h, as indicated, according to surgical procedure

    Avoid sudden movements or twisting of extremities or neck

    Involve physical therapist as indicated

Expected Outcomes

Moves from one bed position to another

Verbalizes understanding of progression from dependent to independent repositioning in bed

▼ Impaired physical mobility related to musculo-skeletal impairment and pain

Ambulate with assistance when allowed

    Assist with and reinforce teaching of method for sitting up and getting out of bed

    Have patient wear supportive shoes

    Disconnect sequential compression device during ambulation

    Assist patient in walking

        Observe for vertigo, nausea, and hypotension

        Observe gait

        Avoid shuffling feet

    Place patient in straight-backed chair with feet on floor

    Increase ambulation to tolerance; have patient avoid standing, sudden movements, and twisting

Encourage self-care as tolerated; assist with and teach modified ADLs as needed

Expected Outcomes

Regains mobility to optimal level

Maintains proper body alignment

Participates in rehabilitation plan

▼ Pain related to surgical intervention

Assess location, type, and intensity of pain; use pain rating scale and medicate as needed for continuous comfort

Administer analgesics; avoid morphine for cervical surgery patients; monitor for effectiveness, side effects

Assist patient with changing position frequently, maintaining correct body alignment *to promote comfort*

Provide and teach use of TENS unit if applicable

Discuss and teach alternative pain relief measures: back rubs, imaging

Instruct patient in use of PCA

Encourage diversional activities *to decrease attention on pain*

Expected Outcomes

Reports that pain is at tolerable level

Appears relaxed and comfortable

Cooperates and attempts use of alternate pain management techniques

PATIENT/FAMILY TEACHING

Stress importance of prescribed activity, exercises, and restrictions

    Degree of activity and self-care allowed; ways to avoid overdependence

    Need to maintain good body alignment

    No heavy lifting, strenuous exercise, automobile driving or riding, stooping, or bending

    Methods of knee bending

    Need to avoid fatigue; exercise to tolerance with frequent rest periods

    ROM exercises as allowed

    Straight-backed chair for sitting; no knee crossing

    Convalescent period (may be an extended length of time: 2 to 9 months)

    Need to wear immobilization device as ordered: method of application, care, and removal of device; observance of device for areas that may cause skin irritation or breakdown

    Firm mattress with bedboard (essential)

Provide and review instructions on diet and fluid intake; explain ways to avoid weight gain and constipation

Discuss and demonstrate incisional care

    Signs and symptoms of wound infection

    Need to shower daily with mild soap and observe skin for signs of irritation; apply lotion as needed

Discuss signs and symptoms to report to physician

    Decreased motor activity and/or sensation in extremities

    Increased pain in surgical area

    Elevated temperature

Discuss medications: name, schedule, purpose, dosage, and side effects

Encourage follow-up visits with physician

DISCHARGE/HOME CARE PLANNING

Assess and continue with patient/family teaching and monitor the following:

    Environmental/safety status

        Caregivers' ability to perform needed tasks

        Accessible telephone and emergency numbers: physician, pharmacy, home health care team

        Emergency call device to summon outside help

Absence of scatter rugs, unbacked carpets

Presence of stairs with hand rails

Grab bars at tub and toilet

Nonskid strips in tub

Adequate lighting for safe movement

Wide doorways to accommodate wheelchairs/walkers

Height of chair and bed for easy transfer on and off of each

Flashlights near bed and chair

Medications accessible and labeled

Availability of transportation to needed appointments

Needed supplies: what and where to purchase

Mobility status

Ability and desire to follow prescribed rehabilitation plan and exercises

Correct transfer techniques

Amount of weight bearing; reinforce wearing low-heeled, comfortable shoes

Correct use of walkers, canes, crutches

Ability to apply brace, corset, removable cast

Status of immobilizing device

Neurovascular status of each affected extremity

Condition of device: wet, loose, clean, soiled

Condition of skin under device: clear, red, tender

Status of wound

Incision for healing, infection

Signs of infection: redness, pain, swelling, fever, drainage

Ability to care for wound: correct supplies and handwashing technique

Knowledge of where and what supplies to purchase

Nutritional status

Understanding of basic food groups and what to eat to provide nutrition with no weight gain

Signs of weight loss, dehydration

Ability to prepare meals; refer to social agency to provide meals

Elimination status

Presence of elevated toilet seat

Use of stool softeners, natural laxatives, bulk in diet

Ability to be active

Amount of fluids taken per day; increase to upper limits for age and weight

Use of fracture pan/urinal/female urinal

■ FRACTURE OR DISLOCATION OF CERVICAL SPINE

A condition of the cervical spine in which one or more vertebrae are fractured or dislocated; either condition may cause pressure on the spinal cord resulting in neurovascular dysfunction

ASSESSMENT

SUBJECTIVE DATA

Neck pain, headache

OBJECTIVE DATA

Signs of spinal cord compression

Loss of mobility and sensation below compression

Urinary retention

Paroxysmal hypertension

Bradycardia

Dyspnea

DIAGNOSTIC TESTS

Radiologic examination of cervical spine

Baseline CBC, urinalysis, electrolytes

POTENTIAL COMPLICATIONS

Respiratory distress

Abdominal distention, paralytic ileus

Decreased bowel and urine function

Complete paralysis of all extremities and trunk

MULTIDISCIPLINARY MANAGEMENT

THERAPEUTIC MANAGEMENT

Immobilization devices: halo traction, Crutchfield tongs, skeletal traction

Analgesics, muscle relaxants, stool softeners

Parenteral fluids with electrolytes

Diet, activity, rest

Physical therapy

Rehabilitation planning

Use of immobilizing devices and tilt table

PATIENT PROBLEMS—NURSING DIAGNOSES/INTERVENTIONS

▼Impaired physical mobility related to musculoskeletal impairment and bed rest

Maintain bed rest in correct body alignment; have patient avoid lifting or twisting head; use sandbags until immobilization device is applied

Maintain and monitor immobilization device: halo traction, cervical head halter, skeletal traction, Stryker frame, or CircOlectric bed; maintain cervical spine in extension

Perform passive or assist with and teach active ROM exercises for all extremities q2h

Promote isometric exercises q2h to 4h

As fracture heals, traction is replaced with casts (halo, Minerva) or neck brace; it is worn continuously; monitor for comfort and correct fit

Ambulate with assistance; monitor for vertigo and weakness; progress slowly

Expected Outcomes

Participates in rehabilitation plan and activity schedule

Regains mobility to optimal level

Performs ROM exercises accurately

▼Altered peripheral tissue perfusion related to injury, trauma

Assess neurovascular status q2h; monitor pulses, color, temperature, sensation, and mobility of all extremities

Monitor vital signs q2h to 4h

Apply antiembolic stockings; remove daily and monitor skin integrity

Encourage lower leg movement *to promote venous return*

Monitor extremities for edema and capillary refill

Expected Outcomes
Vital signs are stable

Extremities are warm and of normal color

Capillary refill is normal

Motor activity and sensation are within normal limits

▼Risk for impaired skin integrity related to pressure resulting from physical immobilization

Provide alternating pressure, gel, foam, air mattress *to maintain skin integrity*

Administer skin care q2h without turning if necessary

Change positions in small ways q1h to 2h *to decrease amount of pressure*

Apply lotions and provide massage and back rubs; *do not massage reddened areas*

Maintain wrinkle-free bottom sheets

Monitor bilateral skull dressings and tong placement of skeletal traction; observe amount of drainage and cleanse areas q4h with normal saline, apply Betadine ointment; allow to dry and redress

Monitor weights for correct amount and placement; *never release traction and keep weights off floor*

Expected Outcomes
Maintains skin integrity around insertion sites

Moves about in bed frequently and maintains body alignment

Verbalizes understanding of needed immobilizing device

▼Self-care deficit: feeding, bathing, toileting related to restricted positioning and trauma

Assess level of dependency

Plan care to meet needs as identified (e.g., provide total care only for those areas of self-care in which patient cannot participate)

Feeding
Maintain parenteral fluids with electrolytes until oral intake is adequate for patient

Collaborate with physician and provide well-balanced diet when tolerated

Initiate clear-to-full liquids and progress to soft or regular diet

    Provide foods easily chewed and swallowed

    Assist with feeding or feed prn

    Observe for signs of dysphagia

Encourage patient to make own food selections *to promote independence*

Serve food attractively arranged *to stimulate appetite*

Provide oral hygiene before and after meals

Bathing
Discuss and plan daily care and routines with patient

Encourage self-care; instruct to avoid overexertion or fatigue

Provide needed equipment for patient comfort and ADLs

Assist as needed or perform total care if patient is dependent

Promote increasing self-care as tolerated by patient

Toileting
Measure intake and output; monitor for urine retention

Offer bedpan regularly or keep close at hand; fracture pan may be more comfortable

Encourage fluid intake of 2500 ml/day if not contraindicated

Provide privacy and perform perineal care as needed

Monitor bowel sounds: observe for decreased sounds, distention (paralytic ileus)

Prevent constipation with stool softeners, natural laxatives, high-fiber diet

Expected Outcomes
Regains independence as activity and mobility increase

Participates in self-care to optimal level

Maintains weight normal for age, height

Experiences normal elimination patterns

▼Pain related to fracture, trauma, edema

Assess location, type, and intensity of pain; use pain rating scale

Report any increase in pain to physician

Monitor devices for comfort

Administer analgesics and muscle relaxants; avoid morphine; assess effectiveness of pain relief measures

Collaborate with physician about PCA

Administer back rubs and massages *to promote comfort*

Encourage patient to change position slightly at frequent intervals *to promote comfort*

Reinforce correct body alignment

Provide diversional activities *to decrease attention on discomfort*

Discuss and teach alternative pain relief measures

Expected Outcomes
Reports reduced level of discomfort

Seems relaxed; rest and sleep are adequate

Participates in diversional activities

Additional Nursing Diagnoses to Consider
Impaired transfer ability

Impaired bed mobility

Ineffective breathing pattern related to location of fracture and frank spinal cord injury (see Spinal cord injury, p. 547)

Self-care deficit related to frank injury

PATIENT/FAMILY TEACHING

Stress importance of prescribed activity and
    immobilization device
    Avoiding fatigue with planned rest periods
    Signs and care of pressure points from device
    Length of time device is to be worn
Demonstrate application and care of immobilization
    device
Discuss/explain the importance of good skin care around
    immobilization device
Explain importance of well-balanced diet; avoid weight
    gain
Avoid constipation with use of stool softeners; discuss
    importance of activity, exercise, and fluids
Discuss maintaining a safe environment *to prevent
    accidents and falls*
Provide information on resuming activities slowly and
    avoiding strenuous exercise
Encourage diversional activities
Provide phone numbers of home health care team
Encourage follow-up visits with physician

DISCHARGE/HOME CARE PLANNING

Assess and continue with patient/family teaching and
    monitor the following:
    Environmental/safety status
        Caregivers' ability to perform needed tasks
        Accessible telephone and emergency numbers:
            physician, pharmacy, home health care team
        Emergency call device to summon outside help
        Absence of scatter rugs, unbacked carpets
        Presence of stairs with hand rails
        Grab bars at tub and toilet
        Nonskid strips in tub
        Adequate lighting for safe movement
        Wide doorways to accommodate
            wheelchairs/walkers
        Height of chair and bed for easy transfer on and off
            of each
        Flashlights near bed and chair
        Medications accessible and labeled
        Availability of transportation to needed
            appointments
        Needed supplies: what and where to purchase
    Mobility status
        Ability and desire to follow prescribed rehabilitation
            plan and exercises
        Correct transfer techniques
        Correct use of walkers, canes, crutches
        Ability to apply brace, corset, removable cast
    Status of immobilizing device
        Neurovascular status of each affected extremity
        Condition of device: wet, loose, clean, soiled
        Condition of skin under device: clear, red, tender
    Status of wound
        Incision for healing, infection
        Signs of infection: redness, pain, swelling, fever, drainage
        Ability to care for wound; correct supplies and
            handwashing technique
        Knowledge of where and what supplies to purchase

Nutritional status
    Understanding of basic food groups and what to
        eat to provide optimal nutrition with no weight
        gain
    Signs of weight loss, dehydration
    Ability to prepare meals; refer to social agency to
        provide meals
Elimination status
    Presence of elevated toilet seat
    Use of stool softeners, natural laxatives, bulk in diet
    Ability to be physically active
    Amount of fluids taken per day: increase to upper
        limits for age and weight
    Use of fracture pan/urinal/female urinal

■ ANKYLOSING SPONDYLITIS

*A progressive inflammatory disease of the vertebral
column and surrounding tissues that begins in the lower
back and eventually causes ankylosing (hardening or
fusing) and deformity of the entire spinal column; etiology is unknown but a hereditary factor (histocompatibility antigen HLA B27) is linked to the disease; more common in males in third decade of life*

ASSESSMENT
SUBJECTIVE DATA
Vertebral pain and stiffness on arising; may radiate to
    other joints (knees, heels, sacroiliac,
    temporomandibular)
Fatigue
Malaise
Anorexia

OBJECTIVE DATA
Loss of normal lumbar lordosis
Paravertebral muscle spasm
Limited mobility
Malaise, chest discomfort
Weight loss
Conjunctivitis, urethritis, polyarthritis
Kyphosis
Painful, tender peripheral joints

DIAGNOSTIC TESTS
Radiologic examination of spine: degeneration,
    calcification, and inflammation
MRI
Histocompatibility antigen HLA B27 (positive) but not
    specific
CK and alkaline phosphatase
ESR: elevated
IgM rheumatoid factor: negative

POTENTIAL COMPLICATIONS
Neurologic damage
Respiratory dysfunction, depending on stage of
    progression

Thrombophlebitis
Fractured vertebrae
Polyarthritis
Aortic insufficiency, uveitis
Colitis
Anemia
Temporomandibular joint (TMJ) disease

MULTIDISCIPLINARY MANAGEMENT
THERAPEUTIC MANAGEMENT
Medications
  Analgesics, antipyretics
  NSAIDs
  Steroids
  Phenylbutazone
  Methotrexate
Supportive care
  Bedboard, firm mattress, small pillow
  Back brace, corset
Surgical intervention
  Cervicospinal fusion
  Osteotomy
  Laminectomy
  Arthroplasty
Rest periods
Physical therapy
  Axial loading precautions
  Postural training
  Traction/back brace
Exercise program
Occupational therapy
Social medicine: job change, assistance at home

PATIENT PROBLEMS—NURSING DIAGNOSES/INTERVENTIONS

▼ Impaired physical mobility related to musculo-skeletal impairment and pain

Assess present mobility and observe for increased impairment
Assist with and reinforce prescribed exercise program
  ROM exercises, ambulation, self-care, and ADLs as tolerated
  Discuss importance of taking rest periods between activities and exercise
  Provide diversional activities
Prepare bed with bedboard, firm mattress, and small pillow; administer frequent back rubs and massages
Assess baseline vital signs
Assess neurovascular status: monitor peripheral pulses and check extremities for color, warmth, sensation, edema, and weakness q4h
Assist with and teach deep breathing exercises *to promote respiratory and peripheral-vascular function*
Monitor skin and mucous membranes for irritation, rashes, or breaks

Encourage Hubbard tank immersions *to relieve muscle spasms and increase strength*
Administer antiinflammatory agents; observe for side effects: gastric discomfort, diarrhea, constipation
Maintain elimination patterns *to promote normalcy*
  Stool softeners
  Adequate fluid intake
Promote ambulation; assist as needed

Expected Outcomes
Participates in exercise program
Seeks assistance as needed
Maintains coordination and mobility at optimal level

▼ Pain related to inflammation/edema

Assess location, intensity, and type of pain; observe for progression of pain to new areas
Administer analgesics; assess effectiveness of pain relief measures
Maintain back brace or corset in correct position
Encourage frequent, small position changes *to increase comfort*
Administer soothing backrubs
Promote diversional activities *to decrease attention on pain*
Teach and assist with alternative pain management techniques

Expected Outcomes
Reports a reduction in discomfort
Presents a more relaxed behavior
Demonstrates learned pain-reducing skills with increasing success

▼ Body image disturbance related to altered body structure/function disturbance

Allow time for and encourage verbalization of feelings and concerns
Reinforce physician's explanation of disease process, treatment, and expected outcome; clarify misconceptions
Provide a supportive environment and assist patient with identifying positive coping styles
Provide realistic hope and set short-term goals to be attained; praise patient for each task accomplished or attempted
Encourage communication with significant other(s) and socialization with family and friends
Encourage self-care as tolerated *to promote independence*
Promote adherence to treatment plan *to postpone further development of deformities*

Expected Outcomes
Verbalizes feelings/concerns and uses adaptive coping skills in dealing with altered image
Participates in treatment regimen and seeks assistance appropriately
Performs ADLs at optimal level

Additional Nursing Diagnosis to Consider
Self-care deficit related to increasing musculoskeletal impairment

PATIENT/FAMILY TEACHING
Stress importance and benefits of maintaining prescribed exercise program including swimming and other non–weight-bearing exercises as tolerated

Discuss medications: name, schedule, purpose, dosage, and side effects

Promote physical therapy activities: ROM, deep breathing; avoid excessive rest

Demonstrate application and care of brace or corset

Encourage nutritious diet and adequate fluid intake

Stress importance of safe environment *to prevent fractures*

Discuss signs and symptoms of disease progression: increased pain and immobility

Encourage follow-up visits with physician

DISCHARGE/HOME CARE PLANNING
Assess and continue with patient/family teaching and monitor the following:

Environmental/safety status
Caregivers' ability to perform needed tasks
Accessible telephone and emergency numbers: physician, pharmacy, home health care team
Emergency call device to summon outside help
Absence of scatter rugs, unbacked carpets
Presence of stairs with hand rails
Grab bars at tub and toilet
Nonskid strips in tub
Adequate lighting for safe movement
Wide doorways to accommodate wheelchairs/walkers
Height of chair and bed for easy transfer on and off of each
Flashlights near bed and chair
Medications accessible and labeled
Availability of transportation to needed appointments
Needed supplies: what and where to purchase

Mobility status
Ability and desire to follow prescribed rehabilitation plan and exercises
Correct transfer techniques
Amount of weight bearing; reinforce wearing low-heeled, comfortable shoes
Correct use of walkers, canes, crutches
Ability to apply brace, corset, removable cast

Status of immobilizing device
Neurovascular status of each affected extremity
Condition of device: wet, loose, clean, soiled
Condition of skin under device: clear, red, tender

Nutritional status
Understanding of basic food groups and what to eat to provide nutrition with no weight gain
Signs of weight loss, dehydration
Ability to prepare meals; refer to social agency to provide meals

Elimination status
Presence of elevated toilet seat
Use of stool softeners, natural laxatives, bulk in diet
Amount of fluids taken per day: increase to upper limits for age and weight
Use of fracture pan/urinal/female urinal

■ OPEN REDUCTION WITH INTERNAL FIXATION
internal fixation: Surgical repair of bones and spine using such devices as a nail, pin, screw, wire, plate, rod, or a combination thereof. These surgeries include the following:

osteotomy: Alteration of bone structure to provide stability, straighten abnormal curvatures, or change weight-bearing surfaces

arthroplasty: Repair or remodeling of bones, cartilage, ligaments, or tendons to relieve pain, rectify traumatic injuries, or remove torn tissues

Harrington rod insertion: Procedure for correcting scoliosis

spinal fusion: Solidification of several vertebrae to strengthen, repair, or correct deformities

PREOPERATIVE ASSESSMENT AND CARE
Assess respiratory, neurovascular, nutritional, and integumentary status

Assess hearing, visual status and presence of other diseases

Monitor traction, braces if applicable

Discuss with and teach patient
Method of coughing and deep breathing and use of incentive spirometer
ROM exercises to unaffected extremities
Postoperative position to be maintained
Gluteal and abdominal contractions and quadriceps setting if applicable
Dorsiflexion and plantar flexion of foot if applicable
Monitor medications; especially be certain antiinflammatories and corticosteroids have been discontinued before admission if possible
Method of log rolling
Importance of leg abduction postoperatively; avoidance of adduction if applicable
Use of trapeze, abduction brace, and pillow
Method of bladder and bowel elimination
Method of pain management
Use of PCA (p. 40)

Discuss and assist patient in dealing with fears and anxieties

Reinforce physician's explanation of surgical procedures and follow-up care

Encourage communication with significant other(s)

Older adult patients may need instructions repeated with each task or procedure

Provide praise or encouragement for tasks attempted and completed

POSTOPERATIVE ASSESSMENT
SUBJECTIVE DATA
Location and character of pain

OBJECTIVE DATA
Correct placement of affected extremity, cast or brace
Neurovascular status of each affected extremity
Urinary output, vital signs
Color and amount of wound drainage
Mental alertness
Respiratory status

DIAGNOSTIC TESTS
CBC, electrolytes, blood gases PT/INR
Radiologic examination of extremity/spine

POTENTIAL COMPLICATIONS
Hemorrhage
Shock
Urinary retention, infection
Confusion if older adult
Pressure ulcers
Atelectasis
Thrombophlebitis
Wound infection
Pin or prosthesis slippage
Extreme internal or external rotation
    Severe pain
    Localized edema of extremity
Malunion of fracture
    Severe pain
    Elevated tempreature
    Severe muscle spasms
Fat embolus
    Decreased oxygen saturation
    Difficulty in breathing
    Cough
    Chest petechiae
    Tachycardia
Compartment syndrome (p. 490)

MULTIDISCIPLINARY MANAGEMENT
THERAPEUTIC MANAGEMENT
Supportive care
    Position to be maintained
    Immobilization devices
Medications
    Analgesics
    Muscle relaxants
    Antibiotics
Parenteral therapy with electrolytes
Urinary catheter
O_2 therapy, incentive spirometer
Social medicine
    Postdischarge placement if indicated
    Home care assistance
Physical therapy
    Rehabilitation plan
    Exercises
Occupational therapy

PATIENT PROBLEMS—NURSING DIAGNOSES/INTERVENTIONS

▼ Impaired physical mobility related to surgical incision and temporary inability to bear weight

Maintain bed rest in prescribed position with firm
    mattress and trapeze
Assist and teach patient to cough and deep breathe qh
    Auscultate chest for breath sounds q8h
    Provide incentive spirometer q1h while awake
    Observe for dyspnea and chest pain
Turn patient on unaffected side q2h; maintain body
    alignment with pillow between knees and at back;
    turn on affected side if ordered
Ambulate with assistance; help patient with dangling legs
    at bedside, then with standing and pivoting on
    unaffected leg into chair (no weight bearing); involve
    physical therapy department if available
Maintain bed rest for 24 to 48 hours on spinal fusion
    patients; when allowed out of bed, must wear brace
Assist with and teach ROM exercises to unaffected
    extremities q4h, and with ROM exercises to knee,
    foot, and ankle of affected leg; passive continuous
    ROM machine may be ordered (p. 498)
Encourage and teach use of walker and increase
    ambulation and weight bearing as tolerated
Assist with ADLs as needed
Promote self-care as soon as patient is able
Balance rest periods with activity

Expected Outcomes
Regains mobility and weight bearing to optimal level
Participates in rehabilitation plan
Progressively participates in own care

▼ Altered peripheral tissue perfusion: related to surgical procedure and interruption of arteriovenous (A/V) flow

Monitor vital signs q2h to 4h
Perform neurovascular checks on all extremities; monitor
    color, temperature, pulse, capillary refill, sensation,
    movement q2h to 4h
Monitor intake and output q4h
Administer parenteral fluids with electrolytes
Apply antiembolic stockings *to enhance venous return;*
    remove at least once daily to inspect skin
Encourage frequent movement of feet and legs *to*
    promote venous return
Administer anticoagulants as prescribed

Expected Outcomes
Vital signs are stable and within normal limits
Neurovascular status and intake and output are within
    normal limits

▼ Risk for infection related to invasive procedure and lowered primary defenses

Assess incision for Hemovac placement; observe for increased drainage

Monitor incision for drainage q2h to 4h

Change dressings as needed; report bleeding, increased drainage to physician

Observe for signs of infection; obtain culture for suspicious drainage

Monitor temperature q4h

Provide well-balanced diet *to promote healing*

Monitor laboratory tests for increased WBC

Expected Outcomes

Temperature is normal

Incision is healing

Surrounding tissue is clean, dry, and intact

Leukocyte count is within normal limits

▼Pain related to surgical procedure and impaired mobility

Assess location, intensity, and character of pain using pain scale

Assess neurovascular status, especially for calf pain (thrombophlebitis)

Administer analgesics; assess effectiveness of pain relief measures

Reinforce instructions in use of PCA

Be alert for severe increase in pain caused by prosthetic slippage or malunion of fracture; report immediately

Provide frequent skin care and back rubs; change position slightly *to prevent skin breakdown and to provide comfort*

Monitor dosage of analgesics for the older adult patient because confusion and disorientation may result with normal dosage

Encourage and increase self-care activities as tolerated; medicate before activity

Provide diversional activities *to decrease attention on pain*

Teach and assist with alternate pain relief measures

Expected Outcomes

Reports a reduction in pain level

Appears more relaxed and calm

Participates in self-care with less discomfort

Additional Nursing Diagnoses to Consider

Risk for altered perfusion: cardiopulmonary, cerebral tissue related to fat embolus

Impaired skin integrity related to mechanical factors and/or physical immobilization

Risk for impaired transfer ability

PATIENT/FAMILY TEACHING

Stress importance of following prescribed rehabilitation plan: amount of weight bearing, activities allowed, and correct body alignment; provide written material as a reference source

Discuss need for nutritious diet and fluids *to facilitate bone union and to maintain optimal circulation and elimination*

Prevent constipation with natural laxatives, stool softeners

If patient had arthroplasty surgery, discuss need to take antibiotics when having invasive procedures performed

Discuss signs and symptoms to report to physician: increased incision or leg pain, fever, decreased urinary output, signs of wound infection

Demonstrate incision care

Promote increasing self-care and ADLs as tolerated

If hip involved, discuss need to use hip precautions: use raised toilet seat and abductor pillow

Encourage follow-up visits with physician and physical therapist

DISCHARGE/HOME CARE PLANNING

Assess and continue with patient/family teaching and monitor the following:

Environmental/safety status

Caregivers' ability to perform needed tasks

Accessible telephone and emergency numbers: physician, pharmacy, home health care team

Emergency call device to summon outside help

Absence of scatter rugs, unbacked carpets

Presence of stairs with hand rails

Grab bars at tub and toilet

Nonskid strips in tub

Adequate lighting for safe movement

Wide doorways to accommodate wheelchairs/walkers

Height of chair and bed for easy transfer on and off of each

Flashlights near bed and chair

Medications accessible and labeled

Availability of transportation to needed appointments

Needed supplies: what and where to purchase

Mobility status

Ability and desire to follow prescribed rehabilitation plan and exercises

Correct transfer techniques

Amount of weight bearing; reinforce wearing low-heeled, comfortable shoes

Correct use of walkers, canes, crutches

Ability to apply brace, corset, removable cast

Status of immobilizing device

Neurovascular status of each affected extremity

Condition of device: wet, loose, clean, soiled

Condition of skin under device: clear, red, tender

Status of wound

Incision for healing, infection

Signs of infection: redness, pain, swelling, fever, drainage

Ability to care for wound: correct supplies and handwashing technique

Knowledge of what supplies are needed and where to purchase them

Nutritional status
  Understanding of basic food groups and what
    to eat to provide adequate nutrition with no
    weight gain
  Signs of weight loss, dehydration
  Ability to prepare meals; refer to social agency to
    provide meals
Elimination status
  Presence of elevated toilet seat
  Use of stool softeners, natural laxatives, bulk in diet
  Ability to be active
  Amount of fluids taken per day: increase to upper
    limits for age and weight
  Use of fracture pan/urinal/female urinal

■ TOTAL JOINT ARTHROPLASTY: HIP, KNEE, ANKLE, SHOULDER, WRIST, FINGER

Replacement of a total joint with a prosthesis to provide stability and motion and to eliminate pain thereby improving functional status and quality of life

PREOPERATIVE ASSESSMENT AND CARE

Assess medication history; be certain that
  antiinflammatories and corticosteroids were
  discontinued at least 10 days before admission,
  if possible

Assess respiratory, neurovascular, nutritional, and
  integumentary status
Assess hearing and visual status and presence of
  other diseases (diabetes, arthritis, coronary artery
  disease (CAD), chronic obstructive pulmonary disease
  (COPD); history of deep vein thrombosis (DVT),
  pulmonary embolism (PE)
Review x-rays of diseased joints
Medication being taken, including iron supplements
Prepare for autologous blood donation
Discuss implant device
Discuss with and teach patient the following:
  Presence of drains and Hemovac postoperatively
  Pain management (epidural/PCA)
  Method of coughing and deep breathing; use of
    incentive spirometer
  ROM exercises to unaffected extremities
  Postoperative restrictions or limitations; these may
    differ according to physician preference
Total hip arthroplasty (Fig. 8-2)
  Gluteal and abdominal contractions and quadriceps
    setting
  Pneumatic compression stocking
  Need to avoid bending hip beyond 90 degrees
  Dorsiflexion and plantar flexion of foot
  Hip hiking, isometric exercises
  Use of trapeze and continuous passive motion
    (CPM) device to prevent rotating hip in bed
  Importance of leg abduction postoperatively

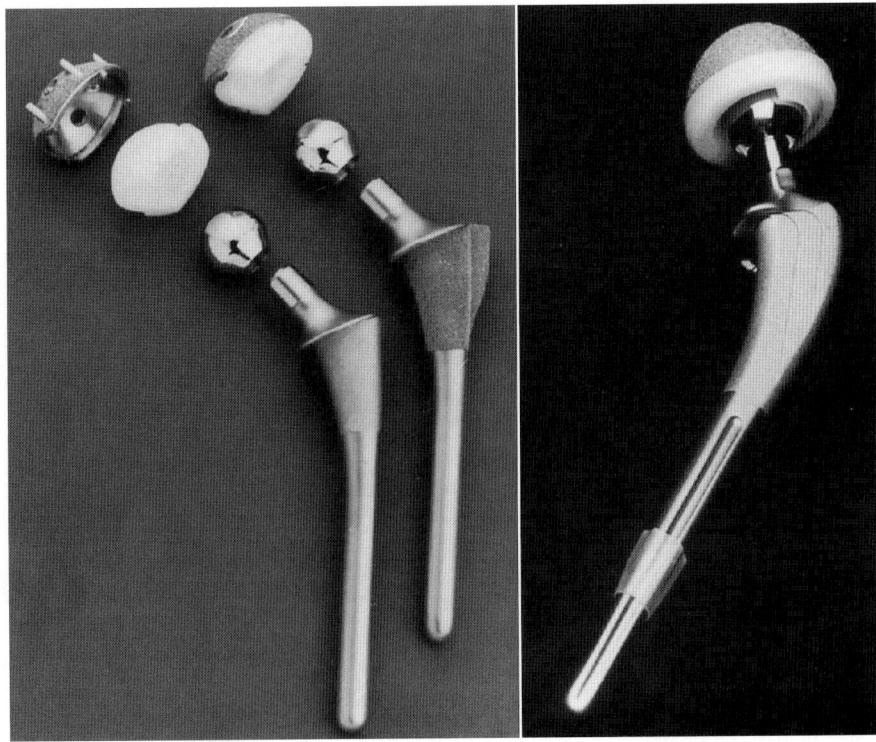

Fig. 8-2 Several types of total hip replacement prostheses.
(***A,*** *Courtesy Zimmer, Warsaw, Ind.* ***B,*** *Courtesy Biomet, Warsaw, Ind. From Mourad LA:* Mosby's clinical nursing series: orthopedic disorders, *St Louis, 1991, Mosby.)*

Physical therapy to begin 1 to 2 days
    postoperatively
Total knee arthroplasty (Fig. 8-3)
    Discuss implant device
    Quadriceps setting, gluteal contractions, and
        flexion-extension exercises
    Straight leg lifts
    Use of CPM device
Total shoulder arthroplasty
    Teach Codman pendulum exercises
    Presence of sling to support affected arm; no side
        elevation of arm
    Presence of drain/dressing
    Prescribed exercises of fingers, wrist, and elbow
Total wrist arthroplasty
    Presence of volnar splint to prevent wrist flexion
    Prescribed finger and arm exercises
Total thumb replacement
    Presence of immobilizing splint or brace to provide
        wrist and thumb support but allow movement
        of fingers
    Prescribed finger and arm exercises
Total finger arthroplasty
    Presence of immobilizing splint or brace that
        provides involved finger support but allows
        movement of other fingers
    Prescribed exercises for arm and unaffected
        fingers
Total ankle arthroplasty
    Presence of plaster splint, soft bulky dressing and
        Hemovac suction apparatus
    Method of crutch walking
    Short leg cast
    Prescribed exercises for toes and knee

Involvement of physical therapy department in planning
    rehabilitation goals
Methods of bladder and bowel elimination
Methods of pain management: PCA (p. 40) or continuous
    epidural analgesia (CEA) (p. 41)
Administer antibiotics and anticoagulants
Measure for antiembolic stockings
Discuss sequential compression devices
Administer surgical scrub as prescribed
Discuss and assist patient in dealing with fears and
    anxieties
    Reinforce physician's explanation of surgical
        procedure and follow-up care
    Encourage communication with significant other(s)
    Repeat instructions as needed with each procedure or
        task for older adult patients
    Provide praise and encouragement for tasks attempted
        or completed

POSTOPERATIVE ASSESSMENT
SUBJECTIVE DATA
Location and character of pain
Nausea/vomiting

OBJECTIVE DATA
Neurovascular status of involved extremity
    Peripheral pulse, pallor, cyanosis, edema
    Sensation, temperature, mobility
Site of incision; wound drains
    Hemovac
    Excessive bleeding or drainage
Respiratory status
Position of affected joint and extremity
Mental alertness

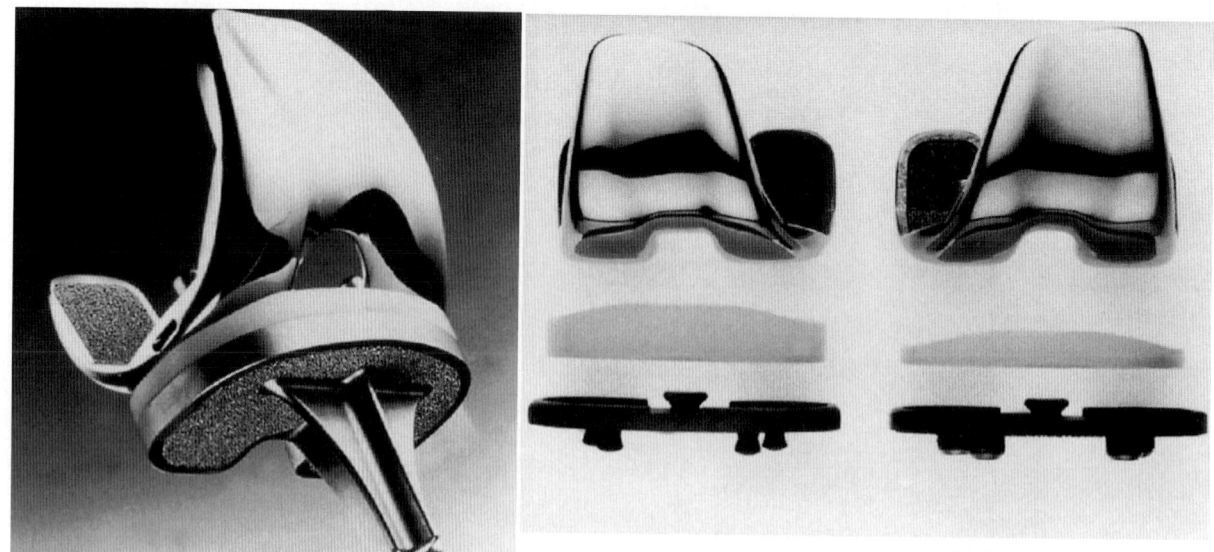

Fig. 8-3   Several types of total knee replacement prostheses.
(Courtesy Zimmer, Warsaw, Ind. From Mourad LA: Mosby's clinical nursing series: orthopedic disorders, *St Louis, 1991, Mosby.)*

DIAGNOSTIC TESTS

Electrolytes, CBC, PT/INR
Joint radiologic study

POTENTIAL COMPLICATIONS

Disorientation (older adult patient)
Tachycardia
Tachypnea
CHF/MI
Chest pain
Atelectasis
Pneumonia
Thrombophlebitis
Pulmonary embolus
Hemorrhage
Shock
Fat embolus
Wound infection
Compartment syndrome (knee, elbow) (p. 490)
Implant failure

MULTIDISCIPLINARY MANAGEMENT
THERAPEUTIC MANAGEMENT

Postoperative position of involved extremity
Parenteral fluids with electrolytes initially
Incision and draining apparatus care
Cast, splint, brace, sling: device depends on joint replaced
Medications
    Analgesics
    NSAIDs
    Antibiotics
    Sedatives, antipyretics
    Anticoagulant
    Stool softeners, laxatives
Epidural/PCA analgesia
Oxygen therapy, incentive spirometer
Antiembolic stockings, sequential compression device, foot pumps
Diet, rest, activity
Physical therapy
    Rehabilitation plan: inpatient/outpatient therapy
    Occupational therapy
    Crutch walking
Social medicine: follow-up placement, if needed

PATIENT PROBLEMS—NURSING DIAGNOSES/INTERVENTIONS

▼Impaired physical mobility related to surgical implant of joint involved and pain

Encourage proper positioning and use of trapeze when in bed
Maintain bed rest with affected joint in prescribed position
Provide firm mattress, trapeze, and overhead frame
Assist to chair 2 to 4 times/day as tolerated
Maintain support of joint through use of splint, brace, sling, cast, or pillows

Perform passive or assist with and teach active ROM exercises to unaffected joints
Reinforce restrictions and limitations on affected joint *to prevent dislocation*
Assist with ADLs as needed
    Turn patient as ordered; support joint to maintain immobilization and body alignment
    Monitor skin for reddened areas; massage bony prominences prn
    Maintain wrinkle-free linens
Promote quadriceps, gluteal muscle sets and isometric exercises as indicated
Ambulate patient with assistance (duration of bed rest depends on joint replaced)
    Provide ambulatory aids as needed
    Observe weight-bearing restrictions
    Monitor for vertigo, weakness, and nausea
Continuous passive ROM machine may be ordered for affected extremity of hip and knee arthroplasty patients

Expected Outcomes

Maintains proper body alignment in bed and while ambulating
Increases weight bearing as prescribed
Expresses understanding of and participates in rehabilitation regimen
Progresses toward self-care

▼Altered tissue perfusion: peripheral related to reduced blood flow, tissue edema secondary to immobilization

Administer parenteral fluids with electrolytes *to increase tissue perfusion*
Monitor vital signs q2h to 4h and prn
Assess neurovascular status of affected extremity qh for 12 hours, then q4h; observe color, temperature, pulse, sensation, and mobility; observe for signs of venous thrombosis (p. 77) and compartment syndrome (p. 490)
Encourage early mobilization and ambulation
Monitor antiembolic stocking or sequential compression device; remove stockings q2d to observe skin for redness, monitor pulses
Encourage use of ankle pumps, quadriceps and gluteal sets q2h to 4h while awake *to promote venous return* if applicable
Apply ice bags to affected joint
Monitor CBC, electrolytes, and PT/INR
Maintain indwelling urethral catheter; monitor intake and output; observe for urinary retention; output may be less than intake for 24 to 48 hours
Administer anticoagulants *to prevent phlebitis;* assess effectiveness and for side effects

Expected Outcomes

Vital signs are stable and within normal limits
Laboratory values are within normal limits

Extremities are warm and normal color, and pulses are palpable

▼Risk for infection (wound, pneumonia) related to surgical intervention, immobility, and decreased primary defenses

Monitor incision and dressings for drainage and presence of drain or Hemovac *to keep surgical site clear of fluids*

    Monitor output for color and amount q4h; report excessive bleeding to physician

    Reinforce and change dressings prn; observe for signs of healing and wound infection

    Administer parenteral antibiotics for 24h to 48h after surgery as ordered

    Obtain culture for any suspicious drainage

Assess respiratory status q4h; observe for pain, dyspnea, and tachypnea

Monitor temperature q4h; report any elevation to physician

Auscultate chest for breath sounds q4h; observe for diminished breath sounds

Initiate use of incentive spirometer q1h to 2h

Change position q2h while in bed *to prevent stasis of lung secretions*

Expected Outcomes
Incision is clean, dry, intact
Temperature is normal
Respiratory rate and rhythm are regular
Breath sounds are normal

▼Pain related to surgical intervention and impaired mobility

Assess location, intensity, and character of pain using pain rating scale

Administer analgesics, sedatives, and/or antiinflammatory agents; assess effectiveness of pain relief measures; monitor dosage for older adult patients *because prescribed dose may cause disorientation*

Monitor PCA or continuous epidural analgesia (CEA) as indicated

Change position frequently *to prevent fatigue and pressure on bony prominences;* administer back rubs as indicated

Provide diversional activities *to reduce attention on pain*

Discuss and teach alternate pain relief techniques

Promote self-care activities as tolerated

Monitor for severe chest or affected joint pain; may indicate emboli or displacement of joint

Expected Outcomes
Displays more relaxed affect
States pain is at tolerable level
Participates in diversional activities

Additional Nursing Diagnoses to Consider
Risk for injury, related to dislocation of prosthesis
Self-care deficit
Impaired transfer ability

PATIENT/FAMILY TEACHING
Stress importance of and provide written instructions for prescribed rehabilitation program: daily exercises and/or ROM for affected joint, activity allowed, and position to be maintained; no adduction of extremity or >90 degree flexion

Discuss and demonstrate incision care

Provide medication schedule including name, purpose, dosage, and side effects; if patient is taking anticoagulants, explain need to have PT checked regularly, observe for bleeding, and avoid aspirin use

Explain need to use soft toothbrush, electric razor while on anticoagulant

Discuss need to take prophylactic antibiotics before invasive procedure including dental cleaning or procedure

Explain importance of high-protein, high-fiber diet and increased fluid intake *to facilitate healing and prevent constipation*

Discuss need for a safe environment

Discuss signs and symptoms of wound infection, dislodgment to report: fever, inflammation, pain, immobility

Encourage follow-up visits with physician

DISCHARGE/HOME CARE PLANNING
Assess and continue with patient/family teaching and monitor the following:
    Environmental/safety status
    Caregivers' ability to perform needed tasks
    Accessible telephone and emergency numbers: physician, pharmacy, home health care team
    Emergency call device to summon outside help
    Absence of scatter rugs, unbacked carpets
    Presence of stairs with hand rails
    Grab bars at tub and toilet
    Nonskid strips in tub
    Adequate lighting for safe movement
    Wide doorways to accommodate wheelchairs/walkers
    Height of chair and bed for easy transfer on and off of each
    Flashlights near bed and chair
    Medications accessible and labeled
    Availability of transportation to needed appointments
    Needed supplies: what and where to purchase
    Mobility status
        Ability and desire to follow prescribed rehabilitation plan and exercises
        Correct transfer techniques
        Ability to apply brace, corset, removable cast
    Status of wound
        Incision for healing, infection
        Signs of infection: redness, pain, swelling, fever, drainage

Ability to care for wound: correct supplies and
  handwashing technique
Knowledge of where and what supplies to purchase
Nutritional status
  Understanding of basic food groups and what to eat
    to provide nutrition with no weight gain
  Signs of weight loss, dehydration
  Ability to prepare meals; refer to social agency to
    provide meals
Elimination status
  Presence of elevated toilet seat
  Use of stool softeners, natural laxatives, bulk in diet
  Ability to be active
  Amount of fluids taken per day: increase to upper
    limits for age and weight
  Use of fracture pan/urinal/female urinal

■ AMPUTATION OF LEG: ABOVE OR BELOW KNEE

*Surgical removal of part of the leg because of trauma,
disease, tumors, or congenital anomalies; a skin flap is
generally constructed to facilitate healing and use of prosthetic equipment*

PREOPERATIVE ASSESSMENT AND CARE

Monitor neurovascular status, both extremities
Observe affected extremity for ulcerations, edema,
  necrosis
Obtain baseline vital signs, ECG, chest x-ray, Doppler
  studies, angiography, transcutaneous oxygen pressures
  as ordered
Administer skin preparation as ordered; wound care,
  antibiotics, analgesia as ordered
NPO after midnight
Encourage and allow time for verbalization of fears and
  anxieties
  Reinforce physician's explanation of operative
    procedure and phantom limb sensation
  Begin to deal with body image change, loss, and grief;
    listen carefully and support positive coping
    behaviors; assist patient with expressing feelings
    to significant other(s)
Explain process of and preparation for rehabilitation
  Strengthen muscles of upper extremities for crutch
    walking
    Push-ups from prone position
    Alteration of flexing and extending arms holding
      weights
    Sit-ups from seated position
  Practice crutch walking
  Practice quadriceps setting exercises, gluteal
    contraction exercises, and leg lift of affected
    extremity unless contraindicated
Practice use of overhead trapeze attached to frame
Explain types of prostheses available if appropriate
  Immediate postoperative prosthetic fitting (IPOP): for
    immediate or early ambulation and weight bearing;

cast is applied to stump and prosthesis is attached
  to cast
Delayed: dressing and elastic bandage are applied to
  stump; prosthesis is not made for 2 to 3 months

POSTOPERATIVE ASSESSMENT
SUBJECTIVE DATA
Location, intensity, and type of pain

OBJECTIVE DATA
Type of dressing or rigid plaster cast
Position of stump
Stump dressing, amount and color of drainage, presence
  of drains, Hemovac, Jackson-Pratt
Respiratory status, vital signs
Presence of phantom pain: cramping, burning, stabbing
  feeling of amputated limb/foot

DIAGNOSTIC TESTS
CBC, fasting blood sugar (for diabetics)
Electrolytes

POTENTIAL COMPLICATIONS
Hemorrhage, dehiscence
Wound infection
Phantom pain
Contractures
Abduction deformity
Scar formation

MULTIDISCIPLINARY MANAGEMENT
THERAPEUTIC MANAGEMENT
Wound care
Position of stump postoperatively
Type of dressing and/or postsurgical fitting applied
Analgesics, PCA, antibiotics, antipyretics, sedatives
Diet, activity, rest
Physical therapy
  Prescribed exercises and rehabilitation plan
  Occupational therapy for lifestyle changes
Orthotic technician: cast and prosthesis management
Social medicine: assist with home health care, placement
  as needed

PATIENT PROBLEMS—NURSING DIAGNOSES/INTERVENTIONS

▼Impaired physical mobility related to pain and
musculoskeletal impairment

Maintain bed rest in prescribed position
Elevate residual limb *to prevent edema,* for first 24 hours.
  Subsequently the limb is fully extended *to prevent hip
  and knee contractures*
Elevate head of bed no more than 30 degrees *to
  maintain alignment*
Turn from side to back to abdomen (after 24 hours) q2h
  to prevent contractures

Avoid excess hip abduction, flexion and external rotation for patients with above-the-knee (AK) amputations

Avoid prolonged knee flexion in patients with below-the-knee (BK) amputations

Assist and teach patient to exercise bid in supine and prone position to increase strength and flexibility of the hip extensors, abductors, and adductors; and knee flexors and extensors (for BK amputation)

Assist with and teach adduction and extension exercises to affected extremity q4h

Assist with ambulation

    Without prosthesis

        Avoid long periods of chair sitting *to prevent stasis of venous return*

        Provide ambulation devices: crutches, walker

        Encourage use of good walking shoes and maintain stump in normal position—relaxed and downward; involve physical therapy department

    With prosthesis

        Assist with measuring for prosthesis

        Provide ambulation device: crutches, walker

        Increase ambulation with prescribed amount of weight bearing; involve physical therapy department

        Assist and teach patient/family proper application and use of shrinkage device (elastic bandages, shrinker socks, elastic stockinette, rigid dressing)

Assist with and reiterate postoperative conditioning exercises: trunk flexion, sit-ups, hopping in place, hopping with walker *to maintain mobility*

Encourage participation in group exercise/pool program if applicable

Expected Outcomes

Expresses understanding of treatment and exercise plan

Cooperates/participates in needed activities

Maintains correct body alignment

Exhibits no contractures

▼ Risk for fluid volume deficit related to increased drainage or bleeding at surgical site

Administer parenteral fluids and anticoagulants as indicated *to sustain hydration*

Monitor vital signs q2h to 4h

Measure intake and output q8h

Monitor dressings and incision for color and amount of drainage and for presence of drains or Hemovac; observe for bleeding; outline bleeding area on dressing with pen and write date and time

Apply pressure and elevate stump in case of hemorrhage; follow with use of tourniquet if hemorrhage not controlled

Monitor Hgb, Hct, PT/INR, and electrolytes

Monitor postsurgical cast for bleeding and mark area as discussed previously; observe for cast slippage and report to physician

Expected Outcomes

Vital signs are within normal limits

Wound is healing

Skin is warm, dry

▼ Risk for infection related to surgical procedure and lowered primary defenses

Change stump dressing and elastic bandage *to produce shrinkage and prepare for prosthesis*

Wash and dry area; expose it to air before reapplying dressing

    Perform at least qod

    Observe for signs of infection and increasing edema

    Begin stump strengthening and conditioning; push against pillow and increase to firmer surface as tolerated

Change postsurgical cast dressing bid; wash and dry area; allow it to air-dry

    Apply properly fitting stump sock prn *to provide support*

    Observe incision and surrounding area for increasing edema and signs of wound infection

    Massage stump toward suture line as ordered: usually 1 week postoperatively

    Reapply postsurgical cast

Maintain dry dressing; cover with plastic while using bed pan or if incontinent *to prevent soiling*

Begin teaching dressing change procedure

Monitor temperature q4h

Provide high-protein diet and encourage fluids to upper limits for age and weight *to promote healing*

Administer antibiotics and/or antipyretics: monitor for effectiveness, side effects

Expected Outcomes

Participates in maintaining aseptic techniques

Remains afebrile with adequate wound healing

▼ Pain related to surgical intervention and immobility

Assess character, intensity, and location of pain; observe for compartment syndrome in BK amputation (p. 490)

Administer analgesics (PCA) and sedative; assess effectiveness of pain relief measures

Explain sensation of phantom limb pain; often precipitated by contact, urination, angina, defecation

Manage phantom limb pain as ordered: beta blocker, anticonvulsants, tricyclic antidepressants, neuroleptics; biofeedback, TENS, early prosthetic use may be helpful

Assist patient with changing position slightly at frequent intervals *to reduce fatigue and pressure;* provide back rubs

Provide diversional activities *to reduce attention on pain*

Teach and assist with alternative pain relief measures

Monitor use of TENS unit (p. 42) or PCA (p. 40)

Discuss and explain phantom pain and that it is normal and usually temporary

Coordinate care to provide rest periods

Expected Outcomes

Verbalizes that pain is at a tolerable level

Appears calm, relaxed; is able to sleep and rest adequately

Denies presence of phantom pain

▼ Body image disturbance related to loss of body part

Assess value patient places on altered body part

Encourage and allow time for patient to express feelings of loss and grief, mutilation, anger, and avoidance of looking at stump

Assist in identifying positive coping behaviors and provide encouragement and praise for strengths observed

Provide praise for attempted and/or completed tasks

Encourage patient to discuss and view stump

Encourage patient to perform self-care activities and involve patient in stump care as soon as able; promote independence

Allow patient to wear own clothing *to increase self-esteem*

Demonstrate positive regard for patient and acceptance of changed physical appearance

Promote communication with family and significant other(s)

Explain all procedures and treatments

Provide a supportive environment

Encourage socialization with another amputee

Expected Outcomes

Begins using positive coping skills in dealing with loss of body part

Begins expressing feelings of acceptance of altered self

Participates in self-care activities, ADLs and stump care

▼ Alteration in skin integrity related to surgical procedure

Protect heel of remaining extremity with padding and encourage use of overhead trapeze/arms for position changes

Provide meticulous skin care of remaining extremity to preserve function (skin softeners, trimming toenails)

Assess wound for healing q shift: erythema, edema, pain, approximation of wound edges, drainage characteristics; culture if indicated

Change/reinforce dressing q shift as prescribed

Teach patient/family stump care:
  Clean daily with soap/water or prescribed solution
  Inspect skin daily for redness, abrasion and dermatologic lesions associated with prosthetic wear

Massage stump end to prevent scar formation and desensitize residual limb

Demonstrate proper stump wrapping technique, application, and care

Expected Outcome

Stump scar will be well-healed

Stump fits onto prosthesis

Additional Nursing Diagnosis to Consider

Risk for injury related to imbalance caused by loss of leg

PATIENT/FAMILY TEACHING

Stress importance of and review rehabilitation program; involve physical therapy department in daily exercises and stump strengthening and conditioning

Demonstrate and teach care of patient's intact lower extremity: avoid using heel on intact lower extremity to push up in bed; use trapeze; protect heel with padding; stress importance of careful foot care including keeping toenails trimmed, applying softeners, keeping toes dry

Demonstrate dressing changes and stump care: cleanse daily with soap and water, drying thoroughly before replacing shrinkage device; inspect incision daily for redness, abrasion, irritation; change stump sock and elastic wrap every day and wash with mild soap and water; skin care, and technique for massage of stump

Discuss and demonstrate care of IPOP as indicated; consult physical therapy department or provide referral for permanent prosthesis

Promote safe home environment; instruct patient to wear rubber-soled shoe as indicated

Discuss signs and symptoms to report to physician: fever, inflammation of incision, prolonged phantom pain, increasing edema of stump

Discuss phantom limb sensation: self-limiting nature, precipitating factors, treatment including drugs, TENS, stump desensitization

Discuss importance of well-balanced diet, avoiding weight gain

Refer to support group

Encourage follow-up visits with physician/physical therapist

DISCHARGE/HOME CARE PLANNING

Assess and continue with patient/family teaching and monitor the following:
  Environmental/safety status
    Caregivers' ability to perform needed tasks
    Accessible telephone and emergency numbers: physician, pharmacy, home health care team
    Emergency call device to summon outside help
    Absence of scatter rugs, unbacked carpets
    Presence of stairs with hand rails
    Grab bars at tub and toilet
    Nonskid strips in tub
    Fall precautions

Adequate lighting for safe movement

Wide doorways to accommodate wheelchairs/ walkers

Height of chair and bed for easy transfer on and off of each

Flashlights near bed and chair

Smoke detector and evacuation plan

Medications accessible and labeled

Availability of transportation to needed appointments

Needed supplies: what is required and where to purchase it

Mobility status

Ability and desire to follow prescribed rehabilitation plan and exercises

Correct transfer techniques

Reinforce wearing low-heeled, comfortable shoes

Correct use of walkers, canes, crutches

Status of wound

Incision for healing, infection

Signs of infection: redness, pain, swelling, fever, drainage

Ability to care for wound: correct supplies, handwashing technique, and application of bandage(s)

Knowledge of what supplies are required and where to purchase them

■ ARTHROSCOPY

The examination of the interior of a joint with a small fiberoptic tube called an arthroscope; allows a means for diagnosing and performing needed surgery; most frequently scoped joints are the knee, elbow, and shoulder

PREOPERATIVE ASSESSMENT AND CARE

Obtain preoperative lab work: Hgb, Hct, PT/PTT, urinalysis

Obtain history of medications, presence of underlying diseases, infection

Perform neurovascular assessment, including presence of both pulses distal to the joint

Discuss with and teach patient

ROM exercises to unaffected extremities

Restrictions and limitations postoperatively

These will vary with physicians and according to extent of surgery

Bulky dressings with elastic wraps

Usually patient returns home the same day of surgery if stable and supports are in place

Method of crutch walking if applicable

Methods of pain management

Purpose of NPO

Administer antiseptic scrub to affected joint

Reinforce physician's explanation of procedure

Obtain consent form

POSTOPERATIVE ASSESSMENT
SUBJECTIVE DATA

Location and character of pain

OBJECTIVE DATA

Position of joint and degree of elevation

Character and amount of drainage

Type of immobilization device

Neurovascular status of affected extremity: pulse, color, temperature, sensation, mobility

POTENTIAL COMPLICATIONS

Edema

Hemorrhage

Thrombophlebitis (p. 77)

Infection

DVT

Postoperative arthrosis

Compartment syndrome (p. 490)

MULTIDISCIPLINARY MANAGEMENT
THERAPEUTIC MANAGEMENT

Medications

Analgesics, antibiotics, sedatives

Position of joint postoperatively; exercises, ambulation

Activity

Partial weight bearing or crutches 24 to 48 hours postoperatively

Physical therapy (done on outpatient)

ROM on second or third postoperative day

Muscle strength training

Diet: regular

PATIENT PROBLEMS—NURSING DIAGNOSES/INTERVENTIONS

▼Altered peripheral tissue perfusion: related to arthroscopy and risk of altered arteriovenous flow

Elevate extremity *to promote venous return*

Monitor neurovascular status of affected extremity for 4 hours, then q4h; check pulse, color, temperature, sensation, and mobility

Monitor vital signs q4h

Apply ice pack to joint *to reduce swelling*

Monitor pressure dressing and observe for bleeding

Expected Outcomes

Affected extremity is warm, dry, mobile

Vital signs are stable

Distal pulses are palpable

▼Impaired physical mobility related to postoperative pain discomfort

Maintain bed rest in position of comfort with involved joint elevated in slight flexion

Avoid excessive use of joint for 24 to 48 hours

Ambulate with assistance, usually on evening of surgery

Assist patient with getting out of bed, keeping affected extremity elevated until standing; no weight bearing until ordered

Assist patient with use of crutches, walker as indicated

Increase ambulation as tolerated

Provide rest periods between ambulations

Initiate and assist with prescribed exercises; these depend on physician's preference and extent of surgery

Involve physical therapy department if applicable

Teach dorsiflexion and plantar flexion of foot or wrist and increasing flexion of knee, elbow

Expected Outcomes

Demonstrates increasing mobility and ROM

Participates in exercise program

Ambulates correctly with crutches

▼Pain related to invasive procedure

Assess location, intensity, and type of pain; *severe unrelenting pain and edema may indicate compartment syndrome*

Administer analgesics and/or sedatives: assess effectiveness and for side effects

Provide diversional activities

Change position in small ways *to promote comfort*

Apply ice bag *to decrease edema/pain*

Expected Outcomes

Reports a reduced level of discomfort

Exhibits relaxed facial expressions

Sleeps for longer periods at night

Additional Nursing Diagnosis to Consider

Risk for infection related to surgical procedure

PATIENT/FAMILY TEACHING AND DISCHARGE/HOME CARE PLANNING

Stress importance and goals of prescribed rehabilitation program

ROM exercises to begin second or third day

Muscle strengthening (quadriceps sets)

Knee

Amount of weight bearing and knee flexion allowed

Elevation of leg while sitting

Avoiding twisting knee

Dorsiflexion and plantar flexion exercises of feet

Ambulation with crutches

Swimming should be encouraged

Elbow/shoulder

Amount of flexion allowed

Type of arm support needed (sling, cast) and care of device

Activity permitted; avoid excessive use of joint

Discuss signs of wound infection to report to physician: fever, redness, pain, odor, edema at operative site; explain that small effusion is common

Importance of rest periods between exercises

Dates and times of physical therapy visits if applicable

Return to work approximately 1 week

Swimming/biking permitted as tolerated

Limited sports activities usually to week 4

Encourage follow-up care with physician approximately 7 to 10 days postoperatively

■ EXTERNAL FIXATION FOR COMPLICATED FRACTURES

A surgical procedure to immobilize and reduce complicated fractures; percutaneous pins or wires are inserted into and/or through the bone and attached to an external metal frame (Fig. 8-4); may be applied to jaw, arm, leg, ribs, pelvis, fingers, or toes; one type of fixator is the Ilizarov external fixator (Fig. 8-5, Box 8-2)

PREOPERATIVE ASSESSMENT AND TEACHING

Preoperative teaching may be limited depending on urgency of needed treatment

Assess neurovascular and respiratory status

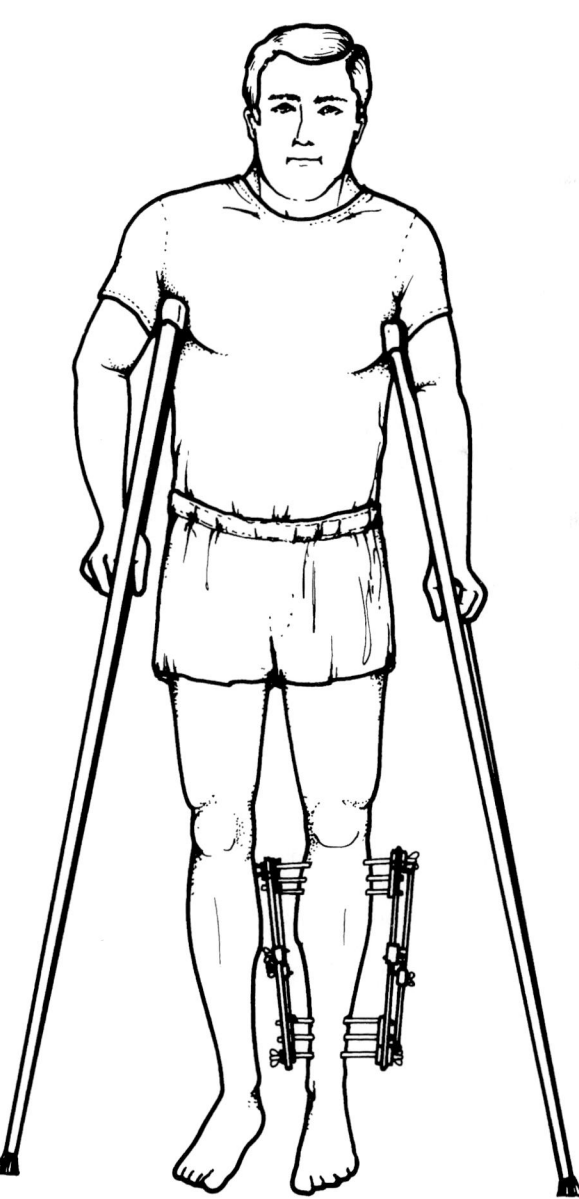

Fig. 8-4 External fixation for complicated fractures.

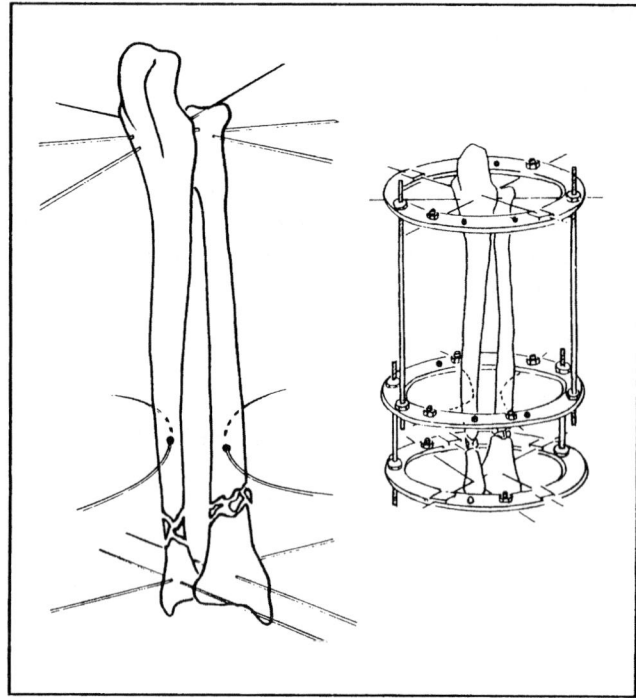

Fig. 8-5 Treatment of fracture of the ulna with dislocation of the head of the radius using Ilizarov external fixator.
(From Ilizarov external fixator general surgical technique brochure, Richards Medical Co, Memphis, Tenn, 1990.)

Assess impact on lifestyle, employment, ability to perform ADLs

Discuss with and teach patient the following:

Methods of coughing and deep breathing and/or use of incentive spirometer

Necessary ROM exercises, quadriceps setting, and gluteal contractions according to location of fracture

Use of trapeze

Necessary movement limitations and activities allowed

Importance of external fixator

Reinforce physician's explanation of procedure

Fixator usually causes little pain or discomfort and allows for early ambulation

Device is unsightly, but long-range results are the primary goal

Explain that extremity will be elevated postoperatively to reduce edema

Involve physical therapy department, if available, for crutch walking and exercises

Administer prescribed antibiotics and skin prep

POSTOPERATIVE ASSESSMENT
SUBJECTIVE DATA
Location, intensity, and character of pain
Nausea, vomiting

OBJECTIVE DATA
Elevation and position of extremity
Edema of extremity at operative site and below

Box 8-2 Ilizarov External Fixator

An external fixator, developed by Gauril Ilizarov, that allows control over a variety of bone disorders including rotation, angulation, translation, lengthening, and shortening. It preserves limb function and blood supply and promotes healing. Also known as a *compression-distraction apparatus,* it can be assembled in more than 600 different ways and therefore is very versatile (Fig. 8-5).

Indications

Open, closed fractures

Nonunion, pseudoarthrosis of long bones

Limb lengthening, shortening

Correction of deformities, defects of bony or soft tissue

Postoperative care is essentially the same as for the external fixator on this page.

Presence of supportive dressings

Character and amount of drainage from wound and pin sites

Neurovascular status of affected extremity: color, sensation, mobility, peripheral pulse, temperature, and other vital signs

DIAGNOSTIC TESTS
CBC, PT/INR, chemistries
Radiologic examination of affected bone
Cultures: wound and pin sites

POTENTIAL COMPLICATIONS
Pin loosening and drainage
Loss of bone stabilization
Pin tract or wound infection
Nonunion, malunion
Cutaneous nerve injury
Compartment syndrome (p. 490)
DVT, hemorrhage

MULTIDISCIPLINARY MANAGEMENT
THERAPEUTIC MANAGEMENT
Position of affected extremity
Schedule for tightening nuts on fixator if applicable
Analgesics, antibiotics, antipyretics, sedatives, antibacterial cream
Diet, activity, ambulation, rest
Physical therapy: exercises and rehabilitation plan
Pin site care per institutional policy

PATIENT PROBLEMS—NURSING DIAGNOSES/INTERVENTIONS

▼ Impaired physical mobility related to musculoskeletal impairment and pain

Assess and teach active ROM exercises to unaffected extremities q2h to 4h; initiate quadriceps setting, gluteal contractions, or palmar or dorsal flexion as needed

Ambulate when edema of soft tissues has decreased
  Move extremity and fixator as a unit
  Assist patient to ambulate with crutches or sling as indicated

Do not change or adjust fixator bars (can cause misalignment)
  No weight bearing until ordered
  Physical therapy department should be involved where available
  Elevate extremity while sitting up

Provide high-protein diet and fluids *to maintain muscle mass* for possible long rehabilitation

Expected Outcomes
Demonstrates mobility returning to optimal level
Cooperates with and participates in exercise program
Uses supporting devices correctly

▼ High risk for peripheral neurovascular dysfunction

Assess neurovascular status (color, temperature, capillary refill, sensation, mobility, pulses)
Elevate affected extremity *to prevent edema*
Pain assessment: location, duration, and severity; presence of pain during active/passive ROM

Expected Outcomes
Vital signs are within normal limits
Extremity is warm and normal color
Neurovascular checks are within normal limits

▼ Risk for infection related to pins and fixator insertion

Monitor pin sites, incision, and supportive dressing q1h to 2h for drainage, edema, loosening, and skin tension
Initiate pin site and incision care as prescribed
  Assess for pain, tenderness, redness, and tension around each pin site
  Obtain culture for drainage suggestive of infection
  Pin site care per institutional policy or as prescribed
  Assist with and teach patient wound, pin site, and fixator care as soon as patient is physically and emotionally able
  Change incision dressings as necessary; observe for wound healing
Apply ice bags to areas *to reduce edema*
Antibiotic therapy as prescribed

Expected Outcomes
Tissue around pin sites remains clean and dry
Incision and surrounding area are healing
Demonstration of incision and pin care is adequate
Temperature is normal

▼ Pain related to surgical intervention and immobility

Elevate extremity to prevent edema and promote comfort
Assess location, intensity, and character of pain; observe proximal joint for compartment syndrome signs: unrelenting pain, edema (p. 490)
Administer analgesics and sedatives: assess effectiveness of pain relief measures; encourage use of PCA (p. 40)
Assist patient with changing position frequently while in bed *to prevent fatigue and pressure*
Provide diversional activities *to decrease focus on discomfort*
Discuss and teach alternative pain management techniques
Unrelieved pain and pain out of proportion to injury suggests compartment syndrome

Expected Outcomes
States pain is at a tolerable level
Appears more relaxed and calm
Reports ability to sleep and rest for increasing length of time

▼ Body image disturbance related to external fixator

Provide supportive environment *to allow for expression of feelings*
Promote and allow time for expression of feelings; encourage communication with significant other(s)
Encourage patient to regain as much control as possible for care of fixator
Promote self-care activities and praise tasks attempted or completed

Expected Outcomes
Attempts to express concerns/feelings
Begins to use positive coping skills in dealing with altered self-image
Seeks assistance appropriately

PATIENT/FAMILY TEACHING
Provide and review written goals, restrictions, and activities of rehabilitation program as outlined by physician and/or physical therapist
Demonstrate care of pins, fixator, and incision
  Observe return demonstration
  Stress importance of not tampering with fixator, which may alter alignment of fracture
  Explain that showering is permitted but that patient should avoid swimming because chlorine and salt corrode metal
Stress importance of diet and elimination
Discuss signs and symptoms of wound infection to report to physician
Encourage follow-up visit with physician/physical therapy department

DISCHARGE/HOME CARE PLANNING

Assess and continue with patient/family teaching and monitor the following:

Environmental/safety status

Caregivers' ability to perform needed tasks: patient may require short-term rehabilitation

Accessible telephone and emergency numbers: physician, pharmacy, home health care team

Emergency call device to summon outside help

Absence of scatter rugs, unbacked carpets

Presence of stairs with hand rails

Grab bars at tub and toilet

Nonskid strips in tub

Adequate lighting for safe movement

Wide doorways to accommodate wheelchairs/walkers

Height of chair and bed for easy transfer on and off of each

Flashlights near bed and chair

Medications accessible and labeled

Availability of transportation to needed appointments

Needed supplies: what is required and where to purchase

Mobility status

Ability and desire to follow prescribed rehabilitation plan and exercises

Correct transfer techniques

Amount of weight bearing; reinforce wearing low-heeled, comfortable shoes

Correct use of walkers, canes, crutches

Status of wound

Incision for healing, infection

Signs of infection: redness, pain, swelling, fever, drainage

Ability to care for fixator: correct supplies and handwashing technique

Knowledge of what supplies are required and where to purchase

■ DIGITAL REPLANTATION OF FINGERS, THUMB

Surgical reconnection of severed digit(s) after trauma by a sharp object, crushing blow, or avulsion; general criteria for replantation include thumb replacement, multiple digit replacement, or replacement if patient is a child or patient's occupation requires manual skills; surgery must be performed within 24 hours

PREOPERATIVE ASSESSMENT AND CARE

Preservation of digit(s)

Wrap digit(s) in gauze or dry cloth soaked with normal saline if available

Place in double plastic bags and seal

Place bags in ice

Never place digit directly on ice

Care of amputated stump: apply sterile pressure dressing and elevate hand as ordered

Administer parenteral fluids with antibiotics as ordered

Administer anticoagulant and tetanus toxoid as ordered

Assess respiratory, cardiovascular, and neurologic status

Determine presence or absence of further trauma or injury

Assess medication and medical history: diseases such as diabetes, chronic obstructive pulmonary disease (COPD), vascular disease, rheumatoid arthritis, osteoarthritis, and bleeding tendencies inhibit replantation success

Determine dominant hand

Assess emotional status where possible

Be alert for maladaptive behavior because functional return depends on patient's motivation, emotional acceptance, and willingness to adapt to alterations in body image and lifestyle

Reinforce physician's explanation of surgical procedure

Discuss and deal with fears and anxieties

Encourage communication with significant other(s)

Discuss with and assist patient to understand that nicotine and caffeine are potent vasoconstrictors and therefore are prohibited

POSTOPERATIVE ASSESSMENT

SUBJECTIVE DATA

Location and character of pain

OBJECTIVE DATA

Neurovascular status of digit

Sensation, color, temperature

Capillary refill, skin turgor

Edema

Anatomic position of digit, wrist, and elbow and elevation of each

Presence or absence of skin graft and graft site

Character and amount of drainage from incision

DIAGNOSTIC TESTS

CBC, PT/INR, chemistries

Radiologic examination of replantation

POTENTIAL COMPLICATIONS

Hemorrhage

Shock

Vascular thrombosis or occlusion

Wound infection

Inappropriate or maladaptive behavior

Nonunion or malunion of digit(s)

MULTIDISCIPLINARY MANAGEMENT

THERAPEUTIC MANAGEMENT

Position and immobilization of extremity and digits

Analgesic, antibiotics, anticoagulants

Leech therapy (Box 8-3)

Fluorometry

Diet, activity, rest

Box 8-3 Leech Therapy

After microsurgery for digital replantation, a leech is introduced to the digit where venous congestion is present to drain the engorgement and restore normal venous circulation. The saliva of the leech contains an anticoagulant, a vasodilator, and an anesthetic to assist it in sucking out the blood. The procedure may be repeated every 4 hours until the digit returns to normal. A new leech is used for each treatment to prevent infection.

PRETHERAPY ASSESSMENT OF DIGIT

Venous congestion
    Skin color: pink, dusky purple
    Capillary refill: brisk
    Skin turgor: swollen, distended
    Temperature: cool

PRETHERAPY PREPARATION

Cleanse area with warm water
Explain procedure
Warn patient not to touch leech after it is applied
Place gauze or towels around site to prevent leech from
    escaping
Physician will apply leech to skin

INTRATHERAPY ASSESSMENT/CARE

After application of leech, monitor continually until leech
    is fully distended (10 to 15 minutes)
Leech will usually drop off once this occurs
If leech does not drop off, gently stroke it with an alcohol
    sponge
Never grasp leech with forceps because regurgitation might
    occur, resulting in a wound infection

POSTTHERAPY ASSESSMENT/CARE

Once the leech has dropped off the digit, gently pick it up
    and place it in alcohol-filled container and send it for
    disposal
Cleanse site and apply dressing because site will continue
    to drain and ooze for 24 to 48 hours
Assess digit for improved color, turgor, temperature

Apply heat *to promote vasodilation*
Elevate affected arm on pillow above heart level
Wrist and hand elevated 30 degrees
Forearm in prone position
Elbow flexion of no more than 10 to 15 degrees
    because further flexion may impair venous return
Maintain prescribed position of affected arm during
    repositioning
Assess neurovascular status of digit(s) qh
    Check sensation, temperature, color, pulse, skin turgor,
        and capillary refill qh
    Digit is pinker and capillary refill is faster immediately
        after surgery; accurate assessment and recording are
        imperative
    Report alterations in color to physician immediately
        Normal color to white or mottled: arterial
            occlusion
        Normal to dusky purple: venous congestion
        Leech therapy is used for venous congestion
        Initiate fluorometry readings as indicated
        Both nurses should assess status at change of shift
Monitor vital signs q4h for 24 hr, then qid; monitor BP on
    unaffected arm
Check dressing qh for drainage; report excess bleeding to
    physician; change dressing as indicated
Monitor Hgb, Hct, and PT/INR
Maintain parenteral fluids with antibiotics and
    anticoagulants: assess effectiveness and monitor for
    side effects of medications
Observe for occult bleeding: gums and injection sites if
    patient is on anticoagulants
Measure intake and output

Expected Outcomes

Arteriovenous flow is maintained
Digit is warm and of normal color
Capillary refill, skin turgor, and sensation are within
    normal limits
Vital signs are normal
Laboratory values are within normal limits

▼ Risk for disuse syndrome related to surgical procedure with prescribed immobilization of hand

Teach active ROM exercises q4h to unaffected
    extremities while patient is in bed
Ambulate with assistance
    Maintain forearm and hand in sling
    Observe for vertigo and nausea
Involve patient and physical and occupational therapy
    departments in establishing rehabilitation goals
    according to physician's order
Individualize goals according to the following:
    Healing process and progress
    Patient's motivation to master manual skills
    Patient's willingness to use replanted digit
    Patient's acceptance of replanted digit into body
        image

Physical therapy: rehabilitation plan, exercises
Occupational therapy for change in lifestyle
Psychologic social worker to evaluate and assist in
    acceptance of altered body image

PATIENT PROBLEMS—NURSING DIAGNOSES/INTERVENTIONS

▼ Altered peripheral tissue perfusion related to interruption of arteriovenous flow

Maintain bed rest in position of comfort within confines
    of prescribed position of affected arm
Maintain warm environment *to prevent vasoconstriction;*
    avoid topical pressure on affected limb

Assist patient with and teach modified ADLs according to prescribed limitations dictated by surgery and if affected arm is dominant

Begin exercise program as planned

Encourage use of nondominant hand if appropriate

Allow time for completion of tasks

Encourage adequate fluid and food intake *to maintain normal elimination patterns*

Provide a supportive environment

Promote diversional activities *to increase focus on use of nondominant hand*

Encourage visitation *to promote feeling of well-being*

Expected Outcomes

Undertakes using nondominant hand

Participates in activities, ADLs, rehabilitation program

Sets realistic goals for self and strives to complete tasks

▼Pain related to trauma and surgical procedure

Assess location, intensity, and character of pain; use pain rating scale

Administer analgesic; assess effectiveness of pain relief measures; encourage use of PCA

Assist patient with changing position frequently *to prevent pressure and fatigue;* maintain elbow flexion at prescribed amount

Discuss and teach alternative pain relief measures if applicable

Provide diversional activities *to reduce attention to pain*

Expected Outcomes

Reports a tolerable level of pain

Presents a calm, relaxed facial affect

Sleeps/rests for longer periods

▼Body image disturbance related to replanted digit

Assess degree of acceptance of replanted finger

Provide time for and assist patient in expressing feelings, encourage communication with significant other(s)

Explain all procedures and treatments

Assess present and past coping behaviors and reinforce positive coping patterns that helped in the past

Stress positive aspects of replantation

Reinforce physician's explanation of expected outcome of surgical procedure; clarify misconceptions

Involve patient in self-care as soon as physically and emotionally able

Involve psychologic social worker to evaluate needs and provide counseling

Expected Outcomes

Begins to incorporate replanted digit into body image

Verbalizes concerns/feelings and begins to understand expected outcome

Participates appropriately in self-care

PATIENT/FAMILY TEACHING

Stress and review importance of prescribed rehabilitation program

Degree of movement of digit allowed and duration and times of exercise

    Exercises for wrist, elbow, and arm

    Position of arm, elbow, and hand during rest and ambulation

Stress that using and wanting to use the digit are the most important factors in function return

Paresthesia may last 4 to 6 months, whereas return of function may take a year

Replanted digit(s) may be shorter than opposing digit(s)

Demonstrate incision care and discuss signs of wound infection

Stress importance of well-balanced diet, fluid intake, rest, and daily exercise

Explain symptoms to report to physician

    Changes in color and temperature of digit

    Increased incision pain and/or edema

    Wound infection

Discuss importance of physical therapy and follow-up visits with physician

DISCHARGE/HOME CARE PLANNING

Assess and continue with patient/family teaching and monitor the following:

    Rehabilitation/exercise plan

        Correct positioning of hand

        Willingness to perform exercises

    Status of wound

        Incision for healing, infection

        Signs of infection: redness, pain, swelling, fever, drainage

        Neurovascular status of replaced digit

        Ability to care for wound: correct supplies and handwashing technique

        Knowledge of what supplies are required and where to purchase

■ COMPARTMENT SYNDROME

Increased arterial pressure in compartments of the forearm or lower leg after trauma; within compartments are muscles, blood vessels, and nerves, and any internal pressure (trauma, surgery, edema, bleeding) or external pressure (tight casts or dressings, IV infiltrations) can cause impaired circulation, nerve damage, and muscle weakness; if left unchecked, necrosis with loss of extremity and renal failure, acidosis, and shock (crush syndrome) can occur (Fig. 8-6)

ASSESSMENT
SUBJECTIVE DATA

Assess risk factors for compartment syndrome

Pain in compartment area: increasing, unrelenting, and unrelieved by narcotics

Pain on passive stretch of compartment

Paresthesias

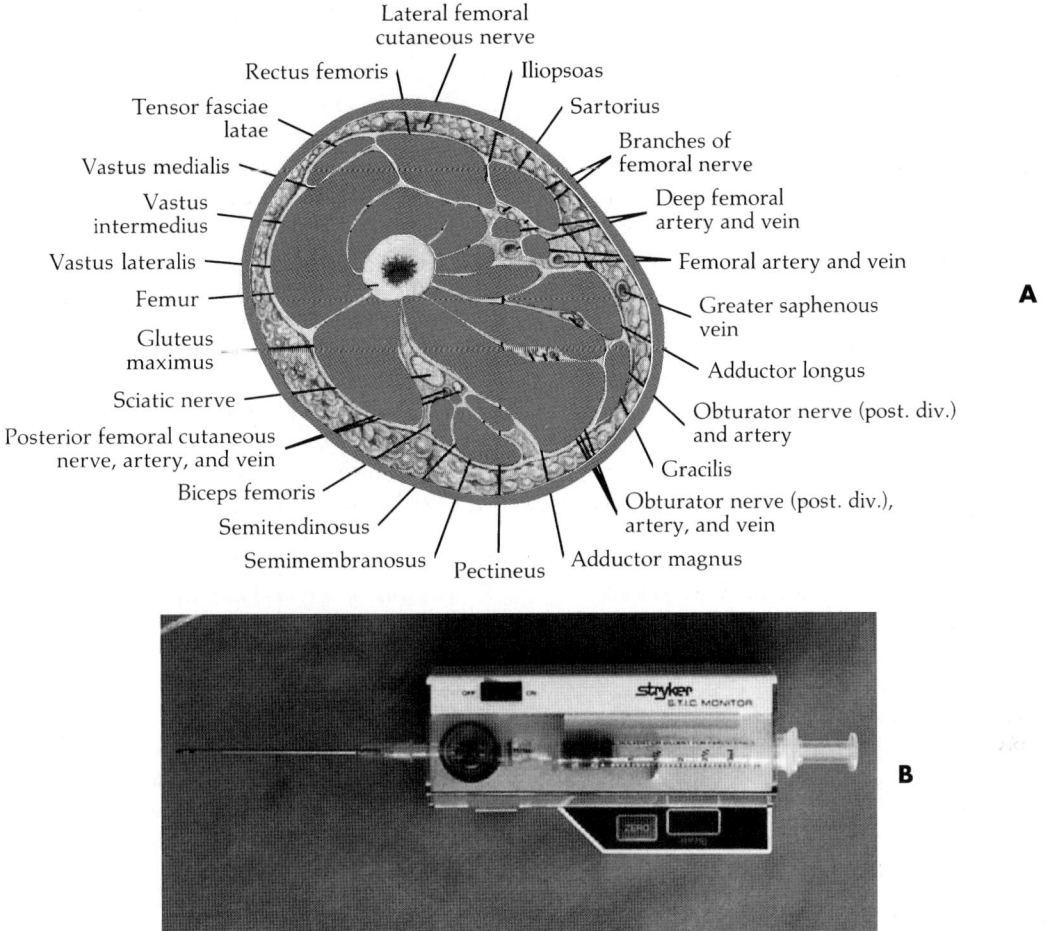

Lateral femoral cutaneous nerve
Rectus femoris
Iliopsoas
Tensor fasciae latae
Sartorius
Branches of femoral nerve
Vastus medialis
Vastus intermedius
Deep femoral artery and vein
Vastus lateralis
Femoral artery and vein
Femur
Greater saphenous vein
Gluteus maximus
Adductor longus
Sciatic nerve
Obturator nerve (post. div.) and artery
Posterior femoral cutaneous nerve, artery, and vein
Obturator nerve (post. div.), artery, and vein
Biceps femoris
Gracilis
Semitendinosus
Adductor magnus
Semimembranosus
Pectineus

A

B

Fig. 8-6 **A,** Compartments and cross section of the thigh. Each compartment contains muscle(s), nerve, artery, and vein. **B,** Equipment for measurement of interstitial venous pressure.
(*A From Thompson JM et al:* Mosby's clinical nursing, *ed 4, St Louis, 1997, Mosby.* **B** *Courtesy Stryker, Inc., Kalamazoo, Mich.*)

OBJECTIVE DATA
Increased compartment pressure
Swelling and localized redness
Pulselessness
Progressive loss of motor function
Sensory deficits
Skin tense, shiny

DIAGNOSTIC TESTS
MRI
DVT studies
Ankle or brachial index
Vascular occlusion studies
CBC, PT/INR
Serum chemistry, myoglobin
AST/lactate dehydrogenase (LDH) and creatine kinase (CK)
Measurement of intracompartmental pressure

POTENTIAL COMPLICATIONS
Neurovascular dysfunction of extremity
Muscle weakness
Necrosis, amputation, infection
Renal failure, acidosis

Shock
Delayed union or nonunion of fractures

MULTIDISCIPLINARY MANAGEMENT
THERAPEUTIC MANAGEMENT
Medication
    Analgesics, antibiotics
    NSAIDs
Dressing and cast removal; cast window made
Tissue pressure monitoring, fasciotomy

PATIENT PROBLEMS—NURSING DIAGNOSES/INTERVENTIONS

▼High risk for peripheral neurovascular dysfunction

Assess neurovascular status and pain at least every 1 to 2 hours in high-risk patients; every 4 to 8 hours in all orthopedic patients
Notify physician immediately if pain in extremity is any of the following:
    Increasing
    Unrelenting

Unrelieved by narcotics

Occurring during passive motion

NOTE: Be aware that this type of pain is the primary indicator of compartment syndrome; other symptoms may take longer to appear

Remove dressing or have windows cut in cast immediately as ordered

Assess neurovascular status of foot or hand bilaterally q15min to 30min

Measure forearm or calf bilaterally for presence of or increase in edema q1h to q2h

Monitor intake and output

If no improvement is noted, prepare for and assist with interstitial venous pressure monitoring (p. 491), a means to measure interstitial pressure (normal pressure is about 0 to 30 mm Hg, and when this pressure nears 30 mm Hg, capillaries and arteries will close, causing occlusion)

Prepare for fasciotomy as ordered (longitudinal incision into fascia surrounding compartment to release pressure), if interstitial pressure is >30 mm Hg

Postoperatively, extremity will be immobilized in posterior cast or splint

Be aware that wound may be left open, with future grafting required; there may be more than one incision, depending on the number of affected areas in the compartment

Change dressings as needed; observe for altered alignment of extremity

Continue neurovascular monitoring qh; observe for return of color, temperature, and capillary refill

Assess pain and monitor effectiveness after analgesic administration

Expected Outcomes

Compartment pressure is reduced as evidenced by palpable peripheral pulses, reduced muscle edema, minimal discomfort

Extremity is warm and dry, capillary refill is normal

Mobility is intact

▼ Anxiety/fear related to lack of knowledge of the syndrome and situational crisis

Simple explanation of syndrome, procedure, outcome, and rehabilitation plan

Allow time for verbalization of fears and explain all treatments as much as possible

After procedure assist patient in identifying coping strengths and discuss ways of dealing with wound and possible skin grafting

Encourage communication with significant other(s)

Promote self-care activities

Implement comfort measures (medications, positioning)

Expected Outcomes

Begins to observe wound and discuss feelings about it

Participates in own care

Verbalizes understanding of treatment and rehabilitation plan

PATIENT/FAMILY TEACHING

Discuss and teach dressing change technique, neurovascular assessment

Provide information on where to purchase needed supplies

Reinforce prescribed rehabilitation program

Promote return visits with physical therapist and physician

■ BUNIONECTOMY

Surgical correction of hereditary or acquired hallux valgus: lateral deviation of the first metatarsophalangeal joint; operation involves procedures to realign the great toe and includes adjustment of soft tissues (contracted tendons, stretched ligaments) and lateral wedge osteotomy of the first metatarsal

PREOPERATIVE ASSESSMENT AND CARE

Pain and enlargement at first metatarsal head

Evidence of gout

Callous formation under second and third metatarsal head

Assess mobility, neurovascular status of toes, footwear evaluation, occupation, skin integrity

Assess gait, stance and mobility during weight bearing and non-weight bearing

Provide instruction and discussion with patient/family

    Crutch walking

    Use of walker

    Slipper cast

    Weight-bearing status and activity restriction

    Orthotics

    Toe flexing

    Quadriceps setting

    ROM exercises

POSTOPERATIVE ASSESSMENT
SUBJECTIVE DATA

Location and character of pain

OBJECTIVE DATA

Neurovascular status of affected toes: color, temperature, sensation, edema

Site of incision for drainage and bleeding

Placement of cast or splint

Ice cap to operative site

POTENTIAL COMPLICATIONS

Fever

Soft tissue problems (infection, delayed wound healing, skin scarring)

Recurrence of the deformity

Limitation of motion of metatarsophalangeal joint

Paresthesias of the great toe

Overcorrection of the deformity

Dorsal nerve impingement

MULTIDISCIPLINARY MANAGEMENT
THERAPEUTIC MANAGEMENT
Medications
    Narcotic analgesics
    Antipyretics
    NSAIDs
    Antiemetics
Ice/elevation of the operative foot
Activity: ambulation, positioning, weight-bearing status
Type of immobilization device/positioning
Diet, activity, rest
Physical therapy

PATIENT PROBLEMS/NURSING DIAGNOSES

▼ Impaired physical mobility related to surgery

Maintain bed rest until fully reactive
Elevate foot of bed
    Place bed cradle over feet
    Monitor immobilization device for pressure areas and circulatory constriction
Assist with crutch walking
Assist patient with performing ROM exercises q4h while in bed
Apply plaster walking boot if ordered
Encourage activities as strength with cast or splint permit

Expected Outcomes
Performs rehabilitation exercises correctly
Participates in self-care activities
Has satisfactory physical mobility

▼ Altered tissue perfusion: peripheral related to surgical procedure and immobilizing device

Assess pain and change dressings as ordered
Assess neurovascular status of toes q1h to 2h; check color, temperature, capillary refill, sensation, and mobility
Apply ice bags *to decrease edema*
Monitor toes for increasing edema
Encourage movement of legs *to increase venous return*
Elevate leg on pillow

Expected Outcomes
Vital signs are normal
Extremity is warm and of normal color
Pulse, sensation, and mobility are normal

▼ Pain related to surgical intervention

Assess location, intensity, and character of pain; use pain rating scale
Administer analgesics; assess effectiveness of pain relief measures and monitor for side effects
Apply ice bag *to lessen bleeding/edema*
Assist with position changes and skin care
Elevate foot/leg *to lessen edema*

Provide diversional activities *to lessen concentration on discomfort*

Expected Outcomes
States that pain is at tolerable level
Appears relaxed and calm

PATIENT/FAMILY TEACHING
Stress importance of and review foot and incision care and prescribed exercises
    Demonstrate dressing change
    Discuss care of plaster boot if applicable
    Demonstrate toe and foot ROM exercises
    Explain importance of proper fitting footwear
Discuss activities allowed; encourage self-care and ADLs
Discuss signs of wound infection to report to physician: fever, pain, edema, redness
Encourage follow-up care with physician

DISCHARGE/HOME CARE PLANNING
Assess and continue with patient/family teaching and monitor the following:
    Environmental/safety status
        Caregivers' ability to perform needed tasks
        Accessible telephone and emergency numbers: physician, pharmacy, home health care team
        Emergency call device to summon outside help
        Absence of scatter rugs, unbacked carpets
        Presence of stairs with hand rails
        Grab bars at tub and toilet
        Nonskid strips in tub
        Adequate lighting for safe movement
        Wide doorways to accommodate wheelchairs/walkers
        Height of chair and bed for easy transfer on and off of each
        Flashlights near bed and chair
        Medications accessible and labeled
        Availability of transportation to needed appointments
        Needed supplies: what and where to purchase
    Mobility status
        Ability and desire to follow prescribed rehabilitation plan and exercises
        Correct transfer techniques
        Amount of weight bearing
        Wearing proper fitting shoes
        Correct use of walkers, canes, crutches
        Ability to apply plaster boot if applicable
    Status of immobilizing device
Neurovascular status of each affected extremity
Condition of boot if applicable: wet, loose, clean, soiled
Condition of skin under device: clear, red, tender
Status of wound
    Incision for healing, infection
    Signs of infection: redness, pain, swelling, fever, drainage
    Ability to care for wound: correct supplies and handwashing technique

Knowledge of what supplies are required and where to purchase them

■ TRACTION MANAGEMENT

Application of force to skin, muscles, and bone to reduce and align fractures, relieve muscle spasms, and exert pull to relieve pressure on peripheral nerves (Table 8-1 and Figs. 8-7 through 8-10)

■ CAST MANAGEMENT

Casts are applied to immobilize musculoskeletal tissues after trauma; they are made of plaster, fiberglass, plastic, or cast tape

ASSESSMENT

SUBJECTIVE DATA

Location, intensity, and character of pain
Level of anxiety

OBJECTIVE DATA

Presence or absence of drainage
Type of cast applied, moistness
Neurovascular status of affected extremity

Integumentary status at edges and under cast
GI, renal, and/or respiratory dysfunction (body or cervical cast)
Alignment/position of affected body part
Integrity of immobilization device

POTENTIAL COMPLICATIONS

Neurovascular impairment
Skin impairment/pressure ulcers
Compartment syndrome (see p. 490)
Cast syndrome (reduced circulation through mesenteric artery caused by unnatural kinking from cast; may cause intestinal ileus)

MULTIDISCIPLINARY MANAGEMENT
THERAPEUTIC MANAGEMENT

Type of cast applied
Positioning of cast
Ambulation
Ice bags to affected part
Diet, activity, rest
Analgesics, antibiotics
Physical therapy: rehabilitation plan if indicated
Occupational therapy if applicable

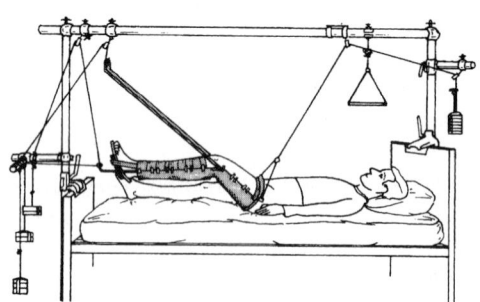

Fig. 8-7 Balanced suspension with Thomas's splint and Pearson's attachment.

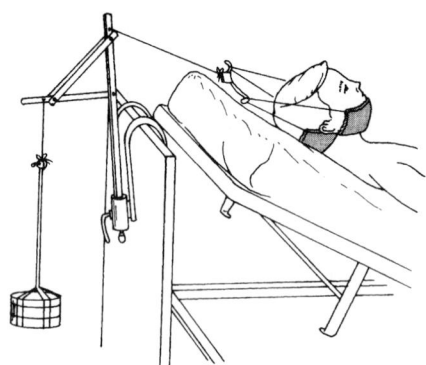

Fig. 8-9 Cervical traction.

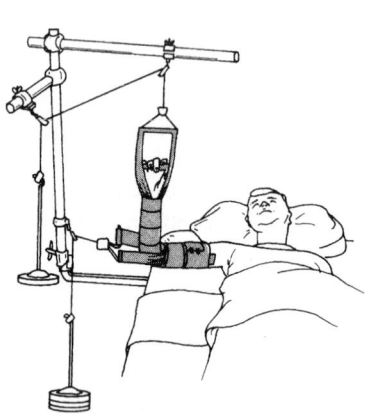

Fig. 8-8 Traction of humerus.

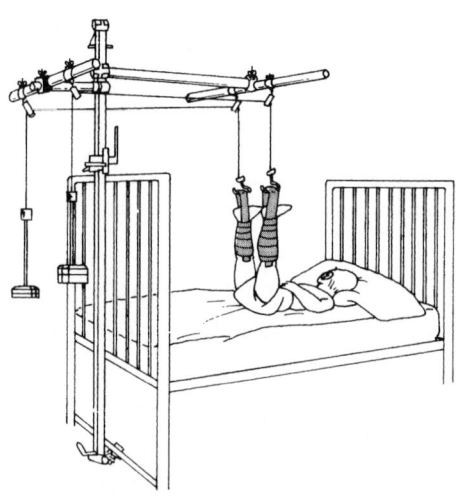

Fig. 8-10 Bryant's traction.

PATIENT PROBLEMS—NURSING DIAGNOSES/INTERVENTIONS

▼Impaired physical mobility related to disuse syndrome

Teach exercises to strengthen muscles before surgery if possible
Maintain bed rest in position of comfort with extremity elevated
Assist with and teach ROM exercises to unaffected joints every 4 hours to maintain strength
Assist with and teach exercise to joints above and below immobilizer
Collaborate with physical therapist to develop and teach exercise program for affected extremity after immobilizer is removed
Explain that muscle atrophy and an accumulation of dead skin cells is common after cast removal
Begin ambulation as prescribed
    Assist and teach crutch walking, use of cane, walker
    Observe for vertigo or disequilibrium
    Monitor use for correctness to prevent further injury
Involve patient in own physical care as tolerated to promote independence

Expected Outcomes
Activity level increases
Performance of ROM exercises is adequate
Unaffected extremities maintain strength

▼High risk for peripheral neurovascular dysfunction

Check tightness of immobilizer
Apply ice/elevate casted tissues
Perform neurovascular checks
Have cast cutter, spreader, and large scissors available on unit

Expected Outcomes
Vital signs are within normal limits
Neurovascular status is stable: color, temperature, capillary refill are normal and pulses are present; motion and sensation are adequate

▼Risk for impaired skin integrity related to pressure from immobilizer

Assess area to be enclosed prior to immobilization, if possible
Expose cast to air until dry; use only palms of hands when handling wet cast
Ensure that edges of immobilizer are well padded
Massage under edges *to stimulate circulation and prevent skin breakdown*
Explain that skin under cast will feel warm until cast dries
Assist with and encourage small position changes *to relieve pressure*

Monitor cast for drainage: check stockinette, wadding beneath cast; call physician if drainage excessive

Expected Outcomes
Skin under edges of cast is warm and dry
Cast is dry and intact

▼Pain related to cast application and/or trauma
Administer analgesics as ordered *to promote comfort*
Monitor severity of pain to avoid complications, compartment syndrome (p. 490)
Elevation and cold therapy *to promote comfort and reduce swelling*
Encourage small movements and position changes *to promote comfort*
Administer back rubs *to increase circulation and promote comfort*
Discuss alternative pain management techniques

Expected Outcomes
Verbalizes a reduction in discomfort at desired level
Able to rest, sleep, and perform activities adequately
Appears relaxed and talkative

Additional Nursing Diagnoses to Consider
Altered elimination patterns related to cast and bed rest
Constipation related to inactivity
Body image disturbance related to changes in appearance caused by immobilizer
Knowledge deficit related to immobilizer care

PATIENT/FAMILY TEACHING
Provide information on and stress importance of prescribed activities and rehabilitation exercises
Demonstrate turning procedure for patient in spica cast and reiterate crutch-walking procedure where appropriate
Discuss need to keep cast out of water; use plastic bag for showering
Notify physician immediately if cast becomes wet
Suggest clothing that can be put on easily
Discuss measures to ensure warmth of affected digits
Demonstrate neurovascular monitoring of each affected extremity as needed
Discuss signs and symptoms to report to physician
    Fever; foul odor from cast, edema
    Increasing pain or decreased sensation
Demonstrate skin care around cast
Teach signs and symptoms of compartment syndrome

DISCHARGE/HOME CARE PLANNING
Assess and continue with patient/family teaching and monitor the following:
    Environmental/safety status
        Caregivers' ability to perform needed tasks
        Accessible telephone and emergency numbers: physician, pharmacy, home health care team

Table 8-1	**Traction Management**		
Type	**Balanced Suspension**	**Skin**	**Skeletal**
Definition	Skeletal or skin traction applied to a lower extremity while weights and a splint simultaneously provide countertraction to and suspension of that extremity	Light or temporary traction applied directly to the skin to align fracture and reduce muscle spasm	Insertion of a pin or wire directly into the bone to provide continuous traction

General interventions (same for all types of traction listed in this table)	Maintain constant pull in line with deformity
	Assess and maintain ropes and pulleys
	    Taut
	    Riding freely over pulleys
	    Free of bedding
	    Knots secure
	    Adequate space between pulley and traction
	Monitor and maintain weights
	    Hanging free
	    Off floor
	    Away from bed
	    NOTE: *Never remove weights; never lift weights*
	Monitor and maintain countertraction
	    Elevation of bed under part to which traction is applied
	    Pull exerted against fixed point
	    Pull exerted against traction in opposite direction		

Interventions for specific type of traction	Maintain anatomic position of extremity Maintain 20-degree angle between thigh and bed Have heel clear of sling under calf Maintain abduction of extremity Monitor femoral and popliteal pulses	Observe carefully for slippage and bunching up of bandage Replace bandage prn Observe for pressure areas at distal end of bandage (wrist or heel), especially if weight is >7 lb Check neurovascular status q2h to 4h	Cover ends of pin with cord Observe site of insertion for redness, swelling, discharge, odor, bleeding Clean skin around puncture sites q8h with hydrogen peroxide soaked cotton swabs; allow to air-dry; apply antibacterial ointment if ordered Monitor neurovascular status q2h to 4h

Table 8-1	**Traction Management—cont'd**			
Pelvic	**Side Arm**	**Cervical**	**Bryant's**	**Halo**
Traction provided to lower back to reduce low back pain from fracture, herniated disks, muscle spasms	Skin or skeletal traction to the humerus to maintain alignment after open reduction procedure	Application of cervical halter with traction to relieve neck pain or when a cervical fracture is suspected	Treatment of fractures of femur shaft in young children	Metal brace inserted in the skull and iliac crest or femur with pins attached to four metal posts and a shoulder brace or body cast provides spinal support after spinal fusion or for preoperative treatment of scoliosis
Ensure that pelvic girdle is proper size for patient and that pelvic girdle fits snugly over iliac crests and pelvis Inspect skin areas over iliac crests for pressure points q4h Pelvic straps must be equal in length and unrestricted	Maintain position as directed by physician Check neurovascular status of affected arm q2h to 4h Notify physician immediately if any change is noted Apply chest restraint sheet for counter-traction prn	Position without pillows Monitor so weight and pulley are free of wall Observe for pressure areas Jaws, chin, and ears Side of head Back of head Pad as necessary for comfort	Raise buttocks slightly from mattress Observe bandages carefully for slippage and bunching over heel cords Observe for skin sloughing on both legs Check feet for color, P, T, and sensation q2h to 4h Use harness restraint to prevent turning over Avoid thick, wide diapers between legs	Cover ends of pins with cork to prevent injury Observe pin insertion sites for redness, swelling, drainage, odor, bleeding Clean skin around pin sites q8h with hydrogen peroxide soaked swabs; allow to air dry; apply antibacterial ointment if ordered Monitor straps for areas of constriction Pad pressure points as necessary for comfort Do not alter amount of traction applied Advise patient not to bend over; use reaching device

Emergency call device to summon outside help
Absence of scatter rugs, unbacked carpets
Presence of stairs with hand rails
Grab bars at tub and toilet
Nonskid strips in tub
Adequate lighting for safe movement
Wide doorways to accommodate
    wheelchairs/walkers
Height of chair and bed for easy transfer on and off
    of each
Flashlights near bed and chair
Medications accessible and labeled
Availability of transportation to needed
    appointments
Needed supplies: what and where to purchase
Mobility status
    Ability and desire to follow prescribed rehabilitation
        plan and exercises
    Correct transfer techniques
    Amount of weight bearing
    Correct use of walkers, canes, crutches
Status of cast
    Neurovascular status of each affected extremity
    Condition of cast: wet, loose, clean, soiled
    Condition of skin under cast: clear, red, tender
Skin care after cast removal
Nutritional status
    Understanding of basic food groups and what to eat to
        provide nutrition with no weight gain
    Signs of weight loss, dehydration
    Ability to prepare meals; refer to social agency to
        provide meals
Elimination status
    Presence of elevated toilet seat
    Use of stool softeners, natural laxatives, bulk in
        diet
    Ability to be active
    Amount of fluids taken per day: increase to upper
        limits for age and weight
    Use of fracture pan/urinal/female urinal

■ CONTINUOUS PASSIVE MOTION (CPM) DEVICE

An electrically driven apparatus that consists of a frame, supportive padding, and a control box to continuously move an extremity through its ROM. Devices are available for both upper and lower extremities

PURPOSE

Facilitates early movement and increased flexion
    of joint
Prevents stiffness of joint, tissue contraction, and joint
    effusions
Enhances circulation and healing
Reduces pain of or psychologic resistance to flexion and
    edema

ASSESSMENT/PROCEDURE

Physician's order to include the following:
    Initial degree of flexion; number of degrees to increase
        flexion per hour and number of hours per day to
        use
    Restrictions or special instructions for use
Assess patient's ability to operate and manage device
Explain purpose of machine and its advantages
Remove any splints before applying device as ordered
After machine is set up by physical therapist or cast or
    traction technician
Place extremity on device and check the following:
    Lower buttock is against femur support
    Knee is directly over center of frame
    Foot is firmly against foot plate
Apply Velcro safety straps to extremity; check that they
    do not interfere with gear assembly
Set automatic flexion and/or extension motion as ordered
    by physician
Increase flexion as ordered
Assess patient's tolerance before increasing flexion
Adjust speed as prescribed (maximum speed to flex joint
    from 0 to 110 degrees is about 1 minute 40 seconds;
    minimum speed is approximately 12 minutes; slow
    speeds are used initially and at night to facilitate
    sleep)
Set ROM limits as ordered by physician
Instruct patient in use of controls
Control has three settings: flexion, stop, and extension
Once device is operating, patient can control movement,
    stop, or reverse at any point within preset range limits
Encourage patient to use machine as much as possible
    and as tolerated

PATIENT PROBLEMS—NURSING DIAGNOSES/INTERVENTIONS

Assess risk factors for impaired skin integrity
Assess pressure points q4h to 8h (sacrum, unaffected
    extremity's heel, elbows)
Encourage patient to shift weight and change positioning
    frequently to decrease pressure
Assess pressure areas supported by CPM (heel, pelvis) at
    least q shift

PATIENT/FAMILY TEACHING AND DISCHARGE/HOME CARE CONSIDERATIONS

Explain procedure to patient/family: proper application
    of device, how to use the control, how to set
    parameters of the CPM device. If at home, check
    pressure areas with mirror, or have someone
    check them
Instruct patient/family regarding proper diet: drink plenty
    of fluids, consume foods high in fiber to prevent
    constipation
Encourage activity within prescribed restrictions:
    exercise unaffected extremity while using CPM
    device; shift CPM body weight frequently or ask for
    assistance; follow prescribed times for getting out of
    bed and physical therapy prescription

Procedure
    Proper application of device
    How to use control
    How to set parameters of CPM device
    If at home, check pressure areas with mirror, or have someone check them
Diet
    Drink plenty of fluids
    Consume foods high in fiber *to prevent constipation*
Activity
    Exercise unaffected extremity while using CPM
    Shift body weight frequently or ask for assistance
    Follow prescribed times for getting out of bed and physical therapy

BIBLIOGRAPHY

Arnaud C: Osteoporosis: using bone markers for diagnosis and monitoring, *Geriatrics* 51(4):24-30, 1996.

Bailey MM, Michalski J: Close-up on clavicle fracture, *Nursing '92* 22(8):41, 1992.

Bailey MM, Michalski J: Close-up on posterior shoulder dislocation, *Nursing '93* 23(10):43, 1993.

Bailey MM, Michalski J: Close-up on radial head fracture, *Nursing '93* 23(9):43, 1993.

Bailey MM, Michalski J: Close-up on scaphoid fracture, *Nursing '93* 23(3):49, 1993.

Barkett PA: Obstructed airway with wire jaws, *Nursing '91* 21(12):33, 1991.

Botstein GR: Soft tissue rheumatism of the upper extremities: diagnosis and management, *Geriatrics* 45(11):30, 1990.

Bryant GA: When your patient needs back surgery, *RN* 55(7):46, 1992.

Canobbio MM: *Mosby's patient teaching,* ed 2, St Louis, 2000, Mosby.

Doenges ME et al: *Nursing care plans: guidelines for planning and documenting patient care,* ed 3, Philadelphia, 1993, FA Davis.

Gluchacki BK: Recognizing compartment syndrome, *Nursing '91* 21(10):33, 1991.

Grossman A et al: *Cost effective diagnostic imaging: the clinician's guide,* ed 3, St Louis, 1995, Mosby.

Harris C: Osteoarthritis: how to diagnose and treat the painful joint, *Geriatrics* 48(8):39, 1993.

Joseph, J, McGrath, H: Gout or pseudogout: how to differentiate crystal-induced arthropathies, *Geriatrics* 50(40):33-39, 1995.

Kim MJ et al: *Pocket guide to nursing diagnoses,* ed 7, St Louis, 1997, Mosby.

Licata AA: Therapies for symptomatic primary osteoporosis, *Geriatrics* 46(11):62, 1991.

Maher A, Salmond S, Pellino T: *Orthopaedic nursing,* ed 2, Philadelphia, 1998, WB Saunders.

McCance KL, Huether SE: *Pathophysiology: the biological basis for disease in adults and children,* ed 3, St Louis, 1998, Mosby.

McFarland GK, McFarlane EA: *Nursing diagnosis and intervention: planning for patient care,* ed 3, St Louis, 1997, Mosby.

Monk HL: Fractures are never simple, *RN* 56(4):30, 1993.

Mourad LA: *Mosby's clinical nursing series: orthopedic disorders,* St Louis, 1991, Mosby.

Mulvey MA, Sharma PK: Traumatic amputation, *RN* 54(9):26, 1991.

North American Nursing Diagnosis Association: *NANDA nursing diagnosis, definitions and classification, 1999-2000,* Philadelphia, 1999, The Association.

North B et al: Living in a halo, *Am J Nurs* 92(4):55, 1992.

Nussman DS, Poole RC: Traumatic hip dislocation, *Am J Nurs* 91(11):34, 1991.

Peel K: Making sense of leeches, *Nurs Times* 89(27):34, 1993.

Pellino TA: How to manage hip fractures, *Am J Nurs* 94(4):46, 1994.

Present D, Shaffer B: Disease-associated fractures: detection and management in the elderly, *Geriatrics* 45(3):48, 1990.

Prestwood K, Kenny A: Osteoporosis: pathogenesis, diagnosis and treatment in older adults, *Clin Geriatr Med* 14(3):577-599.

Rogers-Seidle FF: *Geriatric nursing care plans,* St Louis, 1991, Mosby.

Strangio L: Leeches—when bleeding is exactly what you want, *RN* 54(9):31, 1991.

Thompson JM et al: *Mosby's clinical nursing,* ed 4, St Louis, 1997, Mosby.

Urrows ST et al: Profiles in osteoporosis, *Am J Nurs* 91(12):33, 1991.

Wainwright ST, Bacon ES: Traumatic amputation, *Nursing '93* 23(10):33, 1993.

USC UNIVERSITY HOSPITAL

1500 San Pablo
Los Angeles, CA 90033

MULTIDISCIPLINARY PLAN

NAME _____
ALLERGIES _____
MR# _____

DIAGNOSIS

SURGERY Total Hip Replacement (209)
Bilateral/Multiple Major Joint LE (471)

DISCHARGE OUTCOMES	DRG 209/471 ALOS 9.4/11.9	ADMIT DATE:
PHYSIOLOGICAL	Independent household ambulator. Absence of pain. Good/adequate circulation to affected extremity. Maintain total hip precautions.	
COGNITIVE	Demonstrates independence in home activity, hip precautions, and use of adaptive devices. Verbalizes follow-up medical plan.	
PSYCHOLOGICAL	Demonstrates realistic expectations of rehabilitation and adaptive coping patterns as evidenced by ability/willingness to participate in perioperative/recovery care activities.	

DISCIPLINE	PRE-OP/ PRE-ADMIT	D.O.S. DATE ___ / DAY 1	P.O.#1 DATE ___ / DAY 2	P.O.#2 DATE ___ / DAY 3	P.O.#3 DATE ___ / DAY 4	P.O.#4 DATE ___ / DAY 5	P.O.#5 DATE ___ / DAY 6
LOCATION		OR/Surgical	Surgical	Surgical	Surgical	Surgical	Surgical
LABS	CBC, PT, PTT U/A C+S Type & Cross V on Autologous units	CBC in PAR	CBC Chem 7		CBC		
CARDIO-PULMONARY	ECG	I.S. Instruction & use q° WA	Continue I.S.	Evaluate for self I.S. use			
IMAGING/ NUCLEAR MEDICINE	CXR	AP and Lateral hip x-ray in PAR					
SOCIAL SERVICES D/C PLAN REHAB. SERVICES	P.T. eval Instruct hip precautions, equipment, crutch training. Initiate D/C planning.	Continue D/C planning. Assess home care needs. Initiate total hip precautions. Consider Rehab eval. P.T. hip protocol wt bearing/fixation. Consult MSW prn	P.T. eval and exercise. Confer with patient for activity instruction. Assess home environment	Start progressive ambulation. Wt bearing status per MD. O.T. eval & issue adaptive device. Demonstration of usage of adaptive equipment	Re-evaluate home care needs. Consider Acute rehab transfer. Arrange D.M.E. needs. Include S/O in education to environment, i.e., stairs, rugs, pets, furniture, transfers. P.T. training with lower extremity mgmt using equipment	Prepare for discharge. Required minimal (25% or less) cues to maintain hip precautions. Progress to crutches. Demonstrates transfers. Complying with lower extremity management	Reassess compliance with all activities. Demonstrates energy conservation, work simplification. Independent in activities, hip precautions, stairclimbing, car transfers. Shower eval. Discharge planning
PHARMACY		IV TKO when fully awake & when taking po fluids well. Epidural/PCA-pain mgmt. Antibiotics x48°. DO NOT DC until all drains/catheters DC'ed		Give one more dose of antibiotics after Foley is discontinued			
DIETARY/ NUTRITION	NPO after midnight	Post-op clear liquids. Advance diet as tolerated					

Used by permission of USC University Hospital, Los Angeles, California.

page 2 of 4

USC UNIVERSITY HOSPITAL

1500 San Pablo
Los Angeles, CA 90033

MULTIDISCIPLINARY PLAN

NAME _____
ALLERGIES _____

MR# _____

DIAGNOSIS _____

SURGERY Total Hip Replacement (209)
Bilateral/Multiple Major Joint LE (471)

DRG _209/471_   ALOS _9.4/11.9_   ADMIT DATE: _____

DISCHARGE OUTCOMES
PHYSIOLOGICAL
COGNITIVE
PSYCHOLOGICAL

DISCIPLINE	PRE-OP/ PRE-ADMIT	P.O.#6 DATE	DAY 7	P.O.#7 DATE	DAY 8	P.O.#8 DATE	DAY 9	P.O.#9 DATE	DAY 10	P.O.#10 DATE	DAY 11	P.O.#11 DATE	DAY 12
LOCATION													
LABS													
CARDIO-PULMONARY													
IMAGING/ NUCLEAR MEDICINE													
SOCIAL SERVICES D/C PLAN REHAB. SERVICES													
PHARMACY													
DIETARY/ NUTRITION													

Continued

PATIENT NAME: _____

MULTIDISCIPLINARY PLAN

MEDICAL RECORD # _____

DISCIPLINE	PRE-OP/ PRE-ADMIT	D.O.S. DAY 1 DATE	P.O.#1 DAY 2 DATE	P.O.#2 DAY 3 DATE	P.O.#3 DAY 4 DATE	P.O.#4 DAY 5 DATE	P.O.#5 DAY 6 DATE
PATIENT ACTIVITY	Betadine Shower. TED hose apply to unoperative extremity.	HOB <45° Slings & Springs to operative leg. Avoid peroneal nerve pressure. TED hose/sequentials encourage performance of isometric exercises, gluteal/ quad sets. Ankle/toe pumps. Encourage use of OHT	Activity to edge of bed, dangle & stand. Any hip drainage-bedrest until clearance	Evaluate for ability to lift leg, get in and out of bed with minimal assist, stand to walk, and transfer to chair. Encourage up in chair for meals	Ambulate or strengthening/ toilet transfer. If pt active, DC sequentials, and slings & springs BRP with assist	Ambulate/transfer maintaining hip precautions. Shower	Stairs, climbing
EDUCATION	Video. Pre-op clinic. Pre-op teach D/C instructions. Begin Admission Assessment. Educational booklet provided to pt.	Hip Precautions: • Keep operative leg elevated • Do not cross legs • Do not use low chairs/toilets • No flexion >60° • No twisting • Instruct on use of OHT to turn		Explain stress/wt bearing restrictions. Reinforce techniques on how to use ambulatory devices	D/C Training: • Hip precautions/activity restrictions • Sleep with pillow between legs. Sleep on back or on either side - teach why each side may be better for individual pt. • Sex education • Hygiene - use raised toilet seat. Lean toward operative side when performing toileting hygiene. BATHING - DO NOT sit in tub. • Signs & symptoms to report: wound infection, increase in pain, persistent swelling of leg (does not disappear after one hour of elevation), calf tenderness, sudden shortening of affected extremity.		

1. To initiate a problem or intervention, document under corresponding date.

2. Document outcomes under appropriate date for achieving the goal.

3. To discontinue an intervention, or resolve a patient problem, highlight date and initial.

KEY
mgmt = management
OHT = overhead trapeze

DATE	DC DATE INIT	COLLABORATIVE PROBLEMS	DATE	DC DATE INIT	COLLABORATIVE PROBLEMS	DC DATE INIT
		1. Impaired physical mobility R/T disease/surgery.			7. Self care deficit R/T surgical procedure.	
		2. Alteration in comfort, pain R/T surgical procedure.				
		3. Potential for injury, i.e. displacement of prosthesis, infection, DVT R/T surgical procedure.				
		4. Tissue perfusion, alteration in R/T surgical procedure.				
		5. Fear/anxiety R/T hospitalization.				
		6. Knowledge deficit R/T activity/hip precautions.				

OUTCOMES

1. Demonstrates wt bearing status and use of ambulatory devices.	1. Demonstrates ambulation & transfers with assistive device.	1. Independent in activity, hip precautions, stairs, transfers, shower. Independent home exercise program initiated.
2. Pain controlled as evidenced by participation in activity.	7. Minimal assistance required for self-care.	7. Independent in self-care/or support system identified/able to provide for deficit.

1. Demonstrates leg exercises as instructed by P.T.

5. Apprehensions regarding hospitalization, continuum of health verbalized/controlled anxiety.

2. Verbalizes pain control within 30 min of intervention.

3. No injury/infection throughout hospitalization.

4. Tissue perfusion to affected extremity maintained throughout hospitalization.

PLAN OF CARE DISCUSSED WITH	D.O.S. DAY 1	P.O.#1 DAY 2	P.O.#2 DAY 3	P.O.#3 DAY 4	P.O.#4 DAY 5	P.O.#5 DAY 6
	DATE _____	DATE _____	DATE _____	DATE _____	DATE _____	DATE _____
	INTERVENTIONS					
DATE INIT SO/P _____ _____ _____ _____ _____	Orient to room/environment. Explain purpose of equipment in use.	Transfuse 1 unit of autologous blood as ordered.	Monitor use of crutches/walker to determine proper use of aid/wt bearing activities.	Assess level of ability to participate in ADL.	Ensure home D.M.E. has been arranged prn.	Discharge Instructions: • Continue wearing TEDs for 1 month post surgery • Take ASA BID times 1 month • Continue exercise regimen • Reinforce hip precautions • Driving restrictions
	Assess location, type, severity of pain. Maintain Epidural/PCA.	Continued pain management.	Encourage isometrics & quad sets.	Assess level of support from family/friends.	Reinforce hip precautions.	
	Monitor respiratory status. Encourage use of I.S.	Reinforce hip precautions. Increase activity as ordered.	Nursing to assist pt in/out of bed maintaining hip precautions.	Ensure ADL equipment available.		
CASE MANAGER:	Monitor color, warmth, sensation, pulses of affected extremities.		Ensure po intake adequate to promote healing/maintain hydration.	BRP or BSC privileges by nursing maintaining hip precautions.		
CONSULTING MD. _____	Ice packs at surgical site to decrease edema daily after P.T.		Dietary consult as needed.	Discontinue sequential compression boots.		
	Observe hip wrap dressing every 2° for drainage. Reinforce prn.		Offer pain med 30 min prior to therapy. Encourage use as needed.	Discontinue springs & slings if pt able to SLR.		
SOCIAL SERVICE:	Reinforce hip precautions. Record Hemovac output every 8°.		Discontinue foley 4 hrs after Epidural Catheter/PCA is removed.			
ANOINTING OF THE SICK DATE: _____	Maintain foley.		May I&O catheterize every 8° if no void.			
	Apply TED hose. Remove BID x 30 min.					
	Sequentials.					
	Assess for signs & symptoms of DVT.					
	Assess bowel/bladder output. Consider laxative.					
	Encourage expressions of fears/anxiety.					
	Ensure initiation of P.T.					

MULTIDISCIPLINARY PLAN UPDATE

DATE	SIGNATURES	DATE	SIGNATURES	DATE	SIGNA

USC UNIVERSITY HOSPITAL
1500 San Pablo
Los Angeles, CA 90033 ©1991

SIDE 1   **MULTIDISCIPLINARY PLAN**

DIAGNOSIS _____
SURGERY **Orthopedic Service-LAMINECTOMY**
General Anesthesia

NAME _____
ALLERGIES _____
ADMIT DATE _____

DISCHARGE OUTCOMES   DRG 215   ALOS 6.0

PHYSIOLOGICAL	Patient will have pain controlled at level < 3 on 1 - 10 scale c̄ p.o. meds, will ambulate c̄ steady gait independently, VS within normal limits & wound will be healing c̄ redness or edema.
COGNITIVE	Patient will verbalize spine precautions-no lifting, twisting, flexion, brace compliance & sitting only for meals & commode. Will verbalize s/sx of infection & when to call M.D.
PSYCHOLOGICAL	Patient will verbalize acceptance of lifestyle change to incorporate spine precautions into activities of daily living.

DISCIPLINE	PRE-OP/ PRE-ADMIT	DOS DAY 1	P.O.#1 DAY 2	P.O.#2 DAY 3	P.O.#3 DAY 4	P.O.#4 DAY 5	P.O.#5 DAY 6
LOCATION	OP CLINIC	SURGERY/PAR/DOU	MED/SURG	MED/SURG	MED/SURG	MED/SURG → HOME	
LABS	CBC Chem 20 UA PT PTT		H & H				
CARDIO-PULMONARY	ECG May require PFT's ABG	I.S.					
IMAGING/ NUCLEAR MEDICINE	CXR						
SOCIAL SERVICES D/C PLAN REHAB. SERVICES	Psycho-social eval. P.T. eval & treat measure for brace	Initiate discharge planning Trapeze Rehab eval, if indicated	P.T. eval & teach bed mobility, logrolling, prone to stand transfer. Spine precautions	Home health eval if indicated Progressive ambulation	Identify D.M.E. requirements Instruct in stairs	Clearance by P.T. for discharge	
PHARMACY	General anesthesia	PCA in PAR - no pain management consult Ancef or Vanco IV TKO when taking po well. Decadron Zantac Vitamin C, Ferrous gluconate	D/C PCA D/C antibiotics when drains are out	Laxative or suppository prn			
DIETARY/ NUTRITION		NPO	Clear liquids Advance as tolerated				

PATIENT NAME: _____

MULTIDISCIPLINARY PLAN

DISCIPLINE	PRE-OP/ PRE-ADMIT	DOS DAY 1	P.O. #1 DAY 2	P.O. #2 DAY 3	P.O. #3 DAY 4	P.O. #4 DAY 5	P.O. #5 DAY 6
PATIENT ACTIVITY		DATE ____ BR TED hose in PAR Bilateral leg squeezers in OR.	DATE ____ High rise toilet seat/BSC	DATE ____	DATE ____	DATE ____	DATE ____
EDUCATION	Spine pre-cautions Review pathway goals	Orient to room, unit & hospital routine. Teach &/or reinforce spine precautions	Reinforce lack of sitting (or as ordered by MD), except for meals & commode			Shower instructions: Water to flow on front of body only, no direct flow on back	

COLLABORATIVE PROBLEMS

DATE			DATE			DC DATE/INIT
❶ Alteration in comfort, pain R/T surgery.			❼ Potential alteration in coping, anxiety R/T discharge planning.			▧
❷ Potential for infection R/T surgical procedure.			❽ Alteration in mobility R/T surgical procedure.			▧
❸ Potential alteration in elimination, bowel ileus R/T surgery.						▧
❹ Knowledge deficit R/T surgical procedure & spine precautions.						▧
❺ Potential for neurosensory impairment R/T surgery.						▧
❻ Potential alteration in coping, anxiety R/T hospitalization.						▧

OUTCOMES

					DC DATE/INIT
❶ Pt. will have pain controlled at 4-5 on 1-10 scale by 4° postop.	❶ Pt. will verbalize pain controlled at 3-4 on 1-10 scale.	❶ Pt. will verbalize pain controlled at 3-4 on 1-10 scale c̄ p.o. pain meds.	❹ Consistently demonstrates spine precautions.	❼ All DME equipment available.	▧
❷ Pt. will remain free from s/sx of infection throughout stay.		❸ Pt. will resume bowel function.	❽ Supervised bed mobility, transfers. Independent self-care except shower.	❽ Independent ambulation all surfaces & stairs.	▧
❹ Pt. will verbalize spine precautions by 4° post-op.		❼ Pt. will verbalize feelings of assurance c̄ discharge plans within 8° of initiation.		❽ Independent shower.	▧
❺ Pt. will remain free from neurosensory deficits during hospitalization.	❽ Ambulate to BR & hall c̄ assistance. Assisted self-care.				▧
❻ Pt. will verbalize feelings of assurance c̄ hospital routine within 4° post-op.					▧

❶ To initiate a problem or intervention, document under corresponding date.

❷ Document outcomes under appropriate date for achieving the goal.

❸ To discontinue an intervention, or resolve a patient problem, highlight date and initial.

KEY

S/O	=	Significant Other
Pt.	=	Patient
A/E	=	As evidenced by
I.S.	=	Incentive spirometer
△	=	Change
S/Sx	=	Signs & Symptoms
D.M.E.	=	Durable medical equipment

Continued

INTERVENTIONS

PLAN OF CARE DISCUSSED WITH			DOS — DAY 1	P.O. #1 DAY 2	P.O. #2 DAY 3	P.O. #3 DAY 4	P.O. #4 DAY 5	P.O. #5 DAY 6
DATE	INITIAL	S.O.	Pt.					
			DATE ___	DATE ___	DATE ___	DATE ___	DATE ___	DATE ___
			— Maintain patent IV c̄ PCA started in PAR. — Assess for edema & pain location, quality & duration.	— Encourage use of po pain meds at pain scale mid-point.				
			— Notify M.D. if not controlled. — Orient to surroundings, unit & hospital routine.	— D/C foley. Assess bladder distension, urinary retention. I & O cath q̄4° PRN.				
			— Assess for drainage, bleeding at surgical site. Notify M.D. if present & immediately if CSF noted.	— Reinforce spine precautions: • sit only for meals/commode (or as MD orders) • avoid twisting, flexion	— Reinforce spine precautions.			
			— Cold packs to surgical site x48°.	or bending. • maintain back alignment when OOB.				
			— Assess bowel sounds, abdominal distension, flatus.	— Nursing to ambulate pt. c̄ back brace & continue p̄ cleared by P.T.	— Assess bowel function & need for laxative or suppository.	— Assess bowel function & need for laxative or suppository.		
			— Neuro ✓'s q1° x 12°, q4° x 12°. Notify M.D. if Δ occurs.	— Maintain sequential compression bilaterally while in bed.		— Reinforce discharge plans. — Sitting per MD instructions.		
			— Log roll q2°. Keep spine in correct alignment c̄ pillow between legs.	— Maintain TED hose per policy.				
			— Notify M.D. if T > 101°.	— Assess orthostatic hypotension.	— Introduce home health liaison for needs assessment.			
Case Manager: _____			— Teach s/sx of infection, aseptic wound techinque & good hand washing.					
Consulting MD: _____			— Teach or reinforce spine precautions.					
Social Service: _____								
Anointing of The Sick Date: _____			— Assess & record I & O until Regular diet tolerated along c̄ drains & foley out.					
			— Check drains q̄4° & empty when ½ full.					

MULTIDISCIPLINARY PLAN UPDATE

DATE	SIGNATURES	DATE	SIGNATURES	DATE	SIGNATURES

USC UNIVERSITY HOSPITAL
1500 San Pablo
Los Angeles, CA 90033 ©1991

MULTIDISCIPLINARY PLAN

SIDE 1

NAME _____
ALLERGIES _____
ADMIT DATE _____

DIAGNOSIS _____

SURGERY **Orthopedic Service-LUMBAR FUSION WITH INSTRUMENTATION**

DRG 214   ALOS 10.1

DISCHARGE OUTCOMES

PHYSIOLOGICAL: Patient will have pain controlled at level < 3 on 1 - 10 scale c̄ po meds, will ambulate c̄ steady gait independently, or c̄ D.M.E., VS within normal limits, improved neuro-sensory status & wound will be healing s̄ redness or edema.

COGNITIVE: Patient will verbalize spine precautions-no lifting, twisting, flexion & sitting as per M.D. instructions. Will verbalize s/sx of infection & when to call M.D.

PSYCHOLOGICAL: Patient will verbalize acceptance of lifestyle changes to incorporate spine precautions into activities of daily living.

DISCIPLINE	PRE-OP/PRE-ADMIT	D.O.S. DAY 1	P.O.#1 DAY 2	P.O.#2 DAY 3	P.O.#3 DAY 4	P.O.#4 DAY 5	P.O.#5 DAY 6
LOCATION	OP CLINIC	SURGERY/PAR/SICU DATE	SICU → MED/SURG DATE	MED/SURG DATE	MED/SURG DATE	MED/SURG DATE	MED/SURG DATE
LABS	CBC Chem 20 PT PTT UA		Hgb & Hct Lytes	Hgb & Hct			
CARDIO-PULMONARY	ECG	I.S.					
IMAGING/NUCLEAR MEDICINE	CXR				AP & lat lumbar/sacral spine x-ray.		
SOCIAL SERVICES D/C PLAN REHAB SERVICES	Psycho-social eval. R.T. eval, teach measure for brace; Orthomedics ☐ Lerman & Sons ☐	No Trapeze	P.T. for all extremity ROM, passive assisted SLR Back brace fitting.	P.T. eval & teach bed mobility, logrolling, prone to stand transfer. OOB c̄ back brace If indicated, Home Health or D/C Planner for placement	Progressive ambulation c̄ assistive device prn	Continue ambulation Assess D.M.E. needs	
PHARMACY		MS PCA; No pain management consult		Laxative or suppository prn		D/C Decadron, Zantac & PCA Begin po pain meds Ancef or Vanco D/C'd when drains are removed	
DIETARY/NUTRITION		NPO until passing flatus	NPO until passing flatus	Clear liquids Advance diet as tolerated			

Continued

Used by permission of USC University Hospital, Los Angeles, California.

MULTIDISCIPLINARY PLAN

PATIENT NAME: _____

DISCIPLINE	PRE-OP/ PRE-ADMIT	D.O.S. DAY 1 DATE___	P.O. #1 DAY 2 DATE___	P.O. #2 DAY 3 DATE___	P.O. #3 DAY 4 DATE___	P.O. #4 DAY 5 DATE___	P.O. #5 DAY 6 DATE___
PATIENT ACTIVITY		BR Logroll q2° / TED hose in PAR / Bilateral leg squeezers begun in OR / Gatch prn to any angle		OOB c̄ back brace / High rise toilet seat			❽ Ambulates to BR & hall c̄ assistance. Assisted self-care.
EDUCATION	Spine precautions Review pathway goals	Spine precautions orient to room, unit & hospital routine	Instruct pt on rationale for I & O cath until complete return of bladder function	Reinforce sitting activity as per M.D. orders.			Shower instructions: Water to flow on front of body only, no direct flow on back

COLLABORATIVE PROBLEMS

Instructions:

❶ To initiate a problem or intervention, document under corresponding date.

❷ Document outcomes under appropriate date for achieving the goal.

❸ To discontinue an intervention, or resolve a patient problem, highlight date and initial.

Collaborative Problems (DAY 1, DATE___):

❶ Alteration in comfort, pain R/T surgery.

❷ Potential for infection R/T surgical procedure.

❸ Potential alteration in elimination, bowel ileus R/T surgery.

❹ Knowledge deficit R/T surgical procedure & spine precautions.

❺ Potential for neuro-sensory impairment R/T surgery.

❻ Potential alterations in coping, anxiety R/T hospitalization.

Collaborative Problems (DAY 4, DATE___):

❼ Potential alteration in coping, anxiety R/T discharge planning.

❽ Altered mobility R/T surgical procedure.

OUTCOMES

DAY 1:

❶ Pt. will have pain controlled at 5-6 on 1-10 scale by 4° post-op.

❷ Pt. will remain free from s/sx of infection throughout stay.

❹ Pt. will verbalize spine precautions by 4° post-op.

❺ Pt. will remain free from neuro-sensory impairment during hospitalization.

❻ Pt. will verbalize feelings of assurance c̄ hospital routine within 4° post-op.

P.O. #1 DAY 2:

❶ Pt. will verbalize pain controlled at 4-5 on 1-10 scale.

❸ Pt. will resume bowel function.

P.O. #3 DAY 4:

❼ Pt. will verbalize feelings of assurance c̄ discharge plans within 8° of initiation.

P.O. #4 DAY 5:

❶ Pt. will verbalize pain controlled at 3-4 on 1-10 scale c̄ po pain meds.

KEY

S/O = Significant Other
Pt. = Patient
A/E = As evidenced by
△ = Change
S/SX = Signs & Symptoms
D.M.E. = Durable Medical Equipment
SLR = Straight leg raises
I.S. = Incentive spirometer

INTERVENTIONS

D.O.S. DAY 1	P.O.#1 DAY 2	P.O.#2 DAY 3	P.O.#3 DAY 4	P.O.#4 DAY 5	P.O.#5 DAY 6
DATE ___	DATE ___	DATE ___	DATE ___	DATE ___	DATE ___
— Maintain patent IV c̄ PCA started in PAR.	— Assess bladder distension once Foley D/C'd. I & O cath q 4° prn.	— Reinforce spine precautions. — Teach back brace compliance when OOB.	— Introduce discharge planner, Home Health liaison for needs assessment.	— Encourage use of po pain meds at pain scale mid-point.	
— Orient to surroundings, unit & hospital routine.	— Reinforce spine precautions: • Sit only for meals & commode or as M.D. orders.	— Nursing to ambulate pt. c̄ back brace & continue p̄ cleared by P.T.		— Reinforce discharge plans.	
— Assess for edema & pain location, quality & duration. Notify M.D. if not controlled.	• Teach Pt. to avoid twisting, flexion or bending.	— Assess orthostatic hypotension.		— Reinforce mobility c̄ brace Reinforce Spine Precautions • No bending • No twisting	
— Assess for drainage, bleeding at surgical site. Notify M.D. if present & immediately if CSF noted.	• Maintain back brace compliance when OOB.	— Assess bowel function & need for laxative or suppository.		• No lifting • Keep spine in good alignment.	
— Cold packs to surgical site x 48°.	— Maintain leg squeezers bilaterally when in bed until discharge.			— D/C Foley I & O cath q̄ 4° PRN.	
— Assess bowel sounds, abdominal distension, flatus.	— Maintain TED hose per policy.				
— Neuro ✓'s q2° x 12°, q4° x 12°. Notify M.D. if Δ occurs.					
— Logroll q2°. Keep spine in correct alignment c̄ pillow between legs. Notify M.D. if T > 101°.					
— Teach s/sx of infection, aseptic wound technique & good hand washing.					
— Teach & reinforce spine precautions.					
— Assess & record I & O until Regular diet tolerated along c̄ drains & foley out.					
— Check drains q4° & empty when 1/2 full.					

PLAN OF CARE DISCUSSED WITH

DATE	INITIAL	S.O.	Pt.

Case Manager: ___

Consulting MD: ___

Social Service: ___

Anointing of The Sick Date: ___

MULTIDISCIPLINARY PLAN UPDATE

SIGNATURES	DATE	SIGNATURES	DATE	SIGNATURES

Continued

MULTIDISCIPLINARY PLAN

PATIENT NAME: _____

DISCIPLINE	PRE-OP/ PRE-ADMIT	P.O. #6 DAY 7	P.O. #7 DAY 8	P.O. #8 DAY 9	P.O. #9 DAY 10	P.O. #10 DAY 11	P.O. #11 DAY 12
		DATE	DATE	DATE	DATE	DATE	DATE
PATIENT ACTIVITY		OOB c̄ back brace. High rise toilet seat					
EDUCATION		Reinforce no direct spray from shower					

COLLABORATIVE PROBLEMS

DATE

❶ Alteration in comfort, pain R/T surgery.

❷ Potential for infection R/T surgical procedure.

❹ Knowledge deficit R/T surgical procedure & spine precautions.

❼ Potential alteration in coping, anxiety R/T discharge planning.

❽ Altered in mobility R/T surgical procedure.

COLLABORATIVE PROBLEMS — DATE / INIT / D.C. DATE

OUTCOMES

❷ Pt. will remain free from s/sx of infection throughout stay.

❹ Pt. will consistently verbalize/ demonstrate spine precautions.

❼ Pt. will verbalize/demonstrate feelings of assurance c̄ discharge plans.

❽ Supervised bed mobility, transfers. Independent self-care except shower.

❶ Pt. will verbalize pain controlled at <3 on 1-10 scale c̄ po pain meds.

❼ All D.M.E. available.

❽ Independent ambulation all surfaces & stairs. Independent shower.

❶ To initiate a problem or intervention, document under corresponding date.

❷ Document outcomes under appropriate date for achieving the goal.

❸ To discontinue an intervention, or resolve a patient problem, highlight, date, and initial.

KEY

S/O = Significant Other
Pt. = Patient
A/E = As evidenced by
Δ = Change
S/SX = Signs & Symptoms
D.M.E. = Durable Medical Equipment
SLR = Straight leg raises
I.S. = Incentive spirometer

USC UNIVERSITY HOSPITAL
1500 San Pablo
Los Angeles, CA 90033 ©1991

SIDE 2

MULTIDISCIPLINARY PLAN

DIAGNOSIS _____

SURGERY **Orthopedic Service-LUMBAR FUSION WITH INSTRUMENTATION**

NAME _____
ALLERGIES _____
ADMIT DATE _____

DRG 214   ALOS 10.1

DISCHARGE OUTCOMES	
PHYSIOLOGICAL	Patient will have pain controlled at level < 3 on 1 - 10 scale c̄ p.o. meds, will ambulate c̄ steady gait independently or c̄ D.M.E., VS within normal limits, improved neuro-sensory status & wound will be healing c̄ redness or edema.
COGNITIVE	Patient will verbalize spine precautions-no lifting, twisting, flexion & sitting as per M.D. instructions. Will verbalize s/sx of infection & when to call M.D.
PSYCHOLOGICAL	Patient will verbalize acceptance of lifestyle change to incorporate spine precautions into activities of daily living.

DISCIPLINE	PRE-OP/ PRE-ADMIT	P.O. #6 DAY 7 DATE	P.O. #7 DAY 8 DATE	P.O. #8 DAY 9 DATE	P.O. #9 DAY 10 DATE	P.O. #10 DAY 11 DATE	P.O. #11 DAY 12 DATE
LOCATION		MED/SURG	MED/SURG → HOME				
LABS							
CARDIO-PULMONARY	I.S.						
IMAGING/ NUCLEAR MEDICINE							
SOCIAL SERVICES D/C PLAN REHAB. SERVICES	Clearance by P.T. for D/C.						
PHARMACY	PO pain medications						
DIETARY/ NUTRITION	Diet as tolerated						

Continued

PLAN OF CARE DISCUSSED WITH			P.O. #6 DAY 7	P.O. #7 DAY 8	P.O. #8 DAY 9	P.O. #9 DAY 10	P.O. #10 DAY 11	P.O. #11 DAY 12
DATE	INITIAL	S.O.	Pt.	DATE ___	DATE ___	DATE ___	DATE ___	DATE ___	DATE ___

INTERVENTIONS

— Reinforce discharge plans.

— Reinforce proper body mechanics, no lifting.

— Reassess pt understanding of S/SX of infection & when to notify M.D.

— Limit sitting as per M.D. order.

— Encourage use of po pain meds at <3 on 1-10 pain scale.

Case Manager: ___

Consulting MD: ___

Social Service: ___

Anointing of
The Sick
Date: ___

MULTIDISCIPLINARY PLAN UPDATE

DATE	SIGNATURES	DATE	SIGNATURES	DATE	SIGNATURES	DATE	SIGNATURES

CHAPTER 9

Neurologic System

■ NEUROLOGIC ASSESSMENT (Fig. 9-1)

SUBJECTIVE DATA

Dizziness
Muscle weakness (bilateral or unilateral)
Inability to move
Headaches
Numbness
Bowel and/or bladder dysfunction
Pain
Memory loss
Tremors
Nervousness
Irritability
Drowsiness
Drooping face
Disturbances in the following:
    Smell
    Taste
    Vision
    Hearing
Insomnia
Difficulty speaking
Difficulty walking
Fatigue

OBJECTIVE DATA

General
    Level of consciousness (LOC) (Table 9-1)
        Orientation to person, time, and place
        Best motor response, verbal response, eye opening
            (Table 9-2)
        Delirium, hallucination
        Dementia
    Behavior: general appearance, social adaptation,
        attitude, personal grooming, facial expression, ability
        to concentrate
    Speech pattern: verbal expression, verbal response,
        fluency, sound and flow of words.
    Emotional status: affect, mood, feeling
    Thought and perception: thought processes, thought
        content, perception, insight, judgment
    Intellectual or cognitive function
        Memory: immediate, recent, past
        Attention span
        Calculation: simple and complex calculation

        Abstract thinking: by asking clients proverbs or
            difference of two given objects
        Judgment and insight
    Age: see Gerontologic Considerations box
Specific
    Sensory discrimination: visual, tactile, auditory, body
        part agnosia
    Cortical motor integration: motor and cortical
        apraxia
    Language: Broca's (expressive), Wernicke's (receptive),
        combined (conductive) aphasia.
    Spatial disorientation (dizziness): vertigo, presyncope,
        disequilibrium
    Pain symptoms: Onset, duration, severity, location,
        frequency, aggravating factors, relieving factors,
        and character—freezing/burning, throbbing/
        shooting, spreading/radiating, tingling/itchy
    Skin
        Temperature
        Color, discolored areas
        Turgor
        Rashes
        Angiomatous lesions
        Moles
Vital signs
    Blood pressure (BP)
        Both arms; standing, sitting, lying
        Increased
        Decreased
        Widening pulse pressure
    Arterial pulses
    Respirations (R) (Table 9-3)
        Rate
        Rhythm
        Quality
        Type of breathing pattern
        Chest movements
        Breath sounds
Eyes
    Pupils (Figs. 9-2)
        Shape
        Equality
        Size
            Pinpoint
            Dilation
        Reaction to light, to accommodation

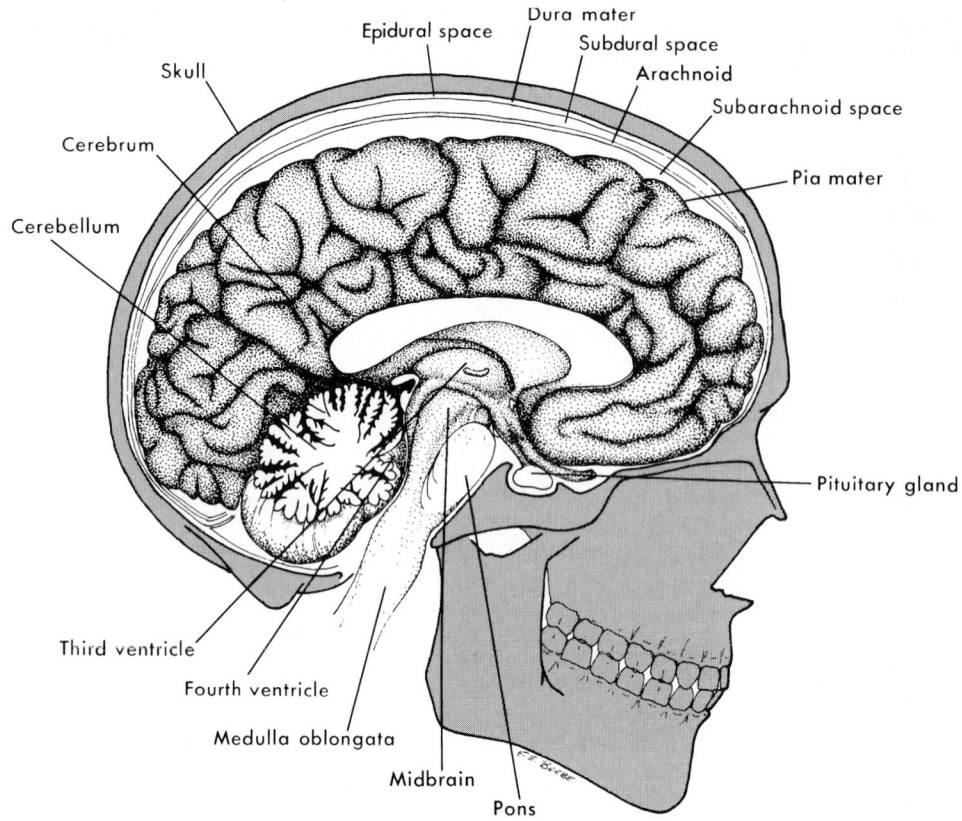

Fig. 9-1 Nervous system.

Table 9-1	**Continuum of Level of Consciousness**

Full consciousness ⇨ Confusion ⇨ Lethargy ⇨ Obtundation ⇨ Stupor ⇨ Light coma (Semicoma) ⇨ Coma ⇨ Deep coma

Level of Consciousness	Description
Full consciousness	Oriented to time, place, and person, alert; aware of one's own cognition and mental processes
Confusion	Disturbed orientation in regard to time, place, and person; shortened attention span and memory; inability to follow commands; may accompany with hallucination, irritation, agitation, and restlessness
Lethargy	Oriented to person, time, and place; responds slowly to stimulation, sluggish in speech, mental processes, and motor activities; able to follow commands; appears drowsy
Obtundation	Appears extremely drowsy; arousable with stimulation; responds to one or two words; able to follow simple commands
Stupor	Appears to be in a sleeping state with minimal spontaneous movement; responds to only vigorous and repeated stimuli and painful stimuli by making incomprehensible sounds and/or opening eyes
Light coma (also called *semicoma***)**	Unconscious; no verbal sounds; no spontaneous movement; withdraws purposefully to pain stimulation; brainstem reflexes intact
Coma	Unarousable; no verbal sounds; no spontaneous movement; withdraws nonpurposefully to pain stimulation; brainstem reflexes may or may not be intact; decorticate or decerebrate postures present
Deep coma	Unarousable; no verbal sounds; unresponsive to pain stimulation; brainstem reflexes absent

Table 9-2	Glasgow Coma Scale (GCS)			
Items	**Factors**	**Scores**	**Description**
Best motor response	Obeys verbal command	6	To painful stimuli, record best upper
	Localizes pain	5	extremities response
	Withdraws from pain	4	
	Flexion-decorticate rigidity	3	
	Extension-decerebrate rigidity	2	
	No response	1	
Verbal response	Oriented to person, place, time	5	Record *T* if tracheostomy tube in place;
	Confused	4	*E* if endotracheal tube in place
	Inappropriate words	3	
	Incomprehensible sounds	2	
	No response	1	
Eye opening	Spontaneous	4	Record *C* if the patient's eyes are
	To speech	3	unable to open because of swelling
	To pain	2	
	No response	1	Range score from 3 to 15

Modified from Christensen BL, Kockrow EO: Foundations of nursing, ed 3, St Louis, 1998, Mosby.

Gerontologic Considerations

- As neurons are lost with aging, there is a deterioration in neurologic function, resulting in slowed reflex and reaction time.
- Tremors that increase with fatigue are commonly observed in adults.
- The sense of touch and the ability for fine motor coordination diminish with aging.
- Most older persons possess the ability to learn, but the speed of learning is slowed. Short-term memory is more affected by aging than long-term memory.
- The incidence of physiologic dementia or organic brain syndrome, including Alzheimer's disease, Pick's disease, and multiinfarct dementia, increases with aging.
- The incidence of cerebrovascular accident increases with age. The prognosis is affected by the location and extent of the cerebral damage. Rehabilitation potential after a stroke is often reduced by advanced age and coexisting medical problems.
- Nerve irritation resulting from arthritis, joint injuries, or spinal cord compression can cause chronic pain or weakness.
- Dementia is not a normal consequence of aging but may be a result of many reversible conditions, including anemia, infection, fluid and electrolyte imbalance, malnutrition, hypothyroidism, metabolic disturbances, drug toxicity, and hypotension.

Ptosis
Nystagmus
"Doll's eyes" (see Figure 9-3, *A*)
Caloric test (Fig. 9-3, *B*)
Diplopia
Visual acuity

Visual fields
Eye movement
Ophthalmoscopic assessment
Motor function
    Balance
    Coordination of body movements
    Posture and gait (Table 9-4, Fig. 9-4)
    Strength
        Hands, arms
        Hips, legs, ankles, and neck
    Muscle mass
        Size
        Tone
        Strength
        Symmetry/asymmetry
Involuntary movement
    Tremors: resting tremor and postural tremor
    Tics
    Myoclonus
    Athetosis
    Dystonia
    Ballismus
    Chorea
Seizure activity
    Partial seizures
    Generalized seizures
Reflex responses (Table 9-5; Box 9-1)
Autonomic functions
    Bowel and/or bladder dysfunctions
    Sexual dysfunction
Cranial nerve abnormalities (Table 9-6)
Nutritional assessment
    Weight, height
    Anthropometric measurements
    Triceps skinfold (TSF)
    Arm muscle circumference (AMC)
    Mid-upper arm circumference (MUAC)
Abnormal posturing

Table 9-3	**Patterns of Respiration in Neurologic Dysfunction**	
Terms	**Description**	**Selected Neurologic Causes**
Eupnea	Normal breathing	
Cheyne-Stokes respirations	Breathing characterized by regular, alternating periods of hyperpnea and apnea; breathing builds from respiration to respiration in a smooth crescendo and, as peak is reached, declines in an equally smooth decrescendo; ordinarily, hyperpneic phase endures longer than apneic phase	Deep bilateral diencephalic lesions, hypertensive encephalopathy, uremia, anoxia, or imminent transtentorial herniation
Central neurogenic hyperventilation	Sustained regular, rapid hypocapnic hyperpnea	Midbrain lesions
Biot's respirations	Regular periods of hyperventilation and irregular periods of apnea	
Apneustic respirations	Ataxic, gasping, shallow breathing	Infarction at midpontine or caudal pontine level, usually as a result of basilar artery occlusion
Posthyperventilation apnea	Respirations interrupted for up to 30 seconds after five voluntary breaths in wakeful patients	Diffuse metabolic or structural forebrain disease
Cluster breathing	Breaths follow each other in disorderly sequence with irregular pauses between them	Low pons or high medulla lesion; may be result of expanding lesion in posterior fossa (cerebellar hemorrhage)
Ataxic breathing	Completely chaotic pattern with deep and shallow breaths occurring randomly; progressively leads to apnea	Dorsomedial medulla dysfunction; may appear in relation to meningitis or acute parainfectious demyelination

From Barber JM, Stokes LG, Billings DM: Adult and child care: a client approach to nursing, *ed 2, St Louis, 1977, Mosby.*

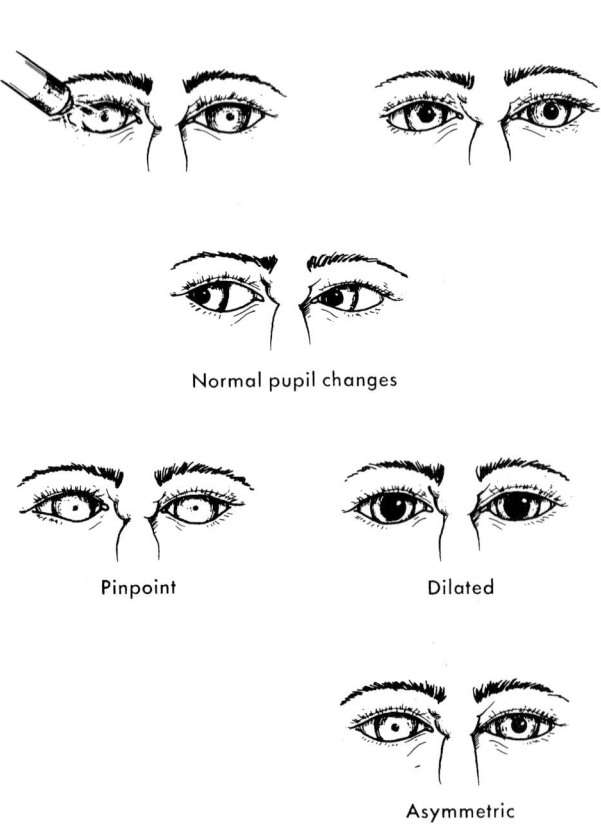

Normal pupil changes

Pinpoint   Dilated

Asymmetric

Fig. 9-2 Variations in pupil response.

PERTINENT BACKGROUND INFORMATION

Description of past or concurrent neurological or muscular disorders
Recent operations or hospitalization
Epilepsy
LOC
Headaches
Hypertension
Cancer
Coronary artery disease
Atrial fibrillation
Hyperlipidemia
Pernicious anemia
Diabetes
Coarctation of aorta
Allergies
Prenatal history
Diseases in childhood
Infections
Motor, sensory disturbances
Behavioral or emotional changes
Head trauma, spinal trauma
Drug abuse
Shock
Dietary restrictions
Pregnancies

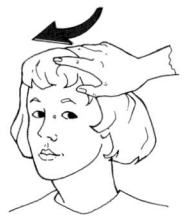
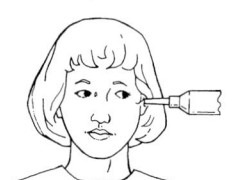

A

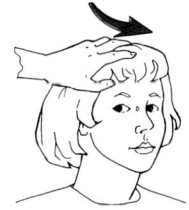
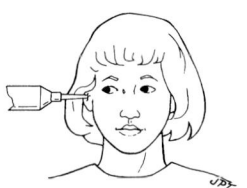

Doll's eyes   Ice water calorics

BRAINSTEM INTACT

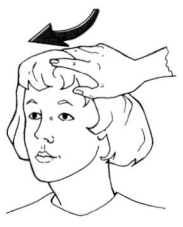
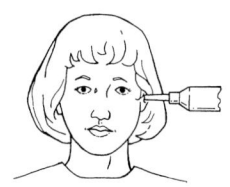

B

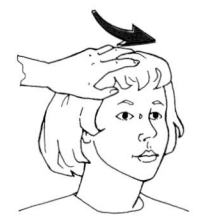
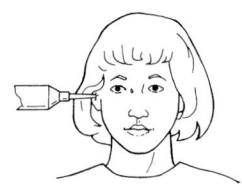

Doll's eyes   Ice water calorics

BRAINSTEM NOT INTACT

Fig. 9-3 Ocular reflexes at different levels of consciousness. **A,** Response when brainstem is intact; eyes move in opposite direction of head movement. Nystagmus is present with ice water calorics. **B,** Response when brainstem is not intact; gaze remains fixed in direction of head movement. Nystagmus is not present with ice water calorics.
(From Beare PG, Myers JL: Adult health nursing, ed 3, St Louis, 1998, Mosby.)

FAMILY HISTORY
Hypertension
Seizure disorders
Neurologic disorders
Cancer
Strokes
Tremors/Parkinson's disease
Dementia/Alzheimer's disease
Migraine

Mental retardation
Mental illness
Sudden, unexplained death

SOCIAL HISTORY
Sleep patterns
Exercise and activity level
Occupation: work patterns, exposure to toxic substances
Travel history, recent
Leisure activities
Dietary preferences
Smoking
Alcohol consumption
Psychosocial patterns
    Personality changes
    Relationships with family and friends
Social support system
School history; learning disorders
Sexual activity

MEDICATION HISTORY
Prescription medications
Over-the-counter medications
Use of controlled substances
Oral contraceptives
Hormone therapy
Chemotherapy
Radiotherapy

KEY ASPECTS OF NEUROLOGIC EXAMINATION*
Mental status
    LOC
        Glasgow Coma Scale (GCS)
    Information obtained regarding mental status during
        history and physical examination
        Appearance
        Cognitive abilities
        Emotional stability
        Speech and language
Cranial nerves: II to XII commonly tested
Cerebellar function and proprioception
    Coordination and fine motor skills
    Balance
    Gait
    Posture
Sensory function
    Perception of position sense
    Two-point discrimination
    Superficial touch and superficial pain
    Vibratory response to tuning fork
    Ability to identify familiar object by touch
        (stereognosis)
    Ability to identify number or letter drawn on body part
        (graphesthesia)
Superficial and deep tendon reflexes (DTR)
    Biceps

Modified from Seidel HM et al: Mosby's guide to physical examination, ed 4, St Louis, 1999, Mosby.

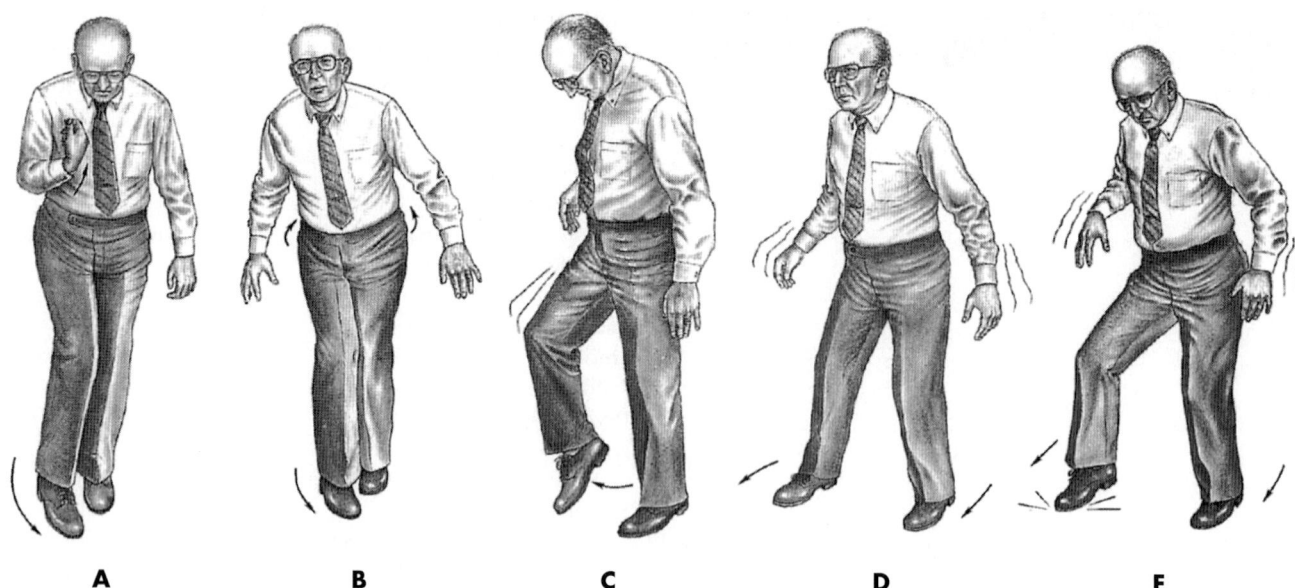

A   **B**   **C**   **D**   **E**

Fig. 9-4 Unexpected gait patterns. **A,** Spastic hemiparesis. **B,** Spastic diplegia (scissoring). **C,** Steppage gait. **D,** Cerebellar ataxia. **E,** Sensory ataxia.
(From Seidel HM et al: Mosby's guide to physical examination, ed 4, St Louis, 1999, Mosby.)

Table 9-4	**Characteristics of Unexpected Gait Patterns**
Gait Pattern	**Characteristics**
Spastic hemiparesis	The affected leg is stiff and extended, with plantar flexion of the foot. Movement of the foot results from pelvic tilting upward on the involved side. The foot is dragged, often scraping the toe, or it is circled stiffly outward and forward (circumduction). The affected arm remains flexed and adducted and does not swing (see Fig. 9-4, *A*).
Spastic diplegia (scissoring)	The patient uses short steps, dragging the ball of the foot across the floor. The legs are extended, and the thighs tend to cross forward on each other at each step (see Fig. 9-4, *B*).
Steppage	The hip and knee are elevated excessively high to lift the plantar flexed foot off the ground. The foot is brought down to the floor with a slap. The patient is unable to walk on the heels (see Fig. 9-4, *C*).
Dystrophic	The legs are kept apart, and weight is shifted from side to side in a waddling motion. The abdomen often protrudes, and lordosis is common.
Tabetic	The legs are positioned far apart, lifted high and forcibly brought down with each step. The heel stamps on the ground.
Cerebellar ataxia	The patient's feet are wide-based. Staggering and lurching from side to side are often accompanied by swaying of the trunk (see Fig. 9-4, *D*).
Sensory ataxia	The patient's gait is wide-based and unsteady. The feet are lifted high and brought down with a slap. The patient watches the ground to guide his or her steps. A positive Romberg sign is present (see Fig. 9-4, *E*).
Dystonia	Jerky dancing movements appear nondirectional.
Ataxia	Uncontrolled falling occurs.

Modified from Seidel HM et al: Mosby's guide to physical examination, ed 3, St Louis, 1999, Mosby.

Brachioradialis
Triceps
Patellar
Achilles
Abdominal reflexes
Plantar reflex
Ankle clonus
Cremasteric reflex (in males)

■ DIAGNOSTIC TESTS

Blood tests
    Complete blood cell count (CBC) and platelet count
    Erythrocytes sedimentation rate (ESR)
    Arterial blood gases (ABGs)
    Anticardiolipin antibodies
    Lipid panel test
    Antiphospholipid antibody test

Table 9-5	Reflexes	
Reflexes	**Associated Nerve Function**	
SUPERFICIAL		
Upper abdominal	T-8, T-9, T-10	
Lower abdominal	T-10, T-11, T-12	
Cremasteric	T-12, L-1, L-2	
Gluteal	L-4 to S-3	
DEEP TENDON		
Biceps	C-5, C-6	
Triceps	C-6, C-7, C-8	
Finger flexion	C-7 to T1	
Brachioradialis	C-5, C-6	
Patellar	S1 to S-2	
Achilles	S-1, S-2	
PATHOLOGIC REFLEXES (IN ADULTS)		
Babinski sign (plantar)		
Chaddock sign		
Grasp reflex		
Hoffmann		
Palmomental response		
Sucking reflex		

Box 9-1	Grading of Tendon Reflexes
4+	Hyperactive, brisk; muscle contractions, clonus; indicative of a lesion in upper motor neuron
3+	Hyperactive; may be normal or indicative of diseases
2+	**Normal**
1+	Diminution or weakening of reflexes; often found in patients with neuropathies
0	No response

Plasma C proteins and S proteins
Dilute Russell viper venom time
Electrolytes
Glucose
Endocrine testing (e.g., thyroid function tests, growth hormone)
Metabolism end-product tests (e.g., liver function tests, kidney function tests)
Drug monitoring (e.g., phenytoin [Dilantin] level)
Toxicology screening panel; ETOH level
Coagulation tests: bleeding time, prothrombin time (PT), partial thromboplastin time (PTT), and thrombin time International Ratio (INR)
Hemostasis tests
Serum fasting homocysteine
Enzyme tests

Human immunodeficiency virus (HIV) test
Venereal Disease Research Laboratories (VDRL) test for syphilis
Apolipoprotein E (APOE)
Urine studies
 Urine analysis
 Toxicology screening panel for suspected substance abuse
Lumbar puncture
 Test of cerebral pressure
 Cerebrospinal fluid analysis
 VDRL test for syphilis
Radiology studies
 Skull/facial x-rays
 Spinal x-rays
 Chest x-ray
Neuroimaging
 Cerebral angiography
 Brain computed tomography (CT)
 Spinal computed tomography
 Brain magnetic resonance imaging (MRI)
 Spine magnetic resonance imaging
 Magnetic resonance angiography (MRA)
 Xenon computed tomography (Xenon CT)
 Single photon emission computed tomography (SPECT)
 Positron emission tomography (PET)
 Cerebral blood flow studies
Studies to determine the source of stroke
 Cardiac studies
  Echocardiogram
  Transesophageal echocardiography (TEE)
  Electrocardiogram (EKG)
  Carotid studies
  Duplex and transcranial doppler
  Venous bolus angiography
  Digital subtraction angiography
Stereotactic technologies
 Stereotactic brain biopsy
Spinal studies
 Myelography
Nervous system electrical activity and conduction studies
 Electromyogram (EMG)
 Nerve conduction velocity studies (NCV)
 Evoked potentials
 Visual evoked potentials
 Brainstem auditory evoked responses
 Electroencephalogram (EEG)
Autonomic studies
 Temperature test
 Sweat testing
 Sympathetic adrenergic function test
 Cardiovagal parasympathetic function test
 Cardiac and blood pressure (BP) monitoring
 Postural BP testing
 Neurobehavioral assessment
 Anesthetic nerve/ganglia blocks

Table 9-6	**Cranial Nerve Function**

Nerve	Findings
I. Olfactory	Smell
II. Optic	Visual acuity, visual fields; examination of fundi
III. Oculomotor	Pupillary reflex, external ocular muscles inducing upward, downward, and medial movements; involvement will cause ptosis, dilation of pupils
IV. Trochlear	Ocular movements; involvement will cause inability to look downward and laterally; nystagmus
V. Trigeminal	Sensory function: corneal reflex, skin of face and forehead, mucosa of nose and mouth; motor function: maxillary "jaw" reflex
VI. Abducens	Ocular movements; involvement will cause inability to look downward and laterally; nystagmus
VII. Facial	Motor function of upper and lower face; involvement will cause asymmetry of face and paresis; sensory function is tested by taste
VIII. Vestibulocochlear	Cochlear nerve test: hearing, lateralization, air and bone conduction; involvement will cause tinnitus, decreased hearing, or deafness
IX. Glossopharyngeal	Motor function: pharyngeal gag reflex, swallowing; vocal cord assessment: speak clearly without hoarseness
X. Vagus	Rise of uvula
XI. Accessory	Strength of trapezius and sternocleidomastoid muscle; involvement will cause inability to elevate shoulder
XII. Hypoglossal	Motor function of tongue; involvement will cause lateral deviation, atrophy, tremor, inability to extend or move tongue from side to side

Polysomnography
 Multiple sleep latency test
 Nocturnal polysomnogram
Ophthalmologic evaluation

■ DIAGNOSTIC PROCEDURES

Numerous procedures, both invasive and noninvasive, performed for neurologic diagnostics; general guidelines for preprocedure preparation and postprocedure observations/interventions are listed

PREPROCEDURE PREPARATION

For all tests or procedures patient and family or significant others should be fully informed of the nature of the procedure, its rationale, and risks involved

Reinforce physician's explanation

Explain procedure and any sensations or discomforts that will be experienced during and after procedure

Reinforce importance of cooperation and immobility of patient for appropriate procedures

Determine patient's allergies to iodine or procaine, or kidney function when indicated

Whenever possible, be present to provide physical and emotional support during procedure

Obtain signed informed consent as indicated

POSTPROCEDURE OBSERVATIONS/INTERVENTIONS

Changes in vital signs

Changes in LOC or orientation

Changes in any neurologic functions: speech, range of motion (ROM), visual acuity, sensory function, pupils (shape, equality, size, reaction to light)

For vascular procedures: observe for hemorrhage, bleeding, and stability in vital signs

Maintain positioning postprocedurally as indicated

Restrict fluids and/or foods as ordered *to prevent aspiration*

Maintain bed rest as ordered

Measure intake and output *to monitor fluid status*

Control pain as indicated

Palpate the arterial pulses, (e.g., dorsalis pedis pulse)

■ COMA AND IMPAIRED CONSCIOUSNESS

altered consciousness (lowered): The state in which alteration in the interaction of the cerebral hemisphere and the reticular activating system (RAS) results in an inability of the individual to relate to self and environment

ASSESSMENT

SUBJECTIVE DATA

Agitation, restlessness

OBJECTIVE DATA

(See also Objective Data under Neurologic Assessment)

LOC: Glasgow Coma Scale (see Table 9-2, p. 515)

Agitation, restlessness, disorientation, coma

(see Continuum of Level of Consciousness under Neurologic assessment, p. 514)

Motor function assessment

Motor function abnormalities
 Flaccidity
 Contractures
 Spasticity
 Abnormal posturing: decortication, decerebration (Fig. 9-5)

Teach the patient to change positions slowly *to prevent untoward postural changes in blood pressure*

Stress importance of implementing and maintaining daily exercise program with planned rest periods; active ROM exercises should be maintained

Diet

Stress the need to continue monitoring intake and output to prevent further cerebral edema and neurologic deficits; family may need to monitor urine osmolarity

Continue high-calorie, high-protein, high-fiber diet at home

Refer patient/family to community agencies that may provide home meals or nutritional counseling, if indicated

General instructions

Assist family members to recognize the signs and symptoms of seizure activity to report to nurse or physician

Ensure that family members are able to initiate seizure precautions as indicated

Encourage family to support independence but remember that patient may require assistance in maintaining medication regimen

■ EPILEPSY AND SEIZURE DISORDERS

Epilepsy is defined as a paroxysmal transient derangement of the nervous system resulting from sudden excessive abnormal electrical discharge of cerebral neu-rons. The manifestations of epilepsy are episodes of partial or complete loss of consciousness, localized or generalized involuntary motor movement, sensory disorders, or autonomic symptoms (Table 9-7)

ASSESSMENT
SUBJECTIVE DATA

Blackout

Loss of memory

Sensory symptoms

Auditory: buzzing or roaring thunder

Visual: flashing lights, visual hallucination, or distorted vision

Vertiginous: sense of falling, floating, or rotating

Olfactory: unpleasant odors

Gustatory: sweet, sour, salty, bitter, or metallic taste in the mouth

Somatosensory symptoms: pins or needles, numbness, burning or sensation of shock

Difficulty breathing

Nausea, vomiting

Psychic symptoms: depression, anxiety, déjà vu

OBJECTIVE DATA

Cerebral sysmptoms

LOC: fully conscious or impaired consciousness

Behavior: atypical behavior, irritation, restlessness

Cognition: disorientation, loss of memory, inability to follow commands

Table 9-7	International Classification of Epileptic Seizures	
Traditional Terminology	**New Nomenclature**	
	I. Partial seizures (seizures beginning locally)	

Focal motor; jacksonian seizures (occasionally become secondarily generalized)	A. Simple (without impairment of consciousness)
	   1. With motor symptoms
	   2. With special sensory or somatosensory symptoms
	   3. With autonomic symptoms
	   4. With psychic symptoms	

Temporal lobe or psychomotor seizures	B. Complex (with impairment of consciousness)
	   1. Simple partial onset followed by impaired consciousness—with or without automatisms
	   2. Impaired consciousness at onset—with or without automatisms
	C. Secondarily generalized (partial onset evolving to generalized tonic-clonic seizures)	

	II. Generalized seizures (bilaterally symmetric and without local onset)	
Petit mal	A. Absences	
Minor motor	B. Myoclonic seizure	
Limited grand mal	C. Clonic seizure	
	D. Tonic seizure	
Grand mal	E. Tonic-clonic seizure	
Drop attacks	F. Atonic seizure	
	G. Infantile spasm	
	III. Unclassified seizures (because of incomplete data)	
	IV. Status epilepticus (prolonged partial or generalized recovery between attacks)	

From McCance KL, Heuther SE: Pathophysiology: the biological basis for disease in adults and children, *ed 3, St Louis, 1998, Mosby.*

Motor symptoms (body parts may involve unilateral or bilateral activity):

Body motor: clinic, myoclonic, tonic, clonic-tonic, abnormal posturing movement, dystonia, motor arrest, back arch

Eye deviation, blinking, twitching, eye rolling, eye fluttering

Facial jerking, lip smacking, chewing, swallowing, yawning, spitting

Nodding and head turning

Autonomic features

Pupils: dilated/pinpoint and symmetry/asymmetry with or without reaction to light

Heart: tachycardia, arrhythmia

Respiration: dyspnea, airway abstraction, tachypnea, apnea

Gastrointestinal: vomiting, nausea, "butterflies" in stomach, belching, or bloating

Skin: cyanotic, flushed, pale, clammy, or ashen

Vocalization

Speech arrest, moaning, gagging, groaning, humming, snoring, whistling, barking, repetitive words, paraphasia (using wrong words)

Psychic symptoms

Depression, anxiety, depersonalization, or déjà vu (sense of familiarity with current situation)

DIAGNOSTIC TESTS

Intracranial structure evaluation *to rule out a stroke or tumor-caused seizure*

MRI

Brain CT scan

EEG

Lumbar puncture: CSF analysis *to rule out CNS infection cause of seizure*

Metabolic evaluation

Serum electrolytes

Serum glucose

Serum calcium and magnesium

ABGs

Value of pH

Liver function test

Kidney function test

Adrenocorticotropic hormone (ACTH)

Cortisol

ETOH

Prolactin *to distinguish a pseudoseizure from seizure*

Toxicology screening panel (blood and urine)

Drug level monitoring (e.g., phenytoin [Dilantin]) *to rule out subtherapeutic level as cause of seizure*

POTENTIAL COMPLICATIONS

Physical trauma: fracture, head injury, tongue and/or lip laceration

Pulmonary damages: respiratory tract obstruction (food or denture), aspiration pneumonia, lung damage by aspirating acid (gastric juice)

Cerebral ischemia

Increased ICP

Neurogenic pulmonary edema

MULTIDISCIPLINARY MANAGEMENT
THERAPEUTIC MANAGEMENT

Emergency management (seizure is a medical emergency)

Airway

Breathing

Circulation

Anticonvulsants

Medical treatment

Antiepileptic agents (see Table 9-8)

Drugs used to treat systemic disease (e.g., systemic acidosis or electrolyte imbalance)

Continuous EEG monitoring

Surgical treatment

Callosotomy

Dissection of the cortex of one hemisphere (used in young children)

Diet: rich in calcium and magnesium, vitamin B_6 and C; ketogenic diet

Social services

PATIENT PROBLEMS—NURSING DIAGNOSES/INTERVENTIONS

▼Risk for injury/trauma related to rapid onset of altered state of consciousness and seizure activity

Preconvulsive care (preictal stage)

Pad side rails

Maintain bed in low position

When patient is on bed rest, raise padded side rails

If patient is not on bed rest, maintain wheelchair in locked position at all times *to prevent injury and falls*

Assist patient to identify auras

Call light within reach at all times *to promote patient's feelings of security*

Convulsive care

If out of bed during seizure activity, ease patient to floor and remove objects of potential harm; loosen constrictive clothing *to prevent injury to self*

Turn head to side *to prevent aspiration*

Note frequency, time, LOC, body parts involved, and length of seizure activity *to identify type of seizure experienced*

Provide privacy to maintain self-esteem

Administer medications as ordered (Table 9-8)

Have suction equipment at bedside *to prevent airway obstruction*

Administer supplemental O_2 as indicated *to prevent cerebral hypoxia*

Postconvulsive care (postictal stage)

Assess and monitor patient carefully after seizure

Table 9-8	**Drugs Used in Seizure Disorders**		
Drug	**Plasma Therapeutic Levels**	**Average Daily Dose**	**Side and Toxic Effects**
Carbamazepine (Tegretol)	4-10 µg/ml	450-700 mg (maximum dose 1200 mg)	Skin rash, blurred vision, ataxia, bone marrow depression, nausea/vomiting, interference with cognitive function
Clonazepam (Klonopin)	40-100 µg/ml	1.5-20 mg	Drowsiness, ataxia, anorexia, behavior changes
Diazepam (Valium)		8-30 mg	Drowsiness, ataxia
Ethosuximide (Zarontin)	40-90 µg/ml	500-1500 mg	Drowsiness, aplastic anemia, headache, lethargy, nausea/vomiting, leukopenia
Felbamate (Felbatol)	Not established	1200-3600 mg	Dizziness, fatigue, headache, weight gain, insomnia
Gabapentin (Neurontin)	Not established	900-2400 mg	Fatigue, dizziness, ataxia, somnolence
Lamotrigine (Lamictal)	Not established	100-500 mg	Dizziness, headache, nausea/vomiting, drowsiness
Mephenytoin (Mesantoin)	10-20 µg/ml	200-600 mg	Nystagmus, ataxia; skin rashes, serious toxicity common, pancytopenia
Methsuximide (Celontin)		300-600 mg	Drowsiness, ataxia, anorexia, aplastic anemia
Paramethadione (Paradione)		300-900 mg	Nephrotoxicity, neutropenia
Phenobarbital (Luminal)	20-40 µg/ml	90-150 mg	Drowsiness, ataxia, nystagmus
Phenytoin, sodium diphenylhydantoin (Dilantin)	10-20 µg/ml	300 mg or 4-7 mg/kg/day	Drowsiness, ataxia, nausea, rash, gingival hyperplasia, nystagmus, anemia, dizziness
Primidone (Mysoline)	7-15 µg/ml	750-1500 mg	Drowsiness, ataxia, psychotic reaction
Trimethadione (Tridione)		900-1200 mg/day	Bone marrow depression, dermatitis, photophobia, irritability
Valproic acid (Depakene, Depakote)	50-120 µg/ml	1000-3000 mg	Nausea; hepatotoxicity

Maintain effective patent airway *to provide for adequate oxygenation and gas exchange*

Assess patient for injury carefully, inspecting oral cavity

Check BP, pulse (P), respirations (R) and do neurologic check immediately after seizure and prn

Assess for the following:
　　Altered LOC
　　Malaise
　　Nausea, vomiting
　　Muscular soreness, backache, or back weakness
　　Aspiration
　　　　Choking, difficulty in breathing, cyanosis
　　　　Decreased or absent breath sounds
　　　　Tachycardia
　　　　Tachypnea
　　　　Suction as indicated *to prevent aspiration*

Provide emotional support *to decrease anxiety and minimize feelings of shame or guilt*

Inform patient of seizure and reorient if necessary

Resume routine activity

Administer oral care as indicated

Assist patient to a position of comfort and turn head to side to maintain patent airway

Expected Outcome
Free of injury

▼Ineffective breathing pattern related to neuromuscular impairment associated with seizure

Preconvulsive care
　　Keep oral airway at bedside
　　Have suction equipment readily available
　　Administer oxygen *to prevent cerebral hypoxia and decrease work of breathing*
Convulsive care
　　Do not force artificial airway into mouth or nose
Postconvulsive care
　　Maintain patent airway
　　Suction oropharynx as indicated to maintain patent airway
　　Administer oxygen as ordered *to minimize cerebral hypoxia*

Expected Outcomes
Demonstrates patent airway

Lungs are clear

Respiration rate and depth are clear

▼Social isolation related to an altered state of wellness associated with lack of friends, groups because of stigmatization associated with seizure (epilepsy) disorders

Assess past experiences with social contacts, degree and amount of discrimination, ostracism of patient by family, friends, classmates, co-workers
Establish trust
Discuss feelings of loneliness; validate normality of feelings *to improve self-esteem and decrease sense of isolation*
Assist patient to identify barriers, actual or perceived, in establishing meaningful relationships
Offer support and encouragement to engage in social activities *to minimize feelings of isolation*
    Assist in identifying diversional activities
    Refer to and encourage participation in support groups

Expected Outcomes
Verbalizes feelings of isolation
Identifies barriers to interaction with others
Seeks participation in social groups
Engages in conversation

Additional Nursing Diagnoses to Consider
Ineffective airway clearance
Self-esteem disturbance related to repeated negative interpersonal experiences

PATIENT/FAMILY TEACHING
Assist patient and family to recognize auras, type of seizure activity involved, and course of action to take
Discuss importance of not restraining or interrupting behavior
Observe and record behaviors exhibited during preictal and convulsive phases
Instruct patient and family about the nature of disorder and need to attempt to adopt positive attitude toward patient's life and treatment
Dispel and clarify common fears and myths about convulsive disorders
    Epilepsy is not a form of insanity
    Epilepsy does not get progressively worse
Emphasize importance of communication between patient and family regarding feelings of shame and humiliation associated with epilepsy
Explain importance of identifying aura and course of action to take
Explain need to identify and avoid stimuli that can stimulate onset of seizure activity
    Flickering lights
    Certain sounds
    Certain types of food
    Full bladder
Discuss medications: name, dosage, frequency of administration, purpose, side effects, and toxic effects

---

| Box 9-2 | **Seizure Prevention Strategies** |

- Regulation of physical and mental activity: get enough sleep, avoid alcohol and recreational drugs, engage in a moderate amount of physical exercise, and participate in relaxation classes
- Avoid excessive visual stimulation, especially flashing light (e.g., video games, three-dimensional movies)
- Awareness of aura to prevent injury following seizure
- Take antiepileptic drug(s) regularly and maintain therapeutic level by checking blood regularly
- Carry a medical card that records history of seizure, type of antiepileptic being taken, and physician's name and phone number

---

Stress importance of taking medication as ordered, not skipping dose
Explain need to avoid taking over-the-counter medications without physician approval
Explain importance of maintaining regular diet, exercise, and activity
Explain importance of well-balanced diet; avoid use of alcohol
Discuss importance of avoiding overexertion
Explain to family the following:
    Need to encourage patient to continue with normal routines such as work, recreation, and other outside interests
    Need to avoid being overprotective; assure patient and family that activity often inhibits seizure occurrence
Discuss need to avoid excessive physical and emotional excitement or stress; need to avoid stimulants
Instruct patient to wear or carry medical alert band or card
Discuss available agencies for use as references
    Epilepsy Foundation of America
    4351 Garden City Drive, Suite 500
    Landover, MD 20785
    (301) 459-3700
    1-800-332-1000
    fax (301) 577-4941
    www.efa.org
Educate patient regarding possible limitations or restrictions of driving privileges
Instruct patient on seizure prevention strategy (Box 9-2)
Discuss the risk of different sports (Table 9-9)
Refer patient and family to a support group

DISCHARGE/HOME CARE PLANNING
Activity
    Seizure precautions are implemented as indicated
        Assist patient to sit or lie down
        Do not attempt to restrain patient or stop the seizure activity
        Protect patient from physical injury
        Provide privacy

Table 9-9	Risks for Different Sports—What's Right for Me?	
Low Risk, Little or No Supervision	Medium Risk, Low to Moderate Supervision	High Risk, Generally Prohibited Unless You've Been Seizure-Free and Off Medicine for 5 Years
Aerobics	Archery	Boxing (prohibited at all times)
Badminton	Basketball (H)	Mountain Climbing
Baseball (H)	Bicycling (H)	Rock Climbing
Bowling	Bobsledding (H)	Sky Diving
Cricket	Canoeing (S)	Scuba Diving
Croquet	Diving (S—low board only)	Hang Gliding
Cross-Country Skiing (no long, steep hills)	Downhill Skiing (H)	Bungee Jumping
Curling	Fishing	Surfing
Dancing	Football (H)	Wind Surfing
Discus	Horseback Riding (H)	
Fencing	Hunting	
Field Hockey (H)	Ice Hockey (H)	
Golf	Ice skating (H)	
High Jump	Orienteering	
Hiking	Parallel Bars (H—low only)	
Jogging	Rollerblading (H)	
Long Jump	Roller skating (H)	
Ping Pong	Rugby (H)	
Running	Sailing (S—no one-person boats)	
Soccer (H)	Sledding (H)	
Softball (H)	Snorkeling (S)	
	Tennis	
	Snowmobiling (H—if okay to drive)	
	Swimming (S)	
	Tumbling	
	Volleyball	
	Wrestling	
	Waterskiing (S)	

From Gumnit RJ: The epilepsy handbook: the practical management of seizures, *ed 2, Raven Press, 1995, New York.*
H, *Must wear a helmet.* S, *swim precautions: Swim with a buddy and make sure there is a lifeguard present and/or use a life preserver.*

Observe and record involved body parts, time and duration of the seizure activity

Report all seizure activity to the physician and home health nurse

Do not place a spoon or other object in the patient's mouth to prevent tongue biting during siezure

Maintain regular exercise program

Maintain normal routine and avoid overprotection and social isolation

Diet

Avoid excessive use of stimulants

Avoid alcohol ingestion

Maintain a well-balanced diet; incorporate dietary restrictions as indicated

Maintain ketogenic diet if prescribed

General instructions

Stress the need for correct body mechanics when transferring patient or assisting during seizure activity

Assist family in making home environment as accessible and risk free as possible

■ CEREBRAL VASCULAR DISEASES (CVD)

Abnormalities of the brain resulting from occlusion of cerebral vessel lumen, rupture of the vessel, and any lesion or permeability of the cerebral vessel wall disrupting the quality of cerebral blood flow. Causes of CVD include various diseases (Box 9-3); CVD may be classified as ischemic or hemorrhagic (Table 9-10).

ASSESSMENT

The signs and symptoms of CVD depend on the size of ischemic area, collateral circulation, territory of blood supplied by specific cerebral vessels

affected, and degree of the cerebral ischemia
(Table 9-11)

SUBJECTIVE DATA
Sudden severe headache
Dizziness
Nausea
Stiff neck

Box 9-3	**Causes of Cerebral Vascular Diseases (CVD)**

- Ischemic stroke (infarction)
- Hemorrhagic stroke
- Ruptured or unruptured saccular aneurysm
- Ruptured or unruptured arteriovenous malformation (AVM)
- Arteritis: menigovascular syphilis, tuberculous meningitis, and connective tissue diseases
- Traumatic or spontaneous dissection of cervicocerebral arteries
- Transient ischemic attacks (TIAs)
- Reversible ischemic neurologic deficits (RIND)
- Amyloid angiopathy
- Neurologic migraine with persistent neurologic deficits
- Children and young adults: moyamoya, multiple progressive intracranial arterial occlusions, and complications of oral contraceptives and high-dose estrogen therapy

OBJECTIVE DATA
Hemorrhagic (Symptoms Generally Abrupt in Onset)
Intracranial hemorrhage (ICH)
Deteriorating consciousness, progressing to coma
Dilated pupil on the ipsilateral of the hemorrhage
Hemiparalysis on the contralateral side of the hemorrhage
Increased ICP
Syndromes of brainstem compression—changes of vital signs and respiratory pattern, if brain herniation develops and/or hemorrhage in inferior tentorial area

Subarachnoid hemorrhage
Signs of meningeal irritation—Brudzinski's sign and Kernig's sign
Nuchal rigidity
Deteriorating consciousness, progressing to coma
Abrupt severe headache
Hemiparesis
Hemiplegia
Ipsilateral dilated pupil

Ruptured arteriovenous malformation (AVM) and aneurysms
Deteriorating consciousness, progressing to coma
Progressive neurologic deficits—motor/sensory deficits (depends on the specific area of cerebral tissue deprived of adequate blood supply)
Seizure
Neuropsychiatric manifestations

Table 9-10	**Classification of Stroke**

Ischemic Strokes (Infarction)	Hemorrhagic Strokes

I. Cerebral vessel occlusion
  A. Large vessel occlusion
    1. Atherosclerosis
    2. Dissection of carotid and basilar arteries
    3. Embolism
      • Cardiac sources
      • Proximal artery sources
      • Paradoxical embolism
  B. Small penetrating vessel occlusion
    1. Lacunar stroke
    2. Cardiogenic embolism
    3. Hypertension
  C. Reduced cerebral perfusion
    1. Watershed cerebral infarction
    2. High-grade carotid stenosis
    3. Hypotension caused by pump failure
    4. Dissection of cervicocerebral arteries
	I. Intracerebral hemorrhage
	  A. Primary intracerebral hemorrhage
	    1. Hypertension
	  B. Secondary intracerebral hemorrhage
	    1. Bleeding disorders
	    2. Ruptured aneurysms
	    3. Ruptured vascular malformations
	    4. Trauma
	    5. Intracranial tumors
	    6. Drugs
	    7. Vasculitis and other angiopathies
	  C. Subarachnoid hemorrhage
	    1. Berry aneurysms

Signs of meningeal irritation, nuchal rigidity, if the subarachnoid is irritated by blood

Ischemic
Ischemic stroke
Deteriorating consciousness, stupor, confusion, agitation, or progressing to coma
Malaise
Hemiparalysis
Sensory loss of one or more limbs
Aphasia
Dysarthria

Dysphagia
Vertigo
Nausea/vomiting
Acoustic phenomena (e.g., tinnitus, hearing loss)
Visual disturbances—blurred vision, double vision, visual loss of one or both eyes, photophobia, phonophobia
Difficulty keeping balance, ataxia, and difficulty walking
Facial paralysis (ipsilateral or contralateral to limb weakness)
Episodic attacks of epilepsy: focal seizure and general seizure

Table 9-11	Signs and Symptoms Related to Specific Affected Cerebral Vessels
Specific Affected Cerebral Vessels	**Signs and Symptoms**
Anterior cerebral artery (ACA)	Hemiparesis affects legs and feet more often than upper extremities. Sensory deficits, particularly in the lower extremities. Transient loss of consciousness. Language difficulty. Amnesia. Abulia or akinetic mutism
Middle cerebral artery (MCA) Main truck Upper division Lower division	Hemiplegia, hemianesthesia, and hemianopia. Hemiparesis, sensory loss, Broca's aphasia and hemineglect. Wernicke's aphasia, global aphasia, and hemianopia
Posterior cerebral artery	Isolated hemianopia, alexia, color anomia. Cerebral blindness, anesthesia dolorosa with spontaneous thalamic pain. Hemiballism and tremors. Amnesia. Oculomotor palsy
Internal carotid artery (ICA)	Ipsilateral blindness. Hemianopia. Aphasia. Contralateral hemiparesis and hemianesthesia. Hemineglect
Vertebrobasilar artery	Medial syndromes: Ipsilateral hemiparalysis of tongue, Paralysis gaze, Ophthalmoplegia. Lateral syndromes: Dysphagia, Hoarseness, Ipsilateral vocal cord paralysis, Ipsilateral loss of pharyngeal reflex, Vertigo, Nystagmus, Ipsilateral facial analgesia, Taste loss, Deafness, tinnitus, Ipsilateral jaw weakness, Ipsilateral facial numbness, Ataxia, Difficulty with coordination, gait

Transient ischemic attack (TIA) versus reversible ischemic neurologic deficits (RIND)

Episodic attacks of syncope

Symptoms are same as ischemic stroke, but in a TIA the symptoms resolve within 24 hours and in a RIND the symptoms will resolve within 1 week

Dissection of cervicocerebral arteries

Tinnitus

Vertigo

Cervical bruit

Hemiparalysis

Lingual paresis

Horner's syndrome—sinking in of the eyeball, ptosis of the upper eyelid, constriction of the pupil, and anhidrosis

DIAGNOSTIC TESTS

Imaging

   Brain CT scan without contrast (initial assessment)

   MRI

   Intracranial and extracranial arteries MRA

   Conventional cerebral angiography

Cerebral blood flow technique

   Xenon CT scan

   Regional cerebral blood flow

Blood tests

   Antiphospholipid antibody test

   Plasma C proteins and S proteins

   Coagulation and hemostasis tests

   Blood glucose

   Blood urea nitrogen (BUN) creatinine

   CBC, platelet count

   ESR

   Serum fasting homocysteine

   VDRL test

   Dilute Russell viper venom time

   Anticardiolipin antibodies

   Lipid panel test

Cardiac studies

   Chest x-ray

   Echocardiogram

   Transesophageal echocardiography (TEE)

   ECG

Carotid studies

   Duplex and transcranial Doppler

   Carotid duplex

EEG (if seizures are suspected)

Lumbar puncture (if subarachnoid hemorrhage suspected and CT scan negative)

X-ray

   Chest x-ray

   Lateral cervical spine x-ray (if the patient is comatose or has cervical spine pain)

POTENTIAL COMPLICATIONS

Acute care stage

   Vasospasm

   Hemorrhagic transformation

   ICP

   Cerebral edema: both cytotoxic and vasogenic edema

   Brain herniation

   Neurogenic pulmonary edema following elevated ICP

   Seizures

   Hydrocephalus

   Stroke-associated cardiac dysfunction

   Pulmonary embolism

   Aspiration following oropharyngeal dysfunction

   Aspiration pneumonia

   Nosocomial infections

   Hypoventilation

   Myocardial ischemia

   Cardiac arrhythmia

   DVT

   Constipation

   Pressure ulcer

Post CVD stage

   Dementia

   Pulmonary infection: Aspiration pneumonia caused by dysphagia

   Amnesia

   Incontinence

   Thalamic pain following CVD in thalamus

   Movement disorders following CVD in subthalamus and thalamus

   Bowel movement dysfunction: constipation or diarrhea

   Depression

   Headache

   Impaired mobility

   Muscle contracture and joint stiffness

   Urinary tract infection and urine retention

   Malnutrition

MULTIDISCIPLINARY MANAGEMENT
THERAPEUTIC MANAGEMENT
General Management

Ventilator and oxygen support

Cardiovascular hemodynamic monitoring

ICP monitoring (see p. 583)

Laboratory studies: coagulants, serum electrolytes, blood glucose, and ABGs

Fluid management: avoid hypotonic IV fluid

BP regulation: avoid hypotension (NOTE: American Heart Association recommends withdrawal of antihypertensive drugs until systolic BP > 220 mm Hg or mean arterial pressure > 130 mm Hg)

Medicines

   Anticonvulsants

   Antipyretics

   Steroids

   Diuretics: osmotic diuretic

   Sedatives

   Analgesics

   Antacids

   Laxatives

   Insulin if blood glucose elevates

Respiratory therapy
Physical therapy
Occupational therapy
Dietitian consult as indicated
Social services
Spiritual support as indicated
Treatment of vasospasm
    Ventilator and oxygen support
    Hypertension/hypervolemia/hemodilution (HHH):
        "triple H therapy"

Calcium channel antagonists: nimodipine
Sedatives
Neurologic function, ICP, hemodynamic
    monitoring

Specific Management
Hemorrhagic
Intracranial hemorrhage (ICH)
Surgical consultation when cerebellar hematoma,
    brainstem compression, hydrocephalus occurs

Subarachnoid hemorrhage (SAH)
Surgical repair if SAH caused by ruptured aneurysm or
    AVM
Subarachnoid precautions (Box 9-4)

Ruptured/unruptured arteriovenous malformation (AVM) and aneurysms
Surgery: clipping, ligation
Embolization: Guglielmi detachable coil (GDC)
    embolization
Stereotactic radiosurgery

Ischemic
Ischemic stroke
Anticoagulants: aspirin 325 mg qd, heparin, ticlopidine,
    warfarin, clopidogrel
Thrombolysis: t-PA (Boxes 9-5 and 9-6)
Neuroprotective therapy

TIAs versus RIND
Endarterectomy
Anticoagulants: aspirin 325 mg qd

Dissection of cervicocerebral arteries
Anticoagulants: aspirin 325 mg qd, heparin, ticlopidine,
    warfarin, clopidogrel
Thrombolysis t-PA
Surgery (reserved for patients with accessable and
    localized dissection who experience further cerebral
    ischemia)

Box 9-4 | **Subarachnoid Precautions**

Provide private room with dim artificial lighting
Ensure complete bed rest
Maintain quiet environment
Reduce environmental stimuli
Limit visitors
Provide all nursing care
Administer stool softeners

Box 9-5 | **Key Points for Pre-Hospital Care of Stroke Patients**

- What was once called *stroke* is now called *brain attack*. This term was chosen to convey not only the severity of the problem, but also the urgency.
- Saving time means saving brain cells. People should be instructed to activate EMS by calling 911 if a stroke is suspected.
- The therapeutic window for ischemic stroke is short. Treatment must be provided within 30 minutes to 6 hours after onset of stroke.
- t-PA, considered the best medicine for ischemic stroke, must be delivered within the first 3 hours after onset of stroke, so patients must arrive at the emergency room within 2 hours of onset.

Box 9-6 | **Precautions for Administering t-PA**

- T-PA 0.9 mg/kg total or maximum 90 mg
- Administer 10% of t-PA dose as a bolus and 90% of t-PA as a continuous infusion over 1 hour
- **STOP** any anticoagulants for 24 hours from start of t-PA administration
- **STOP** any antiplatelet agents for 24 hours from start of t-PA administration
- **AVOID** central venous line replacement and arterial puncture for 24 hours
- **AVOID** insertion of nasogastric tube for 24 hours after t-PA administration
- **AVOID** insertion of bladder catheter tube for 30 minutes after t-PA administration
- **AVOID** hypotension; maintain systolic BP under 180 mm Hg and diastolic BP 105 mm Hg
- When newly developed hypertension is observed, consider intracranial hemorrhage, stop t-PA infusion and obtain a brain CT scan stat
- Admit to intensive care unit
- Monitor BP for 24 hours after administering t-PA: every 15 minutes for 2 hours; every 30 minutes for 6 hours; hourly for next 16 hours
- Monitor any newly developed neurologic deficits

PATIENT PROBLEMS—NURSING DIAGNOSES/INTERVENTIONS

▼ Altered cerebral tissue perfusion: related to vasospasm secondary to hemorrhagic injury

Assess neurologic status q 15 min to 30 min or as indicated

Monitor for increased ICP *to prevent changes in cerebral circulation*

Monitor for changes or signs of cerebral ischemia

Maintain bed rest with head of bed elevated 15 to 40 degrees *to facilitate cerebral venous drainage*

Check BP, P, and R q15min to 30min

Report any sudden changes in BP (>20 mm Hg with widened pulse pressure), pupillary, or neurologic status immediately

Assess and monitor respirations and ventilation; provide oxygen as indicated *to decrease work of breathing*

Monitor ABGs as ordered to assess acid-base balance

Check rectal temperature q2h to 4h; hypothermia or cooling measures may be indicated

Initiate subarachnoid precautions (see Box 9-4) if needed

Initiate treatment for vasospasm as ordered *to prevent further cerebral ischemia and injury*

Auscultate lung sounds q4h to 8h *to detect adventitious breath sounds*

Monitor pulmonary capillary wedge pressure (PCWP), pulmonary artery pressure (PAP), systemic venous resistence (SVR), central venous pressure (CVP), and BP to achieve and maintain within prescribed parameters

Expected Outcomes

Demonstrates effective cerebral perfusion; is oriented to time, person, place

No alteration in consciousness

Vital signs are within normal limits

▼ Altered cerebral tissue perfusion related to increased intracranial pressure caused by brain edema secondary to cerebral ischemia

Assess neurologic status q15min to 30min or as indicated

Initiate monitoring of ICP as ordered; report increase >15 mm Hg lasting 15 to 30 minutes or >20 mm Hg lasting 5 minutes

Monitor for signs and symptoms of increasing ICP (p. 583; maintain patency and sterility of ICP monitoring devices, if used

Avoid positions that increase intraabdominal or intrathoracic pressure (e.g., prone position, extreme hip flexion)

Maintain head and neck in midline position

Administer medications as ordered

If steroids are administered: check stools, urine, and gastric contents for occult blood

Expected Outcomes

Demonstrates effective cerebral perfusion; is oriented to time, person, place

No alteration in consciousness

ICP ≤15 mm Hg

No clinical signs of increased ICP

▼ Pain (headache, nuchal rigidity) related to irritation of meninges secondary to subarachnoid hemorrhage

Assess type, location, and severity of pain

Monitor for signs of increasing pain or discomfort; report any changes in character of pain

Administer medications as ordered: analgesics *to minimize discomfort*

Maintain quiet environment; remove or modify any stimuli that may heighten pain or discomfort; dim lights

Explain all procedures and treatments *to minimize anxiety and facilitate understanding*

Organize care *to maximize periods of quiet and rest to allow for sufficient REM sleep*

Move or reposition patient gently; avoid excessive movement

Implement relaxation techniques

Pace activities and plan ahead

Encourage open communication about feelings of discomfort

Expected Outcomes

Reports pain relief

Achieves comfort level

Appears comfortable; sleeps and rests quietly

▼ Ineffective airway clearance related to impaired cough and inability to handle secretions

Assess and monitor respirations, cough reflex, and secretions

Position body and head *to prevent obstruction of airway and provide optimal secretion removal*

Suction secretions prn: hyperoxygenate in 100% O_2 for 60 seconds before and after suctioning *to minimize hypoxemia;* limit suctioning to <15 seconds at a time

Insert oropharyngeal or nasopharyngeal airway *to maintain airway patency*

Auscultate chest for breath sounds q2h to 4h *to detect adventitious breath sounds*

See Care of patient with coma and impaired consciousness (p. 520)

Administer oxygen/humidification as ordered *to decrease work of breathing and minimize potential for drying of mucous membranes*

Provide mechanical ventilation as ordered *to prevent/minimize respiratory distress*

Monitor serial ABGs, pulse oximetry, hemoglobin (Hgb) as indicated *to assess oxygenation status*

Expected Outcomes

Demonstrates patent airway

Chest expansion is symmetric

Breath sounds are clear to auscultation

ABGs and vital signs are within normal limits

No signs of respiratory distress

▼Impaired physical mobility related to impaired neurophysiologic function

Assess functional ability and extent of impairment; record and monitor changes and improvements

Maintain body alignment; use bedboard, air mattress, or footboard as indicated (Fig. 9-7) *to lessen muscle fatigue*

Turn and reposition q2h *to facilitate comfort*

Elevate affected limbs on pillows *to prevent swelling*

Use pull sheet when indicated *to minimize tissue trauma*

When patient is on side, support with pillows; may use hand rolls and arm splints *to maintain patient in functional position* (see Fig. 9-7)

Perform active and/or passive ROM exercise to all extremities q2h to 4h and prn (Figs. 9-8 and 9-9) *to help relieve muscle soreness, weakness, and deep vein embolism*

Assist and encourage patient to perform quadriceps setting and gluteal exercises q4h

Encourage hand, finger, and foot exercises

Have patient squeeze rubber/sponge ball

Perform flexion

Perform extension of fingers, legs, and feet

Assist patient with using supportive devices as indicated: overhead trapeze, braces, wheelchair, canes, walker

Apply antiembolic stockings *to prevent venous stasis*

Encourage use of involved side when possible

Instruct patient to use healthy extremity to support weaker side (e.g., lift involved left leg with good right

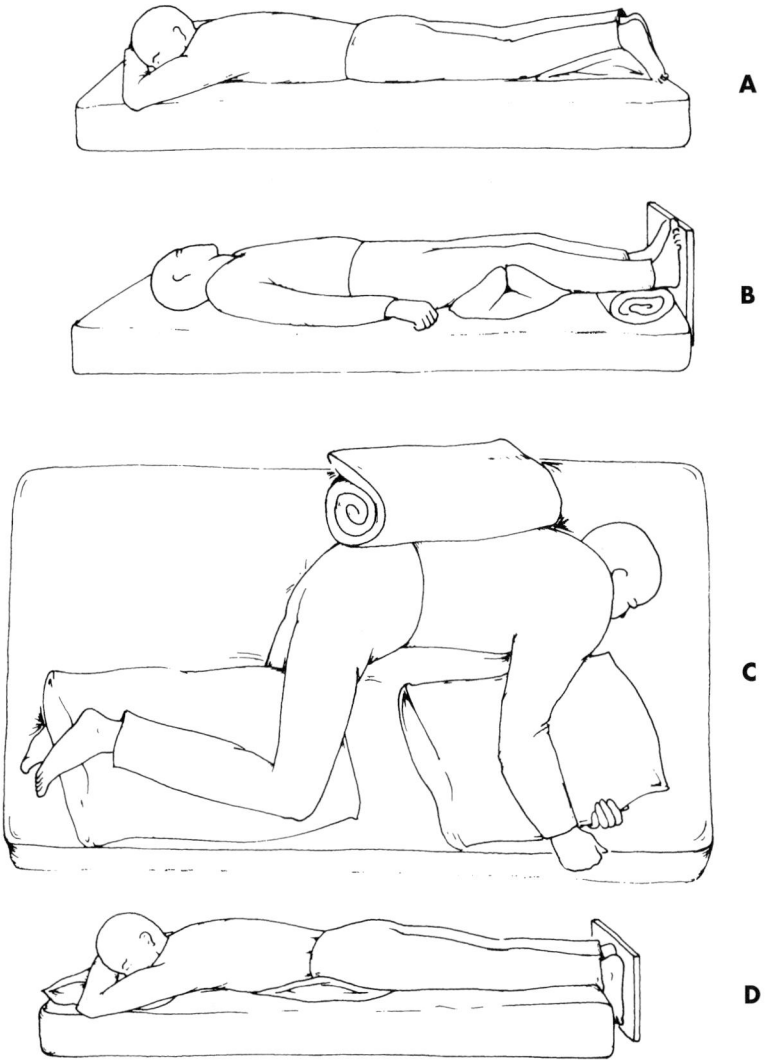

Fig. 9-7   Various body positions to maintain correct alignment. **A,** Prone position. **B,** Supine position. **C,** Side-lying position. **D,** Prone position with support of feet.

leg or lift involved left arm with good right arm) to increase mobility

Encourage patient to perform basic ADLs as soon as possible using unaffected side *to increase self-sufficiency*
    Bathing
    Brushing teeth
    Combing hair
    Eating

Begin progressive ambulation as ordered; assist to balanced sitting position; begin with transfer procedure from bed to chair to regain position sense

Consult with physical and occupational therapy departments regarding activity program to establish effective team approach

Expected Outcomes

Demonstrates optimal physical mobility and function within physiologic limitations

Exhibits behaviors and skills necessary for resumption of activities

▼ Unilateral neglect related to right/left cerebral hemisphere lesions secondary to neurologic illness and trauma

Assess degree of neurologic deficit and patient's perception and awareness of deficit

Orient patient to environment on regular basis *to reestablish reality orientation*

Provide realistic feedback

Provide a safe environment *to minimize potential for injury*
    Remove unnecessary furniture and equipment
    Place call bell, bedside stand, and personal items on unaffected side within reach
    Keep side rail up on affected side; lock rails up if patient is impulsive
    Observe and anticipate needs
    Structure environment to decrease environmental hazards

Approach and speak to patient from unaffected side

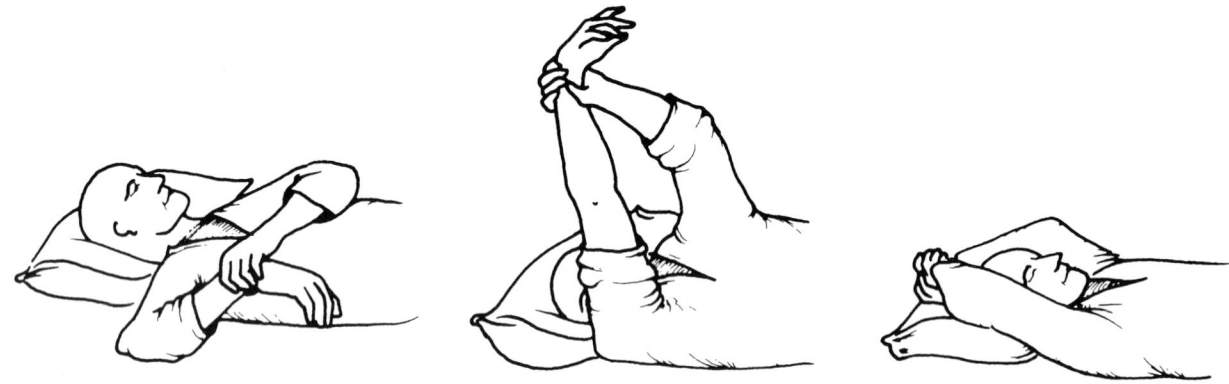

Fig. 9-8   Range of motion of affected shoulder and elbow.

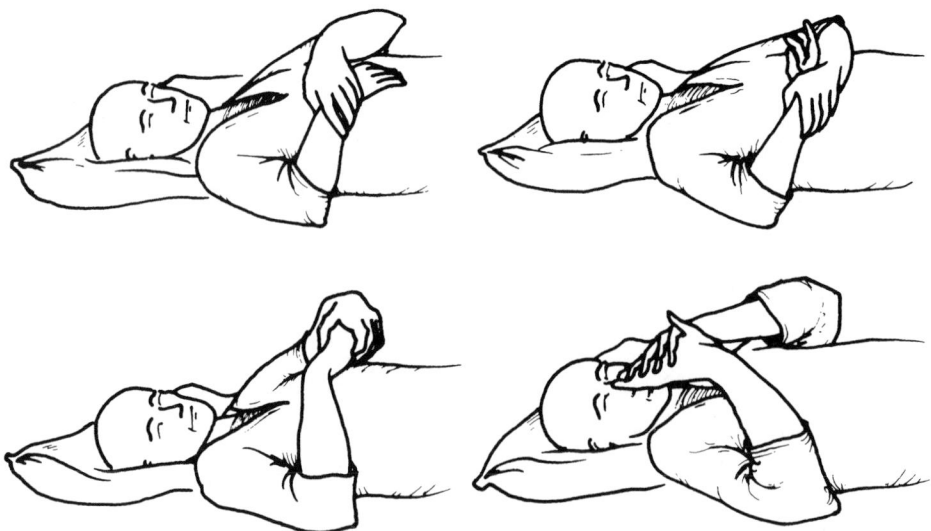

Fig. 9-9   Range of motion of affected wrist and hand.

Assist patient to recognize and deal with perceptual deficit

Initially: arrange environment within perceptual field

After initial stress: promote increased attention to neglected side

Encourage patient to look at affected side *to assist in recovery*

Stay with patient, touching or stroking affected side; encourage patient to handle affected limbs

Instruct and remind patient to include affected limbs when performing simple tasks *to decrease weakness on affected side*

Use tactile stimulation to reintroduce patient to affected limbs; use scented lotions or differently textured materials *to stimulate different sensations*

Consult with rehabilitation team to design a rehabilitation program

Encourage patient to participate in ADLs; begin by teaching individual components of an activity; later, integrate components into total activity

Encourage activities that will force patient to look at or involve affected side (e.g., place food closer to affected limb)

Expected Outcomes
Free of injury
Demonstrates a realistic perception of deficit

▼Self-care deficit: hygiene, feeding, and/or toileting related to impaired physical mobility and alteration in cognitive process

Assess degree of disability in performing self-care activities (bathing, feeding, toileting) *to determine realistic amount of required assistance*

Administer skin care q4h to 5h *to increase circulation*

Use oil-based lotions

Inspect area over bony prominences daily for any breakdown *to prevent pressure ulcer formation*

Provide for total physical hygiene as indicated

Comb hair daily; shampoo every week as indicated

Keep nails clipped and clean to prevent self-injury

Administer oral hygiene q4h to 8h; brush teeth; clean mucous membranes with water and/or alkaline mouthwash *to prevent drying of mucous membranes*

Assess and monitor nutritional status

Administer tube feedings as ordered; check tube placement to prevent aspiration

Initiate oral feedings as indicated to maintain caloric intake

Begin with clear liquids *to prevent nausea*

Assist with feedings as necessary

Observe for difficulty in swallowing *to prevent aspiration*

Position on side with head of bed elevated *to prevent aspiration* if feeding patient in bed

Encourage fluid intake to 2000 ml/day unless contraindicated to aid in elimination

Ensure regular elimination

Connect indwelling catheter to closed gravity drainage system as ordered; provide catheter care q8h and prn *to prevent infection and possible urosepsis*

Use external catheters as ordered

Offer bedpan/urinal q2h to 4h if catheter is not used

Monitor daily bowel movement; if none, check for impaction q2d to 3d

Give stool softeners or enema as ordered *to prevent impaction*

Expected Outcome
Needs for hygiene, nutrition, elimination, and toileting are met

---

▼Risk for aspiration caused by dysphagia

Perform swallow evaluation and assess LOC before each meal (see "Swallowing evaluation," Box 9-7).

Assess function of cranial nerves V, VII, IX, and X, which are involved in swallowing (Table 9-12)

Watch for the warning signs of dysphagia—decreased alertness, dysarthria, difficulty controlling oral secretions, difficulty controlling the head, difficulty controlling the jaw, reduced gag/cough reflexes, wet gurgle voice, decreased tongue and mouth movement

For patients without feeding tubes (Box 9-7)
Avoid feeding and report if patient is weak or lethargic or suffers extreme fatigue or reduced LOC

Select food that can easily form a bolus, *to prevent aspiration* (Tables 9-13 and 9-14)

Provide safe feeding techniques

Never pour liquids into patient's mouth

For patients with feeding tubes
Check gastric residual before feeding; if gastric residual is more than 150 ml or twice the hourly infusion rate, withhold one feeding and recheck residual

---

Box 9-7	**Tips for Patients Without Feeding Tubes**

SWALLOWING EVALUATION
The movement of swallowing can be felt by placing a finger on the thyroid notch between the hyoid bone and the larynx and feeling the larynx move up and forward during swallowing.

SAFE FEEDING TECHNIQUES
While feeding, the patient must be alert, able to concentrate on eating, and sitting upright, with his or her head slightly down and in the midline. The caregiver faces the patient and sits lower than patient to watch for signs of choking.

Table 9-12	**Process for Assessing Function of Cranial Nerves (CN) Related to Swallowing**
Cranial Nerve	**Assessment**
V, Trigeminal	Inspect face for muscle atrophy and tremors Palpate jaw muscles for tone and strength with patient's teeth clenched
VII, Facial	Inspect symmetry of facial features with various expressions (smile, frown, puffed cheeks, wrinkled forehead, etc.)
IX, Glossopharyngeal	Test gag reflex Test ability to identify sour and bitter tastes
X, Vagus	Inspect palate and uvula for symmetry with speech sounds and gag reflex

Table 9-13	**Food Selection for Patients With Dysphagia**
Component	**Suggestions**
Carbohydrate	Thinned oatmeal, cream of wheat, cream of rice, moist mashed white or sweet potatoes with thick gravy, farina, soft noodles with sauce, moist bread dressing with gravy
Protein	Soft scrambled eggs with gravy or melted cheese, thick puréed meat with gravy, plain yogurt, thickened milk, ice cream, pudding, sherbet, flavored gelatin, milkshakes
Fiber	Thick puréed vegetables, thick puréed fruits, thickened juice

Table 9-14	**Foods to Avoid for Patients With Dysphagia**
Problem Foods	**Rationale**
Thin liquids: water, juice, soft drinks	Thin liquids are difficult to control in the mouth and easily aspirated
Particulate foods: hamburger, corn, nuts, seeds	These foods require more chewing or do not easily form a bolus. They need too much oral preparation and easily fall over into the base of the tongue and into the respiratory system
Sticky foods: white bread, peanut butter	
Stringy foods: fresh fruits and vegetables	
Dry foods: dry muffins, dried fruits, toast, crackers	

Box 9-8	**Communication Deficit**

Expressive aphasia (Broca's aphasia): inability to express oneself verbally

Receptive aphasia (Wernicke's aphasia): inability to understand the spoken word

Global aphasia: combination of expressive and receptive aphasia

Measure abdominal girth at least q8h to prevent vomiting caused by abdominal distension

Elevate the head of the bed 30 to 45 degrees during feeding

Expected Outcome

Airway clearance is maintained

Adequate nutrition and fluid supply

▼Impaired verbal communication related to cerebral ischemia or hemorrhage

Assess type of communication deficit (Box 9-8)

Assess patient's ability to speak, comprehend, read, or write

Stand within patient's line of vision; when speaking, allow patient to observe lips and hands

Speak in normal voice; do not shout or speak loudly; maintain calm environment

Speak slowly using simple sentences and common vocabulary; use vocabulary that patient understands

Ask questions that can be answered with a *yes* or *no* response *to minimize patient's frustration level*

Allow time for patient to respond to questions

Be supportive and accepting of behavior *to assist in improving self-esteem if patient shows signs of frustration*

Provide flash cards with pictures or words of common objects to which patient can point

Consult with speech therapist to identify an appropriate means of communication

Perform swallow evaluation before each meal to prevent aspiration

Expected Outcome
Able to communicate basic needs

Additional Nursing Diagnoses to Consider
Risk for impaired skin integrity
Self-esteem disturbance: body image
Powerlessness
Anxiety related to perceived and actual biologic threat
Ineffective breathing pattern related to neurologic impairment
Unilateral neglect secondary to cerebrovascular accident

PATIENT/FAMILY TEACHING
Assess level of understanding of disability
Explain to family the following:
  Need to encourage as many independent activities as possible; be alert to limitations
  Need to set realistic, achievable goals
  Need to avoid being overprotective
  Need to praise any tasks accomplished
  Importance of dealing with body image changes and behavioral changes
  Need to allow patient to be expressive
Encourage diversional activities
  Reading to patient
  Watching television
  Listening to radio, book recordings
Plan regular rest periods *to prevent fatigue*
Encourage verbalization and communication between patient and family to promote acceptance and understanding
Be sympathetic to emotional upsets but firm in following regimen
Stress importance of ongoing outpatient care and follow-up visits
Stress importance of continuation of rehabilitation program
Instruct patient and significant other in proper dietary and fluid needs
Stress importance of safety measures: side rails, ramps, low-heeled shoes, removal of scatter rugs *to prevent injury*
Provide explanation of primary clinical disorder, causes, and treatment as indicated
Encourage questions; correct any misconceptions
Discuss medications: name, dosage, frequency of administration, purpose, side effects, and toxic effects
Explain need to avoid taking over-the-counter medications without consulting physician
Explain need to increase activities as ordered; physical activity as tolerated
Discuss symptoms of progression of condition to report to physician
If patient is taking multiple medications, suggest the purchase of a small, portable, multidose medications container
Stress the importance of wearing a medical alert tag at all times

Alert the patient to change positions slowly *to prevent postural changes in blood pressure*
Provide patient/family with discharge instructions, time and date of next outpatient appointment
Encourage patient and family to join the support groups:
  The National Institute of Neurological Disorders and Stroke
  (301) 496-5751
  American Heart Association, Stroke Connection
  1-800-553-6321
  Web site: www.americanheart.org

DISCHARGE/HOME CARE PLANNING
Activity
  Stress the importance and proper use of mobility devices (wheelchair, cane, walker) to patient/family
    Assist family to identify local community agencies that can help in providing such devices
    Assist family to learn ways of adapting the home for accessibility
    Stress the need for initial home health referral to do the following:
      Teach family members proper body mechanics and how to protect their backs
      Assist in learning safety measures *to prevent falling*
  Maintain regular exercise program including active and passive ROM exercises to all joints
  Continue planned rest periods *to prevent fatigue and agitation*
Diet
  Offer small portions frequently and supplemental feedings if indicated
  Avoid foods such as soft breads, mashed potatoes, semicooked vegetables, and large pieces of meat that may cause choking
General instructions
  Assist family, as indicated, to develop competency in the following:
    Home ventilation
    Suctioning
    Tracheostomy care
    Parenteral or enteral home nutrition therapy
    Positioning techniques
  Assist family to recognize and report signs and symptoms of stroke including the following:
    Headaches
    Nausea and vomiting
    Restlessness and lethargy
    Changes in LOC
    Feelings of impending doom
    Pupillary changes
    Changes in vital signs
      Increased systolic BP
      Decreased pulse
Implement speech exercises on a regular basis

■ BRAIN TUMORS

A brain tumor is a neoplasm in the intracranial portion of the CNS. Primary brain tumors originate in the brain, whereas secondary (metastatic) brain tumors are transferred from a distant origin (Table 9-15)

ASSESSMENT

The signs and symptoms of brain neoplasms in a patient depend on the size, type, and location and the compression and infiltration of specific cerebral tissue

SUBJECTIVE DATA

Persistent severe headache
Drowsiness
Blurred vision
Emotional ups and downs
Forgetfulness
Lack of coordination
Nausea
Dizziness
Difficulty speaking

OBJECTIVE DATA

Changes in behavior and mental function
General seizure activity or focal seizure
Signs and symptoms of increased ICP (projectile vomiting, drowsiness, and pressure headache)
Papilledema
Obstruction of cerebrospinal fluid flow

Specific Symptoms Associated With Tumor Locations

Frontal lobe: inappropriate behavior, inattentiveness, inability to concentrate, emotional lability, inappropriate social behavior, impaired recent memory, headache, expressive aphasia, abulia, hemiplegia, hemiparesis, focal seizure, conjugate eye deviation
Temporal lobe: psychomotor seizure, symptoms of increased ICP, receptive aphasia
Occipital lobe: contralateral homonymous hemianopia, visual hallucinations, focal seizure
Parietal lobe: hyperesthesia, paresthesia, agraphia, loss of right-left discrimination, loss of two-point discrimination
Cerebellum: vomiting, nausea, nystagmus, vertigo, poor coordination, loss of equilibrium
Pituitary adenomas: visual disorder (complete or partial bitemporal hemianopia), abnormalities of endocrines (Cushing's disease, vegetative disturbance, or diabetes insipidus), amenorrhea-galactorrhea syndrome, acromegaly (acral growth and prognathism combining with visceromegaly, headache, hypermetabolism, or diabetes mellitus)
Anterior part of the base of the skull: unilateral/bilateral anosmia, psychiatric disturbances, and seizure

Cerebellopontine angle (C-P angle): Loss of 8th cranial nerve function (hearing loss, nystagmus, or vertigo), difficulty keeping balance, dyssynergia, loss of 5th and 7th cranial nerve function (abnormalities of sensation in face or asymmetry of the face), symptoms of raised ICP, and brainstem symptoms
Cavernous sinus: ophthalmoplegia, exophthalmos, and vegetative disturbances
Superior orbital fissure: exophthalmos; vegetative disturbance; dysfunction of 3rd, 4th, and 6th cranial nerves (abnormalities in gaze or ptosis); and pain and sensory disturbance in the V_1 area of the face

DIAGNOSTIC TESTS

MRI
Brain CT scan
Cerebral angiography
EEG
Visual field and funduscopic examination
Audiometric studies
Chest x-ray (detects lung cancer metastasis)
Endocrine studies
Stereotactic brain biopsy or brain cyst aspiration
Examination of CSF

POTENTIAL COMPLICATIONS

Brain herniation
Cerebral edema
Cerebral necrosis
Hydrocephalus
Increased ICP

COLLABORATIVE MANAGEMENT
THERAPEUTIC MANAGEMENT

Chemotherapy
Conventional radiotherapy
Conventional surgery: craniotomy
Stereotactic radiosurgery (see p. 581)
Combined craniotomy and stereotactic radiosurgery
Combined craniotomy and chemotherapy/or conventional radiotherapy
Combined stereotactic radiosurgery and conventional radiotherapy
Supportive therapy
    Decrease ICP: steroid therapy and osmotic diuretics
    Prevent seizure: anticonvulsants
    Inhibit nausea and vomiting: antiemetics
    Prevent gastric (pressure) ulcer: antiacid and H_2 blocker
    Narcotic analgesics
    Antidepressants
    Antianxiety
    Nutrition
    Rehabilitation
    Family counselling
    Spiritual support

Table 9-15	**Brain and Spinal Cord Tumors**		
Neoplasm	**Location**	**Characteristics**	**Cell of Origin**
GLIOMAS			
Astrocytoma	Anywhere in brain or spinal cord	Slow-growing, invasive	Astrocytes
Glioblastoma multiforme	Predominantly in cerebral hemispheres	Highly invasive and malignant	Thought to arise from mature astrocytes
Oligodendro-cytoma	Most commonly in frontal lobes deep in white matter; may arise in brainstem, cerebellum, and spinal cord	Relatively avascular, tends to be encapsulated; more malignant form an oligo-dendroblastoma	Oligodendrites
Ependymoma	Intramedullary: wall of the ventricles; may arise in caudal tail of the spinal cord	More common in children, variable growth rates; more malignant, invasive form is called *ependymoblastoma;* may extend into the ventricle or invade brain tissue	Ependymal cells
NEURONAL CELL			
Medulloblastoma	Posterior cerebellar vermis, root of fourth ventricle	Well-demarcated, rapid-growing, fills fourth ventricle	Embryonic cells
MESODERMAL TISSUE			
Meningioma	Intradural, extramedullary: sylvian fissure region, superior parasagittal surface of frontal and parietal lobes, olfactory groove, wing of sphe-noid bone, superior surface of cerebellum, cerebellopontine angle, spinal cord	Slow-growing, circumscribed, encapsulated, sharply demarcated from normal tissues, compressive in nature	Arachnoid cells, may be from fibroblast
CHOROID PLEXUS			
Papillomas	Choroid plexus of the ventricular system, lateral ventricle in children, fourth ventricle in adults	Usually benign, slow expansion inducing hemor-rhage and hydrocephalus; malignant tumor is rare	Epithelial cells
CRANIAL NERVES AND SPINAL NERVE ROOTS			
Neurilemmoma	Cranial nerves (most com-monly vestibular division of cranial nerve VIII)	Slow-growing	Schwann cells
Neurofibroma	Extramedullary—spinal cord	Slow-growing	Neurilemma, Schwann cells
PITUITARY TUMORS	Pituitary gland; may extend to or invade floor of the third ventricle	Age-linked, several types slow-growing, macro-adenomas and micro-adenomas	Pituitary cells, pituitary chromophobes, basophils, eosinophils

From McCance KL, Huether SE: Pathophysiology: the biologic basis for disease in adults and children, *ed 3, St Louis, 1998, Mosby.*

Continued

Table 9-15	**Brain Tumor Classification According to Cell of Origin—cont'd**		
Neoplasm	**Location**	**Characteristics**	**Cell of Origin**
PINEAL REGION	Pineal region; pineal parenchyma	Several types (germinoma, pineocytomas, teratoma	Several types with different cell origins
BLOOD VESSEL TUMORS			
Angioma	Predominantly in posterior cerebral hemispheres	Slow-growing	Arising from congenitally malformed arteriovenous connections
Hemangioblastomas	Predominant in cerebellum	Slow-growing	Embryonic vascular tissue

PATIENT PROBLEMS—NURSING DIAGNOSES/INTERVENTIONS

▼Altered cerebral tissue perfusion related to increased intracranial pressure secondary to tumor

Obtain and record baseline history of signs and symptoms, monitor for signs of progression

Assess LOC q2h and prn

Use Glasgow Coma Scale for rapid assessment (see Table 9-2, p. 515)

Monitor BP, P, R, and size, shape, and light reaction of pupils, and do neurologic check q1h or as indicated

Monitor for and intervene at signs of increasing ICP q1h (p.583)

Calculate CPP q1h or as indicated

Maintain seizure precautions

Maintain safe environment
    Use side rails with padding
    Use soft restraints

Maintain quiet environment

Check rectal temperature q2h to 4h; hypothermia or cooling measures may be indicated

Monitor ABGs q2h or as indicated

Administer medications as ordered

Monitor for signs of mental and personality changes

Expected Outcomes

Demonstrates improved or normal cerebral tissue perfusion

Neurologic signs and LOC are within acceptable limits

No signs of ICP

▼Self-care deficit: hygiene, feeding, toileting, and/or mobility related to perceptual, cognitive, and/or neurologic impairment

Assess for degree of disability in performing ADLs: bathing, feeding, toileting, and mobility

Monitor for signs of progressive disability

Assist with daily physical hygiene care as indicated
    Administer oral hygiene prn *to prevent infection*
    Administer skin care *to minimize potential for pressure ulcer formation*

Assess neurologic function *to detect newly developed neurologic deficits*

Familiarize patient with surroundings *to decrease anxiety if eyesight and/or visual fields are impaired*

Ensure elimination
    Use external or indwelling catheter as indicated
    Initiate voiding measures prn
    Have patient avoid constipation and straining through use of stool softeners or mild laxatives

Maintain diet as ordered *to maintain nutritional status*

Feed and assist with nutritional intake as needed

Ambulate as tolerated; assist as necessary with wheelchair, walker, or cane

If patient is unable to ambulate, assist and teach patient to turn, cough, and deep breathe q2h and prn

Elevate head of bed 30 to 45 degrees

Perform active and passive ROM exercises to all extremities q4h to 5h *to prevent fixed joints*

Expected Outcome

Self-care needs are met

▼Anxiety related to actual or perceived biologic or psychologic threat

Assess for signs and symptoms of fear and anxiety, noting verbal and nonverbal expressions

Explore feelings, encouraging patient to discuss fears and concerns regarding diagnosis and prescribed therapies

Provide emotional support

Offer simple explanations to questions

Assist patient to deal with anxiety, providing alternative methods for dealing with stress: guided imagery, relaxation techniques, music therapy

Encourage patient to join The Brain Tumor Society Support Group (818) 362-3428

Expected Outcomes

Anxiety level is reduced

Appears calm and is able to verbalize feelings and concerns

Additional Nursing Diagnoses to Consider

Pain (headache)

Impaired verbal communication

Risk for injury secondary to seizure activity

PATIENT/FAMILY TEACHING

Assess level of understanding regarding disease process and prescribed treatments

Reinforce physician's explanation of the disease and its causes, symptoms, and treatment

Encourage questions; assess for any misconceptions

Discuss medications: name, dosage, frequency of administration, purpose, side effects, and toxic effects

Explain need to avoid taking over-the-counter medications without consulting physician

Teach importance of well-balanced diet

Explain need for ongoing rehabilitation therapy as ordered

Stress importance of follow-up clinical visits

Provide patient/family with information on the brain tumor resources

The Brain Tumor Society (617) 783-0340

National Brain Tumor Foundation (800) 934-2873

American Brain Tumor Association (800) 886-2282

DISCHARGE/HOME CARE PLANNING

Activity

Stress the importance and proper use of mobility devices (wheelchair, cane, walker) to patient/family

Assist family to identify local community agencies that can help in providing such devices

Assist family to learn ways of modifying the home for accessibility

Stress the need for initial home health referral to do the following:

Teach family members proper body mechanics and how to protect their backs

Assist in learning safety measures to prevent falling

Alert the patient to change positions slowly to prevent postural changes in BP

Maintain a regular exercise program with planned rest periods

Implement safety measures such as side rails and ramps as indicated

Diet

Maintain well-balanced diet

Offer small portions; instruct patient to chew slowly

Offer supplemental feedings

Monitor intake and output

General instructions

Encourage independent activities to tolerance

Encourage socialization with friends and family members

Develop competence of family members, as indicated, in the following:

Home ventilation

Suctioning

Tracheostomy care

Chest physiotherapy

Coughing and deep-breathing exercises

Home parenteral or enteral nutrition therapy

Bowel/bladder management

Refer to home health agencies as indicated

Table 9-16	Classification of Traumatic Brain Injury Based on Glasgow Coma Scale	
Classification of Brain Injury		Glasgow Coma Scale
Mild brain injury		13-15
Moderate brain injury		9-12
Severe brain injury		3-8

Develop knowledge base regarding signs and symptoms of seizure activity

Implement seizure precautions as indicated

Report potential signs and symptoms of increasing ICP including the following:

Restlessness, lethargy

Changes in LOC

Nausea and vomiting (may be projectile)

Pupillary changes

Changes in vital signs

Seizures

Changes in breathing patterns

Stress importance of informing the neurosurgeon of change on LOC or new neurologic deficits found, because the brain tumor may recur

■ CRANIOCEREBRAL TRAUMA

Any sudden impact or blow to the head with or without LOC; the following are types of head injuries (Table 9-16):

linear fracture: *A break in the continuity of bone without displacing bone tissue*

comminuted fracture: *Multiple breaks leading to fragmentation of bone*

depressed fracture: *Bone fragments displaced below the surface of the skull*

compound fracture: *A fracture complicated by laceration of surrounding scalp or membranes*

concussion: *Shock to brain soft tissue without bruising or lacerations; accompanied by temporary memory loss and amnesia lasting approximately 48 hours*

contusion: *Shock to brain soft tissue with bruising and laceration; accompanied by loss of consciousness and amnesia; patient may exhibit varying degrees of consciousness: stupor, agitation, disorientation, coma*

coup-contrecoup phenomenon: *Brain injury resulting from acceleration type of injury causing contusion and laceration in areas remote or opposite from the site of impact (Fig. 9-10)*

subdural hematoma: *An accumulation of blood between the arachnoid and dura mater resulting from contusion or laceration of subdural blood vessels; symptoms (headaches, increasing drowsiness, seizures, unilateral pupil dilation) may not occur for weeks or months (Table 9-17)*

intracranial hematoma: *Shearing of the bridging veins or of a cortical artery results in bleeding within the cerebral parenchyma. Intracranial hemorrhage is commonly located in frontal lobes, temporal lobes, and*

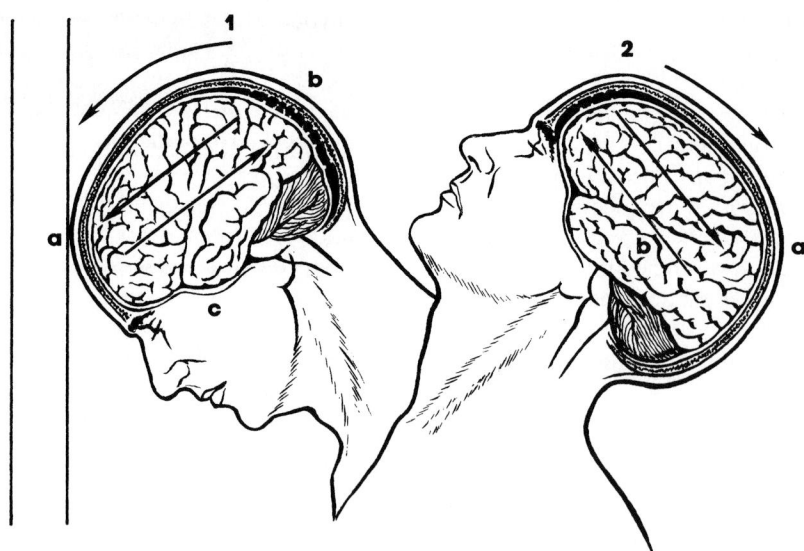

Fig. 9-10 Coup and contrecoup head injury following blunt trauma. *1,* Coup injury: impact against object. *a,* Site of impact and direct trauma to brain. *b,* Shearing of subdural veins. *c,* Trauma to base of brain. *2,* Contrecoup injury: impact within skull. *a,* Site of impact from brain hitting opposite side of skull. *b,* Shearing forces through brain. These injuries occur in one continuous motion—the head strikes the wall (coup), then rebounds (contrecoup).
(From Rudy EB: Advanced neurological and neurosurgical nursing, *St Louis, 1984, Mosby.)*

Table 9-17	Classification of Subdural Hematomas
Type	**Time Interval of Hematoma Developed**
Acute SDH	Within 48 hours
Subacute SDH	2 days to 2 weeks
Chronic SDH	2 weeks to months

SDH, *Subdural hematoma.*

deep hemispheres. Intracranial hematomas are space-occupying lesions and are surrounded by edema, so all hematomas are potentially life threatening

   subarachnoid hemorrhage: *Subarachnoid hemorrhage is often seen in severe head injury cases. Intraventricular hemorrhage occurs secondary to subarachnoid hemorrhage*

   epidural hematoma: *Bleeding in the epidural space between the skull and dura mater; usually involves a temporoparietal fracture, which results in a lacerated middle meningeal artery; transient loss of consciousness occurs and is followed by lucid periods; patient then lapses into unconsciousness again with signs of rapidly developing increased ICP; this is usually a surgical emergency*

ASSESSMENT
   SUBJECTIVE DATA
Headache
Dizziness, vertigo
Drowsiness
Vomiting/nausea

OBJECTIVE DATA
Altered LOC; periods of consciousness followed by
   unconsciousness
Posturing
   Decorticate rigidity (see Fig. 9-5)
   Decerebrate rigidity
   Motor and/or sensory movement of extremities:
      unilateral, bilateral
   Muscle weakness, paresis, paralysis, stimulus, response
Mental changes
   Irritability
   Restlessness
   Confusion
   Delirium
   Stupor
   Coma
Pupillary response
   Size, equality, response to light
Corneal reflex
Brainstem integrity: extraocular movement (EOM), gag or
   swallow reflex
Airway patency
   Rate and rhythm of respirations
   Breathing pattern
   Secretion management
Unequal pupils and uncoordinated eye movement
Periocular edema, ecchymosis
Seizure activity
Hematemesis
Projectile vomiting
Lacerations and abrasions around head and face
Drainage from ears and nose
Elevated temperature

Elevated or decreased BP
Increased weakness
Facial asymmetry
Aphasia
Nuchal rigidity
Dehydration
Polyuria
Bruit over carotid artery

DIAGNOSTIC TESTS

Radiology
    Skull x-ray
    Cervical spinal x-ray (rules out cervical fracture)
    Chest x-ray
Neuroimaging
    Brain CT (gold standard for head injury)
    Brain MRI
Blood tests
    CBC, platelet count
    ESR
    ABGs
    Coagulation tests: Bleeding time, PT, PTT, thrombin
       time
    Electrolytes
    Glucose
    Drug level monitoring (if indicated by patient's history
       [e.g., phenytoin level, digoxin level])
    Toxicology screening panel; ETOH level
Urine
    Toxicology screening panel
Transcranial Doppler, cerebral blood flow studies

POTENTIAL COMPLICATIONS

Respiratory system: aspiration pneumonia, hypostatic
    pneumonia, atelectasis, ARDS, neurogenic pulmonary
    edema, pulmonary embolism, respiratory
    dysfunction
Cardiovascular system: deep vein embolism, cardiac
    dysfunction (tachycardia/bradycardia or
    hypertension/hypotension secondary to
    increased ICP)
Genitourinary system: urinary tract infection, retention of
    urine
Gastrointestinal system: malnutrition, dehydration,
    constipation, bleeding stress ulcer
Musculoskeletal system: articular contracture, muscle
    atrophy, posttraumatic tremor, drop foot
Skin: skin infection, pressure ulcer (for comatose patients)
Hematopoietic system: disseminated intravascular
    coagulopathy (DIC)
Endocrine system: diabetes insipidus, syndrome of
    inappropriate secretion of antidiuretic hormone
    (SIADH)
Immune system: infection secondary to use of steroids
    and nosocomial infections
Central nervous system: impaired consciousness, cerebral
    edema (both cytotoxic and vasogenic edema), cerebral

hypertension, hydrocephalus, posttraumatic headache,
seizure, brain herniation, neurologic deficits, cerebral
ischemia following increased ICP and hyperthermia/
hypothermia

MULTIDISCIPLINARY MANAGEMENT
THERAPEUTIC MANAGEMENT

Oxygenation/mechanical ventilation
Surgical repair
    Craniotomy
    Ventriculostomy
    Burr holes
    Cranioplasty
    Shunting procedures
    Tracheostomy
Medications
    Anticonvulsants
    Histamine antagonists
    Antibiotics
    Antacids
    Diuretics
    Steroids
    Analgesics/antipyretics
    Artificial tears
    Barbiturates
    Muscle relaxants and paralyzers
    Stool softeners
    Antianxiety agents
    Sedatives
    Antihistamines
Jugular bulb catheterization *to monitor venous oxygen*
    saturation
ICP monitoring
CSF drainage
Cardiac/hemodynamic monitoring
Continuous EEG monitoring
Fluid and electrolyte management monitoring
Nutritional support
Rehabilitation
    Occupational therapy
    Physical therapy
    Speech therapy
    Spiritual support
Temperature control
Barbiturate coma therapy

PATIENT PROBLEMS—NURSING DIAGNOSES/INTERVENTIONS

▼Altered cerebral tissue perfusion related to increased intracranial pressure secondary to acute head injury

Assess neurologic status q15min to 30min as indicated;
    establish baseline parameters
Monitor and record signs of improvement or
    deterioration: change in LOC; seizure activity
Assess for signs of increased ICP (p. 583)

Check BP, P, and R q15min to 30min, decreasing
frequency as condition stabilizes

Initiate ICP monitoring as ordered; report increase of >15
mm Hg lasting 15 to 30 min or >20 mm Hg lasting 5
min

Elevate head of bed 30 degrees; maintain head in midline
position *to promote venous drainage*

Maintain quiet environment

Avoid or minimize activities known to precipitate Valsalva
maneuvers (e.g., prolonged suctioning)

Administer medications as ordered

Maintain normothermia

Monitor serial ABGs and pulse oximetry

Maintain strict intake and output *to monitor hydration
status;* monitor specific gravity and color of urinary
output

See also ICP monitoring (p. 589)

Expected Outcomes

Oriented to time, place, situation

Demonstrates no signs of increased ICP

No alteration in LOC

ICP of ≤15 mm Hg

No clinical signs of increased ICP

▼Ineffective airway clearance related to impaired
sensorimotor function

Avoid flexion of neck until cervical x-rays rule out neck
injury

Assess and monitor respiratory function and secretions
q30min to 60min

Maintain patent airway: endotracheal tube or
tracheostomy as ordered; suction prn (hyperoxygenate
with 100% O_2 for 60 seconds before and after
suctioning; suction <15 seconds)

Monitor oxygen saturations *to ensure adequate
oxygenation*

Position head *to prevent obstruction of airway and
provide optimal secretion removal;* maintain neck in
neutral position

Administer oxygen, humidification, or mechanical
ventilation as ordered *to decrease work of
breathing*

Auscultate lungs q2h to 4h *to detect adventitious breath
sounds*

Obtain and monitor serial ABGs; maintain $Paco_2$ as
ordered *to prevent hypoxia and hypercapnia*

Assist in coughing and deep breathing when patient is
conscious *to prevent atelectasis*

Maintain emergency airway equipment at bedside

Elevate head of bed 30 degrees if patient is unconscious,
unless contraindicated, *to maximize airway patency
and control secretions*

Check BP, P, R, and Glasgow Coma Scale (p. 515) q15min
to 30min; report any pupillary or mental changes
immediately: changes may signal respiratory
embarrassment

Maintain NPO status to prevent aspiration

Expected Outcomes

Demonstrates effective breathing pattern

Clear breath sounds

ABGs and vital signs within normal limits

No sign of respiratory distress

▼Sensory/perceptual alteration: cognitive, visual,
auditory, kinesthetic related to neurologic trauma

Assess LOC, orientation, mood/affect, and thought
process; monitor and record changes

Assess for any sensory deficits: responses to pain,
touch; changes in vision including blurred
vision, changes in visual field, depth and
perception

Assess and monitor motor coordination, ability to locate
body parts

Orient to reality: environment, situation, individuals
interacting with patient *to decrease uncertainty*

Interpret sights, sounds, smells in environment *to prevent
sensory overload*

Speak in calm voice with normal tone

Maintain eye contact

Provide meaningful stimuli: clocks, calendars

Place patient near window *to differentiate day and
night*

Structure daily activities and routines

Place common and familiar object within field of vision
to assist in reality orientation

Maintain safety precautions

    Bed in low position, side rail up *to prevent injury and
falls*

    Assist with ambulation

    Remove potentially dangerous objects

Encourage decision making, exploration of environment
to enhance competence and feelings of self-worth

Expected Outcome

Demonstrates improved LOC, appropriate perceptual
functioning

▼Self-esteem/body image disturbance related to
perceived changes in physical and personal self-
image

Assess perception of body image and relate to degree of
disability

Provide emotional support; allow patient to verbalize
needs and participate in planning care

Encourage verbalization of feelings about body image and
functional changes

Acknowledge and praise attempts to improve body image
(e.g., wearing make-up, selecting clothing)

Assist patient to accept physical disability; assist patient
to identify other physical characteristics that remain
unchanged

Offer supportive counseling

Encourage participation in counseling and/or self-help
group

Expected Outcomes

Verbalizes positive expression of body image

Demonstrates signs of decreasing body image disturbance

Additional Nursing Diagnoses to Consider

Impaired physical mobility related to neurophysiologic function (see Cerebrovascular diseases, p. 529)

Risks of infection

Risk for unilateral neglect related to right cerebral hemisphere lesions secondary to neurologic trauma (see Cerebrovascular diseases, p. 529)

Altered body temperature related to hypothalamus compression or injury

Aspirations risk related to decreased LOC, depressed gag/cough reflexes, impaired swallowing, surgery, and tracheotomy/endotracheal tube or feeding tube

PATIENT/FAMILY TEACHING

Discuss nature of disorder, treatment, and procedures; explain as they occur

Explain to family need to encourage verbalization about any body image change or limitations

Explain need to ambulate as tolerated

Teach about importance of planned rest periods

Discuss possible residual effects such as dizziness, headache, and memory loss, which may persist for 3 to 4 months after trauma

Discuss medications: name, dosage, frequency of administration, purpose, side effects, and toxic effects

Explain need to avoid over-the-counter medications without physician approval

Discuss symptoms of progression of condition to report to physician

Explain importance of ongoing outpatient care
  Physician's visits
  Physical therapy

Explain importance of diet as ordered; need to chew and swallow slowly

Discuss care of abrasions or lacerations as indicated

Discuss injury prevention (e.g., safety helmets, seatbelts)

Stress importance of informing the physician if change of LOC, severe headache, or new neurologic deficits are found

DISCHARGE/HOME CARE PLANNING

Activity
  Stress the importance and proper use of mobility devices (wheelchair, cane, walker) to patient/family
    Assist family to identify local community agencies that can help in providing such devices
    Assist family to learn ways of adapting the home for accessibility
    Stress the need for initial home health referral to the following:
      Teach family members proper body mechanics and how to protect their backs
      Assist in learning safety measures to prevent falling

Alert the patient to change positions slowly to prevent postural changes in BP

Implement safety measures such as side rails and ramps as indicated

Maintain as much independence in ADLs as possible

Maintain a regular exercise program with planned rest periods

Refer to home physical therapy as indicated

Maintain socialization activities with friends and family

Diet
  Maintain well-balanced diet
  Maintain fluid intake of 2000 ml/day unless contraindicated
  Maintain intake and output
  Avoid use of alcohol

General instructions
  Check stools for occult blood if patient takes corticosteroids
  Report any seizure activity; maintain seizure precautions as appropriate
  Report signs and symptoms of increasing ICP (see list in Discharge/home care planning for intracranial tumors, p. 583)

■ SPINAL CORD INJURIES (SCI)

cord injuries: Injuries to the spinal cord include contusion, ischemia, or compression caused by fractured or displaced vertebrae, bleeding, edema, or tumors (Fig. 9-11; Table 9-18)

cervical cord injuries: Level of injury is located in the cervical spine C-2 to C-6

thoracic cord injuries: Level of injury is located in the thoracic spine T-1 to T-12

lumbar cord injuries: Level of injury is located in the lumbar spine L-1 to L-2

quadraplegia: Preferred term is tetraplegia; refers to impairment or loss of motor and/or sensory function in the cervical segments, but does not refer to peripheral nerve injuries. There is complete or partial loss of function in the arms, trunk, legs, and pelvic organs

paraplegia: Refers to impairment or loss of motor and/or sensory function in thoracic, lumbar, or sacral segments of the cord but does not refer to peripheral nerve injuries outside the spinal cord. Arm functioning is intact, depending on level of injury, but the trunk, leg, and pelvic organs may be involved. It also refers to cauda equina injuries

complete spinal cord injury: Absence of motor and sensory function, which includes the lowest sacral segment

spinal shock: A state of areflexia that occurs following SCI. There is interruption of sympathetic nervous system (SNS) activity, which is different from autonomic hyperreflexia (SNS hyperactivity manifested by HTN). The signs/symptoms are flaccid paralysis, lack of autonomic function and tendon reflexes, loss of sensation, loss of

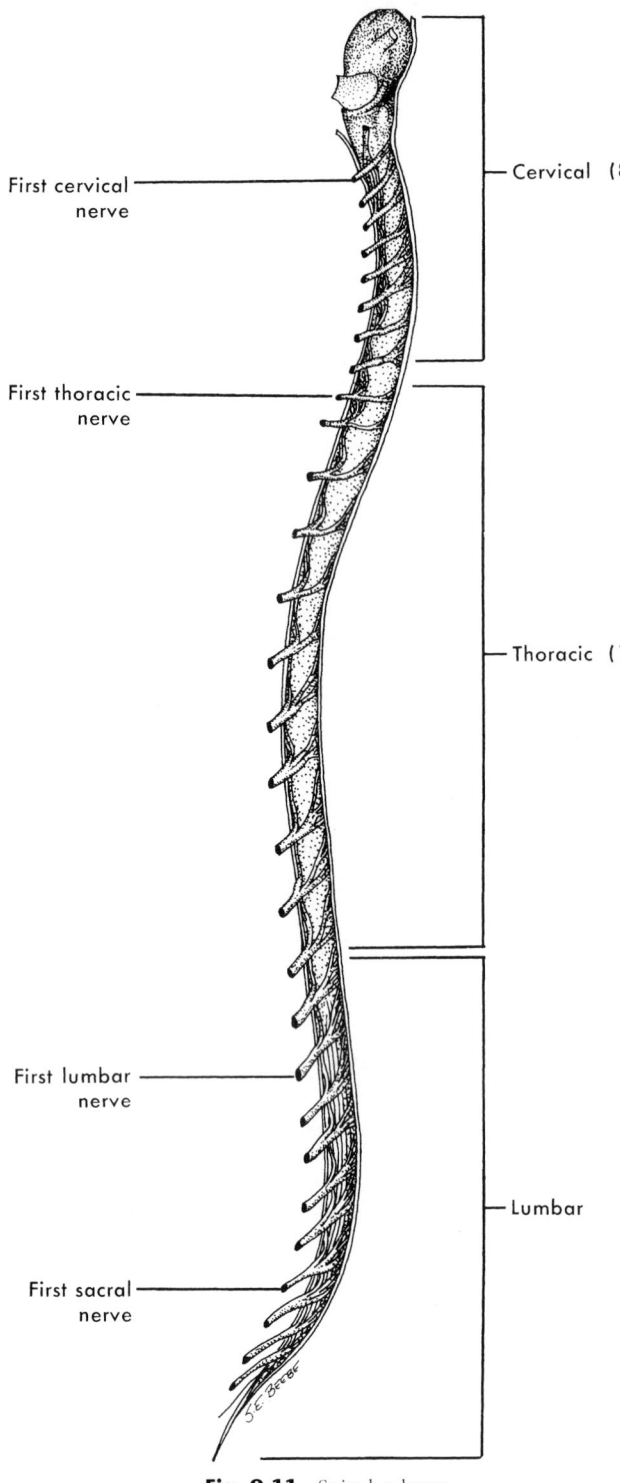

First cervical
nerve

Cervical (8)

First thoracic
nerve

First lumbar
nerve

Thoracic (12)

Lumbar

First sacral
nerve

Fig. 9-11   Spinal column.

thermoregulation, loss of bladder and bowel function, possible hypotension, and bradycardia. Spinal shock may last for minutes, hours, days and emerge up to 1 week after the injury

incomplete spinal cord injury: *Partial preservation of motor or sensory function is found below the level of injury. It presents in a variety of patterns but can be*

grouped into certain syndromes that describe the predominant area of the cord that is involved (see Table 9-20). It includes central cord syndrome, anterior cord syndrome, Brown-Séquard syndrome, cauda equina syndrome, and posterior cord syndrome

NOTE: *Clinical descriptions of spinal cord injuries generally refer to deficits in terms of upper motor neuron (UMN) and lower motor neuron (LMN): UMN injuries involve the corticobulbar or corticospinal tract and result in muscle spasticity and increased tendon reflexes; LMN injuries involve anterior horn cells or nerve fibers which exit the spinal cord to innervate the skeletal muscles, and result in muscle flaccidity, loss of reflexes, loss of tone, and muscle atrophy (Figs. 9-12 and 9-13 and Table 9-19)*

ASSESSMENT
SUBJECTIVE AND OBJECTIVE DATA
NOTE: Assessment findings depend on: spinal level of injury, degree of involvement (complete or partial) (see Fig. 9-12 and Table 9-18)

DIAGNOSTIC TESTS
Blood
  Serial ABGs
  CBC with differential
  Electrolytes
  Glucose
Urine
  Culture and sensitivity
  Routine urinalysis
Imaging
  X-rays of spine
  CT scan
  MRI
  Myelography
Electromyography (EMG)
Pulmonary function tests

POTENTIAL COMPLICATIONS
Respiratory arrest: hypoxia
Pneumonia
Atelectasis
Aspiration
Pulmonary embolus
Spinal shock
  Complete transection
    Flaccid paralysis below level of injury
    Loss of reflexes below level of injury
    Loss of proprioception, sensations of touch, temperature, and pressure below level of injury
    Orthostatic hypotension
  Paralytic ileus
  Loss of somatic and visceral sensations
  Loss of ability to perspire below level of injury
  Decreased BP
  Urinary retention
  Bowel dysfunction
  Possible priapism

Table 9-18	**Functional Level of Spinal Cord Disruption and Rehabilitation Potential**	
Autonomic	**Movement Remaining**	**Rehabilitation Potential**
QUADRIPLEGIA		
C1-C3		
Usually fatal injury, vagus nerve domination of heart, respiration, blood vessels, all organs below injury	Movement in neck and above, loss of innervation to diaphragm, absence of independent respiratory function	Ability to drive electric wheelchair equipped with portable respirator by using chin control or mouth stick, headpiece to stabilize head, lack of bowel and bladder control
C4		
Vagus nerve domination of heart, respirations, and all vessels and organs below injury	Sensation and movement above neck	Ability to drive electric wheelchair by using chin control or mouth stick, lack of bowel and bladder control
C5		
Vagus nerve domination of heart, respirations, and all vessels and organs below injury	Full neck, partial shoulder, back, biceps; gross elbow, inability to roll over or use hands; decreased respiratory reserve	Ability to drive electric wheelchair with mobile hand supports, ability to use powered hand splints (in some patients), lack of bowel and bladder control, feed self with setup and adaptive equipment
C6		
Vagus nerve domination of heart, respirations, and all vessels and organs below injury	Shoulder and upper back abduction and rotation at shoulder, full biceps to elbow flexion, wrist extension, weak grasp of thumb, decreased respiratory reserve	Ability to assist with transfer and perform some self-care, feed self with hand devices, push wheelchair on smooth, flat surface; lack of bowel and bladder control
C7-C8		
Vagus nerve domination of heart, respirations, and all vessels and organs below injury	All triceps to elbow extension, finger extensors and flexors, good grasp with some decreased strength, decreased respiratory reserve	Ability to transfer self to wheelchair, roll over and sit up in bed, push self on most surfaces, perform most self-care; independent use of wheelchair; ability to drive car with powered hand controls (in some patients); lack of bowel and bladder control
PARAPLEGIA		
T1-T6		
Sympathetic innervation to heart, vagus nerve domination of all vessels and organs below injury	Full innervation of upper extremities, back, essential intrinsic muscles of hand; full strength and dexterity of grasp; decreased trunk stability, decreased respiratory reserve	Full independence in self-care and in wheelchair, ability to drive car with hand controls (in most patients), ability to use full body brace for exercise but not for functional ambulation, lack of bowel and bladder control
T6-T12		
Vagus nerve domination only of leg vessels, GI and genitourinary organs	Full, stable thoracic muscles and upper back; functional intercostals, resulting in increased respiratory reserve	Full independent use of wheelchair; ability to stand erect with full body brace, ambulate on crutches with swing (though gait difficult); inability to climb stairs; lack of bowel and bladder control
L1-L2		
Vagus nerve domination of leg vessels	Varying control of legs and pelvis, instability of lower back	Good sitting balance, full use of wheelchair
L3-L4		
Partial vagus nerve domination of leg vessels, GI and genitourinary organs	Quadriceps and hip flexors, absence of hamstring function, flail ankles	Completely independent ambulation with short leg braces and canes, inability to stand for long periods, bladder and bowel continence

From Lewis SM, Collier IC: Medical surgical nursing: assessment and management of clinical problems, ed 4, St Louis, 1996,
Mosby.
GI, *Gastrointestinal.*

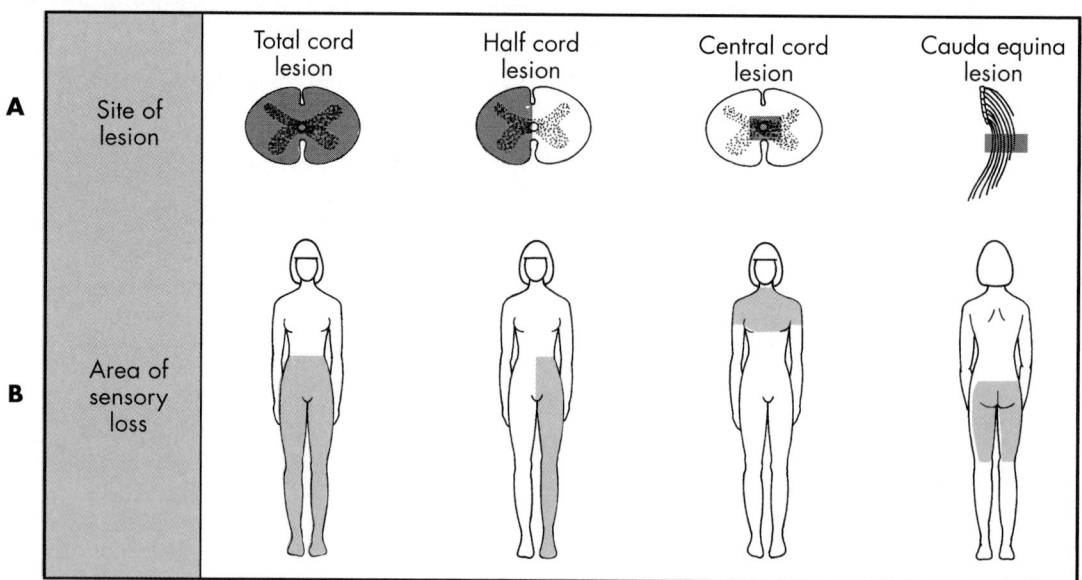

Fig. 9-12 Common patterns of sensory abnormality. **A,** Site of lesion. **B,** Distribution of corresponding sensory loss. *(From Thelan LA et al:* Critical care nursing: diagnosis and management, *ed 2, St Louis, 1994, Mosby.)*

Table 9-19	**Clinical Manifestations of Upper and Lower Motor Neuron Lesions**
Upper Motor Neuron	**Lower Motor Neuron**
Muscle spasticity, possible contractures	Muscle flaccidity
Little or no muscle atrophy	Muscle atrophy
Hyperreflexia	Loss of muscle tone
	Hyporeflexia or areflexia
	Fasciculations
Damage above level of brainstem will affect opposite side of the body	Muscle changes will be in muscles supplied by that nerve— usually muscle on same side as lesion

From Rudy EB: Advanced neurological and neurosurgical nursing, *St Louis, 1984, Mosby.*

Bladder dysfunction
Fecal incontinence
Urinary tract infection
Autonomic dysreflexia
Sexual dysfunction
Malnutrition: acute or chronic
Pressure ulcer
Contractures, ankylosis
Spasms
Foot drop, wrist drop
Behavioral changes
   Anxiety
   Grief reaction
   Acute depression
Heterotopic ossification
Severe bradyarrhythmia
DVT
Osteoporosis
Superior mesenteric artery syndrome

MULTIDISCIPLINARY MANAGEMENT
THERAPEUTIC MANAGEMENT
Surgical
   Decompression: laminectomy
   Stabilization: spinal fusion, Harrington rods
   Skull tongs (Crutchfield, Vinke, Cone, Gardner-Wells)
   Halo traction
   Tracheostomy
   Myotomies, tenotomies, neurectomies, rhizotomies, and
      muscle transplants
Ventilatory support; V_T measurements
Respiratory therapy
Physical therapy
Occupational therapy
Speech therapy as indicated
Spiritual support
Medication
   Muscle relaxants
   Tranquilizers

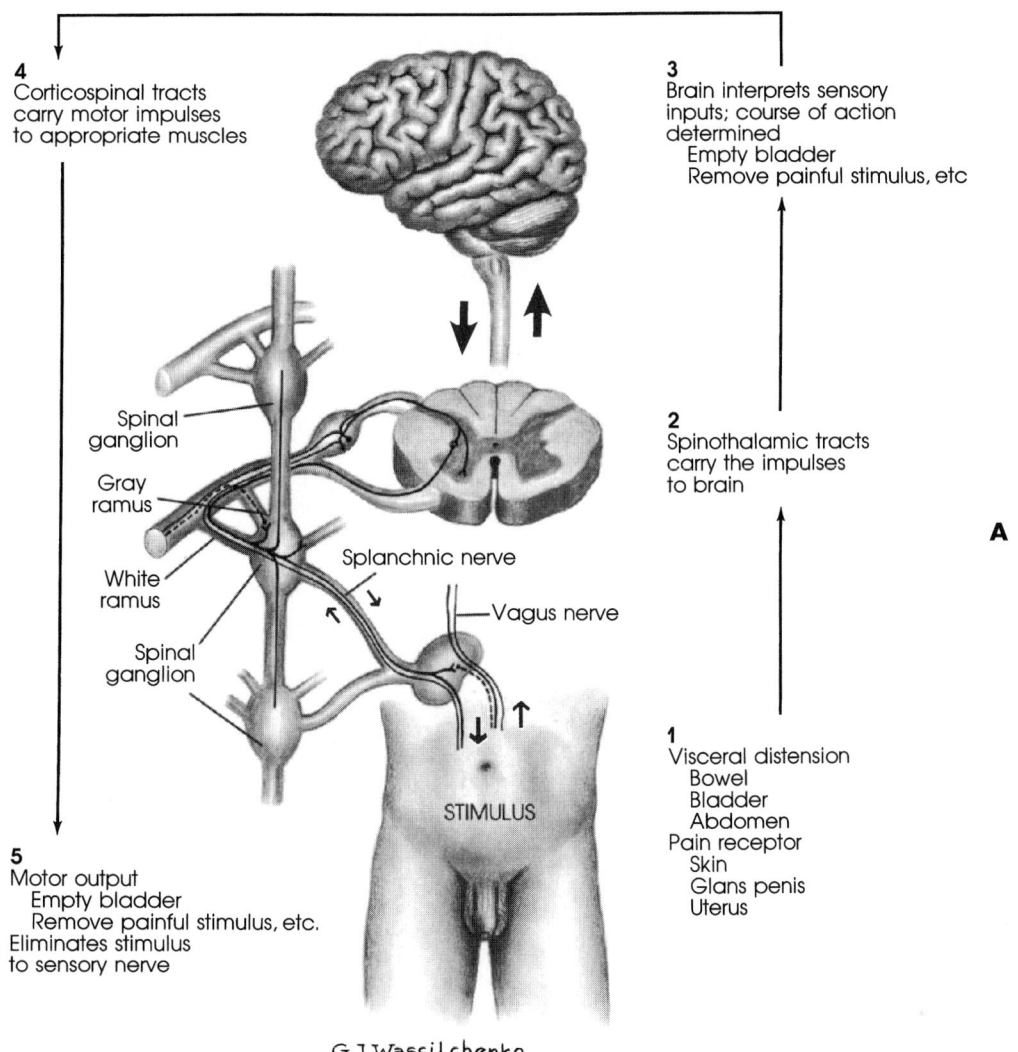

Fig. 9-13 A, Normal response pathway.
(From Rudy EB: Advanced neurological and neurosurgical nursing, *St Louis, 1984, Mosby.)*   *Continued*

Anticoagulants
Laxatives
Antacids
Steroids
Antianginals
Vasodilators
Anticholinergics
Spasmolytics
Antihypertensive agents
Parathyroid agents
Histamine antagonists
Stool softeners
Antidepressants
Antibiotics
Stryker or Foster frame or kinetic treatment
   table
Cervical collar
Splints, braces
Cardiac monitoring/hemodynamic monitoring

Arterial pressure line/management
Fluid/electrolyte management
Nutrition consult, calorie count
Intake and output
Urinary catheterization
Neurologic rehabilitation
Hypothermia/hyperthermia management
Seizure precautions
Pressure ulcer prevention
Chest physiotherapy

PATIENT PROBLEMS—NURSING DIAGNOSES/INTERVENTIONS

▼ Ineffective breathing pattern related to neurogenic or traumatic injury

Maintain patent airway; avoid flexion of the neck *to prevent airway obstruction*

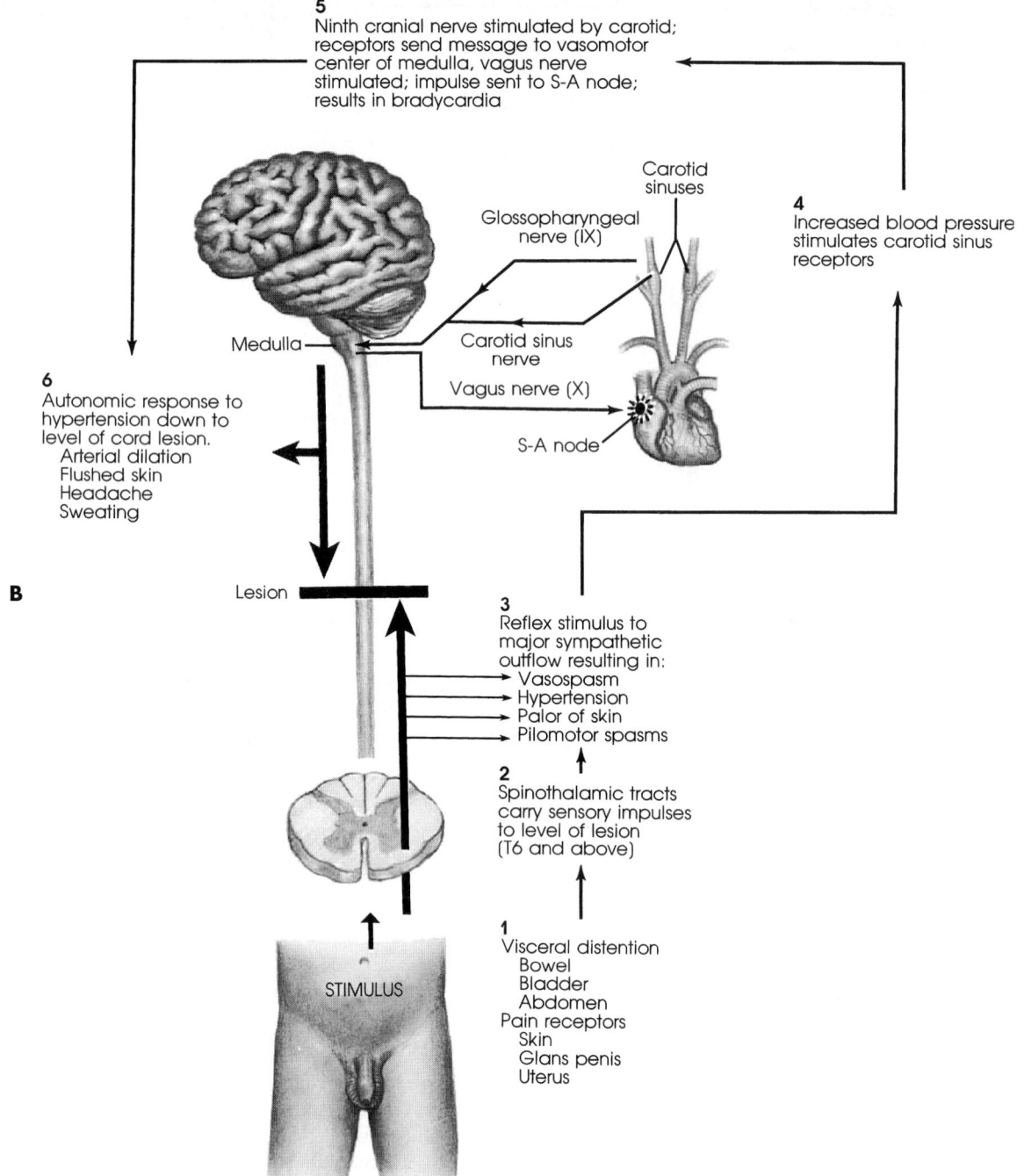

5
Ninth cranial nerve stimulated by carotid; receptors send message to vasomotor center of medulla, vagus nerve stimulated; impulse sent to S-A node; results in bradycardia

Carotid sinuses

Glossopharyngeal nerve (IX)

4
Increased blood pressure stimulates carotid sinus receptors

Medulla

Carotid sinus nerve

Vagus nerve (X)

S-A node

6
Autonomic response to hypertension down to level of cord lesion.
Arterial dilation
Flushed skin
Headache
Sweating

B

Lesion

3
Reflex stimulus to major sympathetic outflow resulting in:
→ Vasospasm
→ Hypertension
→ Palor of skin
→ Pilomotor spasms

2
Spinothalamic tracts carry sensory impulses to level of lesion (T6 and above)

STIMULUS

1
Visceral distention
Bowel
Bladder
Abdomen
Pain receptors
Skin
Glans penis
Uterus

Fig. 9-13, cont'd   **B,** Autonomic dysreflexia pathway.
(From Rudy EB: Advanced neurological and neurosurgical nursing, *St Louis, 1984, Mosby.)*

Assess respiratory function noting rate, quality, and depth of *respirations to determine adequacy of gas exchange*

Assess ability and quality of cough

Maintain NPO status if indicated

Aspiration precautions

Monitor character of sputum

Monitor CBC to determine hemoglobin (Hgb) available to carry oxygen and *to detect inflammation or infection*

Assess sensorimotor function *to ensure adequate rhythm or pattern of respiration*

Auscultate breath sounds q1h to 2h and prn to detect adventitious breath sounds

Administer assisted ventilation and oxygenation as ordered; measure vital capacity and minute ventilation *to ensure adequate ventilation and oxygenation*

Be aware that tracheostomy or endotracheal intubation may be indicated

Table 9-20	Incomplete Spinal Cord Injuries: Syndromes, Area of Injury, and Functional Loss	
Syndrome	**Area of Injury**	**Functional Loss**
Central cord syndrome	Central gray or white matter of the spinal cord; occurs mostly with cervical hyperextension injuries	Upper motor neuron loss of arms
Anterior cord syndrome	Anterior two thirds of the spinal cord; occurs mostly with flexion and compression injuries Corticospinal tracts (motor) Spinothalamic tracts (Sensory)	Complete motor function loss below level of injury Loss of pain, touch, and temperature sensation Preservation of light touch, proprioception, and position sense
Posterior cord syndrome	Rare Associated with cervical hyperextension trauma	Loss of motor function depends on whether injury was caused by compression of cord, dislocation of disk, fracture, or dislodgment of bone fracture
Brown-Séquard syndrome	Hemisection of the anterior and posterior cord (e.g. caused by stab wound) Corticospinal tract on ipsilateral side Spinothalamic tract on contralateral side	Complete loss of motor function below level of lesion, on ipsilateral side Loss of pain, touch, and temperature on contralateral side for all areas below the lesion
Cauda equina syndrome	Below L2	Motor and sensory loss

Provide nasopharyngeal or oropharyngeal airway as needed

Suction as needed (preoxygenate with 100% O_2 for 60 seconds before and after suctioning; suction <15 seconds)

Oral suctioning as needed

Monitor vital signs with neurologic check q1h to 2h as indicators of impaired ventilatory status

Obtain and monitor serial ABGs *to determine acid-base balance, hypercapnia, hypoxia*

Report decrease of Po_2 of 10 to 15 mm Hg

Report increase of Pco_2 > 10 to 15 mm Hg

Monitor oxygen saturation by oximetry *to determine peripheral oxygenation*

Teach diaphragmatic cough when indicated

Expected Outcomes

Demonstrates effective breathing pattern

Chest expansion is symmetric

Breath sounds are clear to auscultation

ABGs and vital signs are within normal limits

No sign of respiratory distress

Secretions adequately managed

▼Self-care deficit: hygiene, feeding/nutrition, toileting, and/or mobility related to neurophysiologic impairment

Assess level of injury and related disability in performing self-care needs

Maintain NPO until chewing, swallowing, and GI function is established and *to prevent aspiration*

Advance diet as tolerated

Provide nutritional support as ordered; consult with dietitian *to establish nutritional needs*

Assist with feedings as necessary *to ensure adequate caloric intake*

Encourage fluid intake to 2000 ml/day unless contraindicated

Connect indwelling catheter or condom catheter to closed gravity drainage system as ordered

Check urine for presence of calculi, occult blood

Administer catheter care bid *to prevent infection*

Give colon lavage or enemas q3d as ordered *to prevent fecal impaction*

Perform passive ROM exercises to extremities; check with physician before starting exercises

Assist and teach muscle-building exercises as indicated
  Squeeze toys
  Rubber balls
  Clay

Use trapeze and pulleys if not contraindicated

Apply antiembolic stockings *to prevent venous stasis*

Administer oral hygiene q2h to 4h; brush teeth

Administer skin care q2h to 4h *to prevent breakdown*
  Incontinence care devices
  Give back rubs
  Use footboard, foot splints, boots
  Use log-roll technique when turning
  Use heel and/or elbow guards *to prevent pressure point irritation and possible skin breakdown*

Provide for total physical hygiene as indicated: comb hair daily; shampoo weekly as indicated

Explain importance of skin care
Position change q2h to 4h

Expected Outcomes
Self-care needs are met
Fluid and nutritional needs are met
Elimination needs are met
Skin, oral, and eye hygiene needs are met
Passive or active ROM exercise is performed

▼Dysfunctional grieving related to loss of physiopsychosocial well-being

Assess and monitor patient's and significant others' perceptions of medical condition and prognosis
Assess stage of grieving that patient is experiencing
    Shock and disbelief
        Provide simple but honest explanations to questions regarding diagnosis, treatments, and prognoses; identify and correct misconceptions
        Permit and encourage expressions of emotions *to minimize frustration*
        Allow use of denial; avoid confronting patients when experiencing distorted perceptions
        Point out reality in nonthreatening manner
        Refrain from judgmental responses
        Avoid reinforcement of denial
        Provide encouragement and supportive counseling
Anger
    Accept expressions of emotion; avoid arguing
    Identify manipulative and disruptive behavior; set limits on acting-out when necessary
Depression
    Encourage participation of significant others
    Outline progressive steps towards a goal; minimize frustration

Expected Outcomes
Able to express thoughts and feelings related to loss
Demonstrates beginning of resolution of feelings
Participates in prescribed treatment
Patient and significant others have realistic, positive goals

Additional Nursing Diagnoses to Consider
Risk for autonomic dysreflexia
Impaired physical mobility
Impaired walking
Impaired wheelchair ability
Impaired wheelchair transfer ability
Impaired bed mobility
Sensory/perceptual alterations
Powerlessness
Impaired skin integrity
Reflex incontinence
Constipation

PATIENT/FAMILY TEACHING
Ensure that patient and significant other are informed about disease and prognosis

Prepare for chronicity and duration of rehabilitative process
Discuss medications: name, purpose, dosage, route, time of administration, and side effects
Refer to appropriate rehabilitative and counseling resources
Stress importance of follow-up care
Provide education material from National Spinal Cord Injury Association (1-800-962-9629)

DISCHARGE/HOME CARE PLANNING
Activity
    Stress the importance and proper use of mobility devices (wheelchair, cane, walker) to patient/family
    Assist family to identify local community agencies that can help in providing such devices
    Assist family to learn ways of adapting the home for accessibility
    Stress the need for initial home health referral to do the following:
        Teach family members proper body mechanics and how to protect their backs
        Assist in learning safety measures to prevent falling
        Implement safety devices such as side rails and ramps as indicated
    Maintain regular ROM exercise program to all joints
    Maintain regular turning schedule (side-back-side) if indicated
    Provide skin care on a regular basis to prevent breakdown
    Encourage mobility to tolerance
    Encourage self-care activities to tolerance
    Maintain planned rest periods
Dietary
    Provide diet that is high in roughage, protein, and bulk
    Maintain fluid intake of 2000 ml/day unless contraindicated
    Monitor intake and output
    Obtain home nutritional referral if needed
    Institute regular bowel evacuation program
    Perform intermittent urinary catheterization as indicated
    Maintain bladder retraining program
    Acidify urine by encouraging patient to drink cranberry juice and take ascorbic acid if ordered
    Include foods high in calcium
    Avoid alcoholic beverages, coffee, tea, and soft drinks with caffeine
    Avoid bananas, beans, and cabbage
Medications
    Establish routine medication regimen
General instructions
    Refer for psychologic and sexual counseling as needed
    Provide wound care on an established basis if surgical intervention was implemented
    Monitor closely for any signs of skin breakdown or decubitus ulcer formation

Administer antibiotics, if ordered, until all medication is gone

Monitor for signs and symptoms of autonomic hyperreflexia if lesion is at T6 or above; autonomic hyperreflexia is a medical emergency and requires immediate intervention

■ ALZHEIMER'S DISEASE
Progressive deterioration of intellect, memory, personality, and self-care, leading to severe dementia from degeneration of nerve cells in the cerebral cortex

ASSESSMENT
SUBJECTIVE DATA
Forgetfulness
Anxiety
Fear
Confusion
Tiredness
Depression

OBJECTIVE DATA
Early
Memory loss
  Loss of orientation to time and location
  Inability to recognize family and friends
  Lack of recent memories but able to recall early life events
Personality changes
  Apathy, loss of initiative
  Belligerence, stubbornness
  Suspicion progressing to paranoia
  Loss of sense of humor
  Insensitivity to others
Intellectual changes
  Difficulty in making decisions or plans
  Inability to calculate (e.g., money transactions)
  Inability to learn new material
  Loss of train of thought during conversations
  Requiring repetitive directions
  Inattentiveness
Conversation changes: slow speech, loss of words, use of clichés
Fatigues easily
Mood
  Reactive depression
  Crying spells
  Lethargy
  Neglect of self-care
Nocturnal wandering

Advanced
Progressive increase in early symptoms
Apathetic, mute
Inability to recall recent or remote events
Disorientation/confusion
Inability to perform ADLs

Incontinence
Decreased appetite; weight loss

POTENTIAL COMPLICATIONS
Physical and/or psychologic dependence
Social isolation
Injury
Dehydration/malnutrition
Seizures (rare)

MULTIDISCIPLINARY MANAGEMENT
THERAPEUTIC MANAGEMENT
Supportive management; social services
Physiologic and psychologic support measures for patient and family to enhance coping with progressive deterioration

PATIENT PROBLEMS—NURSING DIAGNOSES/INTERVENTIONS*

▼Risk for injury related to deterioration of physiologic and cognitive function

Maintain safety precautions *to minimize risks of falls and patient injury*
  Have attendant with patient during any treatment or procedure
  Remove or disconnect door locks
  Avoid having patient use razors without assistance
  Avoid potentially dangerous tasks (e.g., smoking, cooking)
  Assist with ADLs

Expected Outcomes
Free of injury
Demonstrates no signs of physical injuries

▼Altered thought processes related to loss of memory

Explain to patient and family the nature of this disorder and that it is progressive
Assist with reality orientation
  Introduce all caregivers by name each time; repeat on regular basis
  Writing instructions and directions may be helpful
  Provide large-face clock and current calendar
  Orient patient to day, hour, and location frequently
  Provide familiar objects and memory aids (e.g., photos of family members) *to facilitate memory*
Speak in quiet tones
Maintain calm atmosphere; avoid rushing
Use consistency and repetition with patient
Give singular, simple instructions

Care and teaching are combined to provide nurse and family with consistent approach.

Expected Outcomes
Demonstrates enhanced interpretation of reality
Oriented to environment, self, time
Makes wants and needs known

▼ Self-care deficit: hygiene, nutrition, and/or toileting related to physiologic and/or psychologic dependence

Assess degree of self-care needs *to establish baseline for caregiver assistance*
Provide for physical hygiene needs: bathing, shampooing, skin and oral care
Provide properly balanced diet *to maintain adequate nutritional status*
Administer diet as ordered; present one course at a time (e.g., salad first, then entrée)
Assist patient in cutting food as needed *to facilitate adequate dietary intake*
Establish regular bowel habits *to minimize potential for constipation or diarrhea*
    Determine patient's normal bowel patterns
    Encourage bowel movement on schedule *to aid in timing of defecation*
    Recognize signs of impaction
        No formed stool for 3 days
        Semiliquid stools
        Distention
        Restlessness
    Discuss treatment for impaction: laxative, suppository, enema *to prevent bowel obstruction*
Establish routine voiding measures
    Remind patient q2h to void
    Avoid giving fluids before bedtime *to minimize potential for nocturnal incontinence*
Administer medications as ordered

Expected Outcomes
Self-care needs are met
Nutritional intake is adequate
Elimination needs are met

▼ Ineffective family coping related to long-term deteriorating effects of disease process

Provide emotional support *to minimize anxiety and stress*
Refer family to support groups
Refer to social services for financial concerns and potential placement
Refer to home care services for potential in-home assistance for home maintenance and management problems
Ensure that self-care needs of patient's primary caregivers are met (e.g., elderly spouse)
Ensure that family and significant other(s) are informed about disease process and physician's instructions for supportive care

Expected Outcomes
Family and significant other(s) are coping effectively with home management, and proper resources are being used for patient care needs, counseling, and financial assistance

Additional Nursing Diagnoses to Consider
Caregiver role strain
Sleep pattern disturbance
Anticipatory grieving: family

DISCHARGE/HOME CARE PLANNING
Activities
    Institute safety measures such as removing or nailing down area rugs to prevent falling
    Stress the importance and proper use of mobility devices (wheelchair, cane, walker) to patient/family
        Assist family to identify local community agencies that can help in providing such devices
        Assist family to learn ways of adapting the home for accessibility
        Stress the need for initial home health referral to do the following:
            Teach family members proper body mechanics and how to protect their backs
            Assist in learning safety measures *to prevent falling*
    Maintain quiet environment, reducing environmental stimuli to minimum if patient is confused or agitated
    Assist with reality orientation as indicated
    Refer to home care services for potential in-home assistance
    Remove or disconnect door locks
    Avoid potentially dangerous tasks such as cooking, smoking, driving, using power tools
    Assist with daily hygiene as needed
    Maintain regular exercise program with planned rest periods
Diet
    Provide high-protein, low-calcium diet
    Encourage fluid intake to 2000 ml/day unless contraindicated
    Assist in cutting food as needed
    Present one course of diet at a time (i.e., salad, then entrée)
    Establish routine voiding measures
    Establish regular bowel habits
    Avoid giving fluids before bedtime
    Monitor intake and output
General instructions
    Provide instructions on reporting any seizure activity
    Discuss need to maintain seizure precautions
    Provide skin care
    Encourage focus on remaining strengths and intact roles
    Encourage a sense of control
    Facilitate expression of emotions, but advise family that patient may exhibit depression, anger, anxiety

Provide educational resources:
    Alzheimer's Hotline (1-800-621-0379)
    Alzheimer's Disease and Related Disorders Association
      (1-800-272-3900)

■ PARKINSON'S DISEASE (PARALYSIS AGITANS)

A progressive, degenerative disease of the brain's dopamine neuronal system, most commonly idiopathic in nature

ASSESSMENT
SUBJECTIVE DATA
Shaking of hand or arm; tremors
Depression
Nervousness
Urinary incontinence
Constipation
Uncoordinated and/or loss of muscular ability: impaired writing (micrographia)

OBJECTIVE DATA
Rigidity of limbs: arms lose natural swing and remain at side of body
Tremors
    Exaggerated by stress and anxiety
    Most severe when limb is resting; absent during sleep
    Fingers: pill-rolling movement
    Head: to-and-fro tremor; "yes-yes" or "no-no" patterns
Movements
    Voluntary body movements become slower (bradykinesia)
    Starting activities becomes difficult (akinesia)
Posture (Fig. 9-14)
    Bent forward, head bowed
    Walking with slow, short, shuffling steps (festination)
    Breaking into run if pushed
    Propulsion
    Retropulsion
Blank facial expression (masked facies)
    Wide-eyed
    Infrequent blinking of eyes
Speech
    Slowed, soft, monotonous
    Dysarthric
    Slurred
    Voice tremors
Dysphagia
Excessive salivation and drooling
Emotional changes
    Generalized apathy
    Mood swings
    Social withdrawal
    Hallucinations
    Paranoia
    Dementia

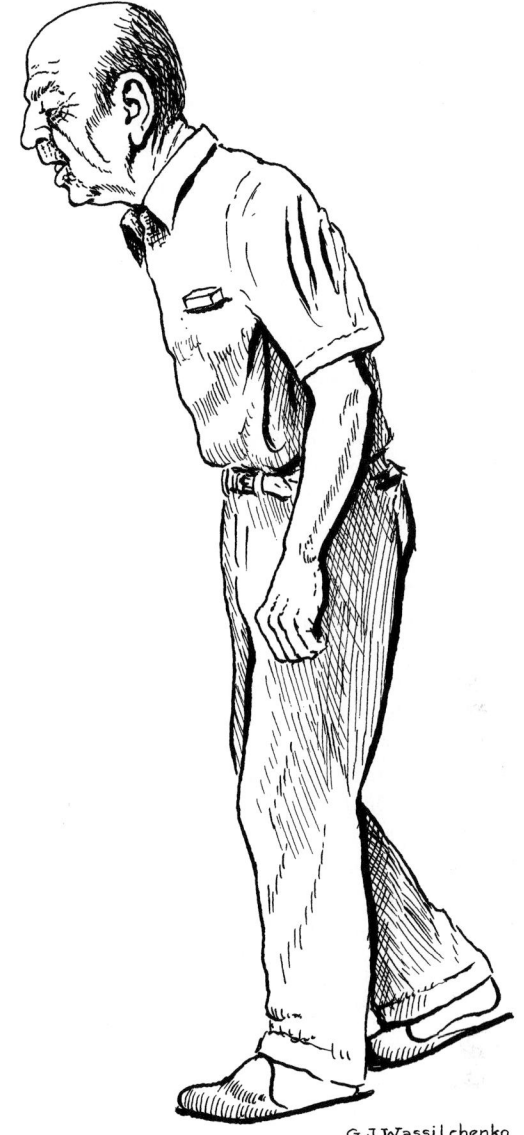

Fig. 9-14 Posture and shuffling gait associated with Parkinson's disease.
(From Rudy EB: Advanced neurological and neurosurgical nursing, *St Louis, 1984, Mosby.)*

Side effects of drugs
Orthostatic hypotension

DIAGNOSTIC TESTS
CSF
    Usually within normal limits
    May show slight increase in protein concentration
Imaging
    CT scan: normal results or may show cerebral atrophy
    MRI *to rule out other causes*
Blood
    CBC: mild microcytic anemia
    Serum drug levels *to rule out drug-induced dopamine-blocking parkinsonism*

GI studies
    Hypomotility
    Delayed emptying of stomach
    Varying degrees of bowel distention
EEG
    Normal with minimal slowing
    Marked or moderate slowing and/or disorganization
        (with marked dementia or bradykinesia)
Skull x-rays
Cineradiographic study of swallowing

MULTIDISCIPLINARY MANAGEMENT

THERAPEUTIC MANAGEMENT

Surgical
    Surgical stereotactic thalamotomy to relieve
        contralateral tremor and rigidity: neurotransplants
    Pallidotomy
    Deep brain stimulation
Medications
    MAO inhibitors
        Selegiline (Eldepryl)
    Dopamine agonists
        Bromocriptine (Parlodel)
        Pramipexole (Mirapex)
    Dopaminergics
        Levodopa-carbidopa (Sinemet)
        Amantadine hydrochloride (Symmetrel)
    Anticholinergics
        Benztropine mesylate (Cogentin)
        Trihexphenidyl (Artane)
    Antiparkinsonian and antihistamine: diphenhydramine
        (Benadryl)
    Muscle relaxant and anticholinergic: orphenadrine
        hydrochloride
Nutrition therapy
Physical therapy
Occupational therapy
Speech therapy

PATIENT PROBLEMS—NURSING DIAGNOSES/INTERVENTIONS

▼Impaired physical mobility related to neurologic degenerative disorder

Assess level of disability
Encourage ambulation to tolerance *to improve mobility*
Assist to chair
Perform active or passive ROM exercises q4h to all
    extremities *to increase muscle mass, tone, and
    strength*
    Neck
    Hands and fingers
    Wrists
    Elbows
    Knees
Evaluate effectiveness of drug therapy
Initiate gait-retraining program; consult with physical
    therapy department to increase ambulation

Provide physical therapy as ordered: massage and
    stretching exercises
Have patient practice lifting legs while walking rather
    than shuffling; try to maintain erect position
Maintain planned rest periods
Conduct occupational therapy as indicated by amount of
    tremors
Assist patient with turning q2h to 4h if unable to move
    self
Provide raised toilet seat with side rails *to facilitate
transfer from sitting to standing*

Expected Outcome

Demonstrates optimal level of mobility appropriate for
physical disability

▼Self-care deficit: feeding/nutrition, toileting, hygiene

Assess functional ability related to self-care needs
Assess nutritional needs; consult with dietitian
Maintain well-balanced, soft diet
Avoid foods and medications that contain pyridoxine
    hydrochloride (vitamin B_6), which reverses effect
    of levodopa
Maintain frequent, small feedings as indicated
Maintain fluid intake to 2000 ml/day unless
    contraindicated *to maintain adequate hydration*
Maintain supplemental high-calorie fluids such as eggnog,
    milk shakes, and malts
Use bibs and straws as indicated; place food and drinks
    within easy reach of patient
Initiate voiding measures as necessary
Institute bladder control program as indicated
Have patient avoid constipation through use of high-
    residue foods, stool softeners, and/or enemas
Provide or assist with general hygiene as indicated
Administer oral hygiene q4h to 6h and prn
Encourage self-care as tolerated: bathing, mouth care

Expected Outcomes

Self-care needs are met
Optimal nutritional intake maintained
Demonstrates skin integrity

▼Self-esteem disturbance related to actual or perceived changes in physical and personal self-image

Provide emotional support; allow patient to verbalize
    needs and participate in planning care *to foster
    feelings of self-worth and to reduce
    powerlessness*
Encourage verbalization of feelings about body image and
    functional changes
Acknowledge and support attempts to improve
    appearance
Permit expression of emotions
Encourage use of support groups

Expected Outcomes
Experiences self-respect and self-confidence
Achieves goals that reflect awareness of abilities and limitations
Acknowledges and supports attempts to improve appearance
Permits expression of emotions
Uses support groups

Additional Nursing Diagnoses to Consider
Impaired verbal communication
Risk for injury
Social isolation

PATIENT/FAMILY TEACHING
Assess level of understanding regarding disease and treatments prescribed
Reinforce physician's explanation of disease and its causes, symptoms, and treatment
Discuss importance of verbalization about loss of body function, self-esteem, and sexuality
Explain that behavioral changes may be part of disease process or caused by medications
Emphasize need to discuss feelings about symptoms
    Tremors
    Drooling
    Slurred speech
Explain to family
    Need to provide psychologic support
    Need to emphasize capabilities rather than limitations
    Need to encourage active participation in family activities
    Need to encourage socialization
    Need to encourage independence; avoid overprotection
    Need to permit patient to do things for self
        Self-care
        Feedings
        Dressing
        Ambulation
Explain that although patient may be physically disabled, he or she is intellectually normal
Discuss need for family to show security, love, need for patient, and patience with and understanding of patient's slowness and clumsiness
Explain that frustration over tremors and dependence may be source of patient's irritability and loss of self-interest
Discuss agencies available for use as resources such as:
    American Parkinson Disease Association
        116 John St.
        New York, NY 10038
    National Parkinson's Foundation Hotline:
        1-800-327-4545
Explain importance of daily exercise to delay progression of disease
Explain importance of performing any physical task that is difficult 5 to 10 times a day

Explain importance of ongoing outpatient care
    Physician's visits
    Physical therapy
Discuss medications: name, dosage, frequency of administration, purpose, side effects, and toxic effects
Explain need to avoid taking over-the-counter medications without physician approval
Encourage patient to participate in activities to decrease attention on symptoms
    Reading
    Watching television
    Listening to radio or stories on audio cassettes
    Engaging in hobbies
    Painting
Prevent falls and injuries by clearing walkways of furniture and scatter rugs; build side rails on stairs and in tub or shower
Provide supports as indicated when patient is ambulating with walker or cane
Provide speech therapy
    Instruct patient to speak slowly and practice reading aloud slowly in an exaggerated manner
    Provide electronic amplifiers as ordered for weak voice
Explain need for oral hygiene q2h to 4h and prn to control drooling
    Have tissues easily accessible to patient (e.g., in pockets)
    Have patient use bib while eating
    Clean corners of mouth after eating and prn
    Apply ointment if necessary
Explain importance of proper elimination
    Conduct voiding measures as necessary
    Conduct bladder control program as necessary
    Provide raised toilet seat with side rails in home to facilitate sitting and standing

DISCHARGE/HOME CARE PLANNING
Activity
    Explain need for activity
        Plan rest periods
        Perform passive or active ROM exercises to all extremities
    Encourage family or significant other(s) to participate in physical therapy exercise of stretching and massaging muscles
    Give warm baths
    Encourage daily ambulation outdoors except during extremely hot or cold weather
    Encourage patient to practice lifting feet, using heel-toe gait, and swinging arms deliberately while walking
    Place head of bed or back of chair on blocks to facilitate getting out of bed or chair; use pulleys such as sheets tied to end of bed
    Have patient avoid sitting for long periods
    Encourage patient to dress daily
        Avoid clothing with buttons; use zippers or Velcro fasteners instead
        Avoid shoes with laces or small buckles

Provide diversional activities depending on extent of
tremors or disability

Apply splints and braces as indicated

Diet

Explain need for well-balanced, soft diet; limit high-
protein food, which may block effects of drugs

Cut foods for patient

Place all utensils within easy reach

Use blender for thick foods

Use braces for severe tremors occurring during meals

Maintain fluid intake to 2000 ml/day unless
contraindicated

Serve frequent, small meals

Serve supplemental high-calorie fluids such as eggnog
and milkshakes

Use straws and bibs for excessive drooling

Avoid food high in vitamin B_6 (reverses effects of
levodopa)

Instruct patient to swallow slowly and take small bites
of food

Maintain intake and output

General instructions

Focus on strengths and intact roles

Reorient to time, person, and place as needed

Protect patient privacy

Monitor urinary and bowel habits

■ MULTIPLE SCLEROSIS (DISSEMINATED SCLEROSIS)

A chronic, progressive disease characterized by scattered demyelinating lesions in the central nervous system (CNS) that affect the white matter of the brain and spinal cord

ASSESSMENT
SUBJECTIVE DATA
Shakiness
Difficulty walking
Fatigue
Muscle weakness
Numbness, tingling
Visual disturbances
Difficulty swallowing and chewing
Difficulty speaking
Urinary or fecal incontinence

OBJECTIVE DATA
Cerebellar
Ataxia
Staggering gait
Loss of position sense
Cognitive
Mood swings
Depression
Euphoria
Irritability
Apathy
Inattention

Lack of judgment
Memory deficits

Visual
Diplopia
Blurred vision
Dilation of affected pupil when light is shined into eye
(Marcus Gunn's phenomenon)
Nystagmus
Optic neuritis
Scotoma (dark spots in visual field)

Sensory/motor/reflexes
Spasticity of extremities
Tremors
Muscular spasms
Weakness of throat muscles; difficulty in chewing and
swallowing; dysphagia
Facial palsy
Speech impairment
Positive Babinski sign
Fatigue (may be increased by heat [e.g., hot bath or
shower])
Decreased to absent superficial reflexes

Gastrointestinal/genitourinary
Fecal and/or urinary incontinence or retention
Impotence

DIAGNOSTIC TESTS
CSF
Usually normal
Normal or low protein concentration
Increased white blood cell count (WBC)
Increased gamma globulin level
Imaging
MRI
CT scan
PET scan
Evoked responses
Myelography
Urodynamic studies

POTENTIAL COMPLICATIONS
Neurologic deficit: paralysis, quadriplegia
Visual disturbances; blindness
Sexual dysfunction
Spastic bladder, urinary retention
Bowel dysfunction
Respiratory failure; pneumonia; aspiration
Infection
Pressure ulcers
Thrombus formation
Speech deficits
Dementia

MULTIDISCIPLINARY MANAGEMENT
THERAPEUTIC MANAGEMENT
Medications
Antiinflammatory agents
ACTH
Corticosteroids

Muscle relaxants
Immunosuppressive agents
Vitamin B
Anticholinergics (for urinary frequency)
Cholinergices (for urinary retention)
Antidepressants
Antianxiety drugs/tranquilizers
β-Adrenergic blocking agents
Respiratory therapy
Physical therapy, hydrotherapy
Occupational therapy
Speech therapy
Rehabilitation
Psychotherapy/counseling
Social services
Nutritional therapy
Surgical
    Cordotomy, rhizotomy, neurectomy (for spasticity)
    Stereotaxic thalamotomy
Consultation with Wound, Ostomy, and Continence/ET
    Nurse specialist for bowel and bladder management

PATIENT PROBLEMS—NURSING DIAGNOSES/INTERVENTIONS

▼Impaired physical mobility related to neuromuscular impairment

Assess and monitor degree of physical disability
NOTE: Limit activity level when patient is unduly tired,
    during periods of exacerbation
Maintain quiet, relaxing, and cool environment
Institute activity
    Massage and stretch muscles *to increase circulation
        and joint mobility*
    Perform resistive exercises to all extremities and joints
    Perform active or passive ROM exercises q4h to 5h
        and prn
    Instruct patient to avoid exercising when tired and on
        hot days
    Encourage ambulation to tolerance
    Encourage self-care activities *to promote perception of
        positive body image*
    Avoid use of heating pad; measure bathwater
        temperature (heat reduces muscle strength)
    Plan all activities *to prevent fatigue*
    Plan rest periods *to minimize fatigue*
    Encourage diversional activities during periods of
        exacerbation
        Reading
        Watching television
        Listening to radio and/or book recordings
If patient is confined to bed rest
    Apply air or foam mattress to bed
    Position comfortably
    Turn q2h to 4h and prn *to prevent skin breakdown*
    Perform active or passive ROM exercises q2h to 4h *to
        promote circulation and joint mobility*
    Perform dorsiflexion of ankles and quadriceps q2h to 4h

Help patient out of bed and into chair two or three times
    daily if allowed
Observe for signs of thrombophlebitis
    Use antiembolic stockings
    Administer anticoagulation therapy as ordered *to
        minimize thrombus formation*
Feed as necessary; hand braces may be indicated
Administer skeletal muscle relaxants to reduce spasticity
    (NOTE: Use with caution—may exacerbate general
    weakness and decrease mobility)

Expected Outcomes
Demonstrates improved mobility or minimal degree of
    physical immobility
Participates in activities that promote improved function
Verbalizes understanding of conditions that may
    exacerbate symptoms

▼Altered elimination: bowel and bladder related to neuromuscular impairment

Assess degree of functional disability
Initiate bladder program as indicated
    Assess bladder function and voiding pattern (urgency,
        frequency, incontinence, nocturia)
    Teach perineal (Kegel) exercise *to improve tone of
        urinary sphincter*
    Measure intake and output
    Catheterize intermittently as indicated
    Teach self-catheterization whenever possible
    Plan bladder dysfunction program as appropriate for
        spasticity or flaccidity
Institute bowel control program/consult with Wound,
    Ostomy, Continence/ET Nurse
    Establish regular bowel routines
    Prevent constipation
Maintain high-fiber diet
Encourage fluids to 3000 ml/day, unless contraindicated,
    to promote adequate hydration

Expected Outcomes
Maintains bladder and bowel elimination
Has stable intake and output
Evidences no bladder distention
Has regular bowel evacuation pattern
Does not experience fecal impaction

▼Activity intolerance related to generalized weakness secondary to neuromuscular disease

Assess energy level and ability to carry out activities
Assess sleep and rest patterns; determine when patient
    feels strongest
Schedule nursing care, procedures, and tests *to permit
    maximal periods of rest*
Plan periods of uninterrupted rest *to facilitate REM sleep*
Assist patient to plan activities at level of ability
Instruct patient to avoid activities when tired or on days
    that are hot *to minimize fatigue*

Expected Outcomes

Demonstrates improved activity tolerance

Verbalizes understanding of activity allowance and limitations

Verbalizes understanding of need to balance activities and periods of rest

▼ Self-esteem disturbance related to altered perception of self

Assess patient's perception of illness and physical disabilities

Encourage questions and verbalization of feelings *to promote understanding and acceptance*

Provide accurate explanation of disease process

Acknowledge and permit discussion related to actual and perceived changes *to facilitate normal grieving process*

Acknowledge concerns about body image *to enhance healthy adjustment to body changes*

Be supportive of patient's emotional changes and needs for improving image and self-esteem

Encourage expression of emotion *to facilitate normal grieving process*

Expected Outcomes

Experiences self-confidence and demonstrates beginning of adaptation to physical changes

▼ Ineffective airway clearance related to motor weakness and/or immobility

Assess respiration: rate, depth, and pattern; assess degree of respiratory effort and cough reflex

Monitor serial ABGs *to determine acid-base balance*

Suction oropharynx as needed *to maintain patent airway*

Assist and teach patient to cough and deep breathe q2h to 4h and prn *to minimize risk for atelectasis*

Maintain patent airway and avoid flexion of patient's neck if immobile

Monitor oxygen saturation *to control peripheral oxygenation*

Auscultate breath sounds q2h to 4h and prn *to detect adventitious breath sounds*

Position patient for maximal respiratory expansion and control of respiratory secretions

Administer oxygen as indicated *to improve gas exchange and decrease work of breathing*

Maintain aspiration precautions, especially while eating

Expected Outcomes

Demonstrates effective breathing pattern and patent airway

Chest expansion is symmetric

Breath sounds are clear to auscultation

ABGs and vital signs are within normal limits

No signs of respiratory distress

Additional Nursing Diagnoses to Consider

Sensory/perceptual alterations: visual

Altered role performance

Ineffective individual coping

Impaired verbal communication

PATIENT/FAMILY TEACHING

Assess level of understanding regarding disease process

Explain nature of disease

Explain factors that may precipitate exacerbation of symptoms
- Heat
- Hot baths
- Cold
- Fever
- Emotional stress
- Overexertion
- Pregnancy
- High humidity

Explain need to do muscle stretching exercises daily

Explain need for ROM exercises for patient with spasticity

Explain importance of daily routines for activities, regular exercise, and rest periods

Discuss need for patient support when ambulating with walker, cane, or braces as indicated

Instruct patient to walk with a wide base, keeping feet apart

Emphasize importance of speech therapy; instruct patient to speak slowly and practice reading aloud

Emphasize need for diversional activities
- Reading
- Watching television
- Listening to radio/book recordings
- Knitting
- Playing quiet games

Explain importance of decubitus care if patient is confined to bed rest or wheelchair

Explain importance of regulating bathwater temperature; need to avoid extremes of hot and cold because of loss of temperature-change sense

Discuss symptoms of disease progression to report to physician

Explain importance of avoiding persons with infections, especially URIs

Discuss symptoms of cold or influenza to report to physician
- Elevated temperature
- Chills
- Cough
- Extreme fatigue

Discuss symptoms of urinary tract infection to report to physician
- Fever
- Burning with urination
- Cloudy urine

Encourage activity as long as patient is able
- Recreational activities
- Work
- Household chores

Encourage verbalization

Allow time for patient to complete all activities and deal with any body image changes and loss of self-esteem

Encourage socialization with friends and family

Encourage independence and self-care to point of tolerance

Family planning counseling for women of childbearing age

DISCHARGE/HOME CARE PLANNING

Activities

Institute safety measures such as removing or nailing down area rugs *to prevent falling*

Stress the importance and proper use of mobility devices (wheelchair, cane, walker) to patient/family

Assist family to identify local community agencies that can help in providing such devices

Assist family to learn ways of adapting the home for accessibility

Stress the need for initial home health referral to do the following:

Teach family members proper body mechanics and how to protect their backs

Assist in learning safety measures to prevent falling

Alert the patient to change positions slowly *to prevent postural changes in BP*

Encourage diversional activities such as the following:

Reading

Watching TV

Listening to stereo, radio, recorded books

Maintain regular exercise program with planned rest periods

Encourage daily ambulation outdoors except during particularly hot or cold weather

Support patient during ambulation if needed

Assist to walk with a wide base

Encourage patient to dress daily

Avoid clothing with buttons if possible

Avoid shoes with laces or small buckles

Assist with daily hygiene as indicated

Administer skin care on regular basis *to stimulate circulation and prevent skin breakdown*

Home speech therapy should continue as appropriate

Apply splints or braces to minimize tremors

Avoid individuals with respiratory infections

Diet

Maintain well-balanced diet

Offer small portions

Offer supplemental feedings

Monitor intake and output

Weigh on a weekly basis

Maintain daily fluid intake up to 2L if not contraindicated

Administer oral hygiene before and after meals

Monitor and maintain routine elimination program: bowel and urinary output

Maintain regular bowel evacuations

Provide 8 oz cranberry or orange juice daily *to acidify urine*

■ MYASTHENIA GRAVIS

A neuromuscular disorder characterized by muscular weakness and fatigue resulting from a defect in transmission of motor impulses at the neuromuscular junction; probably a result of an autoimmune response

ASSESSMENT

SUBJECTIVE DATA

Fatigue

Weakness

Difficulty chewing and swallowing

Difficulty with ADLs

Difficulty walking

OBJECTIVE DATA

Expressionless facies/facial droop

Generalized weakness

Increased with exercise

May be confined to one area

Weakness of face, jaw, neck, arms, hands, and/or legs

Difficulty in raising arms above head or extending fingers outward

Dysphagia/drooling

Choking; aspiration

Impaired swallowing

Difficulty in chewing

Weak, high-pitched, soft voice, progresses to whisper

Ptosis of one or both eyelids

Ocular palsy

Diplopia

Inability to walk on heels; may walk on toes

Strength decreases as day progresses

Stress incontinence

Anal sphincter weakness

Respirations

Shallow

Decreased vital capacity (VC) and tidal volume (TV)

Use of accessory muscles

Muffled cough

Normal or brisk reflexes

DIAGNOSTIC TESTS

Chest x-ray, CT scan and MRI of chest *to assess for thyoma*

Tensilon test (edrophonium chloride)

Single-fiber electromyogram

Nerve conduction studies

Antiacetylcholine receptor antibody test (curare test)

T_3, T_4 levels *to rule out thyroid etiology*

POTENTIAL COMPLICATIONS

Myasthenia crisis

Cholinergic crisis

Neuromuscular deficit: mild to severe

Respiratory

Atelectasis

Aspiration

Pneumonia

Respiratory failure

Sepsis

MULTIDISCIPLINARY MANAGEMENT
THERAPEUTIC MANAGEMENT

Plasmapheresis
Thymectomy
    Suprasternal approach
    Transsternal approach
Tracheostomy
Mechanical ventilation/oxygen therapy
Bronchoscopy
Respiratory therapy
Physical therapy
Occupational therapy
Speech therapy
Medications
    Anticholinesterase
    Pyridostigmine (Mestinon)
    Neostigmine (Prostigmin)
    Corticosteroids
    Pituitary hormones
Nutritional support
Social services

PATIENT PROBLEMS—NURSING DIAGNOSES/INTERVENTIONS

▼Impaired verbal communication related to neuromuscular disease

Assess degree of speech impairment
Avoid rushing patient: provide sufficient time to respond *to minimize patient anxiety and frustration*
Provide for alternative communication methods if vocalization is impaired
    Magic Slate*
    Pencil and pad
Provide handkerchief or tissues
Stand close to patient; listen carefully

Expected Outcomes
Accepted method of communication is established
Verbalizes understanding of alternative methods of communicating needs

▼Self-care deficit: feeding/nutrition, hygiene related to decreased motor function

Assess severity of deficits
Initiate a self-care plan that permits maximal patient participation
Maintain well-balanced, high-roughage regular diet *to optimize nutrition and prevent constipation*
Provide frequent, small feedings
Maintain aspiration precautions especially during eating
Manage tube feedings, if indicated, for persistent dysphagia

Western Publishing Co, Inc, Racine, Wis.

Change to semisolid/soft diet if chewing becomes difficult
Administer oral hygiene q2h to 4h, after meals, and prn
Meet physical hygiene needs as indicated
Administer skin care q4h to 6h
    Turn patient q2h to 4h if patient is unable to ambulate
    Rub back
Administer eye care q4h to 5h
    Remove any formed crusts
    Place eye patch over affected eye *to prevent diplopia*
    Administer eyedrops as ordered

Expected Outcome
Self-care needs are met as evidenced by optimal nutritional status and skin integrity

▼Impaired physical mobility related to neuromuscular weakness

Assess degree of physical limitations
Assess medications: check dosage, times taken
Work with patient to determine time of day patient is weakest
Increase activity to tolerance; plan treatments and major activities early in day or 30 minutes after medication is taken
Perform passive or active ROM exercises q4-5h and prn *to increase circulation and joint mobility*
Maintain planned rest periods *to minimize fatigue*
Administer medication as ordered
    Anticholinesterase: to be given 20 to 30 minutes before meals *to make chewing easier;* note increase in muscular strength within 30 minutes of taking medication
    Medication should always be taken at scheduled time; never miss a dose (rationale: anticholinesterase maximizes physical mobility)

Expected Outcome
Experiences optimal mobility

▼Self-concept deficit: body image related to actual or perceived changes in physical and personal self-image

Assess patient's understanding and feelings about disease, and the effect it has had on physical appearance
Provide emotional support; allow patient to verbalize needs and participate in planning care
Encourage verbalization of feelings about body image and function changes
Support efforts to optimize physical appearance

Expected Outcome
Demonstrates positive strategies to deal with body image and functional changes

Additional Nursing Diagnosis to Consider
Ineffective breathing pattern related to neuromuscular impairment

PATIENT/FAMILY TEACHING

Assess level of understanding regarding disease process

Explain to family the following:

Need to encourage patient to deal with body image changes and fears of permanent disability, dying, or loss of body function

Need to encourage verbalization

Need to encourage independence and continued socialization

Discuss medications: name, dosage, time of administration, purpose, side effects, and toxic effects

Anticholinesterase

Importance of dosage

Take at scheduled times

Do not miss doses

Take with milk, crackers, or bread

Avoid taking with coffee, fruit or tomato juice

Avoid taking with sedatives or tranquilizers

Toxic side effects: muscular weakness, abdominal cramps, diarrhea, respiratory depression

Discuss symptoms and first signs of drug toxicity to report to physician

Explain need to avoid taking over-the-counter medications without physician approval

Explain need to wear medical alert band

Discuss symptoms of recurrence or progression of disease or any complications, such as respiratory failure, to report to physician

Discuss precipitating factors to myasthenic crisis

Alcohol

Infection

Inadequate drug levels

Fatigue

Pregnancy, menses

Physical or emotional stress

Prolonged exposure to hot or cold weather

Explain importance of avoiding persons with infections, especially URIs

Discuss symptoms of URI to report to physician

Increased weakness

Low-grade fever

Chills

Cough

Explain importance of ongoing outpatient care

Explain need to maintain regular diet according to patient's status

Serve soft or solid food as tolerated

Arrange foods and utensils so as to be easily managed by patient

Instruct patient to chew small pieces of food well and eat slowly

Explain need for exercise to tolerance; to avoid strenuous activity

Plan activities when maximal effect of medication is seen; patient will usually exhibit most strength in morning or after nap

Assist in planning ADLs in a manner in which patient will accomplish tasks without too many motions

Explain need for active or passive ROM exercises to all extremities

Explain need for planned rest periods and at least 8 hours of sleep at night

Emphasize need for diversional activities

Reading

Watching television

Listening to radio/book recordings

Working puzzles

Discuss need for speech therapy; instruct patient to speak slowly and practice reading aloud

Explain need to use eye patch over affected eye or frosted lens to increase clear vision if diplopia persists

Explain importance of avoiding constipation; may need to use stool softeners or mild laxatives

Explain need for adequate fluid intake: up to 2000 ml/day unless contraindicated

Discuss available agencies for use as references such as:

Myasthenia Gravis Foundation

222 South Riverside Plaza, Suite 1540

Chicago, IL 60606

1-800-541-5454

Refer patient and/or significant other to Visiting Nurses Association (VNA) or social service worker for obtaining any necessary equipment, such as suctioning equipment, for home use

Family planning counseling for women of childbearing age

DISCHARGE/HOME CARE PLANNING

Activities

Institute safety measures such as removing or nailing down area rugs to prevent falling

Stress the importance and proper use of mobility devices (wheelchair, cane, walker) to patient/ family

Assist family to identify local community agencies that can help in providing such devices

Assist family to learn ways of adapting the home for accessibility

Install safety devices such as side rails, ramps, raised toilet seats as indicated

Stress the need for initial home health referral to do the following:

Teach family members proper body mechanics and how to protect their backs

Assist in learning safety measures to prevent falling

Alert the patient to change positions slowly to prevent postural changes in BP

Continue gait-training program and encourage patient to walk on heels

Continue regular exercise program with planned rest periods

Encourage self-care activities to tolerance

Encourage patient to dress self daily

Diet

Maintain well-balanced, regular diet as tolerated; administer tube feedings as ordered if dysphagia persists

Offer small portions

Offer supplemental feedings

Provide oral hygiene before and after meals and as indicated

Maintain bowel and bladder programs

General instructions

Provide skin care q4h to 6h to prevent breakdown

Administer eye care as indicated

Remove formed crusts

Place patch over affected eye

Administer eyedrops as ordered

Test stool for occult blood if corticosteroids are being administered

Report any symptoms of cholinergic or myasthenia crisis; keep emergency equipment (airway, supplemental oxygen, atropine) readily available

■ MYASTHENIA GRAVIS CRISIS, CHOLINERGIC CRISIS

myasthenia gravis crisis: Acute exacerbation of myasthenic process resulting in increased generalized weakness and respiratory failure; usually a result of infection, surgery, or emotional upset

cholinergic crisis: Acute exacerbation of muscle paralysis resulting from an overdose of anticholinesterase, which produces increased parasympathetic nervous system activity

ASSESSMENT
Myasthenia Gravis Crisis
SUBJECTIVE DATA

Difficulty breathing

Severe weakness

Fatigue

Anxiety

Difficulty swallowing

OBJECTIVE DATA

Respiratory distress progressing to periods of apnea and respiratory failure

Tachypnea

Extreme muscular weakness

Restlessness

Irritability

Difficulty in handling secretions

Dysphagia

Inability to chew or move jaws

Facial weakness

Speech impairment

Elevated temperature

Ptosis of one or both eyelids

Cholinergic Crisis
SUBJECTIVE DATA

Dizziness

Blurred vision

Abdominal cramps

Nausea

Difficulty swallowing

Muscle cramps

Weakness

OBJECTIVE DATA

Respiratory distress progressing to periods of apnea and respiratory failure

Bradycardia, hypotension

Dyspnea and wheezing

Vertigo

Lacrimation

Salivation

Anorexia

Nausea and vomiting

Dysarthria

Dysphagia

Muscular cramps and spasms (fasciculations)

Extreme weakness

Toxic effects of anticholinesterase

Anorexia

Abdominal cramps

Nausea, vomiting

Excessive salivation

Sweating

Diarrhea

DIAGNOSTIC TESTS

Tensilon test to distinguish between cholinergic crisis and myasthenic crisis

POTENTIAL COMPLICATIONS

Aspiration

Respiratory failure

Respiratory arrest

MULTIDISCIPLINARY MANAGEMENT
THERAPEUTIC MANAGEMENT

Respiratory therapy

Oxygen therapy; possible intubation and mechanical ventilation

Tracheostomy

Intake and output

Medication therapy: reduce or withdraw anticholinergic drugs

NPO as indicated

Cardiac/hemodynamic monitoring

PATIENT PROBLEM—NURSING DIAGNOSIS/INTERVENTIONS

▼ Ineffective breathing pattern related to neuromuscular (respiratory) impairment

Assess respirations: rate, depth, pattern, and respiratory effort

Maintain patent airway and aspiration precautions

Administer oxygen with assisted ventilation as ordered

Inspect and auscultate chest frequently *to monitor for adequate ventilation*

Monitor VC q2h to 4h as ordered

Assist and teach patient to turn, cough, and deep breathe q2h as possible

Suction oropharynx q2h and prn

Suction via tracheostomy, endotracheal tube, nasopharyngeal tube q1h to 2h and prn with 100% O_2 before and after suctioning; suction < 15 seconds

Monitor consciousness until breathing pattern is stabilized

Check rectal temperature q2h to 4h; cooling measures may be ordered *to decrease work of breathing*

Maintain bed rest to maximize effective breathing

    Elevate head of bed 30 degrees as tolerated

    Maintain body alignment

Maintain neck in neutral position

Administer medication *to optimize ventilatory muscular activity*

    Reduce or withdraw anticholinergic drugs as ordered; may be given to differentiate type of crisis

        Myasthenia gravis crisis: patient worsens

        Cholinergic crisis: patient improves

    Keep atropine at bedside; *avoid use of morphine*

Maintain ventilatory support until crisis is resolved, then resume noncrisis management

Expected Outcomes

Demonstrates effective breathing pattern without ventilatory support

Respiratory rate, rhythm, and pattern are within normal limits without mechanical support

Additional Nursing Diagnoses to Consider

Risk for injury related to neurologic deficit

Anxiety relate to fear of respiratory distress

Impaired swallowing related to dysphagia

PATIENT/FAMILY TEACHING AND DISCHARGE/HOME CARE PLANNING

See Myasthenia Gravis (p. 563)

■ AMYOTROPHIC LATERAL SCLEROSIS

A progressive degenerative disease of the motor neurons of the spinal cord, brainstem, and motor cortex; unknown etiology; results in muscular wasting and atrophy; commonly known as "Lou Gehrig disease"

ASSESSMENT
SUBJECTIVE DATA

Weakness

Difficulty swallowing

OBJECTIVE DATA

Involvement of upper and/or lower motor neurons (see Table 9-18)

Uncoordination of movement of hands and fingers

Muscle wasting involving hands, arms, shoulders

Spastic gait

Progressive weakness, flaccidity, atrophy of legs

Dysarthria

Dysphagia

Excessive drooling

NOTE: Extraocular movements, bowel and bladder function, sensory function, and mental capacity remain intact

DIAGNOSTIC TESTS

Blood

    Creatinine phosphokinase (CPK): elevated

    CBC

    Sedimentation rate

    T_3, T_4 to rule out thyroid cause

Urine

    Toxicology, heavy metals to rule out other causes

Imaging

    CT scan: cerebral atrophy or normal

    MRI

Other

    CSF: elevated protein

    Myelography

    Muscle biopsy

    Electromyelogram

    Nerve conduction studies

POTENTIAL COMPLICATIONS

Neuromuscular deficit: mild to severe

Respiratory infection

Aspiration, atelectasis

Injury

Respiratory failure

MULTIDISCIPLINARY MANAGEMENT
THERAPEUTIC MANAGEMENT

Cricopharyngeal myotomy to alleviate dysphagia

Percutaneous endoscopic gastrostomy tube to provide nutrition

Transtympanic neuroectomy to decrease drooling

Medications

    Anticholinesterase

    Antibiotics

    Muscle relaxants

Respiratory therapy

Oxygenation/ventilatory support

Cardiac monitoring

Dietary consultation

Parenteral fluids/nutritional support

Physical therapy

Occupational, speech therapy

Social services

PATIENT PROBLEMS—NURSING DIAGNOSES/INTERVENTIONS

▼ Ineffective airway clearance related to progressive neuromuscular impairment

Assess respiratory function and ability to handle secretions

Assess ability to swallow; maintain NPO if reflexes are weak

Maintain patent airway by the following:

     Proper body and head positioning

     Suction oropharyhx q2h and prn

     Aspiration precautions especially while eating

     Suctioning q2h to 4h as indicated; hyperoxygenating with 100% O_2 before and after suctioning; suctioning <15 seconds

     Encouraging coughing and deep breathing as patient's condition permits

Observe for alterations in respiratory rate and pattern

Auscultate chest for adventitious sounds q2h to 4h

Administer oxygen, humidification, and ventilatory support as ordered *to promote oxygenation and decrease work of breathing*

Perform chest percussion and vibration *to loosen secretions*

Test muscular strength for respiratory effort by monitoring tidal volume and vital capacity

Expected Outcomes

Demonstrates effective breathing pattern

Chest expansion is symmetric

Breath sounds are clear to auscultation

ABGs and vital signs are within normal limits

No signs of respiratory distress

▼Self-care deficit: feeding, hygiene, and/or toileting related to progressive neuromuscular deterioration

Assess degree of self-care deficit

Encourage self-care as long as possible

     Bathing

     Feeding

Direct nursing care to promote self-care and prevention of complications according to severity of symptoms

Administer oral hygiene q4h to 5h

Provide physical hygiene as indicated

Check gag reflex

Modify eating patterns as gag reflex diminishes

Maintain high-calorie, high-protein, soft diet as tolerated

Initiate tube feedings as indicated

Administer skin care q4h and prn

     Use air mattress *to prevent breakdown at pressure points*

     Use footboard or multipodus boots *to prevent foot-drop*

     Rub back *to stimulate circulation*

Anticipate and manage elimination needs

Help patient avoid constipation

     Encourage drinking fluids

     Use daily suppositories or stool softeners

Expected Outcomes

Self-care needs are met

Fluid and nutritional needs are met

Elimination needs are met

Skin, oral, and eye hygiene needs are met

▼Impaired physical mobility related to muscle weakness and wasting secondary to neuromuscular deterioration

Assess and document level of motor function

Consult with physiotherapist *to outline an appropriate exercise program*

Perform active or passive ROM exercises q4h to all extremities *to maintain joint mobility*

Apply necessary braces or splints *to support ankles and hands*

Apply soft cervical collar prn *to support neck muscles*

Turn q2h to 4h and apply air or foam mattress to bed if patient is confined to bed *to prevent skin breakdown and mobilize respiratory secretions*

Encourage ambulation to tolerance

Avoid strenuous exercise to prevent fatigue

Administer or supervise physical therapy as ordered: massage and stretching exercises

Maintain planned rest periods

Test muscular strength of extremities q4h and prn

Expected Outcomes

Maintains full ROM to affected limbs

Motor function is optimized

Demonstrates use of support devices

▼Powerlessness related to perceived and/or actual lack of control over body function

Assess feelings and perceptions of physical deterioration

Assess expressions of dissatisfaction and frustration over inability to perform tasks

Provide emotional support; be aware that there is no cure

     Focus and support use of motor functions that still exist

     Encourage expression of feelings *to facilitate open communication*

Assist family and patient with accepting reality of progressive loss of bodily functions

Be supportive; encourage active listening and expression of feelings by patient and family members

Permit patient to participate in care as long as possible

Provide opportunity for patient and family to discuss issue of life-sustaining measures

Expected Outcomes

Experiences an increased sense of control over life situation and prescribed activities

Verbalizes feelings of increased control

Participates in decisions regarding physical care and activities

Additional Nursing Diagnoses to Consider

Ineffective breathing pattern related to neuromuscular degeneration

Impaired verbal communication

Risk for injury/trauma

PATIENT/FAMILY TEACHING

Assess level of understanding regarding disease

Reinforce physician's explanation of disease, symptoms, progression, and management

Emphasize that although activity is impaired, cognitive processes are not affected

Emphasize importance of verbalization of feelings about progressive muscular wasting and weakness

Emphasize need to discuss feelings about the following:

Excessive salivation

Weakening voice, hoarseness

Dysphagia

Life-support issues (e.g., mechanical ventilation)

Emphasize need for family to encourage active participation in family activities

Demonstrate use of electrolarynx to facilitate vocalization as tolerated

Discuss need to develop alternative methods of communication when voice becomes nonfunctional: use of eyes and eyelid blinking

Explain importance of ongoing outpatient care and physician's visits

Explain need for oral suctioning as disease progresses

Explain need for oral hygiene q2h to 4h and prn

Have tissues easily accessible to patient

Have patient use bib while eating

Clean corners of mouth after eating and prn

Provide educational resources:

Amyotrophic Lateral Sclerosis Association (1-800-782-4747)

DISCHARGE/HOME CARE PLANNING

Activities

Discuss use of braces, splints, and/or cervical collars as indicated for support of hands, ankles, and neck to increase self-care activities

Maintain gait-retraining program

Maintain regular exercise program to tolerance

Maintain planned rest periods

Maintain home physical therapy

Encourage ambulation to tolerance

Stress the importance and proper use of wheelchair, cane, walker, raised toilet seat

Assist family to learn ways of adapting the home for accessibility

Explain need to avoid strenuous exercise/activity

Explain need to perform ROM activities as tolerated

Discuss agencies available for use as resources

Explain importance of providing skin care frequently, turning patient q2h to 4h to alternate potential pressure areas

Explain need to provide for and anticipate elimination needs

Encourage regular coughing and deep breathing exercises

Perform regular percussion and chest vibration *to mobilize secretions*

Provide diversions/recreation:

Radio

Book recordings

Videos/television

Diet

Explain need for high-calorie, high-protein, soft diet as tolerated; assess swallowing reflex before feeding

Assist patient in dealing with problems of swallowing

Place puréed foods on posterior aspect of tongue

Cut foods for patient

Use wrist and hand braces

May need to consider nasogastric or gastrostomy feedings

Offer small, frequent feedings

Instruct patient to swallow slowly to prevent aspiration

Administer oral hygiene before and after meals

Administer tube feedings as ordered if patient is unable to take oral nutrition

Check tube feedings q4h or as ordered

Elevate head of bed during tube feeding administration

Elimination

Encourage fluid intake to 2000 ml/day unless contraindicated

Avoid constipation

Encourage fluid intake

Use stool softeners or suppositories as ordered

Maintain urinary elimination program

Perform intermittent catheterization

Provide regular hygiene care for indwelling catheter

General instructions

Encourage expression of emotions about changing body functions

Direct care to permit for maximal participation by the patient

Modify activities, diet, and care as symptoms increase

Maintain social interactions with family and friends

■ GUILLAIN-BARRÉ SYNDROME (ACUTE INFECTIOUS POLYNEURITIS; POLYRADICULITIS)

A neurologic syndrome of acute ascending paralysis; etiology is unknown, but syndrome generally follows a recent infection; onset is rapid, and symptoms are generally reversible; characterized by widespread inflammation and demyelination of ascending or descending nerves in the peripheral nervous system (Fig. 9-15)

ASSESSMENT

SUBJECTIVE DATA

Symmetric muscular weakness of lower extremities, progressive to arms, trunk, head, and face

Dyspnea

Ascending paresthesia, pain, paralysis

OBJECTIVE DATA

Paralysis of upper extremities may be partial, or complete quadriplegia may develop

Absent or diminished deep tendon reflexes

Unstable BP: hypertension (during acute phase)

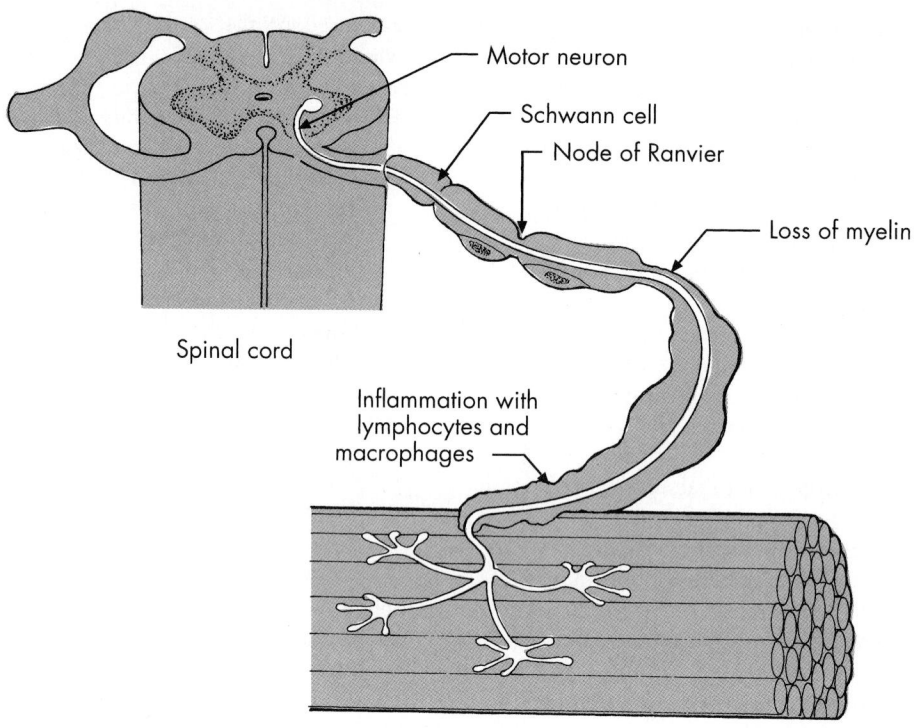

Fig. 9-15 Demyelination of nerve segments in Guillain-Barré syndrome. *(From Chipps E et al: Mosby's clinical nursing series: neurologic disorders, St Louis, 1992, Mosby.)*

Postural hypotension
Sinus tachycardia, bradycardia
Choking, tachypnea
Decreased or absent breath sounds
Dysphagia, difficulty in swallowing
Speech impairment
Low-grade fever
Urinary retention or infection

DIAGNOSTIC TESTS
Lumbar puncture: CSF
    Increased protein concentration
    Normal WBC
Electromyography
Nerve conduction studies
Pulmonary function tests

POTENTIAL COMPLICATIONS
Autonomic dysfunction
    Postural hypotension
    ECG changes: dysrhythmias
    Urinary, bowel incontinence
Aspiration, atelectasis
Respiratory failure
    Decreased V_T
    Hypercapnia
Respiratory arrest
Neuromuscular deficit
    Atrophy
    Contractures

Infection: sepsis
Cardiac failure
Venous thrombosis
Pulmonary embolus
SIADH

MULTIDISCIPLINARY MANAGEMENT
    THERAPEUTIC MANAGEMENT
Endotracheal intubation; tracheostomy
Oxygen/mechanical ventilation
Serial ABGs
Chest physiotherapy
Respiratory therapy consultation
Physical and/or occupational therapy
Speech therapy
Medications
    Antibiotics
    Immunosuppressive agents
    Prophylactic antibiotics
    Analgesics (not opiates)
    Anticoagulant agents
    Pituitary hormones
Bed rest; monitoring of muscular strength
Percutaneous endoscopic gastrostomy tube to provide
    route for nutrition
Cardiac monitoring: hemodynamic monitoring
Plasmapheresis
Bowel and bladder management
Social services

PATIENT PROBLEMS—NURSING DIAGNOSES/INTERVENTIONS

▼Ineffective breathing pattern related to neuromuscular impairment (ascending paralysis)

Assess respiratory function noting rate, depth, and pattern q1h to 2h and prn

Maintain patent airway, neck in neutral position

Administer oxygen, humidification, and assisted ventilation as ordered *to increase oxygenation and decrease work of breathing*

Assess and monitor V_T and VC

Provide tracheostomy care if indicated (p. 278)

Monitor closely for signs of impending respiratory failure; do not leave patient unattended during periods of respiratory distress

Auscultate chest q2h to 4h *to detect adventitious breath sounds*

Elevate head of bed 30 degrees

Maintain body alignment and position *to increase comfort and maximize respiratory effort*

Monitor peripheral oxygenation with pulse oximetry q1h to 2h and prn

Monitor vital signs with neurologic signs q1h to 2h and prn for change

Test muscular strength q4h to 8h *to establish baseline and monitor for changes*

Maintain patent airway; suction oropharynx q2h and prn

Suction prn: hyperoxygenate with 100% O_2 before and after suctioning; suction <15 seconds

Assist and teach coughing and deep breathing as appropriate

Keep intubation equipment and mechanical ventilator available in acute phase

Expected Outcomes

Demonstrates effective breathing pattern and patent airway

Chest expansion is symmetric

Breath sounds are clear to auscultation

ABGs and vital signs are within normal limits

No signs of respiratory distress

▼Sensory/perceptual alterations related to neuromuscular paralysis and paresthesia: tactile, communication, visual

Assess and monitor signs of sensory alterations: inability to differentiate hot and cold, dull and sharp

Record changes/improvement daily

Establish and maintain means of communication

　Call bell within reach *to increase patient's feelings of security*

　Magic Slate, pad and pencil, or word board at bedside

Administer eye care q2h to 4h; remove crusts, apply eye shields, and administer artificial tears *to prevent corneal ulceration*

Provide prescription eyeglasses: optometry consult if needed

Administer analgesics as indicated

Assist patient to differentiate tactile sensations: hot or cold

Protect patient from injury

　Test bath water and foods for appropriate temperature

　Keep all sharp objects out of reach

　Assist patient to turn q2h; observe for pressure points

Expected Outcomes

Demonstrates increase in sensory stimulation

Sustains no injuries

Able to communicate needs

▼Impaired physical mobility related to progressive weakness and paresthesia secondary to neuromuscular disease

Assess and document degree of functional ability

Maintain bed rest; place patient in position of comfort

Support extremities with pillows and footboards or multipodus boots *to prevent edema and foot-drop*

Change position q2h to 4h; administer skin care q2h to 4h as indicated *to prevent skin breakdown*

Apply air or foam mattress to bed

Perform passive ROM exercises to all extremities

Increase frequency of nursing functions as patient's condition requires

Monitor for signs of thrombophlebitis

Encourage ambulation as tolerated

　Begin by having patient sit on bedside with support, progressing to chair bid to tid

　Later have patient walk in room or hall for 15 min qid

Administer analgesics as indicated

Administer anticoagulants as ordered

Consult with physical therapy department for structured exercise program

Maintain planned rest periods

Apply antiembolic stockings

Maintain aspiration precautions, especially during eating

Expected Outcomes

Experiences optimal level of mobility

Performs passive and active ROM exercises

No complications related to immobility (e.g., contractures, pressure sores)

▼Altered nutrition: less than body requirements related to neuromuscular weakness

Assess and record ability to chew, swallow, and cough on daily basis *to prevent aspiration*

Monitor daily caloric intake

Consult with dietitian as indicated

Weigh patient daily *to establish baseline and detect any potential deleterious changes*

Administer diet as tolerated; progress from soft to solid foods

Offer frequent, small feedings

Supplement feedings with high-calorie, high-protein fluids such as eggnog and milkshakes

Administer enteral feedings as indicated

Encourage fluids to 2000 ml/day unless contraindicated

Maintain parenteral fluids as indicated and ordered *to maintain hydration status*

Expected Outcomes

Nutritional and fluid needs are met

Weight is maintained or increased

▼Powerlessness related to perceived/actual loss of body function imposed by progressive physical deterioration

Assess feelings of frustration, anxiety, and fear over loss of body function

Provide emotional support, thorough explanations, and reassurance

Be alert to emotional changes and mood swings

Encourage patient's expression of needs and feelings

Encourage participation in self-care activities *to facilitate in increasing self-esteem*

Support and focus on existing body function (eating, dressing, shaving) as indicated

Consult and provide physical, occupational, and psychosocial support

Expected Outcomes

Feels in control of or participates in as many routine activities as possible

Participates in decision making and activities related to care

Identifies need areas

Participates in self-care

Participates in diversional activities

Optimal communication is established

Additional Nursing Diagnoses to Consider

Functional incontinence

Altered urinary elimination

Risk for injury

PATIENT/FAMILY TEACHING

Ensure that patient and/or significant other understands that recovery may take up to 1 year or longer

Stress importance of dealing with body image changes and fears of permanent disability, loss of function, and dying

Explain to family the following:

Need to encourage verbalization

Need to encourage independence and socialization

Need to encourage self-care as a strategy for health maintenance

Importance of allowing patient to take meals with family

Discuss medications: name, dosage, frequency of administration, purpose, and side effects

Explain need to avoid over-the-counter medications without physician approval

Stress need to avoid individuals with infections, especially URIs

Encourage diversional activities: TV, reading, radio, book recordings

Discuss alternative methods of communication as patient condition changes (e.g., word board, hand signals)

DISCHARGE/HOME CARE PLANNING

Activity

Alert patient to change positions slowly to minimize orthostatic changes in BP

Stress the importance and proper use of mobility devices (wheelchair, cane, walker) to patient/family

Assist family to identify local community agencies that can help in providing such devices

Assist family to learn ways of adapting the home for accessibility

Stress the need for initial home health referral to do the following:

Teach family members proper body mechanics and how to protect their backs

Assist in learning safety measures *to prevent falling*

Implement safety measures such as side rails, and ramps, raised toilet seats

Maintain regular exercise program with planned rest periods; perform regular passive ROM exercises to all extremities if patient is unable to exercise

Encourage maximal participation in self-care activities

Maintain home physical therapy program if indicated

Provide regular skin care to promote circulation

Use warm baths to alleviate/minimize stiffness and discomfort

Diet

Maintain high-calorie, high-protein, regular or soft diet as tolerated

Assess swallowing reflex before feeding/meals

Modify diet if swallowing reflex diminishes

Supplement diet with small, additional, high-calorie, high-protein snacks

Encourage fluid intake to 2000 ml/day unless contraindicated

Monitor intake and output

Weigh patient weekly

Obtain home nutrition referral

Maintain bowel and bladder programs

General information

Encourage emotional expressions of anxiety, frustrations, and fears

Maintain focus on remaining body functions

■ NEUROLOGIC INFECTIONS

Conditions in which a microorganism has gained entry into the body, producing a reaction, brain abscess, or meningitis

brain abscess: *Secondary to systemic infections or may be introduced through trauma; results in space-occupying lesions causing a potential for increased ICP*

meningitis: *Infection of the meninges, causing inflammatory reaction in the pia-arachnoid membrane; may be caused by bacteria or virus (acute aseptic meningitis)*

encephalitis: *Infection of the brain parenchyma*

ASSESSMENT

(NOTE: See Box 9-9 for specific findings)

SUBJECTIVE DATA

Headache
Diplopia
Malaise
Anorexia

OBJECTIVE DATA

History of recent URI, sinus or ear infection, penetrating trauma, or basal skull fracture
Elevated temperature
Meningeal irritation
  Nuchal rigidity
  Positive Kernig and Brudzinski signs
  Photophobia
Altered LOC: irritability, disorientation to coma
Vomiting
Cranial nerve dysfunction (III, IV, VI, VII, VIII)
  Ocular palsies
  Facial paresis
Deafness
Vertigo
Seizures: focal, generalized

DIAGNOSTIC TESTS

Lumbar puncture (contraindicated if increased ICP is suspected): CSF
  Protein level and pressure
  Glucose level
Serum blood, urine, stool cultures *to identify source of pathogenic organism*
CBC with differential
EEG
CT scan (serial)
MRI
X-ray examination
  Chest
  Skull
  Sinus
Brain tissue biopsy

POTENTIAL COMPLICATIONS

Increased ICP
Seizures
Neurologic deficit: paresis
Hydrocephalus
Herniation
Altered mentation
Pneumonia
Respiratory failure
Sepsis

Box 9-9	**Specific Findings Associated With Bacterial Meningitis, Viral Encephalitis, Brain Abscess**

BACTERIAL MENINGITIS	**VIRAL ENCEPHALITIS**	**BRAIN ABSCESS**
Elevated temperature (101° to 103° F [38° to 39.5° C])	Altered LOC	**Acute**
Altered LOC	Aphasia	Chills and fever
Memory loss, disorientation to delirium to coma	Hemiparesis	Confusion
	Ataxia	Drowsiness
Meningeal irritation	Nystagmus	Seizures: local or generalized
Oligenia	Ocular paralysis	Motor or sensory deficits
Muscle hepatoma, flaccid paralysis	Facial weakness	
Deafness		**Second Stage**
Petechial hemorrhage		Headache, recurrent and severe
Increased ICP		Confusion to stupor
		Increased ICP
DIAGNOSTIC TESTS		
CSF	CSF	CSF
Turbid	Increased WBC with mononuclear cells	Increased WBC (lymphocytes)
Increased WBC	Increased (slightly) protein	Increased (high) protein
Increased protein	Normal glucose	Normal glucose
Decreased glucose		Elevated CSF pressure
Elevated CSF pressure (>180 mm H$_2$O)		(200-300 mm H$_2$O)

MULTIDISCIPLINARY MANAGEMENT
THERAPEUTIC MANAGEMENT
Institutional protocol for isolation or infection control as indicated by organism (identified)

Medications
  Antibiotic therapy specific to the organism
  Antiviral therapy
  Analgesics
  Glucocorticosteroids
  Anticonvulsants
  Antipyretics
Respiratory therapy
Ventilatory/oxygenation support
ICP monitoring
Fluid/electrolyte therapy
Serial CT scans
Temperature control/hypothermia
Bowel/bladder management
Nutritional support
Physical therapy
Stereotactic-guided drainage of abscess

PATIENT PROBLEMS—NURSING DIAGNOSES/INTERVENTIONS

▼Ineffective thermoregulation related to infectious process

Monitor temperature q2h to 4h or as indicated
Administer antipyretic medications as ordered
Maintain room temperature to 68° F or 20° C
Initiate cooling measures as indicated
  Give tepid sponge bath
  Remove excess bed linens
  Use hypothermia blanket
Encourage fluid intake
Monitor WBC as ordered

Expected Outcome
Normothermic; temperature is 98.6° F or 37° C

▼Pain: headache related to cerebral tissue irritation

Maintain quiet environment; darken room if photophobia occurs
Maintain bed rest; assist patient in assuming position of comfort
Administer analgesics as ordered; monitor neurologic status
Administer comfort measures
  Elevate head of bed 30 degrees
  Put cool cloth over eyes
  Apply ice cap to head

Expected Outcomes
Verbalizes absence of or improved headache
Appears to be resting quietly

▼Ineffective breathing pattern related to increased ICP and depressed cerebral functioning

Assess and monitor respirations: rate, depth, and breathing pattern
Assess respiratory status q1h to 2h as indicated
Auscultate breath sounds
Monitor pulse oximetry *to assess peripheral oxygenation*
Monitor serial ABGs as ordered
Administer oxygen/ventilatory support as ordered
Position patient for optimal ventilation
Assist and instruct patient to turn and deep breathe q2h to 4h
Maintain patent airway
Suction prn; hyperoxygenate with supplemental 100% O_2 before and after suctioning; suction <15 seconds
Check BP, P, R, and LOC to indicate neurologic and respiratory stability
Maintain aspiration precautions

Expected Outcomes
Demonstrates effective breathing pattern
Chest expansion is symmetric
Breath sounds are clear to auscultation
ABGs and vital signs are within normal limits
No signs of respiratory distress

Additional Nursing Diagnoses to Consider
Impaired physical mobility
Sensory/perceptual alterations

PATIENT/FAMILY TEACHING
Discuss medications: name, dosage, frequency of administration, purpose, side effects, and toxic effects
Explain need to avoid taking over-the-counter medications without consulting physician
Explain to family need to encourage verbalization; help patient understand nature of disorder
Discuss symptoms of progression of condition to report to physician
Explain importance of ongoing outpatient care
Explain isolation protocols as indicated for specific organism

DISCHARGE/HOME CARE PLANNING
Activity
  Encourage self-care to tolerance
  Maintain regular exercise program with planned rest periods
  Report and record any seizure activity
  Maintain seizure precautions
  Assist patient to cough and deep breathe regularly
  Encourage ambulation to tolerance
  Maintain home physical therapy program if indicated
Diet
  Encourage fluid intake to 2000 ml/day unless contraindicated
  Monitor intake and output
  Weigh weekly
  Maintain well-balanced diet

General instructions
    Report any temperature elevations
    Administer antipyretics as ordered
    Administer antibiotics until all medication has been
       taken
Monitor stools for occult blood if glucocorticosteroid
    therapy is continued at home
Report any new or increased neurologic deficits

■ SUBSTANCE ABUSE (DRUG ABUSE AND ALCOHOL INTOXICATION)

NOTE: Care of the intoxicated patient will depend on the amount and type of drug ingested (Box 9-10) and on the effect it has on other organ systems (e.g., respiratory, hepatic); for severe drug overdose or intoxication refer to Care of patient with altered consciousness, shock syndrome, respiratory failure, and seizures

■ ALCOHOL INTOXICATION

ASSESSMENT
SUBJECTIVE DATA
Weakness
Confusion
Anxiety
Nausea, vomiting
Loss of appetite

OBJECTIVE DATA
Acute intoxication
    Confusion
    Slurred speech
    Ataxia
    Depressed deep tendon reflexes
    Nystagmus
    Anxiety, restlessness
    Dilated pupils
    Stupor
    Coma
    Gastric irritation: vomiting
Withdrawal
    Anxiety
    Tremors
    Diaphoresis
    Nausea, vomiting
    Anorexia
    Confusion
    Moroseness
    Confabulation
    Delirium tremens
    Seizure activity
    Uncontrolled rage
    Hallucination
    Insomnia
    Toxic psychosis
Chronic intoxication
    Mental confusion

Box 9-10	**Drugs Commonly Abused**

NARCOTICS Opium Heroin (horse, smack) Oxycodone Codeine Methadone Hydromorphone (Dilaudid) Meperidine (Demerol) Morphine **HALLUCINOGENS** LSD (acid) Mescaline DMT Scopolamine Atropine Phencyclidine: PCP (angel dust, crystal, dust mist, peace pill, superweed) Psilocybin Peyote **ORGANIC SOLVENTS** Glue Cleaning fluid Paint thinner Freons Marker pens	**DEPRESSANTS/SEDATIVES** Alcohol Barbiturates Meprobamate Chloral hydrate Glutethimide (Doriden) Quaaludes Benzodiazepines (Valium, Dalmane, Xanax) **STIMULANTS** Cocaine (coke, rock, crack) Amphetamines Methamphetamine (crank) Methylphenidate (Ritalin) **CANNABIS** Marijuana (grass, weed, joints) Hashish (weed oil, hash)

Cerebellar degeneration
   Ataxic gait
   Nystagmus
   Dysarthric speech
  Nutritional deficiencies
  Myopathy
  Hepatic coma
Seizure disorders
Marchiafava-Bignami syndrome (progressive organic dementia)
Wernicke's syndrome
  Ophthalmoplegia
  Apathy, apprehension
  Confusion
  Coma
Korsakoff's syndrome
  Disorientation to time and place
  Peripheral neuropathy
  Confabulation

DIAGNOSTIC TESTS

Serum ETOH (see Table 9-21)
Serum chemistries
CT scan (to screen for head trauma [e.g., subdural hematoma])

POTENTIAL COMPLICATIONS

Aspiration
Hypertension
Severe stages
  Hypoventilation
  Hypotension
  Hypothermia
  GI hemorrhage
  Myocardial infarction (MI)
  Hepatic failure
  Metabolic encephalopathy

MULTIDISCIPLINARY MANAGEMENT
THERAPEUTIC MANAGEMENT

Acute
  Ventilatory, airway, and oxygenation support and management

Fluid/electrolyte therapy
Respiratory therapy
Nutritional consultation
Social services
Medications during withdrawal
  Antianxiety
   Chlordiazepoxide (Librium)
  Phenothiazines
  Tranquilizers
  Barbiturates
  Anticonvulsants
  Thiamine, folate
Seizure precautions

PATIENT PROBLEMS—NURSING DIAGNOSES/INTERVENTIONS

▼ Ineffective breathing pattern (potential) related to CNS depression

Maintain patent airway; assisted ventilation as indicated
See Coma and Impaired consciousness (p. 520) and Respiratory failure (p. 268)
Position to optimize respiratory excursion, airway patency, and secretion removal
Monitor BP, P, and R q2h to 4h and prn
Provide oropharyngeal or nasopharyngeal tube as indicated to maintain patent airway
Suction prn: hyperoxygenate with 100% O_2 before and after suctioning; suction <15 seconds
Auscultate breath sounds prn to detect adventitious breath sounds
Provide oxygenation/respiratory therapy
Monitor serial ABGs as indicated
Avoid use of sedatives, which may potentiate effects of alcohol
Provide soft restraints as indicated to protect patient from self-injury
Maintain aspiration precautions

Expected Outcomes

Demonstrates effective breathing pattern and patent airway
Chest expansion is symmetric
Breath sounds are clear to auscultation
ABGs and vital signs are within normal limits
No signs of respiratory distress

▼ Ineffective individual coping related to inadequate coping methods

Maintain quiet, supportive environment; avoid punitive approach
Maintain safety precautions for anxious and restless patients
Provide supportive counseling services to patient when receptive
Ensure that patient and/or significant other is knowledgeable about effects of alcohol abuse

Table 9-21	Serum Alcohol Levels	
Serum Alcohol Levels	**Effects**
Mild: 0.5 to 1.5 mg/ml	Muscular uncoordination, personality changes: talkative, morose, noisy
Moderate: 1.5 to 3 mg/ml	Marked ataxia, mental impairment, uncoordination, prolonged reaction time, nausea, vomiting, diplopia
Severe: 3 to 5 mg/ml	Dysarthria, amnesia, hypothermia, hypoventilation, coma

Expected Outcomes

Demonstrates effective coping strategies

Discusses effects of alcohol abuse

Attends counseling/educational support groups

Additional Nursing Diagnoses to Consider

Sensory/perceptual alterations

Altered family proceses

▌ CHEMICAL SUBSTANCE ABUSE

Intermittent or chronic use of stimulants or depressants resulting in alterations in mental and physiologic function

NOTE:*Level of intoxication and signs/symptoms depend on amount of substance ingested, route, prior history of abuse, and whether the substance was mixed with another drug (e.g., PCP mixed with marijauna). Signs/symptoms are primarily cardiopulmonary and CNS manifestations. Refer to Chapters 3, Cardiovascular System, and Chapter 5, Respiratory System, for management of specific alterations in these systems (e.g., cardiac dysrhythmias secondary to cocaine abuse or respiratory insufficiency related to sedative overdose)*

ASSESSMENT

SUBJECTIVE AND OBJECTIVE DATA
Depressants: Narcotics, Opiates*

LOC

  Impaired intellectual function

  Lethargy

  Apathy

  Withdrawal

  Euphoria

  Coma

Airway obstruction

Dysarthria

Stridor

Decreased BP

Tachycardia or bradycardia

Pupillary changes

  Pinpoint (opiates)

  Dilated (barbiturates)

Depressed gag and swallow reflexes

Respiratory distress, respiratory rate <8/min or
  >30/min

Seizure activity

Hypothermia

Method of administration

  Oral

  Subcutaneous:"skin popping"

  Nasal insufflation:"snorting"

  Intravenous

Signs of withdrawal

  Abdominal and muscular pain

  Severe cramping

  Insomnia

Refers to all drugs that possess some morphine-like activity.

Hallucinogens, Stimulants

Anxiety progressing to pain

Paranoid reaction

Combativeness progressing to violence

Insomnia

Hallucinations

  Auditory

  Visual

Grand mal seizures

Rapid speech

Confusion

Ataxia

Depression: mild to severe

Suicidal tendencies

Anorexia

Nausea

Headache

Elevated BP

Elevated temperature

Tachycardia, palpitations

Hypertension progressing to crisis

Pupillary changes: dilated

Photophobia

Diplopia

Horizontal and vertical nystagmus

Hot flashes

ECG changes

  Dysrhythmias

  ST-T wave changes

Decreased urine output

LSD, Mescaline

Hyperactivity

Pupil dilation

Increased vital signs

Low doses: euphoria

High doses: hallucinatory psychosis

PCP: "Angel Dust"

Low-to-moderate doses: effect begins within 5 minutes
  and peaks within 30 to 60 minutes

  Elevated systolic and diastolic pressures

  Tachycardia

  Increased deep tendon reflexes

  Small pupils

  Nystagmus: horizontal and vertical (persists for
    4 days)

  Tremors, clonus

  Muscle rigidity

  Euphoria

  Amnesia

  Agitation, violent outbursts

  Image distortion

  Illusions of superhuman strength

  Increased urine output

High doses

  Slurred speech

  Drowsiness

  Depressed deep tendon reflexes

Seizures
Opisthotonos
Bradypnea
Decreased BP
Disordered thought processes, hallucinations
Coma

DIAGNOSTIC TESTS

Serum chemistries and toxicology screening
Urine toxicology screening
ABGs
ECG
Chest x-ray

MULTIDISCIPLINARY MANAGEMENT
THERAPEUTIC MANAGEMENT

Depressants
  Respiratory support with oxygenation or ventilation
  Fluid/electrolyte therapy
  Emetics
  Gastric lavage
  Activated charcoal for ingested opiates
  Naloxone for opioid overdose
  Peritoneal dialysis
  Vitamins
Stimulants
  Decreased external stimuli
  Medications
    General
      Barbiturates, phenothiazines
      Sedatives, anticonvulsants
      Vitamins
    For LSD, mescaline
      Diazepam (oral)
      Avoid phenothiazine, which may potentiate
        psychotic action
    For PCP
      Haloperidol
      Diazepam
      Activated charcoal (high doses)
      Acidify urine; increase diuresis
    Parenteral fluids
    Gastric suction for PCP
Nutritional support and concentration
Psychiatric liaison
Social services
Suicide precautions if indicated

PATIENT PROBLEMS—NURSING DIAGNOSES/INTERVENTIONS

If patient arrives in coma refer to p. 520. If patient arrives in respiratory failure, refer to p. 268
Assess respirations q2h to 4h, noting rate, quality, and depth *to detect adventitious breath sounds*
Assess LOC and monitor q2h to 4h
Report any changes in consciousness or vital signs to physician to prevent further decline in neurologic status

Administer parenteral fluids as ordered *to maintain adequate hydration and electrolyte balance*
Understand that peritoneal dialysis may be indicated for long-acting barbiturates
Obtain accurate and detailed history regarding drug ingested: type, amount, time of ingestion, method of administration
Administer emetics as ordered; contraindicated in presence of depressed gag reflex, seizures, or coma
Administer gastric lavage as ordered (within 2 hours of ingestion); endotracheal tube is usually inserted before lavage in comatose patient
Provide patient with positive reassurance about condition; avoid punitive approach
Be firm, patient, and understanding
Administer medication as ordered: naloxone (Narcan) for opiate overdose; effects can be noted within 1 to 2 minutes if given intravenously
Give activated charcoal orally for ingested opiates
Check BP and P on admission and q4h as indicated by condition
Assist patient to monitor cardiac status for dysrhythmias
Assist patient to meet self-care needs as indicated

Expected Outcomes

Demonstrates effective breathing pattern
Chest expansion is symmetric
Breath sounds are clear to auscultation
ABGs and vital signs are within normal limits

▼ Risk for violence self-directed or directed at others related to drug toxicity

Admit to private room when possible
Decrease external stimuli
  Use low lighting
  Avoid loud voices and rapid movements *to minimize further agitation*
NOTE: Administration of the following care may heighten patient's paranoid state and cause increased agitation; approach patient quietly, using friend to assist if required
Allow friend or family member to remain in room during all procedures to assist in "talking down"
Provide patient with support, reassurance, and reality-defining information
Instruct patient to avoid trying to differentiate between real perceptions and effects of drug; remind patient that effects of drug will end
Avoid mechanical restraints if possible
Approach cautiously; avoid whispering to others
Explain all procedures; allow same person to care for patient at all times *to provide consistent approach in interactions and care*
Administer medications as ordered
Avoid phenothiazine (may potentiate effect or produce anticholinergic crisis)
Administer parenteral fluids as ordered
Monitor BP, P, and R q2h to 4h or as indicated by level of consciousness

Expected Outcome
Demonstrates calm and nondestructive behavior
Does not experience accidental or intentional self-injury

Additional Nursing Diagnoses to Consider
Withdrawal related to decreased intake of drug/alcohol after long-term use
Ineffective individual coping related to chemical substance abuse
Altered nutrition: less than body requirements related to chronically poor dietary intake
Self-care deficit related to depressed mood or altered reality orientation
Altered family processes related to dysfunctional family relationships

PATIENT/FAMILY TEACHING
Explore patient's willingness to participate in self-help and support group experiences
Provide supportive, nonjudgmental approach to patient
Provide opportunity for participation in counseling and group support

DISCHARGE/HOME CARE PLANNING
Consult social services if further assessment needed of home environment (e.g., care of minor children, elderly)

■ INTRACRANIAL SURGERY
Surgical repair of conditions involving the brain
craniotomy: *Surgical revision, resection, or removal of growths or abnormalities within the cranium; consists of removing and replacing bones of the skull to provide access to intracranial structures*
　　craniectomy: *Removal of a portion of the skull; includes burr hole performance*
　　NOTE: *For preoperative assessment, nursing management, and patient/family teaching, refer to the specific condition requiring surgery (e.g., Brain Tumors)*

ASSESSMENT
POSTOPERATIVE SUBJECTIVE AND OBJECTIVE DATA
LOC; see Glasgow Coma Scale for rapid assessment (see Table 9-2)
Pupillary response; ocular movement
Cranial nerves III through XII
Visual disturbances
Periocular edema
Focal neurologic deficits
Pain: headache
Personality changes
Respirations: rate, pattern
Motor-sensory function
　　Paresthesia
　　Paralysis
Signs of increased ICP

POSTOPERATIVE DIAGNOSTIC TESTS
Blood
　　CBC
　　Electrolytes, glucose
　　Creatinine
　　Osmolarity
Imaging
　　CT scan
　　Transcranial Doppler, cranial blood flow studies

POTENTIAL COMPLICATIONS
Seizure activity
Increased ICP
Diabetes insipidus
Hemorrhage
Infection of bone graft
Cardiac dysrhythmias
Meningitis
Thrombophlebitis
ARDS
Permanent or transient loss of motor, sensory, and/or cranial nerve function

MULTIDISCIPLINARY MANAGEMENT
THERAPEUTIC MANAGEMENT
Oxygenation/ventilatory support
Medications
　　Corticosteroids
　　Anticonvulsants
　　Antiemetics
　　Antipyretics
　　Analgesics
　　Diuretics
　　Antibiotics
　　Antacids
　　Histamine-blocking agents
　　Stool softeners
Parenteral therapy
Diet
ICP monitoring
Cardiac/hemodynamic monitoring
Physical therapy

PATIENT PROBLEMS—NURSING DIAGNOSES/INTERVENTIONS

▼Ineffective breathing pattern related to sensori-motor depression

Maintain NPO status until cough/gag reflexes return *to prevent aspiration*
Assess spontaneous respiratory function: monitor rate, quality, and depth of respirations
See Care of patient in recovery room (p. 10)
Maintain patent airway
　　Maintain neck in neutral position
　　Position on side with head of bed elevated 30 degrees
Monitor CBC *to determine amount of Hgb available to carry oxygen and to detect inflammation or infection*

Immediately report any change in vital signs, LOC, or restlessness

Administer oxygen with assisted ventilation as ordered

Monitor serial ABGs to determine acid-base balance

Maintain parenteral therapy as indicated *to maintain adequate hydration*

Assess ventilatory status

    Auscultate chest for breath sounds q1h to 2h and prn *to detect adventitious breath sounds*

    Maintain optimal positioning *to promote ventilatory status and mobilize secretions*

    Assist and teach patient to turn and deep breathe q2h *to prevent atelectasis*

Expected Outcomes

Demonstrates effective breathing pattern

Chest expansion is symmetric

Breath sounds are clear to auscultation

ABGs and vital signs are within normal limits

No signs of respiratory distress

▼ Altered cerebral/peripheral tissue perfusion related to interruption of arterial flow

Maintain bed rest with head of bed elevated 15 to 30 degrees or as ordered

Check BP, P, and R and do neurologic check q15min to 30min

Monitor ICP and report sustained elevations or trends to elevation immediately *to minimize risks of cerebral ischemia and brain herniation*

Report immediately any sudden changes in BP, pupillary or neurologic status, numbness, tingling, weakness, or loss of pulses

Assess for restlessness and seizure activity

Check rectal temperature q2h to 4h; hypothermia or cooling measures may be indicated

Monitor oxygen saturation *to determine adequacy of ventilation and oxygenation*

Maintain parenteral fluids as ordered to support hydration

Maintain bed rest; use firm mattress or bedboard

Provide cervical collar or traction as ordered

Keep head in neutral or slightly flexed position *to maintain patent airway*

Observe skin color and peripheral pulse *to monitor adequacy of peripheral circulation*

Expected Outcomes

Alert and oriented

Maintains adequate tissue perfusion

Cognitive processes are intact

Evidences sensory-motor integrity

▼ Self-care deficit: feeding, hygiene, toileting, and/or mobility related to physical postoperative limitations

Assess degree of functional disability

Maintain proper positioning as indicated by surgical restrictions

Limit activities and perform nursing functions as indicated

Maintain quiet environment to decrease stressors

Administer skin care q4h to 5h *to prevent breakdown*

    Give back rubs *to increase circulation and comfort*

    Use air mattress (for patient in traction)

Check for redness, irritation, and pressure areas q2h to 4h when patient is in traction *to prevent skin breakdown*

Provide additional padding and pressure reduction if indicated *to prevent skin breakdown*

Keep skin dry

Meet all physical hygiene needs as indicated

Provide passive or active ROM exercises to nonoperative extremities *to prevent contractures*

Maintain NPO status until otherwise ordered *to prevent aspiration*

Provide fluids and/or diet within restrictions as ordered; assess for swallowing and chewing ability

Maintain adequate elimination *to prevent constipation*

    Initiate voiding measures as appropriate

    Monitor time and amount

Expected Outcomes

Self-care needs are met

Medications are administered as ordered

Fluid and nutritional needs are met

Elimination needs are met

Skin, oral, and eye hygiene needs are met

Passive or active ROM exercises are performed

Planned rest periods are maintained

PATIENT/FAMILY TEACHING

Assess cognitive and motor skills; assess level of understanding regarding diagnosis and prescribed treatment

Explain nature of disorder, symptoms, and importance of maintaining traction, corset, or braces at home

Explain to family need to encourage verbalization to deal with body image changes and anxieties over disability and loss of work

Teach principles of body mechanics

    Avoid bending from waist: keep back straight, bend knees, and lower body to pick up objects

    Use straight, flat chairs; avoid soft-cushioned chairs

    Avoid crossing knees

    Avoid lifting while back is flexed or twisted

Explain need to avoid constipation through use of stool softeners, mild laxatives, and/or fruit juices and roughage in diet

Explain need to avoid extremes of hot and cold to lower extremities because of possible sensory nerve loss

Explain need to avoid hyperextension of spine while sleeping, sleeping in prone position or straight supine position

Explain need to sleep on side with knees and hips in flexion

Explain need to wear corset or brace support as ordered

Explain need for exercise as ordered; instruct patient to stop exercises if pain is unrelieved or worsens

Explain importance of maintaining diet as ordered

Discuss medications: name, dosage, time of administration, purpose, and side effects
Explain need to avoid taking over-the-counter medications without physician approval
Explain importance of ongoing outpatient care
  Physician's visits
  Physical therapy
Ensure that patient and/or significant other demonstrates proper use and maintenance of traction and corsets

DISCHARGE/HOME CARE PLANNING
Activity
  Stress the importance and proper use of mobility devices (wheelchair, cane, walker) to patient/family
    Assist family to identify local community agencies that can help in providing such devices
    Assist family to learn ways of adapting the home for accessibility
    Stress the need for initial home health referral to
      Teach family members proper body mechanics and how to protect their backs
      Assist in learning safety measures to prevent falling
  Alert the patient to change positions slowly *to prevent postural changes in BP*
  Elevate head of bed if patient is still immobile
  Install side rails and ramps *to maintain patient safety*
  Monitor and report all seizure activity
  Institute seizure precautions as indicated
  Maintain regular exercise program with planned rest periods
  Initiate home physical therapy referral
Diet
  Maintain fluid intake of 2000 ml/day unless contraindicated
  Maintain well-balanced diet
  Monitor intake and output
  Administer oral hygiene as indicated
  Check stools for occult blood if steroids are being administered

General instructions
  Support and protect head
  Provide wound care to incision site
  Administer skin care to stimulate circulation and prevent skin breakdown
  Maintain quiet environment, reducing external stimuli to a minimum

■ STEREOTACTIC APPLICATIONS

Stereotactic *means pertaining to precise localization in the brain. Stereotactic applications are broadly applied to morphologic and functional procedures (Table 9-22)*

Stereotactic biopsy is performed under MRI guidance. Brain CT and MRI are requested. The stereotactic frame is attached to the patient's head under local anesthesia. Stereotactic biopsy is necessary for patients with intracranial lesions that cannot be removed safely or with multiple lesions without an etiologic diagnosis. The same principle applies to stereotactic cyst aspiration and abscess aspiration

Stereotactic radiosurgery is a technique designed to deliver a pinpoint dose of high-energy radiation to a targeted abnormality in the patient's brain while allowing only a low dose of radiation to be delivered to the surrounding normal brain tissue

Two types of stereotactic radiosurgery:

single-dose stereotactic radiosurgery: *patient receives a single high-dose radiation treatment*

fractionated stereotactic radiotherapy: *patient receives several lower-dose radiation treatments*

NOTE: *The patient receives either single-dose or fractionated radiosurgery based on the following criteria: (1) The maximum tolerance dose for various brain structures. If the lesion is situated near brain structures sensitive to radiation (e.g., cranial nerve II), fractionated radiosurgery is preferred because it minimizes risk of damage. (2) The location of the lesion*

Table 9-22	**Stereotactic Applications in Both Morphologic and Functional Procedures***		
Morphologic Procedures		**Functional Procedures**	
INTERVENTIONS	**INDICATIONS**	**INTERVENTIONS**	**INDICATIONS**
Stereotactic biopsy/aspiration	Diagnosis	Pallidotomy	Parkinson's disease
Stereotactic radiosurgery	Arteriovenous malformation (AVM), brain metastases, benign brain tumors, and primary malignant brain tumors	Thalamotomy	Parkinson's disease, tremor, dystonia
Stereotactic craniotomy	Deep-seated brain tumors	Depth electrode	Seizure
Interstitial radiation	Brain tumors	Deep brain stimulation	Parkinson's disease, tremor
		Internal capsule stimulation	Interrupt the pathways to control pain

Functional interventions are applied to interrupt functional pathways in brain; used in treatment of movement disorders, epilepsy, pain symptoms.

Box 9-11	**Patient Selection and Complications of Stereotactic Radiosurgery**

PATIENT SELECTION

The brain lesion is not greater than 30 mm in diameter.

Surgical resection has already been attempted and failed or is considered unsafe.

The lesion is in a deep-seated or functionally critical area of the brain.

COMPLICATIONS

Cerebral edema

Brain necrosis

Nausea/vomiting

Headache

Seizures

New neurologic deficits

Local hair loss

Pin site infections (The stereotactic ring is attached to the patient's head with four screws.)

For complications and patient selection of stereotactic radiosurgery (Box 9-11 Patient selection and complications of stereotactic radiosurgery)

PATIENT PROBLEMS—NURSING DIAGNOSES/INTERVENTIONS
Preprocedure

Explain the procedure to the patient

Introduce the therapists to the patient

Allow the patient to visit the treatment room

Make sure the patient is comfortable staying in an isolated room

Inform patients that they may experience temporary, local hair loss

Assure patients that nurses and therapists will monitor them during the procedure

     Patients wishing to stop the procedure for any reason need only wave their hands to get the nurses' attention

     Therapists will stop the radiation treatment and enter the room to see the patient

During the Procedure

Postpone procedure if patient is experiencing nausea or vomiting

     When vomiting, the patient is unable to turn his or her head because it is attached to the stereotactic ring and fixed to the table; respiratory tract obstruction or aspiration may result

Observe the patient for signs and symptoms of impaired airway clearance

Postprocedure
Pain

Inform patients that mild headache and pin site pain are common symptoms following radiosurgery

     Narcotics, such as Tylenol No. 3, will be prescribed

Cerebral tissue perfusion

Watch closely for development of new neurologic deficits

Instruct patients' families that it is essential to call their physicians if LOC changes

Inform patients of the importance of calling their physicians for severe persistent headache

Risk of infection

Instruct patients to watch the pin sites for redness, discharge, and swelling

Instruct patients to monitor their body temperature

Other nursing managements are as for patients undergoing stereotactic craniotomy

■ GENERAL REHABILITATIVE CARE OF NEUROLOGIC PATIENT

May involve minimal to long-term chronic rehabilitative care; specialized settings have programs designed to meet special need areas; the following discussion describes general guidelines for observation and intervention in the care of the neurologically impaired patient

CONDITIONS REQUIRING REHABILITATIVE APPROACH

Cognitive impairment

     Alteration in memory

     Alteration in speech, auditory, or visual function

Sensory-perceptual impairment

Impaired physical mobility

Paralysis

Behavioral changes

Spinal cord injuries

Alteration in elimination function

Self-care deficit

Ineffective individual coping

Chronic pain

REHABILITATIVE APPROACH

Reinforce physician's explanation of disorder and its limitations and allowances

Deal with behavioral response

     Allow patient to go through stages of grief over loss of body function

     Be supportive but firm dealing with patient

Encourage verbalization of feelings and fears

Use positive and reassuring approach to patient

Encourage independence when possible; be alert to limitations

Involve family or significant other in care and instructions

Establish program for ADLs; collaborate with physical and occupational therapy plans of care

Encourage patient's participation in developing a program

If patient on mechanical ventilator

     Coordinate activity/rest with weaning trials

     Maintain respiratory plan of care (e.g., tracheostomy care)

Establish daily routines of activity and rest periods

Sample

7:00 to 7:30	Morning care
7:30 to 8:30	Breakfast
9:00 to 9:30	Commode (bowel training)
9:30 to 10:30	Bath
10:30 to 11:00	Chair, stretcher
11:00 to 12:00	Bed rest; turn and position
12:00 to 12:30	Lunch
12:30 to 2:30	Bed rest; turn and position
2:30 to 3:00	Exercises
3:00 to 5:00	Bed rest
5:00 to 6:00	Chair, stretcher, dinner
6:00 to 9:00	Bed rest
9:00 to 9:30	Exercises
9:30 to 10:00	Evening care
10:00 PM to 7:00 AM	Bed rest

Turn and reposition to the following:
  Right side
  Left side
  Prone position
  Supine position
Attempt to avoid sensory deprivation by providing the following:
  Calendars
  Clocks
  Pictures
  Include schedule for favorite television or radio programs, hobbies, and visiting hours
Explain all treatments and procedures as they occur
Alert staff to patient's emotional changes and mood swings
Allow patient time to express needs
Refer to social service, VNA, and/or local rehabilitation centers as ordered
Report symptoms of urinary tract infection to physician
  Foul odor of urine
  Sedimentation, pus, or blood in urine
  Decreased output
  Low-grade fever
  Chills
Encourage participation in bowel and bladder training
Avoid constipation
Cleanse perineal region; wipe from front to back after urination
Cleanse perineal region with soap and water after each bowel movement
Give high-calorie, high-protein diet as ordered; avoid high-calcium foods

ACTIVITIES
Explain importance of exercise programs
Exercise to tolerance; avoid fatigue
Assist and instruct patient to use assistive devices as ordered
Plan rest periods
Encourage patient to participate in self-care as indicated

NUTRITION
Assess daily caloric needs
Maintain high-calorie, high-protein, low-residue diet as ordered
Limit high-calcium and gas-producing foods
Maintain aspiration precautions

ELIMINATION
Encourage fluids to 3000 ml/day unless contraindicated
Have patient avoid constipation through use of stool softeners, mild cathartics, suppositories, and/or enemas
Check for bowel movement q3d
Institute bowel and bladder programs
Avoid overdistention of bladder and bowel
Initiate intermittent catheterization as indicated

PATIENT/FAMILY TEACHING
Ensure that patient and significant other(s) know and understand the following:
  Importance of exercise programs
  Need to exercise to tolerance; avoid fatigue
  Importance of fluid intake; measure intake and output
  Importance of turning q2h to 4h while in bed
  Need to inspect skin and bony prominences for detection of skin breakdown
  Importance of skin care q2h to 4h while in bed
  Need to avoid constrictive clothing below level of lesion (e.g., garters, belts)
  Need to avoid UTIs
  Need to avoid overdistention of bladder; empty on regular basis
  Need for fluid to 3000 ml/day
Need to ensure daily bowel evacuation *to avoid fecal impaction;* encourage participation in bowel training
Need for ongoing support and counseling services
  Sexual counseling: patients can engage in some form of satisfying sexual activity; limitations depend on site of injury; incomplete injuries and high cord injuries allow for varying amounts of sensation and sexual function—even if spinal reflexes are absent, sensation of genital organs may endure
  Female reproductive system usually remains intact; patient can bear children—refer for family planning counseling
Refer to appropriate support services
  Vocational rehabilitation
  Recreational rehabilitation
  Home care

■ INCREASED INTRACRANIAL PRESSURE
Slow or sudden elevation in CSF pressure caused by edema, hemorrhage, or trauma; caused by increase in CSF or obstruction to outflow

ASSESSMENT
SUBJECTIVE DATA
Headache
Anxiety
Confusion

Vision difficulties
Nausea

OBJECTIVE DATA
Deterioration in mental status
   Restlessness
   Instability
Deterioration in LOC
   Lethargy
   Obtunded/stupor
   Semicoma
   Coma
Headache: location, duration, severity
Visual disturbances
   Diplopia
   Blurring
   Decreased acuity
Motor weakness
Paresis
Progressive weakness or paralysis of extremities
Pupil dysfunction (ipsilateral to edema or lesion)
Papilledema
Vomiting (projectile)
ICP $\geq$20 mm Hg for 5 minutes
Changes in respiratory rate; Biot's or Cheyne-Stokes
   respirations
Elevated BP (systolic); widened pulse pressure
Pulse rate decreased to 50 beats/min or below
Elevated temperature
Seizure activity
After cranial surgery
   Swelling around surgical site
   Elevation of bone flap

DIAGNOSTIC TESTS
Lumbar puncture (contraindicated if ICP
   elevated)
Continuous ICP monitoring
CPP/hemodynamic monitoring
Cerebral blood flow studies/transcranial Doppler
Serial ABGs
Serum studies
   Osmolarity
   Electrolytes
   Coagulation studies
   Anticonvulsant drug levels
Imaging
   CT scan
   MRI

POTENTIAL COMPLICATIONS
Deterioration of neurologic function
Infection; sepsis
Respiratory failure/arrest
Cerebral hemorrhage
Herniation
Cardiac arrest
Cerebral hypertension
Neurogenic pulmonary edema

MULTIDISCIPLINARY MANAGEMENT
THERAPEUTIC MANAGEMENT
Management of ventilatory status
   Oxygenation
   Ventilatory support
   Hyperventilation: keep PCO_2 <35 mm Hg or as
      prescribed
Medications
   Diuretics
   Osmotic diuretics
   Muscle relaxants/paralytics
   Volume expanders
   Steroids
   H_2 Blocker
   Anticonvulsants
   Sedatives
   Barbiturate coma
   Antiinfectives
   Stool softeners, laxatives
   Antacids
   Antipyretics
Fluid restriction if indicated
Electrolyte balance
Cardiac monitoring; hemodynamic monitoring
Surgical intervention
Ventricular drainage

PATIENT PROBLEM—NURSING DIAGNOSIS/INTERVENTIONS

▼Altered cerebral tissue perfusion: related to sustained elevations in ICP

Assess and monitor LOC, reporting any changes
   immediately
Maintain patent airway *to facilitate oxygenation*
Elevate head of bed 30 degrees
Maintain bed rest *to minimize energy expenditures*
   Avoid semiprone or prone position
   Avoid flexion of neck
   Avoid compression of neck veins
   Avoid extreme hip flexion
Monitor BP, P, and R q30min; if possible take BP on same
   arm each time
Monitor ICP, CPP q5min to 15min or as indicated by
   patient's condition
Perform neurologic check q30min using Glasgow Coma
   Scale (p. 515); report scores of 8 or less or any
   significant changes
Check rectal temperature q2h to 4h and prn; perform
   cooling measures as indicated
Monitor ABGs q2h to 4h as indicated
Maintain parenteral fluids as ordered; hypertonic
   solutions may be ordered
Measure intake and output *to monitor hydration
   status*
Initiate specific medical management as indicated
Avoid Valsalva maneuvers: vomiting, retching, straining;
   initiate measures *to avoid constipation* as indicated

Avoid isometric muscular contractions; instruct patient to avoid pushing feet against bedboard

Perform passive ROM activities as ordered *to maintain joint mobility and promote circulation*

Avoid stress-producing procedures during rapid eye movement (REM) stages of sleep

Explain and prepare for diagnostic tests and/or return to surgery as ordered

See standard of care for primary condition

Expected Outcomes
Remains free of injury
Demonstrates appropriate orientation and LOC
Demonstrates vital signs within normal limits
Demonstrates an effective breathing pattern
Demonstrates normal ICP
Demonstrates normal ROM

Additional Nursing Diagnosis to Consider
Ineffective breathing pattern related to altered cerebral perfusion

PATIENT/FAMILY TEACHING AND DISCHARGE/HOME CARE PLANNING
Refer to standard based on patient's primary condition

■ PARAPLEGIA
Partial or complete paralysis of the lower extremities resulting from injury to the spinal cord (thoracic and/or lumbar regions)

ASSESSMENT
SUBJECTIVE AND OBJECTIVE DATA
Partial or complete loss of sensory and motor function below level of injury
See Musculoskeletal assessment (p. 453)
Bladder distention
Dysuria
Bowel incontinence, impaction
Skin integrity problems

MULTIDISCIPLINARY MANAGEMENT
Physical therapy
Occupational therapy
Social services
Wound, Ostomy, Continence/ET Nurse to consult on skin integrity

REHABILITATION PLAN
COMMUNICATION
Give praise for tasks completed
Avoid tasks that patient cannot complete
Provide diversional activities as indicated
    Reading
    Watching television
    Listening to radio
    Working puzzles
    Listening to tape cassettes

Establish means of communication
    Call bell within reach
    Calling out to nurse

BED ACTIVITIES
Perform weight-bearing exercises
    Begin elevating head of bed, progressing to high-Fowler's position as tolerated when condition stabilizes
    Use tilt bed as ordered
        Begin elevating patient's head at 10 degrees for 10 to 15 minutes tid, progressing to 15 degrees for 1 hour bid or tid
        Keep legs wrapped with elastic stockings as ordered
        Take BP before tilting patient and every 5 minutes at 10 degrees; in absence of hypotension or dizziness, progress to 15 degrees as tolerated
        Gradually progress to 90-degree elevation as tolerated
Change position qh: maintain body alignment
    Prone position
    Supine position
    Rolling to side
    Sitting up
    Moving forward and backward
Check placement of lower extremities with each movement
Administer skin care q2h to 4h *to promote circulation*
    Use air mattress
    Give back rubs with lanolin-based lotions
    Put foam rubber pads on chairs
    Keep bed linen dry and wrinkle free
    Place rubber sheet under bath blanket
    Use body corset as ordered
Perform muscle-building exercises
    Active ROM exercise to support extremities
    Dumbbells: extending and flexing of arms
    Overhead trapezes
    Push-ups
    Sit-ups
    Hand-finger exercises
        Rubber sponge balls
        Extension and flexion
Teach method of turning self and pulling up in bed
Teach use of overhead trapeze, if appropriate

WHEELCHAIR ACTIVITIES
Get patient out of bed bid or tid
Demonstrate method of transferring from bed to wheelchair and from wheelchair to toilet or shower
Demonstrate management of wheelchair: moving forward, backward, turning, stopping, and locking

SELF-CARE ACTIVITIES
Encourage self-care as tolerated
    Bathing
    Dressing
    Combing hair

Shaving

Oral hygiene

Encourage patient to wear own clothing: pajamas, slippers, or shoes

MOTION ACTIVITIES

Use long leg braces as ordered

Perform physical therapy as ordered

Weight-bearing exercises

Parallel bar exercises

Balancing exercises

Crutch-walking exercises

To relieve spasticity

Perform active or passive ROM exercises

Wear long leg braces

Give medications as ordered

ELIMINATION

Perform urinalysis weekly as indicated

Check urine output for sedimentation or presence of renal calculi

Perform intermittent catheterization as ordered

Initiate bowel and bladder programs

Teach self-catheterization when appropriate

PATIENT/FAMILY TEACHING

Refer to General rehabilitative care of neurologic patient, p. 582

■ QUADRIPLEGIA

Partial or complete paralysis of the upper and lower extremities resulting from injury to the spinal cord (thoracic and cervical regions)

ASSESSMENT

SUBJECTIVE AND OBJECTIVE DATA

Partial or complete loss of motor and sensory function below level of injury

Loss of sweating reflex

Bladder distention and incontinence

Mass reflex of bladder

Muscular spasms

Diaphoresis

Elevated BP

Headache

Skin integrity problems

Ventilatory problems

REHABILITATION PLAN

COMMUNICATION

Encourage staff to allow time for patient care; do not rush patient

Provide diversional activities as indicated

Television/videos

Reading

Socializing with nursing staff

Provide means of communication

Calling out to nurse

Whistling

Maintain respiratory plan of care as indicated (e.g., mechanical ventilation, tracheostomy care, suctioning)

BED ACTIVITIES

Maintain good body alignment to promote comfort

Turn and position patient q1h to 2h *to stimulate circulation and improve muscle mass, tone, and strength*

Use supports: sandbags and pillows

Avoid external rotation of lower extremities

Position patient: supine, prone, and on side

Cough and deep breathe q1h to 2h *to prevent atelectasis*

Respiratory support as indicated

Administer skin care q1h to 2h *to promote circulation and prevent skin breakdown*

Use air mattress

Use footboard

Keep bed linen dry and wrinkle free

Rub back and heels with lanolin-based lotions *to promote circulation*

Change bed clothing prn

Place rubber sheet under bath blanket to be used as draw sheet

Assist with or provide perineal care after each voiding or bowel movement

Begin elevating head of bed as condition stabilizes, progressing to high-Fowler's position as tolerated

Tilt table as ordered; begin raising head to 10 degrees for 10 to 15 minutes tid, progressing to 20 degrees for 1 hour bid to tid, on to 90 degrees for 1 hour bid to tid, on to 90 degrees as tolerated

Take BP before tilting patient and at 5 to 10 minutes intervals as head is being raised; in absence of hypotension or dizziness progress to 90 degrees

Apply elastic bandages or stockings as ordered

WHEELCHAIR ACTIVITIES

Use three or four persons to transfer patient to stretcher chair or stretcher for 15 to 30 minutes bid to tid as ordered

Encourage wheelchair activity as ordered as condition stabilizes

Provide braces, splints, and other supports as ordered

Take safety measures

Soft jacket restraints

Soft abdominal binders

Siderails when indicated

SELF-CARE ACTIVITIES

Encourage patient to wear clothing from home and make selections

MOTION ACTIVITIES

To relieve spasticity

Perform gentle, passive ROM exercises

Have patient wear braces

Give medications as ordered

Prepare for rhizotomy or chordotomy as ordered

NUTRITION

Give tube feedings as indicated
Position patient with head of bed at 30 to 45
degrees
Feed patient
Allow 30 to 45 minutes for feeding time
Give small bites of food
Perform oral hygiene q4h and after meals
Clean with hydrogen peroxide and water
Gargle and mouthwash
Brush teeth

ELIMINATION

Provide indwelling or external catheter to closed gravity
drainage as ordered
Instruct patient to develop exercise or signals that may
help to stimulate urge to defecate
Smoking
Pressure on inner thigh
Stroking anus
Digital rectal stimulation
Drinking coffee
Massaging abdomen downward or right to left
Instruct patient to respond to "cues" promptly
Discuss importance of established, well-balanced diet that
includes bulk and roughage
Discuss foods to avoid
Bananas
Beans
Cabbage
Foods that previously have been constipating
Encourage fluids to 3000 ml/day unless
contraindicated
Include prune and orange juice and coffee in daily diet as
preferred
Discuss possible programs to develop
Instruct patient to take 8 to 10 oz of prune juice 12
hours before time set for defecating; insert glycerin
suppository high in rectum 15 to 20 minutes before
set time, then place patient on bedpan, toilet, or
commode
Insert lubricated glycerin suppository 2 hours before
set time and position patient in sitting position or
transfer to bedpan or commode
Instruct patient to drink 4 to 8 oz of prune juice each
night
Instruct patient to drink a warm drink 30 minutes
before set time
Water
Coffee
Milk
Insert laxative suppository for 2 to 4 days, then glycerin
suppository for 2 to 4 days; note length of time
between insertion and defecation; place patient on
bedside commode at appropriate time; if no bowel
movement, give small tap water enema
Instruct patient to recognize signs of impaction
No formed stool for 3 days
Semiliquid stools
Restlessness and increased feeling of discomfort

Discuss treatment for impaction
Laxative suppository
Tap water or oil-retention enemas
Manual clearing of bowel followed by enema

◼ BOWEL TRAINING
Method of bowel evacuation by reflex conditioning

ASSESSMENT
SUBJECTIVE AND OBJECTIVE DATA
Abdominal distention
Impaction
Diarrhea
Bowel incontinence
Dehydration
Autonomic hyperreflexia (dysreflexia)
Restlessness
Chills
Hypertension
Diaphoresis
Headache
Elevated temperature
Bradycardia
Flushing

PATIENT/FAMILY TEACHING
Explain purpose and necessity of developing bowel
regulation
Encourage patient's participation in developing a
program
Assess previous bowel habits
Establish regular bowel habits
Time of day that will be convenient for patient once
discharged: after breakfast
Development of program to have bowel evacuation at
same time each day or q3d
Administer medications as indicated
Stool softeners
Mild laxatives
Teach exercises that will help develop abdominal and
pelvic floor muscles and tone
Pushing up
Bearing down
Contracting abdominal muscles
Ensure privacy
Provide bedside commode rather than bedpan when
possible; encourage sitting position rather than
lying
Keep equipment easily available at bedside
Teach patient to recognize signals or "cues" that may
indicate full bowel
Goose pimples
Perspiration
Raising of hair on arms or legs
Sense of fullness
Instruct patient to eat diet high in fiber

■ ELECTROENCEPHALOGRAM (EEG) MONITORING

Recording of the electrical activity generated by the brain cortex by means of electrodes that are placed on the scalp surface in specific locations

PREPROCEDURE

Explain purpose of EEG monitoring to patient and family

Save cut hair, if patient/family requests

Cleanse scalp—must be free of lotion, oils

Inform patient and family that EEG wires do *not* deliver electrical shock

EEG wires may limit patient's range of ambulation because of attachment of wall monitor

Assess patient for possible need for sedation during application of electrodes so that optimal placement can be obtained

DURING EEG MONITORING

Provide call light and other necessary articles within reach of patient (EEG monitor wires may limit the patient's range of ambulation around the room)

Hygiene for hair: keep scalp free of lotion, oils; do not immerse scalp, hair in water; comb and disentangle hair bid

If patient needs to be disconnected from EEG monitoring (e.g., for transport to radiology department), notify EEG technician before disconnection and upon patient's return to the room so that EEG monitoring can be maintained as nearly continuous as possible

Minimize electrical equipment around patient and use only electrically grounded equipment; instruct patient and family to use battery-powered radios, shavers— *to prevent electrical interference with EEG monitoring*

Assess patient for seizure activity and document carefully. Notify physician and EEG technician so that EEG waveforms can be correlated with the observation of seizure activity in the patient. NOTE: Patients may have "subclinical seizures" in which motor signs are *not* evident or are very subtle, but the EEG tracing indicates that seizure activity is occuring

Be prepared to administer anticonvulsants, sedatives, as prescribed, if seizure activity is observed in the patient and/or on the EEG tracing

NURSING DIAGNOSES TO CONSIDER

Risk for injury related to seizures

Altered tissue perfusion: cerebral related to seizures

Altered body image related to EEG monitor apparatus, loss of hair

■ HYPOTHERMIA: CARE OF PATIENT

Controlled reduction and maintenance of body temperature to decrease the metabolic rate; patients with neurologic disorders may require control of fever resulting from infectious or neurogenic cause

ASSESSMENT

SUBJECTIVE AND OBJECTIVE DATA

Patient

Complications of hypothermia

Shivering

Decreased BP

Bradycardia

Bradypnea

Altered LOC

Medication reactions

Pupil inequality

Equipment

Cooling solution; amount in unit

Patency of connections

Pads

POTENTIAL COMPLICATIONS

Dysrhythmias

Increased ICP

Respiratory failure

Decreased urinary output

Intestinal ileus

Frostbite and burns

IMMEDIATE CARE

Take and record temperature before starting treatment and q5min until desired temperature is reached, then q15min

Check BP, P, and R and do neurologic check q5min to 10min while temperature is stabilizing

Observe for any change in skin color or presence of edema and induration; report any changes to physician immediately *to prevent peripheral ischemia*

Assist and teach patient to turn, cough, and deep breathe q1h to 2h *to facilitate ventilation*

Measure intake and output; measure output qh; report output <30 ml/hr to physician; specific gravity test may be ordered

Connect indwelling catheter to closed gravity drainage as ordered

Auscultate chest for breath sounds q1h to 2h

Administer medication for shivering as ordered

Test gag reflex before administering any oral fluids or food to patients with temperatures <90° F (32.2° C)

Perform naso-oral suction as indicated *to maintain patent airway*

Administer skin care q1h to 2h *to promote circulation*
  Lubricate skin before and during procedure with oil or lotion *to prevent dryness*
  Place bath blankets over thermal blankets

Maintain good body alignment

Perform passive or active ROM exercises q4h *to maintain joint mobility*

Monitor ABGs to monitor $Paco_2$

Administer oral hygiene q1h to 2h; keep lips well lubricated *to prevent dryness*

Administer nose care q1h to 2h

Provide emotional support
  Remain with patient when anxious
  Anticipate needs

ONGOING CARE
PATIENT
Check BP,T, P, and R and do neurologic check q30min ×
  4, then q4h for 24 hours, then as ordered
Check any dressing and all skin surfaces q1h to 2h until
  patient's temperature is stable
Measure intake and output
Assist and teach patient to turn, cough, and deep breathe q2h
Resume care of disease as ordered

EQUIPMENT
Check for leaks or punctures in pads before applying to
  patient
Check for proper temperature probe placement q1h to
  ensure accurate temperature readings

■ INTRACRANIAL PRESSURE MONITORING (TABLE 9-23)
Insertion of a catheter into epidural, subdural, sub-arachnoid, parenchymal, or ventricular space to measure the intracranial pressure (ICP) (see Increased intracranial pressure, p. 583)

ASSESSMENT (PREPROCEDURE, AS APPLICABLE, AND DURING ONGOING CARE OF PATIENT WITH ICP MONITORING)
OBJECTIVE DATA
LOC, score of Glasgow Coma Scale
Calculate cerebral perfusion pressure (CPP)
  $CPP = MAP - ICP$
  $MAP = (\text{systolic BP} - \text{diastolic BP}) \div 3 + \text{diastolic BP}$
  The normal range of CPP = 50 to 85 mm Hg
    (Table 9-24)
  The normal range of ICP = 4 to 15 mm Hg
    (Table 9-25)
Cardiopulmonary hemodynamic measurements and
  calculations
  Cardiac output, cardiac index
  Pulmonary capillary wedge pressure
  Pulmonary artery diastolic pressure
  CVP
  BP, HR
  Mean arterial pressure
  Respiratory pattern and rate
  TV
  ABGs, pulse oximetry, end-tidal CO_2
Cerebral hemodynamics
  Cerebral blood volume (CBV)
  CPP
  ICP and waveform (Fig. 9-16)
  Cerebrovascular resistance (CVR)

Table 9-23	Comparison of ICP Monitoring Systems	
System	**Advantages**	**Disadvantages**
Ventricular catheter	Reliable measurement within CSF Access for CSF drainage and sampling Access for determination of volume-pressure curve	Difficulty locating lateral ventricle Risk of intracerebral bleeding or edema at cannula track Risk of infection Need for transducer repositioning with head movement
Subarachnoid bolt/screw	Useful if ventricles are small No penetration of brain Decreased risk of infection	Unable to drain CSF Unreliable pressure when high ICP herniates brain into bolt Requires intact skull Need for transducer repositioning with head movement
Epidural sensor	Ease of insertion No dural penetration Lower risk of infection No adjustment of transducer needed with head movement	Unable to drain CSF Unable to recalibrate or rezero after placement Separate, large monitoring system required Questionable accuracy of sensing ICP through dura
Fiberoptic transducer-tipped catheter	Versatile system that can be placed in ventricle, subarachnoid space, or brain tissue Able to monitor intraparenchymal pressure Access for CSF drainage with ventricular system No adjustment of transducer needed with head movement	Catheter relatively fragile Unable to recalibrate or rezero after placement Separate monitoring system required

From Thelan LA et al: Critical care nursing: diagnosis and management, *ed 3, St Louis, 1998, Mosby.*

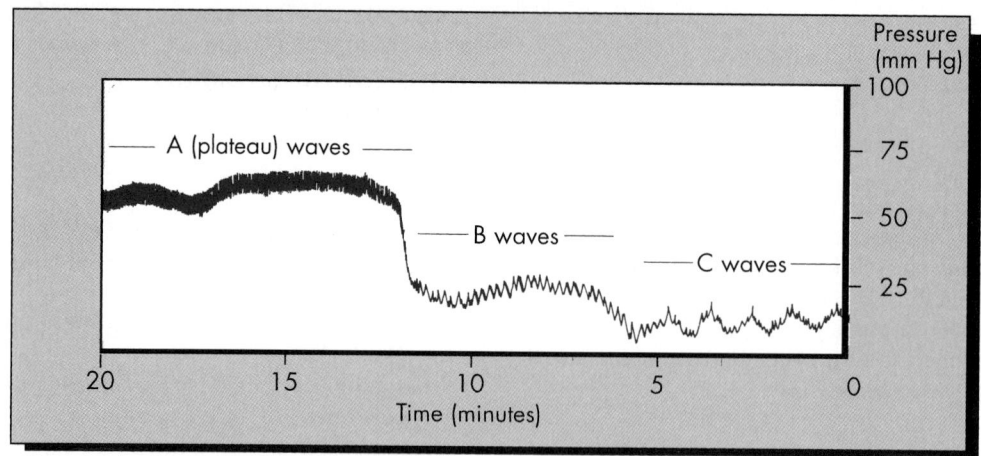

Fig. 9-16 Intracranial pressure waves. Composite drawing of A (plateau) waves, B waves, and C waves. (*From Chipps E et al:* Mosby's clinical nursing series: neurologic disorders, *St Louis, 1992, Mosby.*)

Table 9-24	Significance of Cerebral Perfusion Pressure (CPP) Measurements	
Level of CPP Measurements		**Description**
50-85 mm Hg		Normal CPP
<50 mm Hg		Cerebral ischemia
<20-30 mm Hg		Irreversible cerebral ischemia

Table 9-25	Significance of Intracranial Pressure (ICP) Measurements	
Level of ICP Measurements		**Description**
4-15 mm Hg		Normal ICP
16-20 mm Hg		Slightly elevated ICP
21-39 mm Hg		Moderately elevated ICP
40 mm Hg or greater		Severely elevated ICP

Cerebral blood flow (CBF)
Cerebral metabolism
Balance of cerebral oxygen delivery and consumption: $SjvO_2$ monitor
EEG monitor waves
Neurologic function
Pupils: size, shape, equality, and reaction to light
CSF: color (clear, light yellow, cloudy, bloody) and the drainage status (amount; frequency of drainage required)
Body temperature

POTENTIAL COMPLICATIONS
Infection: local skin infection, osteomyelitis, meningitis, ventriculitis, encephalitis, empyema, and abscess
Hemorrhage: catheter insertion site or intracranial hemorrhage
Iatrogenic hypertension
Catheter dislodgment

PREPARATION FOR ICP MONITOR PLACEMENT
Patient
Pre-ICP monitor placement
Explain the purpose, procedure, and benefits, risks to the patient and family
Help the patient and family express their fear and feelings
Perform a comprehensive neurologic and cardiopulmonary assessment and record baseline results
Obtain the coagulation profile and the most recent lab results
Obtain the files of brain CT scan and/or MRI scan
Document baseline vital signs
Explain the tubes and the devices that will be attached to the patient's head

ICP monitor placement
Position the patient supine; immobilize the head with rolled towels on either side
Sedate the patient if necessary
Observe the patient's cardiopulmonary hemodynamic and respiratory pattern and rates
Assist the neurosurgeon and/or advanced nurse practitioner to incise down to the skull; maintain sterile field
Attach the ICP device to the ICP monitoring system
Apply a topical antibiotic and sterile dressing
Document the initial ICP waveform and reading
Document the date, time, the kind of ICP monitoring system inserted, the patient's reaction during the procedure
Document the color of CSF and drainage status if intraventricular ICP monitoring system inserted

Equipment
Before insertion, calibrate all equipment including transducer and recording display unit
Position transducer so it is level to the patient's tragus for ventricular ICP monitoring

Be aware that insertion must be done under sterile conditions

Ongoing Care
Patient
Post-ICP monitor placement
Position the patient supine with head of bed elevated about 30 degrees

Avoid neck flexion, prone position, and extreme hip flexion

Evaluate neurologic function, LOC, vital signs, CPP, ICP and ICP waveform, and rectal temperature q1h or as indicated by patient's condition

Never flush or irrigate ventricular catheter

Observe the insertion site and dressing for bleeding, signs of infection, loosened attachment

Report immediately any abnormal changes of vital signs, any newly developed neurologic deficits, and change of LOC

Report immediately any sudden stoppage of CSF drainage or lost ICP waveform

Observe the color of CSF if intraventricular ICP monitor inserted and report immediately if CSF turns bloody

If the patient is uncooperative, restrain upper extremity to prevent patient from dislodging ICP monitor

Check for leaks to prevent introduction of microorganisms and air bubbles

Use sterile technique to change the CSF drainage bag and dressing

Equipment
Avoid kinking, compression, or tension on tubing

Position transducer so it is level to the patient's tragus for ventricular ICP monitoring

Check patency of tubing at least q2h

Calibrate and zero transducer q4h to q6h as indicated by manufacturer and protocol

Never apply direct pressure to diaphragm of transducer

Removal of Monitor
Apply a sterile dressing to the wound and avoid getting it wet

Report immediately any CSF leak from the wound

Report immediately any redness, swelling, heat, or pain surrounding the wound

Report immediately fever or change of LOC and vital signs

■ Lumbar Puncture (Spinal Tap)
Puncture usually made at the junction of the third and fourth lumbar vertebrae to obtain CSF for purposes of measuring CSF pressure and laboratory examination

Preprocedure Preparation
Obtain results of coagulation studies (lumbar puncture contraindicated if patient is coagulopathic)

Explain procedure

Have patient empty bowel and bladder

Position patient on side with spine close to edge of bed; support soft mattress with bedboards

Maintain aseptic technique throughout procedure
    Handle specimen with care
    Verify specimen delivery to laboratory within 30 minutes to ensure diagnostic accuracy

Explain to patient that procedure may be uncomfortable

Explain importance of immobilization during procedure

Instruct patient to breathe normally; not to hold breath

Provide patient with physical and emotional support during procedure

Postprocedure Assessment
Subjective and Objective Data
Assess for complications
    Altered LOC
    Headache: mild to severe
    Nuchal rigidity
    Hypotension
    Tachycardia
    Tachypnea
    Bleeding from site of puncture
    Elevated temperature

Diagnostic Tests
Normal adult CSF
    Pressure: 70 to 200 mm H_2O
    Color: colorless, clear
    Glucose level: 45 to 75 mg/100 ml or 60% to 70% of blood glucose
    Protein level (total): 20 to 45 mg/100 ml
    RBCs: none
    WBCs: 0 to 5 cells/mm^3
    Microorganisms: none

Potential Complications
Transient back pain

Paresthesia in legs

Headache

Infection

Elevated ICP

Coagulation abnormalities

Brain herniation with increased ICP

Immediate Postprocedure Care
Maintain bed rest; place patient in supine position, keeping head of bed flat for 4 to 8 hours as ordered; if headache occurs, elevate feet 10 to 15 degrees above bed

Assist and teach patient to turn and deep breathe q2h to 4h

Check BP, P, and R q15min × 4, then qh × 4, then as ordered

Control pain as ordered

Observe site of puncture for redness, swelling, ecchymosis, or drainage and report any symptoms to physician

Maintain diet as ordered; aspiration precautions while head of bed flat

Force fluids unless contraindicated
Explain importance of keeping head and body position flat in bed

ONGOING CARE
Resume activities as ordered
Ambulate to tolerance

■ SKULL TONGS AND HALO TRACTION
Methods of immobilizing the neck and stabilizing the spine

ASSESSMENT
SUBJECTIVE AND OBJECTIVE DATA
Site of insertion of tongs
  Redness
  Swelling
  Drainage
Skin condition: pressure sores of scapula, coccyx, occipital scalp, clavicles, and heels
Alignment of head, pulleys, and weights: do not allow patient's head to touch head of bed
Weights
  Pounds ordered
  Off floor, hanging freely
Position of bed

ONGOING CARE
Educate all caregivers: how to unfasten halo vest *to provide access to chest for CPR if needed*
Inspect and clean site of insertion q1h to 2h; remove *any* formed crusts with hydrogen peroxide q6h to 8h and prn; apply antibiotic ointment to insertion sites q6h to 8h
Administer skin and scalp care q2h to 4h
  Use air mattress
  Give back rubs
  Keep bed linen dry and wrinkle free
  Avoid powders
  Keep hair clean
Perform passive ROM exercises to all extremities q4h
Apply antiembolic stocking
Check alignment of pulleys and weights q4h to 6h; sandbags may be indicated for restlessness as ordered
Turn patient q2h as ordered
Avoid pulling/pushing on skull tongs when repositioning patient
Maintain safety precautions
Assist and teach patient to deep breathe q2h
Establish means of communication and keep within easy reach of patient: call bell
Provide diversional activities
Assist with ambulation as indicated for patient with halo traction

PATIENT/FAMILY TEACHING
Explain purpose of tongs
Explain methods of turning when possible
Explain importance of keeping head straight

■ STRYKER FRAME OR ROTATIONAL THERAPY BED
Stryker frame: Metal frame bed used to facilitate administration of nursing care to patient with spinal cord injuries

rotational therapy bed: A bed with the combined features of kinetic air mattress, adjustable degrees of lateral rotation, and cervical/pelvic immobilization

ASSESSMENT
OBSERVATIONS/FINDINGS
Patient
Body position: straight body alignment
Place in center of frame
Body parts not resting on metal frame
Skin
  Temperature
  Color
Pressure areas
Pulse
Respirations
Lightheadedness
Numbness

Equipment
Canvas supports
Arm and foot supports
Locks
Frame
  Anterior
  Posterior

PREPARATION OF UNIT
Check unit for security of bolts, locks, and frame before placing patient on Stryker frame or rotational therapy bed
Prepare bed with linens, foam mattress, arm rests, and footboards before receiving patient

ONGOING CARE
Turn patient q2h during day
Adjust degree of lateral rotation on rotational therapy bed as appropriate to patient's condition
Turn patient q4h during night
Check pulse and respirations before and after turning
Free all excess tubing before turning
Secure all bolts and safety straps tightly before turning
Reassure patient when turning
Administer skin care q2h to 4h and prn
Inspect pressure points q2h to 4h
Prevent sensory deprivation when patient must be prone or supine (e.g., provide radio, visitors)

BIBLIOGRAPHY
Adams RD et al: *Principles of neurology*, New York, 1997, McGraw-Hill.
Avery-Smith W: Treatment of mechanical swallowing disorders. In Groher ME, ed: *Dysphagia: diagnosis and management*, ed 3, Boston, 1997, Butterworth-Heinemann.

Awadalla S et al: Neurologic emergencies in internal medicine. In Ewald GA, McKenzie CR, eds: *The Washington manual,* ed 28, Boston, 1995, Little, Brown.

Barker E: *Neuroscience nursing,* St Louis, 1994, Mosby.

Beare PG, Myers SL: *Principles and practice of adult health nursing,* ed 2, St Louis, 1998, Mosby.

Biller J, Patrick JT: Management of medical complications of stroke, *J Stroke Cerebrovasc Dis* 6(4):217, 1997.

Buchholz DW: Neurologic disorders of swallowing, In Groher ME, ed: *Dysphagia: diagnosis and management,* ed 3, Boston, 1997, Butterworth-Heinemann.

Campbell VG: Neurological system. In Thompson JM et al, eds: *Mosby's clinical nursing,* ed 4, St Louis, 1997, Mosby.

Chandler CL, Cummins B: Initial assessment and management of the severely head-injured patient, *Br J Hosp Med* 53(3):102, 1995.

Freeman JM et al: *Seizures and epilepsy in childhood: a guide for parents,* London, 1990, The Johns Hopkins University Press.

GlaxoWellcome Inc: *Living with epilepsy: special concerns of adults,* Research Triangle Park, 1997, GlaxoWellcome Inc.

Gummit R: *The epilepsy handbook: the practical management of seizures,* ed 2, New York, 1995, Raven.

Hickey J: *The clinical practice of neurological and neurosurgical nursing,* ed 5, Philadelphia, 1997, JP Lippincott.

Kinney M et al: *AACN's clinical reference for critical care nursing,* ed 4, St Louis, Mosby.

Kunkel J et al: *Intracranial pressure monitoring,* Chicago, 1997, American Association of Neuroscience Nurses.

Label L: *Injuries and disorders of the head and brain,* St Louis, 1997, Mosby.

Lang EW, Chesnut RM: Intracranial pressure monitoring and management, *Neurosurg Clin North Am* 5(4):573-605, 1994.

Lewis S, Collier J: *Medical-surgical nursing: assessment and management of clinical problems,* ed 3, St Louis, 1992, Mosby.

Mathewson-Kuhn M: *Pharmacotherapeutics: a nursing process approach,* ed 3, Philadelphia, 1994, FA Davis.

Nadeau SE: Transient ischemic attacks: diagnosis, and medical and surgical management, *J Fam Pract* 38(5):495-564, 1994.

Ozuna J et al: *Seizure assessment,* Chicago, 1997, American Association of Neuroscience Nurses.

Phipps WJ et al: *Medical-surgical nursing: concepts and clinical practice,* ed 6, St Louis, 1998, Mosby.

Robertson CS et al: SjvO$_2$ monitoring in head-injury patients, *J Neurotrauma,* 12(5):891, 1995.

Saver J: State of the art medical management of acute ischemia stroke, *J Stroke Cerebrovasc Dis* 6(4):189-194, 1997.

Seidel HM et al: *Mosby's guide to physical examination,* ed 3, St Louis, 1995, Mosby.

Thelan LA et al: *Critical care nursing: diagnosis and management,* ed 2, St Louis, 1994, Mosby.

Thompson J et al: *Mosby's clinical nursing,* ed 4, 1997, St Louis, Mosby.

Young, GB et al: *Coma and impaired consciousness: a clinical perspective,* New York, 1998, McGraw-Hill.

USC UNIVERSITY HOSPITAL
1500 San Pablo
Los Angeles, CA 90033   ©1991

SIDE 1   NAME _____   ALLERGIES _____

MULTIDISCIPLINARY PLAN

ADMIT DATE _____

DIAGNOSIS ____ Acoustic Neuroma ____

SURGERY ____ CRANIOTOMY ____

DISCHARGE OUTCOMES

PHYSIOLOGICAL: Patient will have ADL needs met by self or c̄ assistance of other(s). Will be able to explain surgical site care, verbalize precautions to take for medication use. Complications/injury will be prevented or minimized, discomfort relieved/controlled & infectious process(es) resolving/absent.

COGNITIVE: Patient will be able to verbalize disease process/prognosis & therapeutic regimen & state the s/sx to report to health care team.

PSYCHOLOGICAL: Patient will verbalize acceptance of potential lifestyle changes & incorporate into ADLs. Able to verbalize fears/anxieties & demonstrate effective coping mechanisms A/E ability to participate in self-care decisions.

DRG __001__ ALOS __12.4__

DISCIPLINE	PRE-OP/ PRE-ADMIT	DOS DAY 1 DATE	POD#1 DAY 2 DATE	POD#2 DAY 3 DATE	POD#3 DAY 4 DATE	POD#4 DAY 5 DATE	POD#5 DAY 6 DATE
LOCATION		SURGERY/PAR/NSICU	NSICU	NSICU→DOU	DOU	DOU → MED/SURG	MED/SURG
LABS	CBC Chem 20 UA PT PTT T & C 2u PRBCs	Chem 7 Hct (on arrival to unit)	CBC Chem 7	CBC Chem 7	CBC Chem 7	CBC Chem 7	
CARDIO-PULMONARY	ECG R/O Arrhythmias	I.S. Pulse oximetry O₂ 40% face mask A-Line	DC A-Line	DC face mask & pulse oximetry			
IMAGING/ NUCLEAR MEDICINE	CXR 2 Views						
SOCIAL SERVICES D/C PLAN REHAB. SERVICES			Assess need for speech/ swallowing consult. Consider need for OT evaluation—self-care	Assess need for PT consult. Consider need for social worker services	Asses need for home health evaluation if indicated. Support adaptive group OT	Assess need for Rehab consult	
PHARMACY	IV of LR	IV fluids Corticosteroid Ocular lubricants Analgesics H₂ antagonist Antibiotic Vestibular Sedative		Stool softener Antiemetic	Convert IV to SL DC antibiotics		
DIETARY/ NUTRITION	NPO	NPO until awake, then ice chips	Advance to diet as tolerated if no swallowing difficulty, otherwise refer to speech/ swallow consult recommendations				

Used by permission of USC University Hospital, Los Angeles, California.

MULTIDISCIPLINARY PLAN

PATIENT NAME: _____

DISCIPLINE	PRE-OP/ PRE-ADMIT	DOS DAY 1	DAY 2	POD#1	POD#2 DAY 3	POD#3 DAY 4	POD#4 DAY 5	POD#5 DAY 6
		DATE ___		POD #1 DATE ___	POD #2 DATE ___	POD #3 DATE ___	POD #4 DATE ___	
PATIENT ACTIVITY		BR HOB ↑ 30 – 45° Leg squeezers begun in OR	OOB TO chair c̄ assistance only BID	Ambulate c̄ assist TID			DC leg squeezers	
EDUCATION Baseline vestibular testing/pt education done re: dizziness Basic audiogram, c̄ air, bone, speech, middle ear testing	I.S. instruct C & DB. Teach reason for surgery, post-op restrictions & expected LOS	Orient to room, unit & hospital routine Pre-optic moisture eye chamber to affected eye Monitoring of dressing for drainage Discuss need for Foley	DC Foley I & O cath q 6° prn Review s/sx of CSF leak Discuss c̄ pt/family need for safety precautions due to pt's balance disturbances (up c̄ assist only). Move slowly when getting up & keep eyes open. May experience difficulty c̄ reading (nystagmus)	Review disease process, prognosis & understanding of therapeutic regimen during hospitalization. Teach self-application & care of eye moisture chamber	Review all previous teaching. Consult for placement of spring or gold weight by ophthalmology may be indicated.	Balance visit	Shower instructions: • Staples may become wet • Towel dry throughly p̄ showering • Avoid hot curls until hair has regrown Postop audiogram, balance lab visit, vestibular rehab will begin q d

COLLABORATIVE PROBLEMS

DATE		DATE	
❶ Potential for altered level of consciousness R/T postop cerebral edema &/or bleeding.		❼ Knowledge deficit R/T lack of exposure to hospitalization, misinterpretation of information received or limitation of cognitive ability; discharge planning.	
❷ Potential for infection R/T supressed inflammatory response secondary to steroids or exposure to pathogens.		❽ Potential for inadequate corneal lubrication R/T facial nerve involvement.	
❸ Potential for injury R/T possible postop weakness, paresthesia, ataxia or vertigo.		❾ Impaired hearing R/T manipulation of cranial nerve VIII.	
❹ Alteration of comfort; pain R/T surgical procedure.			
❺ Potential for impairment physical mobility R/T ↓ strength, perceptual/cognitive impairment, pain or restriction in activity.			
❻ Potential anxiety/fear R/T situational crisis of hospitalization or change in health status & separation from support system.			

OUTCOMES

❶ Pt. will maintain usual or improved LOC & motor-sensory function.	❺ Pt. will regain &/or maintain optimal physical mobility.	❽ Pt. will be able to apply care for & remove eye moisture chamber independently or c̄ S/O assistance.
❷ Pt. will demonstrate timely healing free from infectious spread.	❼ Pt. will verbalize understanding of condition/disease process.	❼ Pt. will be able to correctly perform procedures & explain reasons for actions.
❸ Pt. will remain free from injury during hospitalization.	❾ Pt. will verbalize understanding of hearing loss & will take measures to optimize present hearing.	❹ Pt. will verbalize pain controlled c̄ po pain medications.
❹ Pt. will verbalize pain controlled c̄ ordered medications. Displays relaxed posture & able to sleep &/or rest.		❾ Pt. will verbalize understanding of discharge plans.
❻ Pt. will acknowledge & discuss fears. Will appear relaxed & reports anxiety reduction to a manageable level.		

KEY

❶ Document outcomes under appropriate date for achieving the goal.

❷ To discontinue an intervention, or resolve a patient problem, highlight date and initial.

Continued

PLAN OF CARE DISCUSSED WITH

DATE | INITIAL | S.O. | Pt.

	DOS / DAY 1	POD#1 / DAY 2 / DOS	POD#2 / DAY 3	POD#3 / DAY 4	POD#4 / DAY 5	POD#5 / DAY 6
	DATE____	DATE____	DATE____	DATE____	DATE____	DATE____

INTERVENTIONS

DOS / DAY 1
- Assess neuro status per MD order, report Δs to MD
- Strict I & O
- Monitor temp per unit routine
- Assess respiratory status q 1° x 24°
- Reposition frequently & encourage use of I.S.
- Evaluate for s/sx of ↑ ICP:
  - decreased response to stimuli
  - Δs in VS
  - restlessness
  - weakness/paralysis of extremities
  - changes in vision or pupillary Δs
  - worsening of headache
- Monitor urine characteristics - color, odor, clarity
- Assess for clinical signs of infection & report to MD if present
- Note c/o pain location, intensity & duration
- Medicate for pain as ordered & assess pain relief
- If pt has headache, reduce bright lights & room noise if possible
- Provide eye patch as ordered to ↓ eye strain
- Assess pt &/or S/O level of anxiety
- Answer questions & explain all procedures prior to initiation
- Clarify misunderstandings of info & involve pt & S/O in decision making, care planning & evaluations
- Assess ability to close eyelid. Notify MD if unable to do so
- Avoid nose blowing or sneezing if preventable

POD#1 / DAY 2
- Assess for factors that impair physical mobility:
  - pain &/or nausea
  - fear of falling
  - vertigo
  - dislodging tubes
  - compromising surgical wound
- Treat those items present above &/or educate pt as needed
- Assure pt that activity ordered will enhance rather than compromise healing process
- Provide praise & encouragement for all efforts to ↑ mobility
- Reinforce need for assistance when getting OOB
- Provide pt c̄ safe environment (seizure precautions may also be indicated)
- Provide info to pt & S/O in short segments
- Discuss expected length of recovery
- Assess pt ability to swallow prior to advancing diet
- If pt has hearing loss, speak distinctly. Note side of hearing loss & speak to unaffected ear
- Discuss c̄ pt the need to verbalize lack of hearing
- Discuss need for eye moisture chamber, apply as ordered
- Assess respiratory status q 2°

POD#2 / DAY 3
- Increase activity & participation in ADLs
- Encourage S/O to assist c̄ ↑ activity
- Assess for need of stool softener
- Assess pt & S/O understanding of disease process, prognosis & understanding of therapeutic regimen
- Discuss application, care for & removal of eye moisture chamber
- Assess affected eye for irritation & drainage
- Apply cool compresses to affected eye if ordered
- Change VS c̄ neuro √'s to q 4° p̄ transfer
- Continue strict I & O
- Assess resp status q 4°
- Continue use of I.S.
- Assess for s/sx of CSF leak:
  - Worsening headache upon standing
  - Ask if pt experiencing frequent swallowing or feels fluid in the back of the throat
  - Have pt bend over & note drainage presence
  - If drainage noted, place a sterile pad under nose & observe for halo of blood surrounding clear or yellow colored ring of spinal fluid
  - If above present, notify MD immediately
  - Temp elevation may indicate meningitis
  - Reassess frequently

POD#3 / DAY 4
- Reassess pt &/or S/O level of anxiety
- Support planning for realistic lifestyle p̄ hospitalization within limitations but fully using capabilities
- Explore sources of support:
  - S/O
  - Clergy
  - Social Worker
- Encourage use of po pain meds
- Assess need for home health evaluation & outpatient therapies
- Continue to monitor for CSF leakage

POD#4 / DAY 5
- DC leg squeezers once pt fully ambulatory
- Reassess pt need for stool softener
- Encourage increased activity
- Continue to monitor for CSF leakage

POD#5 / DAY 6
- Instruct in showering technique

Case Manager: ____

Consulting MD: ____

Social Service: ____

Anointing of The Sick Date: ____

DATE	SIGNATURES

MULTIDISCIPLINARY PLAN UPDATE

DATE	SIGNATURES	DATE	SIGNATURES	DATE	SIGNATURES

USC UNIVERSITY HOSPITAL
1500 San Pablo
Los Angeles, CA 90033   ©1991

SIDE 2

NAME _____
ALLERGIES _____

MULTIDISCIPLINARY PLAN

ADMIT DATE _____

DIAGNOSIS ___ Acoustic Neuroma ___

SURGERY ___ CRANIOTOMY ___

DISCHARGE OUTCOMES	DRG _001_ ALOS _12.4_
PHYSIOLOGICAL	Patient will have ADL needs met by self or c̄ assistance of other(s). Will be able to explain surgical site care, verbalize precautions to take for medication use. Complications/injury will be prevend or minimized, discomfort relieved/controlled & infectious process(es) resolving/absent.
COGNITIVE	Patient will be able to verbalize disease process/prognosis & therapeutic regimen & state the s/sx to health care team.
PSYCHOLOGICAL	Patient will verbalize acceptance of potential lifestyle changes & incorporate into ADLs. Able to verbalize fears/anxieties & demonstrate effective coping mechanisms A/E ability to participate in self-care decisions.

DISCIPLINE	PRE-OP/ PRE-ADMIT	POD #6 DAY 7 DATE ___	POD #7 DAY 8 DATE ___	POD #8 DAY 9 DATE ___	POD #9 DAY 10 DATE ___	POD #10 DAY 11 DATE ___	POD #11 DAY 12 DATE ___
LOCATION	MED SURG	MED SURG	MED SURG → HOME				
LABS							
CARDIO-PULMONARY							
IMAGING/ NUCLEAR MEDICINE							
SOCIAL SERVICES D/C PLAN REHAB. SERVICES	Ordered therapies to assess pt discharge needs						
PHARMACY	DC S.L.		To be discharged c̄ po pain medications				
DIETARY/ NUTRITION	Regular diet						

Continued

MULTIDISCIPLINARY PLAN

PATIENT NAME: _____

DISCIPLINE	PRE-OP/PRE-ADMIT	POD #6 DAY 7	POD #7 DAY 8	POD #8 DAY 9	POD #9 DAY 10	POD #10 DAY 11	POD #11 DAY 12
		DATE	DATE	DATE	DATE	DATE	DATE
PATIENT ACTIVITY		Ambulate as much as tolerated					
EDUCATION		Teach s/sx to report to health care team. Instruct pt in care of surgical site. Discuss discharge medications. Reinforce safety precautions at home.	Staples to be removed 7-10 days postop. Discuss follow-up care regimen.				

COLLABORATIVE PROBLEMS

	DATE		DATE	
❶ Potential for altered cerebral tissue perfusion R/T cerebral edema altering or interrupting cerebral blood flow.			❾ Impaired hearing R/T position of tumor.	
❷ Potential for infection R/T suppressed inflammatory response (medication induced) or exposure to pathogens.				
❸ Potential for injury R/T seizure activity, weakness, paralysis, paresthesia, ataxia or vertigo.				
❹ Alteration in comfort, pain R/T headache &/or surgical procedure.				
❼ Knowledge deficit R/T lack of exposure to hospitalization, misinterpretation of information received or limitation in cognitive ability; discharge planning.				
❽ Potential impaired corneal tissue integrity R/T inadequate lubrication.				

OUTCOMES

❶ Pt will maintain usual or improved LOC & motor-sensory function.	❼ Pt & S/O will describe follow-up care regimen.
❷ Pt will continue to demonstrate healing free from infectious spread.	
❸ Pt will demonstrate absence of seizure or injury.	
❹ Pt will verbalize pain controlled c̄ po pain medications.	
❽ Pt will be able to apply, care for & remove eye moisture chamber independently or c̄ S/O assistance.	
❾ Pt will verbalize if unable to hear any conversation involved in.	

KEY

❶ Document outcomes under appropriate date for achieving the goal.

❷ To discontinue an intervention, or resolve a patient problem, highlight date and initial.

PLAN OF CARE DISCUSSED WITH	POD #6 DAY 7	POD #7 DAY 8	POD #8 DAY 9	POD #9 DAY 10	POD #10 DAY 11	POD #11 DAY 12
DATE INITIAL S.O. Pt.	DATE ___	DATE ___	DATE ___	DATE ___	DATE ___	DATE ___
	INTERVENTIONS					

INTERVENTIONS — POD #6 DAY 7:

- Teach s/sx that need to be reported to the health care team:
  - rhinorrhea
  - changes in vision
  - elevated temp
  - intense headache
  - drainage from surgical site
  - balance △s
- Teach pt how to care for surgical site:
  - Avoid scrubbing
  - Dab very dry
  - Keep hair off wound × 72°
  - Avoid sun exposure
  - OK to shampoo p̄ staples out × 24°
- Instruct pt & S/O regarding discharge meds. Include name & purpose, route, dosage, frequency, time of administration & side effects.
- Explain safety precautions to maintain at home:
  - Assistance when ambulating in the dark
  - Assistance in performing ADLs as needed
- Continue to monitor for CSF leakage

INTERVENTIONS — POD #7 DAY 8:

- Reinforce those s/sx that need to be reported to the health care team
- Encourage tips to recovery:
  - Return to normal social & physical activity
  - Verbalization of concerns c̄ health care team
- Emphasize the importance of ongoing outpatient care & follow-up visits
- Review those medications pt will take home

Case Manager: ___

Consulting MD: ___

Social Service: ___

Anointing of The Sick Date: ___

MULTIDISCIPLINARY PLAN UPDATE

DATE	SIGNATURES	DATE	SIGNATURES	SIGNATURES

Genitourinary/Renal System

■ GENITOURINARY/RENAL ASSESSMENT

▉ SUBJECTIVE DATA

Reported changes in voiding pattern
    Anuria
    Diurnal frequency
    Hesitancy or intermittent
    Force of urinary stream, straining
    Frequency of urination
    Burning
    Nocturia
    Oliguria
    Polyuria
    Urgency
    Incomplete emptying
    Incontinence (type/containment devices used)
    Bladder spasm
    Pain (location of)
        Back
        Flank
        Groin
        Colicky
        Dysuria
        Lumbar
        Urethral
        Genital
        Perineal
        Abdominal
Sexual history
    Decreased libido
    Dyspareunia
    Impotence/erectile dysfunction
Gastrointestinal (GI) status
    Anorexia
    Nausea, vomiting
    Constipation, diarrhea
    Thirst
    Hiccups
    Metallic taste in mouth
Fatigue, malaise, weakness
Restlessness
Headache
Inability to concentrate
Pruritus
Muscle cramps

Paresthesias of lower extremities
Visual disturbances, changes
Lost sense of smell
Chills

▉ OBJECTIVE DATA

See Fig. 10-1
Physical examination
    Kidney (abdominal mass, flank mass, costovertebral
        angle tenderness) (Fig. 10-2)
    Bladder (presence of distention, pain)
    External genitalia (redness, sores, ulcers/lesions,
        masses, rash, inflammation, pain) (Fig. 10-3, 10-4, and
        10-5)
    Urethra (drainage, pain, inflammation)
    Vagina (drainage, discharge, redness,
        inflammation)
    Testes/scrotum (enlargement, mass, tenderness)
        (Fig. 10-6)
    Prostate via rectum (size, consistency, induration)
Character of urine
    Color (clear, yellow, red, pink, rusty brown, tea,
        cola)
    Odor
    Amount
    Specific gravity
Indwelling catheter (type, date of insertion)
Vital signs
    Fever
    Tachycardia, bradycardia
    Hypotension, hypertension
Respiratory status
    Decreased breath sounds
    Crackles
    Rales
Mental status, behavior
    Disorientation, confusion
    Agitation
Gastrointestinal status
    Absent/decreased bowel sounds
    Abdominal distention/rigidity
    Melena
Weight (recent loss or gain > 10 lb)
Hematemesis
Urinelike/ammonia odor to breath

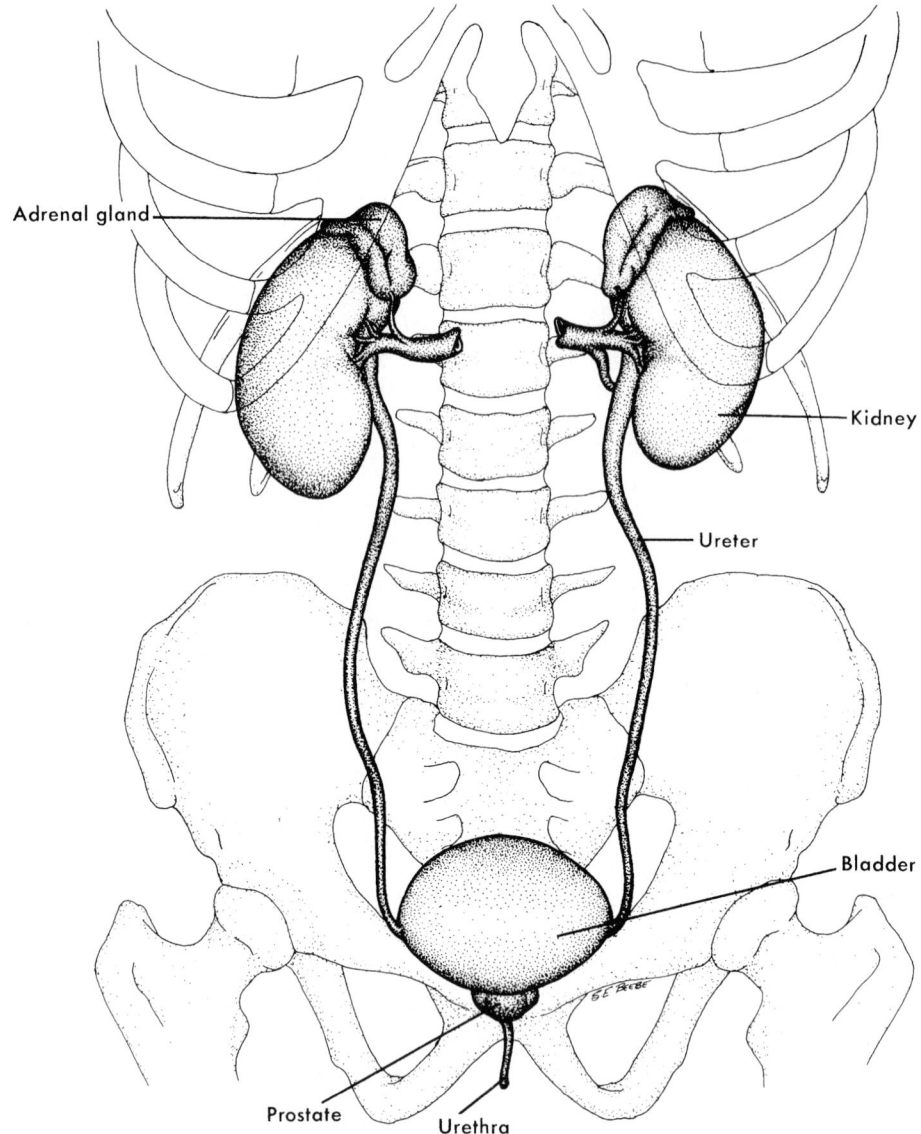

Fig. 10-1 Genitourinary system.

Edema
  Generalized
  Positional
  Pitting
  Nocturnal
  Periorbital
Mucous membranes
Jugular venous distention, flat neck veins
Skin
  Pallor
  Petechiae, ecchymoses
  Uremic snow
  Tophi in ear cartilage
  Turgor
  Dry, scaly, pale, black, yellow-tan
Brittle nails

▌ PERTINENT BACKGROUND INFORMATION

CONCURRENT DISEASES AND CONDITIONS
Anemia
Amenorrhea
Impotence/erectile dysfunction
Infertility
Diabetes
Tuberculosis
Hormonal, endocrine imbalance
Systemic lupus erythematosus
Vascular disease, polyarteritis
Sickle cell disease
Amyloidosis
Gout

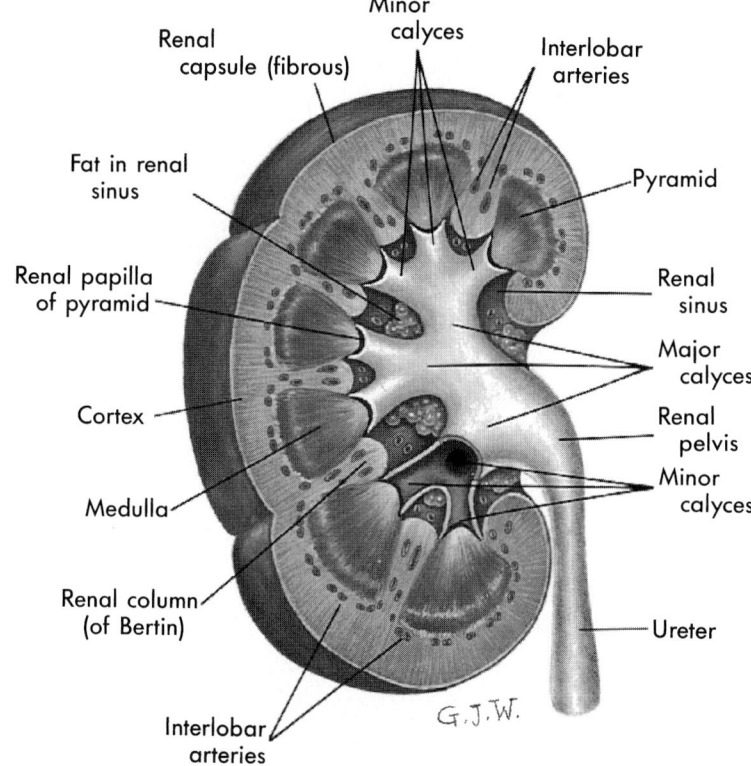

Fig. 10-2 Cross section of the kidney showing basic structures.
(From Brundage DJ: Mosby's clinical nursing series: renal disorders, St Louis, 1992, Mosby.)

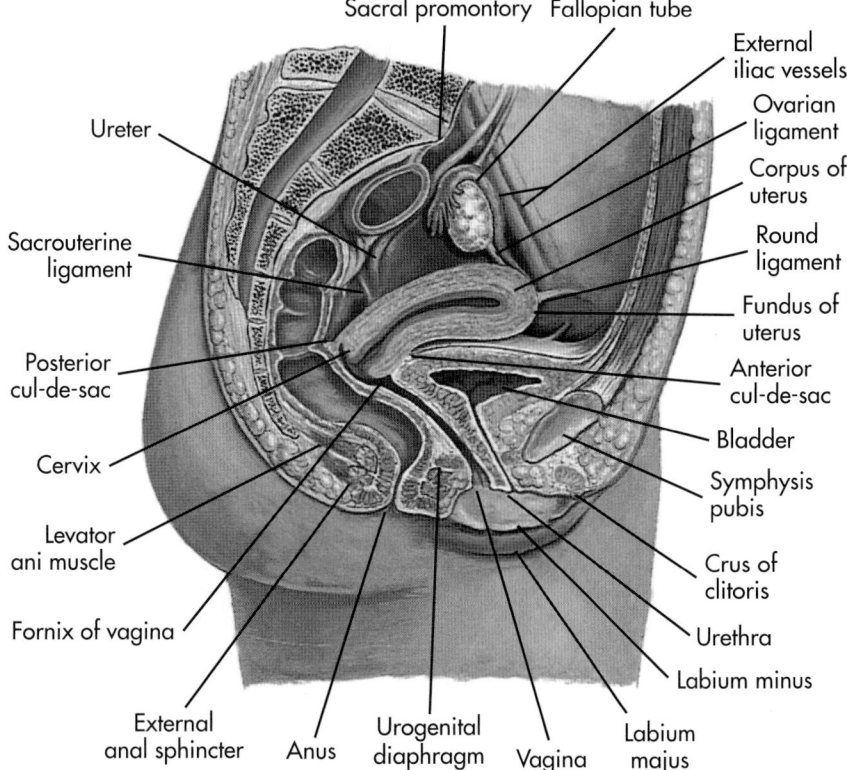

Fig. 10-3 Midsagittal view of the female pelvic organs.
(From Seidel HM et al: Mosby's guide to physical examination, ed 4, St Louis, 1999, Mosby.)

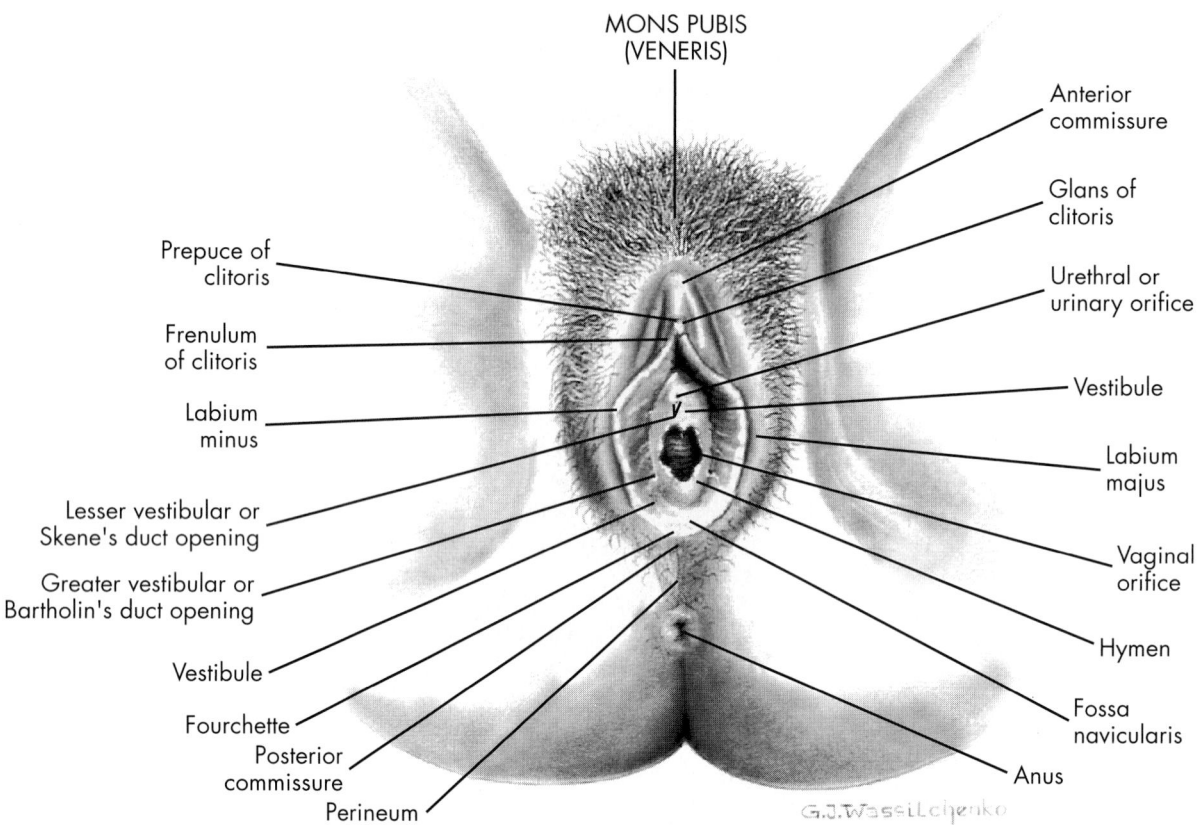

Fig. 10-4 External female genitalia.
(From Lowdermilk DL, Perry SE, Bobak IM: Maternity and women's health care, *ed 6, St Louis, 1997, Mosby.)*

Hyperparathyroidism
Cerebrovascular accident (CVA)
Traumatic brain injury
Alzheimer's disease
Spinal cord injury
Transverse myelitis
Guillain-Barré syndrome
Hepatitis
Acquired immunodeficiency syndrome (AIDS)
Cancer, leukemia (chemotherapy, radiation)
Renal failure
Dialysis (continuous ambulatory peritoneal dialysis [CAPD], hemodialysis)
Allergies (food, medication, environmental)

PREVIOUS SURGERY OR ILLNESS
Genitourinary (trauma, injury)
Urologic or renal surgery
Urinary tract, vaginal infections
Gynecologic/obstetric history (LMP, gravida para, forceps delivery)
Hepatitis
Tuberculosis
Neurologic disorders
Spinal cord disorders
Peripheral nervous system disorders

FAMILY HISTORY
Renal and other types of cancer
Congenital anomalies/urologic disorders
Diabetes mellitus
Hypertension
Renal disease
Polycystic kidney disease
Lupus erythematosis

SOCIAL HISTORY
Marital status
Family structure
Employment status
Occupation
Exposure to chemicals
Sexual history (exposure to sexually transmitted diseases [STDs])
Products used or hygiene (e.g., feminine sprays, soaps)
Use of caffeine, alcohol, cola drinks
Use of illegal drugs
Smoking history
Age (Gerontologic Considerations box)

MEDICATION HISTORY
Current prescribed and over-the-counter medications
    Adrenergic blockers to diminish bladder resistance
    Antibiotics to prevent or treat infection

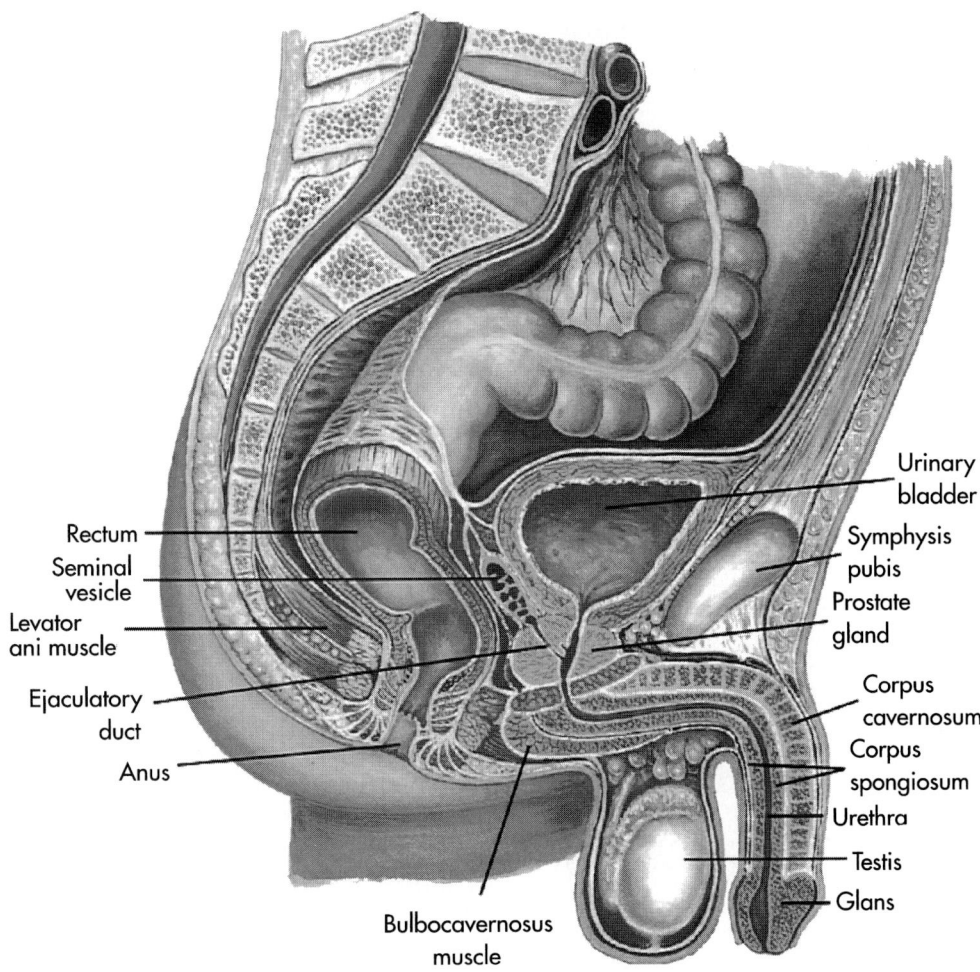

Fig. 10-5   Male pelvic organs.
(From Seidel HM et al: Mosby's guide to physical examination, *ed 4, St Louis, 1999, Mosby.)*

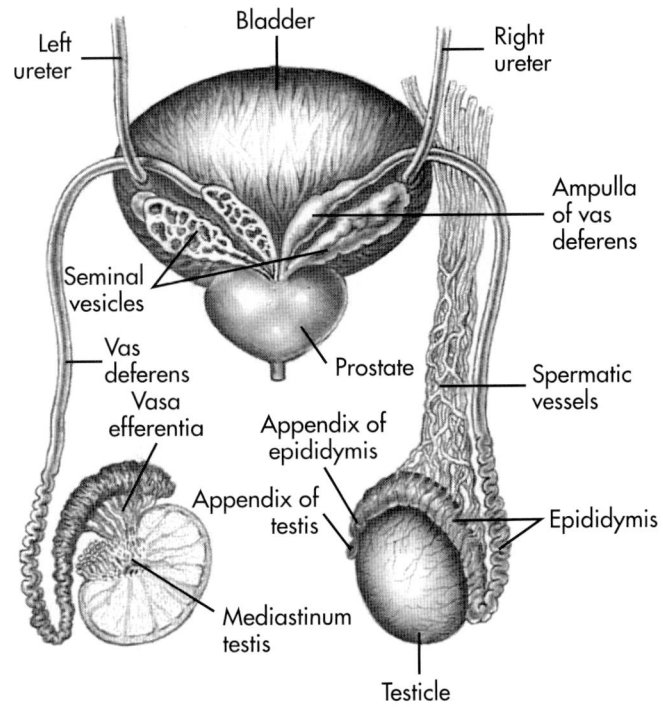

Fig. 10-6   Testes.
(From Thompson JM et al: Mosby's clinical nursing, *ed 4, St Louis, 1997, Mosby.)*

Gerontologic Considerations

- Urinary frequency, urgency, nocturia, and incontinence are common with aging. These occur because of weakened musculature in the bladder and urethra, reduced renal blood supply, diminished neurologic sensation combined with decreased bladder capacity, effects of medications, allergic reactions, and environmental toxins.
- Urinary incontinence is a leading reason for institutional placement of older adults.
- Urinary incontinence can lead to a loss of self-esteem and result in decreased participation in social activities.
- Older women are particularly at risk for stress incontinence because of hormonal changes and weakened pelvic musculature.
- Older men are particularly at risk for urinary retention because of prostatic hypertrophy.
- Urinary tract infections in older adults are often associated with invasive procedures such as catheterization, diabetes, and neurologic disorders.
- Inadequate fluid intake, immobility, and conditions that lead to urinary stasis increase the risk of infection in the older adult.
- Frequent toileting and meticulous skin care can reduce the risk of skin impairment secondary to urinary incontinence.

Modified from Christensen BL, Kockrow EO: Foundations of nursing, *ed 3, St Louis, 1998, Mosby.*

Anticholinergics/antispasmodics to relax smooth muscle in the bladder resulting in decreased involuntary contraction

Anticoagulants to decrease consistency of or thin blood

Antigout drug (xanthine oxidase inhibitor); allopurinol

Analgesics (narcotic or nonnarcotic to control pain)

Alpha-adrenergic blockers to decrease bladder outlet resistance, manage symptoms of benign prostatic hypertrophy (BPH)

Adrenergic agents to manage stress incontinence, enuresis, retrograde ejaculation

Antidysrhythmics to regulate heart rate

Antidepressants to manage depression associated with acute or chronic genitourinary conditions or diseases; bicyclic and tricyclic antidepressants also used to manage incontinence

Antihypertensives to manage blood pressure (BP)

Chemotherapeutic agents to treat various types of cancer

Cholinergic agents to stimulate bladder contraction

Diuretics to increase renal excretion of water and solutes

Decongestants to decrease urinary output, manage incontinence

Erythrocyte-stimulating hormone to treat anemia resulting from chronic renal failure

Hormones to increase or decrease existing levels of hormones (such as estrogens and androgens)

Immunosuppressive agents to reduce graft rejection after renal transplantation

Muscle relaxants to promote regular bladder emptying

Papaverine hydrochloride to manage erectile dysfunction

Stool softeners to decrease straining with bowel movements and therefore reduce pressure on genitourinary organs

Vasodilators to diagnose and treat impotence

Vitamins to replace or augment existing levels of vitamins/iron

Intravenous fluid/total parenteral nutrition (TPN) therapy to replace or maintain necessary fluid volume, electrolyte levels

Blood transfusions to replace or maintain appropriate circulating blood volume

DIAGNOSTIC TESTS

Urinalysis

Color
Clarity
Odor
pH
Specific gravity
Osmolality
Sediment
Red blood cells (RBCs)
Pus
Bacteria
White blood cells (WBCs)
Nitrites
Casts
Crystals/calculi
Blood
Protein
Glucose
Creatinine
Urea
Uric acid
Electrolytes
    Sodium
    Potassium
    Chloride
    Calcium
Urine culture and sensitivity
Urine collection (24 hour)
    Aldosterone
    17-Hydroxycorticosteroids
    17-Ketosteroids
    Catecholamines
        Norepinephrine
        Epinephrine
        Dopamine
    Vanillylmandelic acid (VMA)
    Calcium

Phosphorus
Uric acid
Urine clearance tests
    Inulin
    Creatinine
    Phenolsulfonphthalein (PSP)
Stone analysis
    Oxylate
    Calcium
    Uric acid
    Cystine
Voiding diary
Urine cytology

Blood analysis

Osmolality
Electrolytes
    Sodium
    Potassium
    Chloride
    Calcium
Magnesium
Phosphorus
Alkaline phosphatase
Blood urea nitrogen (BUN)
Creatinine
Uric acid
Total protein
Albumin
Glucose
Prostate-specific antigen (PSA)
Complete blood cell count (CBC)
Coagulation factors
    Prothrombin time/International Normalized Ratio
        (PT/INR)
    Activated partial thromboplastin time (APTT)
Blood type and antibody screen
Tissue compatibility testing
Serum complement
Antistreptolysin O titer
Hepatitis B and C antigens
Human immunodeficiency virus (HIV) antigen
Tumor markers
    Prostatic specific antigen
    Alpha-fetoprotein (AFP)
    Human chorionic gonadotropin (HCG)
    Wound or throat cultures

Imaging studies

Flat plate of abdomen
Kidney, ureters, bladder (KUB)
Excretory urogram
Nephrotomogram
Captopril renal scan
Intravenous pyelography (IVP)
Antegrade pyelogram
Retrograde pyelogram
Retrograde cystogram, voiding cystourethrogram

Retrograde urethrogram
Renal angiogram (renogram)
    Renal arteriogram
    Renal venogram
Renal computed tomography (CT) scan
Renal and prostate ultrasonography
Scrotal nuclear imaging
Scrotal ultrasonography
Magnetic resonance imaging (MRI)
Chest x-ray

Other tests

Whitaker test
Penile temescence tests
Radionuclide imaging
Endoscopies
    Cystoscopy
    Cystourethroscopy
    Ureteroscopy
    Percutaneous renal endoscopy (nephroscopy)
Renal biopsy
Prostate biopsy
Urodynamic studies
    Cystometrogram
    Uroflowmetry
    Pressure flow study
    Urethral pressure profile
    Electromyography and electromyogram
    Dynamic infusion cavernosometry and
        cavernosography (DICC)
Electrocardiogram (ECG)
Pulmonary function tests

■ URINARY TRACT INFECTION

Infection, with or without symptoms, that occurs in the lower or upper urinary tract (Table 10-1); most urinary tract infections (UTIs) (85% to 90%) are caused by Escherichia coli; asymptomatic UTI is most common for persons over the age of 65; the percentage is increased for those in long-term care facilities or hospitals; risk and severity may increase with conditions such as vesicoureteral reflux, urinary tract obstruction, urinary stasis, recent urethral instrumentation, septicemia, pregnancy, diabetes, and spinal cord injury

ASSESSMENT
See Table 10-1

DIAGNOSTIC TESTS
Urinalysis
    Cloudy
    Bacteria
    Pyuria
    WBCs
    RBCs may be present
Positive urine culture and sensitivity

Table 10-1	Symptoms of Urinary Tract Infection	
	Subjective	**Objective**
Lower UTI (cystitis, urethritis, prostatitis)	Suprapubic discomfort Lower back pain Bladder spasm Dysuria Urinary urgency Urinary frequency Nocturia	Hematuria Pyuria Malodorous urine Fever
Upper UTI* (pyelonephritis)	Flank pain Malaise Anorexia Nausea	Enlarged kidney Costovertebral tenderness Abdominal rigidity Chills Vomiting Decreased urinary output

Findings are in addition to those for lower UTI.

Radiography
   KUB
   Excretory urography
   Cystoscopy
CBC: elevated WBC; often left shift (increase in band cells)

POTENTIAL COMPLICATIONS
Dehydration
Bacteremia
Renal involvement
Parenchymal scarring
Urinary calculi
Abscess formation

MULTIDISCIPLINARY MANAGEMENT
THERAPEUTIC MANAGEMENT
Medications
   Antibiotics: ampicillin, amoxicillin, cephalosporins, ciprofloxacin (Cipro), sulfonamides
   Urinary tract antiseptics: cinoxacin (Cinobac), methenamine mandelate (Mandelamine), nalidixic acid (NegGram), nitrofurantoin (Furandantin, Macrodantin)
   Urinary tract analgesics: phenazopiridine (Pyridium)
   Antipyretics: acetaminophen, ibuprofen, aspirin
Acid-ash diet may be indicated
Rest with gradual return to activities as tolerated
Oral or IV fluids
Cystoscopy, intravenous pyelogram (IVP)
Urology consult
Infectious disease consult
Surgical intervention for obstruction

Follow-up cultures may be ordered
   Weeks 1 and 4
   Every 3 to 4 months for 1 year for chronic UTI

PATIENT PROBLEMS—NURSING DIAGNOSES/INTERVENTIONS

▼ Infection related to presence of bacteria in the urinary tract

Assess temperature (T) q4h and report if > 101° F (38.5° C), *which may indicate progressing infection*
Monitor character of urine and report if cloudy and malodorous, *which may indicate that present medication therapy is ineffective*
Collect repeat midstream urine for culture and sensitivity when no evidence of improvement is noted
Encourage high oral fluid intake *to promote systemic flushing of some bacteria* (unless fluid restriction is ordered/appropriate)
Offer cranberry juice *to prevent bacteria from adhering to bladder wall*
Instruct patient to void as soon as urge is felt and completely empty bladder *to prevent overdistention of and decreased blood supply to the bladder and decrease chance for bacteria to colonize*
Encourage patient to shower rather than bathe *to promote good hygiene without allowing bacteria to enter the urethra*
Encourage good perineal hygiene by keeping perineal area clean and dry *to discourage growth of bacteria*
Teach female patient to wipe perianal area from front to back *to decrease ability of bacteria to enter urinary tract*

Expected Outcomes
Exhibits no signs or symptoms of UTI (see Table 10-1)
Urine culture and sensitivity negative for bacteria

▼ Altered urinary elimination related to UTI

Monitor urinary output and report if < 30 ml/hr, *which may indicate inadequate fluid volume*
Provide opportunities for patient to void q2h and prn (assist to bathroom and/or with urinal/bedpan)
Promote ability of patient on bed rest *to completely empty bladder* by assisting to upright position before patient voids
Advise patient to avoid drinking fluid for 2 to 3 hours before bedtime *to decrease nocturia*
Advise patient to avoid caffeine and alcohol, *which exacerbate irritative symptoms*

Expected Outcomes
Maintains balanced fluid intake and output
Usual voiding pattern is resumed by patient
Reports absence of dysuria, urinary frequency and urgency, nocturia

▼ Pain related to bladder spasm and mucosal irritation

Assess nature, intensity, location, duration, and precipitating and alleviating factors of pain *to establish baseline condition*

Provide bed rest *to promote healing and comfort;* increase activities as ordered/tolerated

Institute comfort measures (relaxation techniques/guided imagery, diversional activities)

Encourage high oral fluid intake *to dilute urine and decrease dysuria*

Monitor and document response to efforts aimed at decreasing discomfort

Notify physician of unrelieved or increasing pain *to collaborate on alternative approaches*

Expected Outcomes
Takes analgesics as needed
Verbal and nonverbal evidence of decrease in pain

Additional Nursing Diagnosis to Consider
Altered sexuality patterns related to UTI

PATIENT/FAMILY TEACHING
Teach methods of preventing recurrence of UTI
   Force fluids to 2000 to 2500 ml/day unless restricted
   Avoid fluids that aggravate urinary tract (caffeinated beverages) and drink fluids that promote systemic flushing (e.g., water and cranberry juice)
   Empty bladder every q2h to 3h
   Shower rather than bathe and use antibacterial soap
   Avoid using perfumed products in perineal area and colored toilet tissue
   Avoid douching unless ordered by physician
   Keep perineal area clean and dry
   Wipe from front to back when cleansing perineal area
   Void before and after sexual intercourse
   Wear cotton underpants; avoid nylon underpants
   Wear loose, nonrestrictive clothing
Teach about ordered medications: names, dosages, schedules, purposes, and side effects; remind patient taking phenazopyridine (Pyridium) that urine may be orange

DISCHARGE/HOME CARE PLANNING
Emphasize importance of ongoing outpatient care because of high incidence of recurrent infection
Teach symptoms of recurring UTI (e.g., dysuria, urgency, and frequency) and importance of reporting to physician
Reinforce importance of completing prescribed medication therapy (patient with chronic infections may be prescribed prophylactic medication after completion of present antibiotic therapy)
Teach method and importance of obtaining midstream specimen for culture and sensitivity after completion of antibiotic therapy

Teach method of self-monitoring urine test for bacteria (Microstix) (patient with chronic infections may be asked to test frequently)
Advise patient to avoid taking over-the-counter medications without physician approval

■ URINARY CALCULI (UROLITHIASIS)
Formation of stones in the kidney (pelvis or calyx) and their passage in the path of urine flow; renal calculi are classified according to their composition (usually calcium, uric acid, cystine, phosphate, oxalate, or struvite); urinary calculi may vary from a few millimeters up to a size that occupies the entire renal pelvis (Fig. 10-7)

ASSESSMENT
SUBJECTIVE DATA
Pain (back, flank, abdominal, groin, colicky)
Nausea, vomiting
Chills
Dysuria
Frequency/urgency of urination

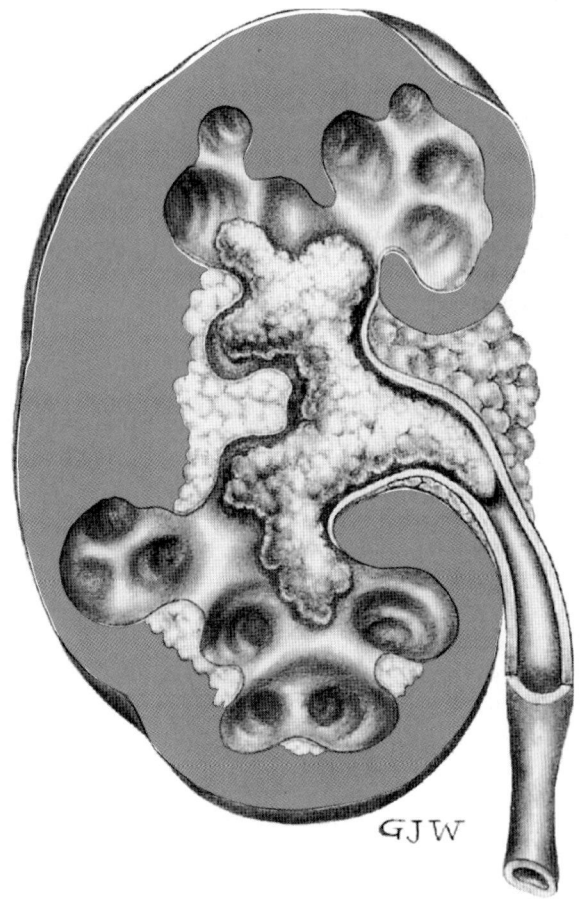

Fig. 10-7 Staghorn calculus.
(From Brundage DJ: Mosby's clinical nursing series: renal disorders, *St Louis, 1992, Mosby.)*

OBJECTIVE DATA
Anxiety/distress
Hematuria (microscopic or gross)
Oliguria
Fever

DIAGNOSTIC TESTS
Serum BUN, creatinine, calcium, phosphorus, uric acid: elevated results
Urinalysis: WBC, hematuria, abnormal color, bacteria, crystals
Urine culture and sensitivity
Urine collection (24 hour): abnormal creatine clearance/abnormal excretion of calcium, phosphorus, magnesium, uric acid, cystine, and oxalate
KUB: radiopaque stone
Renal ultrasound: stones identified
Renal CT scan: abnormalities of kidneys
Intravenous (IV) urogram: filling defects; ureteral dilation; hydronephrosis
Analysis of stones: constituents such as cystine, calcium, oxalate, uric acid

POTENTIAL COMPLICATIONS
Infection
Obstruction
Sepsis
Hydronephrosis
Renal failure
Kidney loss

MULTIDISCIPLINARY MANAGEMENT
THERAPEUTIC MANAGEMENT
See Table 10-2 for treatment plan based on type of stone
Medications
 Analgesics
 Antispasmodics

IV or oral fluids
Catheterization
Straining of all urine for stones and analysis
Urology consult
Endocrinology consult (to assess parathyroid function)
Dietary consult
Surgical interventions (Box 10-1)

Table 10-2	Therapeutic Management for Renal Calculi
Type of Stone	**Treatment Plan**
Calcium	Nonthiazide diuretics / Low-calcium diet / Oral phosphates
Uric acid	Allopurinol / Sodium bicarbonate / Sodium citrate / Potassium phosphate / Low-purine diet
Cystine	D-Penicillamine / Sodium bicarbonate / Low-animal protein diet
Oxalate	Low-oxalate diet / Pyridoxine
Struvite	Penicillin / Drugs to acidify urine

Box 10-1 Interventions for Urinary Calculi

STONE DISINTEGRATION
Extracorporeal Shock Wave Lithotripsy (ESWL), Transcutaneous Shock Wave Lithotripsy
Carefully directed shock waves enter the body and disintegrate the calculus

Laser Lithotripsy
Endoscopy tube is threaded up the ureter to the stone, and laser energy is passed via a thin wire into the stone, breaking it into fine pieces

Percutaneous Stone Dissolution
Chemical agents are injected into the nephrostomy tube to dissolve the stone

Percutaneous Ultrasonic Lithotripsy (PUL)
Ultrasonic probe is inserted into renal pelvis, and pulses of ultrasound are administered to disintegrate the stone

STONE EXTRACTION
Endoscopic Removal of Stone
After a tube is inserted via flank incision through the parenchyma into renal calyx, an endoscope is passed and the stone is extracted

Ureteroscopy and Stone Basket Extraction
A flexible ureteroscope is passed transurethrally into ureter; a special collapsible wire basket instrument is inserted to snare the stone, which is then pulled out with the instrument

Pyelolithotomy
Removal of stone through an incision into the renal pelvis

Nephrolithotomy
Removal of stone through a longitudinal incision across the middle two thirds of the kidney

Ureterolithotomy
Removal of stone by incision into the ureter

Cystolithotomy
Removal of stone by incision into the bladder

Nephrectomy/Partial Nephrectomy
Removal of a kidney when extensive renal damage occurs

PATIENT PROBLEMS—NURSING DIAGNOSES/INTERVENTIONS

▼Pain related to presence or passage of renal stone(s) and/or surgical incision

Assess type, intensity, location, and duration of pain; document *so changes may be noted*
  Report intensified pain *indicating impaction of calculus or obstruction of urine flow*
  Report sudden relief in pain *indicating that stone has passed through narrow junction*
  Report colicky pain *indicating movement of calculus*
Identify verbal and nonverbal responses to pain
Monitor for syncopal episodes associated with renal colic
Offer analgesics, document effectiveness and tolerance *so treatment plan can be altered as needed*
Apply external heat to painful flank *to promote comfort*
Institute nonpharmacologic comfort measures
  Optimal positioning
  Restful environment
  Relaxation techniques/guided imagery
  Diversional activities

Expected Outcomes
Relaxed with no other evidence of pain
Reports increase in comfort level

▼Altered urinary elimination, related to stone in path of urinary flow

Assess patient's usual voiding pattern and begin voiding diary *so changes can be noted*
Monitor for signs and symptoms of UTI (dysuria, frequency, urgency) and report to physician *for evaluation and treatment*
Maintain patency of catheters to *promote optimal flow of urine*
  Tubing below level of bladder *to allow for gravity flow*
  Assess for clamping, kinks in tubing
  Secure catheters while still allowing for patient movement
  Irrigate as ordered
Label each tube clearly and record drainage from each tube separately *to allow for accurate assessment of output from each system*
If nephrostomy tube in place
  Tape to flank
  Do not clamp
  Irrigate only with physician's order (may be continuous or intermittent)
  Have extra tube available at bedside
  Notify physician immediately if nephrostomy tube becomes dislodged
If double-J ureteral stent in place, check that suture from urinary meatus to stent is present (suture will be used to remove stent)

After urinary catheter is removed, institute measures *to facilitate voiding*
  Privacy
  Comfortable positioning
  Running tap water
  Placing patient's hand in warm water
  Pouring warm water over perineum
  Relaxation techniques
  Applying oil of peppermint (a few drops in bedpan/urinal or on cotton ball in front of urinary meatus)
  Stroking inner aspect of thigh gently with ice
  Offering analgesic
  Voiding 1 to 2 hours after fluid intake
  Double voiding (to empty bladder more completely)
Strain all urine for stones and send for analysis if found
Report, describe, and document passage of all stones
Encourage patient to drink at least 2500 ml/day (unless contraindicated) *to flush stones from system*
Monitor and report signs and symptoms of urinary retention (e.g., bladder distention) and report to physician
Monitor intake and output frequently *to identify imbalance requiring treatment*

Expected Outcomes
Intake and output are balanced
All stones are passed
Regular voiding pattern is resumed

▼Altered nutrition: less than body requirements related to nausea and vomiting

Identify factors contributing to nausea and vomiting; relieve as possible
Remove noxious sights, smells from room if possible
Monitor and document effectiveness, tolerance of ordered antiemetics
Instruct patient to change position slowly *to decrease GI upset*
Provide frequent oral hygiene *to decrease acidic taste in mouth, throat*
Encourage small, frequent meals *to prevent overdistention of the stomach*
Encourage patient to eat easily digestible foods (e.g., toast, crackers)
Encourage patient to eat slowly *for optimal digestion*
If emesis occurs, assess and document character and amount for physician evaluation
Request dietitian as needed

Expected Outcome
Exhibits no nausea, vomiting

▼Risk for impaired skin integrity related to wound drainage

Assess incisional site for signs and symptoms of infection (erythema, edema, pain, drainage) and report to physician

Change surgical dressings using sterile technique as ordered

Inspect skin surrounding catheters and tubes and report redness, breakdown

Apply ostomy pouch and skin barrier around wounds exposed to prolonged or copious urinary drainage *to prevent excoriation*

Expected Outcome

Skin is intact

PATIENT/FAMILY TEACHING

Explain purpose, procedure of ordered diagnostic tests

Teach patient/family to care for incision and perform ordered dressing changes; refer to home health agency if needed

To help prevent UTI

Empty bladder every q2h to 3h

Drink 2000 to 3000 ml/day unless contraindicated; (e.g., water, cranberry juice)

Avoid fluids that aggravate urinary tract (caffeinated beverages)

Shower rather than bathe and use antibacterial soap

Keep perineal area clean and dry

Wipe from front to back when cleansing perianal area

Explain special diets (low calcium, purine, or oxalate) and provide written food list

Teach about ordered medications: names, dosages, schedules, purposes, and side effects

DISCHARGE/HOME CARE PLANNING

Emphasize importance of ongoing outpatient care

Teach patient and those in contact to use good handwashing techniques

Advise patient to take frequent rest periods during the day and sleep 6 to 8 hours per night; increase activity as ordered and tolerated

Encourage patient to avoid contact with persons who have infections (e.g., colds, flu)

Encourage patient to report signs and symptoms of incisional infection (redness, swelling, pain, drainage) to physician

Teach symptoms of UTI (dysuria, urgency, frequency, foul-smelling urine, fever > 101° F [38.5° C]) and encourage patient to report these findings to physician

Instruct patient to maintain ordered diet at home

Teach patient how to measure, strain urine; advise patient to save any passed stones or gravel and notify physician when stones are passed

Advise patient to report abnormalities of urine to physician (e.g., frank hematuria)

Instruct patient how to collect 24-hour urine at home

Advise patient to avoid taking over-the-counter medications without physician approval

■ ACUTE URINARY RETENTION

A condition in which the bladder becomes distended with urine and the patient is unable to empty the blad-der; potential causes of acute urinary retention are medications, infection, detrusor function deficit, obstruction, constipation/fecal impaction, anxiety, immobility from acute illness, trauma, postoperative complications, and muscle tension

ASSESSMENT
SUBJECTIVE DATA
Cessation of urination
Dribbling
Urinary frequency/urgency
Inability to start stream; straining
Decrease in force of stream
Interruption of flow
Dysuria
Nocturia
Bladder/suprapubic pain
Restlessness
Anxiety

OBJECTIVE DATA
Postvoid residual > 100 ml
Output less than intake
Bladder distention
Diaphoresis

DIAGNOSTIC TESTS
Urinalysis: WBCs/RBCs, bacteria
Urine culture and sensitivity: bacteria
Serum electrolytes, BUN, creatinine: abnormal, or elevated results
KUB: abnormalities with kidneys, ureters, or bladder
Urodynamic studies: evidence of obstruction
Cystogram: obstruction, deficient contractility
IVP: obstructive uropathy
Cystoscopy: bladder changes, strictures

POTENTIAL COMPLICATIONS
UTI
Vesicoureteral reflex
Compromised/insufficient renal function

MULTIDISCIPLINARY MANAGEMENT
THERAPEUTIC MANAGEMENT
Catheterization
Voiding schedule/program
Urology consult
Medications
Antibiotics (if infection present)
Cholinergics to stimulate bladder contraction
Adrenergic-blocking drug to diminish bladder resistance
Analgesics
IV fluids (for postobstructive diuresis syndrome)
Pharmacology consult
Surgical resection or laser ablation of obstructive lesion
Dilation of stricture or surgical repair of pelvic descent

PATIENT PROBLEMS—NURSING DIAGNOSES/INTERVENTIONS

▼Urinary retention related to obstruction or neuro-muscular dysfunction

Catheterize patient as ordered using sterile technique *to minimize risk of infection*

If unable to pass catheter (sign of obstruction) remove and report to physician

If bright red urine occurs after decompression (sign of tissue damage, irritation, or inflammation), notify physician

Monitor for and report postobstructive diuresis; urine output > 200 ml/hr

Assess bladder frequently for distention, tenderness and document changes *so collaborative treatments can be instituted*

Monitor intake and output *to determine imbalances requiring interventions*

Institute measures that facilitate bladder emptying
  Privacy
  Comfortable positioning
  Running tap water
  Placing patient's hand in warm water
  Applying heat to suprapubic area (if ordered)
  Pouring warm water over perineum
  Relaxation techniques
  Applying oil of peppermint (a few drops in bedpan/urinal or on cotton ball in front of urinary meatus)
  Stroking inner aspect of thigh gently with ice
  Offering analgesic
  Voiding 1 to 2 hours after fluid intake
  Double voiding (to empty bladder more completely)

Monitor and document effectiveness, tolerance of medications *so changes can be made when required*

Apply ice to perineum *to decrease swelling when ordered*

Check postvoid residual *to determine whether bladder is emptying effectively;* report if >100 ml

Vital signs, intake and output, and serum and urine electrolytes must be assessed frequently *for evidence of abnormalities*

Expected Outcomes
Intake and output are balanced
Regular voiding pattern is established

▼Pain related to bladder fullness and inability to void

Assess and document type, intensity, location, and duration of pain

Identify factors that precipitate and alleviate pain

Offer analgesics, documenting effectiveness and tolerance *to determine need for treatment plan change*

Institute nonpharmacologic comfort measures
  Optimal positioning
  Sitz baths, warm perineal soaks
  Relaxation techniques/guided imagery
  Diversional activities

Expected Outcome
Relaxed, without other evidence of pain, and reports increased comfort

Additional Nursing Diagnoses to Consider
Risk for infection related to frequent home catheterization
Self-esteem disturbance related to need for home self-catheterization

PATIENT/FAMILY TEACHING
To help prevent UTI
  Empty bladder q2h to 3h
  Encourage patient to take fluids to 2000 to 3000 ml/day (unless contraindicated) to flush bacteria from system
  Avoid fluids that aggravate urinary tract (e.g., caffeinated beverages) and drink fluids that promote systemic flushing (e.g., water and cranberry juice)
  Shower rather than bathe and use antibacterial soap
  Keep perineal area clean and dry
  Wipe from front to back when cleansing perianal area
Teach technique of intermittent self-catheterization if ordered (Box 10-2)
Teach about ordered medications: names, dosages, schedules, purposes, and side effects

DISCHARGE/HOME CARE PLANNING
Reinforce method of self-catheterization
Teach care of Foley catheter and drainage units
Emphasize importance of ongoing outpatient care
Teach symptoms of UTI (dysuria, urgency, frequency, foul-smelling urine, fever > 101° F [38.5° C]) and encourage patient to report these findings to physician
Instruct patient to measure urine after voiding and note character of urine, time, amount, and force of stream (use voiding diary if appropriate)
Advise patient to avoid taking over-the-counter medications without physician approval

■ INDWELLING URETHRAL CATHETER MANAGEMENT
A catheter inserted through the urethra into the bladder to drain urine (Fig. 10-8)

ASSESSMENT
SUBJECTIVE DATA
While catheter is in place
  Bladder spasms
  Sensation of needing to void
  Discomfort, pulling at catheter insertion site

Box 10-2	Instructions for Self-Catheterization

EQUIPMENT
Catheter
Soap/water
Water-soluble lubricant
Washcloth
Mirror
Pan/toilet
Measuring container
Storage container

PREPARATION
Try to urinate (measure output)
Wash hands thoroughly with soap and water
Assume appropriate/comfortable position
Position mirror if needed

PROCEDURE

Men

Wash and rinse end of penis with soap and water (pull back foreskin if not circumcised)
Lubricate first 2 inches of catheter
Hold penis in nondominant hand and extend out from body
Slowly insert catheter into urethra (7 to 10 inches) until urine begins flowing
Allow all urine to drain into measuring container
Slowly remove catheter; if urine begins to flow again, stop until drainage ends, then continue to remove catheter
Replace foreskin to normal position
Measure/record amount

Women

Separate vaginal folds with fingers of nondominant hand and cleanse perineal area with soap
Lubricate tip of catheter
Hold catheter in dominant hand
Using nondominant hand to keep vaginal folds open, insert catheter into urethra (about 3 inches) until urine begins flowing
Press down with abdominal muscles to help empty bladder into measuring container
Allow all urine to drain
Remove catheter when urine flow stops
Measure/record amount

AFTER PROCEDURE

Wash penis/perineal area to remove lubricant
Wash catheter in soap and water, rinse well
Dry catheter and wrap in clean towel
Place in clean container for storage in clean area
Wash hands

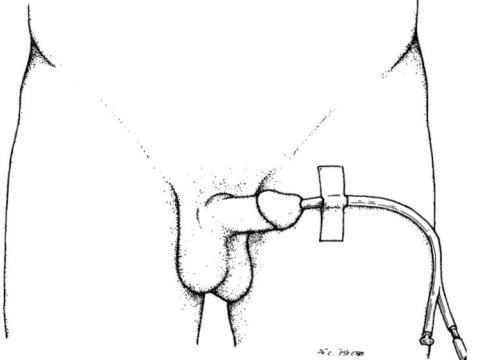

Fig. 10-8   Indwelling urethral catheter.

After catheter removal
  Inability to urinate
  Difficulty initiating urine stream
  Small urinary stream
  Dysuria
  Frequency/urgency with urination

OBJECTIVE DATA
While catheter is in place
  Distended bladder
  Fever
  Chills
  Pyuria
  Hematuria
  Edema of urethral meatus
After catheter removal
  Urinary retention with overflow
  Hematuria
  Dribbling
  Incontinence

DIAGNOSTIC TESTS
Urinalysis: cloudy, malodorous, WBC, RBC, bacteria
Urine culture and sensitivity: bacteria

POTENTIAL COMPLICATIONS
Recurrent and/or progressive UTI
Septicemia
Urinary tract calculi

Strictures
Urethral erosion
Epididymitis
Difficulty in voiding after removal

MULTIDISCIPLINARY MANAGEMENT
THERAPEUTIC MANAGEMENT
Medications
　Antibiotics
　Local anesthetic agents
　Stool softeners
Periodic catheter change

PATIENT PROBLEM—NURSING DIAGNOSIS/INTERVENTIONS

▼Altered urinary elimination related to presence of indwelling urethral catheter

Monitor intake and output frequently *to determine imbalances that require treatment*
Palpate bladder *to determine whether distention is present*
Maintain patency of catheter *to promote optimal drainage*
　Avoid clamping or occluding catheter
　Irrigate catheter as ordered
　Keep catheter drainage unit and tubing below level of bladder
Maintain integrity of closed gravity drainage system at all times *to decrease risk of infection;* change system per policy
Maintain tension-free catheter
　Tape drainage tubing to inner aspect of lateral thigh or use catheter strap (female)
　Tape catheter to abdomen or upper thigh or use catheter strap (male)
Cleanse periurethral area bid to promote hygiene and comfort
Apply anesthetic ointment to urethral meatus if ordered
Collect urine specimens only by aspirating urine through catheter collection port with sterile 10-ml syringe and 25-gauge needle
After urinary catheter is removed, institute measures to facilitate voiding
　Privacy
　Comfortable positioning
　Running tap water
　Placing patient's hand in warm water
　Applying heat to suprapubic area (if ordered)
　Pouring warm water over perineum
　Relaxation techniques
　Applying oil of peppermint (a few drops in bedpan/urinal or on cotton ball in front of urinary meatus)
　Stroking inner aspect of thigh gently with ice
　Offering analgesic

Box 10-3	**Instructions for Care of Indwelling Urethral Catheter**

- Wash hands with soap and water before and after handling catheter or drainage unit.
- Do not open the closed drainage system except to empty the bag.
- Obtain urine samples using a syringe after cleaning the aspiration port.
- Use gloves when draining the system to protect from contamination.
- Tape the catheter securely to prevent traction on the meatus.
- Empty drainage bag once q8h or as soon as it fills.
- Avoid clamping or kinking tubing.
- Empty the bag by loosening the clamp on the end of the leg or bedside bag.
- Always keep the drainage bag lower than the bladder.
- Change catheter when it becomes obstructed or falls out or drainage tubing is coated with grit and sediment (some policies indicate q4wk).

Voiding q1h to 2h after fluid intake
Double voiding (to empty bladder more completely)
Report abnormalities in urine, residual volume > 100 ml and/or retention of urine with overflow to physician

Expected Outcomes
Experiences no symptoms of infection while catheter is in place or after removal
Voids without evidence of complications after removal of catheter

Additional Nursing Diagnoses to Consider
Body image disturbance related to presence of indwelling urethral catheter at discharge
Anxiety related to ability to care for indwelling urethral catheter

PATIENT/FAMILY TEACHING
Explain to patient that presence of catheter may cause urge to urinate
To help prevent UTI
　Encourage patient to maintain fluid intake of 2000 to 3000 ml/day (unless contraindicated) to flush bacteria from system
　Avoid fluids that aggravate urinary tract (caffeinated beverages) and drink fluids that promote systemic flushing (e.g., water and cranberry juice)
　Teach about ordered medications: names, dosages, schedules, purposes, and side effects

DISCHARGE/HOME CARE PLANNING
Teach/reinforce method of caring for indwelling urinary catheter (Box 10-3)
Emphasize importance of ongoing outpatient care

Teach patient how to cleanse periurethral area

Advise patient to report absence of urine, persistent leaking around catheter, accidental removal of catheter, and back pain to home health nurse or physician

Teach signs and symptoms of UTI (dysuria, urinary urgency and frequency, foul-smelling urine, fever > 101° F [38.5° C]) and encourage patient to report these findings to physician

Advise patient to avoid taking over-the-counter medications without physician approval

■ URINARY INCONTINENCE

Urinary incontinence is the involuntary loss of urine; incontinence affects more than 13 million people in this country: at some time, 10% to 30% of women between ages 15 and 64 are incontinent, 15% to 35% of the non-institutionalized population ages 60 and older are incontinent; risk and severity of incontinence may be related to existing medical conditions and diseases, urinary or vaginal infections, surgical history, childbearing history, hormonal changes, sexual history, age, obesity, physical condition, and certain medications; a variety of mechanisms may be involved, and incontinence may be classified into five types: functional, stress, reflex, urge, and total

functional incontinence: The involuntary loss of urine that is unpredictable and occurs when continent people are unable or unwilling to get to the bathroom on time; there is no impairment of the urinary system

stress incontinence: The involuntary loss of 50 ml or less of urine occurring with increased intraabdominal pressure; this type of incontinence is associated with decreased tone of the pelvic floor muscles, damage to the internal sphincter bladder neck caused by surgery, trauma, or radiation, decreased estrogen levels, or UTI

reflex incontinence: The involuntary loss of urine at fairly predictable intervals; the detrusor contraction is stimulated by a full bladder; the bladder empties, but a large residual usually remains; this type of incontinence is associated with spinal cord lesions above S-2 to S-4, traumatic injuries, tumors, multiple sclerosis, other demyelinating diseases, and some cerebral lesions

urge incontinence: The involuntary loss of urine occurring after a strong urge is felt, but the patient is unable to hold the urine long enough to reach the bathroom or receptacle; this type of incontinence is associated with detrusor instability caused by disorders of the central nervous system such as CVA, Parkinson's disease, Alzheimer's disease, or brain tumors or trauma; bladder irritation caused by infection or ingestion of irritating fluids or overdistention of the bladder related to increased fluid intake or decreased intervals between voiding may also result in urge incontinence

total incontinence: The involuntary, unpredictable, or continuous loss of urine; this type of incontinence is asso-ciated with neurologic diseases or conditions, anatomic deficits such as fistulae or damage from surgery, trauma, or radiation

ASSESSMENT (ALL TYPES)

Urinary incontinence is considered a symptom of an underlying problem or condition rather than a disease process in itself; Table 10-3 compares the five types of urinary incontinence

DIAGNOSTIC TESTS

Voiding diary
  Nocturia
  Urinary frequency (more often than q2h)
  Urinary urgency
  Leakage of urine after coughing, lifting, or exercising

Postvoid residual: urine remaining in the bladder (>50 ml) immediately after voiding

Urodynamic testing: reduced bladder and urethral sphincter function

Voiding cystourethrogram: bladder distends below inferior margin of symphysis pubis when patient is upright

IVP: normal unless complicated by other condition such as ectopic ureter

Cystoscopy: abnormalities in bladder and lower urinary tract

Urinalysis culture and sensitivity: infection, hematuria

Bladder biopsy: abnormal bladder cells

MULTIDISCIPLINARY MANAGEMENT

THERAPEUTIC MANAGEMENT

See Table 10-3 for a comparison of the five types of urinary incontinence

Urology consult

Wound, Ostomy, Continence/ET Nurse consultation

Pharmacology consult/evaluation

Occupational therapy consult

Physical therapy consult: general and pelvic exercise programs

Dietary consult: weight reduction if necessary

Psychologic consult/support

PATIENT PROBLEMS—NURSING DIAGNOSES/INTERVENTIONS

INCONTINENCE, ALL TYPES

▼ Impaired skin integrity related to urinary incontinence

Assess perineal area for redness, irritation, swelling, or breakdown and document initial findings *so subsequent changes may be identified and treated*

Cleanse skin with mild soap and water or nonrinse cleaners and dry well after each incontinent episode *to prevent irritation of skin surfaces*

Apply skin barrier, protective spray, or sealant q8h to 12h and after each episode of incontinence *to prevent breaks in integrity*

Table 10-3	Incontinence Assessment and Therapeutic Management				
Factors	**Functional Incontinence**	**Stress Incontinence**	**Reflex Incontinence**	**Urge Incontinence**	**Total Incontinence**
SPECIFIC ASSESSMENT					
Character of voiding urge	Usually strong	Sudden, associated with increased abdominal pressure	None	Very strong with inability to delay voiding	None
Amount voided	Moderate to large	Small, usually <50 ml	Moderate	Small to large	Constant leakage
Nocturia (more than two times)	May be present	Not usual	Always	Common	Always
Frequency of urination (more than q2h)	Variable	Increased	Regular intervals related to volume	Increased	Constant, unpredictable
Awareness of incontinence	Aware	Aware	Unaware; however, sympathetic response may be present: diaphoresis, flushing of skin, "gooseflesh," nausea	Aware	Unaware
Precipitating factors	Inability to reach receptacle Environmental problems (e.g., lack of privacy, side rails up on bed) Physical, mental disabilities	Increased intra-abdominal pressure Obesity Laughing Coughing Sneezing Lifting Exercise	Full bladder Bladder contraction or spasm	Sensation of full bladder and inability to reach receptacle on time Catheter use Increased fluids Increased urine concentration Alcohol, caffeine use	Unpredictable
THERAPEUTIC MANAGEMENT					
	Evaluate medication regimen and change as necessary and possible Behavioral therapy Evaluate and change environmental factors	Surgery Vesicourethral suspension Artificial urinary sphincter Periurethral injection Alpha-adrenergics Estrogen therapy Anticholinergics Skin care management Behavioral therapy	Intermittent catheterization External catheter drainage Surgery; continent diversion Indwelling catheter (last resort) Skin care management	Medications Anticholinergics Antispasmodics Treatment of infections Evaluate diuretic therapy and change when possible (e.g., schedule) Reduced-calorie diet if obese Skin care management Behavioral therapy	Surgery Repair fistulas Correct congenital defect Artificial sphincter Urinary diversion External collecting devices Skin care management

Modified from McFarland GK, McFarlane EA: Nursing diagnosis and intervention: planning for patient care, *ed 3, St Louis, 1997, Mosby.*

Keep bed linen dry and wrinkle free *to decrease shearing effect on skin surfaces*

Use absorbent products, briefs, shields, or underpants if incontinent episodes are frequent *to provide optimal protection from urine on skin surfaces*

Be certain plastic does not touch skin and *cause maceration from increased perspiration*

Apply external collection device to further protect skin if incontinence continues and skin shows signs of breakdown

  Males

    Condom catheter with drainage bag

      Check penis regularly *for excoriation or constriction* and condom *for twisting and pooling of urine*

    Retracted penis pouch with drainage bag

      Clip pubic hair and apply skin protective barrier film before applying

      Check regularly for excoriation and adherence

  Females

    Prepare skin and apply external device

    Check regularly for excoriation

    Connect external devices to collection system

    Coil tubing *to prevent dependent loops and urine stasis*

Keep drainage bag below bladder at all times *to promote gravity drainage*

Expected Outcome

Skin remains intact

▼Body image disturbance related to urinary incontinence

Provide an accepting and supportive atmosphere *to maintain patient's self-esteem and promote verbalization of feelings, fears, concerns, and questions*

Determine how incontinence has affected patient's daily activities and sexual activity in order *to provide emotional support* and suggest methods of problem management

Identify positive features of patient's life *to promote feelings of self-worth*

Offer assistance from other professionals (psychologist, sexual counselor) *to assist with the management of emotional changes*

Encourage communication with significant other(s) and/or members of support group *to decrease feelings of isolation*

Expected Outcomes

Participates in ADLs at optimal level

Comfortably discusses feelings, fears, concerns, and questions

Identifies approaches for making positive changes in daily activities

Accepts assistance from professionals and support group

FUNCTIONAL INCONTINENCE

▼Functional incontinence related to sensory, cognitive, or motor deficits or altered environment

In collaboration with physician and pharmacist, assess effect of medications and determine whether changes may decrease risk of incontinence

Monitor intake and output *to determine whether appropriate fluid balance is maintained*

Adjust fluid intake so that largest amounts are taken at time of day when patient feels attempts at continence will be successful

Advise patient to maintain fluid intake of at least 2000 ml/day (unless contraindicated) *to ensure adequate fluid intake and output*

Cognitive deficit

Assess and document cognitive deficit *so that individualized and appropriate voiding program may be established*

Plan a fixed voiding schedule (q2h) *to eliminate incontinence and assist patient with voiding as needed*

Document times of voiding *so that accurate records may be referred to as needed to update plan of care*

Positively reinforce successes in maintaining continence *to promote self-esteem and motivation*

Motor/sensory deficits

Identify and document sensory or motor deficits that may inhibit patient from reaching bathroom or receptacle in time to void *so that necessary assistance may be provided*

Provide equipment to enable patient to eliminate alone: bedpan or urinal within reach, trapeze or walkers for easy movement, bedside commode, elevated toilet seats, bar in bathrooms

Determine optimal interval between voiding to prevent incontinence *to establish individualized and appropriate voiding program*

Slowly increase intervals between voidings; optimal time to reach is q3h to 4h

Assess pain and comfort level so that analgesics or nonpharmacologic methods of pain control may be employed before established voiding times

Altered environment

Assess environment *to determine obstacles that may inhibit patient's ability to reach toileting facilities in adequate time*

Institute safety measures

  Orient to location of bathroom and/or placement of toileting equipment

  Remove obstacles (e.g., furniture, belongings) from path to bathroom

  Keep bed in low position

  Use night light or keep bathroom door ajar with light on

Maintain privacy so patient will be comfortable voiding

Place call light within reach and answer promptly *to promote success with voiding program*

Suggest bed clothes that permit easy removal before voiding

Expected Outcomes

Exhibits no sign of injury

Fluid intake is at least 2000 ml/day (unless contraindicated)

Intake and output are balanced

Establishes and maintains voiding program

Remains continent

STRESS INCONTINENCE

▼Stress incontinence related to weak pelvis and structure supports, overdistention between voidings, or high intraabdominal pressure

Assist with diagnostic measures as indicated

Observe urinary meatus to check for leakage when patient has a full bladder and document/report findings to determine effectiveness of treatment plan

Instruct patient to cough while in lithotomy position; if no leakage, repeat with patient at 45-degree angle; continue with patient standing if no previous leakage

Weak pelvic and structural supports

Instruct in techniques aimed at strengthening pelvic muscles (pubococcygeus)

Pelvic muscle exercises (PME) (Kegel exercises)

Identify pelvic muscles by doing the following:

Tightening muscles around anus while sitting or standing

Starting and stopping urine flow while voiding *to identify pelvic muscles*

Keeping buttocks, thigh, and abdominal muscles relaxed

Perform quick pelvic muscle/Kegel exercises: tighten and relax pelvic muscles as quickly as possible

Perform slow pelvic muscle/Kegel exercises: tighten muscle group and hold for count of 10 and then relax for same count

Push in—pull out exercises

Use pelvic and abdominal muscles to pull up pelvic floor as though trying to suck water

Push or bear down to push imaginary water out

Daily schedule

Week 1: do 10 of each exercise (quick and slow pelvic muscle/Kegel exercises and pull in—push out exercises) qid

Each succeeding week increase exercises by five, completing four sets a day

Results should be seen in about 3 months

Teach method for using weighted cones *to increase muscle tone*

Insert weighted cone into vagina

Contract pelvic muscles to retain cone for 15 minutes

Perform bid

Increase weight of cone as ordered

Instruct patient to tighten pelvic muscles before coughing, laughing, or any activity that increases abdominal pressure to prevent leakage

Encourage patients with chronic obstructive pulmonary disease (COPD) to avoid smoking, use inhalators as prescribed *to avoid repetitive coughing*

Overdistention

Assess factors leading to overdistention: increased fluid intake, use of diuretics, or decreased frequency of urination resulting from immobility, unwillingness to ask for assistance

Assess abdomen for bladder distention immediately after an episode of incontinence *to determine whether urine is being retained*

Discuss reasons for voiding frequently (preventing bladder irritation, decreasing potential for UTI)

Plan a fixed voiding schedule

Set interval shorter than that in which incontinence occurs, such as q2h, to ensure sufficient time in which to prepare for voiding; assist with voiding as needed

Teach to double or triple void

Identify factors that may interfere with patient's attempts to maintain continence to amend plan of care as needed

Provide positive reinforcement for continent behavior

High intraabdominal pressure

Discuss with patient that weight reduction may decrease incidence of incontinence by reducing pressure on the bladder

Dietitian to counsel patient

Institute nutritionally sound weight-loss program

Patient to make daily menu selections within restrictions

Physical therapist to coordinate appropriate exercise regimen

Weigh weekly to determine effectiveness of reduction plan

Promote motivation and compliance by praising efforts to comply with treatment plan

Expected Outcomes

Performs pelvic muscle exercises daily and experiences fewer episodes of incontinence

Voids on a regular schedule without bladder distention

Complies with diet/exercise program

REFLEX INCONTINENCE

▼Reflex incontinence related to neurologic impairment

Assess for signs and symptoms patient may experience before incontinence (e.g., diaphoresis, flushing, pilomotor response, or nausea)

In collaboration with physician, identify acceptable residual urine volume

Perform catheterization with sterile technique *to decrease occurrence of UTI and bladder changes*

Report residual volume more than that determined acceptable and amend plan of care as needed (e.g., intermittent catheterization)

Before expected voiding, place patient in optimal voiding position

Assess for autonomic dysreflexia (hyperreflexia): pounding headache, blurred vision, hypertension, profuse diaphoresis above level of spinal injury, severe pilomotor response and pale skin appearing below injury level, nausea, restlessness, and nasal congestion; *if these findings exist,* elevate head of bed, empty bladder (to alleviate symptoms), and immediately notify physician

Help patient to identify activities that may stimulate voiding *so that these may be avoided or used to initiate voiding when needed* (e.g., stroking inner thigh, anal stimulation, stroking vulva or glans penis)

Encourage patient to initiate voiding or perform self-catheterization before social activities, trips

Advise patient to carry self-catheterization equipment for use when unplanned delays occur

Expected Outcomes

Intake and output are balanced

Uses triggering mechanism to initiate voiding; residual volume is within prescribed limits *or*

Empties bladder via self-catheterization with a volume not > 300 ml

URGE INCONTINENCE

▼Urge incontinence related to decreased bladder capacity, bladder irritability, overdistention of the bladder, or neurologic deficits

In collaboration with physician and pharmacist, assess effect of medications and determine whether changes may decrease risk of incontinence

Motor/sensory deficits
See Functional incontinence p. 618

Overdistention
See Stress incontinence p. 619

Irritable bladder
Assess for symptoms of UTI (e.g., dysuria, cloudy urine); obtain culture and report to physician

Discuss need to avoid irritating fluids such as drinks with caffeine or alcohol

Expected Outcome
Remains continent and is able to increase interval between voidings without episodes of incontinence

TOTAL INCONTINENCE

▼Total incontinence related to neurologic dysfunction; independent contraction of detrusor reflex caused by surgery, trauma, or radiation; or anatomic problems such as fistulae

Assess type of incontinence in collaboration with physician using voiding diary and checking for residual

Provide absorbent briefs, undergarments, and underpads; plan schedule for routine changes q1h to 2h during period when most fluids are being taken, q2h to 3h during sleep periods

Encourage patient to increase level of self-care when able

Expected Outcomes
Wet garments are changed on a regular basis

Assumes increased responsibility for self-care

Additional Nursing Diagnoses to Consider (for All Types of Incontinence)
Altered role performance related to inability to engage in usual ADLs

Isolation related to inability to communicate feelings and relate to others

PATIENT/FAMILY TEACHING
Assist patient in identifying urinary elimination pattern by explaining how to organize voiding diary and evaluate findings

Help patient identify how voiding schedule will be incorporated into daily activities

Discuss methods for preventing and managing unexpected incontinence

    Void before social activities, trips

    Carry a change of clothing for use when unexpected episodes of incontinence occur

    Plan sexual activity for times when bladder is empty to decrease chances of incontinence during this time

    Discuss availability of undergarments or shields with absorbent materials

Teach about ordered medications: names, dosages, schedules, purposes, and side effects

DISCHARGE/HOME CARE PLANNING
Encourage patient to maintain voiding diary and schedule at home

Discuss need to perform ADLs and resume self-care within capabilities

Teach symptoms of UTI and encourage patient to report these to physician

Teach signs of skin impairment, early action to take, and when to report to physician

Encourage patient with weakened pelvic muscles to perform appropriate exercises (e.g., Kegel exercises) daily

Review techniques to control odor of urine

Discuss importance of maintaining fluid intake at 2000 to 2500 ml/day (unless contraindicated); explain that decreased fluid intake does not reduce episodes of incontinence

Reinforce need to evaluate episodes of incontinence for precipitating factors and to make changes as necessary; report continued incontinence

Encourage patient to continue communicating with others who are supportive: significant other(s) or support group

Emphasize need to keep regular laboratory and follow-up appointments

Reinforce need to continue weight reduction (if needed) and exercise program

Discuss care and storage of equipment: catheters, external collection devices

Help patient evaluate home environment for necessary modifications

Provide information about available resources for individuals with incontinence (Box 10-4)

■ SURGERY FOR FEMALE URINARY INCONTINENCE

Marshall-Marchetti-Krantz procedure: A surgical procedure for correcting stress incontinence; the urethra and vesical neck of the bladder are suspended to restore the normal vesicourethral angle by suturing the paraurethral anterior vaginal wall to the periosteum of the symphysis pubis and the lower rectal fascia via suprapubic incision

Pereya-Raz procedure: A surgical procedure performed vaginally to restore the normal vesicourethral angle, thus decreasing stress incontinence; the urethra and vesical neck are suspended by suturing the anterior vaginal wall to the rectal fascia

Other procedures include Stamey and Burch

ASSESSMENT
SUBJECTIVE DATA (POSTOPERATIVE)
After urinary catheter removal
  Dysuria
  Urinary frequency/urgency
  Inability to start urine stream
  Incisional pain

OBJECTIVE DATA (POSTOPERATIVE)
Decreased urinary output
Unbalanced fluid intake and output
Cloudy, foul-smelling urine
Incisional erythema or edema

DIAGNOSTIC TESTS (PREOPERATIVE)
Urinalysis: WBCs, RBCs, bacteria
Urine culture and sensitivity
Cystoscopy: abnormalities with bladder/urethra
Urodynamic testing: reduced bladder and urethral sphincter function
Urine flow rate measurement: abnormal urinary flow patterns

Box 10-4	**Incontinence Information and Support**

Alliance for Aging Research
2021 K Street, NW
Suite 305
Washington, DC 20006
202-293-2856

Bladder Health Council
American Foundation for Urologic Diseases
300 West Pratt, Suite 401
Baltimore, MD 21201
800-242-2383

SIMON Foundation for Continence
P. O. Box 835
Wilmette, IL 60091
800-23SIMON

Agency for Health Care Policy and Research (AHCPR)
    Publications Clearinghouse
P. O. Box 8547
Silver Spring, MD 20907
800-358-9295
301-495-3453

National Kidney and Urologic Diseases of National
    Institute of Health
Information Clearinghouse
3 Information Way
Bethesda, MD 20892-3580
301-654-4415

Urethral pressure profile: abnormal urethral pressure during bladder filling/micturition

POTENTIAL COMPLICATIONS
UTI and postoperative complications
  Atelectasis
  Thrombophlebitis
  Pulmonary embolism
  Paralytic ileus
  Wound infection

MULTIDISCIPLINARY MANAGEMENT
THERAPEUTIC MANAGEMENT
Medications
  Antibiotics
  Analgesics
  Stool softeners
  IV fluids
NPO until bowel sounds present
Indwelling urethral catheter and/or suprapubic catheter
Voiding schedule/program (after catheter removed)
Intermittent self-catheterization if indicated

PATIENT PROBLEMS—NURSING DIAGNOSES/INTERVENTIONS

▼Pain related to surgical incision and manipulation of organs

Assess and document type, intensity, location, and duration of pain *so changes can be noted and interventions implemented*

Identify verbal and nonverbal responses to pain

Ensure that urethral catheter and/or suprapubic tube are patent *to promote optimal drainage and prevent pressure from urinary backflow*

Tape catheters securely *to prevent pulling sensation and irritation*

Apply anesthetic ointment to swollen urethral meatus if ordered

Offer analgesics, document effectiveness and tolerance *so that pharmacologic changes may be made as needed*

Institute nonpharmacologic comfort measures
  Optimal positioning
  Relaxation techniques/guided imagery
  Restful environment
  Diversional activity
  Splint incision when turning, coughing, and deep breathing

Expected Outcome
Relaxed and verbalizes increased comfort

▼Altered urinary elimination related to presence of urethral catheter and/or suprapubic catheter

Maintain patency of catheter *to promote optimal flow of urine*
  Tubing below level of bladder *to allow for gravity flow*
  Assess for clamping/kinks in tubing *to prevent urine stasis*
  Secure catheters *to prevent dislodging*
  Irrigate catheters as ordered

Monitor intake and output frequently *so that abnormal balance will be identified and treated*

Assess for bladder distention and report to physician

Cleanse periurethral area bid and prn *to prevent infection and promote patient comfort*

Document tolerance of clamping routine if ordered for residual checks and amend treatment plan as needed

After urinary catheter is removed, institute measures to facilitate voiding
  Privacy
  Comfortable positioning
  Running tap water
  Placing patient's hand in warm water
  Applying heat to suprapubic area (if ordered)
  Pouring warm water over perineum
  Relaxation techniques

Applying oil of peppermint (a few drops in bedpan/urinal or on cotton ball in front of urinary meatus)
  Stroking inner aspect of thigh gently with ice
  Offering analgesic
  Voiding 1 to 2 hours after fluid intake
  Double voiding (to empty bladder more completely)

Report to physician abnormalities in urine; residual volume > 100 ml; and/or retention of urine with overflow *so that collaborative changes can be instituted*

Expected Outcomes
Intake and output are balanced

Urethral catheter and suprapubic catheter are patent

Able to void after catheter removal without evidence of urinary retention

▼Risk for infection related to potential for UTI resulting from presence of indwelling urethral catheter and/or suprapubic catheter

Report temperature > 101° F (38.5° C) to physician

Maintain clean technique during catheter care *to decrease risk of bacteria entering urethra*

Order urine culture and notify physician if cloudy and/or malodorous urine is noted; monitor results

Expected Outcomes
Temperature is within normal limits for patient

Urine is clear and of normal color

▼Impaired skin integrity related to surgical incision

Assess incision q4h for presence of erythema, edema, tenderness, and drainage; document findings *so that changes can be identified and treated*

Report signs and symptoms of infection (fever, chills) to physician

Obtain wound culture as ordered to identify presence of bacteria *so that presence of bacteria may be identified*

Monitor for elevation of WBC, *which indicates presence of infection*

Administer and monitor tolerance of ordered antibiotics

Expected Outcome
Incision is clean and dry

Additional Nursing Diagnoses to Consider
Altered tissue perfusion: peripheral, cardiopulmonary, or gastrointestinal related to risk of stasis of blood as evidenced by thrombophlebitis, pulmonary embolism, or parlytic ileus

Body image disturbance related to need for continued urethral catheter and/or suprapubic catheter at discharge or dissatisfaction with surgical outcome

PATIENT/FAMILY TEACHING

Explain postoperative procedures/routines to patient; encourage questions

Develop plan with patient to increase participation in ADLs

Teach/demonstrate proper body mechanics (e.g., bend knees to pick up items from the floor)

Explain to patient that an urge to urinate may be felt when catheter is in place and not to be concerned about sensation

Reinforce importance of keeping hands clean and not touching incision *to prevent infection*

To prevent UTI

Empty bladder q2h to 3h

Encourage patient to maintain fluid intake of 2000 to 3000 ml/day (unless contraindicated) to flush bacteria from system

Avoid fluids that aggravate urinary tract (caffeinated beverages) and drink fluids that promote systemic flushing (water and cranberry juice)

Shower rather than bathe and use antibacterial soap

Keep perineal area clean and dry

Wipe from front to back when cleansing perianal area

Teach about ordered medications: names, dosages, schedules, purposes, and side effects

DISCHARGE/HOME CARE PLANNING

Emphasize importance of ongoing outpatient care

Advise patient to avoid interacting with persons who have infections (e.g., colds, influenza) during recuperation period

Reinforce need to rest and increase activity as tolerated; avoid sitting or standing for long periods

Instruct patient to avoid heavy lifting (>5 lb) and heavy housework as indicated by physician

Encourage patient to ask physician when sexual activity may be resumed

Teach patient to perform wound care and dressing change as ordered

Teach symptoms of wound infection (fever, chills, redness, swelling, tenderness, and purulent and/or malodorous drainage from incision) to report to home health nurse or physician

Teach/reinforce method of self-catheterization as needed (see Box 10-2)

Teach symptoms of UTI (dysuria, urgency, frequency, foul-smelling urine, fever > 101° F [38.5° C]) and encourage patient to report to physician

Advise patient to avoid taking over-the-counter medications without physician approval

Advise patient to avoid straining during bowel movements; ask physician to prescribe stool softeners/laxatives as needed

■ URINARY DIVERSION

A method of diverting urine away from the bladder so that it leaves the body through another route; urinary di-

version may be used to manage bladder tumors, strictures or trauma of ureters and urethra, pelvic malignancy, neurogenic bladder, chronic infection, and advanced cases of cystitis

Urinary diversion may either be incontinent or continent. There is a higher risk for skin integrity problems with incontinent diversions (Box 10-5)

ASSESSMENT

SUBJECTIVE DATA

Pain

Anxiety

OBJECTIVE DATA

Decreased urinary output

Unbalanced fluid intake and output

Cloudy, foul-smelling urine

Skin excoriation surrounding stoma

Incisional erythema, edema

DIAGNOSTIC TESTS

Urinalysis: WBCs, RBCs, bacteria

Urine culture and sensitivity

Serum electrolytes, BUN, creatinine: abnormal/elevated results

---

Box 10-5	**Common Urinary Diversion Procedures**

INCONTINENT URINARY DIVERSION
Ileal Conduit (Fig. 10-9)
Ureters are anastomosed to an isolated section of the terminal ileum (ileal conduit) and brought to the abdominal wall

Ureterosigmoidostomy
Ureters are introduced into the sigmoid colon

Cutaneous Ureterostomy (Fig. 10-10)
One or both ureters are implanted into an opening in the abdominal wall

Nephrostomy
Catheter is inserted into the renal pelvis

CONTINENT URINARY DIVERSION
Continent Ileal Urinary Reservoir, Kock's Pouch (Fig. 10-11)
Ureters are anastomosed into a prepared segment of the ileum, forming a pouch that contains two nipple valves

Vesicostomy
Bladder is sutured to the abdominal wall, and a stoma is created through the abdominal and bladder walls

Other Continent Diversion Procedures
Mainze reservoirs, Indiana pouches, Camey procedure

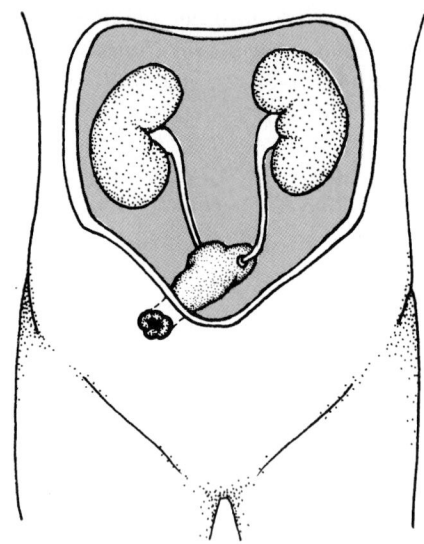

Fig. 10-9   Ileal conduit.

POTENTIAL COMPLICATIONS

Hemorrhage
Shock
Atelectasis
Thrombophlebitis
Pulmonary embolism
Electrolyte imbalance
Paralytic ileus
Peritonitis
UTI
Hydronephrosis
Renal failure

MULTIDISCIPLINARY MANAGEMENT

THERAPEUTIC MANAGEMENT

Preoperative bowel preparation (enemas, laxatives, restricted diet)
Medications
    Antibiotics
    Analgesics
    Antipyretics
    Antiemetics
    Local antiinfective ointment/cream
    Stool softeners
    IV fluids
NPO until bowel sounds present
Wound, Ostomy, Continence/ET Nurse
Dietitian
Psychologic consult
Pharmacology consult
Sex therapist

PATIENT PROBLEMS—NURSING DIAGNOSES/INTERVENTIONS

▼ Pain related to surgical incision and/or urinary obstruction

Assess type, intensity, location, and duration of pain and document changes *so that changes can be reported and treatment initiated*
Identify verbal and nonverbal responses to pain
Ensure catheters/drains are patent and not causing discomfort related to obstruction of flow
Offer analgesics, documenting effectiveness and tolerance *so that needed pharmacologic changes can be made*
Institute nonpharmacologic comfort measures
    Optimal positioning
    Relaxation techniques/guided imagery
    Restful environment
    Diversional activity
    Splint incision when turning, coughing, and deep breathing

Expected Outcome

Relaxed and verbalizes increased comfort

▼ Altered urinary elimination related to urinary diversion

Monitor urine from all sources (ureteral stents, conduit catheters, reservoir catheters) and record color, clarity, and volume
Label each collecting container/catheter/stent (type, left or right) *to avoid errors when recording output*
Report urinary output of < 30 ml/hr, *which may indicate altered fluid balance or impaired renal function*
Pink-colored urine and mucus from conduit and continent diversions is expected for the first 24 hours postoperatively; report frank bleeding
Maintain patency of catheters/stents *to prevent backflow*
    Avoid kinking drainage tubing
    Keep drainage bag below level of patient's kidneys
    Position so that flow of urine is not impeded
    Tape ureteral stents securely
Assess size, shape, color, type, and placement of stoma/ureteral buds and record *so that changes can be reported promptly*

Expected Outcomes

Urinary output is > 30 ml/hr
Intake and output are balanced
Urine is clear

▼ Impaired skin integrity related to incision/ostomy

Keep skin surfaces clean and dry
Change position *to prevent breakdown of skin surfaces*
Change dressings as ordered using sterile technique *to prevent infection*
Change dressings when wet *to decrease risk of excoriation;* use skin barrier around stoma; apply antiinfective ointments as ordered

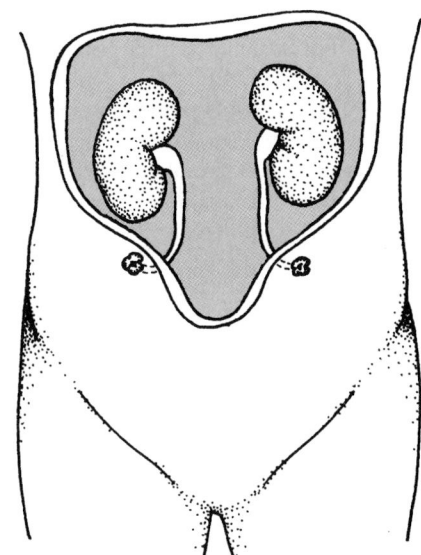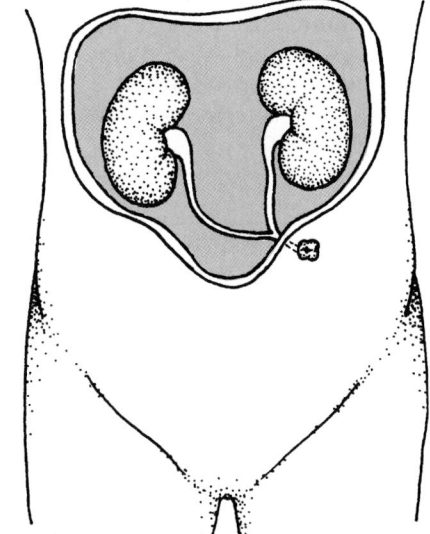

Fig. 10-10 Cutaneous ureterostomies.

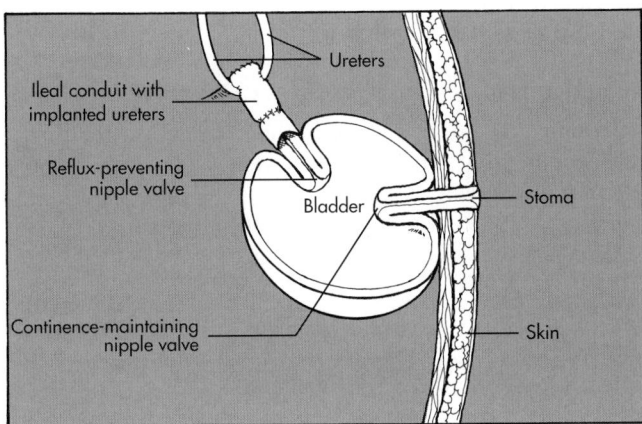

Ureters

Ileal conduit with
implanted ureters

Reflux-preventing
nipple valve

Bladder

Stoma

Continence-maintaining
nipple valve

Skin

Fig. 10-11 Kock pouch (continent ileal reservoir).
(From Belcher AE: Mosby's clinical nursing series: cancer nursing, *St Louis, 1992, Mosby.)*

Inspect skin around stoma and report signs of erythema, breakdown, and/or excoriation *so that any change can be evaluated and treated promptly*

Check color of stoma; report if other than pink

Check for leakage around appliance and, if noted, confer with enterostomal therapist to institute methods *to prevent urine contact with skin surfaces*

Change temporary appliance as needed in accordance with institutional policy and advice from Wound, Ostomy, Continence/ET Nurse; reapply/remeasure as needed

Monitor for signs and symptoms of incisional infection (fever, erythema, edema, malodorous drainage, pain) and report to physician for treatment; order culture of suspicious drainage and check results

Expected Outcomes
Skin surfaces are dry and intact
Stoma buds are pink and swelling is decreasing

▼Body image disturbance related to loss of normal body function and presence of urinary stoma/bud on abdomen

Provide an accepting and supportive atmosphere *to maintain patient's self-esteem and promote verbalization of feelings, fears, concerns, and questions*

Assist patient in identifying coping measures used effectively in the past *so that these behaviors may be used to help patient to adapt to ostomy*

Offer opportunities to look at and touch ostomy; encourage participation in care

Explore how presence of ostomy may affect patient's normal activity and sexual functioning

Discuss activities that may be prohibited (e.g., heavy contact sports)

Identify types of clothing that will not draw attention to ostomy (e.g., loose-fitting garments)

Identify positive features of patient's life *to promote feelings of self-worth*

Offer assistance from other professionals (Wound, Ostomy, Continence/ET Nurse, psychologist, sexual counselor) *to assist with management of emotional changes*

Encourage communication with significant other(s) and/or members of support group *to decrease feelings of isolation*

Expected Outcomes
Participates in ADLs and care of ostomy at optimal level
Comfortably discusses feelings, fears, concerns, and questions and identifies approaches for making positive changes in daily activities
Requests assistance from professionals and support group appropriately

Additional Nursing Diagnoses to Consider
Ineffective breathing pattern related to pain or fatigue
Altered tissue perfusion: GI related to peritonitis
Altered urinary elimination related to UTI
Risk for fluid volume deficit related to potential for excessive losses and electrolyte imbalances
Ineffective individual coping related to fear of diagnosis, prognosis
Sexual dysfunction related to postoperative condition and self-consciousness about stoma

PATIENT/FAMILY TEACHING
PREOPERATIVE
Encourage verbalization of fears, concerns, and questions related to upcoming surgery
Provide information about equipment, tubes, and drains to expect postoperatively (depending on type of diversion)
Discuss purpose and type of bowel preparation
Determine whether significant other(s) will be involved in care postoperatively
Request Wound, Ostomy, Continence/ET Nurse consult (determines location of stoma in collaboration with patient and physician)
Offer visit from Ostomy Visitation Program (through American Cancer Society)

POSTOPERATIVE
Encourage verbalization of fears, concerns, and questions related to ability to care for appliance
Include significant other(s) in teaching sessions
Wound, Ostomy, Continence/ET Nurse meets with patient *to address special needs*
Explain/reinforce importance of thorough handwashing before and after caring for ostomy
Include patient in care of appliance early in postoperative period *to promote optimal level of self-care and independence*
Advise patient that stoma will decrease in size approximately 3 to 6 weeks after surgery
Instruct patient about purpose of prescribed diet; dietary consult for special needs
Identify liquids that have diuretic effect (e.g., alcoholic beverages, tea, and coffee)
Encourage patient to maintain fluid intake of 2000 to 3000 ml/day (unless contraindicated) *to maintain adequate level of hydration*
Teach about ordered medications: names, dosages, schedules, purposes, and side effects

DISCHARGE/HOME CARE PLANNING
Teach/reinforce method of changing, managing appliance
Emphasize importance of ongoing outpatient care
Reinforce need for rest and increased activity as tolerated
Provide patient with a list of instructions that includes places to purchase supplies and type and size of appliance needed
Instruct patient to shower daily *to promote hygiene;* avoid bathing *to prevent loosening of bag*

Instruct patient to empty appliance q2h to 3h or when > 100 ml of urine accumulates to prevent bag from leaking or separating
Explain to ureterostomy patients importance of not irrigating urethral buds
Ensure that patient is proficient in the application of appliances before hospital discharge
Instruct patient to attach appliance to bedside closed gravity system at night, keeping drainage apparatus lower than ostomy
Schedule follow-up care for patient with physician and Wound, Ostomy, Continence/ET Nurse
Offer to refer patient to sexual counselor as needed
Instruct patient to report the following symptoms to home health nurse and/or physician
Absence of urine
Hematuria; cloudy, foul-smelling urine
Pain in back or abdomen
Fever > 101° F (38.5° C)
Incisional redness, pain, swelling, or drainage
Severe skin excoriation
Retraction of stoma
Malaise
Nausea, vomiting
Abdominal distention, pain
Encourage patient to avoid straining during bowel movements, call physician to order stool softeners and/or laxatives
Advise patient to avoid taking over-the-counter medications without physician approval

ARTIFICIAL URINARY SPHINCTER (AUS)
A urologic prosthetic device used to manage incontinence caused by sphincter incompetence; it consists of three major components: an abdominal reservoir, a periurethra cuff, and a pump mechanism (Fig. 10-12)

The movement of fluid through a tubing network from the cuff to the abdominal reservoir operates the device; fluid normally remains in the cuff, promoting continence, until pumped into the reservoir; this action deflates the cuff and allows urine to pass through the urethra; the cuff automatically refills with fluid through hydraulic action. In females, the cuff is located near the bladder neck; in males, near the bladder neck or bulbous urethra

ASSESSMENT
SUBJECTIVE DATA (POSTOPERATIVE)
Bladder spasm
Pain

OBJECTIVE DATA (POSTOPERATIVE)
Incontinence
Leakage of urine
Scrotal swelling
Labial swelling

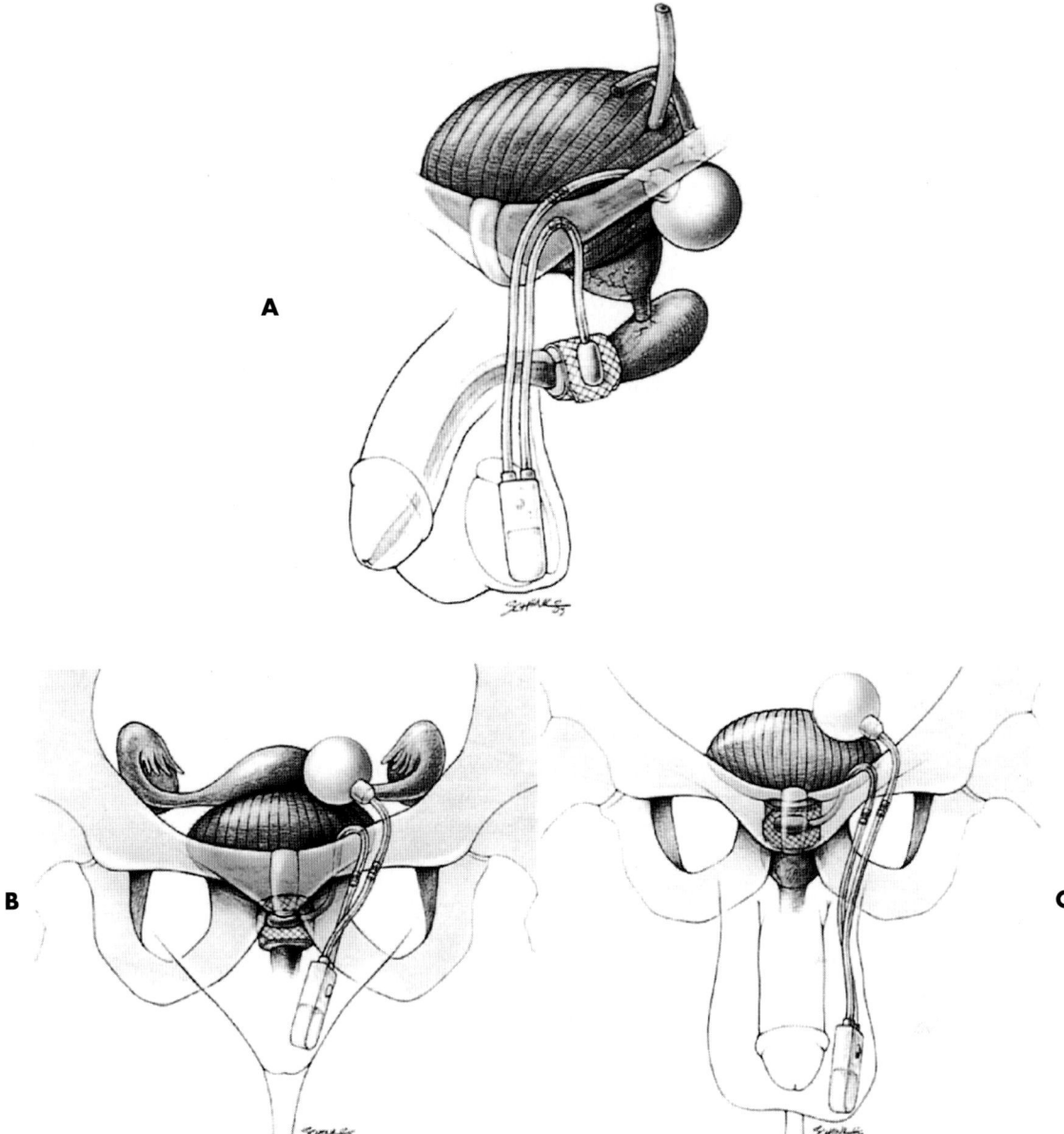

Fig. 10-12 **A,** Placement of AUS cuff around bulbous urethra in male. **B,** Placement of AUS in female. Cuff is placed around bladder neck, balloon is placed in prevesical space, and pump is placed in labia. **C,** Placement of AUS in male. Cuff is placed around bladder neck, balloon is placed in prevesical space, and pump is placed in scrotum.
(Courtesy American Medical Systems, Inc., Minnetonka, Minn. From Doughty D: Urinary and fecal incontinence: nursing management, *St Louis, 1991, Mosby.)*

DIAGNOSTIC TESTS
Urinalysis: cloudy, malodorous, WBC, RBC, bacteria
Urine culture and sensitivity
See Urinary incontinence, p. 616

POTENTIAL COMPLICATIONS
Patient's inability to operate AUS
UTI
Infection
Compromised bladder wall compliance
Progressive renal deterioration

MULTIDISCIPLINARY MANAGEMENT
THERAPEUTIC MANAGEMENT
Urology consult
Medications
    Antibiotics
    Analgesics
    Stool softeners
    IV fluids
NPO until bowel sounds present
Psychologic consult/support

PATIENT PROBLEMS—NURSING DIAGNOSES/INTERVENTIONS

▼ Pain related to low, transverse, deep surgical incision and bladder spasm

Assess type, intensity, location, and duration of pain and document *so that changes are noted and treatment plan altered*

Identify verbal and nonverbal responses to pain

Notify physician if scrotum/labia are swollen *so that care can be collaboratively initiated* (e.g., Trendelenburg position, ice)

Offer analgesics, document effectiveness and tolerance *so needed changes can be implemented*

Institute nonpharmacologic comfort measures
  Optimal positioning
  Relaxation techniques/guided imagery
  Restful environment
  Diversional activity

Expected Outcome
Relaxed and verbalizes increased comfort

▼ Altered urinary elimination related to presence of artificial urinary sphincter and bladder spasms

Locate pump qh and document findings; notify physician *immediately* if unable to palpate pump, *which may indicate its movement into inguinal canal*

Activate pump when ordered
  Provide privacy while palpating or activating pump
  Pump bulb q2h during the day and once midway through the night or as scheduled by physician
  Deflate device when patient is asleep when ordered and connect to an external urine collecting device; may use pads for female, changing as necessary to maintain dryness
  Report any leakage of urine to physician *so that source of leakage may be identified and treated*

Monitor intake and output frequently *to identify and treat imbalances*

Expected Outcomes
AUS operates successfully without leakage
Intake and output are balanced

▼ Risk for infection (urinary and/or wound), and rejection of artificial sphincter related to implantation of foreign body surrounding urinary tract

Report signs and symptoms of infection to physician for treatment
  Fever > 101° F (38.5° C)
  Erythema, edema, pain of wound or surrounding area
  Purulent/malodorous drainage from wound

Obtain urine culture and notify physician if cloudy and/or malodorous urine is noted; monitor results

Report signs and symptoms of AUS rejection to physician for treatment
  Erosion
  Increasing pain
  Abdominal tenderness
  Swelling
  Urinary retention

Monitor tolerance and effectiveness of antibiotics and document *so that pharmacologic changes are made when needed*

Expected Outcome
Does not exhibit signs and symptoms of infection/rejection

Additional Nursing Diagnoses to Consider
Body image disturbance related to presence of AUS
Anxiety related to concern about care of AUS

PATIENT/FAMILY TEACHING
Explain surgical procedure; encourage questions and verbalization of concerns and feelings

Explain that urethral catheter will be removed as ordered by physician

Teach about ordered medications: names, dosages, schedules, purposes, and side effects

DISCHARGE/HOME CARE PLANNING
Teach and reinforce method of caring for AUS (Box 10-6)
Emphasize importance of ongoing outpatient care

Box 10-6	**Instructions for Care of AUS**

PROCEDURE
Palpate pump and activate AUS
  Locate AUS in labia or scrotum with thumb and forefinger of dominant hand
  Locate and gently support tubing above pump with nondominant hand to prevent pump from slipping away
  Using thumb and forefinger of dominant hand, squeeze pump until it reaches decompressed state, which allows urine to flow
  Within 1 to 3 minutes cuff will refill and compress urethra

TROUBLE SHOOTING
If urine does not flow
  Move from supine to sitting or standing position
  Cough
  NOTE: Pump may need to be deflated twice to fully empty bladder

REMINDERS
Follow prescribed pumping schedule
  Do not leave AUS completely inflated while asleep unless ordered
  Report leakage of fluid to physician
  Report if AUS goes flat
  Some incontinence may occur with certain physical activities

To prevent UTI

   Encourage patient to maintain fluid intake of 2000 to 3000 ml/day (unless contraindicated) to flush bacteria from system

   Avoid fluids that aggravate urinary tract (e.g., caffeinated beverages) and drink fluids that promote systemic flushing (e.g., water and cranberry juice)

Teach signs and symptoms of UTI (dysuria, urgency, frequency, foul-smelling urine, fever > 101° F [38.5° C]) and encourage patient to report to physician

Teach signs and symptoms of wound infection (fever, chills, redness, swelling, tenderness, and purulent and/or malodorous drainage from incision) and encourage patient to report to physician

Teach symptoms of AUS rejection (erosion, increasing pain, abdominal tenderness, swelling, urinary retention)

Instruct patient to wear a medical alert tag at all times *so that if patient is ever unconscious, the pump may be activated and urine eliminated*

■ BENIGN PROSTATIC HYPERTROPHY/HYPERPLASIA

The enlargement of the prostate gland, associated with endocrine changes of aging, which may prevent the bladder from emptying appropriately

ASSESSMENT
SUBJECTIVE DATA
Hesitancy in starting flow of urine
Diminished force, amount of urine stream
End-stream dribbling
Urinary frequency, urgency
Dysuria
Sense of not emptying bladder
Nocturia
Incontinence
Fatigue
Nausea, vomiting
Weight loss
International Prostate Symptom Score (American Urological Association): high

OBJECTIVE DATA
Enlarged prostate gland
Hematuria
Bladder distention

DIAGNOSTIC TESTS
Urinalysis: WBC, RBC, sediment, bacteria
Urine culture and sensitivity
Serum BUN, creatinine: elevated
Serum WBC: elevated
PSA: elevated
Voiding diary: frequency, urgency, nocturia, incontinence

IVP, intravenous urogram (IVU): dilation of ureters with hydronephrosis; delayed excretion contrast medium; parenchymal thinning
Cystoscopy
Urinary flow study: poor flow pattern; prolonged voiding time; large postvoid residual
Prostatic ultrasound: bilateral enlargement of gland with no hypoechoic areas suspicious of malignant tumor

POTENTIAL COMPLICATIONS
Acute urinary retention
UTI
Pyelonephritis
Hydronephrosis
Compromised renal function
Detrusor decompensation

MULTIDISCIPLINARY MANAGEMENT
THERAPEUTIC MANAGEMENT
Medications
   Analgesics
   Antibiotics
   Antispasmodics
   Alpha-adrenergic blocking drugs (antagonists)
   Androgen hormone inhibitor: finasteride (Proscar)
   Estrogens, androgen antagonists, luteinizing hormone
   Stool softeners/laxatives
Catheterization: intermittent or long term
Surgeries
   Transurethral resection of prostate (TURP)
   Open prostatectomy for very large gland
   Balloon dilation of prostate
   Transurethral needle ablation of the prostate (TUNA)
   Laser prostatectomy
   Transurethral microwave therapy
   Implantation of intraurethral prostatic stent
Restriction of rapid intake of fluids (especially alcohol)

PATIENT PROBLEMS—NURSING DIAGNOSES/INTERVENTIONS

▼ Altered urinary elimination related to benign prostatic hypertrophy

Monitor intake and output frequently *so that imbalances can be reported and treated*
Implement voiding diary *to identify abnormal elimination requiring specific interventions*
Monitor serum BUN, creatinine levels for evidence of increase
After urinary catheter is removed (if used), institute measures to facilitate voiding
   Privacy
   Comfortable positioning
   Running tap water
   Placing patient's hand in warm water
   Applying heat to suprapubic area (if ordered)
   Pouring warm water over perineum
   Relaxation techniques

Applying oil of peppermint (a few drops in
   bedpan/urinal or on cotton ball in front of urinary
   meatus)
Stroking inner aspect of thigh gently with ice
Offering analgesic
Voiding 1 to 2 hours after fluid intake
Double voiding (to empty bladder more completely)
If postvoid residual ordered, record/report findings

Expected Outcomes
Intake and output are balanced
Voiding pattern is established

▼ Pain related to hypertrophy of prostate

Assess type, intensity, location, and duration of pain and
   document *so changes can be made in plan of care*
Identify verbal and nonverbal responses to pain
Ensure that catheter is patent *to promote optimal
   drainage, prevent pressure from backflow*
Secure catheter *to prevent pulling sensation*
Offer analgesics, documenting effectiveness and
   tolerance *so changes in pharmacologic plan can
   be made*
Institute nonpharmacologic comfort measures
   Optimal positioning
   Relaxation techniques/guided imagery
   Restful environment
   Diversional activity

Expected Outcome
Relaxed and verbalizes increased comfort

▼ Risk for infection (urinary tract infection related to
benign prostatic hypertrophy

See UTI, p. 607

Additional Nursing Diagnoses to Consider
Body image disturbance related to BPH
Sexual dysfunction related to BPH
Anxiety related to fear of cancer, embarrassment about
   symptoms, and concerns about effect on ADLs

PATIENT/FAMILY TEACHING
Explain method and reasons for voiding diary
Explain reasons for checking postvoid residual
Teach about ordered medications: names, dosages,
   schedules, and side effects

DISCHARGE/HOME CARE PLANNING
Emphasize importance of ongoing outpatient care
Teach/reinforce method of self-catheterization (see Box
   10-2)
Instruct patient to measure urine after each void and note
   character of urine, time, amount, and force of stream
   (use voiding diary if appropriate)
Reinforce methods of preventing UTI (see UTI, p. 607)
Teach symptoms of UTI (dysuria, foul-smelling urine, fever
   > 101° F [38.5° C]) and encourage patient to report to
   physician
Provide accurate information concerning sexual function
   to dispel myths
Advise patient to avoid taking over-the-counter
   medications without physician approval
Advise patient to avoid straining during bowel
   movements and ask physician for stool
   softeners/laxatives as needed

■ PENILE IMPLANT
*Surgical implantation of a prosthesis in the penis to
restore erectile function; the two common types are semirigid (which maintains a continuous state of erection)
and inflatable (which allows a flacid or erect penis); procedure performed when use of Viagra is not indicated
(Figs. 10-13, 10-14, 10-15, and 10-16)*

ASSESSMENT
SUBJECTIVE DATA (POSTOPERATIVE)
Pain
Spasm
Anxiety

OBJECTIVE DATA (POSTOPERATIVE)
Scrotal edema, discoloration
Incision: redness, swelling, drainage

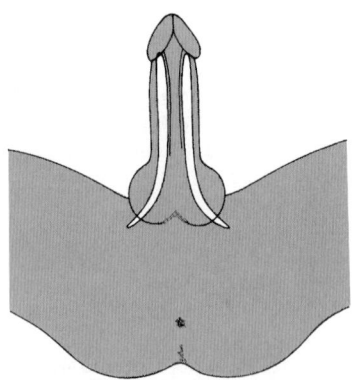 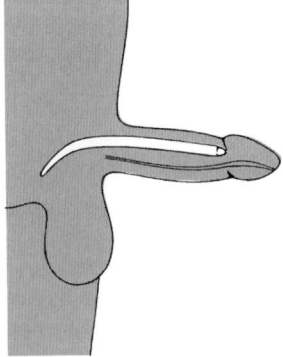

Fig. 10-13 Semirigid intrapenile prosthesis.
(From Beare PG, Myers JL: Adult health nursing, *ed 3, St Louis, 1998, Mosby.)*

Function of prosthesis
Change in character of urine (e.g., hematuria)
Fever

DIAGNOSTIC TESTS (PREOPERATIVE FOR ERECTILE DYSFUNCTION)
Medical, sexual history
Nocturnal penile tumescence tests
    Snap gauge device: evaluates rigidity of a single tumescent episode
    Nocturnal penile tumescence (NPT) monitor: continuous monitoring tumescence
Rigiscan monitor: computer-based tumescence monitor that records penile tumescence and provides information on rigidity of tumescent episodes
Doppler studies for penile blood flow

Dynamic infusion cavernosometry/cavernosography (DICC): erectile dysfunction
Penile arteriogram: insufficient blood flow
Urinalysis: hematuria, WBC, RBC, sediment, bacteria
Urine culture and sensitivity
Glucose
Testosterone
Prolactin

POTENTIAL COMPLICATIONS
Rejection
Mechanical failure
Extravasation of fluid from prosthesis reservoir into surrounding tissue
Urethral or glans erosion
Infection

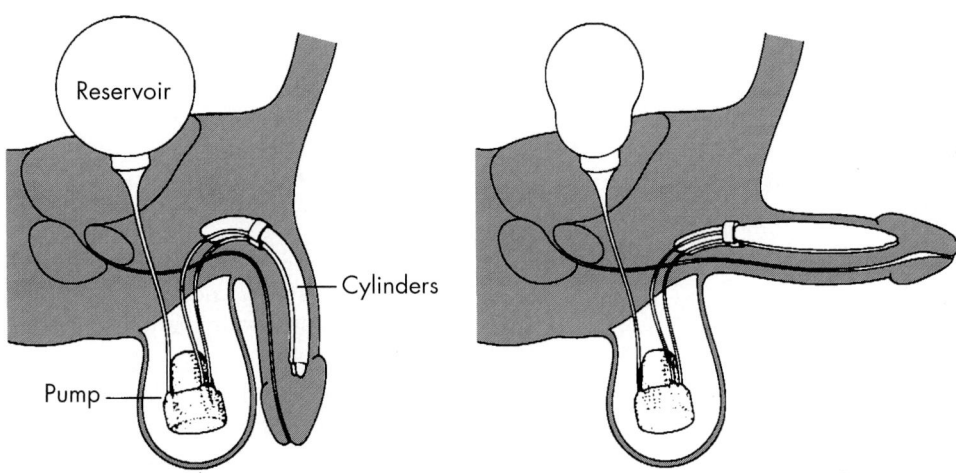

Fig. 10-14   Scott inflatable penile prosthesis.
(From Beare PG, Myers JL: Adult health nursing, *ed 3, St Louis, 1998, Mosby.)*

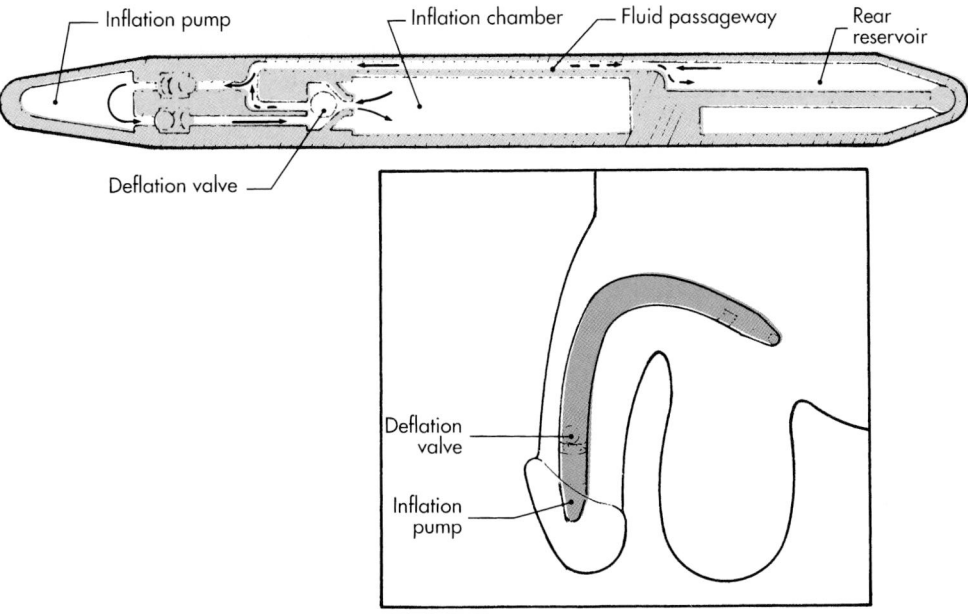

Fig. 10-15   One-piece inflatable penile prosthesis.
(From Gray M: Mosby's clinical nursing series: genitourinary disorders, *St Louis, 1992, Mosby.)*

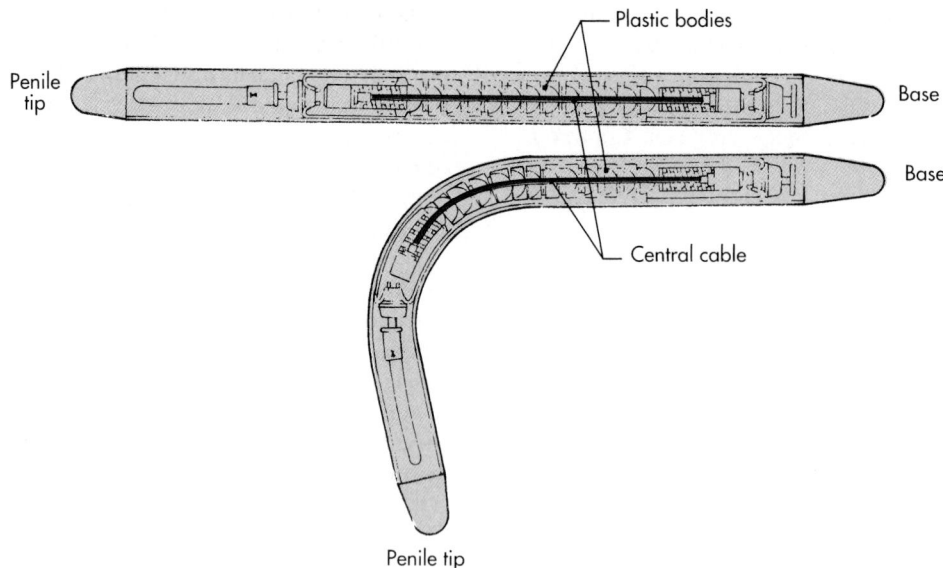

Penile tip

Plastic bodies

Base

Base

Central cable

Penile tip

Fig. 10-16 One-piece prosthesis with central cable that shortens plastic bodies to produce erection. *(From Gray M:* Mosby's clinical nursing series: genitourinary disorders, *St Louis, 1992, Mosby.)*

MULTIDISCIPLINARY MANAGEMENT
THERAPEUTIC MANAGEMENT
Medications
  Analgesics
  Antispasmodics
  Antianxiety agents
  Antibiotics
  Hormonal therapy
  Stool softeners/laxatives
  IV fluids
Ice to scrotal area
Psychologic consult
Sexual counseling

PATIENT PROBLEMS—NURSING DIAGNOSES/INTERVENTIONS

▼ Pain related to surgical incision

Assess type, intensity, location, and duration of pain and document *so changes are noted and treated*
Identify verbal and nonverbal responses to pain
Offer analgesics, documenting effectiveness and tolerance *so pharmacologic interventions are updated*
Institute nonpharmacologic comfort measures
  Optimal positioning
  Restful environment
  Relaxation techniques/guided imagery
  Diversional activities
Elevate scrotum as ordered *to decrease discomfort from edema*
Apply ice to scrotal area as ordered *to decrease edema*
Use bed cradle *to decrease pressure from bed linen on surgical area*

Expected Outcome
Relaxed and verbalizes increased comfort

▼ Risk for infection and/or rejection related to surgical incision and implantation of foreign object

Assess incision for presence of erythema, edema, tenderness, and drainage; document findings *so that changes are identified and treated*
Use sterile technique for dressing changes *to prevent introduction of microorganisms*
Report signs and symptoms of infection (fever, chills) to physician *for immediate intervention*
Report signs and symptoms of rejection (stretched skin, appearance of device outline, pain over implant site, urinary retention) to physician **for immediate intervention**
Obtain wound culture as ordered *to identify bacteria*
Monitor for elevation of WBC, *which indicates presence of infection*
Administer and monitor tolerance of ordered antibiotics

Expected Outcomes
Temperature is within normal range for patient
Incision is dry and without evidence of redness or swelling
Outline of implant is not visible on penis

▼ Altered sexuality patterns related to penile implant

Provide an accepting and supportive atmosphere *to maintain patient's self-esteem and promote verbalization of feelings, fears, concerns, and questions*
Explore how penile implant may affect patient's sexuality

Encourage patient to look at and participate in care of dressings, location of pump

Offer assistance from other professionals (sexual counselor, clergy) *to assist patient to manage emotional changes*

Encourage communication with significant other(s) and/or persons with implants *to decrease feelings of isolation*

Expected Outcomes

Verbalizes fears, feelings, and concerns related to sexuality

Participates in care and activation of penile implant

Additional Nursing Diagnoses to Consider

Body image disturbance related to presence of penile prosthesis

Depression related to unrealistic expectations after penile implant

PATIENT/FAMILY TEACHING

Explain surgical procedure; encourage questions and verbalization of concerns, feelings

Teach name and type of prosthesis

Teach/reinforce care of prosthesis

Use model or picture for demonstration

Practice inflating, deflating pump as ordered by physician

Explain prescribed inflation schedule

Explain that prosthesis restores erectile capability but has no effect on ejaculation, fertility, or orgasm

Explain that penile and scrotal swelling may last 3 to 5 days, with hematoma persisting for about 2 weeks

Provide for privacy when inflating or teaching patient to use prosthesis

Teach patient appropriate method for perineal care after bowel movement

Teach about ordered medications: names, dosages, schedules, purposes, and side effects

DISCHARGE/HOME CARE PLANNING

Emphasize importance of ongoing outpatient care

Reinforce importance of good handwashing technique for patient and others in contact with patient

Reinforce need for rest, sleep

Advise patient to discuss with physician when sexual intercourse may be resumed

Explain that wearing loose clothing will disguise appearance of semirigid implants

Reassure patient that mechanical failure of pump usually can be corrected under local anesthetic

Advise patient to avoid strenuous activity, heavy lifting, jogging, or sports until approved by physician

Avoid sexual contact for approximately 21 days to allow sufficient healing

Encourage patient to report the following findings to physician

Incisional redness, pain, swelling, drainage

Elevated temperature

Inability to urinate

Penile pain

Symptoms of UTI

Advise patient to carry medical identification in case of emergency

Advise patient to avoid taking over-the-counter medications without physician approval

Instruct patient to avoid straining during bowel movements and ask physician for stool softeners/laxatives as needed

■ PROSTATECTOMY

Removal of part or all of the prostate gland. Indications for prostatectomy include cancer, obstructive uropathy, acute urinary retention, bladder complications, or urinary infections related to BPH; surgery is usually done transurethrally, but the prostate gland may also be removed via open procedure (Table 10-4)

ASSESSMENT
SUBJECTIVE DATA

Pain

Bladder spasms

OBJECTIVE DATA

Change in character and volume of urine (hematuria)

Distended bladder

Incision if present

Redness

Swelling

Drainage

Removal of catheter

Incontinence

Frequent urination

Small urinary stream

Retention with overflow

Inability to urinate

DIAGNOSTIC TESTS

Urinalysis: hematuria, WBC, RBC, sediment, bacteria

Urine culture and sensitivity

Serum BUN, creatinine: elevated

Serum electrolytes: abnormal

CBC: decreased Hct, Hgb, elevated WBC

Cystoscopy: obstruction

IVP: obstructive uropathy

POTENTIAL COMPLICATIONS

Hemorrhage

Acute urinary retention

Stress incontinence

Erectile dysfunction

Fistula

Bladder neck contracture

Epididymitis

Infection

Deep vein thrombosis (DVT)

Table 10-4	**Types of Prostate Procedures**
Name	**Description**
Transurethral resection of prostate (TURP) (Fig. 10-17)	Removal of part or most of the prostate gland via resectoscope inserted through the urethra
Transurethral incision of the prostate (TUIP)	Removal of part of the prostate via a cold or hot knife incision made through a cystoscope
Suprapubic prostatectomy (Fig. 10-18, *A*)	Removal of the prostate gland through an incision made into the bladder
Retropubic prostatectomy (Fig. 10-18, *B*)	Removal of the prostate gland via an incision in the lower abdomen through the anterior prostatic fossa without entering the bladder
Visual laser ablation of the prostate (VLAP)	The destruction of obstructive prostate tissue by yttrium-aluminum-garnet (YAG) laser energy
Transurethral electrovaporization of the prostate (Vaportrobe)	Application of electrocautery energy to vaporize prostate tissue via a grooved probe inserted into the urethra through a rigid cystoscope
Perineal prostatectomy	Radical removal of prostate gland through an incision between the scrotum and rectum
Radical retropubic prostatectomy	Removal of the prostate gland including the capsule, seminal vesicles, and adjacent tissue through an incision in the lower abdomen; the urethra is anastomosed to the bladder neck for prostatic cancer

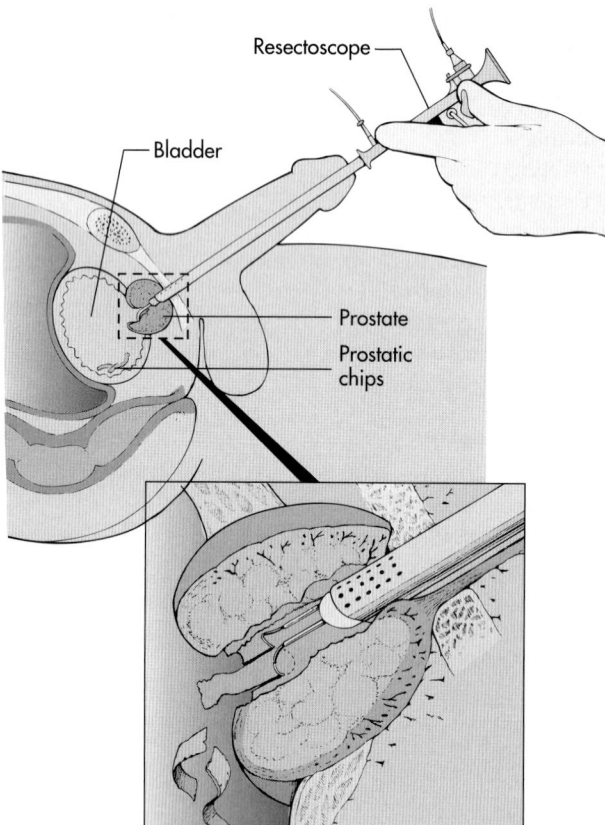

Fig. 10-17 Transurethral resection of the prostate (TURP). *(From Beare PG, Myers JL: Adult health nursing, ed 3, St Louis, 1998, Mosby.)*

Paralytic ileus
Pelvic abscess

MULTIDISCIPLINARY MANAGEMENT
  THERAPEUTIC MANAGEMENT
Medications
    Analgesics
    Antispasmodics
    Antibiotics
    Stool softeners
    IV fluids
Blood transfusion
Antiembolic stockings or sequential compression device (SCD)
Psychologic consult
Sexual counseling

  PATIENT PROBLEMS—NURSING DIAGNOSES/INTERVENTIONS

▼Altered urinary elimination related to prostatectomy and bladder irrigation (Fig. 10-19)

Monitor intake and output frequently *so that imbalances are noted for early treatment*

Monitor for signs and symptoms of dilutional hyponatremia (change in behavior, mental status, muscles twitching, nausea, vomiting, shortness of breath (SOB), elevated blood pressure (BP), decreased serum sodium) and report these findings to physician for evaluation

Stop irrigation *if fluid excess is suspected* and notify physician

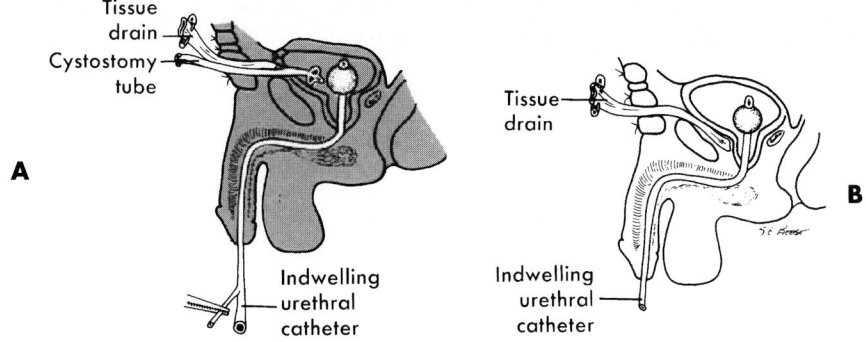

Fig. 10-18 A, Suprapubic prostatectomy (incision made into the bladder) with cystostomy tube. **B,** Retropubic prostatectomy (incision made in abdomen) with tissue drain.

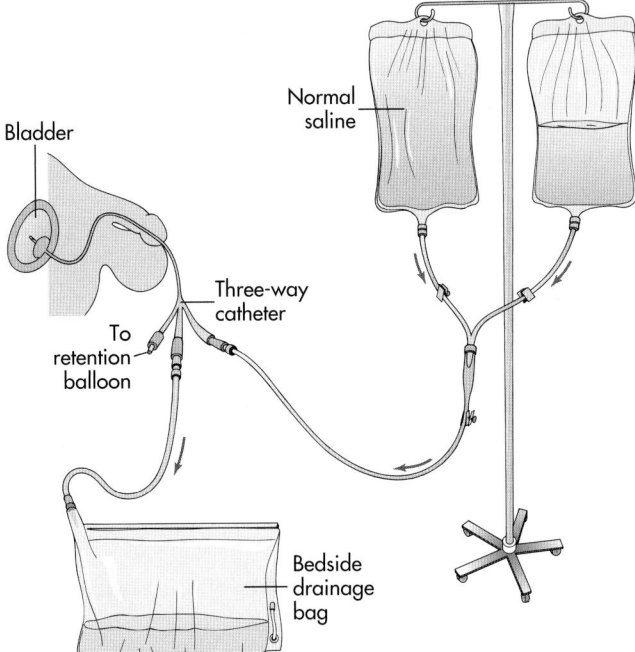

Fig. 10-19 Continuous irrigation of bladder requires a three-way Foley catheter that allows simultaneous infusion and drainage of an irrigating solution (normal saline) through bladder. Solution is infused rapidly into bladder, and bedside drainage bag is assessed for evidence of excessive bleeding and then drained every 1 to 2 hours. *(From Beare PG, Myers JL: Adult health nursing, ed 3, St Louis, 1998, Mosby.)*

Maintain patency of catheters *to promote optimal flow of urine*
    Tubing below level of bladder to allow for gravity flow
    Assess for clamping/kinks in tubing
    Secure catheters while still allowing for patient movement
    Irrigate tubes as ordered
Avoid Fowler's position for long periods *to prevent vascular stasis in lower extremities*
Label each tube clearly and record drainage from tube separately *to allow for accurate assessment of output from each system*
Record amount of irrigant and urine output; subtract irrigant from output and record

Maintain continuous bladder irrigation (CBI) if ordered
    Use sterile technique, sterile normal saline for irrigation
    Instill irrigant through irrigating port of catheter
    Regulate flow of solution at 40 to 60 drops/min or enough *to establish and maintain clear urinary flow*
Maintain suprapubic catheter
    Keep area surrounding insertion site covered with dry, sterile dressing
    Clamp catheter only when ordered so patient can attempt to void; unclamp and measure residual urine
    Monitor tolerance and document
After urinary catheter is removed, institute measures to facilitate voiding
    Privacy
    Comfortable positioning
    Running tap water
    Placing patient's hand in warm water
    Pouring warm water over perineum
    Relaxation techniques
    Applying oil of peppermint (a few drops in bedpan/urinal or on cotton ball in front of urinary meatus)
    Stroking inner aspect of thigh gently with ice
    Offering analgesic
    Voiding 1 to 2 hours after fluid intake
    Double voiding (to empty bladder more completely)
    Monitor and report signs and symptoms of urinary retention (e.g., bladder distention) and report to physician
    Explain to patient that small burgundy colored clots (scabs) may shed 7 to 10 days after catheter removal and they should clear in 1 to 2 days
    Assure patient that irritative voiding symptoms will diminish
Encourage fluid intake of 2000 to 2500 ml/day unless contraindicated

Expected Outcomes
Intake and output are balanced
Catheters remain patent while in place
Establishes regular voiding pattern after catheter is removed (usually within 6 weeks)

▼Altered peripheral tissue perfusion related to hypovolemia

Monitor for signs and symptoms of hemorrhage (hypotension; tachycardia; dyspnea; cool, clammy skin; syncope; hematuria) and report to physician for evaluation

Monitor abdominal/suprapubic dressing q2h *to assess whether bleeding has occurred or increased*

Monitor urethral and suprapubic catheter drainage *to assess whether color indicates bleeding* (i.e., change from pink to red, bright red clots)

Maintain traction on catheter as ordered *to decrease risk of hemorrhage;* release intermittently as ordered to decrease risk of bladder neck damage

Avoid manipulating rectum (e.g., taking rectal temperature), *which may place increased pressure on surgical area*

Monitor Hct, Hgb for evidence of decrease

Monitor blood transfusions according to institutional policy

Expected Outcomes

Vital signs, Hct, Hgb are stable and within patient's normal range

Incision is clean and dry when present

Catheter drainage remains pink-tinged changing to clear yellow

▼Risk for infection (urinary tract infection/incisional) related to prostatectomy

Monitor for signs and symptoms of UTI (e.g., dysuria, frequency, urgency) and report to physician for evaluation and treatment

Obtain urine culture if urine is cloudy or malodorous *to identify bacteria*

Assess incision for presence of erythema, edema, tenderness, and drainage; document *findings so changes may be identified and treated*

Use sterile technique when changing dressing *to decrease risk of infection*

Report signs and symptoms of infection (fever, chills) to physician

Obtain wound culture as ordered *to identify bacteria*

Monitor for elevation of WBC, *which indicates presence of infection*

Administer and monitor tolerance of ordered antibiotics

Expected Outcomes

Temperature is within normal limits for patient

Incision is dry and clean

Urine appears clear (not cloudy)

▼Pain related to bladder spasm/surgical procedure

Assess type, intensity, location, and duration of pain and document changes

Identify verbal and nonverbal responses to pain

Ensure that catheters are patent; irrigate as ordered until urine is free of clots

Offer analgesics, documenting effectiveness and tolerance

Institute nonpharmacologic comfort measures
    Optimal positioning
    Restful environment
    Relaxation techniques/guided imagery
    Diversional activities

Expected Outcome

Relaxed and verbalizes increased comfort

▼Altered sexuality patterns related to prostatectomy

Provide an accepting and supportive atmosphere *to maintain patient's self-esteem and promote verbalization of feelings, fears, concerns, and questions about incontinence, sexuality, and cancer*

Explore how having a prostatectomy has affected patient's sexuality

Offer assistance from other professionals (sexual counselor, clergy) *to assist in management of emotional changes*

Provide opportunities for communication with significant other concerning sexuality *to decrease feelings of isolation*

Expected Outcomes

Seeks psychosocial support when needed

Verbalizes fears, feelings, and concerns related to sexuality

Additional Nursing Diagnoses to Consider

Ineffective breathing pattern related to anesthesia

Body image disturbance related to prostatectomy

PATIENT/FAMILY TEACHING

Explain surgical procedure; encourage questions and verbalization of concerns, feelings

Provide information about expectations of return of sexual functioning

Explain reason for urethral/suprapubic catheters

Explain reason for checking postvoid residual

Explain reason for ordered blood transfusion(s)

Explain importance of turning, coughing, and deep breathing q2h; instruct in use of incentive spirometer and splinting

Explain importance of early ambulation, antiembolic stockings, and activity

Demonstrate appropriate technique for handwashing

Demonstrate dressing change if appropriate

Teach exercises that strengthen pelvic floor muscles *to decrease/eliminate incontinence and enhance sexual function*

Teach about ordered medications: names, dosages, schedules, purposes, and side effects

DISCHARGE/HOME CARE PLANNING

Emphasize importance of ongoing outpatient care

Reinforce importance of good handwashing technique for patient and others in contact with patient

Teach care of catheter and drainage units if present

Advise patient to avoid interacting with persons who have infections (e.g., colds, influenza)

Reinforce importance of adhering to dietary/fluid restrictions

Reinforce need for rest, sleep

Encourage gradual progression of activity and participation in ADLs as tolerated; restrict lifting and driving as advised by physician

Provide information about expectation of return of sexual functioning in collaboration with physician

Erection and orgasm usually the same as preoperatively unless nerves are damaged

Impotence from radical procedures

Retrograde ejaculation

Reinforce restrictions on sexual intercourse as ordered

Explain that urinary control will return, in phases, as surgical site heals

Teach signs and symptoms of UTI (dysuria, foul-smelling urine, fever > 101° F [38.5° C]) and encourage patient to report to physician

Advise patient to report the following signs and symptoms to physician

Heavy urinary bleeding

Difficulty voiding

Incisional redness, swelling, pain, drainage

Elevated temperature

Pain when walking

Advise patient to avoid taking over-the-counter medications without physician approval

Advise patient to avoid straining during bowel movements and ask physician for stool softeners/laxatives as needed

■ GLOMERULONEPHRITIS

A group of diseases that result in an inflammatory reaction and/or necrotizing lesion within the glomeruli; usually caused by an immunologic response

Glomerulonephritis (GN) may be a primary disease of the kidneys or develop secondary to a systemic disease such as systemic lupus erythematosus

ASSESSMENT
SUBJECTIVE DATA

Headache

Malaise

Dyspnea

Low-grade fever

Low back, flank pain

Anorexia

Nocturia

Nausea/vomiting

Chills

Frequent infections

Visual disturbances

OBJECTIVE DATA

Decreased urinary output

Dark brown or rust-colored urine

Fever

Hypertension

Edema (facial, sacral, ankle)

Weight gain

Jugular venous distention

Azotemia

DIAGNOSTIC TESTS

Urinalysis: hematuria, proteinuria, RBC, WBC, granular casts

Urine protein excretion (24 hour): elevated protein excretion

Serum complement: decreased

Antistreptolysin O titer: increased

Hepatitis B antigen: present

Pulmonary function tests: abnormalities in respiratory function, capacity

ECG: abnormalities in cardiac function, capacity

Blood chemistries: decreased serum albumin, elevated BUN/creatinine, abnormal levels of electrolytes

Culture of throat, skin lesion: streptococcal organism

KUB: normal size kidneys, slight bilateral enlargement

Renal biopsy: diffuse endocapillary proliferation

POTENTIAL COMPLICATIONS

Infection

Renal failure

Anemia

Hypertension

Encephalopathy

Cardiac failure

CHF

MULTIDISCIPLINARY MANAGEMENT
THERAPEUTIC MANAGEMENT

Medications

Antibiotics (if infection present)

Corticosteroids/cytotoxic agent *to decrease immune system response and antibody formation*

Antihypertensives *to control BP*

Diuretics *to remove excess fluid*

Antacids

H_2 Blockers

Plasmapheresis to remove antibodies

Hemodialysis, peritoneal dialysis (chronic or rapidly progressive disease)

Increased calories

Fluid replacement according to fluid loss

Bed rest

Dietitian consultation as necessary

Fluid, sodium, potassium, protein restriction
Psychologic consult
Social services

PATIENT PROBLEMS—NURSING DIAGNOSES/INTERVENTIONS

▼Activity intolerance related to protein depletion and/or renal dysfunction

Explain reasons for ordered bed rest
Provide exercise within prescribed activity restriction (e.g., ROM exercises) *to decrease risk of muscle atrophy*
Plan rest periods between activities *to conserve energy*
Monitor blood chemistries for evidence of body depletion of protein (e.g., proteinuria)

Expected Outcomes
Adheres to and tolerates prescribed activity plan
BP remains within patient's normal limits without excessive protein excretion as activity increases

▼Fluid volume excess related to altered renal function

Monitor for signs and symptoms of fluid excess (CHF, hypertension, weight gain, edema, decreased urine output S_3 and S_4 heart sounds, distended neck veins) and report to physician for treatment
Reduce sodium/fluid intake *to decrease fluid retention/edema*
Auscultate breath sounds q4h
Maintain fluid restriction as ordered
Administer diuretics as ordered
Monitor electrolytes and report abnormal laboratory values and signs and symptoms of electrolyte imbalance
  Hypokalemia: abdominal cramps, lethargy, dysrhythmias
  Hyperkalemia: muscle cramps and weakness
  Hypocalcemia: neuromuscular irritability
  Hyperphosphatemia: hyperreflexia, paresthesias, muscle cramps, itching, seizures
  Elevated BUN and creatinine: uremia (confusion, lethargy, restlessness)
Assess effectiveness of electrolytes administered parenterally and orally *to detect and treat changes in condition*

Expected Outcomes
Intake and output are balanced
Heart and breath sounds are within normal limits for patient

▼Altered renal tissue perfusion related to immunologic injury to kidney

Monitor intake and output to determine whether fluid balance is appropriate, report urinary output of < 30 ml/hr to physician
Replace fluids as ordered according to fluid loss
Offer ice chips, if ordered, to control thirst; include in intake measurement
Monitor for signs and symptoms of hypertensive crisis (elevated BP, tachycardia, bradycardia, confusion, decreased LOC, headache, tinnitus, nausea, vomiting, seizures) and report to physician for evaluation and treatment
Monitor BP and note response to and tolerance of antihypertensive medications

Expected Outcomes
BP, P, and weight within normal range for patient
Patient is alert and oriented

▼Risk for infection related to depressed immune system

Assess effectiveness, tolerance of immunosuppressive medications and cytotoxic agents
Monitor serum WBC, antibodies, and T cell values; report abnormal laboratory results to physician
Monitor for signs and symptoms of systemic infection (fever > 101° F [38.5° C]), chills, flushed skin, sore throat, productive cough) and report to physician for evaluation and treatment
Monitor for signs and symptoms of UTI and report to physician for evaluation and treatment
Avoid instrumentation or catheterization of urinary tract if possible; maintain closed gravity drainage system if urethral catheter present *to decrease risk of introducing organisms*

Expected Outcome
Temperature and laboratory studies are within normal range for patient

▼Altered nutrition less than body requirements related to proteinuria

Weigh patient daily (same time, scale, and clothing)
Refer to dietitian *to plan appropriate diet for patient*
  Protein of 0.8 to 1.0 g/kg/day adjusted based on blood level *to decrease excretory load on the kidneys and possible accumulation of potassium and hydrogen ions*
  High-calorie, high-carbohydrate diet

Expected Outcome
Dietary intake meets identified nutritional needs as evidenced by stable weight and laboratory studies

PATIENT/FAMILY TEACHING
Encourage coughing and deep breathing at least q2h *to prevent respiratory tract infections*

Encourage turning, changing position, and ambulating at least q2h *to prevent respiratory tract infections and promote optimal skin integrity*

Reinforce dietary and fluid restrictions (e.g., high-carbohydrate, low-protein, low-sodium diet)

To prevent UTI

Empty bladder every q2h to 3h

Shower rather than bathe and use antibacterial soap

Keep perineal area clean and dry

Wipe from front to back when cleansing perineal area

Teach about ordered medications: names, dosages, schedules, purposes, and side effects

DISCHARGE/HOME CARE PLANNING

Emphasize importance of ongoing outpatient care

Reinforce importance of good handwashing technique for patient and others in contact with patient

Advise patient to avoid interacting with persons who have infections (e.g., colds/flu)

Reinforce need for adequate rest, sleep

Encourage patient to report to physician the following signs and symptoms of recurrence and progression of disease

Edema, puffy eyes, swollen extremities

Lethargy

Decreased urinary output

Instruct patient to weigh self daily (same time, scale, and clothing); report weight gain to home health nurse and/or physician

Encourage patient/significant other to monitor BP daily and report elevation to physician

Encourage patient to report symptoms of infection to physician (e.g., fever, sore throat, flu, cough)

Encourage patient to observe character of urine after each void and report abnormalities (e.g., hematuria) to physician

Teach symptoms of UTI (dysuria, foul-smelling urine, fever > 101° F [38.5° C]) and encourage patient to report to physician

Advise patient to avoid taking over-the-counter medications without physician approval

Advise patient to avoid straining during bowel movements and ask physician for stool softeners/laxatives as needed

■ POLYCYSTIC KIDNEY DISEASE (PKD)

A congenital autosomal dominant disorder in which normal kidney tissue is replaced with grapelike clusters of cysts (Fig. 10-20); surrounding cells are destroyed over time because of compression

ASSESSMENT

SUBJECTIVE DATA

Family history of polycystic kidney disease (PKD)

Abdominal fullness

Flank, abdominal, or lumbar pain

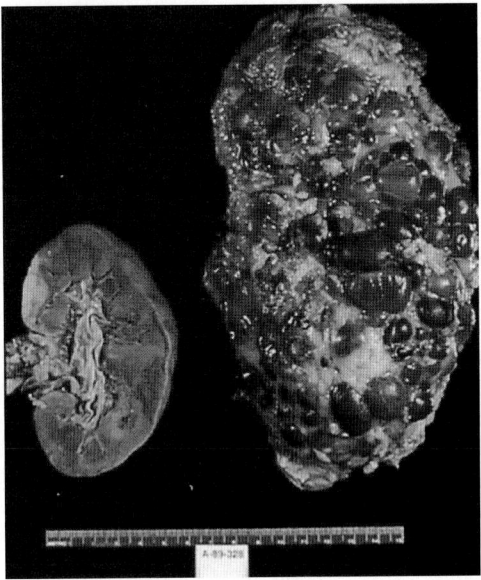

Fig. 10-20 Polycystic kidney. *Left,* Cross-section. *Right,* Whole kidney showing cysts.
(From Brundage DJ: Mosby's clinical nursing series: renal disorders, *St Louis, 1992, Mosby.)*

Frequent infections, UTI

Psychologic problems (e.g., hopelessness, depression)

OBJECTIVE DATA

Palpable abdominal mass

Hypertension

Variable urine output

Hematuria

DIAGNOSTIC TESTS

CBC: elevated WBC, anemia

Urinalysis: WBCs, RBCs, proteinuria, pyuria, bacteria

Urine culture and sensitivity

Serum electrolytes, BUN, creatinine: abnormal/elevated levels

Urine electrolytes: abnormal levels

Urine creatinine clearance: decreased kidney function

KUB/renal ultrasonography: enlarged kidneys

Renal biopsy: abnormal kidney cells, tissue

Renal ultrasound: abnormalities of kidney(s)

IVU: irregular outline and distortion of calyceal pattern; presence of cysts, nephrocalcinosis, or obstruction of the collecting system

POTENTIAL COMPLICATIONS

Ruptured cysts

Infection

Calculi

Liver cysts

Renal bleeding

Obstruction

Malignancy

Salt-wasting defect

End-stage renal disease

MULTIDISCIPLINARY MANAGEMENT
THERAPEUTIC MANAGEMENT
Medications
  Antihypertensives
  Diuretics
  Antibiotics
  Analgesics
Fluid restriction, parenteral IV fluids
Consultation with dietitian
  Dietary restriction of protein and sodium
Dialysis and renal transplant when renal failure occurs
  (see Renal failure, p. 641)
Genetic counseling
Dietitian as recommended
Psychologic consult

PATIENT PROBLEMS—NURSING DIAGNOSES/INTERVENTIONS

▼ Pain related to renal cysts

Assess type, intensity, location, and duration of pain using a pain scale and document *so that changes can be noted and interventions started*
Identify verbal and nonverbal responses to pain
Offer analgesics, documenting effectiveness and tolerance *so that pharmacologic changes can be made as needed*
Heating pads *to relieve discomfort* unless patient is bleeding
Institute nonpharmacologic comfort measures
  Optimal positioning
  Relaxation techniques/guided imagery
  Restful environment
  Diversional activity

Expected Outcome
Appears relaxed and verbalizes increased comfort

▼ Altered renal tissue perfusion related to replacement of normal renal tissue with cysts or incompetence of kidney

Monitor intake and output *to determine whether fluid balance is appropriate*
Monitor for signs and symptoms of fluid deficit (e.g., hypotension, poor skin turgor, decreased urinary output, thirst, dry mucous membranes, weight loss) and report to physician for treatment
Monitor for signs and symptoms of fluid excess (e.g., CHF, hypertension, weight gain, edema, decreased urine output, S_3 and S_4 heart sounds, distended neck veins) and report to physician for treatment
Weigh patient daily (same time, scale, and clothing)
Monitor BP and note response to and tolerance of antihypertensive medications
Monitor for signs and symptoms of hypertensive crisis (e.g., elevated BP, tachycardia, bradycardia, confusion, decreased LOC, headache, tinnitus, nausea, vomiting, seizures, dysrhythmia) and report to physician for treatment
Monitor blood test results *to identify decrease in renal function*

Expected Outcomes
Intake and output are balanced
Weight is stable and within normal range for patient
Vital signs are within normal range for patient

▼ Risk for infection (UTI, local, systemic) related to disease process, depressed immune system, and/or presence and rupture of fluid-filled cysts

Monitor for signs and symptoms of systemic infection (e.g., fever > 101° F [38.5° C], chills, flushed skin, sore throat, productive cough) and report to physician for evaluation, treatment
Monitor for signs and symptoms of UTI and report to physician for evaluation and treatment
Avoid instrumentation or catheterization of urinary tract if possible; maintain closed gravity drainage system if urethral catheter is present

Expected Outcomes
Temperature is within normal range for patient
Urine is clear yellow to amber
Breath sounds are clear

▼ Dysfunctional grieving related to loss of kidney function, changes in lifestyle, decision of having no children, and life-threatening prognosis

Provide an accepting and supportive atmosphere *to maintain patient's self-esteem and promote verbalization of feelings, fears, concerns, and questions*
Explore how having PKD has affected patient's daily activities/lifestyle *to provide support and suggest methods of problem management*
Observe for behavioral and emotional signs of grieving (e.g., denial, anger, crying, withdrawal, noncompliance, dependency) and help patient explore these feelings
Assist patient in identifying coping measures used effectively in the past *so that these may be used to adapt to PKD*
Identify positive features of patient's life *to promote feelings of self-worth*
Reinforce adaptive behaviors and set limits on maladaptive coping mechanisms that interfere with well-being
Provide answers to questions about treatment for PKD
Offer assistance from other professionals (psychologist, sexual counselor, geneticist, clergy) *to help manage emotional changes and decisions concerning pregnancy*

Encourage communication with significant other(s) and/or members of support group *to decrease feelings of isolation*

Expected Outcomes
Participates in ADLs at optimal level
Comfortably discusses feelings, fears, concerns, and questions
Identifies approaches for making positive changes in ADLs, lifestyle
Requests assistance from professionals and support group when needed

Additional Nursing Diagnosis to Consider
Altered family processes related to genetically transmitted disease

PATIENT/FAMILY TEACHING
Encourage coughing and deep breathing using schedule *to prevent respiratory tract infections*
Encourage turning, changing position, and ambulating using a schedule *to prevent respiratory tract infections and promote optimal skin integrity*
Reinforce dietary and fluid restrictions
To help prevent UTI
  Empty bladder q2h to 3h (if able to void)
  Shower rather than bathe and use antibacterial soap
  Keep perineal area clean and dry
  Wipe from front to back when cleansing perianal area
Teach about ordered medications: names, dosages, schedules, purposes, and side effects

DISCHARGE/HOME CARE PLANNING
Emphasize importance of ongoing outpatient care
Reinforce importance of good handwashing technique for patient and others in contact
Advise patient to avoid interacting with persons who have infections (e.g., colds/influenza)
Avoid tight constraints on abdomen such as tight seat belts in cars and planes, tight belt around clothes
Avoid contact sports
Reinforce need for rest, sleep
Advise patient/significant other to monitor BP and report elevation to physician; teach BP procedure
Encourage patient to observe character of urine after voiding and report abnormalities (e.g., hematuria) to physician
Teach symptoms of UTI (dysuria, foul-smelling urine, fever > 101° F [38.5° C]) and encourage patient to report to physician
Advise patient to avoid taking over-the-counter medications without physician approval

■ ACUTE RENAL FAILURE
A sudden and severe impairment of renal function resulting in an acute uremic episode; primary causes of acute renal failure (ARF) are impeded blood flow to the kidney, damage to renal tissue, and disrupted urinary flow

ASSESSMENT
SUBJECTIVE DATA
Change in voiding pattern
Headache
Inability to concentrate
Weakness
Thirst
Metallic taste in mouth
Nausea
Pruritus
Nocturia
Anorexia

OBJECTIVE DATA
Anuria
Oliguria
Bladder distension (in obstruction only)
Anemia
Fever
Hypotension
Hypertension
Dry mucous membranes
Decreased venous filling and skin turgor
Kussmaul respirations
Mental status changes
Edema (eyes, legs, hands)
Jugular venous distention
Bruising
Pallor
Weight loss or gain
Vomiting
Urine (ammonia) breath odor

DIAGNOSTIC TESTS
Urine studies: decreased pH, abnormal findings with osmolality, specific gravity, sodium, creatinine, and urine sediment
CBC: increased WBC, decreased Hgb, Hct, increased BUN and creatinine, phosphate, magnesium, calcium, potassium, sodium, bicarbonate
KUB: normal or enlarged kidney
Renal ultrasound: obstruction, abnormally sized or shaped kidney
Retrograde pyelography: obstruction
IVU: obstruction, strictures, or masses
Renal scan: cysts, tumors, or impaired perfusion
Renal biopsy: abnormal cells, tissue
ECG: dysrhythmias

POTENTIAL COMPLICATIONS
Hypervolemia
Acidosis
Hyperkalemia
Hyperphosphatemia
Hypertension

Anemia
Infection
Cardiovascular/respiratory failure

MULTIDISCIPLINARY MANAGEMENT
THERAPEUTIC MANAGEMENT
Medications
    Alkalinizing agents
    Potassium-lowering agents
    Angiotensin antagonists
    Calcium channel blockers
    Antihypertensives
    Diuretics
    Antiinfective agents
    Phosphate-binding agents
    H_2 Blockers
    Multivitamins
    Ferrous sulfate
    Sodium bicarbonate
    Antiemetics
    Cation exchange resin (for hyperkalemia)
IV fluids
Bed rest
Restraints (only when all other measures fail)
Daily weights
Blood transfusions
TPN
Dialysis
Continuous arteriovenous or venovenous hemofiltration
Transplantation
Dietary consult
Social services

PATIENT PROBLEMS—NURSING DIAGNOSES/INTERVENTIONS

▼Fluid volume excess related to decreased urine output as a result of damage to nephrons

Monitor intake and output frequently *so that abnormal fluid balance is identified and treated*
Monitor for signs and symptoms of fluid excess
    Hypertension
    Weight gain
    Edema
    Breath sounds
    Jugular venous distention
Monitor serum electrolyte levels *for abnormalities associated with fluid volume excess* (hyperkalemia, hyperphosphatemia, hypermagnesemia, hypocalcemia)
Monitor effectiveness and tolerance of medications ordered to decrease fluid volume (e.g., diuretics)
Monitor ECG for dysrhythmias, *which may be associated with increased/decreased levels of serum potassium*

Expected Outcomes
Intake and output are balanced
Weight is stable and within patient's normal range

Heart and breath sounds and electrolytes are within normal limits for patient

▼Altered nutrition: less than body requirements related to GI disturbances and/or restricted dietary intake

Dietitian to assist with developing appropriate meal plan; include patient in planning *to increase compliance*
Encourage small, frequent meals *to promote digestion of foods*
Weigh patient daily (same time, scale, and clothing)
Monitor for conditions that increase loss of needed nutrients (e.g., nausea, vomiting, anorexia)
Monitor effectiveness and tolerance of antiemetics *so pharmacologic changes can be made as needed*
Monitor laboratory studies *that may indicate whether protein intake is adequate* (e.g., serum protein, lipids, potassium, calcium)
Offer oral hygiene regularly *to improve taste in mouth*

Expected Outcomes
Dietary intake meets identified nutritional needs as evidenced by stable weight and laboratory studies
Participates in developing and complies with nutritional plan

▼Fluid volume deficit related to diuretic phase of disease process and/or hemorrhage

Monitor intake and output frequently
Monitor for signs and symptoms of inadequate fluid volume
    Hypotension
    Tachycardia
    Weight loss
    Decreased venous filling and skin turgor
    Dry mucous membranes
    Hemoconcentration; note electrolyte levels (e.g., sodium)
Monitor effectiveness and tolerance of medications ordered *to enhance renal blood flow and systemic circulating volume* (e.g., vasoconstrictors, electrolyte replacements)
Institute measures to decrease hemorrhage
    Use smallest-gauge needle possible for venipuncture, injections
    Apply pressure to all injection sites until bleeding stops
    Advise patient to move slowly and carefully to decrease likelihood of bruising, trauma
Monitor for signs and symptoms of hemorrhage
    Hypotension
    Petechiae
    Prolonged bleeding with venipuncture
    Bleeding gums
    Increased abdominal girth

Expected Outcomes

Intake and output are balanced

Skin turgor is good

Evidence of bleeding is absent

▼Risk for injury related to mental status changes from chemical abnormalities

Assess mental status at admission and document changes

Orient to time, place, and person as needed

Instruct patient to call for assistance when getting out of bed

Observe for changes in behavior *that may indicate alterations in brain function*

Institute seizure precautions

Airway/suction readily available in room

Pad side rails

Restrain only when other measures fail *to protect patient*

Expected Outcome

Patient sustains no injuries

Additional Nursing Diagnoses to Consider

Risk for infection related to compromised immune system

Risk for impaired skin integrity related to decreased activity, uremia, and edema

Self-care deficit related to fatigue, mental status changes

Altered family processes related to health crisis

PATIENT/FAMILY TEACHING

Explain cause of the ARF episode when known

Encourage turning, changing position, and ambulating at least q2h *to prevent respiratory tract infections and promote optimal skin integrity*

Explain reasons for dietary and fluid restrictions

Teach about ordered medications: names, dosages, schedules, purposes, and side effects

Teach about BP procedure

Involve family/significant others in discussions about illness, treatment, prognosis, and discharge plan of care

Support patient/family decisions and use crisis intervention skills as appropriate

DISCHARGE/HOME CARE PLANNING

Emphasize importance of ongoing outpatient care

Reinforce importance of good handwashing technique for patient and others in contact with patient

Advise patient to avoid interacting with persons who have infections (e.g., colds/influenza)

Reinforce need for rest, sleep

Advise patient to weigh self daily (same time, scale, and clothing) and report changes in weight of 2 lb or more to home health nurse and/or physician

Advise patient to measure urine with each void and report to physician decrease in urine or inability to urinate

Instruct patient to check BP at same time each day and report changes to physician; teach procedure for taking BP

Encourage patient to report signs and symptoms of infection to physician (e.g., fever, sore throat, influenza, cough)

Advise patient to avoid taking over-the-counter medications without physician approval

Advise patient to avoid straining during bowel movements and ask physician for stool softeners/laxatives as needed

Refer to resources:

National Kidney Foundation

30 E. 33rd Street, 11th floor

New York, NY 10016

(800) 622-9010

■ CHRONIC RENAL FAILURE

An irreversible, progressive impairment of renal function resulting from damage of nephrons and glomeruli; potential causes of chronic renal failure (CRF) are polycystic kidney disease, chronic glomerulonephritis, chronic pyelonephritis, chronic urinary obstruction, hypertensive nephropathy, diabetic nephropathy, and gouty nephropathy

ASSESSMENT

SUBJECTIVE DATA

Headache

Pruritus

Metallic taste in mouth

Loss of sense of smell

Nocturnal leg cramping

Paresthesia of lower extremities

Blurred vision

Anorexia

Nausea/vomiting

Hiccups

Dyspnea

Diarrhea

Constipation

Thirst

Fatigue

Bone pain

Insomnia

Clouded thinking

Irritability

Depression

Amenorrhea

Decreased libido

OBJECTIVE DATA

Anuria

Oliguria

Anemia

Hypertension

Dysrhythmia

Kussmaul respirations

Urinelike odor to breath (ammonia)
Mental status changes (drowsiness, confusion, stupor, coma)
Edema
Jugular venous distention
Bruising
Pallor
Dry skin
Brittle nails and hair
Uremic frost
Hematemesis
Melena
Weight gain/loss
"Restless legs" syndrome

DIAGNOSTIC TESTS

Urinalysis: acidic pH, WBCs, RBCs, specific gravity
Urine (24 hour): normal volume (early), no or low volume, proteinuria, decreased creatinine clearance
CBC: decreased Hct/Hgb/platelets, increased WBCs
Blood chemistry: abnormal levels of BUN, creatinine, potassium, calcium, phosphorus, sodium, chloride
Imaging studies
  IVP
  Renal ultrasound
  Renal scan
  CT scan
  KUB
    Small/contracted kidneys
    Very large with polycystic disease
  Renal ultrasound: small/contracted kidneys
ECG: dysrhythmias
Stool: occult blood
EEG

POTENTIAL COMPLICATIONS

Anemia
Hypertension
Hyperkalemia
Congestive heart failure
Pulmonary edema
Pericarditis
Accelerated atherosclerosis
Peptic ulcer disease
Osteodystrophy
Metabolic encephalopathy
Peripheral neuropathy

MULTIDISCIPLINARY MANAGEMENT
THERAPEUTIC MANAGEMENT

Medications
  Alkalinizing agents
  Anticonvulsants
  Antihypertensives
  Diuretics
  Antiinfective agents
  Phosphate-binding agents
  H_2-Receptor agents

  Anabolic agents
  Antianemics
  Antiemetics
  Antipruritics
  Laxatives, stool softeners
  Electrolytes, minerals
  Vitamins
Bed rest
Dietary consult
Daily weight
Hemodialysis
Peritoneal dialysis
Hemofiltration
Renal transplantation
Social services
Spiritual support

PATIENT PROBLEMS—NURSING DIAGNOSES/INTERVENTIONS

▼ Fluid volume excess related to inability of kidney to adequately process water and sodium

Monitor intake and output frequently *so that abnormal fluid balance will be identified and treated*
Monitor for signs and symptoms of fluid excess
  Hypertension
  Weight gain
  Edema
  Jugular venous distention
Monitor serum electrolyte levels for abnormalities, *which may be associated with fluid volume excess (hyperkalemia, hyperphosphatemia, hypermagnesemia, hypocalcemia)*
Monitor effectiveness and tolerance of medications ordered to decrease fluid volume (e.g., diuretics if some kidney function is present)
Monitor ECG for dysrhythmias, *which may be associated with increased/decreased levels of serum potassium*

Expected Outcomes
Weight is stable
Breath and heart sounds are normal
Electrolytes are within normal range for patient

▼ Altered nutrition: less than body requirements related to GI disturbances and/or restricted dietary intake

Dietitian to assist with developing appropriate meal plan; include patient in planning *to increase compliance*
Encourage small, frequent meals *to promote digestion of foods*
Weigh patient daily (same time, scale, and clothing) *to ensure accurate and reliable data*
Monitor for conditions that increase loss of needed nutrients (e.g., nausea, vomiting, anorexia) *so that a plan may be implemented to resolve these problems*

Monitor laboratory studies that *may indicate whether protein intake is adequate (e.g., serum protein, lipids, potassium, calcium)*

Offer to provide oral hygiene regularly *to improve taste in mouth*

Expected Outcomes

Dietary intake meets identified nutritional needs as evidenced by stable weight, serum albumin, total protein, iron, Hgb, and Hct

Collaborates in developing and complies with nutritional plan

▼Risk for injury related to mental status changes from chemical abnormalities

Assess mental status at admission and document *so that changes will be noted*

Orient to time, place, and person as needed

Explain procedures, treatments, use of equipment; clarify as needed

Observe for changes in behavior, *which may indicate alterations in brain function*

Provide clutter-free environment

Maintain safety precautions: bed rails up, bed in low position, sharp objects out of reach, call bell in reach *to prevent injury*

Observe frequently if patient is unable to call for assistance

Provide clutter-free environment

Institute seizure precautions

Airway, suction readily available in room

Pad side rails

Restrain only if other measures fail *to protect patient*

Expected Outcome

Patient is free of injury

Additional Nursing Diagnoses to Consider

Risk for infection related to compromised immune system

Altered renal tissue perfusion related to nephron destruction

Risk for impaired skin integrity related to decreased activity, uremia, and edema

Self-care deficit related to fatigue, mental status changes

Altered family processes related to chronic disease process

Sexual dysfunction related to effects of uremia

Body image disturbance related to altered renal function

Ineffective individual coping related to chronic disease process

PATIENT/FAMILY TEACHING

Explain details of CRF to patient/family

Discuss treatments aimed at combating the effects of CRF (e.g., renal dialysis, transplantation)

Encourage turning, changing position, and ambulating at least q2h *to prevent respiratory tract infections and promote optimal skin integrity*

Explain reasons for dietary and fluid restrictions

Teach about ordered medications: names, dosages, schedules, purposes, and side effects

DISCHARGE/HOME CARE PLANNING

Emphasize importance of ongoing outpatient care

Reinforce importance of good handwashing technique for patient and others in contact

Advise patient to avoid interacting with persons who have infections (e.g., colds, influenza)

Reinforce need for rest, sleep

Advise patient to weigh self daily (same time, scale, and clothing); report changes in weight of 2 lb or more to home health nurse and/or physician

Advise patient to measure urine with each void and report decrease in urine or inability to urinate to physician

Instruct patient to check BP at same time each day and report changes to physician

Encourage patient to report signs and symptoms of infection (e.g., fever, sore throat, influenza, cough) to physician

Advise patient to avoid taking over-the-counter medications without physician approval

Advise patient to avoid straining during bowel movements and ask physician for stool softeners/laxatives as needed

Refer to resources:

National Association of Patients on Hemodialysis and Transplantation

505 Northern Blvd.

Great Neck, NY 11021

National Kidney Foundation

30 East 33rd Street, 11th floor

New York, NY 10016

Phone 800-622-9010

Fax 212-689-9261

Web address: www.nephron.com/NKF

■ CARE OF PATIENT AFTER HEMODIALYSIS

Hemodialysis is one form of treatment for acute or chronic renal failure; an external dialyzing system is used to remove toxic wastes and excess water, fluid and correct electrolyte imbalances; types of access for hemodialysis include external (temporary) arteriovenous cannula (shunt) (Fig. 10-21), internal (permanent) arteriovenous fistula, and internal (permanent) arteriovenous graft (Fig. 10-22)

ASSESSMENT

SUBJECTIVE DATA

Muscle cramps

Pruritus

Headache

Nausea/vomiting

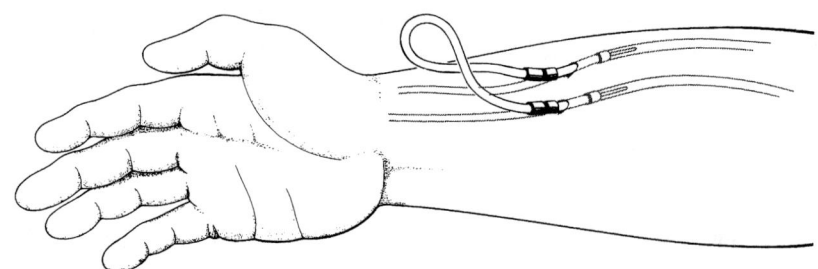

Fig. 10-21 External arteriovenous shunt.
(From Beare PG, Myers JL: Adult health nursing, ed 3, St Louis, 1998, Mosby.)

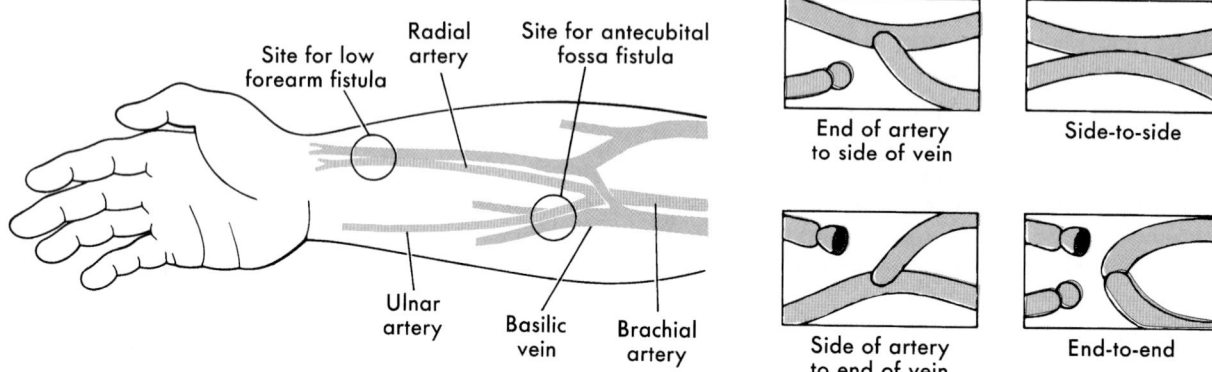

Fig. 10-22 Internal arteriovenous fistula. Types of fistula construction.
(From Beare PG, Myers JL: Adult health nursing, ed 3, St Louis, 1998, Mosby.)

Restlessness
Dizziness

OBJECTIVE DATA
Anuria
Vascular access problems (bleeding, clotting, infection)
Hypervolemia
    Hypertension
    Tachycardia
    Jugular venous distention
    Rales
    Postural edema
    Weight gain
    SOB
Hypovolemia
    Hypotension
    Bradycardia
    Flat neck veins
    Weight loss
    Dry mucous membranes
Confusion
Seizures
Agitation

DIAGNOSTIC TESTS
Serum electrolytes: abnormal levels
Serum BUN, creatinine: elevated levels expected
Coagulation studies: abnormal PT, PTT, platelet count
Hct, Hgb: decreased levels expected
See Chronic renal failure (p. 643)

POTENTIAL COMPLICATIONS
Hemorrhage
Air embolism
Severe hypotension
Hepatitis
Septicemia
Hemodynamic problems
Infection
Metabolic problems
Mechanical problems

MULTIDISCIPLINARY MANAGEMENT
THERAPEUTIC MANAGEMENT
Medications
    Analgesics
    Antacids
    Antibiotics
    Anticoagulants
    Antidysrhythmics
    Antiemetics
    Antihypertensives
    Antiinflammatories
    Antimicrobials
    Sedatives
    Vitamins
    Ferrous sulfate
    Diuretics
    Calcium
    Sodium bicarbonate
Fluid restriction

Daily weight
Dietary restrictions (dietitian consultation)
TPN
Guaiac GI tract fluids
Blood transfusions
Psychologic consult

PATIENT PROBLEMS—NURSING DIAGNOSES/INTERVENTIONS

▼ Altered peripheral tissue perfusion related to risk of vascular access clotting/disconnection

Monitor and document patency of access device frequently *so that changes will be identified* (see Figs. 10-20 and 10-21)
  Auscultate for bruits (use Doppler as needed)
  Palpate for thrills
  Evaluate patency of exposed area of device (shunt should be wrapped securely with gauze, exposing only a portion of loop)
  Observe color of blood and condition of surrounding skin
  Observe for leakage
  Inspect fistula needle puncture sites after dialysis (if bleeding noted, apply pressure until bleeding subsides)
Report signs and symptoms of clotting of access device to physician
  Dark or separated blood within shunt
  Site cool to touch
  Absence of bruits or thrills
Monitor and report signs and symptoms of inadequate peripheral perfusion
  Sudden, unrelieved pain
  Numbness
  Tingling
  Decreased capillary refill time
  Cool skin temperature of extremity distal to access site
Avoid taking BP and performing venipuncture in arm with fistula or cannula *to decrease risk of infection, clotting*
Do not wear jewelry or identification band on extremity with access site
Avoid cutting off dressings at access site *so that puncturing of access will not occur*
Institute measures to manage potentially emergent situations with shunt, subclavian or femoral line
  Keep smooth, rubber-tipped clamps and tourniquet at bedside in case of line disconnection
  If disconnection occurs, clamp tubing and notify physician immediately
  If tubing is pulled out, apply pressure to site and place tourniquet above site; notify physician immediately

Expected Outcomes
Access devices are intact as evidenced by presence of bruits, thrills, and blood circulation
Site of access and distal extremity are warm with capillary refill time of 1 to 2 seconds

▼ Fluid volume excess related to fluid accumulation/inadequate dialysis

Monitor intake and output frequently *so that abnormalities with fluid balance will be identified and treated*
Restrict fluid as ordered
Monitor for signs and symptoms of fluid accumulation (caused by inadequate dialysis)
  Weight gain (check daily [same time, scale, and clothing])
  Elevated BP
  Dyspnea
  Distended neck veins
Monitor blood work *for abnormalities associated with fluid volume excess*
  Elevated BUN, creatinine (nitrogenous waste build-up)
  Elevated sodium, potassium, pH (electrolyte accumulation)
  Anemia (continuing problem with chronic renal failure and blood loss)

Expected Outcome
Does not have symptoms of excess fluid after treatment

▼ Fluid volume deficit related to rapid removal of body fluid during treatment

Monitor intake and output frequently *so that abnormalities with fluid balance will be identified and treated*
Replace fluid as ordered
Monitor for signs and symptoms of fluid deficit
  Weight loss (check daily [same time, scale, and clothing])
  Lowered BP
  Nausea
  Muscle cramps

Expected Outcome
Decreased weight after treatment

▼ Risk for infection related to presence of access site and invasive procedure

Institute measures to decrease risk of infection
  Use sterile technique when caring for access site(s)
  Cleanse access area gently with hydrogen peroxide or alcohol wipes; cover with dry, sterile dressing
Report signs and symptoms of infection to physician for evaluation: temperature elevation above patient's normal, erythema, edema, drainage at access site
Monitor WBCs for elevation (may indicate infection)

Expected Outcomes
Temperature remains within patient's normal range
No signs or symptoms of infection are noted at access site

▼Body image disturbance related to presence of access device for hemodialysis

Provide an accepting and supportive atmosphere *to maintain patient's self-esteem and promote the verbalization of feelings, fears, concerns, and questions*

Explore how having hemodialysis, access catheter has affected daily life and activities *to provide emotional support and suggest methods of problem management*

Identify positive features of patient's life *to promote feelings of self-worth*

Offer assistance from other professionals (psychologist, sexual counselor) *to assist in management of emotional changes*

Encourage communication with significant other(s) and/or members of support group *to decrease feelings of isolation*

Expected Outcomes
Uses psychosocial support systems
Feels comfortable verbalizing fears, feelings, and concerns
Complies with treatment plan

Additional Nursing Diagnoses to Consider
Pain, discomfort related to dialysis process
Altered thought processes related to dialysis disequilibrium syndrome or dialysis dementia
Ineffective individual/family coping related to diagnosis of chronic illness
Noncompliance to prescribed treatment regimen (e.g., dietary restrictions)

PATIENT/FAMILY TEACHING
Explain procedure for surgery to place access device for hemodialysis and hemodialysis procedure; encourage questions, verbalization of concerns and feelings
Explain purpose of prescribed medical regimen
Explain reasons for dietary, fluid restrictions
Teach about ordered medications: names, dosages, schedules, purposes, and side effects

DISCHARGE/HOME CARE PLANNING
Emphasize importance of ongoing outpatient care
Reinforce importance of good handwashing technique for patient and others with whom patient comes in contact; maintain aseptic technique when cleansing access site(s)
Advise patient to avoid interacting with persons who have infections (e.g., colds/flu)
Provide written medication schedule for patient; review which medications should be held until after dialysis treatment (to promote optimal absorption)
Reinforce care of access device
  Palpate for thrill qd; report absence of thrill to physician
  Report presence of dark, separated blood to physician

Report pain, numbness, tingling, change in color of affected extremity to physician
Avoid having blood pressure and/or blood taken from affected extremity
Always carry clamps to stop bleeding in case shunt separates
Advise patient to institute measures that decrease risk of trauma to or bleeding of access device
  Keep sterile dressing on site
  Wear loose sleeves
  No lifting of heavy objects or carrying heavy purse on arm with access
  Wear plastic covering on affected extremity if exposed to water
Encourage patient to report redness, pain, swelling, or drainage from access site(s) to physician
Reinforce importance of adhering to dietary, fluid restrictions; record daily intake and output (if applicable)
Reinforce need for rest, sleep
Encourage gradual progression of activity and participation in ADLs as tolerated
Advise patient to weigh self daily (same time, scale, and clothing); report changes in weight of 2 lb or more to home health nurse and/or physician
Instruct patient to check BP at same time each day and report changes to physician
Teach symptoms of UTI (i.e., dysuria, foul-smelling urine, fever > 101° F [38.5° C]) and encourage patient to report these findings to physician
Advise patient to avoid taking over-the-counter medications without physician approval

■ PERITONEAL DIALYSIS
Perioneal dialysis (PD) is one form of treatment for acute or chronic renal failure; dialysate fluid is introduced into the abdominal cavity, using the peritoneum as a semipermeable membrane between the dialysate and the blood found in abdominal vessels; fluid may be instilled via manual exchanges (Figs. 10-23 and 10-24) or machine

Types of PD include **intermittent peritoneal dialysis (IPD), continuous ambulatory peritoneal dialysis (CAPD),** *and* **continuous cycling peritoneal dialysis (CCPD);** *access devices may be temporary or permanent*

ASSESSMENT
SUBJECTIVE DATA
Abdominal pain, tenderness
Thirst
Headache
Fatigue
Nausea
Anxiety

OBJECTIVE DATA
Abdominal rigidity
Vomiting

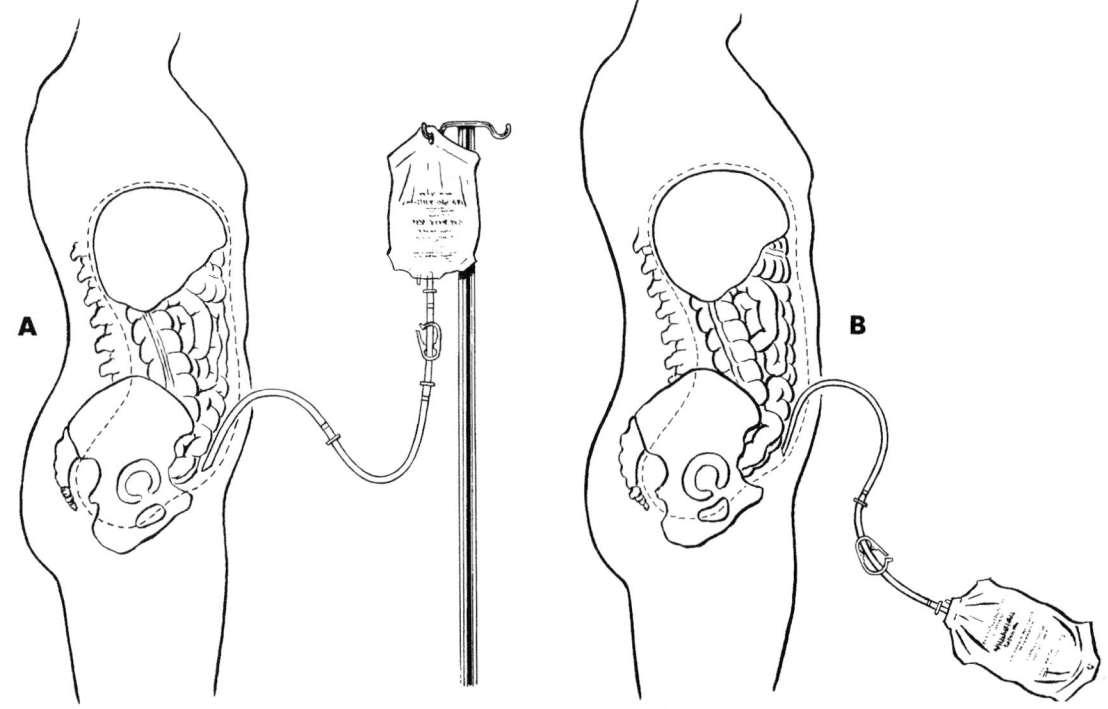

Fig. 10-23   Peritoneal dialysis. **A,** Inflow. **B,** Outflow.
(From Thompson JM et al: Mosby's clinical nursing, *ed 4, St Louis, 1997, Mosby.)*

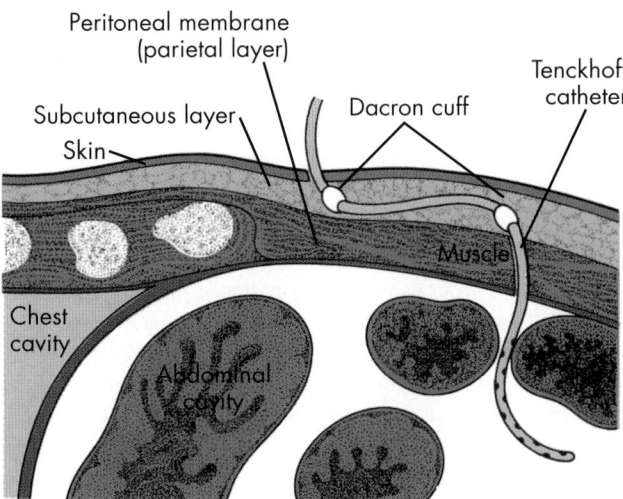

Fig. 10-24   Peritoneal catheter.
(From Lewis SM, et al: Medical-surgical nursing: assessment and management of clinical problems, *ed 4, St Louis, 1996, Mosby.)*

Diarrhea
Decreased/absent bowel sounds
Catheter insertion site
    Redness
    Swelling
    Drainage
Dialysate
    Cloudy
    Red

Fecal colored
Foul smelling
Hypervolemia
    Hypertension
    Tachycardia
    Jugular venous distention
    Tachypnea, rales, crackles
    Postural edema
    Weight gain
Hypovolemia
    Hypotension
    Bradycardia
    Flat neck veins
    Weight loss
    Dry mucous membranes
Confusion
Elevated temperature

Diagnostic Tests

Serum electrolytes: abnormal levels
Serum BUN, creatinine: levels elevated above patient's
    normal range
Glucose
Protein
See Renal failure (p. 641)

Potential Complications

Leakage, extravasation of dialysate
Hyperglycemia
Peritonitis
Bowel adhesions

Hyperosmolar coma
Perforated bladder, bowel
Hemorrhage
Respiratory conditions

MULTIDISCIPLINARY MANAGEMENT
THERAPEUTIC MANAGEMENT
Medications
  Analgesics
  Antacids
  Anticoagulants (history of thrombophlebitis only)
  Antiemetics
  Antihypertensives
  Antimicrobials
  Vitamins
  Ferrous sulfate
  Diuretics
  Calcium
Fluid restriction
Daily weight
Dietary restrictions (dietary consult)
Psychologic consult

PATIENT PROBLEMS—NURSING DIAGNOSES/INTERVENTIONS

▼Fluid volume excess related to fluid accumulation or inability of kidneys to excrete water

Monitor intake and output frequently *so abnormalities will be identified and treated*
Restrict fluid as ordered
Monitor for signs and symptoms of fluid accumulation
  Weight gain (check daily [same time, scale, and clothing] when peritoneal cavity is drained)
  Elevated BP
  Dyspnea
  Increased abdominal girth
Monitor serum blood work for abnormalities associated with the following:
  Fluid volume excess: elevated sodium, potassium, pH (electrolyte accumulation)
  Inadequate dialyzing: elevated BUN, creatinine (nitrogenous waste build-up)
  Failure of kidney to produce erythropoetin: decreased Hct (anemia may be associated with uremia)
Ensure tubing is patent *to allow fluid to drain without obstruction*
Implement and maintain accurate dialysis record *so that treatments may be evaluated, amended as needed*
  Strength of solution: 1.5%, 2.5%, or 4.25% dextrose
  Amount of solution instilled, returned
  Time dialysis cycle begins, ends
  Number of exchanges
  Medication used in dialyzing solution
  Weight before and after treatment
Assess bowel status daily; constipation may cause problem with dialysate inflow or outflow

Expected Outcomes
Weight remains stable
Abdominal girth is unchanged
BP, P, and breath sounds are within patients normal range

▼Fluid volume deficit related to dialysate with high glucose concentration over long periods

Monitor intake and output frequently *so that abnormalities with fluid balance will be identified and treated*
Replace fluid as ordered
Monitor for signs and symptoms of fluid deficit
  Weight loss (check daily [same time, scale, and clothing])
  Lowered BP
  Nausea
  Muscle cramps
Implement and maintain accurate dialysis record *so that treatments may be evaluated, amended as needed*
  Strength of solution: 1.5%, 2.5%, or 4.25% dextrose
  Amount of solution instilled, returned
  Time dialysis cycle begins, ends
  Number of exchanges
  Medication used in dialyzing solution
  Weight before and after treatment

Expected Outcomes
Intake and output are balanced
Weight is stable
Skin turgor is good

▼Risk for infection related to peritoneal dialysis catheter (peritonitis and/or infection at catheter insertion site)

Report any temperature elevation above patient's normal range to physician *for evaluation, treatment*
Monitor WBCs for elevation *(may indicate infection)*
Maintain sterile technique and institutional policy when performing dialysis exchanges and dressing changes
Collect samples of dialysate for culture and sensitivity tests if solution is turbid, bloody, or malodorous per policy
Monitor catheter insertion site for signs and symptoms of infection (e.g., erythema, edema, pain, drainage) and report to physician for evaluation/treatment

Expected Outcomes
Insertion site is clean and dry
Temperature remains within patient's normal range
Outflow dialysate is clear and without odor
Absence of signs of peritonitis: fever, abdominal pain, distention, rebound tenderness, nausea, and malaise

▼Body image disturbance related to presence of peritoneal catheter

Provide an accepting and supportive atmosphere *to maintain patient's self-esteem and promote verbalization of feelings, fears, concerns, and questions*

Explore how having peritoneal catheter has affected daily life, activities *to provide emotional support and suggest methods of problem management*

Identify positive features of patient's life *to promote feelings of self-worth*

Offer assistance from other professionals (psychologist, sexual counselor) *to assist in management of emotional changes*

Encourage communication with significant other(s) and/or members of support group *to decrease feelings of isolation*

Explain that tight pants can cause irritation at exit site and bikinis or girdles may disrupt catheter and should not be worn

Explain that there are no social limitations; patient may participate in sports not requiring direct body contact

Expected Outcomes
Seeks psychosocial support when needed
Comfortably verbalizes fears, feelings, and concerns

Additional Nursing Diagnoses to Consider
Pain, discomfort related to dialysis process
Altered nutrition related to protein loss in the dialysate
Ineffective individual/family coping related to diagnosis of chronic illness
Noncompliance to prescribed treatment regimen related to denial of chronic disease

PATIENT/FAMILY TEACHING
Explain surgical procedure for catheter placement and peritoneal dialysis procedure; encourage questions, verbalization of concerns and feelings
Explain purpose of prescribed medication regimen
Explain reasons for dietary, fluid restrictions
Teach about ordered medications: names, dosages, schedules, purposes, and side effects

DISCHARGE/HOME CARE PLANNING
Emphasize importance of ongoing outpatient care
Reinforce importance of good handwashing technique for patient and others with whom patient comes in contact; maintain aseptic technique when performing dialysis exchanges
Reinforce actions aimed at decreasing infection
 Protect catheter from damage
 Keep sterile cap, dressing in place
 Wash catheter insertion site gently with soap and water, rinse well, and pat dry
Advise patient to avoid interacting with persons who have infections (e.g., colds/flu)
Encourage patient to report any temperature increase to physician
Encourage patient to report turbid, cloudy, malodorous, bloody, or feces-stained dialysate to physician immediately

Encourage patient to report redness, pain, swelling, or drainage from catheter insertion site to physician
Reinforce importance of adhering to dietary, fluid restrictions (e.g., adequate protein, sodium restriction)
Reinforce need for rest, sleep
Encourage gradual progression of activity and participation in ADLs as tolerated
Advise patient to weigh self daily (same time, scale, and clothing); report changes in weight of 2 lb or more to home health nurse and/or physician
Instruct patient to check BP at same time each day and report changes to physician
Teach symptoms of UTI (i.e., dysuria, foul-smelling urine, temperature elevation) and encourage patient to report to physician
Advise patient to avoid taking over-the-counter medications without physician approval
Advise patient to avoid straining during bowel movements and ask physician for stool softeners, laxatives as needed

■ NEPHRECTOMY: TOTAL AND PARTIAL
Total or partial surgical removal of a kidney via a flank, transabdominal, or thoracoabdominal incision; indicated in the treatment of renal malignancy, chronic pyelonephritis, trauma, polycystic kidney disease, renal vascular disease, congenital deformity, or renal calculi, or for the purpose of donation

ASSESSMENT
SUBJECTIVE DATA (POSTOPERATIVE)
Pain

OBJECTIVE DATA (POSTOPERATIVE)
Urine output: character, amount, color
Patent drainage systems
 Ureteral catheter
 Nephrostomy tube stents
Site of incision: redness, swelling, drainage
Fever
Anxiety

DIAGNOSTIC TESTS
Blood typing, cross matching, tissue compatibility testing (done preoperatively)
Serum electrolytes: abnormal results
BUN, creatinine: elevated
Coagulation studies: abnormal clotting patterns
CBC: decreased Hct, Hgb, elevated WBC
Chest x-ray: abnormalities in lung(s): pneumonia, atelectasis
Urinalysis: WBC, RBC, sediment, bacteria
Urine culture and sensitivity
Urine creatinine clearance (24 hour): inadequate processing of waste by kidney(s)
IVP: abnormalities in kidney(s), ureter(s), bladder
Renal arteriogram: inadequate blood supply to kidney(s)

Renal venogram: inadequate venous drainage system of kidney(s)

Renal ultrasound: abnormalities in kidney(s), ureter(s), bladder

POTENTIAL COMPLICATIONS

Pneumonia
Pneumothorax
Hemorrhage/shock
Paralytic ileus
Infection

DISCHARGE/MANAGEMENT

THERAPEUTIC MANAGEMENT

Medications
    Analgesics
    Antiemetics
    Antibiotics
    Stool softeners/laxatives
    IV fluids
Nasogastric tube
NPO until bowel sounds return
Incentive spirometer
Wound, drain management
Social services

PATIENT PROBLEMS—NURSING DIAGNOSES/INTERVENTIONS

▼ Risk for fluid volume deficit related to hypovolemia or hemorrhage

Monitor intake and output frequently *so that abnormalities with fluid balance will be identified and reported*

Assess surgical dressing, tubes, stents, and catheters for patency and bleeding qh and report to physician

Monitor urinary output for evidence of excessive hematuria (urine is expected to be pink tinged not bright red)

Expected Outcomes

Intake and output are balanced
Stents, catheters are patent
Urine is pink to yellow

▼ Pain related to nephrectomy

Assess type, intensity, location, and duration of pain and document *so that changes may be noted*

Identify verbal and nonverbal responses to pain

Ensure that catheters, tubes are patent *to promote optimal drainage, prevent pressure from backflow*

Secure catheters, tubes *to prevent pulling sensation or dislodgement*

Offer analgesics, document effectiveness and tolerance *so that pharmacologic changes may be made as needed*

Institute nonpharmacologic comfort measures
    Optimal positioning

Relaxation techniques/guided imagery
Restful environment
Diversional activity
Splint incision when turning, coughing, and deep breathing

Expected Outcome

Relaxed and verbalizes increased comfort

▼ Altered urinary elimination related to nephrostomy tube, ureteral catheter, and surgical intervention

Assess patient's previous voiding pattern and begin voiding diary *to document changes*

Monitor for signs and symptoms of UTI (e.g., dysuria, frequency, urgency) and report to physician for evaluation and treatment

Maintain patency of catheters *to promote optimal flow of urine*
    Tubing below level of bladder to allow for gravity flow
    Assess for clamping, kinks in tubing
    Secure catheters while still allowing for patient movement
    Irrigate tubes cautiously, using small volume and only when ordered *to prevent damage*

Label each tube clearly and record drainage from each tube separately *to allow for accurate assessment of output from each system*

If nephrostomy tube is in place
    Tape to flank
    Do not clamp
    Irrigate only with physician's order (may be continuous or intermittent)
    Have extra tube available at bedside *for emergency use if tube is dislodged*
    Notify physician immediately if nephrostomy tube becomes dislodged

After urinary bladder catheter is removed, institute measures to facilitate voiding
    Privacy
    Comfortable positioning
    Running tap water
    Placing patient's hand in warm water
    Applying heat to suprapubic area (if ordered)
    Pouring warm water over perineum
    Relaxation techniques
    Applying oil of peppermint (a few drops in bedpan/urinal or on cotton ball in front of urinary meatus)
    Stroking inner aspect of thigh gently with ice
    Offering analgesic
    Voiding 1 to 2 hours after fluid intake
    Double voiding (to empty bladder more completely)

Encourage patient to drink at least 2500 ml/day (unless contraindicated) to promote adequate output

Expected Outcomes

Intake and output are balanced
Regular voiding pattern is established

▼Risk for infection related to surgical incision/ presence of tubes, catheters

Assess incision q4h for presence of erythema, edema, tenderness, and drainage; document findings *so that changes may be identified and treated*

Report signs and symptoms of infection (fever, chills) to physician *so that appropriate interventions may be implemented*

Obtain wound culture as ordered *to identify bacteria*

Monitor for elevation of WBC, *indicates presence of infection*

Administer and monitor tolerance of ordered antibiotics

Expected Outcome
Incision is intact and dry

▼Dysfunctional grieving related to loss of body organ

Provide an accepting and supportive atmosphere *to maintain patient's self-esteem and promote verbalization of feelings, fears, concerns, and questions*

Explore how losing a kidney (or part) or donating kidney for transplantation has affected patient and patient's family

Identify positive features of patient's life *to promote feelings of self-worth*

Offer assistance from other professionals (psychologist, clergy, sexual counselor) *to assist with management of emotional changes*

Encourage communication with significant other(s) and/or members of support group *to decrease feelings of isolation*

Expected Outcomes
Seeks psychosocial support when needed
Comfortably verbalizes fears, feelings, and concerns and uses effective coping measures

Additional Nursing Diagnoses to Consider
Ineffective breathing patterns (postoperatively) related to effects of anesthesia

Altered tissue perfusion: peripheral, cardiopulmonary, and GI related to postoperative complications

Ineffective individual/family coping related to surgical removal of major body organ

PATIENT/FAMILY TEACHING
Explain surgical procedure; encourage questions, verbalization of concerns and feelings

Explain purpose of prescribed medical/surgical regimen

Explain reasons for dietary, fluid restrictions

Explain importance of turning, coughing, and deep breathing q2h; instruct in use of incentive spirometer and splinting postoperatively

Teach about ordered medications: names, dosages, schedules, purposes, and side effects

DISCHARGE/HOME CARE PLANNING
Emphasize importance of ongoing outpatient care

Reinforce importance of good handwashing technique for patient and others with whom patient comes in contact

Advise patient to avoid interacting with persons who have infections (e.g., colds, influenza)

Reinforce need for rest, sleep

Encourage gradual progression of activity and participation in ADLs as tolerated; no heavy lifting until approved by physician

Advise patient to avoid activities (e.g., contact sports) that may endanger remaining kidney

Advise patient to alert other health professionals of presence of nephrostomy or ureteral catheter and history of nephrectomy

Encourage patient to report fever > 101° F (38.5° C) to physician

Reinforce method of caring for incision, dressing, tubes, and drains (refer to home health agency as needed)

Encourage patient to report to physician redness, pain, swelling, or drainage from incisional site

Instruct patient to institute measures to prevent UTI (see p. 607)

Teach symptoms of UTI (dysuria, foul-smelling urine, fever > 101° F [38.5° C]) and encourage patient to report to physician

Advise patient to avoid taking over-the-counter medications without physician approval

Advise patient to avoid straining during bowel movements and ask physician for stool softeners, laxatives as needed

■ RENAL TRANSPLANTATION*

A functioning kidney is removed from a living donor or a human cadaver and is transplanted into the right or left iliac fossa of the recipient; the renal blood vessels of the donor organ are anastomosed to the recipient's iliac artery and vein, and the ureter is transplanted into the bladder or anastomosed to the recipient's ureter to establish urinary tract continuity (Fig. 10-25)

ASSESSMENT
SUBJECTIVE DATA (POSTOPERATIVE)
Pain
Anxiety
Depression

OBJECTIVE DATA (POSTOPERATIVE)
Rejection of kidney (Table 10-5)
Decreased urinary output
Hematuria
Decreased/diminished breath sounds
Tachypnea
Tachycardia
Hemorrhage

---

*See Nephrectomy (p. 651) for care of donor

Table 10-5	Classification of Rejection		
Hyperacute	**Acute**	**Chronic**	
Rejection occurs as soon as new kidney is implanted	Rejection occurs 1 wk to 3 mo after kidney has been implanted	Rejection occurs at any time after surgery	
Rejection is caused by presence of antibodies in recipient that cause polymorphonuclear leukocytes to clot, thus blocking glomerular and peritubular capillaries	Immune response leukocytes and RBCs invade vascular endothelium and intertubular vasculature; renal blood flow is decreased; therefore necrosis of renal tubules occurs	There is gradual decline in kidney function; glomerular filtration is decreased, and serum creatinine and serum urea nitrogen are elevated; proteinuria occurs, and sodium is decreased in urine	
Rejection is usually irreversible	Rejection may be reversible	Early detection and treatment may decrease decline in kidney function	
Transplanted kidney is removed immediately	Attempt is made to save new kidney	Attempt is made to save kidney	
Patient resumes hemodialysis	Patient may need to resume dialysis treatments	Patient may need to resume dialysis treatments	

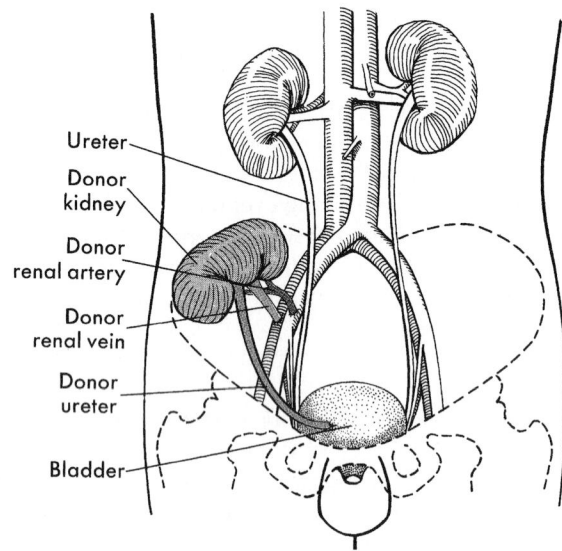

Fig. 10-25 Location of transplanted kidney showing anastomosis of renal artery, renal vein, and ureter.
(From Phipps WJ et al: Medical-surgical nursing: concepts and clinical practice, *ed 6, St Louis, 1999, Mosby.)*

Diagnostic Tests
See Renal Failure, p. 641
Blood typing, cross matching, tissue histocompatibility testing (done preoperatively)
Chest x-ray: abnormalities in lung(s); pneumonia, atelectasis
ECG: dysrhythmias

Potential Complications
Rejection
Acute tubular necrosis
Spontaneous rupture of graft
Ureteral fistula, obstruction
Renal artery stenosis or thrombosis
Perirenal hematoma
Infection
Shock
Paralytic ileus
Diabetes
Cushing's syndrome
GI bleeding
Glaucoma
Reappearance of primary renal disease

Multidisciplinary Management
Therapeutic Management
Medications
    Immunosuppressive agents (cyclosporine, azathioprine)
    Corticosteroids
    Analgesics
    Antacids
    H_2 Blockers
    Antiemetics
    Antibiotics
    Insulin (may be needed if high-dosage steroids used)
    Stool softeners, laxatives
    IV fluids
NPO until bowel sounds return
Incentive spirometer
Wound, drain management
Hemodialysis
Dietitian consultation
Psychologic consult, social services

Patient Problems—Nursing Diagnoses/Interventions

▼ Risk for fluid volume excess or deficit related to postoperative diuresis, changes in renal perfusion

Monitor intake and output frequently *so that abnormalities with fluid balance will be identified and reported*

Weigh patient daily (same time, scale, and clothing) *to ensure accurate and reliable results*

Monitor for signs and symptoms related to fluid balance changes

> Change in skin turgor, mucous membranes
> Change in CVP
> Abnormal serum electrolytes

Restrict/administer fluids as ordered; monitor and document patient response to therapy

Monitor for signs of organ rejection

> Decreased urine output
> Fever
> Anxiety, apathy
> Weight gain
> Proteinuria
> Hypertension

Expected Outcomes

Vital signs and weight are stable and within patient's normal range

Skin turgor is good

There are no signs of rejection

▼ Pain related to surgical incision and bladder spasm

Assess type, intensity, location, and duration of pain and document *so that changes may be noted*

Identify verbal and nonverbal responses to pain

Ensure that catheters, tubes are patent *to promote optimal drainage, prevent pressure from backflow*

Secure catheters, tubes *to prevent pulling sensation*

Offer analgesics, documenting effectiveness and tolerance *so that pharmacologic changes may be made as needed*

Institute nonpharmacologic comfort measures

> Optimal positioning
> Relaxation techniques/guided imagery
> Restful environment
> Diversional activity
> Splint incision when turning, coughing, and deep breathing

Expected Outcome

Relaxed and verbalizes increased comfort

▼ Risk for infection related to immunosuppression, incision, or presence of drains and catheters

Assess incision (transplant site) for presence of erythema, edema, tenderness, and drainage; document findings *so that changes may be identified and treated*

Report signs and symptoms of infection (e.g., fever, chills) to physician *so that appropriate interventions may be implemented*

Obtain wound culture, as ordered, *to identify bacteria*

Obtain urine culture if urine is cloudy or malodorous *to identify bacteria*

Monitor for elevation of WBC, *which indicates presence of infection*

Monitor for decrease in WBC, *which indicates immunosuppressive response*

Administer and monitor tolerance of ordered antibiotics

Expected Outcomes

Patient is afebrile

Incision is clean and dry

WBCs are within normal range for patient

▼ Altered urinary elimination related to renal transplantation

Assess patient's previous voiding pattern and begin voiding diary *to note changes*

Urine may be blood tinged in immediate postoperative period; determine whether irrigation may be performed if needed *to dislodge clots*

Monitor for signs and symptoms of UTI (dysuria, frequency, urgency) and report to physician *for evaluation and treatment*

Maintain patency of catheters *to promote optimal flow of urine*

> Tubing below level of bladder to allow for gravity flow
> Assess for clamping, kinks in tubing
> Secure catheters while still allowing for patient movement
> Irrigate tubes as ordered

Label each tube or catheter clearly and record drainage from each tube separately *to accurately assess output from each system*

Monitor for and report abdominal, bladder distention *to prevent tension on anastomosis*

After urinary catheter is removed, encourage patient to void q1h to 2h *to decrease bladder distention and tension on anastomosis*

Institute measures to facilitate voiding

> Privacy
> Comfortable positioning
> Running tap water
> Placing patient's hand in warm water
> Applying heat to suprapubic area (if ordered)
> Pouring warm water over perineum
> Relaxation techniques
> Applying oil of peppermint (a few drops in bedpan/urinal or on cotton ball in front of urinary meatus)
> Stroking inner aspect of thigh gently with ice
> Offering analgesic
> Voiding 1 to 2 hours after fluid intake
> Double voiding (to empty bladder more completely)

Encourage patient to drink up to 2500 ml/day (unless contraindicated) *to promote adequate output*

Expected Outcomes

Intake and output are balanced

Regular voiding pattern is established

▼Body image disturbance related to new organ

Provide an accepting and supportive atmosphere *to maintain patient's self-esteem and promote verbalization of feelings, fears, concerns, and questions*

Explore how receiving a new kidney and concern for donor have affected patient and patient's family

Explain side effects of immunosuppressants that may cause appearance changes

Identify positive features of patient's life *to promote feelings of self-worth*

Offer assistance from other professionals (psychologist, clergy, sexual counselor) and kidney recipients *to assist in management of emotional changes*

Encourage communication with significant other(s) and/or members of support group *to decrease feelings of isolation*

Expected Outcomes
Seeks psychosocial support as needed
Comfortably verbalizes fears, feelings, and concerns

Additional Nursing Diagnoses to Consider
Ineffective breathing patterns (postoperatively) related to anesthesia

Noncompliance to prescribed treatment plan related to change in condition

Ineffective individual/family coping related to surgical placement of major body organ

PATIENT/FAMILY TEACHING
Explain surgical procedure; encourage questions, verbalization of concerns and feelings

Demonstrate appropriate handwashing technique

Explain reasons for dietary, fluid restrictions

Explain importance of restricting visitors to avoid exposure to infections

Explain importance of turning, coughing, and deep breathing regularly; instruct in use of incentive spirometer and splinting

Explain importance of early ambulation, activity

Teach about ordered medications: names, dosages, schedules, purposes, and side effects

DISCHARGE/HOME CARE PLANNING
Emphasize importance of ongoing outpatient care

Reinforce importance of good handwashing technique for patient and others with whom patient comes in contact

Advise patient to avoid interacting with persons who have infections (e.g., colds, flu)

Reinforce need for rest, sleep

Encourage patient to report signs and symptoms of rejection to physician
  Redness, swelling, tenderness over transplant site
  Fever
  Decreased urinary output
  Edema
  Emotional, mental status changes

Provide written information about potential side effects of immunosuppressive medications and encourage patient to report to physician difficulties in tolerating medication

Encourage patient to wear medical alert/identification bracelet

Advise patient to check BP at same time each day and report changes to physician

Advise patient to weigh self daily (same time, scale, and clothing); report change of 2 lb or more to physician

Encourage gradual progression of activity and participation in ADLs as tolerated; restrict lifting and driving as advised by physician

Advise patient to avoid activities (e.g., contact sports) that may endanger new and remaining kidney

Advise patient to alert other health professionals (e.g., dentist) of presence of new kidney

Reinforce need to comply with dietary, fluid restrictions (e.g., avoiding alcoholic beverages unless approved by physician)

Advise patient to consult with physician regarding resumption of sexual activity, contraception methods

Encourage patient to report fever > 101° F (38.5° C) to physician

Reinforce method of caring for incision, dressing, catheters, and drains (refer to home health agency as needed)

Encourage patient to report to physician redness, pain, swelling, or drainage from incisional site

Instruct patient to institute measures to prevent UTI (see p. 607)

Explain reasons for and importance of having blood drawn as ordered

Encourage eye examinations every 6 months to assess for visual changes; routine physical examination and laboratory follow-up

Teach symptoms of UTI (dysuria, foul-smelling urine, fever > 101° F [38.5° C]) and encourage patient to report to physician

Advise patient to avoid taking over-the-counter medications without physician approval

Advise patient to avoid straining during bowel movements and ask physician for stool softeners/laxatives as needed

BIBLIOGRAPHY
Ackley BJ, Ladwig GB: *Nursing diagnosis handbook: a guide to planning care,* ed 3, St Louis, 1997, Mosby.

Beare PG, Myers JL: *Adult health nursing,* ed 3, St Louis, 1998, Mosby.

Brundage DJ: *Mosby's clinical nursing series: renal disorders,* St Louis, 1992, Mosby.

Gray M: *Mosby's clinical nursing series: genitourinary disorders,* St Louis, 1992, Mosby.

Kim MJ et al: *Pocket guide to nursing diagnoses,* ed 7, St Louis, 1997, Mosby.

Kelly M: Acute renal failure, *Am J Nurs* 97(3):32, 1997.

Lancaster LE: *Core curriculum for nephrology nursing,* ed 3, Pitman, NJ, 1995, American Nephrology Nurses Association.

Marchiondo K: A new look at urinary tract infection, *Am J Nurs* 98(3):34, 1998.

McCance KL, Huether SE: *Pathophysiology: the biological basis for disease in adults and children,* ed 3, St Louis, 1998, Mosby.

McFarland GK, McFarlane EA: *Nursing diagnosis and intervention planning for patient care,* ed 2, St Louis, 1993, Mosby.

Pagana KD, Pagana TJ: *Mosby's diagnostic and laboratory test reference,* ed 3, St Louis, 1998, Mosby.

Peterson KJ, Solie CJ: Interpreting lab values in chronic renal insufficiency, *Am J Nurs* 5:56B, 1994.

Resnick B: Retraining the bladder after catheterization, *Am J Nurs* 11:46, 1993.

Ruth-Sand L: Renal calculi, *Am J Nurs* 95(11):50, 1995.

Scheck DN, Pappas PG: Lower urinary tract infections in women: a pragmatic approach, *Hosp Med* May, 48, 1993.

Schreier RW: *Renal and electrolyte disorders,* ed 5, Boston, 1997, Little Brown.

Sosa-Guerrero S, Gomez NJ: Dealing with end-stage renal disease, *Am J Nurs* 97(10):44, 1997.

Swearingen PL, Ross DG: *Manual of medical-surgical nursing care: nursing interventions and collaborative management,* ed 4, St Louis, 1999, Mosby.

Tanagho E, McAninch J: *Smith's general urology,* ed 14, Los Altos, Calif, 1994, Lange Medical Publications.

Thayer D: How to assess and control urinary incontinence, *Am J Nurs* 10:42, 1994.

US Department of Health and Human Services: Benign prostatic hyperplasia: diagnosis and treatment, pub no 94-0582, Rockville, Md, 1994, US Government Printing Office.

US Department of Health and Human Services: Urinary incontinence in adults, pub no 92-0040, Rockville, Md, 1992, US Government Printing Office.

Willis D: Taming the overgrown prostate, *Am J Nurs* 2:4, 1992.

BARNES
CARE PATH
750 CYSTECTOMY WITH NEOPLASM

①

SERVICE		PHYSICIAN	
PRIMARY NURSE		PRIMARY NURSE	
DC DATE	ADM DATE	DATE OF SURGERY	A-8

PROBLEM NUMBER	PATIENT PROBLEMS / NURSING DIAGNOSES
#1	ALT. IN URINARY ELIMINATION R/T
#2	LACK OF KNOWLEDGE R/T
#3	ALT. IN COMFORT R/T

PROB. NO.		ADM. DAY 1	DAY 2 DOS	DAY 3 POD 1 OU	DAY 4 POD 2 OU	DAY 5 POD 3 OU	DAY 6 POD 4 OU	DAY 7 POD 5
#1 **#2**	**ASSESSMENT/MONITORING**	Adm. work-up	Freq Postop VS;	VS q̄ 4 ×1 ×2 ×3 ×4 ×5 ×6 drsg; NG Stoma viability Stent position Urine output ≥30 cc/hr Monitor labs Pain control Lung sounds Bowel sounds	VS q̄ 4 ×1 ×2 ×3 ×4 ×5 ×6 Stoma viability Stent position Urine output ≥30 cc/hr Monitor labs Pain control Lung sounds Bowel sounds	VS q̄ 4 ×1 ×2 ×3 ×4 ×5 ×6 Stoma viability Stent position Urine output ≥30 cc/hr Monitor labs Pain control Lung sounds Bowel sounds	VS q̄ 4 ×1 ×2 ×3 ×4 ×5 ×6 Stoma viability Stent position Urine output ≥30 cc/hr Monitor labs Pain control Lung sounds Bowel sounds **Hemodynamically stable**	VS q̄ shift ×1 ×2 ×3 Wound open to air Staples intact Stoma viability Stent position Urine output ≥30 cc/hr Monitor labs Pain control Lung sounds Bowel sounds
#2	**CONSULTS**	Surg. CNS	Social Work	Home Health				
#1 **#3**	**PROCEDURE/TEST**	Adm. Labs UA with Micro Urine C & S CXR ECG Mark stoma placement Type & Cross 4 units PRBC	Irrigate NG tube q̄ 4° ×1 ×2 ×3 ×4 ×5 ×6 Check pH CBC, 6 in PAR Check NG pH q̄ 4° ×1 ×2 ×3 ×4 ×5 ×6	CBC, 6 Pulse Oximetry ×1			DC NG tube	IVP Prep
#1 **#3**	**TREATMENT**	Weight TWE till clear. Betadine scrub Measure/order TEDS	TEDS sequential stocking IS / TCDB q̄ 2 ° ×1 ×2 ×3 ×4 ×5 ×6 ×7 ×8 ×9 ×10 ×11 ×12 O₂	D/C sequential TEDS IS/TCDB q̄ 2 ° ×1 ×2 ×3 ×4 ×5 ×6 ×7 ×8 ×9 ×10 ×11 ×12 Weight D/C O₂ Ted Hose	IS / TCDB q̄ 2 ° ×1 ×2 ×3 ×4 ×5 ×6 ×7 ×8 ×9 ×10 ×11 ×12 Weight Ted Hose	**No atelectasis** Using IS independently Ted Hose	Using IS independently Ted Hose	Using IS independently Ted Hose
#3	**ACTIVITY**	UP AD LIB	Bed rest	Up with assist Chair/amb TID ×1 ×2 ×3 Bed bath	Up with assist Chair/amb TID ×1 ×2 ×3 Assist bed bath	Increase amb QID ×1 ×2 ×3 ×4 Assist bath	Amb QID ×1 ×2 ×3 ×4 Assist bath	Amb QID ×1 ×2 ×3 ×4 Assist bath

BARNES

CARE PATH
750 CYSTECTOMY WITH NEOPLASM

②

CNS	DIETARY	RT
HOME HEALTH	OT	OTHER
PT	SW	OTHER

A-8

PROBLEM NUMBER	PATIENT PROBLEMS / NURSING DIAGNOSES

DAY 8 POD 6	DAY 9 POD 7	DAY 10 POD 8	DAY 11 POD 9	POST DC	DC OUTCOMES
VS q̄ shift ×1 ×2 ×3 Wound open to air Staples intact Stoma viability Stent position Urine output ≥30 cc/hr Monitor labs Pain control Lung sounds Bowel sounds	VS q̄ shift ×1 ×2 × Wound open to air Staples intact Stoma viability Stent position Urine output ≥30 cc/hr Monitor labs Pain control Lung sounds Bowel sounds	VS q̄ shift ×1 ×2 ×3 Wound open to air Staples intact Stoma viability Stent position Urine output ≥30 cc/hr Monitor labs Pain control Lung sounds Bowel sounds **No leaking, skin problems with ostomy equipment** **U.O. = ³ prior to stent removal**	VS q̄ shift ×1 ×2 ×3 Wound open to air Staples intact Stoma viability Stent position Urine output ≥30 cc/hr Monitor labs Pain control Lung sounds Bowel sounds		**Afebrile: VSS** **Stoma Viable** **U. O. = ³ than before stent removal** **Wound intact** **Lungs clear** **Labs WNL** **Hemodynamically stable**
					DC with MD/clinic/f/u in 2 weeks home health ref. form completed
DC Urinary stent Modified IVP					
Using IS independently	**Using IS at 90 - 100% of preop level**				**No pulmonary complications** **Loop functioning** **Weight stable** **No thrombophlebitis**
Ted Hose	Ted Hose	Ted Hose	Ted Hose	Ted Hose	
Amb QID ×1 ×2 ×3 ×4 Independent personal hygiene	UP AD LIB	UP AD LIB	**Amb independently**		**As before adm with restrictions involving limited exertional activity**

Continued

(3)

		ADM. DAY 1	DAY 2	DAY 3	DAY 4	DAY 5	DAY 6	DAY 7
#1	MEDS/IVS	IVF Bowel Prep	IVF IV Antibiotics H$_2$ antagonist IV PCA IV Antacid per NG tube	IVF IV Antibiotics H$_2$ antagonist IV PCA IV Antacid per NG tube	IVF IV Antibiotics H$_2$ antagonist IV PCA IV Antacid per NG tube	IVF IV Antibiotics H$_2$ antagonist IV PCA IV Antacid per NG tube	IVF IV Antibiotics H$_2$ antagonist IV DC PCA; oral analgesic DC antacid	IVF IV Antibiotics DC H$_2$ antagonist PO analgesia
#1	NUTRITION	Clear liquid NPO after MN	NPO	NPO	NPO	NPO	Clear liq.	Clear liq.
#1 #2	PATIENT/FAMILY EDUCATION	Preop: IS, Activity Postop goals Intro Ostomy booklet Plan of Care Primary Nsg.	Postop orders, plan of care, pain control Explain ostomy teaching plan	Ostomy Teaching booklet	Demonstrate pouch/valve & connector		Review pouch chg. with pt. Assist pt with flange & pouch chg. Review teaching booklet	Review teaching booklet. Review ostomy/skin care, pouch, flange change. Instruct pt on IVP procedure
#1 #2	DISCHARGE PLANNING	**Pt / family verbalizes understanding of care path.** **Plan of care has been mutually set with pt/ family.**			SW: initial interview regarding: living situation, support systems, resource needs		CNS, SW, HH review DC plan	
#1 #2	PSYCHOSOCIAL / EMOTIONAL NEEDS	Nursing: initial assessment Identify support person(s)	Nursing: Therapeutic emotional care	Nursing: Therapeutic emotional care	SW: initiate support. Assess counseling needs. Provide emotional support	Nursing/SW: Provide emotional support	Nursing / SW: Provide emotional support	Nursing / SW: Provide emotional support
	SIGNATURES							

750

3100-51

	DAY 8	DAY 9	DAY 10	DAY 11	POST DC	DC OUTCOMES
	Heplock IVF PO antibiotics PO analgesia	Heplock IVF PO antibiotics PO analgesia	Heplock IVF PO antibiotics PO analgesia	DC Heplock PO antibiotics PO analgesia	 PO antibiotics PO analgesia	**Pain controlled with oral analgesics** **No gastric distress** **No UTI**
	Full liq.	Soft	Reg prior	Reg as before adm.	Reg as before adm.	**Tolerating diet as before adm.**
	Review night drainage system	Reinforce ostomy education Encourage independence with ostomy care	Pt assist with flange, pouch change. Review home needs. Review community resources available. Instruct on wound care Instruct S/S VTI.	Review disch. needs, Review ostomy care, Review how to order supplies.		**Able to verbalize/demonstrate:** **Use of valve, Application/ removal of pouch/flange.** **Night drainage system** **stoma skin care** **S/S wound infection** **S/S UTI**
	HH: Assess home needs (Barnes) outside home health referral initiated by SW		SW/HH/nursing Finalize DC plans outside home health referral initiated by SW	HH: visit pt to explain services (Barnes) Nursing: inventory ostomy supplies with pt SW/HH/Nursing/MD: plans finalized pt discharged		**Home with appropriate level of care** **HH visit scheduled for next day**
	Nursing/SW: Provide emotional support	Pt able to verbalize, identify lifestyle changes				**Identifies support systems & resources.** **Is able to look at stoma**

3100-51

Female Reproductive System/Women's Health

■ FEMALE REPRODUCTIVE SYSTEM ASSESSMENT

▌ SUBJECTIVE DATA

Lower abdominal pain
Cramps
Bloating
Pressure
Vaginal bleeding: color, amount, and consistency
   Clots
   Spotting
Vaginal discharge
   Mucoid
   Thick, white
   Frothy, watery, yellow-green
   Thick, yellow-green or brown, and bloody
   Yellow
   Gray or green
   Odoriferous
   Duration
Itching
Swelling
Redness
Rash
Painful intercourse
Changes in mood
Fatigue
Urination
   Color and odor
   Stress incontinence
   Burning on urination
   Pain, urgency, or frequency
   Nocturia
Breasts
   Tenderness
   Pain
   Stinging sensation
   Burning

▌ OBJECTIVE DATA

General appearance (Figs. 11-1 and 11-2)
Vital signs, weight
Breasts
   Size

   Symmetry
   Contour
   Lesions
   Lumps, bumps
   "Orange peel" texture
   Venous pattern
   Moles, nevi
   Dimpling or skin retraction
   Fixation, nonmobile
   Erythema
Nipples
   Color
   Discharge (serous, bloody, purulent)
   Inversion
Abdomen
   Contour
   Lesions
   Scars
   Stretch marks
   Symmetry
   Visible pulsations
   Visible peristaltic waves
   Presence of bowel sounds in each quadrant
External genitalia
   Pubic hair
      Hair distribution
      Lice, nits
   Labia majora/minora
      Edema
      Redness
      Leukoplakia
      Lumps
      Lesions, lacerations
      Symmetry
      Pigmentation (nevi)
   Clitoris
      Edema
      Redness
      Adhesions, lesions
   Urethral orifice
      Size
      Redness
      Discharge
   Discharge
      Bloody

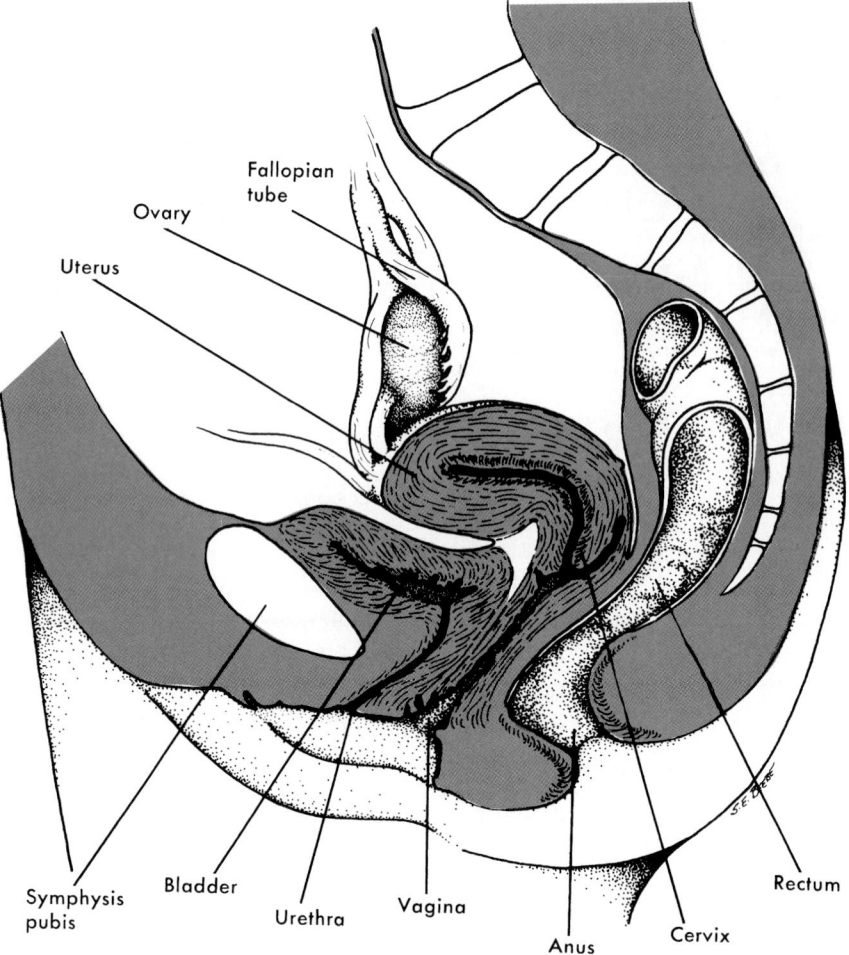

Fig. 11-1 Female reproductive system.

Purulent
Odoriferous
Introitus (vaginal orifice)
  Presence or absence of hymenal ring
  Hymenal tags
  Cystocele, rectocele, enterocele
  Uterine prolapse
  Vaginal prolapse
  Edema
  Redness
  Drainage
    Mucoid (normal)
    Thick, white, cheesy (typical of moniliasis)
    Purulent
    Frothy, watery, yellow-green (typical of
      trichomoniasis)
    Thick, yellow-green or brown, and bloody (typical
      of upper genital tract infection)
    Bloody
    Yellow: thin with odor
    Gray or green
  Perineum
    Scars

Redness
Edema
Excoriation

■ PERTINENT BACKGROUND INFORMATION

CONCURRENT DISEASES OR CONDITIONS

Menstrual cycle
  Age at onset
  Length of cycles (duration)
  Interval between cycles
  Regularity of cycles
  Duration, amount, type of flow
    Number of tampons or napkins used
    Date of most recent douching
  Date of last menstrual period (LMP)
  Associated symptoms (pain, menorrhagia,
    metrorrhagia, breast symptoms)
Pregnancy
  Number of pregnancies and outcome of each
  Complications of pregnancy and delivery and/or
    abortion

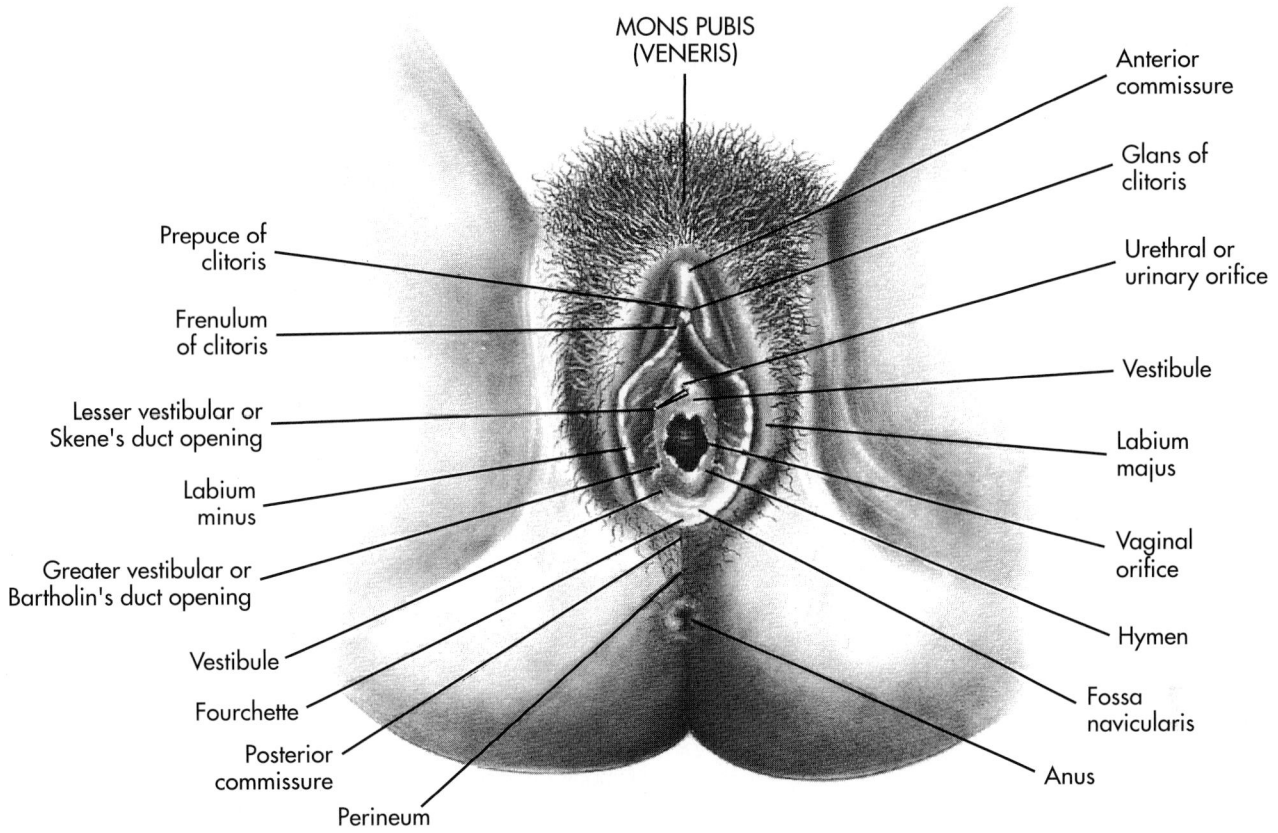

MONS PUBIS
(VENERIS)

Anterior
commissure

Glans of
clitoris

Prepuce of
clitoris

Urethral or
urinary orifice

Frenulum
of clitoris

Vestibule

Lesser vestibular or
Skene's duct opening

Labium
majus

Labium
minus

Greater vestibular or
Bartholin's duct opening

Vaginal
orifice

Vestibule

Hymen

Fourchette

Fossa
navicularis

Posterior
commissure

Anus

Perineum

Fig. 11-2 External female genitalia.
(From Lowdermilk DL, Perry SE, Bobak IM: Maternity and women's health care, *ed 6, St Louis, 1997, Mosby.)*

Lactation history
 Number of infants breast fed
 Duration of breast feeding
 Lactation suppressant medications
Contraceptive history
 Type of method used
 Duration
 Effectiveness
 Side effects
Menopause
 When occurred
 Related symptoms
  Hot flashes, night sweats
  Dry vaginal mucosa
  Insomnia
 (See Gerontologic Considerations box)
Nutrition
 Appetite
 Supplements
 Recent weight gain/loss
Gastrointestinal (GI) system
 Constipation
 Hemorrhoids
Endocrine system
 Hypothyroidism
 Hyperthyroidism
 Stein-Leventhal syndrome
 Cushing's syndrome

Blood dyscrasia
Hypertension
Acquired immunodeficiency syndrome (AIDS)
Sexually transmitted diseases

PREVIOUS SURGERY OR ILLNESS

Gynecologic surgery
Breast surgery
Other major surgery or illness (of abdomen, endocrine
 system)
Sexually transmitted diseases (STDs)
Pelvic inflammatory disease (PID)
Vaginal infections

FAMILY HISTORY

Cancer (ovarian, breast, colon)
Sickle cell disease
Thyroid disorder
Diabetes
Multiple pregnancies
Congenital anomalies
Death resulting from gynecologic-related
 conditions
Maternal diethylstilbestrol (DES) usage

Gerontologic Considerations

- The benefits of hormone replacement therapy should be explored with the woman.
- Many older women are reluctant to seek medical care for problems of the reproductive system. This may be related to cultural factors, embarrassment, or lack of knowledge. Routine gynecologic examination should continue as part of the physical examination even after menopause.
- Certain forms of cancer of the reproductive tract are more common with aging. Any vaginal bleeding should be reported to the physician promptly, as should pelvic pain, pruritus, or skin lesions in the genital region.
- Decreased level of estrogen with aging and systemic disease such as diabetes predispose older women to vaginitis.
- The use of water-soluble lubricant gels can contribute to continued enjoyment of sexual activity. In addition, intercourse on a regular basis can increase the woman's natural secretions.
- Because of earlier deaths in men, a female spouse may date and have sexual relationships with male partners, especially in closed (retirement) communities. Encourage the practice of "safe" sex because sexually transmitted diseases (STDs), including human immunodeficiency virus (HIV) infection, can occur as a result of unprotected sex.
- Breast cancer risk increases for women older than 40 years of age. Breast examination should continue throughout the lifespan. The American Cancer Society recommends an annual mammogram for women over age 50.

Modified from Christensen BL, Kockrow EO: Foundations of nursing, *ed 3, St Louis, 1998, Mosby.*

SOCIAL HISTORY

Sexual activity: number of partners, current relationship, abnormal lesions or discharge in sexual partner, condom use
Contraception
Sexual abuse
Domestic violence/abuse
Douching habits
Clothing habits (cotton or nonventilated underwear)
Patterns of tobacco, alcohol, and prescription/nonprescription drug use
Occupational hazards, radiation, toxins

MEDICATION HISTORY

Oral contraceptives
Hormonal/estrogen replacement therapy
Phenothiazines
Digitalis
Diuretics
Medical management medications

◼ DIAGNOSTIC TESTS

Bimanual examination
Basal body temperature (T)

Cervical mucus testing (Billing's method)
Papanicolaou (Pap) test
Wet mount
Culture
Computed tomography (CT) scan
Magnetic resonance imaging (MRI)
Breast biopsy and aspiration
Cervical biopsy
Endobiopsy
Dilation and curettage (D & C)
Cervical conization (cone biopsy)
Colposcopy
Hysteroscopy
Culdoscopy
Culpotomy
Endoscopy
Laparoscopy
Ultrasound
Insufflation
Mammography
Thermography
Radionuclide imaging
Galactography
Hysterography
Hysterosalpingography
Bone densitometry
Bone scan

LABORATORY STUDIES

Human chorionic gonadotropin (HCG) level
Serum testosterone/dehydroepiandrosterone sulfate (DHEAS)
Estradiol
Progesterone
Serum luteinizing hormone (LH) and follicle-stimulating hormone level (FSH)
Complete blood count (CBC)
CA125
Thyroid function studies
    Thyroid stimulating hormone (TSH)
    Basal metabolic rate (BMR)
    Protein-bound iodine (PBI) level
    T_3 and T_4
Adrenal function
    17-Ketosteroids
    Corticosteroids
Venereal Disease Research Laboratory (VDRL) test

◼ PELVIC INFLAMMATORY DISEASE

An infectious process of the pelvic cavity that may include the fallopian tubes, ovaries, pelvic peritoneum, veins, and pelvic connective tissue (Figs. 11-3 and 11-4)

ASSESSMENT
SUBJECTIVE DATA
Abdominal and pelvic pain
Low back pain

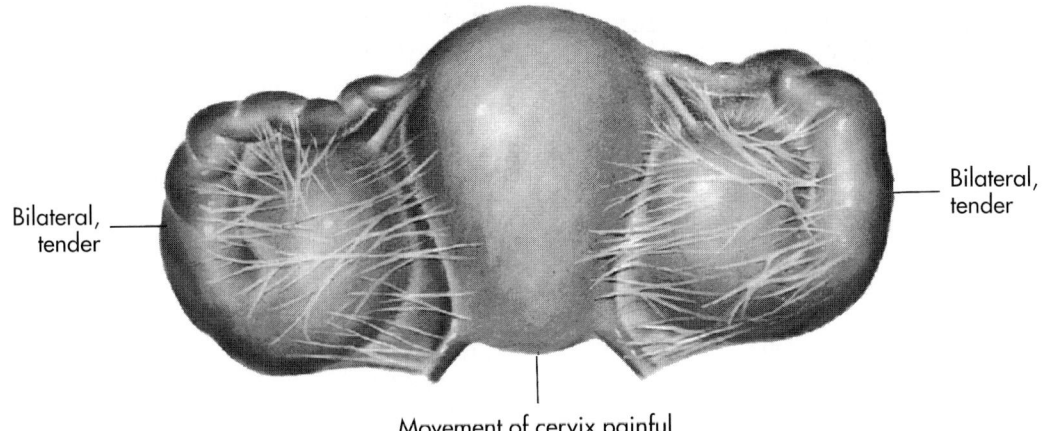

Fig. 11-3 Pelvic inflammatory disease.
(From Seidel HM et al: Mosby's guide to physical examination, *ed 4, St Louis, 1999, Mosby.)*

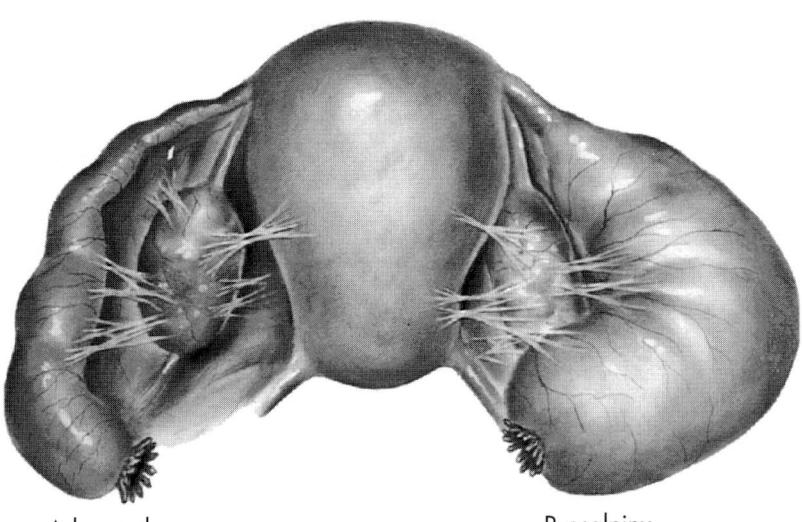

Fig. 11-4 Salpingitis.
(From Seidel HM et al: Mosby's guide to physical examination, *ed 4, St Louis, 1999, Mosby.)*

Dyspareunia (painful intercourse)
Malodorous, purulent vaginal discharge
Malaise, general aching, chills

OBJECTIVE DATA
Fever
Nausea, vomiting
Pruritus or maceration of vulva
Diarrhea
Bloating
Rebound and guarding

DIAGNOSTIC TESTS
Elevated white blood cell count (WBC)
Elevated erythrocyte sedimentation rate
Culture of purulent secretions positive for organisms
Laparoscopic visualization of pelvic inflammation
Ultrasound of tuboovarian abscess, if present
Needle culdocentesis for WBCs or nonclotting blood

POTENTIAL COMPLICATIONS
Urinary tract infection (UTI)
Peritonitis
Tuboovarian abscess
Infertility
Ectopic pregnancy
Paralytic ileus

MULTIDISCIPLINARY MANAGEMENT
THERAPEUTIC MANAGEMENT
Antibiotics as determined by sensitivity
Bed rest in semi-Fowler's position or position of
    comfort
Parenteral fluids
Nasogastric suctioning if ileus is present
Removal of intrauterine device if present
Removal of tampon if present
Analgesics

PATIENT PROBLEMS—NURSING DIAGNOSES/INTERVENTIONS

▼ Pain related to pelvic inflammation and protective guarding

Maintain complete bed rest in semi-Fowler's position or position of comfort *to reduce movement, which can increase the sensation of pain*

Administer analgesics as needed

Increase activity as tolerated

Expected Outcome
States that pain is relieved

▼ Risk for impaired skin integrity secondary to vaginal drainage

Assist and teach patient to perform gentle perineal care q3h to 4h and prn; blot skin dry (avoid rubbing) *to prevent excoriation*

Teach patient to wipe from front to back after elimination *to prevent urethral contamination*

Ensure that bed covers do not result in excessive warmth of perineal area

Explain rationale for wearing cotton underwear

Expected Outcome
Skin integrity is maintained as evidenced by absence of excoriation of perineal area

PATIENT/FAMILY TEACHING

Explain importance of handwashing both before and after contact with perineum

Explain need to use perineal pads, change them as needed, and wrap and properly dispose of them; avoid use of tampons

Explain that a shower is preferred to a tub bath

Promote good nutrition with diet as tolerated

Teach safe sex measures to prevent disease transmission if condition is caused by gonococcus or chlamydia

Explain future risk for infertility and ectopic pregnancy

DISCHARGE/HOME CARE PLANNING

Explain importance of completing antibiotic course as prescribed by physician

Emphasize need for sexual partner to be examined or treated

Discuss condom use

Discuss alternative methods of conception control if condition is related to an intrauterine device (IUD)

Explain importance of avoiding douching, intercourse, or use of tampons for 1 week after antibiotic therapy or as directed by physician

Discuss symptoms of recurrence that should be reported to physician

■ TOXIC SHOCK SYNDROME

An acute bacterial infection caused by penicillinase-resistant Staphylococcus aureus; *may lead to septic shock and release of exotoxins; most often associated with continuous use of super-absorbent tampons during menses*

ASSESSMENT
SUBJECTIVE DATA
Myalgia

Sore throat

Headache

Dizziness

Profound fatigue

OBJECTIVE DATA
Sudden onset of high fever

Vomiting

Watery diarrhea

Macular erythematous rash (sunburnlike) on palms and soles

Eventual desquamation within 1 to 2 weeks after rash appears

Impaired joint mobility

Decreased circulation of fingers and toes

Alterations in level of consciousness (LOC): disorientation, confusion

Vaginal, oropharyngeal, or conjunctival hyperemia

Severe peripheral edema

Diminished urine output

Hypotension

DIAGNOSTIC TESTS
Elevated
    WBC and differential
    Blood urea nitrogen (BUN)
    Creatinine
    Bilirubin
    Aspartate aminotransferase (AST)
    Creatinine phosphokinase (CPK)

Decreased: platelets

POTENTIAL COMPLICATIONS
Pulmonary edema

Adult respiratory distress syndrome (ARDS)

Sudden hypotension progressing to shock

Disseminated intravascular coagulation (DIC)

MULTIDISCIPLINARY MANAGEMENT
THERAPEUTIC MANAGEMENT
Antibiotics

Vital signs monitoring

Parenteral fluids to 3000 ml/day unless contraindicated

Septic shock management as indicated

PATIENT PROBLEM—NURSING DIAGNOSIS/INTERVENTIONS

▼ Altered tissue perfusion related to exchange problems associated with septic shock and/or adult respiratory distress syndrome

For specific desired outcome and interventions, see Shock syndrome (p. 115) and ARDS (p. 270)

PATIENT/FAMILY TEACHING AND DISCHARGE/HOME CARE PLANNING

Explain need to avoid use of tampons until vaginal cultures are negative

Instruct patient to thoroughly wash hands before tampon insertion

Instruct patient to use tampons made of cotton, avoiding the super-absorbent, noncotton type

Explain need to change tampons frequently and rotate using tampons and sanitary napkins (consider wearing napkins at night)

Emphasize importance of avoiding tampons altogether if there is a concurrent skin infection such as a boil caused by *Staphylococcus aureus*

If the following symptoms occur, instruct patient to discontinue use of tampons immediately and report symptoms to physician

Nausea

Vomiting

Diarrhea

Fever

■ HYDATIDIFORM MOLE

Tumor mass of chorionic cells in the uterus that mimics pregnancy; approximately 10% become malignant

ASSESSMENT
SUBJECTIVE DATA
Uterine cramping

OBJECTIVE DATA
Vaginal bleeding (dark brown or bright red; scant or profuse)

Enlarged uterus (larger than pregnant uterus for same date)

Absence of fetal heart tones

Absence of fetal movement

Vaginal expulsion of vesicular tissue

Hypertension

Hyperthyroidism

Nausea, vomiting

Excessive weight loss

Anemia

DIAGNOSTIC TESTS
Ultrasonography

Elevated HCG titer

MULTIDISCIPLINARY MANAGEMENT
THERAPEUTIC MANAGEMENT
Evacuation of mole by suction curettage

Routine preprocedural and postprocedural care

Ongoing ambulatory care

In cases of invasive, persistent, or metastatic mole, methotrexate alone or in combination with other chemotherapeutic agents may be indicated

PATIENT PROBLEM—NURSING DIAGNOSIS/INTERVENTIONS

▼ Anxiety related to situational crisis associated with pseudocyesis

Encourage verbalization about outcome of diagnosis and treatment

Use active listening skills and assist patient and family with use of adaptive coping strategies *to reduce anxiety about pseudocyesis*

Involve bereavement counselor as appropriate

Involve spouse/significant other in dealing with loss/grief

Expected Outcome
Demonstrates a reduction in anxiety and exhibits appropriate coping behaviors

PATIENT/FAMILY TEACHING
Explain condition and related physiology

Provide information about preprocedural and postprocedural care.

Explain preoperative and postoperative vital signs and care routines

DISCHARGE HOME CARE PLANNING
Reinforce physician's explanation of current condition, risk factors, avoidance of pregnancy (usually for 1 year), need for periodic HCG titers, chest x-ray examinations, and follow-up outpatient care

■ DILATION AND CURETTAGE

Expansion of the cervix and scraping of the endometrial lining of the uterus for diagnostic and/or therapeutic purposes; may detect uterine malignancy, evaluate fertility or dysfunctional uterine bleeding, or treat incomplete abortion, dysmenorrhea, or heavy bleeding

ASSESSMENT
SUBJECTIVE DATA
Pelvic and low back pain

OBJECTIVE DATA
Excessive vaginal bleeding

Hematuria

Foul odor of vaginal drainage

Elevated temperature

POTENTIAL COMPLICATIONS
Endometritis

Sepsis

Uterine perforation or rupture

Hemorrhage

MULTIDISCIPLINARY MANAGEMENT
THERAPEUTIC MANAGEMENT
Vital signs
Parenteral fluids
Pad count as indicated
Intake and output for 2 to 4 hours; notation of amount and color of first-voided urine after procedure
Analgesics as indicated

PATIENT PROBLEMS—NURSING DIAGNOSES/INTERVENTIONS

▼Pain related to uterine cramping

Administer analgesics as ordered to reduce sensation of pain and cramping
Maintain bed rest immediately after procedure, progressing to activity as tolerated

Expected Outcome
Experiences minimal discomfort

▼Risk for infection related to traumatized intra-uterine tissue secondary to intrauterine curettage

Administer perineal care after elimination as necessary *to reduce risk of ascending infection*
Monitor temperature and pulse (P) *to identify presence of fever or tachycardia related to infection*
Explain importance of wiping from front to back after elimination *to prevent contamination of urethra with fecal bacteria/matter*
Explain that shower is preferred to tub bath for 3 to 4 days
Note amount, color, and odor of vaginal drainage and change perineal pads as necessary
Understand that vaginal packing, if used, is usually removed by physician because there is a potential for bleeding

Expected Outcome
Does not develop endometritis or vaginitis as evidenced by euthermia and normal drainage

PATIENT/FAMILY TEACHING AND DISCHARGE/HOME CARE PLANNING
Explain that vaginal bleeding or spotting may continue for a week and that mild cramps may continue for 2 to 3 days
Explain that minimal activity is recommended for 2 to 3 days based on personal comfort level
Explain that coitus, douching, and use of tampons should be delayed for 1 to 2 weeks or as indicated by physician *to prevent infection*
Discuss symptoms that should be reported to physician
    Excessive bleeding, heavier than a menstrual period
    Foul odor of vaginal drainage

    Temperature >100° F (37.8° C)
    Severe lower abdominal cramps or pain

■ TUBAL PREGNANCY AND SALPINGECTOMY
tubal pregnancy: Implantation of the fertilized ovum in the fallopian tube is the most common type of ectopic pregnancy; often related to pelvic inflammatory disease (PID) resulting in tubal stricture after salpingitis
    salpingectomy: Removal of the fallopian tube

ASSESSMENT
PREOPERATIVE OBSERVATIONS/FINDINGS
Unruptured Tube
Low abdominal pain and tenderness: unilateral or generalized
Vaginal bleeding: usually scanty and dark brown; intermittent or continuous
Signs of pregnancy
    Amenorrhea
    Nausea, vomiting
    Urinary frequency
    Breast changes

Ruptured Tube (Fig. 11-5)
Severe lower abdominal pain: may be sudden and stabbing
Vaginal bleeding may or may not be present
Dizziness
Fainting
Pallor
Orthostatic hypotension
Progressive supine hypotension
Referred supraclavicular pain

DIAGNOSTIC TESTS
Ultrasonography
Culdocentesis (positive for free blood)
Laparoscopy
Complete blood cell count (CBC), electrolytes, type and screen/cross
Urinalysis
Serum HCG
Serum progesterone

POSTOPERATIVE OBSERVATIONS/FINDINGS
Site of incision
    Redness
    Pain
    Swelling
    Drainage
Elevated temperature
Feelings of loss and grief

POTENTIAL COMPLICATIONS
Incisional infection
Paralytic ileus

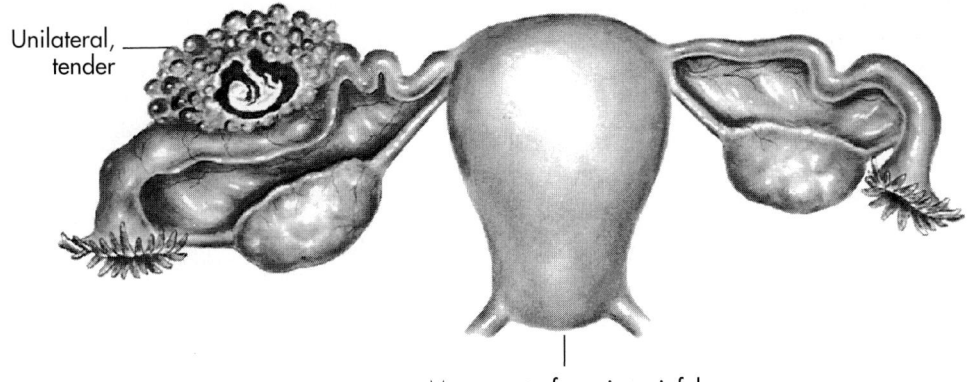

Fig. 11-5 Ruptured tubal pregnancy.
(From Seidel HM et al: Mosby's guide to physical examination, *ed 4, St Louis, 1995, Mosby.)*

Pneumonia
Hemorrhage, anemia
Shock

MULTIDISCIPLINARY MANAGEMENT
POSTOPERATIVE/SURGICAL MANAGEMENT
Parenteral fluids
Analgesics
Antiflatulent medications
Indwelling catheter to closed gravity drainage
Vital signs
Intake and output
Anti-Rh globulin as indicated
Progression of postoperative diet from clear liquids to full meal after return of bowel sounds and expelling flatus

MEDICAL MANAGEMENT/SURGICAL ALTERNATIVE
methotrexate treatment: *Methotrexate interferes with cell multiplication. Tissue most sensitive are those in which cells are rapidly dividing such as pregnancy tissue*
Example protocol
  Day 0: Lab values drawn—HCG, CBC, Rh, AST, BUN, creatinine
  Day 1: Methotrexate 50 mg/m^2 IM
  Day 7: HCG—if <15% decline, give methotrexate
  Weekly titers until HCG <5 mlU/ml
  Patient restrictions: no alcohol, vitamins with folic acid, or intercourse until HCG negative
  Monitor for side effects: nausea, vomiting, diarrhea, and mucosal membrane ulcers
    NOTE: 85% experience HCG rise first few days after treatment; 50% have abdominal pain, which can be severe
    Serial CBCs
    Pain analgesics
    Possible need for hospitalization
Contraindications for use of methotrexate treatment:
  Evidence of impending ruptured ectopic
  Mass >3.5 cm

Cardiac activity (relative contraindication)
Liver or kidney disease

PATIENT PROBLEMS—NURSING DIAGNOSES/INTERVENTIONS

▼Pain related to incision and/or abdominal distention

Assist patient with assuming position of comfort *to minimize sensation of pain*
Administer analgesics as ordered
Auscultate abdomen for bowel sounds and assess for expelling flatus
Splint incision *to avoid discomfort especially when coughing*

Expected Outcome
Reports that discomfort is minimal

▼Anticipatory grieving related to loss of pregnancy

Encourage verbalization of feelings
Assist patient with working through grieving process by using supportive statements *to enable patient to articulate and address feelings*
Involve grief/bereavement counselor as appropriate
Involve spouse or significant other with loss and grief

Expected Outcome
Demonstrates successful progress through grieving process with absence of characteristics of dysfunctional grieving

▼Impaired physical mobility, related to discomfort in the immediate postoperative period

Observe site of incision and reinforce and change dressing as necessary; ensure that patient *understands that incision is secure and to increase activity based on comfort*

Encourage and assist patient as needed with ambulation; increase activity to tolerance

Involve social service worker to assist with planning of child care at home *because mother's emergency surgery prohibits preoperative planning for their care, and temporary limitations in physical mobility may limit mother's ability/responsiveness to manage care of other children*

Expected Outcomes
Fully ambulatory before discharge
Performs self-care activities

PATIENT/FAMILY TEACHING
POST-OP PATIENT
Discuss symptoms of wound infection to report to physician
Explain need for activity to tolerance
Explain importance of planned rest periods

METHOTREXATE RECIPIENT
Explain how methotrexate works, required lab work, and how medication is given
Explain side effects
Instruct, until HCG is <5 mlU/ml, importance of maintaining restrictions and reporting severe abdominal pain or vaginal bleeding

DISCHARGE/HOME CARE PLANNING
POST-OP PATIENT/METHOTREXATE RECIPIENT
Emphasize importance of prevention of pregnancy for 2 to 4 months or as indicated by physician
Explain that childbearing ability can be diminished, especially if tubal pregnancy was a result of PID or anomaly of the tube resulting in bilateral obstruction

METHOTREXATE RECIPIENT
Explain importance of follow-up blood work and possibility of second injection
Explain abdominal pain may occur 5 to 10 days after first injection; however, if pain is severe, contact physician for possible evaluation

■ TOTAL ABDOMINAL HYSTERECTOMY AND BILATERAL SALPINGO-OOPHORECTOMY
Surgical removal of the uterus, cervix, both fallopian tubes, and ovaries through an abdominal incision or laparoscopic procedure to treat malignant neoplastic disease, leiomyomas (Fig. 11-6), chronic endometriosis, and adenomyosis

ASSESSMENT
SUBJECTIVE DATA
Difficulty in voiding
Maladaptive comments related to self-concept

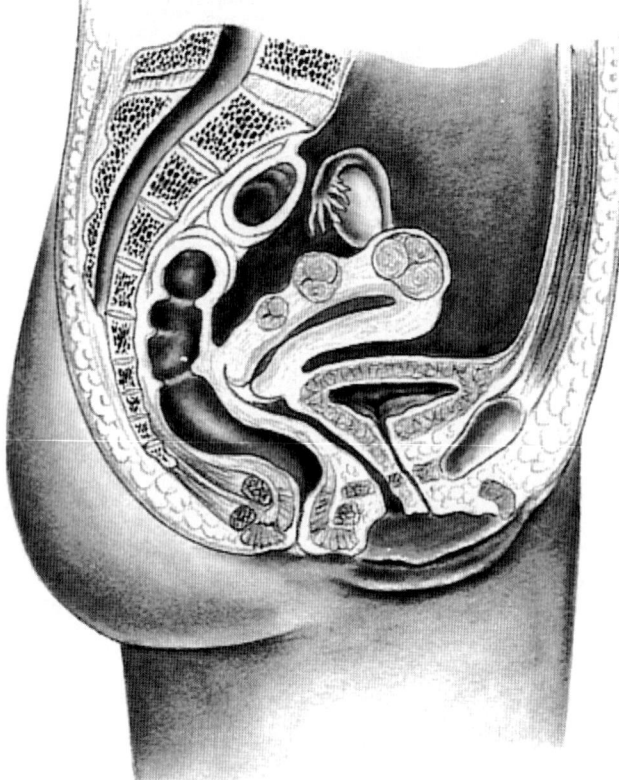

Fig. 11-6 Myomas of the uterus (fibroids).
(From Seidel HM et al: Mosby's guide to physical examination, ed 4, St Louis, 1999, Mosby.)

OBJECTIVE DATA
Vaginal discharge other than serosanguineous and/or with foul odor
Redness, pain, swelling, or drainage at incision site
Fever
Diminished or absent bowel sounds

DIAGNOSTIC TESTS
Urine culture and sensitivity after catheter removal as indicated by symptoms
CBC postsurgically

POTENTIAL COMPLICATIONS
Infection: intraabdominal or incisional
Urinary tract infection
Paralytic ileus
Pneumonia
Hemorrhage
Thrombophlebitis
Pulmonary embolus

MULTIDISCIPLINARY MANAGEMENT
THERAPEUTIC MANAGEMENT
Nothing by mouth (NPO) until bowel sounds are audible
Parenteral fluids until liquids or diet is tolerated
Indwelling catheter to low-gravity drainage system
Intake and output

Blood pressure (BP), T, P, and respirations (R) per postoperative procedure

Patient-controlled analgesia (PCA) pump

Analgesics and stool softeners

Hormone replacement as indicated

PATIENT PROBLEMS—NURSING DIAGNOSES/INTERVENTIONS

▼Altered peripheral tissue perfusion related to interruption in arterial and venous flow secondary to surgical intervention

Monitor vital signs as ordered

Avoid sitting with knees bent and/or crossing legs *to prevent peripheral pooling of blood*

Apply antiembolic stockings/devices as ordered

Auscultate bowel sounds; maintain NPO status until bowel sounds are active *to prevent abdominal distention*

Assist with ambulation as needed

Encourage ambulation and/or leg exercises *to increase peripheral tissue perfusion*

Expected Outcomes

Vital signs remain within normal presurgical limits

Circulation remains normal without evidence of pelvic stasis or peripheral thrombophlebitis

Bowel function is resuming

▼Pain related to surgical incision(s)

Encourage use of PCA pump or administer analgesics as ordered

Assist patient in assuming a position of comfort

Place pillow on abdomen *for support when patient is coughing to reduce sensation of pain*

Assist with personal hygiene as necessary

Expected Outcome

Reports that she is comfortable and pain is reduced

▼Ineffective breathing pattern related to discomfort and postsurgical status

Assist with turning, coughing, and deep breathing, decreasing frequency as patient becomes more active

Assist and teach patient to use incentive spirometer as indicated *to promote adequate ventilation/prevent pooling of secretions*

Auscultate chest for breath sounds

Expected Outcome

Has normal breath sounds on auscultation, and inhalation/exhalation pattern enables adequate ventilation

▼Impaired skin integrity related to surgical incision(s)

Observe incision for condition

Cleanse incision area as indicated; keep clean and dry

Report signs of infection to physician: redness, swelling, or discharge

Change or reinforce dressing as necessary

Explain to patient importance of avoiding lifting or placing strain on abdominal muscles (avoid straining at stool) *to ensure that incisional skin integrity is maintained*

Expected Outcome

Incision remains clean, dry, and intact without signs of infection

▼Constipation related to NPO status and manipulation of pelvic and abdominal structures during surgery

Progress to high-protein or high-residue diet as ordered

Encourage adequate fluid intake *to prevent constipation*

Assist patient with assuming lateral Sims position *if it promotes expulsion of flatus*

Encourage ambulation *to promote muscle activity and bowel motility*

Give stool softeners or mild laxatives as ordered *to prevent constipation*

Expected Outcome

Expells flatus before discharge

▼Altered urinary elimination related to postsurgical sensory motor impairment

Maintain closed gravity drainage system if patient has indwelling catheter *to prevent infection*

Promote micturition at regular intervals when catheter is removed *and monitor/report difficulty in voiding*

Monitor intake and output; encourage fluids

Expected Outcome

Voids qs without difficulty

▼Self-esteem disturbance related to body image change and value of reproductive organs

Encourage patient's comments and questions about surgery, progress, and prognosis *to prevent internalization of negative thoughts*

Reinforce correct information and provide factual information *to correct any misconceptions;* common misconceptions are that after a hysterectomy a woman grows fat and flabby; develops facial hair; becomes wrinkled, old, and masculine appearing; loses her mind; or becomes depressed and nervous; normal concerns to address are fear of death, disfigurement, cancer, loss of femininity, pain, loss of childbearing ability, and changes in sexuality

Encourage verbalization of feelings with significant other *to address and resolve body image and self-esteem issues*

Discuss hormone replacement therapy if appropriate

Expected Outcomes

Demonstrates adaptive responses related to self-concept

Asks appropriate questions

Gives correct information related to procedures and prognosis

Indicates that she has discussed concerns with significant other

PATIENT/FAMILY TEACHING

Instruct patient to ambulate at regular intervals and to avoid sitting for prolonged periods at home or when traveling

Instruct patient to care for incision with general cleanliness and daily bathing; to report signs of infection to physician, including redness, swelling, pain, discharge, increase in vaginal drainage, and foul odor

Instruct patient to report pain or burning with urination or inability to empty bladder

Explain need to avoid constipation and straining at stool

Instruct patient regarding foods that promote postoperative healing and healthy lifestyle

DISCHARGE/HOME CARE PLANNING

Explain need to avoid coitus, douching, tampons, or anything in vagina for 4 to 6 weeks or as indicated by physician

Explain need to avoid heavy lifting and vigorous activity for 6 weeks after surgery

Emphasize importance of maintaining regular outpatient gynecologic examinations

Explain need to take estrogen-progesterone hormones as ordered (if surgical menopause is caused by removal of all ovarian tissue)

■ PERINATAL PERIOD

Time frame beginning with conception and ending 6 weeks after delivery; divided into antepartum, intrapartum, postpartum periods

ASSESSMENT
SUBJECTIVE AND OBJECTIVE DATA

Age

Height

Weight
  Prepregnancy
  Current
  Gain/loss

History of infertility
  Treatment
  Results

Menstrual history
  Menarche
  Intervals
  Regularity
  Length
  LMP

Expected date of confinement or delivery (EDC/EDD)
  Dates
  Ultrasound

Pregnancy history
  Gravida/para
    Full term
    Premature
    Multiples
    Aborts (spontaneous/elective)
    Stillbirths
    Childhood deaths
    Living

Delivery history
  Date of each birth (month/year)
    Infant sex
    Infant weight
    Gestational age at delivery
    Duration of labor (hours)
    Spontaneous/augmented/induced labor
      Method/drug
    Vaginal or cesarean
    Complications (maternal, fetal, neonatal)

Children
  Ages
  Developmental problems

Maternal vital signs
  BP, T, P, R

Fetal heart rate (FHR)

Fetal lie and position

Previous major illnesses, accidents, surgeries

Current health problems
  Diabetes
  Cardiovascular conditions
  Anemia
  Epilepsy
  Asthma or other pulmonary conditions
  Renal disorders
  STDs

Drug allergies/sensitivities

Reproductive system changes
  Uterus
    Fundal height increase of approximately 1 cm per week
  Breasts
    Fullness, tingling, heaviness
    Nipples (extroverted, introverted)
      Nipple, areola (turgid, engorged, darkened)
    Presence of colostrum

Cardiovascular system
  Increased heart rate (HR) of 10 to 15 beats/min from baseline (14 to 30 weeks)
  Slight decrease in BP during second trimester with return to previous baseline BP in third trimester <15 mm Hg in either systolic or diastolic
  Tendency for dependent edema

Basal metabolism
  Increases by 15% to 20% at term
  Lassitude and fatigability in early pregnancy
  Heat intolerance in late pregnancy

Hematologic system

  Blood volume increase, with peak by 30 to 34 weeks

    Hemoglobin decline (11 to 12 g normal)

  Reticulocyte count increase

  WBC count increase of up to 25,000/mm^3

  Total plasma proteins decrease to 3 to 3.5 g/dl

  Sedimentation rate increase

Respiratory system

  Nasal/sinus congestion and increased tendency to nosebleeds

  Increased oxygen consumption

  Decreased functional residual capacity

  Increased minute volume and oxygen uptake

  Compensated respiratory alkalosis

Renal/urinary system

  Increased glomerular filtration rate

  Frequency

  Increased bladder capacity

  Mild glycosuria

Gastrointestinal system

  Tender gums

  Excessive salivation

  Transitory nausea and vomiting

  Unusual food preferences

  Heartburn and acid indigestion

  Delayed gastric emptying

  Hypercholesterolemia

  Decreased gallbladder emptying time

  Tendency to constipation

Neurologic system

  Lightheadedness or faintness

  Sensory changes in legs

Musculoskeletal system

  Decreased abdominal muscle tone

  Increased lumbosacral curve

  Hypermobility of pelvic joints with waddling gait

  Tendency for carpal tunnel syndrome

  Acroesthesia (numbness/tingling of hands)

Integumentary system

  Thickened skin

  Increased subdermal fat

  Hyperpigmentation

    Chloasma (mask of pregnancy)

    Linea nigra

  Increased hair and nail growth

  Thinning and softening of fingernails and toenails

  Increased sebaceous and sweat gland activity

  Increased fragility of cutaneous elastic tissues resulting in striae gravidarum (stretch marks)

  Acne vulgaris (preexisting)

    Aggravated in first trimester

    Improved in third trimester

  Angiomas (vascular spiders) on neck, thorax, face, and arms

Psychosocial

  Patterns of work or employment

  Activity/exercise patterns

  Patterns of nutrient intake

  Desire for participation in prepared childbirth classes

  Planned method of feeding infant

  Plans for postdischarge newborn care at home

  Self-esteem and perceived ability to cope with life situations

  Body image resulting from physiologic changes of pregnancy

  Patterns of tobacco, alcohol, prescription drug, and nonprescription drug use

  Chemical dependency/substance abuse

  Domestic/intimate partner abuse

DIAGNOSTIC TESTING

Pregnancy test confirmation

Blood typing and Rh factor identification

  Irregular antibody screen

Hemoglobin (Hgb) and hematocrit (Hct)

FBS screening (at 26 weeks' gestation if no risk factors for diabetes)

Pap smear (cervical cytology test)

Urinalysis

VDRL or rapid plasma reagin (RPR) test

Rubella antibody titer

Hepatitis BsAg

Gonococcus (GC) culture

Tuberculosis (TB)

HIV (offered)

Abdominal ultrasound

Optional tests as indicated

  Chemistry profile

  Sickle cell test

  Toxoplasmosis, other, rubella, cytomegalovirus, herpes (TORCH) screen

  Alpha-fetoprotein (AFP) (10 to 16 weeks)

  Glucose tolerance test (1 hour glucola at 26 weeks)

  Chorionic villus sampling

  Amniocentesis

  Herpes culture

  Biophysical profile (fetal breathing movements, gross body movements, fetal tone, amniotic fluid index, nonstress test)

POTENTIAL COMPLICATIONS

Pregnancy induced hypertension (PIH)

Hyperemesis gravidarum

HELLP (*H,* hemolysis; *EL,* elevated liver enzymes; *LP,* low platelet count) syndrome

Gestational diabetes mellitus (GDM)

Premature rupture of membranes (PROM)

Prolapsed umbilical cord

Preterm labor (PTL)

Post dates pregnancy

Placenta previa

Abruptio placentae

Hemorrhage

Spontaneous abortion

MULTIDISCIPLINARY MANAGEMENT
THERAPEUTIC MANAGEMENT
Uncomplicated or high-risk pregnancy visit schedule
  Every 4 weeks during first 28 weeks
  Every 2 to 3 weeks until 36 weeks
  Weekly until birth
Genetic counseling as indicated
Fetal well-being assessment
  Nonstress testing (NST)
  Contraction stress testing (CST)
  Oxytocin challenge testing (OCT)
Prenatal vitamins and iron supplementation as indicated
Antibiotic treatment for maternal infection as indicated
Counseling and referral for high-risk situations

PATIENT/FAMILY TEACHING
Discuss danger signals to report immediately to primary
  health care provider
  Vaginal bleeding
  Swelling of face or fingers
  Severe or continuous headache
  Visual changes
  Muscular twitching or seizure activity
  Abdominal or epigastric pain
  Persistent nausea and vomiting
  Diarrhea
  Chills or fever
  Dysuria
  Cramping
  Change in vaginal discharge
  Pelvic heaviness or pressure
  Uterine contractions
  Leakage of fluid from vagina
  Change in fetal activity
Preparation for delivery process
Parent education programs
Community resources
Role of doula as indicated
Emphasize importance of avoiding any nonprescription
  drugs, including aspirin and nose drops without
  consulting healthcare provider
Emphasize need to avoid substance use/abuse (nicotine,
  alcohol, and all street drugs, including marijuana,
  cocaine, amphetamines, benzodiazepines, and
  heroin/related products)
Explain need to check with primary health care provider
  before traveling
Discuss methods to alleviate nausea, hemorrhoids,
  varicose veins
Explain importance of toxoplasmosis precautions (e.g.,
  avoiding cat litter)
Emphasize importance of ongoing outpatient care
Explain need to avoid excessive fatigue when exercising
Explain need to maintain good body mechanics when
  bending, lifting, or walking
Explain need to rest periodically with legs elevated
Encourage rest when feeling fatigued
Explain need to avoid use of constricting garments,
  especially on lower extremities

Explain need to drink adequate amounts of fluid to 3000
  ml/day unless contraindicated
Emphasize importance of well-balanced diet
Explain need to wear well-fitting, supportive brassiere
Explain need to wear only low-heeled shoes if backache
  or unstable balance occurs with higher-heeled shoes
Emphasize importance of maintaining normal bowel
  habits with adequate fluid intake, reasonable exercise,
  and diet high in fiber
  Mild laxatives such as prune juice, milk of magnesia,
    bulk-producing substances, or stool softeners may
    be taken when necessary
  Avoid use of nonabsorbable oil preparations and any
    other nonprescription medications without
    consulting physician
Emphasize importance of avoiding intercourse when
  there is a risk of spontaneous abortion or preterm
  labor
Discuss pros and cons of breast-feeding versus formula
  feeding
Discuss special caretaking considerations for working
  mothers

■ CARE OF MOTHER IN FIRST STAGE OF LABOR
Physiologic process by which the fetus is expelled from the uterus
  early labor: *Dilation of 0 to 4 cm with mild-to-moderate irregular contractions*
  active labor: *Dilation of 4 to 8 cm with moderate-to-strong regular contractions every 2 to 5 minutes*
  transitional labor: *Dilation of 8 cm to complete dilation with strong contractions*

ASSESSMENT
SUBJECTIVE DATA
Behavior
  Surge of energy and activity
  Talking frequently
  Anxious
  Fear of isolation

OBJECTIVE DATA
Rupture of membranes (ROM)
Uterine contractions: regular with increasing intensity
  and frequency
Transitional labor
  Nausea and vomiting
  Hypersensitive abdomen
  Irritability
  Loss of coping mechanisms
  Hiccups, belching
  Trembling, shaking of legs
  Chilling
  Perspiration
  Rectal pressure
  Urge to push

DIAGNOSTIC TESTS

Baseline laboratory tests
   CBC with differential
   Hgb, Hct
   Rubella screen
   Hepatitis screen
   VDRL/RPR serology
   Chemistries
Urinalysis; protein, glucose
Cultures as indicated by history of signs and symptoms
Ultrasound examination as indicated
Electronic fetal monitoring
Vibroacoustic stimulation
Score of biophysical profile (if done before onset of labor
   [Table 11-1])

POTENTIAL COMPLICATIONS

Nonreassuring maternal findings
   Fever
   Hypotension or hypertension
   Dehydration
   Circulatory overload
   Hemorrhage
   Severe pain unrelated to contractions
   Supine hypotension syndrome
   Distended bladder
Nonreassuring fetal findings
   Fetal tachycardia: >160 beats/min
   Fetal bradycardia: <110 beats/min
Fetal hyperactivity or hypoactivity
Monitored labor
   Severe variable decelerations: <70 beats/min for more
     than 30 seconds
   Uncorrectable, repetitive late decelerations of any
     magnitude
   Decreased or absent variability
   Prolonged deceleration
   Unstable FHR; sinusoidal pattern
Inadequate uterine relaxation
   Contractions lasting longer than 90 seconds
   Relaxation between contractions less than 30 seconds
   Tachysystole (>4 contractions in 10 minutes)

Table 11-1	**Biophysical Profile**

DESCRIPTION: A PHYSICAL EXAMINATION OF THE FETUS WITH REALTIME ULTRASOUND MEASUREMENTS

Fetal breathing movements (FBM)
Fetal movement (FM)
Fetal tone (TON)
Amniotic fluid index (AFI)
Nonstress test (NST)

INTERPRETATION

Biophysical Variable	Normal (score = 2)	Abnormal (score = 0)
Fetal breathing movements (FBM)	At least one episode of FBM of at least 30 sec duration in 30-min observation	Absent FBM or no episode of ≥ 30 sec in 30 min
Gross body movements (FM)	At least three discrete body/limb movements in 30 min (episodes of active continuous movement considered as a single movement)	Two or fewer episodes of body/limb movements in 30 min
Fetal tone (TON)	At least one episode of active extension with return to flexion of fetal limb(s) or trunk; opening and closing of hand considered normal tone	Slow extension with return to partial flexion, or movement of limb in full extension, or absence of fetal movement
Amniotic fluid index (AFI)*	AFI ≤1 cm	AFI <1 cm
Nonstress test (NST)	Reactive	Nonreactive

RECORD BIOPHYSICAL PROFILE

Parameter	Score
FBM	_____
FM	_____
TON	_____
AFI	_____
NST	_____
TOTAL:	_____

MANAGEMENT BASED ON INTERPRETATION AND SCORE

Score	Action
8-10	Equivalent to reactive NST; manage per protocol
4-6	If pulmonary maturity is favorable, deliver; if not, repeat test in 24 hr; if score persists, deliver if maturity is certain; otherwise, treat with steroids and deliver in 48 hr
0-2	Evaluate for delivery

*Amniotic fluid index: The summation of deepest vertical pocket of amniotic fluid in each of the four quadrants of the amniotic sac. Measurements are done in centimeters.

Arrest of labor

Meconium-stained amniotic fluid

Foul-smelling amniotic fluid

Intraamniotic infection secondary to prolonged rupture of membranes

MULTIDISCIPLINARY MANAGEMENT
THERAPEUTIC MANAGEMENT

Prenatal chart and previous medical chart ordered to labor and delivery unit

Laboratory tests as indicated

IV fluids as indicated

Analgesia as indicated

Preparation for selected/indicated anesthesia by anesthesiologist/nurse anesthetist

Supportive care to patient and family

PATIENT PROBLEMS—NURSING DIAGNOSES/INTERVENTIONS

▼Risk for injury to mother related to physiologic processes of labor

Assist patient to maintain position of comfort

Encourage ambulation as tolerated if membranes unruptured and or presenting part is well applied to cervix *to avoid prolapse of cord*

Assess temperature q 2 hours after rupture of membranes

Plot cervical dilation and fetal descent on Friedman Graph *to assess progress of labor*

Administer clear liquids as ordered

Encourage frequent voiding and assist patient to bathroom prn if presenting part is well applied to cervix

Measure intake and output

Check urine for protein and glucose

Initiate IV with isotonic solution (lactated Ringer's solution, normal saline) if ordered

Prehydrate with 1000 to 1500 ml of fluid before regional anesthesia

Maintain dosing of prelabor medications as ordered (anticonvulsants, antihypertensives, or methadone)

Expected Outcomes

Experiences no injury related to labor as evidenced by comfort, adequate hydration, absence of hypotensive episodes related to regional anesthesia, absence of distended bladder, and maintenance of prelabor medical status

▼Pain and anxiety related to lack of information physiologic processes of labor

Nursing interventions during active labor

Maintain quiet and calm environment

Avoid conversation during contractions

Avoid having persons in room who are not directly caring for patient or providing support *to decrease anxiety*

Ensure nurse call light accessible

Assist with position changes

Encourage lateral position

Assist with breathing techniques

Encourage significant other to be involved in support activities

Apply cool compresses to forehead prn

Apply sacral pressure prn during contractions *to relieve discomfort*

Change gown and linens prn

Change pad under buttocks prn

Give pain medication as ordered

Assist with administration of local or regional anesthetic

Record vital signs as per unit protocol

Nursing interventions during transitional labor

Palpate abdomen very lightly and only as often as necessary if abdomen is hypersensitive

Prepare for vomiting episodes

Encourage patient to empty bladder

Maintain warmth as necessary

Encourage patient to avoid pushing until cervix completely dilated

Panting or rapid blowing breathing technique

Provide reassurance that transition usually last only 1 to 2 hours

Accept aggression or other coping behaviors and avoid negative comments

Focus on patient and support her by using calm voice, touch, and positive reinforcement

Expected Outcomes

Experiences manageable pain and minimal anxiety as evidenced by verbalization of same

Complies with assistive directions by staff

Has continuing interaction with significant other/family

▼Altered oral mucous membrane related to mouth breathing

Administer oral hygiene qh and prn between contractions

Suck on ice chips, wet washcloths, or sour lollipops unless contraindicated

Rinse mouth with water and/or mouthwash

Apply petroleum jelly or antichapping lipsticks to dry lips prn

Expected Outcome

Does not experience disruption in tissue layers of oral cavity

▼Risk for altered tissue perfusion related to impaired transport of oxygen associated with uterine contractions and/or uteroplacental insufficiency

Note frequency, duration, and strength of contractions according to facility protocols (Box 11-1)

| Box 11-1 | **Maternal-Fetal Assessment Frequencies** |

LOW-RISK PATIENTS

Temperature and pulse q4h (if ROM, then qh)

Blood pressure qh

Evaluate and record the fetal heart rate (FHR) and uterine contractions (UC) q30min in the active phase of the first stage of labor and q15min during the second stage

HIGH-RISK PATIENTS

Temperature, pulse, and blood pressure qh or more frequently if situation necessitates

Evaluate and record the FHR and UC every 15 minutes in the active phase of the first stage of labor and every 5 minutes during the second stage

Auscultate FHR for 1 minute immediately after uterine contractions in unmonitored labor

Every 15 to 30 minutes and prn

Assess FHR immediately after spontaneous or artificial amniotomy *to assess for prolapsed umbilical cord*

Assess maternal vital signs per institutional protocol

T, P, R q2h to q4h hours and prn

BP and P hourly and prn

Initiate intrauterine resuscitation protocols for non-reassuring fetal findings as indicated

Turn mother to lateral position

Increase rate of isotonic IV solution

Administer 100% oxygen by tight face mask at 8 to 10 L/min

Notify physician of situation

Expected Outcome

Gives birth to newborn in good condition with Apgar score ≥8 at 5 minutes of age

PATIENT/FAMILY TEACHING

Allay anxiety as much as possible by doing the following:

Explain reasons for performing all procedures

Encourage spouse or significant other to remain with patient to provide support during labor

Assist spouse or significant other to listen to fetal heart with fetoscope, Doppler, or ultrasound equipment

Provide supportive care based on patient and family's knowledge of labor process

Ask patient if she wants additional support persons present for labor and birth

Inform waiting family and friends about patient's progress and inform patient that they are waiting and interested

Reduce environmental stimuli that may contribute to anxiety and tension; provide relaxed, restful atmosphere

Reassure patient at appropriate intervals that labor is progressing and that both patient and fetus are doing well

■ PROCEDURAL CARE OF MOTHER DURING DELIVERY: SECOND AND THIRD STAGES OF LABOR

The stage of expulsion of the fetus, placenta, and membranes after complete dilatation of the cervix

ASSESSMENT
SUBJECTIVE DATA

Extreme anxiety

Patient stating, "Baby is coming"

Desire to defecate

Fear of losing control

OBJECTIVE DATA

Involuntary bearing down/pushing

Grunting sounds

Vomiting

Involuntary shaking of thighs

Perspiration between nose and upper lip

Increase in bloody show

Prolonged second stage

More than 1 hour for multigravidas

More than 2 hours for primigravidas

Crowning

DIAGNOSTIC TESTS

Electronic fetal monitoring

Cord blood: gases, pH, and other tests as ordered

POTENTIAL COMPLICATIONS

Fetal stress/distress

Birth asphyxia

Difficult birth

Cephalopelvic disproportion (CPD)

Shoulder dystocia

Breech presentation

Forceps delivery

Vacuum extraction

Cesarean birth

Infant bruising, fractures

MULTIDISCIPLINARY MANAGEMENT
CARE DURING DELIVERY

Auscultate FHR q5min and/or after each push if electronic monitor is not used (if electronic monitor was used continuously during labor, then it should be continued in the delivery room until the time of delivery)

Check BP and P q5min to 10min

Pad stirrups if used

Administer oxygen mask at 8 to 10 L/min as ordered

Understand that low- to semi-Fowler's position with lateral tilt is preferred while pushing

Assist with breathing techniques
   Deep ventilation before and after each contraction
   Open-glottis breathing when pushing with
      contractions
Observe perineum while pushing
Notify physician if second stage is prolonged
Prepare perineum according to hospital procedure
Place nurse, spouse, and/or labor coach at head of delivery
   table to encourage patient during delivery process
Encourage long, sustained pushing rather than frequent
   short pushes
Encourage patient to push when she feels urge to push
Encourage complete relaxation between contractions
Reassure patient that she is doing well and is advancing
   fetus with each push
Apply cool, moist cloth to forehead as needed
Keep DeLee suction catheter available and ready to use if
   meconium-stained amniotic fluid is present
Plan for suctioning of nasooropharynx after delivery of
   fetal head and before delivery of thorax to prevent
   meconium aspiration
Assist physician or nurse-midwife as needed

Immediate Postpartum Care (Fourth-Stage Care)

Encourage mother to inspect infant as soon as possible
Place infant on maternal abdomen to provide skin-to-skin
   contact if delivery room is warm
See Care of newborn (p. 696)
Defer neonatal eye therapy for 1 to 2 hours after birth to
   promote eye contact with mother
Assess BP and P q10min to 15min × 4 and prn
Add oxytocic drug as ordered to parenteral fluids
Palpate fundus, noting location and tonus q5min to 10
   min × 4
Administer perineal care before removing legs from
   stirrups *to cleanse and inspect perineum*
Place sterile perineal pad under buttocks before
   transporting patient to recovery area
Place ice pack on episiotomy unless otherwise ordered *to
   reduce swelling*
Assist with infant's warm water bath if newborn's
   temperature is stable
Maintain mother's warmth with blankets as needed
Place radiant heat warmer over upper part of mother's bed
   or place dry, warmly blanketed newborn next to mother *so
   that she can visually inspect, touch, and/or breast-feed
   nude infant while preventing neonatal heat loss*
Encourage mother and spouse and/or labor coach to be
   with infant in delivery area, providing them with as
   much privacy as feasible unless this is contraindicated
   by maternal or neonatal pathologic condition
Encourage mother to freely express her feelings about
   herself and her infant
Explain that behaviors manifested in labor are normal and
   there is no reason to be embarrassed if mother is
   apologetic for behavior
See Postpartum care (p. 685)

■ OXYTOCIN INFUSION: AUGMENTATION OR INDUCTION OF LABOR

Oxytocin infusion may be used to either begin the labor process or to augment a labor that is progressing slowly because of inadequate uterine activity

ASSESSMENT
OBJECTIVE DATA
Dysfunctional labor pattern (Table 11-2)
Absence of CPD
Bishop score (Table 11-3)

DIAGNOSTIC TESTS
FHR, UC monitoring
CPD measurements
Ultrasound

POTENTIAL COMPLICATIONS
Fetal compromise
   Hyperactive fetus
   Fetal tachycardia: >160 beats/min
   Fetal bradycardia: <110 beats/min
   Late decelerations
   Prolonged deceleration
   Severe variable decelerations
Uterine hyperstimulation
   Contractions longer than 90 seconds
   Contractions occurring more frequently than q2min
   Peak pressure of contraction >90 mm Hg pressure
   Inadequate uterine relaxation: less than 30 seconds
      between contractions

Table 11-2	**Dysfunctional Labor Patterns**	
	Nulliparas	**Multiparas**
Prolonged latent phase	>21 hr	>14 hr
Protracted active phase	<1.2 cm hr	<1.5 cm hr
Secondary arrest: *no change*	>2 hr	>2 hr
Prolonged deceleration phase	>3 hr	>1 hr
Protracted descent	<1 cm hr	<2 cm hr
Arrest of descent	>1 hr	>½ hr

Table 11-3	**Bishop Scoring System**			
Score	**0**	**1**	**2**	**3**
Station of presenting part	−3	−2	−1/0	+1/+2
Dilatation in cm	0	1-2	3-4	>5
Effacement in cm	>2.5	2	1	<0.5
Consistency	Firm	Medium	Soft	—
Position of os	Posterior	Central	Anterior	—

Intrauterine resting tone >15 mm Hg pressure
  between contractions
Sustained tetanic uterine contraction
Meconium-stained amniotic fluid
Maternal hypertension
Water intoxication
  Rising BP
  Edema of face, fingers, and around eyes
  Shortness of breath (SOB)
  Difficulty in breathing
  Urinary output <30 to 50 ml/hr
Abruptio placentae: sudden, severe uterine pain
Precipitate delivery
Hemorrhage
Shock
Uterine rupture

MULTIDISCIPLINARY MANAGEMENT
THERAPEUTIC MANAGEMENT
Baseline FHR, UC recording
Oxytocin infusion at a rate of 0.5 mU/min and increasing
  for desired results at 15- to 20-minute intervals in
  increments of 1 to 2 mU/min not to exceed
  20 mU/min or per institutional protocol
Infusion pump or controller
Continuous FHR, UC monitoring
Analgesia
Tocolytic agents for excessive uterine activity that persists
  following oxytocin discontinuation, after supportive
  treatment is provided (lateral position and oxygen by
  mask), and fetal distress is present; terbutaline 0.25 mg
  IV push or magnesium sulfate 4 g, 10% solution IV over
  15 to 20 minutes, or nifedipine per protocol

PATIENT PROBLEM—NURSING DIAGNOSIS/INTERVENTIONS

▼Risk for injury related to augmentation of labor
and potential uterine hyperstimulation

See Care of mother in first stage of labor (p. 677)
Encourage ambulation as tolerated with maternal-fetal
  assessments at prescribed frequencies
Ensure that physician is immediately available
Apply fetal monitoring; obtain baseline strip before start
  of IV oxytocin
Place patient in position of comfort; lateral position is
  preferred *to prevent supine hypotension syndrome*
Always piggyback oxytocin solution into main IV line (10
  U oxytocin in 1000 ml IV fluid = 10 mU/ml) or as per
  institutional protocol
Administer oxytocin via controlled infusion device as
  ordered
Monitor dose in mU/min q15min to 30min and before
  each increase
Increase rate of oxytocic solution as ordered to produce
  contractions every 2 to 3 minutes of 30- to 60-seconds
  duration
Assess BP, P, and FHR q15min to 30min or as ordered

Observe contractions for frequency, duration, strength,
  and relaxation before every dosage increase
Administer analgesics as ordered
Assist in breathing and relaxation techniques
Measure intake and output q2h
Prepare for birth as indicated

Expected Outcome
Patient and fetus are not compromised as a result of
  oxytocin infusion

PATIENT/FAMILY TEACHING
Reinforce physician's explanations
Discuss indications for procedure
Explain administration procedure
Discuss expected effects of oxytocin induction/
  augmentation of labor
Explain differences between induction/augmentation and
  normal, spontaneous contractions

■ FETAL COMPROMISE
*A symptom complex indicative of a critical re-
sponse to stress; may include hypoxemia/hypoxia
and/or acidemia/acidosis*

ASSESSMENT
OBJECTIVE DATA
Fetal tachycardia: >160 beats/min
Fetal bradycardia: <110 beats/min
Meconium-stained amniotic fluid
Fetal hyperactivity or hypoactivity
Monitored fetus
  Nonreassuring FHR patterns
    Progressive increase or decrease in baseline FHR
    Tachycardia: 160 beats/min or greater; progressive
      decrease in baseline variability
    Severe variable deceleration; FHR <70 beats/min
      for longer than 30 to 60 seconds with the
      following:
      Rising baseline FHR
      Decreasing variability
      Slow return to baseline (may be with overshoot)
    Late decelerations of any magnitude that are
      repetitive and uncorrectable
    Absence of variability
    Prolonged deceleration (greater than 60 to 90 seconds)
    Severe bradycardia (fewer than 70 beats/min)
    Unstable FHR; sinusoidal pattern

DIAGNOSTIC TESTS
Electronic fetal monitoring
Amniocentesis
Cord blood studies
Fetal scalp sampling: pH <7.0

POTENTIAL COMPLICATIONS
Hypoxemia
Hypoxia
Acidemia

Acidosis
Asphyxia
Meconium aspiration syndrome
Hypoglycemia
Intracranial hemorrhage
Central nervous system (CNS) disorders
Fetal death
Neonatal death

MULTIDISCIPLINARY MANAGEMENT
THERAPEUTIC MANAGEMENT
Discontinue oxytocic therapy as applicable
Institute lateral position
Administer oxygen to patient: 8 to 10 L/min with face
     mask
IV fluids as indicated
Deliver infant as indicated
Fetal blood sampling as indicated
Laboratory tests as indicated
Continuous fetal evaluation until time of birth
Neonatal resuscitation required at birth

PATIENT PROBLEMS—NURSING DIAGNOSES/INTERVENTIONS

▼Risk for impaired gas exchange due to hypox-
emia/acidemia

Intervene methodically; it is not necessary to proceed
     with subsequent steps if intervention corrects FHR
     pattern
     Change maternal position to allow most improvement
         in FHR pattern
     Correct maternal hypotension: elevate legs; increase
         rate of maintenance intravenous (IV) infusion
     Discontinue oxytocin if infusing
     Administer oxygen by face mask at rate of 8 to 10
         L/min or as ordered
Fetal scalp or acoustic stimulation may be done *to assess
FHR variability* if patient is making good progress
     toward vaginal delivery
Perform vaginal and/or speculum examination *to check
for prolapsed cord*
Prepare for birth as indicated
Explain briefly to patient the reasons for actions
     taken

Expected Outcomes
Fetus has minimal compromise
Fetus/infant is delivered in good condition

▼Anxiety/fear related to uncertain fetal outcome
and unfamiliarity with care required to treat fetal
compromise

Explain all interventions such as the following to mother
     and significant other:
     Reasons for procedure
     How procedures are to be done

     Available options
     Results expected from procedure
Simplify explanations and repeat as necessary
Provide realistic, factual information regarding fetal status
     to allay anxiety
Provide information regarding availability of neonatal
     intensive care unit should infant require this type of
     care
Reassure patient that emergency equipment and
     experienced personnel are available for birth
Encourage patient to express concerns
Offer choices where feasible
Provide information regarding the following:
     Known possible causes of fetal compromise
     Misconceptions
Postdelivery
     Ensure that parents see newborn before transport to
         nursery
     Allow mother to hold and/or stroke newborn if
         possible

Expected Outcome
Patient and significant other verbalize understanding of
     required care and are able to verbalize fears and
     concerns regarding newborn

■ CARE OF MOTHER MONITORED VIA ELECTRONIC FETAL MONITOR
Refer to Care of the mother during labor (p. 677)
The following guidelines relate to patient teaching and
     functioning of the monitor:
Explain that fetal status via FHR can be continuously
     assessed even during contractions
Explain that lower activity on strip chart shows uterine
     activity; upper panel shows FHR
Reassure patient and significant other that prepared
     childbirth techniques can be implemented without
     difficulty
Explain that effleurage performed during external
     monitoring can be done on sides of abdomen or
     upper thighs
Relate that breathing patterns based on timing and
     intensity of contractions can be enhanced by
     observation of uterine activity panel of strip chart
     for onset of contractions
     Note peak of contraction; knowing that contraction
         will not get stronger and is half over is usually
         helpful
     Note diminishing intensity
     Coordinate with appropriate breathing and relaxation
         techniques
Reassure patient/significant other that use of internal
     mode of monitoring does not restrict patient
     movement
Explain that use of external mode of monitoring usually
     requires patient cooperation in positioning and
     movement

Reassure patient and significant other that use of monitor does not imply fetal jeopardy

■ EXTERNAL MONITORING

ULTRASOUND TRANSDUCER
Monitors FHR with high-frequency sound waves

Perform Leopold maneuvers to assess best position for transducer

Apply ultrasound transmission gel to maternal abdomen; clean abdomen and transducer and reapply gel prn

Massage reddened skin areas and reposition belt or adhesive device prn

Auscultate FHR with stethoscope or fetoscope if in doubt as to validity of tracing

Position and reposition transducer prn to ensure clear, interpretable FHR data

TOCOTRANSDUCER
Monitors uterine activity via pressure-sensing device placed on the maternal abdomen

Position and reposition prn on the fundus where least maternal tissue is in evidence

Maintain abdominal strap snugly

Adjust penset *between* contractions to print between 10 and 20 mm Hg on strip chart

Palpate fundus q30min to 60min to gauge strength of contraction; only frequency and duration of contractions can be assessed with tocotransducer

Do not assess patient's need for analgesic based on uterine activity displayed on strip chart

Massage reddened areas under transducer and belt qh and prn

■ INTERNAL MONITORING

SPIRAL ELECTRODE
Obtains fetal ECG from presenting part and converts it to FHR

Ensure that wire(s) is appropriately attached to leg plate

Apply electrode paste to leg plate prn

Observe FHR panel of strip chart for variability

Turn electrode counterclockwise to remove; never pull straight out from presenting part

Administer perineal care after the patient voids as needed

INTRAUTERINE PRESSURE CATHETER
Catheter (may be fluid-filled) that internally monitors intrauterine pressure

Ensure that length line on catheter is visible at introitus

For closed-system catheters: set baseline rate between uterine contractions when uterus is relaxed

Assess proper functioning by asking patient to cough, or applying fundal pressure; observe appropriate inflection on strip chart

Maintain catheter secured to patient's leg to prevent dislodgement

■ NONSTRESS TEST
Basis for nonstress test (NST) is that the healthy fetus will exhibit acceleration of FHR and average FHR variability with fetal movement or in response to vibroacoustic stimulation

ASSESSMENT
OBJECTIVE DATA
Accelerations of FHR

Other periodic changes in FHR

Baseline changes in FHR

Evidence of fetal movement on strip chart
  Blips
  Spikes
  Momentary increases in uterine pressure

DIAGNOSTIC TESTS
Interpretation of Results of Nonstress Test (NST)

Reactive: two or more accelerations of FHR with an amplitude of 15 beats/min lasting 15 seconds or more associated with fetal movement in a 10-minute period *or* five or more FHR accelerations in a 20-minute period

Nonreactive: either less than two accelerations of FHR with an amplitude below 15 beats/min or lasting less than 15 seconds, *or* absence of accelerations associated with fetal movement in a 10-minute period, *or* less than five FHR accelerations in a 20-minute period

Suspicious: definite accelerations of FHR associated with fetal movement; however, number of accelerations or amplitude and duration do not meet criteria of reactive or nonreactive test

Unsatisfactory: quality of FHR recording is not adequate for interpretation

POTENTIAL COMPLICATIONS
Identification of fetal compromise

Detection of uteroplacental insufficiency

MULTIDISCIPLINARY MANAGEMENT
THERAPEUTIC MANAGEMENT
Begun at 32 to 34 weeks in high-risk patients

If nonreactive, proceed to vibroacoustic stimulation test (VAS) and/or CST

If reactive, repeat 1 to 2 times per week until delivery or until nonreactive

NURSING INTERVENTIONS
Explain general use of equipment and procedure to patient and significant other

Give full liquid meal (if not taken before test) to reduce bowel sounds if ordered

Request patient to void

Assist patient to assume semi-Fowler's position with
lateral uterine tilt

Monitor FHR and uterine activity externally until test can
be interpreted

Confirm fetal movement by palpation or patient
confirmation

Reinforce implications of reactive and nonreactive tests

Vibroacoustic Stimulation Test (VAS)

Monitor FHR and uterine activity (UA) until at least 10 to
15 minutes of interpretable data is obtained

Apply artificial larynx firmly to the maternal abdomen
over the fetal head

Depress the button on the artificial larynx from 2 to 3
seconds according to facility procedure

Observe the FHR strip

Reactive test: increase in FHR of at least 15 beats/min
from baseline in response to vibroacoustic
stimulation

Nonreactive test: no response of FHR to vibroacoustic
stimulation; consider proceeding to contraction
stress test

■ CONTRACTION STRESS TEST (CST)

*Assessment of uteroplacental reserve by means of
"stressing" the fetus with contractions and observing the
resultant FHR pattern*

ASSESSMENT
OBJECTIVE DATA

Periodic changes in FHR
  Accelerations
  Decelerations: early, late, variable
Baseline changes in FHR
  Tachycardia
  Bradycardia
  Absent or minimal variability
  Sinusoidal pattern

INTERPRETATION OF RESULTS

Negative: three contractions >40 seconds in a 10-minute
period without late decelerations; there is usually a
good baseline variability and acceleration of FHR with
fetal movement

Positive: persistent and consistent late decelerations
occurring with more than half the contractions

Hyperstimulation: contractions occurring more often
than q2 min and/or lasting longer than 90 seconds
  Uterine hypertonus: rise of baseline uterine tone
  Late decelerations occurring during or after excessive
  uterine activity

Suspicious: late decelerations occurring with less than
half the uterine contractions once an adequate
contraction pattern has been established

Unsatisfactory: inadequate contraction pattern or tracing
too poor to interpret; test is not interpretable and
cannot be used for clinical management

POTENTIAL COMPLICATIONS

Uterine hyperstimulation
Elevated BP
Onset of labor
Supine hypotension syndrome
Fetal compromise
Emergency birth

MULTIDISCIPLINARY MANAGEMENT
THERAPEUTIC MANAGEMENT
After Nonreactive NST

If positive CST, prepare for imminent birth
If negative CST, repeat per hospital protocol until birth or
until CST becomes positive

Preprocedural Care and Teaching

Explain general use of equipment and procedure to
patient and significant other

Give full liquid meal (if not taken before test) to reduce
bowel sounds if ordered

Request patient to void

Assist patient to assume semi-Fowler's or lateral tilt
position

Understand that contractions can be stimulated by dilute
IV oxytocin or nipple stimulation

Nipple-Stimulated Contractions

Monitor FHR and uterine activity externally to determine
baseline until at least 10-minutes of interpretable data
are obtained

Assess BP and P q15min

Defer nipple stimulation if three unstimulated
contractions of greater than 40 seconds occur
within a 10-minute period

Apply warm, moist washcloth to both breasts for several
minutes

Instruct patient to massage and/or roll nipple of one
breast for 10 minutes; if uterine contractions do not
occur, stimulate both breasts for 10 minutes

Restimulate breasts intermittently as needed to maintain
uterine contractions

If nipple stimulation does not produce desired uterine
activity, proceed to oxytocin-stimulated contraction
stress test

Oxytocin-Stimulated Contractions (Oxytocin Challenge Test; OCT)

Administer parenteral fluids with oxytocin piggybacked
into main IV line; deliver with infusion pump in
mU/min

Assess BP and P q15min

Monitor FHR and UC externally to determine baseline
uterine activity until 10 minutes of interpretable data
are obtained before administration of oxytocin

Defer oxytocin infusion if three unstimulated
contractions of greater than 40 seconds duration
occur within a 10-minute period; interpret the results

Increase dosage of oxytocin q15min to 20min as ordered

Discontinue oxytocin when three uterine contractions of greater than 40 seconds have occurred within a 10-minute period

Postprocedure Care
Continue to monitor FHR and uterine contractions until uterine activity is diminished to pretest baseline
Interpret results of test
Teach patient signs of onset of labor; labor almost never begins within 48 hours if fetus is less than 38 weeks' gestational age

Expected Outcomes
Complications are absent or minimized
Complies with procedure instructions

■ POSTPARTUM CARE
Care after birth of a fetus through the vaginal canal throughout the maternal recovery period to 6 weeks after birth

ASSESSMENT
SUBJECTIVE DATA
Uterine cramps
Painful episiotomy
Painful hemorrhoids
Heavy bleeding
Difficulty voiding
Fatigue
Emotional lability
Hunger

Constipation
Tender breasts

OBJECTIVE DATA
Skin
    Mask of pregnancy
    Striae
Breasts
    Colostrum
    Breast milk
Abdomen
    Uterine involution
        Firm (Fig. 11-7)
        Midline
        1 to 2 finger breadths (cm) below umbilicus and decreasing
    Relaxed abdominal muscles
Lochia
    Color: rubra, serosa, or alba
    Flow: heavy, moderate, light, or scant
Perineum: episiotomy clean and intact (Fig. 11-8)
    Hemorrhoids
Appropriate psychoemotional responses to childbirth

DIAGNOSTIC TESTS
Hgb, Hct
CBC with differential if indicated
Electrolytes if indicated

POTENTIAL COMPLICATIONS
Hemorrhage; soft, relaxed fundus
    Retained placental fragments
    Hematoma of episiotomy site

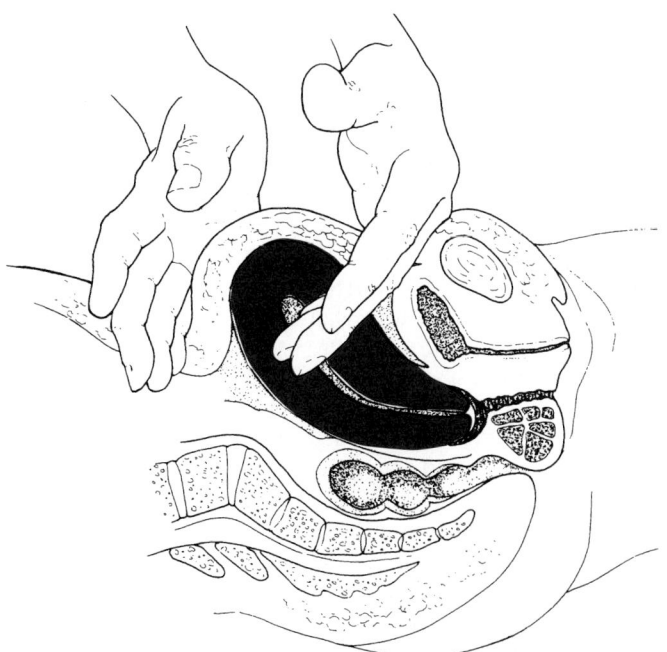

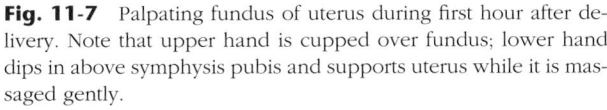
Fig. 11-7 Palpating fundus of uterus during first hour after delivery. Note that upper hand is cupped over fundus; lower hand dips in above symphysis pubis and supports uterus while it is massaged gently.

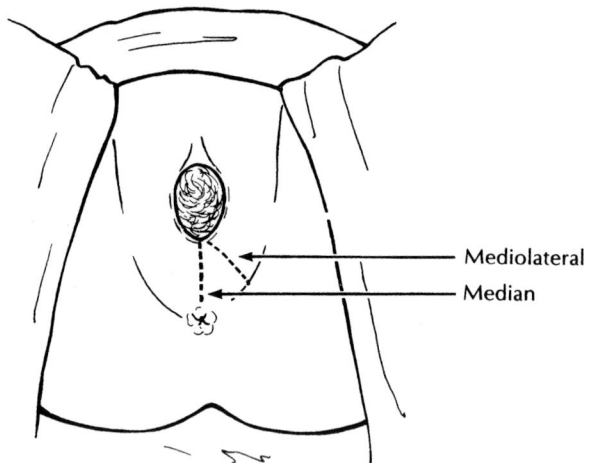

Fig. 11-8 Types of episiotomies.
(From Lowdermilk DL, Perry SE, Bobak IM: Maternity nursing, ed 5, St Louis, 1999, Mosby.)

Infection
    Elevated temperature
    Diaphoresis
    Chilling
    Nausea, vomiting
    Tachycardia
    Foul odor of lochia
    Cramping
    Drainage from episiotomy
    Edema, redness, or discoloration at incisions or
        lacerations
    Gaping sutures at incisions or lacerations
Bladder distention and/or inability to void
Painful hemorrhoids
Constipation
Thrombophlebitis
Pulmonary embolus
Engorged breasts; sore nipples
Behavioral changes
    Depression
    Withdrawal
    Lack of contact with, or care of, newborn
    Newborn abuse or neglect

MULTIDISCIPLINARY MANAGEMENT
THERAPEUTIC MANAGEMENT
Postpartum assessment with vital signs
Neurologic checks and spinal dermatomes check, along
    with vital signs, if regional anesthesia is received
IV fluids
Oxytocics as indicated
Pain medications, stool softeners, antiflatulents as
    indicated
Ice bag to perineum as indicated
Topical anesthetic to episiotomy as needed
Anesthetic ointment for hemorrhoids
Breast binder if indicated
Lactation suppression drugs
Progressive ambulation as tolerated

Laboratory tests as indicated
Regular diet as tolerated; encourage oral fluid and snacks
Intake and output as indicated
Anti-Rh globulin as indicated
Rubella vaccine as indicated
Lactation consultant as indicated

PATIENT PROBLEMS—NURSING DIAGNOSES/INTERVENTIONS

▼ Risk for fluid volume deficit related to active loss
associated with postpartum hemorrhage

Assess the following q15min until stable then q4h to 8h
    per institution policy
    Fundus location and tone
    Episiotomy condition
    Lochia amount, color, and consistency
    BP, T, P
    Level of consciousness (LOC)
If fundus is soft and/or relaxed, massage until firm *to
    prevent excessive blood loss*
Avoid unnecessary massage of fundus, *which can cause
    uterine relaxation and hemorrhage*
Teach mother normal parameters of lochia and instruct
    her to call provider if there is abnormally heavy flow
Change perineal pads q30min to 60min and/or as
    needed; report excessive bleeding to provider
Maintain parenteral fluids with oxytocics *to contract
    uterus,* as ordered
Encourage fluids po unless contraindicated
Measure intake and output for 24 hours or as ordered
Remain with patient during the first time out of bed *in
    case hemodynamic changes or orthostatic
    hypotension results in dizziness/faintness*

Expected Outcome
Does not become hypovolemic as a result of excessive
    blood loss; has vital signs that are within normal limits

▼ Pain related to episiotomy, afterbirth pains, and/
or breast discomfort

Note time when sensation has returned to lower
    extremities after spinal anesthetic
Manage pain; administer medication as ordered
Apply ice bag to perineum as ordered *to reduce swelling
    and sensation of pain*
Maintain warmth with blankets; avoid drafts in patient
    care unit
Administer anesthetic spray to episiotomy and
    hemorrhoids prn *to reduce discomfort*
Apply anesthetic ointment to hemorrhoids prn
Shower or bathe daily; avoid washing nipples of
    breast-feeding mothers at any other time *because it
    removes natural oils and contributes to skin
    irritation and discomfort*
Have mother wear supportive bra at all times *to reduce
    discomfort of heavy breasts*

Assess breasts q4h to 8h and prn

If breast-feeding, place warm, moist towel packs on engorged breasts for 15 to 30 minutes q1h to 3h *to stimulate let-down reflex,* then massage and manually express breasts or have infant nurse

If formula feeding

Never massage or manually express engorged breasts

Have mother wear snug-fitting breast binder over bra and use ice bags q1h to 3h for 15 minutes on each side if breasts are engorged *to reduce circulation and subsequent engorgement*

Stand with back toward water in shower *to avoid stimulation of breasts*

Anticipate need for pain relief

Administer pain medication as ordered and document effectiveness

Instruct mother to squeeze buttocks together when sitting down if episiotomy is painful with ambulation

Encourage mother to use relaxation techniques learned in labor for afterbirth pains during breast-feeding

Expected Outcomes

Pain is relieved or minimized

Uterine fundus is firm and pain free

Demonstrates proper breast care

▼Risk for infection related to incision and/or lacerations

Instruct patient on perineal care per hospital policy

Change perineal pad from front to back after each elimination *to prevent urethral contamination*

Observe condition of episiotomy and document same q8h to 12h

Watch for elevated temperature or other changes in vital sign parameters

Note and report any abnormal, foul-smelling drainage or discharge, *which is indicative of an infectious process*

Administer antibiotics as ordered

Expected Outcome

Episiotomy and/or lacerations heal without infection as evidenced by absence of edema and drainage

▼Urinary retention (potential) related to trauma and subsequent edema associated with childbirth process

Avoid distention of bladder; encourage voiding within 6 to 8 hours after delivery or catheterize as ordered

Encourage daily fluids to 3000 ml unless contraindicated

Encourage patient to void q4h to 6h as able

Employ techniques *to assist voiding as needed,* including voiding in shower or sitz bath if this is the only way the patient can comfortably void

Expected Outcomes

Does not experience bladder distention; voids qs following birth

▼Constipation related to pain of episiotomy and hemorrhoids secondary to childbirth process

Ensure adequate fluid intake

Sitz bath may help *to relax perianal muscles before bowel movement*

Give stool softeners or laxative as ordered

Encourage patient to ambulate as tolerated, increasing progressively

Maintain regular diet with between-meal snacks; increase amount of fruit and roughage

Anesthetic spray/ointment applied to perianal area and episiotomy site may *provide pain relief and subsequently permit bowel movement*

Expected Outcome

Has bowel movement with minimal discomfort

▼Risk for altered parenting related to transition to parenthood and role change

Recover mother and newborn in same bed under radiant heat warmer if possible *to promote visual inspection, skin to skin contact, and attachment*

Assist with holding and inspecting newborn as soon as possible after birth and prn until mother is able to become actively involved in newborn care

Encourage mother to have newborn at bedside as much as she desires *to promote attachment behaviors*

Meet mother's dependency needs during "taking in" phase

Encourage verbalization; mothers are usually extremely talkative, repeatedly relating experience of labor and birth

Understand that enthusiastic listening by nurse helps experience become more meaningful to parents

Meet mother's needs during "taking hold" phase

Reassure mother that she is performing well in all aspects of self-care and newborn care

Avoid intervening between mother and newborn regardless of how awkward her skills seem

Positively reinforce all tasks done well

Avoid negative criticism at all times

Assist and teach mother to perform all newborn care tasks: (e.g., bathing, feeding, diapering, cord care, cuddling)

Teach mother and visitors proper handwashing technique

Involve spouse or significant other in newborn care and teaching

Observe mother-newborn interaction; report to physician or social services

Mother not holding newborn while feeding

Lack of eye contact between mother and newborn

Absence of verbalization of mother to newborn

Lack of physical contact with newborn

Encourage verbalization about role of mothering, effect of new family member, and sibling rivalry, if applicable

Encourage visits by healthy siblings unless contraindicated

See Care of newborn (p. 696)

Expected Outcomes
Demonstrates adequate newborn caretaking skills
Provides an optimal environment for newborn growth and development

▼Situational low self-esteem in response to feelings of inadequacy associated with responsibilities of parenthood related to birth experience

Encourage discussion of real and perceived problems
Help mother validate the reality of her labor and birth experience
Give reassurance concerning her ability *to promote self-perception of adequacy and competency as a mother*
Help patient accept emotional ups and downs of postpartum period and explain that these feelings and changes are common during this time
Encourage rest periods throughout the day *to prevent sleep deprivation*
Provide opportunity for parent-infant interactions and involve father or significant other as possible
Support and encourage parents and/or significant other in interactions and caring for newborn

Expected Outcome
Demonstrates effective emotional adjustment and healthy self-esteem as evidenced by positive statements about self and abilities to care for infant

PATIENT/FAMILY TEACHING
Verify patient's understanding of infant security system
Caution patient to avoid coitus or douching for 4 to 6 weeks or as indicated
Demonstrate breast care and manual expression if infant is breast-feeding
Emphasize importance of nutritious diet
Explain need to carefully clean perineal region
  Wipe from front to back after urinating
  Administer perineal self-care
  Apply perineal pad from front to back
  Wash vulva and perineum, including sutures, before washing anal area when showering
Relate that absorbable sutures do not need to be removed
Instruct patient to use anesthetic spray and/or ointment to treat perineal area and/or hemorrhoids
Caution patient to avoid constipation; stool softeners or mild laxatives may be necessary
Discuss symptoms to report to provider
  Temperature > 100° F (37.8° C)
  Foul odor of lochia
Relate that shower or tub bath may be taken
Explain that lochia may continue for 3 to 4 weeks, changing from red to brown to white
Relate that menses will return 6 to 8 weeks after birth, often despite breast-feeding
  Explain that some nursing mothers do not menstruate until they wean infant from breast, whereas others resume menstruation at various times while nursing

Emphasize that pregnancy is possible 4 to 6 weeks after birth, whether mother is breast-feeding or not; discuss availability of nonprescription methods of contraception

DISCHARGE/HOME CARE PLANNING
Caution patient to avoid lifting anything heavier than the infant for 2 to 3 weeks
Explain need for planned rest periods
Relate that sitz bath may be used at home prn
Explain need for mild exercise initially
  Do not start vigorous exercise until approved by provider
  Explain that Kegel exercises can begin during early puerperium
Discuss normalcy of postpartum "blues"
Discuss need to plan for care of other children at home and discuss possible behavioral changes necessary because of new family member
Teach name of medication, dosage, time of administration, purpose, and side effects
Emphasize importance of ongoing outpatient care, including postpartum checkup
Emphasize the normalcy of feelings that may be disturbing
  Initial lack of feeling of love for infant
  Variations from prenatal expectations of what infant would look like; disappointment in sex, weight, or appearance
  Frustration caused by increased demands on time
  Feelings of being trapped
  Unsettled feelings about being a mother and parent
  Feelings of tension, nervousness, and fatigue
Discuss how to contact available community resources
  Housekeeping agencies
  Nursing care agencies
  Diaper services
  Family planning organizations
  Breast-feeding organizations
    La Leche League International
    9616 Minneapolis Ave.
    Franklin Park, IL 60131
  Parenting groups
  Publications on infant care
    Growth and development
    Parenting
    Health care
    Infant stimulation
Discuss proper principles and practice of infant care

■ CESAREAN BIRTH
Birth of a fetus through a uterine incision; most common is the transverse lower segment incision, with the classic vertical cesarean incision done less frequently

ASSESSMENT
INDICATIONS
CPD in current pregnancy
Fetal compromise
Failure to progress in labor/dystocia

Malposition of fetus
  Breech presentation
  Transverse lie
  Abnormal vertex presentation
Umbilical cord prolapse
Abruptio placentae
Placenta previa

PREOPERATIVE/DIAGNOSTIC TESTS
Fetal monitoring for fetal well-being
ECG monitoring
CBC with differential
Electrolytes
Hgb/Hct
Type and screen or cross match for blood if ordered
Urinalysis
Amniocentesis for fetal lung maturity as indicated
Ultrasound as ordered

SUBJECTIVE DATA
Uterine cramps
Incisional pain
Fatigue
Emotional lability
Hunger
Tender breasts

OBJECTIVE DATA
Skin
  Mask of pregnancy
  Striae
Breasts
  Colostrum
  Breast milk
Abdomen
  Incision clean and intact without redness or drainage
  Uterine involution
    Firm (see Fig. 11-7)
    Midline
    1 to 2 finger breadths (cm) below umbilicus and decreasing
  Relaxed abdominal muscles
Lochia
  Color: rubra, serosa, or alba
  Flow: heavy, moderate, light, or scant
Hemorrhoids
Appropriate psychoemotional responses to childbirth

POTENTIAL COMPLICATIONS
Hemorrhage; soft, relaxed uterine fundus
Shock
Anemia
DIC
Infection
  Elevated temperature
  Tachycardia
  Foul odor of lochia
Site of incision
  Redness

Pain
Swelling
Drainage
Cystitis
Engorged breasts
Pneumonia
Paralytic ileus
Thrombophlebitis
Pulmonary embolus
Behavioral changes
  Guilt
  Depression
  Withdrawal
  Lack of contact with or care of newborn
Anesthesia reaction: malignant hyperthermia
Fetal injury during surgery
Fetal blood loss during surgery
Neonatal depression/resuscitation at birth

MULTIDISCIPLINARY MANAGEMENT
THERAPEUTIC MANAGEMENT
IV fluids as indicated
Diagnostic tests as indicated
Agreement of significant other to attend cesarean birth
Anesthesia: regional or general
Abdominal surgery skin preparation
Foley catheter insertion
Oxytocic administration as indicated after birth
Vital signs per recovery room protocol
See Postpartum care (p. 685) for routine medical management

PATIENT PROBLEMS—NURSING DIAGNOSES/INTERVENTIONS

▼ Knowledge deficit related to lack of information about procedure and precesarean delivery care

Discuss with mother and significant other the reason for cesarean birth
Explain "normal" preoperative procedures and potential variations for current situation
Witness consent form and obtain baseline vital signs
Draw blood for CBC, type, and screen
Obtain urine for urinalysis
Insert Foley catheter
Maintain NPO status
Perform abdominal surgery preparation per hospital policy and aseptic technique principles and explain to patient/family
Administer IV fluids as ordered
Remove contact lenses and jewelry
Discuss presence of significant other in operating room as appropriate
Encourage parents to attend preparatory classes specifically for cesarean birth if cesarean is elective
Inform father that immediately postdelivery, he may hold infant close to mother's face and arms unless contraindicated

Expected Outcome

Verbalizes rationale for cesarean birth and cooperates with presurgical preparations

▼Pain related to postoperative condition

Anticipate need for pain medications and/or additional methods of pain relief

Note, document, and identify the following:

Reports of pain at incisional site: abdomen

Facial grimace of pain

Decreasing mobility

Relief/distraction behavior

Pain scale score

Administer pain medication as ordered, preferably via PCA pump, and evaluate its effectiveness

Monitor effectiveness of epidural if used

Provide other comfort measures that may be helpful such as repositioning or supporting with pillows

Expected Outcome

Pain is minimized/controlled

Verbalizes that she is comfortable

▼Altered cardiopulmonary and peripheral tissue perfusion related to interruption of flow secondary to postoperative immobility

Assess respiratory status with vital signs

Document and report increased respiratory rate, oxygen saturation nonproductive cough, audible rhonchi, rales, or upper airway congestion

Note symptoms of pulmonary embolus

Restlessness

Chest pain

Diaphoresis

Dyspnea

Tachycardia

Change in BP

Abnormal breath sounds

Encourage patient to cough, turn, and deep breathe q2h during first postoperative day, then prn

Encourage patient to cough while splinting *to support incision*

Encourage use of incentive spirometer

Encourage early ambulation *to promote peripheral circulation*

Discuss elevating feet prn and not crossing legs *to avoid constricting circulation*

Check Homan's sign with vital signs: *pain in calf associated with dorsiflexion is indicative of thrombophlebitis*

Note symptoms of deep vein thrombosis formation

Localized tenderness

Calf pain

Redness

Swelling

Elevated temperature

Positive Homan's sign

Expected Outcomes

Does not have respiratory congestion

Shows no signs or symptoms of pulmonary embolism or deep vein thrombosis during hospitalization

▼Altered urinary elimination (postremoval of Foley catheter) and/or constipation related to manipulation or trauma secondary to cesarean birth

Encourage voiding q4h to 6h if possible

Employ techniques to encourage voiding as needed

Explain perineal care procedures per hospital policy

Palpate lower abdomen if patient reports bladder distention and inability to void *to assess for urinary retention*

Encourage mother to do the following:

Ambulate as tolerated

Increase intake of fluids (2000 to 3000 ml/day)

Increase fruit and roughage in diet

Give stool softener/laxative as ordered *to prevent constipation*

Administer antiflatulents as ordered *to reduce discomfort associated with flatus*

Monitor intake and output until eliminating adequately

Expected Outcomes

Voids spontaneously without discomfort

Has a bowel movement within 3 to 4 days after surgery

▼Situational low self-esteem in response to feelings of inadequacy associated with unanticipated cesarean birth and interruption of anticipated childbirth experience

Encourage mother to verbalize fears and feelings of guilt and/or blame

Sense of failure at not giving birth "normally"

Feelings of being cheated or disappointed

Feelings of intrusion caused by surgical procedure

Provide support through reassurance and open communication *to promote feelings of adequacy and competence in self-care and newborn care*

Include significant other in discussions

Provide positive feedback to mother and significant other

Expected Outcomes

Verbalizes feelings of self-worth

Demonstrates appropriate coping skills

▼Risk for infection or injury related to surgical procedure

Monitor for elevated temperature or tachycardia as signs of infection

Observe incision *to identify signs of infection*

Redness

Tenderness

Swelling at incision site

Reports of pain

Unusual discharge

Elevated temperature

Change dressing prn or ordered *to inspect incision and observe for symptoms of infection*

Assess fundus, lochia, and bladder and vital signs as ordered

Evaluate vital signs for symptoms of infection (fever and tachycardia) or hemorrhage q4h and prn

Massage fundus if boggy or does not remain firm

Notify provider of deviations from normal parameters

    Boggy, displaced uterus

    Uterine tenderness at palpation

    Persistent discharge of lochia rubra

    Profuse bleeding

    Foul-smelling lochia

Expected Outcomes

Incision is clean and dry, without any signs or symptoms of infection

Uterine involution progresses normally

PATIENT/FAMILY TEACHING

Verify patients understanding of infant security program

Discuss the following with mother and significant other during the postpartum period

    Need to avoid coitus or douching for 4 to 6 weeks or as indicated by physician

    Breast care and manual expression if breast-feeding

    Need to avoid sitting with knees bent for long periods

    Care of incision

    Symptoms of wound infection to report to provider

    Importance of nutritious diet

    Need to avoid constipation; stool softeners or mild laxatives may be necessary

    Lochia may continue for 3 to 4 weeks, changing from red to brown to white

    Menses will return 6 to 8 weeks after birth unless breast-feeding

        Explain that some nursing mothers do not menstruate until weaning infant from breast

        Explain that others resume menstruation at various times while nursing

        Explain that pregnancy is possible whether mother is breast-feeding or not, 4 to 6 weeks after birth

        Discuss availability of nonprescription methods of contraception

        Name of medication, dosage, time of administration, purpose, and side effects

        Importance of follow-up outpatient care including postpartum checkup

DISCHARGE/HOME CARE PLANNING

Advise patient to avoid lifting anything heavier than infant for 4 to 6 weeks

Encourage planned rest periods

Advise patient that showers may be taken

Explain importance of exercise, need to avoid vigorous exercise until approved by provider

Discuss normalcy of postpartum "blues"

Advise about need to plan for care of other children at home and discuss possible behavioral changes necessary as a result of new family member

Discuss normalcy of feelings that may be disturbing to mother

    Initial lack of feeling of love for newborn

    Variations from prenatal expectations of what newborn would look like: disappointment in sex, weight, or appearance

    Frustration resulting from increased demands on time

    Feelings of being trapped

    Unsettled feelings about being a mother and parent

    Feelings of tension, nervousness, and fatigue

Instruct patient on how to contact available community resources

    Housekeeping agencies

    Nursing care agencies

    Diaper services

    Family planning organizations

    Breast-feeding organizations: La Leche League, lactation institutes

    Cesarean birth groups

    Parenting groups

    Publications on infant care

        Growth and development

        Parenting

        Health care

        Infant stimulation

See Care of newborn (p. 696)

DISCHARGE/HOME CARE PLANNING
FOR BREAST-FEEDING

Discuss, demonstrate, and return-demonstrate breast-feeding principles related to cesarean birth as follows:

    If desired, breast-feeding is possible

    Feed only breast milk to newborn

    Do not supplement with formula or water routinely (see Breast-feeding below)

    Take pain medication 20 to 30 minutes before nursing

    Proper positioning prevents and relieves discomfort (Fig. 11-9)

Instruct mother to do the following:

    When lying on either side

        Put newborn on side facing you

        Pull newborn's buttocks toward abdomen

        Use pillows to support the back and protect abdomen

    When sitting up in bed

        Use pillows under both knees to support them

        Place a pillow under each arm and another over abdomen

        Put newborn on side toward you in "crook" of your arm, with newborn's face and belly facing toward the mother

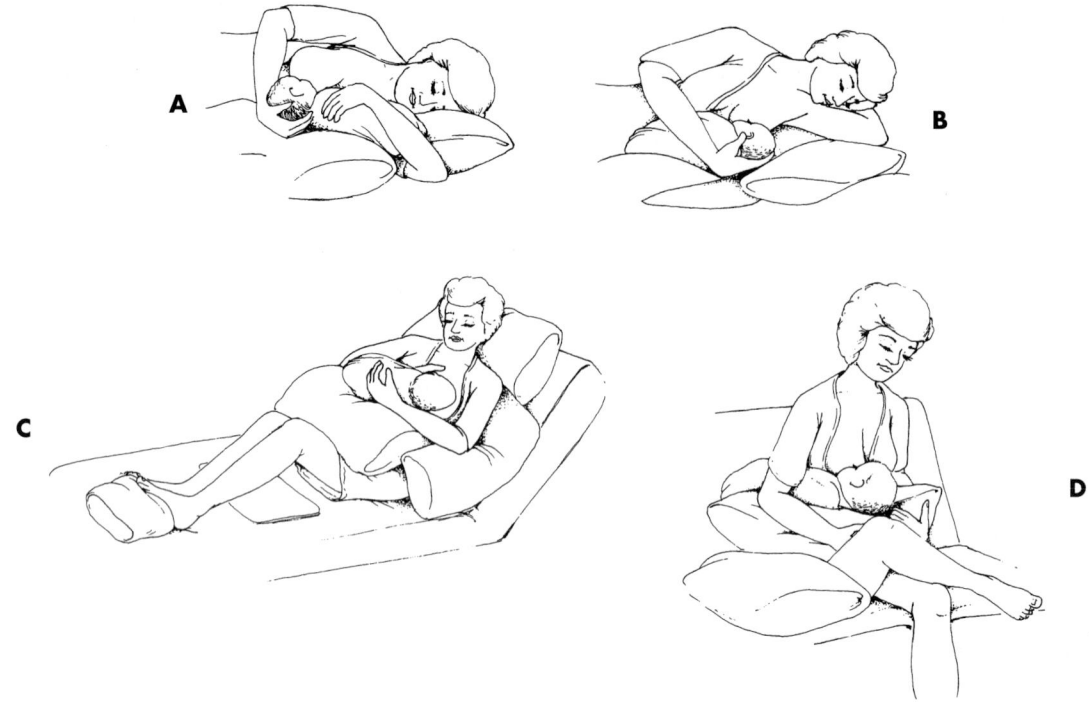

Fig. 11-9 Comfortable breast-feeding positions after cesarean delivery. **A** and **B,** Side-lying position. **C,** Sitting in bed. **D,** "Football" hold.

■ BREAST-FEEDING

ASSESSMENT
SUBJECTIVE DATA
Tenderness
Pain

OBJECTIVE DATA
Breasts
    Hardness
    Redness
    Condition of nipples
Uterine cramping while breast-feeding
Dehydration
Newborn
    Nursing more frequently than q2h
    Voiding less than 6 times daily

POTENTIAL COMPLICATIONS
Engorgement
Nipple problems
    Blistered, cracked nipples
    Inverted nipples
    Sore nipples
Mastitis
Nipple confusion of newborn

MULTIDISCIPLINARY MANAGEMENT
THERAPEUTIC MANAGEMENT
Referral to lactation specialist/consultant
Increase of caloric intake by 500 calories/day
Increase of fluid intake to 3000 ml/day unless
    contraindicated

Antibiotics for mastitis as indicated
Contraception counseling
Family planning counseling referrals as indicated

PATIENT PROBLEMS—NURSING DIAGNOSES/INTERVENTIONS

▼ Risk for fluid volume deficit in newborn related to inadequate breast-feeding

Instruct mother to do the following:
    Feed newborn when hungry
    Begin feeding newborn on one side for 10 to 30 minutes or until rate of sucking begins to slow
    Break suction of newborn's mouth on nipple by placing finger inside mouth between gums
    Avoid pulling newborn off breast without releasing suction
    Burp newborn in a sitting position after nursing at each breast
    Place newborn on opposite breast for 10 to 30 minutes or until sucking begins to slow
    Change back to other breast again until newborn seems satisfied and falls asleep
    Replace nursing bra after nursing is completed *to support breasts*
Remind mother that during newborn period total feeding time can range from 20 to 60 minutes each
Remind mother that best way to tell if newborn is getting enough milk is to listen for swallowing while sucking
Explain that adequate intake and nutrition is judged by six to eight wet diapers per day, newborn sleeping 1 to 2 hours between feedings, and newborn gaining

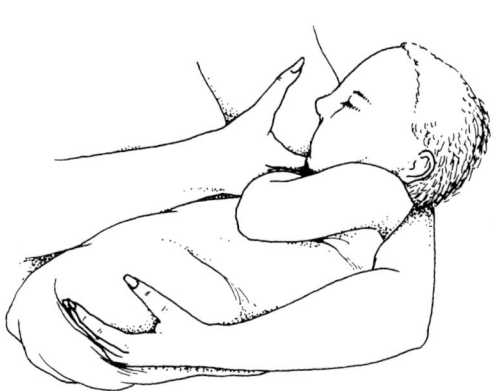

Fig. 11-10 Correct body position for breast-feeding. Head of infant is in crook of mother's arm with front of infant facing front of mother.

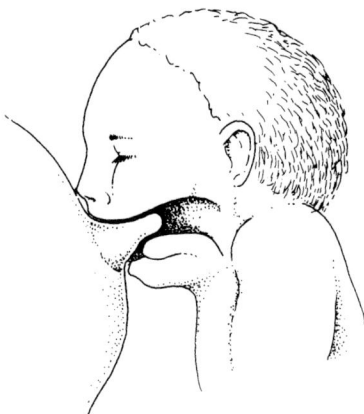

Fig. 11-11 Correct latch-on position. Infant's mouth compresses milk-collecting sinuses in areola.

weight by time of examination with first visit to health care provider

Expected Outcome
Newborn receives adequate intake for appropriate weight gain

▼Ineffective breast-feeding related to any one of multiple factors, including previous history of breast-feeding failure, poor newborn suck reflex, nonsupportive partner, interruption in breast-feeding, and lack of information about appropriate breast-feeding technique

Initiate breast-feeding as soon as mother and newborn are able (may be on delivery table); manually express both breasts q4h until infant can be nursed

See Figs. 11-10 and 11-11 for proper body and nipple positioning

Remain with mother for at least her first two breast-feeding experiences if necessary

Have mother assume most comfortable position for her; may be sitting or lying on side

Alternate breast that is used first at each feeding: place safety pin on bra as reminder

Apply small amount of hydrous lanolin to nipples *to prevent dryness and cracking as ordered;* it does not need to be washed off before next feeding

Have mother shower daily for breast and general cleanliness

Do not wash breasts with any solution except water *to avoid removing protective oils from breasts before each feeding*

Avoid using nipple shield; if necessary, use only long enough to draw nipple out so *that infant may grasp and suckle*

Demonstrate hand expression of milk (Fig. 11-12)
 Wash hands well before starting
 Cup breast with either hand (left hand for left breast, right hand for right breast)
 Place thumb above and fingers below nipple, 1 to 1½ inches behind nipple on areola (forming the letter C)

Press in toward back, then roll fingers down toward nipple, while gently pressing thumb and finger together

Do not let fingers slide on skin

Move fingers completely around areola *to reach all milk sinuses*

Alternate between breasts every few minutes

Instruct patient in appropriate techniques and relate information *to promote a successful breast-feeding experience*

Refer to specific instructions in next section

Expected Outcomes
Demonstrates appropriate breast-feeding skills with minimal discomfort

Expresses satisfaction with the breast-feeding experience

PATIENT/FAMILY TEACHING
Discuss and assist mother with the following:
 Breast-feeding reflex: "let-down" reflex
 Handwashing before breast-feeding
 Body position (see Fig. 11-10)
 Nipple position (see Fig. 11-11)
 Inversion of nipples as indicated

Explain that supply of milk is related to demand
 Giving formula only decreases milk supply
 No need to supplement
 Need for feeding often is on demand (often up to q1½h to 2h; later about q3h; breast-fed newborns usually eat q3h)

Emphasize importance of drinking at least six to eight glasses of liquid each day (water, juice, and milk) and eating a balanced diet including meat, milk, vegetables and fruits, grains and cereals

Relate that milk can be expressed into clean glass containers or into plastic disposable bottle liners

Explain that mother's fluid intake should be a minimum of 3000 ml/day unless contraindicated; a full 8-oz glass of fluid before each nursing session will help ensure adequate maternal hydration

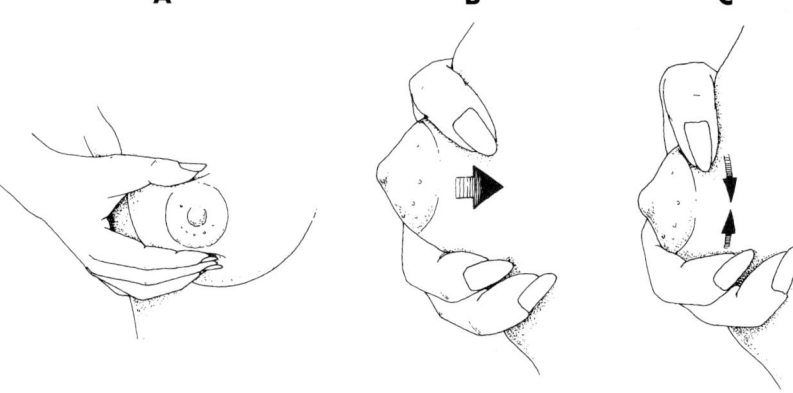

Fig. 11-12 Hand expression of breast milk. **A,** Place thumb and fingers about 1 to 1½ inches behind nipple, forming C shape. **B,** Press in toward body. **C,** Firmly press fingers together on lacteal sinuses to express milk.

Discuss adjustment of dietary intake to meet infant's needs
  Eat well-balanced, high-protein diet
    Avoid foods that cause newborn distress (colicky, crying, wakeful); do not arbitrarily omit foods usually eaten
Explain that breast milk normally has a thin, watery appearance
Explain that milk supply will be adequate if newborn nurses regularly; the more the infant nurses, the more milk is produced
Explain that six wet diapers daily of pale-colored urine is indicative that newborn is properly hydrated
Explain that four to six bowel movements daily is normal in breast-fed newborn
Explain that it may be necessary to keep newborn awake during feedings by unwrapping blanket and gently rubbing back or feet
Tell patient not to give prepared formula routinely
Explain that for several days after birth it is normal to experience uterine cramping while nursing
Explain that milk flowing from opposite breast while nursing is normal
Caution patient to avoid plastic-coated breast shields in bra between feedings; a clean, ironed handkerchief or Woolwich shield from La Leche League is preferred
Discuss treatment for engorged breasts
  Place very warm towel packs on breasts for 15 minutes
  Massage from outer breast to areola
  Manually express milk or nurse newborn
Caution patient that a breast-feeding woman can become pregnant and should be aware of contraceptive methods other than oral contraceptives, which are usually contraindicated for at least the first 3 months after giving birth
Relate that breast milk normally leaks during coitus
Discuss symptoms of complications to be reported to health care provider

DISCHARGE/HOME CARE PLANNING
Advise patient to limit visitors and household duties for the first month postpartum
Suggest that patient have relatives or friends assist with household chores, shopping, and meals prn

Explain need for planned rest periods and napping when able
Discuss how to contact local breast-feeding organizations for further information while at home
  La Leche League
  Lactation Institute
  Lactation specialists/consultants in private practice
  Breast-feeding clinics

■ POSTPARTUM HEMORRHAGE
Maternal postdelivery blood loss resulting from uterine atony, lacerations, or retained products of conception; predisposing factors include overdistended uterus (macrosomic baby, multiple gestation, hydramnios), unusually short (≤4 hours) or prolonged labor, preeclampsia (PIH) treated with magnesium sulfate, chorioamnionitis

ASSESSMENT
SUBJECTIVE DATA
Profuse bleeding
Rapid HR
Faintness
Cold sensation
Thirst

OBJECTIVE DATA
Uterine atony
  Relaxed fundus
  Dark bleeding
  Boggy, distended uterus
  Expulsion of clots
Genital lacerations
  Constant trickle of bright red blood
  Firm fundus
Retained placental tissue
  Dark bleeding
  Boggy, distended uterus
  Abdominal pain
Hematoma
  Bruising
  Edema
  Pain

Tachycardia
Progressive hypotension

DIAGNOSTIC TESTS

Vaginal examination
Clotting studies
Hgb and Hct
Hemodynamic monitoring

POTENTIAL COMPLICATIONS

Shock
    Pallor
    Restlessness
    Weak, rapid pulse
    Decreased BP
    Chills
    Difficulty in breathing
    Air hunger
See Hypovolemic shock (p. 115)
DIC
Postpartum infection
Anemia
Transfusion hepatitis
Hysterectomy (for placenta accreta)

MULTIDISCIPLINARY MANAGEMENT
THERAPEUTIC MANAGEMENT

Dilation and curettage (D & C) as indicated
Repair of lacerations
Manual removal of placental fragments
Insertion of uterine packing as indicated
IV fluids, volume expanders, or blood products
NPO
Strict intake and output
Vital signs as indicated
Antiembolic stockings as indicated
Oxygen therapy as indicated
Medications as indicated (prostaglandin [Hemabate] iron
    therapy)
Oxytocin infusion as indicated
Prostin E_2 (PGE_2) vaginal suppository as indicated
Vaginal packing as indicated
Hysterectomy

PATIENT PROBLEMS—NURSING DIAGNOSES/INTERVENTIONS

▼Fluid volume deficit related to hypovolemia associated with postpartum hemorrhage

Never leave patient unattended during active bleeding
Massage relaxed, boggy fundus until firm; *do not
    overmassage or push hard on a relaxed fundus*
Administer oxygen at 10 to 12 L/min if ordered
Administer parenteral fluids with oxytocics as ordered
    Example: oxytocin 20 to 30 U in 1 L solution infused at
        rate of 200 ml/hr (DO NOT administer an undiluted
        IV bolus of oxytocin)
Administer volume expanders or blood as ordered

Assess BP, P, and R q15min until stable, then as ordered
Palpate fundus and observe amount of vaginal bleeding
    q15min until stable
Measure intake and output
Weigh pads and linens *to estimate blood loss* (1 ml = 1 g)
Apply antiembolic stockings to legs *to enhance venous
    return*
Maintain warmth with blankets
Allay anxiety as much as possible by remaining with
    patient and offering simple, brief explanations of care
Be aware that physician may order prostaglandin IM (or
    PGE_2 vaginal suppository) *to control atony*
Continue with acute care and decrease frequency of
    nursing functions as patient's condition improves
Observe for side effects of iron therapy if ordered
Reinforce primary health care provider's explanation of
    the following, if done
    Vaginal examination
    Insertion of uterine packing
    D & C, hysterectomy

Expected Outcomes

Receives adequate fluid replacement with no untoward
    effects
Does not have symptoms of hemorrhagic/hypovolemic
    shock

▼Pain and discomfort related to uterine massage
and uterine contraction

Explain purpose of frequent postpartum assessments
    Palpation of fundus for height, position, and tone
    Uterine massage if necessary
    Lochia flow
Encourage patient to palpate fundus and learn what firm
    uterine tone feels like
Encourage patient to check fundus periodically and
    massage prn
Apply ice pack to perineum as needed *to reduce pain,
    swelling*
Promote comfort by position changes
Provide emotional support, especially if pain medication
    is contraindicated
Administer medications as ordered by primary health
    care provider and check for any reactions
Minimize other factors that could be contributing to
    discomfort such as distended bladder, episiotomy pain,
    or "afterbirth" pain

Expected Outcomes

Verbalizes symptoms to report
Demonstrates self-care as taught

PATIENT/FAMILY TEACHING

Discuss symptoms to report to primary health care
    provider
    Passage of large or several clots
    Large amount of bleeding: more than a menstrual
        period

Pain
Foul odor of vaginal drainage
See Postpartum care (p. 685)
Teach name of medication, dosage, time of administration,
purpose, and side effects

■ CARE OF NEWBORN

ASSESSMENT
OBJECTIVE DATA
General
Apgar scores
Quality of cry and respirations
Skin color
Apical pulse, HR, respirations
Muscle tone
Reflexes
Thermal control
Cord condition
Feeding and sucking pattern
Stool pattern
Voiding pattern
Congenital defects

Specific
Apgar scores
    HR; presence of murmur
    Respiratory effort
    Muscle tone
    Reflex irritability
    Color
Abnormalities or malformations
Head circumference: normal 33 to 35 cm
Chest circumference: normal 30 to 33 cm
Birth-related trauma: presence of caput,
    cephalohematoma, and forceps marks
Amount of subcutaneous fat
Cry
    Lusty
    Feeble
    High pitched
    Absent
    Asymmetric facies
Umbilical cord
    Drainage
    Bleeding
    Number and type of vessels
    Presence or absence of Wharton's jelly
Unusually high or low temperature: normal, 97.7° F
    (36.5° C) axillary
Edema (except for presenting part)
Color
    Pink
    Jaundice
    Pallor
    Gray, dusky
    Cyanosis
    Plethora

Gastrointestinal system
    Hard and soft palate intact
    Refusal to feed
    Excessive mucus
    Regurgitation; vomiting
    Abdominal distention
    Imperforate anus
    Stools
        Meconium
        Bloody
        Diarrhea
        Absent
Neurologic system
    Moro's reflex: present, absent, asymmetric, or
        hyperactive
    Sucking reflex: strong or weak
    Rooting reflex: good or poor
    Reflexes: grasp (palmar and plantar), tonic neck,
        stepping and Babinski
    Suck/swallow coordination
    Tremors
    Twitching
    Seizure activity
    Loss of motion of an extremity
State of consciousness
    Deep sleep
    Active REM sleep
    Drowsy
    Wide awake (quiet alert)
    Active awake (active alert)
    Crying
Respiratory rate: normal 40 to 60/min
    Tachypnea
    Shallow or periodic breathing
    Nasal flaring
    Retractions
    Expiratory grunt
Cardiovascular rate: normal 110 to 160 beats/min
    Tachycardia
    Bradycardia
    BP: normal 60/30 to 90/50 mm Hg
Musculoskeletal system
    Muscle tone
    Muscle strength
    Limpness
    Weakness
    Rigidity
    Asymmetry
    Swelling of skull or spine
    Abnormal position or posture of extremity
Skin
    Milia
    Birthmarks
    Pustules
    Abrasions
    Rash
    Petechiae
    Ecchymosis
    Condition of circumcision

Genitourinary system
  Hypospadias
  Epispadias
  Undescended testicles
  Indeterminate sex
  Failure to void

DIAGNOSTIC TESTS
Cord blood samples
Phenylketonuria (PKU; newborn screening examination)
Hct; thyroid studies (T_3, T_4)
Bilirubin

POTENTIAL COMPLICATIONS
Altered thermoregulation
Birth injuries
Hyperbilirubinemia
Congenital defects
Need for resuscitation at birth

MULTIDISCIPLINARY MANAGEMENT
THERAPEUTIC MANAGEMENT
Vitamin K IM injection
Newborn screening examination (PKU, thyroid)
Hepatitis B vaccine
Eye prophylaxis
Feeding schedule
Cord care protocol
Circumcision care
Chemstrip as indicated
Hct
Glucose screen
Daily weights
Rectal temperature once, then axillary temperature per protocol

PATIENT PROBLEMS—NURSING DIAGNOSES/INTERVENTIONS
Postbirth Nursing Procedures
Perform stabilization procedures (Fig. 11-13)
Take Apgar scores at 1, 5 (and 10 minutes after birth if 5-minute Apgar is <8)
Apply clamp to umbilical cord
Identify newborn according to facility policy: bracelet, and/or footprints
Perform screening examination for congenital defects
Assist with newborn's warm water bath as indicated
Show warmed newborn to parents; identify sex and check identification bracelets initially and at each visit to mother and at discharge
Encourage parents to hold newborn as condition of newborn and parents permits to promote attachment and family-centered care
Perform the following according to facility policy
  Weigh newborn
  Measure length, head, chest, and abdominal circumference per institution policy

Administer medication as ordered
  Eye prophylaxis
  Vitamin K therapy
Do resuscitation documentation
Do newborn admitting assessment
Perform cord care
Perform neuromuscular maturity and physical maturity assessment (Ballard rating) (Figs. 11-14, 11-15, and 11-16)
Give sponge bath daily until umbilical cord falls off, then bathe daily, washing hair 2 to 3 times per week
Perform neonatal behavioral assessment and share infant responses with parents
Administer circumcision care; apply petrolatum gauze to penis as appropriate
Perform newborn assessments as required by policy and/or newborn condition; perform the following:
  Note time of first voiding and meconium stool
  Auscultate heart rate hourly twice and prn
    Report rate above 180 or below 100 beats/min to primary health care provider
    Report heart sounds heard on right side of chest
    Report murmur
Assess respiratory rate q30min × 4 and prn
Assess quality of respirations and report if abnormal
Perform heel stick for blood glucose testing if newborn is at risk for hypoglycemia or hypothermia
Provide for sucking needs with pacifier as indicated (be aware that homemade pacifiers are unsafe)
Check rectal temperature one time to determine patency of anus
Administer eye prophylaxis and vitamin K therapy as ordered
Administer sterile water to establish adequate sucking/swallowing if this has not been established by infant breast-feeding in the delivery room
Administer feedings as ordered
Apply alcohol or triple dye to cord according to facility policy; remove cord clamp when cord is dry (usually about 24 hours after birth)

PATIENT PROBLEMS—NURSING DIAGNOSES/INTERVENTIONS

▼ Risk for ineffective thermoregulation related to cold stress, hypoglycemia, hypoxemia, or immature thermoregulation mechanism

Recover mother and baby together under radiant heat warmer if possible (e.g., provide neutral thermal environment for infant with warmed blankets)
Observe newborn nude, if possible, for 1 to 2 hours postbirth while maintaining neutral thermal environment
Maintain axillary temperature at 97.7° F (36.5° C); check q30min/2 hr and until stable
Avoid bathing for first hour and until axillary temperature is stable at 97.7° F (36.5° C) and other vital signs are stable *to prevent cold stress*
Return to radiant warmer after bath until axillary temperature restabilizes to 97.7° F (36.5° C)

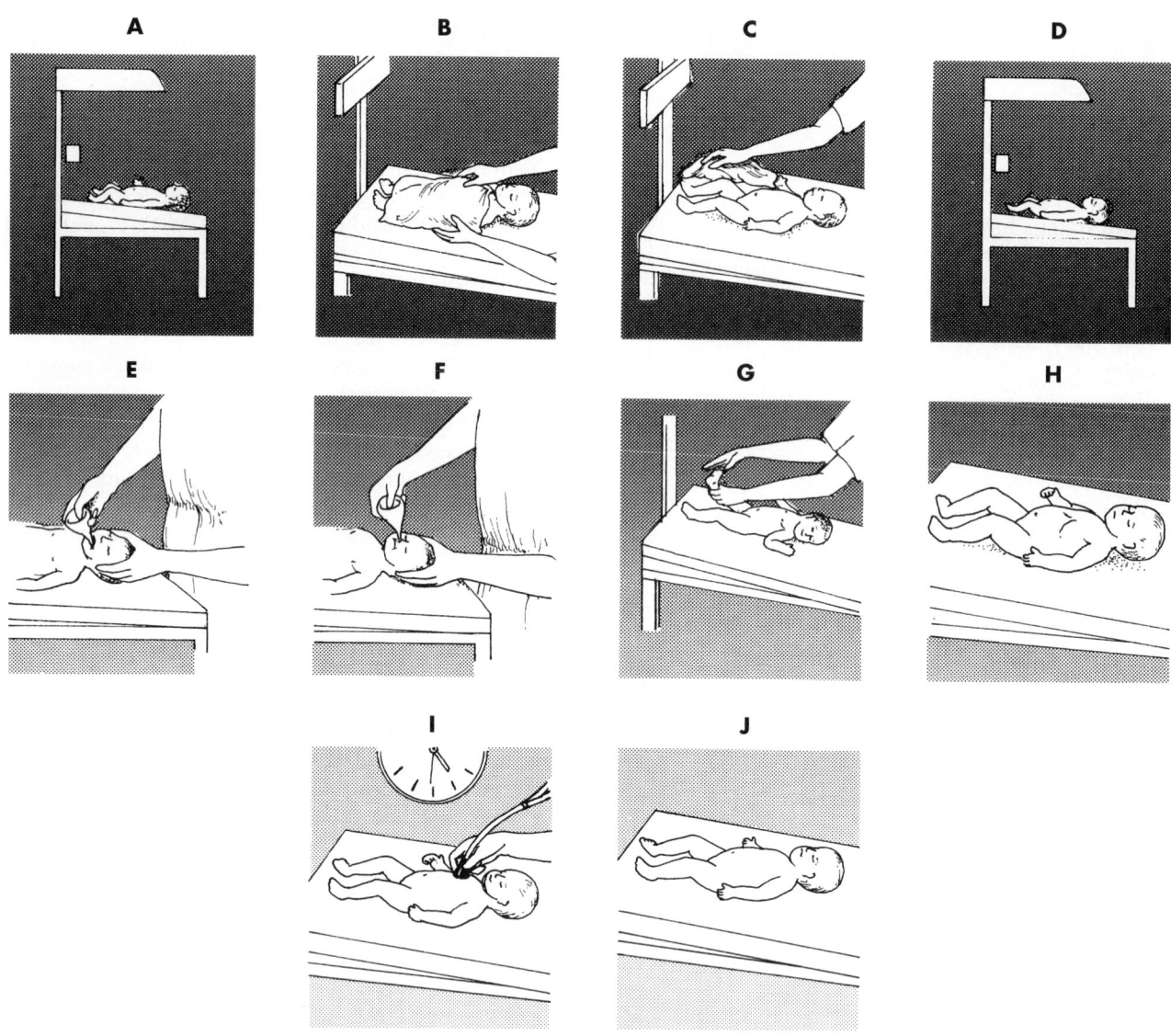

Fig. 11-13 Immediate stabilization of newborn at delivery—sequence of interventions for assessment at birth. **A,** Place newborn under radiant heat warmer in slight Trendelenburg position. **B,** Dry immediately. **C,** Remove wet linens. **D,** Position newborn with head and neck in "sniffing" position. **E** and **F,** Suction oropharynx, then nasopharynx with bulb syringe as needed. Not shown: Suction oropharynx, trachea, and stomach as necessary with No. 10 French catheter connected to wall suction of 80 to 100 mm Hg per gauge. **G,** Tactile stimulate by slapping twice on sole of foot. **H,** Assess respirations. **I,** Assess heart rate by apical pulse. **J,** Assess color. Resuscitate as indicated by assessment.

Expected Outcome

Newborn maintains normal axillary temperature of 97.7° to 98.6° F (36.5° to 37° C)

▼ Ineffective airway clearance related to coordination of suck-swallow-gag reflexes

Keep bulb syringe in crib at all times; suction as needed

Hold newborn for feedings: *never prop bottles* (be aware that although demand feedings are preferred, newborn may need to be awakened if longer than 4- to 5- hour intervals occur between feedings)

Reposition q2h and prn; place on right side or back after feedings

Periodically reassess respiratory rate and rhythm

Perform "football hold" and use obstructed airway maneuvers recommended by American Heart Association as needed for choking

Expected Outcome

Maintains patent airway as evidenced by normal respiratory rate, depth, and rhythm and clear breath sounds

PATIENT/FAMILY TEACHING

Teach principles of, demonstrate and have parents return-demonstrate, and document inpatient teaching plan

Newborn care: bathing, feeding and burping, changing diaper, caring for cord and/or circumcision, taking temperature (rectal and axillary)

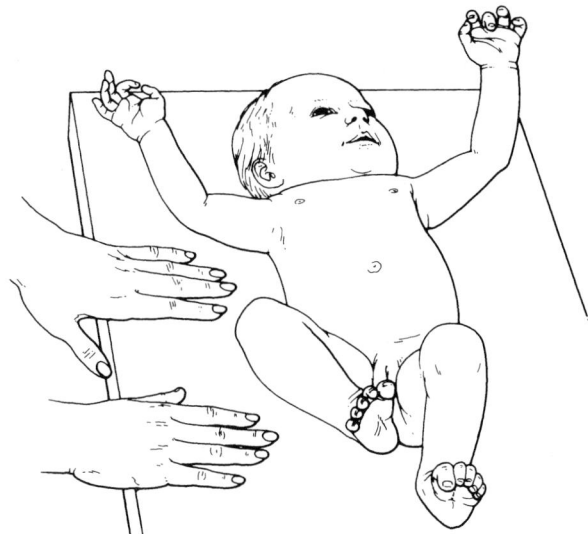

Fig. 11-14 The Moro or startle reflex. Note the position of the arms and the index finger and thumb.
(From Scipien GM et al: Pediatric nursing care, *St Louis, 1990, Mosby.)*

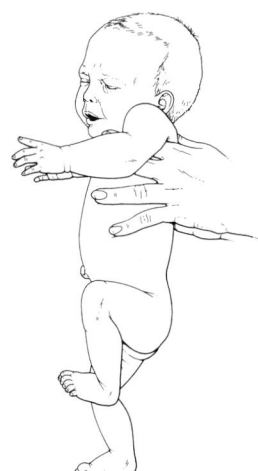

Fig. 11-16 The tonic neck reflex demonstrating the typical asymmetric fencer position.
(From Scipien GM et al: Pediatric nursing care, *St Louis, 1990, Mosby.)*

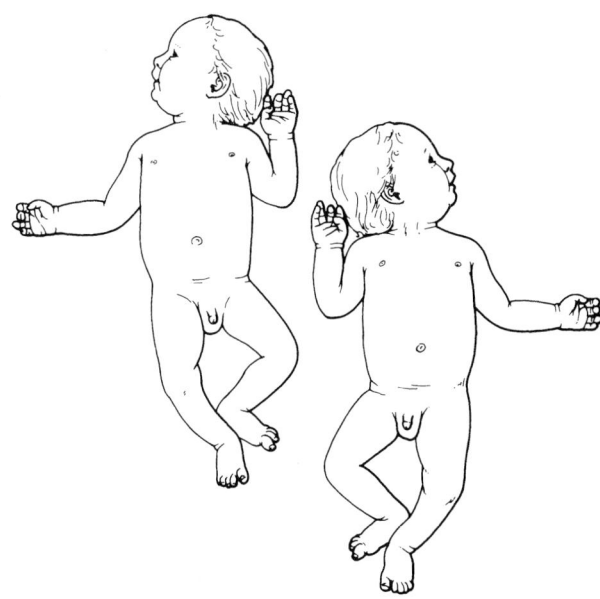

Fig. 11-15 The stepping reflex.
(From Scipien GM et al: Pediatric nursing care, *St Louis, 1990, Mosby.)*

Discuss conflicts of parental roles
    Idealized versus realistic role of parenting
    Love, resentment, or indifference toward newborn
    Personal needs and demands of parenting
Describe how to obtain emergency care if required
Identify abnormal signs and symptoms to report to
    provider
    Jaundice
    Fever lasting longer than 24 hours
    Newborn pulling on ears
    Productive cough
    Vomiting
    Refusal to eat
    Diarrhea
    Lethargy

BIBLIOGRAPHY

American Academy of Pediatrics and American College of Obstetricians and Gynecologists: *Guidelines for perinatal care,* ed 4, Washington DC, 1997, The Academy and the College.

Bajo K, Hager J, Smith J: Clinical focus: keeping moms and babies together, *Lifelines* 2(2):44, 1998.

Beare PG, Myers JL: *Adult health nursing,* St Louis, 1998, Mosby.

Beger D, Cook CAL: Postpartum teaching priorities: the viewpoints of nurses and mothers, *JOGNN* 27(2):161, 1998.

Carlson K et al: *Primary care of women,* St Louis, 1995, Mosby.

Eakes M, Brown H: Home alone: meeting the needs of mothers after cesarean birth, *Lifelines* 2(1):36, 1998.

Grabo TN et al: Uterine myomas: treatment options, *JOGNN* 28(1):23, 1999.

Jarvis C: *Physical examination and health assessment,* Philadelphia, 1992, WB Saunders.

Lambden MP et al: Women's sense of well-being before and after hysterectomy, *JOGNN* 26(5):540, 1997.

Instructions for formula preparation or pumping and
    storage of breast milk
Breast-feeding or formula feeding
Discuss issues related to use of disposable and recyclable
    cotton diapers
Review
    Importance of dressing newborn according to
        temperature of day; avoid overheating
    Importance of natural home environment; avoid
        unnatural quietness and overheating of home
    How to seek assistance for newborn problems and
        concerns of parenthood (e.g., pediatrician's phone
        number, support groups)

Lawrence R: *Breastfeeding: a guide for the medical profession,* ed 5, St Louis, 1998, Mosby.

Lowdermilk DL, Perry SE, Bobak IM: *Maternity and women's health care,* ed 6, St Louis, 1997, Mosby.

Lowdermilk DL, Perry SE, Bobak IM: *Maternity nursing,* ed 5, St Louis, 1999, Mosby.

NANDA Nursing Diagnoses: Definitions and classification 1999-2000, Philadelphia, 1999, North American Nursing Diagnosis Association.

Parer JT: *Handbook of fetal heart rate monitoring,* ed 2, Philadelphia, 1997, WB Saunders.

Ruiz RJ: Mechanisms of full-term and preterm labor: factors influencing uterine activity, *JOGNN* 27(6):652, 1998.

Riordan J: Predicting breast-feeding problems, *Lifelines* 2(6):31, 1998.

Sampselle CM et al: Physical activity and postpartum well-being, *JOGNN* 28(1):41, 1999.

Seidel HM et al: *Mosby's guide to physical examination,* ed 3, St Louis, 1995, Mosby.

Thompson JD, Rock JA: *Te Linde's operative gynecology,* ed 7, Philadelphia, 1992, Lippincott.

Thompson JM et al: *Mosby's clinical nursing,* ed 4, St Louis, 1997, Mosby.

Tucker SM: *Pocket guide to fetal monitoring and assessment,* St Louis, 1996, Mosby.

CATHERINE MCAULEY HEALTH SYSTEM
Ann Arbor, Michigan 48106

Critical Path for: Gynecologic Malignancies

NMP(s): N-K-024: Gynecologic Surgery   Variance Yes_____ No_____

C-P-090: Postoperative Gynecology Patient   DRG/ICD9 Code: DRG - 353, 354, 355, 357

Primary Nurse(s):_____

Case Manager:_____

Page 1 of 3

	Date_____ PPT Appointment	Date_____ ☐ Inpatient Admission (SDA N/A)	Date_____ Surgery ☐ Admission
ACTIVITY	☐ Ambulate as tolerated	☐ Ambulate as tolerated	• Reposition with encouragement q 2-4 hr x 12 hr ☐ Evening: dangle and take steps at bedside ☐ Braden Scale = _____
ASSESSMENT	• History and physical by MD or PA in PPT ☐ Nursing data base by unit RN in PPT (Include assessment psych/social/spiritual needs/feeling r/t sexuality) ☐ Special needs_____ _____ _____ • Describes procedure R/T changes in body function • Opportunity to discuss feeling R/T surgery and recovery • Mutual goal setting initiated	• Complete nursing data base and admission profile • VS q shift • Assess response to bowel prep	• Implement NMP for postop Gyn pt. • Complete nursing data base and admission profile • Assess surgical drsg/incision with VS checks and prn • Assess characteristics of urine and voiding while on I & O • VS q 2 hr x 2, q 4 hr x 4 • LOC c/VS checks x 12 hr • Breath sounds q 8 hr • Bowel sounds q 8 hr until passing gas then BID until first BM • Assess patency tubes/drains
CONSULTS REFERRAL	☐ Cardiology Other:_____ ☐ Anesthesia _____ ☐ Social work ☐ Pastoral care ☐ Home Care	• Follow-up preop referrals • Notify HO with values outside of parameters	☐ Notify HO with values outside of parameters
TREATMENTS (Meds, Diet, etc.)	• Explanation of perioperative procedures • Instruct medications to take day of surgery per anesthesia guidelines • Iron po if donating blood • Stop ASA 10 days or NSAIDS 3 days before OR	• NPO x water, bowel prep, and medications • Start IV per MD order • I & O q shift • Bowel prep per MD order • Measure and order SCD • Medications as ordered	• Strict NPO • IV per MD order ☐ Foley cath to DD ☐ Suprapubic to DD ☐ NG to SX • Other drains_____ or ostomy: _____ • I & O q 4 hr or as ordered ☐ Instruct use of incentive spirometer ☐ C & DB with use IS • SCD • Pain management • Meds as ordered
DC PLANNING	• Assess home; D/C plans/needs	• Continue	• Continue
PATIENT EDUCATION	• MD office/PPT provides Gyn class flier ☐ Attends Preop Gyn class • Implement NMP: K/D R/T Gyn surgery • Initiate PER	• Instruct use of incentive spirometer, leg exercises, C & DB • Reinforce preop education	• Refer to PER, PCIS
DIAGNOSTICS	• Anesthesia guidelines ☐ Autologus or directed donor blood donations		• Labs R/T surgery • CBC
SIGNATURES			
SHIFT/INITIALS			

6111-017 4/94

Continued

CATHERINE MCAULEY HEALTH SYSTEM
Ann Arbor, Michigan 48106

Critical Path for: Gynecologic Malignancies
NMP(s): N-K-024: Gynecologic Surgery   Variance   Yes _____   No _____
C-G-066: Postoperative Gynecology Patient   DRG/ICD9 Code: DRG - 353, 354, 355, 357
Primary Nurse(s): _____
Case Manager: _____

	Date _____ POD 1	Date _____ POD 2	Date _____ POD 3	Date _____ POD 4	Date _____ POD 5	Date _____ POD 6
ACTIVITY	☐ Ambulate BID, progress as tolerated • Assess with AM Care	• Ambulate TID to QID in hallway, progress as tolerated				
ASSESSMENT	• Assess integrity of surgical drsg(s) • Continue to assess characteristics of urine and voiding while on I & O • VS q 4 hr • Breath sounds q 8 hr W/A • Bowel sounds q 8 hr W/A • Assess tubes/drains prn • Weight qd	• Drsg removed per MD; assess incision q 8 hr W/A. Assist with care • VS q 4 hr	• VS q 4 hr to q shift			
CONSULTS REFERRALS	• Continue as applicable					
TREATMENTS (Meds, Diet, etc.)	• Strict NPO • IV per MD order • Foley catheter to DD • NG to sx • Continue drains • Other _____ • I & O q 4° or as ordered • Assist with use IS, C & DB • SCD • Pain management • Other meds	Diet _____ IV: Yes☐ No☐ Foley: Yes☐ No☐ NG: Yes☐ No☐ _____ Yes☐ No☐	Diet _____ IV: Yes☐ No☐ Foley: Yes☐ No☐ NG: Yes☐ No☐ _____ Yes☐ No☐	Diet _____ IV: Yes☐ No☐ Foley: Yes☐ No☐ NG: Yes☐ No☐ _____ Yes☐ No☐	Diet _____ IV: Yes☐ No☐ Foley: Yes☐ No☐ NG: Yes☐ No☐ _____ Yes☐ No☐	Diet _____ IV: Yes☐ No☐ Foley: Yes☐ No☐ NG: Yes☐ No☐ _____ Yes☐ No☐
DC PLANNING	• Continue	• D/C info sheet given to pt. per RN assessment				
PATIENT EDUCATION	• Refer to PER	☐ Pt. instructed in incision care	☐ Pt. participates in incision care • D/C education with pt and/or SO per RN assessment			• Discharge prescriptions per MD
DIAGNOSTICS	• CBC, platelets, BUN, CR, Lytes in AM		• CBC, platelets, BUN, CR, Lytes in AM			
SIGNATURES						
SHIFT/INITIALS						

6111-017 4/94

CATHERINE MCAULEY HEALTH SYSTEM
Ann Arbor, Michigan 48106

Critical Path for: Gynecologic Malignancies

NMP(s): N-K-024: Gynecologic Surgery   Variance Yes_____ No_____

C-G-066: Postoperative Gynecology Patient   DRG/ICD9 Code: DRG - 353, 354, 355, 357

Primary Nurse(s): _____

Case Manager: _____

	Date_____ POD 7	Date_____ POD 8	Date_____ POD 9	Initial box if PATIENT OUTCOMES met. If not, document variance. NA = not applicable
ACTIVITY	☐ Ambulate ad lib			☐ Ambulated as tolerated Date_____
ASSESSMENT	• Assess incision BID prn • Assess characteristics urine voiding pattern prn • VS q shift • Breath sounds BID prn • Bowel sounds BID prn			☐ Collaborative NMP completed Date_____ ☐ Incision clean, dry, & intact Date_____ ☐ Urinating without difficulty Date_____ ☐ BP, HR, & temp at baseline Date_____ ☐ Lungs CTA/baseline Date_____ ☐ Passing flatus Date_____ ☐ Goal setting completed Date_____
CONSULTS REFERRALS	• Continue as applicable _____			Consults completed: ☐ Social service Date_____ ☐ Pastoral care Date_____ ☐ Home care Date_____ ☐ APS Date_____ ☐ Other_____ Date_____
TREATMENTS (Meds, Diet, etc.)	Diet_____ ☐ Foley cath ☐ Suprapubic tube ☐ Other_____ • I & O prn • Pain management • Other meds			☐ General diet Date_____ ☐ Performs ISC Date_____ ☐ D/C'd with Foley-dd; care instructed with demonstration Date_____ ☐ Leg bag use instructed with demonstration Date_____ ☐ Suprapubic tube care Date_____ ☐ Ostomy care: type Date_____
DC PLANNING	• Continue			☐ Discharged Date_____
PATIENT EDUCATION	• Continue prn			☐ Chemotherapy information Date_____ ☐ Radiation therapy information Date_____ ☐ KD NMP completed Date_____ ☐ D/C Education completed (see PER) Date_____ ☐ BSE video viewed Date_____ ☐ Other_____ Date_____
DIAGNOSTICS				
SIGNATURES				
SHIFT/INITIALS				

6111-017 4/94

1

BARNES

**CARE PATH®
702
VAGINAL HYSTERECTOMY**

SERVICE		PHYSICIAN		
PRIMARY NURSE		PRIMARY NURSE		

DC DATE	ADM DATE	DATE OF SURGERY	**A-8**	

Problem Number	PATIENT PROBLEMS/NURSING DIAGNOSES
#1	LACK OF KNOWLEDGE
#2	ALTERATION IN COMFORT
#3	POTENTIAL ALTERATION IN URINARY ELIMINATION
#4	POTENTIAL FOR INFECTION
#5	POTENTIAL ALTERATION IN BOWEL ELIMINATION
#6	POTENTIAL ALTERATION IN BODY IMAGE * IF APPROPRIATE

#	2, 3, 4, 5, 6			3	3, 4, 5
	ASSESSMENT/MONITORING	CONSULTS	PROCEDURES/TEST	TREATMENT	ACTIVITY
PRE ADMIT	Risk factors for surgery Emotional response Comprehension of preop instructions		Type & X Autologous Donation CBC *CXR *ECG		
DAY 1 OP DAY	Pain control I & O S & Ss of shock Vaginal drainage, vaginal packing Bowel sounds Lung sounds Activity level Tolerance of PO fluids N/V VS Fall prevention **VS stable** **Pain controlled w/PCA**	Anesthesia		Foley	TCDB q 2 hr ×1 ×2 ×3 ×4 ×5 ×6 ×7 ×8 ×9 ×10 ×11 ×12 Dangle 6 hr postop Tolerates dangling at bedside
	SIGNATURE	INIT.	SIGNATURE	INIT. SIGNATURE	INIT.

702

Used by permission of Barnes Hospital, St Louis, Missouri.

2

BARNES

CARE PATH®
702
VAGINAL HYSTERECTOMY

CNS	DIETARY	RT	
HOME HEALTH	OT	OTHER	
PT	SW	OTHER	**A-8**

Problem Number	PATIENT PROBLEMS/NURSING DIAGNOSES

2, 4, 5	4	1	1, 2, 3, 4, 5, 6	1	INITIALS (SEE KEY AT BOTTOM)		
MEDS / IVS	NUTRITION	PATIENT/FAMILY EDUCATION	DISCHARGE PLANNING	PSYCHOSOCIAL/ EMOTIONAL/ SPIRITUAL NEEDS			
		Reason & implications of surgery (Loss of fertility) Preop teaching: Tests Procedure NPO after MN Activities before surgery IV Foley Immediate postop activities: TCDB Activity PO intake Pain control **States reason surgery is necessary.** **States organ(s) removed during surgery** **Defines term "sterilization"**		*Social Work for: Needs expressed by pt. High risk for problems with coping (no children, childcare problems during hospitalization)			
IV PCA *ATDs	Clear liquids after surgery Advance Diet as tolerated **Tolerates PO fluids w/o nausea**	Function of PCA Importance of early ambulation, PO intake, and return of bowel and bladder function	*Social Work if advanced age, ≥70 living alone, and/or financial concerns **Pt./family verbalizes understanding of Care Path.** **Estimated length of stay and plan of care mutually set with pt./family**				

SIGNATURE	INIT.	SIGNATURE	INIT.	SIGNATURE	INIT.

Continued

#	2, 3, 4, 5, 6			3	3, 4, 5
	ASSESSMENT/MONITORING	**CONSULTS**	**PROCEDURES/TEST**	**TREATMENT**	**ACTIVITY**
DAY 2 POD 1	Pain control I & O S & Ss of shock Vaginal drainage, vaginal packing Bowel sounds Voiding Tolerance of diet VS Emotional response **Pain controlled with PO meds**		*CBC	d/c foley in AM **Voiding w/o pain, frequency, urgency, or retention**	Up with assistance **Ambulates with assistance**
DAY 3 POD 2	DC Day				Up ad lib Independent in ambulation
DISCHARGE	**Vital signs stable** **H & H WNL** **Vaginal drainage similar to menstrual bleeding in amount and character** **Absence of dysuria, hematuria, burning, frequency, or urgency**			**Voiding w/o pain, frequency, or urgency**	**Able to ambulate and perform self-care as before surgery.**
	SIGNATURE	**INIT.**	**SIGNATURE**	**INIT.**	**SIGNATURE**	**INIT.**

2, 4, 5	4	1	1, 2, 3, 4, 5, 6	1	INITIALS		
MEDS/IVS	NUTRITION	PATIENT/FAMILY EDUCATIONS	DISCHARGE PLANNING	PSYCHOSOCIAL/ EMOTIONAL/ SPIRITUAL NEEDS	(SEE KEY AT BOTTOM)		
IV: Hep lock/KVO in PM PO analgesic d/c PCA in PM if tolerates PO fluids *ATBs *Stool softeners	Regular Diet Tolerates PO intake w/o nausea & vomiting	PO pain meds Begin DC teaching: (S & Ss to report to MD) Increased vaginal discharge Temp ≥101°F (38.5°C) Urinary incontinence, dysuria, painful urination Activity: Up ad lib, no driving for 2 weeks, no heavy lifting for 6 weeks, no douching, intercourse, or tampons until directed by MD Diet: regular as permitted d/c meds: purpose, dosage, route, schedule, side effects of analgesics and laxatives, stool softeners, and other prn.		Provide opportunity to discuss physical, psychosocial, and sexual impact of surgery			
	Regular Diet	Reinforce DC teaching		Provide opportunity to discuss physical, psychosocial, and sexual impact of surgery			
Pain control with PO medication	**Able to tolerate PO intake w/o nausea and vomiting**	**Verbalizes understanding of signs to report to MD, activity limitations, diet, personal hygiene, and medications**	**Able to perform ADLs independently or with assistance of appropriate community resources**	**Able to verbalize concerns about impact of surgery**			
SIGNATURE	**INIT.**	**SIGNATURE**	**INIT.**	**SIGNATURE**			**INIT.**

CHAPTER

12

Integumentary System

■ INTEGUMENTARY SYSTEM ASSESSMENT

■ SUBJECTIVE DATA

Skin
   Pruritus
   Painful
   Rash
   Oily
   Dry
   Rough
   Bumpy
   Thin
   Peeling
   Puffy
   Blisters
   Hot
   Cold
   Changes in skin color
   Liver spots: aging spots
   Boils
   Use of Retin-A, antibiotics

■ OBJECTIVE DATA (Fig. 12-1)

Skin
   Color
      Cyanosis
         Lips
         Circumoral area
         Mucous membranes
         Earlobes
         Nail beds
      Jaundice: sclera, skin
      Pallor: conjunctiva, nail beds
      Pigmentation distribution; freckling, moles
   Turgor
   Elasticity
   Intactness
   Rashes
   Moisture
   Temperature
   Cleanliness
   Odor
   Edema
   Needle marks

Insect bites
Scabies
Acne, calluses, corns
Exudate
Uremic frost: beard, eyebrows
Sclerema
Striae
Pressure areas over bony prominences
Pressure ulcers
Nails
   Cleanliness
   Brittleness
   Condition of surrounding tissue
   Clubbing of fingers and toes
   Lines, pitting
   Ram's horn shape: turning under fingertip
   Spoon shape: concave
Hair
   Distribution and configuration
   Texture
   Color
   Quantity
   Parasites
   Alopecia
Lesions
   Macula (<5 mm) (freckles, moles)
      Flat
      Discolored
   Papule (<5 mm) (warts, eczema)
      Elevated
      Discolored
   Patch (>5 mm) (port wine marks)
      Flat
      Discolored
      Scaly
   Vesicle (blister, varicella)
      Elevated
      Superficial
      Serous exudate
   Pustule (acne, impetigo)
      Elevated
      Purulent exudate
   Bulla (large blister, pemphigus)
      Flaccid
      Tense

709

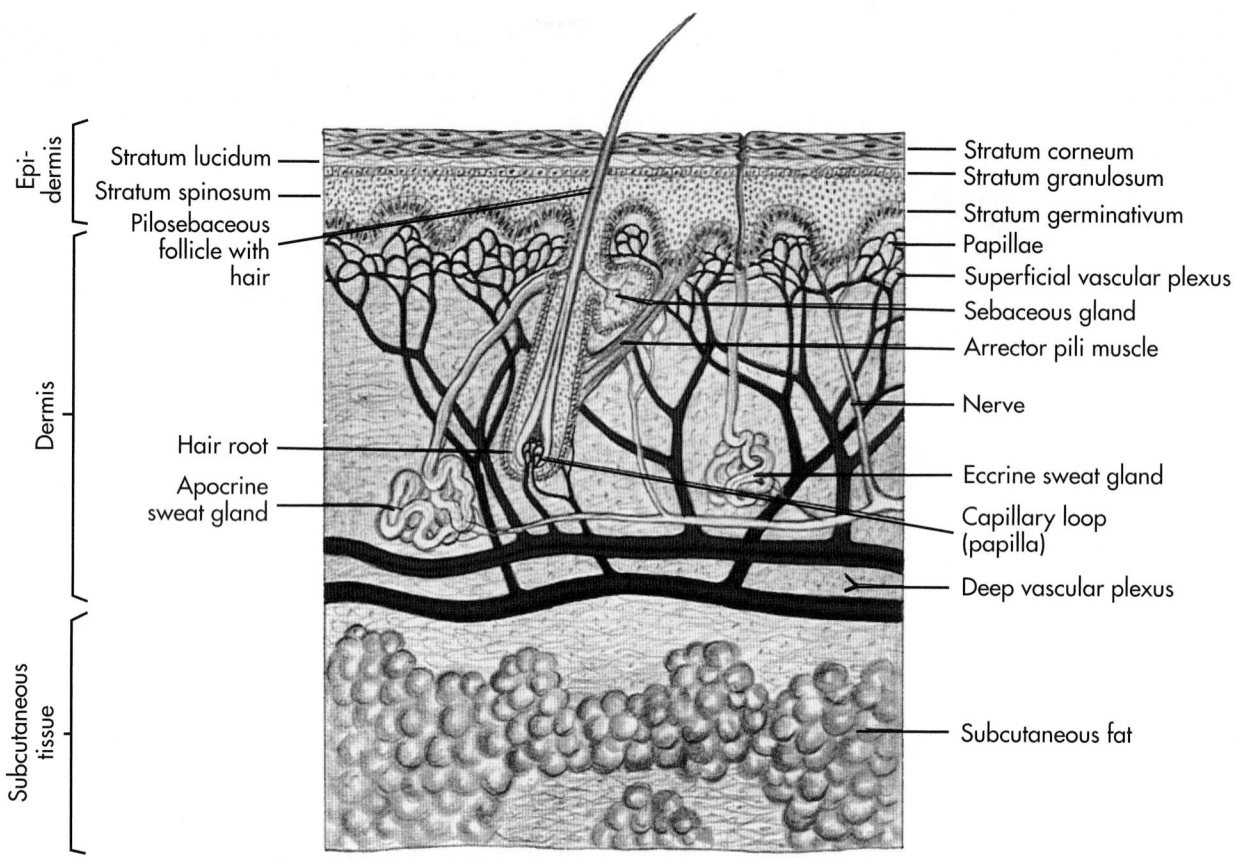

Fig. 12-1 Structures of skin.
(From Thompson et al: Mosby's clinical nursing, *ed 4, St Louis, 1997, Mosby.)*

Plaque (psoriasis, keratosis)
   Thickened
   Coalesced papules
   Elevated
Tumor (>5 cm) (neoplasm)
   Solid
   Elevated
Cyst (sebaceous cyst)
   Semisolid
   Palpable
   Encapsulated
   Serous or purulent exudate
Crust (scab, eczema)
   Dried exudate
   Elevated
Wheal (urticaria, bites)
   Solid
   Irregular shape
   Elevated
   Itchy
   Transient
   Scale (psoriasis, dermatitis)
      Elevated
      Flaky
      Irregular
Nodule (lipoma)
   Elevated
   Firm

   Palpable
   Deep
Comedo: blackhead/whitehead
Chancre
   Small
   Hard or ulcerated
Excoriation (abrasion)
   Loss of epidermis
   Linear
Ulcer (pressure)
   Loss of epidermis, dermis
   Concave
   Exudate
Cicatrix: scar
   Whealed dermis
   Occasionally raised
Keloid: excessive collagen formation around lesion or
   scar
   Irregular shape
   Elevated
   Beyond scar border
Petechia
   Small
   Bright red
   Flat
Fissure (athlete's foot)
   Small
   Deep

Red
Linear
Telangiectasia (rosacea)
Fine red line
Irregular
Erosion (varicella)
Moist
Depressed
Shiny
Lichenification (chronic dermatitis): thick, rough
epidermis

PERTINENT BACKGROUND INFORMATION

FAMILY HISTORY AND CONCURRENT DISEASES
Allergies
Exposures to external allergens
Cosmetics
Soaps
Medication
Plants
Chemicals
Exposures to internal allergens
Drugs
Food
Travel history
Exposure to parasites
Response to sun

MEDICATION PRESENTLY BEING TAKEN
Injectable medication
Prescription medication
Over-the-counter medication
Creams, lotions, ointments
Hygienic practices
Sexual practices

DIAGNOSTIC TESTS
Diagnosis of causative disease
Skin and lesion cultures
Gram stain for organism identification
Electron microscopy
Diascopy
Immunofluorescence (IF)
Lupus erythematosus preparation
Punch biopsies, cytology
Allergy skin testing
Blood culture
Skin scraping: potassium hydroxide (KOH) testing for
fungus
Complete blood count (CBC)

GERONTOLOGIC CONSIDERATIONS
The aging process elicits many alterations in the
integumentary system that can cause physical and
emotional changes in the individual (see Gerontologic
Considerations box)

Gerontologic Considerations

- Physiologic changes make the skin of the older person more fragile and susceptible to impairment.
- Aging changes include decreases in tissue fluid, subcutaneous fat, and sebaceous secretions. This results in dryness, flaking, pruritus, loss of elasticity, altered turgor, and a wrinkled appearance.
- Hyperkeratotic changes are typically seen in the nails, making them thick and difficult to care for. Podiatric care is recommended for older adults, particularly those with circulatory impairment.
- Circulatory changes and decreased mobility increase the risk of senile purpura and pressure ulcers.
- Significant hair and scalp changes can manifest with aging:
  - Loss of pigmentation leading to graying
  - Decreased thickness and increased incidence of balding
  - Increased incidence of seborrheic dermatitis of the scalp requiring special care
  - Growth of facial hair on women, which can be damaging to self-image
  - Localized clusters of melanocytes surrounded by areas of decreased pigmentation resulting in "age spots"
- The incidence of basal and squamous cell carcinoma increases with age, particularly in individuals who have had a high level of sun exposure. Aging skin should be closely inspected for changes in the appearance of moles or warts.

From Christensen BL, Kockrow EO: Foundations of nursing, *ed 3, St Louis, 1998, Mosby.*

PRESSURE ULCER
An area of cellular necrosis usually over a bony prominence that results from tissue hypoxia attributed to pressure, shearing, friction, moisture, poor nutrition, fever, altered circulation; these alone or in combination can contribute to skin frailness and reduce its ability to withstand the irritating factors (Table 12-1)

ASSESSMENT
SUBJECTIVE DATA
Pain, numbness

OBJECTIVE DATA
Risk factor potential (Box 12-1):
Location of pressure area:
Back of head
Ear rims, cheeks
Shoulder blades, acromion process
Elbows, heels, toes
Sacrum, buttocks, coccyx
Hips, greater trochanter, ischial tuberosities
Inner knee; medial, lateral malleolus
Medial, lateral condyles
Breast (women), genitalia (men)
Skin necrosis (Box 12-2)

Table 12-1	**Pressure Ulcer Prevention**
Contributing Factor	**Interventions**
Inactivity	Perform range of motion (ROM) exercises to all extremities Promote self-care activities Provide assistive devices: cane, walker, wheelchair
Immobility	Assess caregivers' ability to provide care Maintain turning schedule Avoid friction, shearing, sliding Institute small, frequent position changes Prop with pillows for comfort Initiate use of pressure-reducing devices: foam, gel, water, air mattress
Incontinence	Assess need for fecal management device Provide perineal, perianal care after each voiding or bowel movement Assess for possible urinary management device: internal, external catheter Offer bedpan or use of commode at scheduled times
Malnutrition	Provide diet high in protein, carbohydrate, vitamins C and E Offer between-meal snacks; Ensure; Carnation Instant Breakfast Offer small, frequent meals (6 per day)
Decreased sensation/mental acuity	Assess neuromuscular function; avoid overexposure to heat, cold Assess caregivers' ability to provide care if needed Maintain warmth without added weight

CHANGE	PATIENT PROBLEM	INTERVENTIONS
Reduced body temperature/ circulation	Cold extremities, pressure ulcers	• Maintain warmth with use of warm stockings, knee and ankle warmers, bed socks, and blankets that provide heat but not extra weight • Encourage use of fleece-lined slippers, mittens, boots, hats • Encourage ambulation, exercises • Provide pressure-reducing devices: air, foam mattress, circulating air mattress • Avoid massaging skin
Decreased moisture retention	Dry, rough, flaky skin	• Encourage use of creams and mild soaps; avoid antibacterial types, which tend to be drying • Maintain and protect skin with emollient application to entire body to prevent dryness • Avoid direct sunlight and wear a sunscreen cream • Encourage fluid intake of 3000 ml/day if allowed • Maintain adequate humidity
Inadequate nutrition/ hydration		• Evaluate knowledge of good nutrition • Maintain diet high in protein, carbohydrates, and vitamins; encourage small, frequent meals • Evaluate ability to chew, encourage to take small bites and chew food well • Provide alternation methods of preparing food to enhance intake: soft, puréed • Refer to community agencies for meals: Meals-on-Wheels

Box 12-1	**Risk Assessment for Pressure Ulcers**

EXTERNAL FACTORS
Immobility
Mechanical factors: shearing forces, friction, pressure, restraint
Moisture: perspiration, incontience,
Chemical substances: excretions, secretions
Hypertermia, hypothermia
Advanced age

INTERNAL FACTORS:
Medical history: e.g., diabetes, AIDS, anemia, carcinoma poor circulation, edema, altered metabolic state
Bony skeletal prominence
Poor nutritional status: emaciation, obesity
Decreased immune state
Altered skin turgor: e.g., loss of elasticity
Mental acuity

DIAGNOSTIC TESTS
Lesion culture
CBC, electrolytes
Serum albumin
Fasting blood sugar, (FBS)

POTENTIAL COMPLICATIONS
Infection
Further necrosis
Amputation

MULTIDISCIPLINARY MANAGEMENT
THERAPEUTIC MANAGEMENT
Wound care
  Biologic: biosynthetic products
    Donor tissue bilayered graft skin (Apligraf)
    Platelet-derived growth factors (Inerpan, Regranex)
  Odor-control dressings (CarboFlex Dressing)
Diet, vitamin, mineral supplements
Surgery
  Debridement: surgical, chemical
  Skin grafting
  Amputation
Systemic and topical antibiotics
Wound, Ostomy, Continence/ET Nurse
  Stage assessment assistance
  Treatment suggestions
  Resources

PATIENT PROBLEMS—NURSING DIAGNOSES/INTERVENTIONS

▼ Risk for impaired skin integrity related to physical immobilization

Assess and monitor pressure area
  Measure length, width, and depth

Box 12-2	**Stages of Necrosis**

I. Erythema only, no break in skin
II. Partial thickness; loss of skin involving epidermis, often into dermis
III. Full thickness; involves epidermis, dermis into or exposing subcutaneous tissue
IV. Deep tissue loss through subcutaneous tissue into fascia, muscle, bone

Preventive measures
  Elevate head of bed only enough to maintain comfort *to prevent sliding and possible shearing*
  Maintain skin integrity by keeping skin clean and dry
  Perform skin care daily and prn
  Bathe with mild soap and warm water; remove powder and ointments
  Rinse skin and pat dry thoroughly
  Apply lotion to feet, elbows, and back and massage very gently; remove excess
  Administer perineal care after elimination
Turn patient q2h: side, back, side *to relieve pressure;* lift patient when turning *to prevent friction;* avoid positioning directly on trochanter when lying on side
Assess and monitor pressure points qid and prn
Assist and teach patient to change position slightly q15min to 30min *to avoid pressure and fatigue*
Maintain clean, comfortable bed with wrinkle-free sheets
Administer back rubs with bland emollient; avoid alcohol-based creams
Prevent and eliminate pressure and friction by placing pillows between pressure areas (knees, ankles)
Prevent pressure with the following devices
  Alternating-pressure mattress
  Foam or static air mattress overlay
  Pressure reduction replacement mattress
  Flotation mattress
  Silicone pads
  Heel and elbow guards *to reduce friction*
Assist with and teach active or perform passive ROM exercises to all extremities q4h
Increase activity as allowed: assist patient out of bed and into chair; avoid sitting for more than 30 minutes; provide pressure relief while in chair; avoid donut-type devices

Expected Outcomes
Verbalizes understanding of procedures needed to prevent tissue breakdown
Participates in treatment/activities
Expresses sense of well-being

▼ Risk for impaired skin integrity related to mechanical factors (shearing factors, pressure, restraint)

Assess skin and identify stage of ulcer development (Table 12-2)

Consult with Wound, Ostomy, Continence/ET Nurse to develop plan of care

Eliminate causative factors

Initiate appropriate ulcer care for stages I and II

Cleanse skin at least q8h with mild soap and water and pat dry

Massage skin gently *to increase circulation;* avoid vigorous rubbing; bathe only as necessary

Do not massage reddened areas *because it may cause deep tissue trauma*

Turn q1h to 2h; use turn sheet or lift patient; avoid sliding *to prevent friction*

Maintain wrinkle-free sheets

Provide special pads, mattresses, beds as indicated

Position patient on unaffected areas

Protect skin surface and affected area with one or combination of the following

Apply Skin Prep/gel around area to prepare skin for dressing

Cover area with transparent dressing (Opsite) or hydrocolloid wafer barrier (Duoderm); bruised skin should not be covered

Continue one type of application, or a combination, for 48 to 72 hours; if improvement is apparent, continue applications; if no improvement is noted, begin another type of treatment

Initiate appropriate ulcer care for stages III and IV

Assess ulcer for size, location, color, odor, and amount and type of drainage

Monitor temperature (T) for elevation

Evaluate ulcer for infection and culture as needed

Administer wound care according to hospital standard of care

If healing is not evident, prepare for debridement as ordered

After debridement, change dressings as ordered; may range from gauze to hydrocolloids to absorbent gel-type dressing

Expected Outcomes

Exhibits skin/tissue color, integrity, and temperature returning to normal

Demonstrates ability to perform exercises/activities to prevent further tissue damage

▼Impaired skin integrity related to altered nutritional state

Assess patient's ability to chew and swallow food, determine dietary preferences, and provide appropriate type of diet; assist with feeding as needed

Explain diet rationale to patient and the need for high-protein, high-carbohydrate foods to promote healing; involve nutritionist/registered dietitian and perform calorie count

Offer frequent, small feedings on attractive trays; provide supplemental feedings

Promote involvement of significant other(s) *to provide support*

Encourage involvement in food selection

Increase fluid intake to 2500 ml/day if not contraindicated

Weigh patient daily (same time, scale, and clothing); report 0.5 kg loss to physician

Monitor CBC, electrolytes, and serum albumin

Measure intake and output q8h; ensure intake equals output

Expected Outcomes

Regains/maintains weight consistent with age/height

Participates in meal planning

Presents normal laboratory values

Table 12-2	**Stages of Pressure Ulcers**	
Stage	Description	Goal of Intervention
I	A reddened area that returns to normal skin color after 15 to 20 minutes of pressure relief (e.g., turning to other side). The skin is intact, but the area may appear pale when pressure first is removed.	To cover and protect.
II	Area in which the top layer of skin is missing. The ulcer usually is shallow with a pinkish-red base, and white or yellow eschar may be present.	To cover, protect, hydrate, insulate, and absorb.
III	Deep ulcers that extend into the dermis and subcutaneous tissues. White, gray, or yellow eschar usually is present at the bottom of the ulcer, and the ulcer crater may have a lip or edge. Purulent drainage is common.	To cover, protect, hydrate, insulate, absorb, cleanse, prevent infection, and promote granulation.
IV	Deep ulcers that extend into muscle and bone. These ulcers have a foul smell and the eschar is brown or black. Purulent drainage is common.	To cover, protect, hydrate, insulate, absorb, cleanse, prevent infection, obliterate dead space, and promote granulation.

From Beare PG, Myers JL: Adult health nursing, *ed 3, St Louis, 1998, Mosby.*

Additional Nursing Diagnoses to Consider
Sleep pattern disturbance
Pain
Risk for infection

PATIENT/FAMILY TEACHING

Discuss underlying causes of pressure ulcer, stage of ulcer development, and means of modifying risk potential
Provide written instructions for pressure ulcer care
Demonstrate cleansing procedure and application of medication and dressings as ordered; observe return demonstrations
Explain dietary regimen and provide written instructions
Stress importance of daily weights
Discuss signs and symptoms to report to physician
Weight loss; elevated temperature
Increased drainage from ulcer
Foul odor from ulcer
Further necrosis around ulcer
Reddened areas at other pressure points
Explain importance of increasing activity as tolerated, changing positions frequently while in bed, and avoiding pressure on affected area
Promote follow-up visits with physician

DISCHARGE/HOME CARE PLANNING

Explain the underlying cause or contributing factors
Identify and review the patient's stage of ulcer development, discussing specific procedures to prevent further progression
Explain that treatment depends on the stage of healing
Instruct the caregiver to recognize and record the signs of healing
Provide instruction for specific stage
Ulcer care, stages I and II
Eliminate causative factors.
Cleanse the skin every 8 hours with mild soap; pat dry
Massage the skin gently to increase circulation; avoid vigorous rubbing; do not massage reddened area
Protect the skin surface of the affected area with protective skin gels, ointment, and porous dressings as ordered; avoid using tape directly on the skin. Demonstrate proper application techniques; use special protective pads and mattresses
If the patient is on bed rest, turn every 1 to 2 hours; demonstrate how to use a turn sheet; instruct not to slide on sheets; keep bedsheets wrinkle free; change linens frequently if the patient is diaphoretic or incontinent
Ulcer care, stages III and IV
After debridement, inspect the wound for size, color, odor, and drainage and record information
Cleanse the wound using prescribed procedure
Explain debridement or skin grafting procedures as indicated

Discuss importance of daily hygiene to prevent infection and skin breakdown
Stress the importance of regular (three times a day or more) inspections of bony prominences and maintaining skin integrity by keeping skin clean and dry
Use mild soap water
Provide perineal care after voiding or bowel movement
Avoid use of skin-damaging products: harsh soaps, alcohol-based lotions, tincture of benzoin, hexachlorophene
Instruct the patient not to use a heat lamp
Instruct the patient and caregiver to gently massage the area around (not on) the bony prominence and administer gentle back rubs with bland emollient; remove any excess and avoid use of alcohol
Discuss importance in protecting the heels, elbows, back of head, iliac crests, sacrum, and coccyx against skin breakdown by using foam rubber pads
Demonstrate wound care, including cleansing procedure and application of medication and dressing changes
Arrange to obtain equipment, such as pressure-reducing mattress, footboard, bed cradle, and wound care supplies, that will be used at home
Explain the function of pressure relief devices and demonstrate how to use the equipment properly
Advise the patient and caregiver on where to buy equipment, such as drugstores and medical supply stores
Consult with Wound, Ostomy, Continence/ET Nurse for specific wound care instruction if necessary
Activity
Explain the importance of increasing activity as tolerated, changing positions every 2 to 3 hours while in bed or in chair, and avoiding pressure on affected area
Instruct the caregiver in assisting the patient out of bed and into a chair
Teach active and passive range-of-motion (ROM) exercises to all extremities and explain that they should be performed every 4 hours

■ CELLULITIS

A diffuse, acute streptococcal, staphylococcal infection of all layers of the skin and subcutaneous tissue, usually caused by bacterial invasion through a broken area in the skin such as skin trauma or ulceration; however, it may occur with no site of entry evident such as in lymphedema; it occurs as a result of a breakdown of tissues by enzymes produced by the invading bacteria

ASSESSMENT
SUBJECTIVE DATA
Localized area of pain, tenderness
Headache

OBJECTIVE DATA
Localized area of infection or open wound
  Redness, heat, swelling
  Purulent discharge
  Lymphangitic streaks
  Skin resembling skin of orange (peau d'orange)
Lymphadenopathy: increased eosinophils, lymphocytes, erythrocyte sedimentation rate (ESR), decreased neutrophils
  Fever, chills, malaise
  Tachycardia

DIAGNOSTIC TESTS
CBC: increased white blood cell count (WBC)
ESR increased
Cultures: lesion and blood

POTENTIAL COMPLICATIONS
Systemic infection
Gangrene
Amputation

MULTIDISCIPLINARY MANAGEMENT
  THERAPEUTIC MANAGEMENT
Medications
  Antibiotics, analgesics, antipyretics
Surgery
  Incision and drainage of abscess
  Debridement of necrotic tissue
  Fasciotomy
Position and immobilization of extremity
Alternate cool/warm compresses
Diet, activity
Wound, Ostomy, Continence/ET Nurse consultation

  PATIENT PROBLEMS—NURSING DIAGNOSES/INTERVENTIONS

▼Impaired skin integrity related to altered impaired circulation, and edema secondary to infectious process

Assess wound, recording changes in size, depth, color, drainage q4h *to monitor progression or improvement of inflammatory process*
Maintain bed rest with affected extremity elevated and immobilized *to decrease edema and promote circulation*
Change dressings using sterile technique *to prevent spread of infection*
Maintain aseptic techniques *to prevent spread of infection*
Apply wet compresses, alternating cold *to reduce discomfort* and warm *to increase circulation*
Instruct patient to avoid scratching *to avoid delay in healing and spread of infection*
Monitor temperature q4h; report elevation to physician
Administer antibiotics *to reduce infection*

Expected Outcomes
Inflammatory/infectious process resolves
  Wound is clean and dry and surrounding area is free of swelling
  Patient verbalizes no pain
No evidence of systemic infection
Remains afebrile

▼Impaired physical mobility related to pain, discomfort

Assess and record degree of immobility and pain of affected limb
Maintain elevation of affected extremity *to reduce swelling and pain*
Assist with use of cane, crutches, walker *to aid in ambulation*
Explain importance of maintaining elevation to just above heart level *to increase circulation*

Expected Outcomes
Mobility improves
Begins to engage in usual activities
Uses appropriate mobilization device correctly

▼Pain related to tissue inflammation

Assess pain for intensity using pain rating scale
Maintain affected extremity in prescribed position *to promote comfort*
Explain need for immobilization for 48 to 72 hours *because it reduces inflammation*
Administer analgesic as appropriate; assess effectiveness
Change position frequently, maintaining alignment, *to prevent pressure and fatigue*
Assist with and teach alternative pain relief measures: imagery, relaxation *to lessen preoccupation with pain*
Promote diversional activities *to decrease attention on pain*

Expected Outcomes
Reports a reduction in pain and discomfort that is at a tolerable level
Appears calm; has relaxed facial expression
Alternates sleep with activity appropriately

PATIENT/FAMILY TEACHING
Explore and discuss cause of disease process
Demonstrate open or draining wound care and dressing-change procedure; stress importance of clean technique
Discuss maintaining prescribed elevation and immobilization of extremity
Encourage activity to tolerance using supportive devices: sling, crutches as indicated
Explain signs and symptoms to report to physician
  Wound pain or increased drainage
  Fever, chills, headache
  Odor from dressings and wound

Discuss medication schedule, including name, purpose, dosage, and side effects

Stress importance of completing all prescribed doses of antibiotics

Stress importance of balanced diet to promote wound healing

Stress importance of follow-up visits with physician

DISCHARGE/HOME CARE PLANNING

Assess and continue with patient/family teaching and evaluate/discuss understanding of the following:

Pressure ulcer prevention (see Table 12-1)

Nutrition and dietary intake

Care of wound; use of clean technique; adequate dressings, medications, correct procedure for disposal of soiled dressings

Discuss activity allowances and limitations (e.g., bathing, exercise)

Review need for safety precautions to protect extremity/site from injury

Use of night light to avoid bumps, falls

Provide referrals for home medical equipment

Knowledge of what items are required and where to purchase them

Importance of changing position, increasing activity

■ PRURITUS

A sensation that evokes the desire to scratch, which can be a symptom of localized primary skin disorders (eczema, irritation, allergic reactions) a systemic disease (renal failure, liver or thyroid disease, opiate drugs, psychologic problems) or malignancy; the sensory nerve endings promote the itching sensation, but exactly how and why are unknown; there are four main areas affected: pruritus ani, occurring usually in men; pruritus vulvae, found in women; otitis externa occurs in the external ear canal; and generalized pruritus may signify a systemic disease

ASSESSMENT

SUBJECTIVE DATA

Pruritus, discomfort

Emotional distress: tension, anxiety, depression

History of liver, renal disease

Pattern of pruritus: at all times, occasional, seasonal

OBJECTIVE DATA

Lesion/affected area

Location, distribution of pruritus

Erythema, scaling, excoriation, fissures

Signs of scratching

DIAGNOSTIC TESTS

Culture of affected area

Biopsy

CBC, blood urea nitrogen (BUN)

FBS

Serum bilirubin, iron

Stool for hemocult, parasites

Sulfobromophthalein retention test

POTENTIAL COMPLICATIONS

Increased excoriation

Fissures

Secondary infection

MULTIDISCIPLINARY MANAGEMENT

THERAPEUTIC MANAGEMENT

Medications

Topical preparations, steroid cream

Antihistamines: diphenhydramine (Benadryl)

Antianxiety agents: hydroxyzine (Atarax, Vistaril)

Psychotherapeutic agents (for antipruritic effect); chlorpromozine (Thorazine)

Cool compresses

Sitz baths

Emollients

Psychologic counseling as needed

PATIENT PROBLEMS—NURSING DIAGNOSES/INTERVENTIONS

▼Impaired skin integrity related to mechanical factors (scratching of affected areas) secondary to inflammatory response

Assess severity and spread of lesion *to monitor progress and/or improvement of irritation*

Encourage patient to maintain excellent hygiene *to prevent secondary infection and further spread*

Apply topical lotions and creams if not contraindicated to reduce sensation to scratch

Administer cooling compresses or baths *to soothe the area*

Advise and discuss importance of keeping nails short *to prevent further tissue damage*

Encourage patient to use tepid water and pat skin dry *to avoid irritating tissues*

Apply mittens if urge to scratch is uncontrollable

Administer antibiotics if skin is infected

Monitor laboratory results *to assist in identifying underlying systemic disease*

Expected Outcomes

Expresses a decreased desire to scratch affected areas

Exhibits no signs of infection

Maintains short fingernails

▼Pain related to biologic, physical factors (itching) secondary to irritation, inflammation, or a systemic condition

Assess degree of pain/discomfort; assist patient to identify irritating factors

Determine area of irritation *to plan appropriate care*

Maintain patient in a position of comfort

Administer antianxietics, antihistamines, psychotherapeutics *to reduce discomfort*

Apply soothing emollients *to decrease itching sensation and increase moisture in the skin*

Provide diversional activities *to decrease attention on discomfort*

For pruritus ani, vulvae offer sitz baths *to alleviate itching*

Change position frequently in small ways *to prevent fatigue*

Offer back rubs *to soothe and promote comfort*

Encourage verbalization of concerns, fears, and stress factors *to prevent further aggravation of pruritus*

Expected Outcomes

Exhibits less discomfort and decreased scratching

Utilizes discomfort-reducing methods successfully

PATIENT/FAMILY TEACHING AND DISCHARGE/HOME CARE PLANNING

Assist patient to identify irritating factors and discuss ways to modify them

Explain and discuss the importance of avoiding the following:

Excess heat/dryness in the home

Clothing that is tight fitting and/or made from rough fabrics

Polyester fabrics that do not allow for ventilation

Irritating soaps, laundry detergents

Explain importance of keeping nails short

Discuss medications schedule and possible side effects

Evaluate procedure for compress application

Discuss signs of infection: redness, pain, drainage, fever; need to promptly report these symptoms to physician

Discuss importance of physician follow-up visits

■ BURN MANAGEMENT

The severity of the physiologic systemic response created in the adult burn patient is directly related to the depth of wound injury and the percentage of total body surface area involved in the injury. Other factors that have an impact on the outcome of the patient with a moderate to major burn include age, the presence of smoke inhalation or associated trauma, and preexisting chronic disease. The minor adult burn or the patient who has experienced 10% to 15% or less total body surface area injury usual has minimal systemic effects and requires little resuscitation. These patients may be treated as an outpatient in some cases.

The causative factors of a burn injury may include the following:

thermal: *Caused by exposure to flame, hot liquids, radiation*

chemical: *Caused by contact, inhalation, ingestion of acids, alkalies, vesicants*

electrical: *Caused by electrical current passing through the body and into the ground*

ASSESSMENT: FULL-THICKNESS BURNS (TABLE 12-3)

OBJECTIVE DATA

Airway, breathing, circulation assessment (ABCs)

Wound assessment, including depth and extent or percentage of body surface involved (Fig. 12-2)

Classification (Table 12-4)

Anatomic location

Pertinent history

Age of patient

Causative agent, source

History of preexisting illness

Inhalation injury

Facial burns

Singed nasal hair

Burns to oropharynx

Hoarseness, stridor, wheezing

Other body trauma

Fractures

Deep tissue destruction

Respiratory tract trauma

Respiratory distress caused by toxic or smoke inhalation

Hypotension, tachycardia, shock

Anxiety, fear

Presence of pain

Fever, chills

Wound infection

Increased erythema

Change in exudate, odor

Increase in pain and wound depth

DIAGNOSTIC TESTS

CBC, electrolytes, serum albumin, oxyhemoglobin, BUN, creatinine, bilirubin, alkaline phosphatase

Arterial blood gases (ABGs) with carbooxyhemoglobin

Type and crossmatch

Urinalysis for Hgb, myoglobin, albumin, glucose, acetone, specific gravity

Chest and body radiology, bronchoscopy, ventilation lung scan

Electrocardiogram (ECG)

POTENTIAL COMPLICATIONS

Initial phase

Hyponatremia (first 24 hours)

Hypernatremia (after 48 hours)

Hyperkalemia (first 48 hours)

Hypokalemia (after 48 hours)

Hypoproteinemia (initial 8 hours)

Dehydration

Hypoxia

Circulatory collapse

Renal failure

Hypovolemic shock

Hematuria, oliguria

Anemia

Adult respiratory distress syndrome (ARDS)

Pulmonary edema

Table 12-3 Burn Wound Classification

Degree of Burn	Cause of Injury	Depth of Injury	Wound Characteristics	Treatment Course
First-degree burn	Prolonged ultraviolet light exposure; brief exposure to hot liquids	Limited damage to epithelium; skin intact	Erythematous, hypersensitive, no blister formation	Complete healing within 3 to 5 days without scarring
Superficial partial-thickness burn (second degree)	Brief exposure to flash, flame, or hot liquids	Epidermis destroyed; minimal damage to superficial layers of dermis; epidermal appendages intact	Moist and weepy, pink or red, blisters, blanching, hypersensitive	Complete healing within 21 days with minimal or no scarring
Deep partial-thickness burn (second degree)	Intense radiant energy; scalding liquids, semi-liquids (e.g., tar), or solids; flame	Epidermis destroyed; underlying dermis damaged; some epidermal appendages remain intact	Pale; decreased moistness; blanching absent or prolonged; intact sensation to deep pressure but not to pinprick	Prolonged healing (often longer than 21 days); may require skin grafting to achieve complete healing with better functional outcome
Full-thickness burn (third degree)	Prolonged contact with flame, scalding liquids; steam; hot objects; chemicals; electrical current	Epidermis, dermis, and epidermal appendages destroyed; injury through dermis	Dry, leatherlike; pale, mottled brown, or red; thrombosed vessels visible; insensate	Requires skin grafting
Full-thickness burn (fourth degree)	Electrical current; prolonged contact with flame (e.g., unconscious victim)	Epidermis, dermis, and epidermal appendages destroyed; injury involves connective tissue, muscle, and possibly bone	Dry; charred, mottled brown, white, or red; no sensation; limited or no movement of involved extremities or digits	Requires skin grafting; amputation of involved extremities or digits likely

From Carrougher GJ, ed: Burn care and therapy, St Louis, 1998, Mosby.

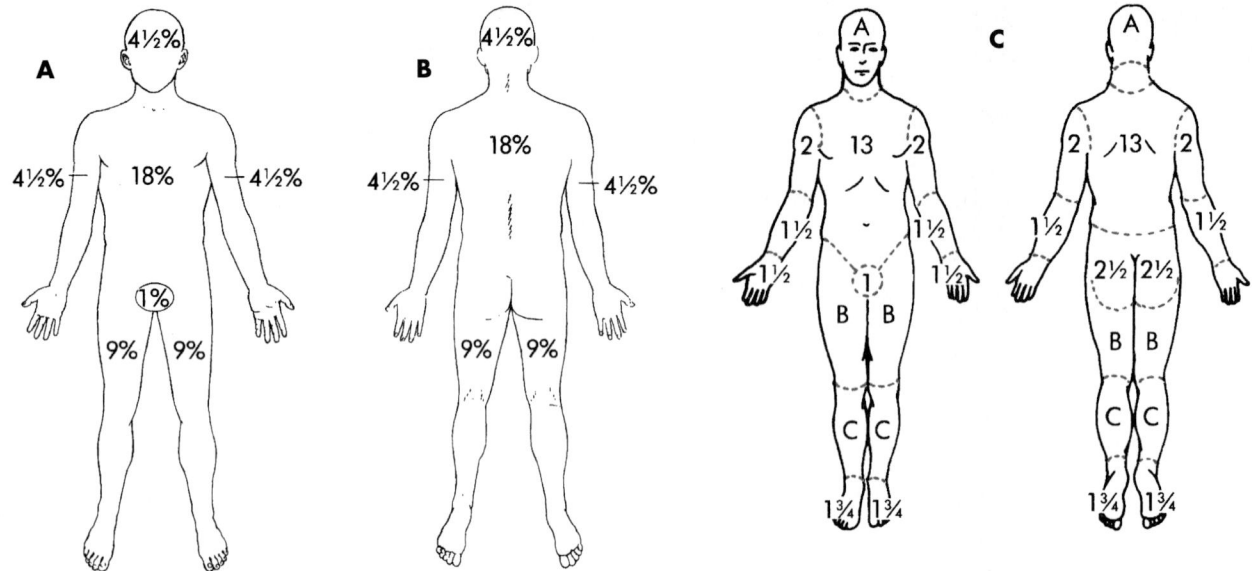

Relative percentages of areas affected by growth (age in years)

	0	**1**	**5**	**10**	**15**	**Adult**
A: half of head	9½	8½	6½	5½	4½	3½
B: half of thigh	2¾	3¼	4	4¼	4½	4¾
C: half of leg	2½	2½	2¾	3	3¼	3½

Second degree _____ and
Third degree _____ =
Total percent burned ___

Fig. 12-2 Estimation of adult burn injury: rule of nines. **A,** Anterior view. **B,** Posterior view. **C,** Estimation of burn injury: Lund and Browder chart. Areas designated by letters (*A, B,* and *C*) represent percentages of body surface area that vary according to age. The accompanying table indicates the relative percentages of these areas at various stages in life. *(From Sabiston DC Jr, ed:* Textbook of surgery: the biological basis of modern surgical practice, *ed 11, Philadelphia, 1977, Saunders.)*

Table 12-4	**American Burn Association Classification of Burn Injury**
Class	**Description**
Major	Full-thickness burns over 10% or more of total body surface area (TBSA)
	Partial-thickness burns over 25% of TBSA
	All burns on face, hands, eyes, ears, feet, or genitalia
	All inhalation and electrical burns
	All burns complicated by trauma
	All burns in poor-risk patients
Moderate	Full-thickness burns <2% to 10% TBSA
	Partial-thickness burns over 15% to 25% of TBSA
Minor	Partial-thickness burns over less than 15% of TBSA
	Full thickness burns over less than 2% TBSA

From Thompson et al: Mosby's clinical nursing, *ed 4, St Louis, 1997, Mosby.*

Gastritis and/or ileus
Local infections
Septic shock
Curling ulcer (as early as first week, as late as ninth week)
Fecal impaction
Emotional shock
Disseminated intravascular coagulation (DIC)
Long term
  Scarring
  Disfigurement
  Disabilities: physical, psychosocial

MULTIDISCIPLINARY MANAGEMENT
THERAPEUTIC MANAGEMENT
Airway management
  Intubation with ventilatory support
  Oxygen therapy
  Humidification (inhalation injuries)

Box 12-3	**Burn Center Referral Criteria**

- Second- or third-degree burns greater than 10% TBSA in patients younger than 10 or older than 50 years of age.
- Second- or third-degree burns greater than 20% TBSA in patients between the ages of 10 and 50 years.
- Third-degree burns greater than 5% TBSA in patients of any age.
- All second- or third-degree burns with the threat of functional or cosmetic impairment to the face, hands, feet, genitalia, perineum, or major joints.
- Electrical burns, including lightning injury.
- Chemical burns with the threat of functional or cosmetic impairment.
- Burns involving inhalation injury.
- Circumferential burns of the extremities and/or chest.
- Burns involving concomitant trauma among which the burn injury poses the greatest risk of morbidity or mortality.
- Burns in patients with preexisting medical conditions that may complicate management and/or prolong recovery, such as coronary artery disease, chronic lung disease, or diabetes.

From Carroucher GJ, ed: Burn care and therapy, *St Louis, 1998, Mosby.*

Medications
    Narcotics, sedatives, analgesics
    Tetanus
    Antibiotics
    Antacids
    H_2 Blocker or protectant: carafate
    Topical antimicrobial agents: bactrin/polysporin, silver nitrate, mafenide acetate cream, silver sulfadizine
Parenteral fluids
    Electrolytes and vitamins
    Transfusion/plasma
Hemodynamic monitoring
    Pulmonary artery pressure catheter
    Arterial line
Nasogastric suction/indwelling urinary catheter
Diet
    Major burns: NPO
    Total parenteral nutrition (TPN)
    Tube feedings
    2 to 4 g protein/kg/d
    3000 to 5000 calories/d
Surgery
    Excision
    Escharotomy
    Fasciotomy
    Skin graft
        Split thickness
        Mesh graft
        Homograft
        Heterograft
        Amputation

Hydrotherapy
Wound care: wet or dry dressing
Chest physiotherapy

COLLABORATIVE MANAGEMENT
Social worker
Case manager
Occupational therapy
Physical therapy
Dietary
Referral to tertiary burn center (Box 12-3)

PATIENT PROBLEMS—NURSING DIAGNOSES/INTERVENTIONS

▼Impaired gas exchange related to altered alveolar-capillary membrane and/or hypovolemia secondary to inhalation injury

Assess respiratory status for signs of inhalation injury, increased airway edema
Monitor breath sounds qh; observe for decreased breath sounds, tachypnea, dyspnea, cough, pallor, and cyanosis
Monitor ABGs and vital signs *to assess hypoxic status*
Assess for signs of hypoxia: tachycardia, altered mental acuity
Maintain patent airway; perform orotracheal suction as needed; position patient for optimal ventilation *to prevent airway obstruction*
Monitor mechanical ventilation and endotracheal tube for correct settings and function *to assist in airway management*
Provide rest periods; avoid overexertion and assist with ADLs as needed *to reduce overtaxation of respiratory system*
Administer oxygen therapy *to reduce hypoxic state*
Administer broncholytic agents *to open alveoli and increase respiratory competency*
Assist/perform chest physiotherapy and incentive spirometer *to drain and expand the lungs*

Expected Outcomes
Respirations are slow, regular
Breath sounds are clear
ABGs are within normal limits

▼Fluid volume deficit related to impaired capillary membrane integrity and osmotic pressure changes secondary to burned skin

Assess and monitor for dehydration, reduced skin turgor, dry mucous membranes, decreased mental acuity
Maintain NPO
Administer parenteral fluids with electrolytes; suture IV in place if placement must be in burned skin
Obtain weight in kilograms, determine percentage of total body surface involved

Calculate IV infusion rate (Table 12-5)

Monitor intake and output q4h *to assess hydration status*

Monitor indwelling catheter and closed gravity drainage system

Measure output qh; report <30 to 50 ml/hr in adults

Observe for hematuria

Monitor CBC, BUN, creatinine, electrolytes

Monitor urine glucose, acetone, and specific gravity q4h to 6h

Monitor mental acuity q8h

Monitor wound drainage and insensible fluid loss and add to output *to establish accurate fluid loss measurement*

Elevate injured extremities *to reduce edema formation*

Expected Outcomes

Intake and output are balanced

Mucous membranes are moist

Electrolytes are within normal limits

▼Risk for infection related to inadequate primary defenses secondary to tissue destruction

Maintain isolation precautions, scrupulous handwashing, and aseptic technique; wear gown, mask, gloves as indicated *to prevent further infection*

Monitor vital signs q2h to 4h to assess for signs of infection: fever and tachycardia

Monitor for signs of wound infection: increased redness and pain, purulent drainage, odor, dark discolored eschar

Monitor invasive hemodynamic monitoring lines and indwelling urethral catheter for infection; culture as indicated

Assess laboratory values: WBC (>10,000/mm) urinalysis, leukocytosis

Limit visitors to patient's *significant* others, especially exclude people with upper respiratory infections (URIs)

Administer tetanus toxoid as indicated

Administer topical/systemic antibiotics as indicated; assess effectiveness, side effects

Monitor for sepsis: fever, tachypnea, altered sensorium, decreased platelets, hyperglycemia

Initiate local burn therapy using the following principles, which are general considerations

Obtain culture for burn areas as needed

Cleanse burn and remove all pieces of detached epithelium; cleanse with saline or mild soap and tap water (hexachlorophene is not recommended)

Debride, using sterile equipment

Remove dirt and blood

Shave surrounding area

Prevent destruction of viable epithelium; prevent burned surfaces from touching viable skin or other burned surfaces

Produce environment unfavorable to bacterial growth

Aid separation of burn slough

Apply skin coverage as soon as possible

Initiate one of the following topical burn agents as ordered

Silver nitrate: antiinfective agent; penetrates burn slowly, is very painful; burn/dressings must be kept saturated; causes electrolyte imbalance and turns all surfaces black

Povidone-iodine (Betadine): broad-spectrum antiinfective; is very painful and may cause increased iodine absorption

Silver sulfadiazine 1% (Silvadene)

Broad-spectrum antibiotic; is slow to absorb but relatively painless; may decrease WBC

Monitor serum chloride and pH; WBC

Mafenide acetate (Sulfamylon): antiinfective agent; penetrates burn well but is painful; may cause rash, decreased $Paco_2$

Examine wounds daily and prn to assess change in odor, appearance, amount of drainage

Apply dressings to prevent skin-to-skin contact: each finger, toe

Table 12-5	**Adult Burn Resuscitation Formulas**	
Formula Name	**Recommended Solutions**	**Formula for Estimating Fluid Needs**
INITIAL 24 HOURS AFTER INJURY		
Modified Brooke*	Lactated ringer's solution	2 ml/kg/% TBSA burn
Parkland	Lactated ringer's solution	4 ml/kg/% TBSA burn
SECOND 24 HOURS AFTER INJURY		
Modified Brooke*	Colloid solution (diluted to physiologic concentration) and 5% dextrose in water	0.3-0.5 ml/kg/% TBSA burn (0.3 ml/kg/% TBSA burn for injuries of 30% to 50%; up to 0.5 ml/kg/% TBSA burn for injuries >50% TBSA)
Parkland	25% albumin and 5% dextrose in water	20% to 60% of calculated plasma volume Volume to maintain desired urine output

Modified from Carrougher GJ, ed: Burn care and therapy, St Louis, 1998, Mosby.
*The total estimated volume is calculated with one half administered over the initial 8 hours after injury and the remaining half over the subsequent 16 hours.

Expected Outcomes

Absence of infection or sepsis
Burned areas begin to heal adequately
Temperature is normal
Laboratory values are within normal limits
Surrounding tissue is clean, dry, and intact

▼Impaired skin integrity related to destruction and skin loss from burn injury

Estimate extent and depth of burn injury
Assess wound characteristics (see Tables 12-3 and 12-4)
Assess for signs of wound infection
Maintain in prescribed position or position of comfort
Assess pressure areas; change position and support with pillows, padding as indicated
Provide bathing and oral care as needed
Monitor mucous membranes if nasogastric tube is in place; keep nares moist
Administer lotions to unaffected areas *to promote comfort and prevent breakdown*
Assess size, depth, color of burned area; observe surrounding tissue for redness or necrosis
Maintain isolation procedures as indicated
Apply prescribed antimicrobial topical agents and redress wound sites:
   Monitor burn covering, dressing prn
   Apply dressings very loosely in anticipation of edema formation
Monitor skin graft sites for adherence of graft, shearing, epithelization
   Homograft: from cadaver skin
   Autograft: from unburned area of patient
   Heterograft: pigskin or synthetic
   Autologous: epithelium cells cultured into sheets
Maintain correct body alignment and elevate affected graft, dressing site if appropriate
Monitor sites for signs of healing
Maintain dressings/grafts as indicated

Expected Outcomes

Healing is progressive
Burn sites are regenerating new tissue
Other tissue/skin areas are free from trauma
No signs of infection, shearing, or breakdown

▼Impaired physical mobility related to decreased strength and endurance

Maintain bed rest in prescribed position *to promote healing*
Monitor neuromuscular status q4h *to prevent contractures*
Maintain body alignment within parameters of treatment
Prevent contractures and/or hypertrophy
   Head and neck: do not use pillows (Fig. 12-3)
   Hand (Fig. 12-4)
   Upper chest, axilla, and arms (Fig. 12-5): maintain arm at 90-degree angle, away from body and slightly above shoulder
   Ankles and feet (Fig. 12-6): use footboard with patient in supine position
   Legs: traction/splints may be used
Encourage active ROM to nonburn areas
Explain necessity of positions, which can be uncomfortable; position of comfort can be position for forming contractures
Administer analgesics before procedures *to reduce pain and enhance movement*
Apply and maintain pressure dressings on graft partial-thickness wounds *to prevent scarring and contractures*
Assist with and teach active or perform passive ROM exercises on unaffected extremities *to maintain muscle strength*
Coordinate care to allow for rest periods *to prevent fatigue*
Encourage patient to perform self-care activities
Change position frequently *to prevent fatigue and pressure;* low-air-loss/air-fluidized beds may be required to promote position changes
Refer patient for physiotherapy and/or hydrotherapy as indicated *to provide individualized activity/exercise program*
Ambulate as soon as possible *to prevent respiratory compromise*

Expected Outcomes

Participates in prescribed activities and therapy
Maintains correct body alignment
Demonstrates ability to balance rest with activities

▼Altered nutrition: less than body requirements related to hypermetabolism

Maintain adequate hydration, nutrition *to replace lost fluids and promote healing* (see Table 12-5)

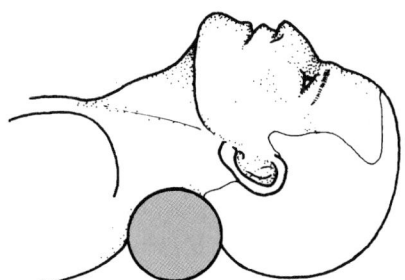
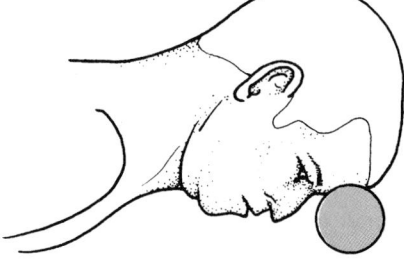

Fig. 12-3   Positioning for head and neck burns to prevent contractures.

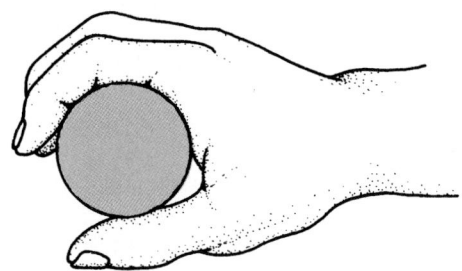

Fig. 12-4 Positioning of hand burn to prevent contractures.

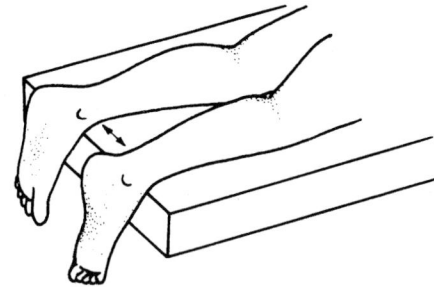

Fig. 12-6 Correct foot and ankle positioning to prevent foot and ankle contractures.

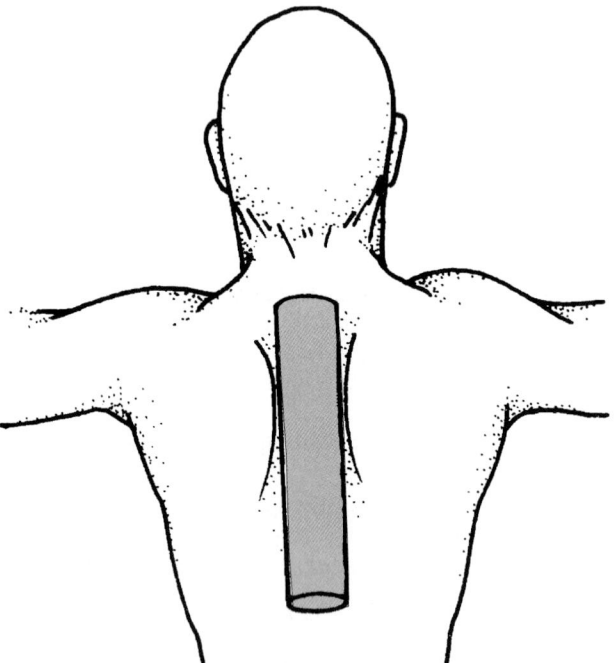

Fig. 12-5 Placement of contracture roll for upper chest, axilla, and arm burns.

Provide TPN (p. 24), tube feedings for burns >40% *to maintain needed calorie intake;* assess bowel sounds q4h

Monitor serum/finger stick glucose, Clinitest/Acetest *to assess for hyperglycemia*

Initiate liquid diet for <40% burns, advancing to high protein/calorie as indicated

Provide high-protein, high-calorie diet as indicated and tolerated:
    Protein: 20% to 23% of calories or 3 g/kg/day
    Fat: 20% of calories
    Carbohydrate: remainder of calories

Provide small, frequent meals; encourage oral fluids: milk, juice *to assure correct intake and prevent gastric distention*

Perform meticulous calorie count after meals *to evaluate/adjust required intake;* tube feeding for nocturnal feeding supplement may be indicated to meet caloric goals

Supplement oral diet with high protein drinks and/or milkshakes

Provide vitamin supplements

Provide H₂ blocker or protectant *to decrease risk of gastritis or ulcer development*

Involve patient in food selection, preferences

Encourage family to provide home-cooked food if permitted

Perform oral hygiene before and after meals *to provide comfort and encourage eating*

Assist with feeding as needed; advance position to sitting in chair for meals when tolerated *to prevent aspiration and promote digestion*

Weigh patient daily (same time, scale, and clothing) *to monitor effectiveness of diet*

Expected Outcomes
Regains lost weight to within 2% to 5% of normal
Wound healing progresses
Participates in food selection and calorie count
Selects foods that increase healing potential

▼Pain related to destruction of tissue

Elevate each extremity periodically *to decrease edema, pain*

Cover burn to decrease discomfort if applicable *because air movement may cause increased pain*

Maintain comfortable temperature/humidity because body temperature regulation may be altered

Assess location, type, and severity of pain; assess intensity with pain rating scale to monitor for increasing intensity, which may indicate complications

Administer analgesics; assess effectiveness of pain relief measures; decrease narcotics as soon as possible *to prevent addiction*

Collaborate with physician and instruct patient in use of PCA

Allow time to discuss feelings about pain

Perform dressing changes only after patient is medicated as needed *to provide comfort*

Offer diversional activities *to decrease attention on pain*

Encourage use of alternative pain relief measures: relaxation techniques, imaging, deep breathing

Encourage small shifts in position *to promote comfort*

Expected Outcomes

Reports a tolerable pain level

Presents calm, relaxed facial affect

Demonstrates use of alternative pain relief measures

▼Body image disturbance related to possible disfigurement from burns

Assess for defining characteristics

Assess feelings of loss, anxiety *to assist patient to work through feelings*

Express acceptance of feelings *to prevent feelings of rejection*

Encourage and allow time for verbalization of concerns/feelings; include significant others; provide privacy

Set realistic short-term goals and acknowledge tasks attempted and/or completed *to inspire confidence*

Allow patient to progress through stages of grief at own pace

Maintain nonjudgmental attitude and avoid nonverbal rejection; discourage maladaptive behavior

Assess present coping attitudes and assist patient with identifying successful past behaviors

Promote self-care activities as soon as possible *to foster self-confidence*

Involve patient with unit routine and other burn patients *to increase support base*

Collaborate with social service and psychiatric services as indicated

Expected Outcomes

Begins to acknowledge altered image

Discusses feelings/anxieties with increasing confidence

Undertakes goal setting for future

Participates in self-care activities

Additional Nursing Diagnoses to Consider

Risk of constipation related to immobility, dehydration, medications

Altered tissue perfusion (renal, cardiopulmonary, gastrointestinal) related to hypovolemia, exchange problems

Fear/anxiety related to risk of disfigurement and/or separation from support groups

Risk for caregiver role strain

PATIENT/FAMILY TEACHING

Review therapeutic plan, discussing discharge care

Nutrition

Provide written dietary instructions; discuss importance of maintaining normal weight and adequate fluid intake

Explain rehabilitation plan; review exercise plan

Discuss maintaining normal activity with planned rest periods; prevent boredom with diversional activities

Demonstrate burn care

Wash hands

Cleanse wound with mild, nonfragrant soap

Rinse well

Pat dry using clean towel

Apply topical ointment/dressing

Discuss care of healing wound/scar management

Apply a water-based moisturizing cream such as Eucerin after washing with mild soap/water and rinsing well

Demonstrate and encourage participation in scar massage; silastic gel sheeting may be used to decrease hypertrophic scarring in conjunction with scar massage and pressure garments if appropriate

Wear nonirritating, loose clothing

Explain use and care of pressure garment if indicated

Wash and rinse well daily with mild soap and water

Allow to dry flat on towels

Observe for signs of skin irritation with initial use; instruct to report appearance of blisters

Have garment checked for correct fit at follow-up appointments

Discuss importance of maintaining meticulous hygiene

Promote use of moisturizers; avoid direct sun: if in sunlight wear protective clothing, use sunscreen

Avoid harsh laundry detergents and fabric softeners

Review symptoms to report to physician

Fever, malaise

Bleeding, odor, and drainage from burn wound, increased redness, swelling, pain

Discuss medication schedule including name, purpose, dosage, and side effects; caution patient to avoid taking over-the-counter medications unless approved by physician

Avoid contact with persons with infections, especially colds or other URIs

Provide names and phone numbers of home health care team

Provide information and prescriptions for follow-up visits with physician, physical, occupational therapist

DISCHARGE/HOME CARE PLANNING

Assess and continue with patient/family teaching and evaluate the following:

Burn site(s)/skin

Healing progress

Signs of infection

Dressing change procedure; aseptic technique

Supplies: what is required and where to purchase them

Pressure garment use if indicated

Pain control

Diversional activities to prevent boredom and decrease attention on pain

Review need for continued physical/occupational rehabilitation program

Discuss need to continue active ROM to maintain function

Discuss need to plan regular rest periods interspersed with activities

Discuss diet therapy

High-caloric, high-protein diet with supplemental vitamins

Bowel function; discuss use of routine stool softeners, natural laxatives as indicated

Emotional

Degree of coping with anxiety/body image change

Knowledge of community resources: homemaker service, counselors, Meals-on-Wheels

BIBLIOGRAPHY

American Burn Association: *Guidelines for burn nursing practice,* Chicago, 1992, American Burn Association.

American Burn Association: *Burn care outcome,* Chicago, 1994, American Burn Association.

Achauer BM (ed): *Management of the burned patient,* Stanford, Conn, 1997, Appleton & Lange.

Barnes HR: Alternating transparent and hydrocolloid dressings, *Nursing '93* 23(3):59, 1993.

Beare PG, Myers JL: *Principles and practice of adult health nursing,* ed 3, St Louis, 1998, Mosby.

Bergstrom N et al: How to predict and prevent pressure ulcers, *Am J Nurs* 92(7):52, 1992.

Blumenfiel M, Schoeps MM: *Psychological care of the burn and trauma patient,* Baltimore, 1993, Williams & Wilkins.

Came RM: Patients with burns. In Clochesy JM et al, eds: *Critical care nursing,* Philadelphia, 1996, WB Saunders.

Canobbio MM: *Mosby's handbook of patient teaching,* St Louis, 1996, Mosby.

Carrougher GJ, ed: *Burn care and therapy,* St Louis, 1998, Mosby.

Cornwell P: *Managed care tools for change,* Davis, Calif, 1995, Regents of the University of California, University of California, Davis, Regional Burn Center.

Demling RH, LaLonde C: *Burn trauma,* New York, 1990, Thieme.

Doenges ME et al: *Nursing care plans: guidelines for planning and documenting patient care,* ed 3, Philadelphia, 1993, FA Davis.

Flory C: Skin assessment, *RN* 55(6):22, 1992.

Greenhalgh DG: The diagnosis of inhalation injury, *Prob Resp Care* 4(3):286-298, 1991.

Greenhalgh DG: The healing of burn wounds, *Dermatol Nurs* 8(1):13-25, 1991.

Kim MJ et al: *Pocket guide to nursing diagnoses,* ed 7, St Louis, 1997, Mosby.

Maklebust J: Pressure ulcer update, *RN* 54(12):56, 1991.

Martyn JA: Acute management of the burn patient, Philadelphia, 1990, WB Saunders.

McCance KL, Huether SE: *Pathophysiology: the biological basis for disease in adults and children,* ed 3, St Louis, 1998, Mosby.

McFarland GK, McFarlane EA: *Nursing diagnosis and intervention: planning for patient care,* ed 3, St Louis, 1997, Mosby.

Motta GJ: How moisture-retentive dressings promote healing, *Nursing '93* 23(12):26, 1993.

NANDA: *Nursing diagnosis: definitions and classification 1999-2000,* Philadelphia, 1999, North American Nursing Diagnosis Association.

Rogers-Seidle FF: *Geriatric nursing care plans,* St Louis, 1991, Mosby.

Schmidtling RE et al: Treating pressure ulcers with a myocutaneous flap, *Nursing '92* 22(7):56, 1992.

Thompson JM et al: *Mosby's clinical nursing,* ed 4, St Louis, 1997, Mosby.

Trofino RB: *Nursing care of the burn-injured patient,* Philadelphia, 1991, FA Davis.

MULTIDISCIPLINARY PLAN OF CARE

Diagnosis: __Cellulitis__

Type of Surgery :_____   DRG #: __277__   Expected Length of Stay: __3 days__

Resuscitation Status   ☐ No Code/DNR   Date: _____   Date of Admission: _____

☐ Other : _____   Date: _____   Date of Surgery: _____

Date/ Initials	Disci- pline	Patient Problem(s)	Patient Goal(s) Met by Discharge	Date Resolved/ Initials
		Impaired skin integrity	Patient will experience initial healing of skin & underlying tissues	
		Pain	Patient will state pain is relieved after appropriate interventions	
		Knowledge deficit	Describe skin care needed to prevent further episodes of cellulitis	
		Impaired physical mobility	Ambulate in hall with assistance, if necessary	

Continued

MULTIDISCIPLINARY PLAN OF CARE

ASPECT OF CARE	Cellulitis	
DISCHARGE OUTCOMES	**DATE:** **Admission Day**	
CONSULTS Consults completed	___ Dietician if diabetic ___ Social Medicine intervention per criteria ___ Diabetic Educator, if Diabetic ___	___ Skin integrity/ET Nurse ___ Home Infusion Program ___
DIAGNOSTIC STUDIES Results within normal limits	___ CBC with differential, Lytes, BUN, Cr, RBS ___ Chemstrips, if Diabetic ___ Blood culture ___ Wound C & S if appropriate ___ X-ray if suspect osteomyelitis ___	___ ___ ___ ___ ___ ___
TREATMENTS, PROCEDURES, & MONITORS Tolerating treatments & procedures well, VSS	___ VS q 4 hrs ___ Skin/wound assessment & care q 8 hrs ___ I & O ___ Elevate affected extremity ___ ___ ___ ___ ___ ___ ___	___ ___ ___ ___ ___ ___ ___ ___ ___ ___ ___
MEDICATIONS/ LINES Pain and/or cellulitis controlled with analgesics & antibiotics	___ IV fluids ___ IVPB antibiotics ___ Oral analgesics PRN ___ Hypoglycemic agent, if Diabetic ___ ___	___ ___ ___ ___ ___ ___
NUTRITION Tolerating diet & understands dietary restrictions	___ Diet as tolerated ___ Diabetic diet, if indicated ___	___ ___ ___
ACTIVITY/ MOBILITY Ambulate with help or device	___ Bedrest with BRP or bedside commode ___ Assist ADLs as appropriate ___ ___ ___	___ ___ ___ ___ ___
PATIENT/FAMILY EDUCATION Patient/SO will describe skin care to prevent further cellulitis	___ Begin/reinforce Diabetic teaching, if appropriate ___ Discuss expected LOS with patient/family ___ Initiate Diabetic MPEPs, if Diabetic ___	___ Begin Skin Care teaching ___ ___ ___
PSYCHO-SOCIAL Coping with illness and/or stressors	___ Psychosocial needs identified: ___ specify _____ ___ _____	___ ___ ___
DISCHARGE PLANNING Adequate support resources identified	___ Discharge Planner for possible SNF placement or Home Health referral ___ Assess family support & resources ___	___ ___ ___

This Plan of Care and guidelines do not purport to reflect all relevant medical considerations and are not intended to replace clinical judgment.
REVISED 6/10/96, Approved by Pharmacy & Therapeutics Committee 8/96, Medical Records Committee 8/96, Executive Committee 9/96

DRG277.DOC

MULTIDISCIPLINARY PLAN OF CARE

ASPECT OF CARE	Cellulitis	
DISCHARGE OUTCOMES	**DATE:** Day 1	
CONSULTS	___ P.T. if necessary for ambulation with assistive device ___	___ ___
DIAGNOSTIC STUDIES	___ FBS - if diabetic ___ Chemstrips, if Diabetic ___ ___ ___	___ ___ ___ ___ ___
TREATMENTS, PROCEDURES, & MONITORS	___ VS q 4 hrs ___ Skin/wound assessment & care q 8 hrs ___ I & O ___ Elevate affected extremity ___ ___ ___ ___ ___	___ ___ ___ ___ ___ ___ ___ ___ ___
MEDICATIONS/ LINES	___ IV fluids ___ IVPB antibiotics ___ Oral analgesics PRN ___ Hypoglycemic agent, if Diabetic ___ ___	___ ___ ___ ___ ___ ___
NUTRITION	___ Diet as tolerated ___ Diabetic diet, if indicated ___	___ ___ ___
ACTIVITY/ MOBILITY	___ Chair BID with affected extremity elevated ___ Assist ADLs as appropriate ___ ___ ___	___ ___ ___ ___ ___
PATIENT/FAMILY EDUCATION	___ Reinforce MPEPs & previous teaching ___ Continue Skin Care teaching ___ ___ ___	___ ___ ___ ___ ___
PSYCHO-SOCIAL	___ Follow-up needs: ___ specify _____ ___ _____	___ ___ ___
DISCHARGE PLANNING	___ Refer to Home Health or SNF as needed ___ ___ ___ ___	___ ___ ___ ___ ___

This Plan of Care and guidelines do not purport to reflect all relevant medical considerations and are not intended to replace clinical judgment.
REVISED 6/10/96, Approved by Pharmacy & Therapeutics Committee 8/96, Medical Records Committee 8/96, Executive Committee 9/96

DRG277.DOC

Continued

MULTIDISCIPLINARY PLAN OF CARE

ASPECT OF CARE	Cellulitis	
DISCHARGE OUTCOMES	**DATE:**	**Day 2**
CONSULTS	___ Home Infusion referral ___ Infectious Disease ___	___ ___ ___
DIAGNOSTIC STUDIES	___ Chemstrips, if Diabetic ___ WBC, if elevated on admission ___ ___ ___	___ ___ ___ ___ ___
TREATMENTS, PROCEDURES, & MONITORS	___ D/C I & O ___ VS q 8 hrs ___ Skin care/wound care q 8 hrs ___ Elevate affected extremity ___ ___ ___ ___ ___ ___	___ ___ ___ ___ ___ ___ ___ ___ ___ ___
MEDICATIONS/ LINES	___ D/C IV - Hep-Lock ___ IVPB antibiotics ___ Oral analgesics PRN ___ Hypoglycemic agent, if Diabetic ___ ___	___ ___ ___ ___ ___ ___
NUTRITION	___ Diet as tolerated ___ Diabetic diet, if indicated ___ ___	___ ___ ___ ___
ACTIVITY/ MOBILITY	___ Ambulate in room with assistive device PRN ___ ___ ___ ___	___ ___ ___ ___ ___
PATIENT/FAMILY EDUCATION	___ Continue diabetic teaching, if needed ___ Begin IV & medication instruction, if needed ___ Continue Skin Care teaching ___ ___	___ ___ ___ ___ ___
PSYCHO-SOCIAL	___ Follow-up needs: ___ specify _____ ___ _____	___ ___ ___
DISCHARGE PLANNING	___ Arrange for dressing supplies, equipment to be used at home PRN ___ ___ ___	___ ___ ___ ___

This Plan of Care and guidelines do not purport to reflect all relevant medical considerations and are not intended to replace clinical judgment.
REVISED 6/10/96, Approved by Pharmacy & Therapeutics Committee 8/96, Medical Records Committee 8/96, Executive Committee 9/96

DRG277.DOC

MULTIDISCIPLINARY PLAN OF CARE

ASPECT OF CARE	Cellulitis	
DISCHARGE OUTCOMES	DATE:	Day 3
CONSULTS	___ ___ ___	___ ___ ___
DIAGNOSTIC STUDIES	___ Chemstrips, if Diabetic ___ ___ ___ ___	___ ___ ___ ___ ___
TREATMENTS, PROCEDURES, & MONITORS	___ VS q 8 hrs ___ Skin care/wound care q 8 hrs ___ Elevate affected extremity ___ ___ ___ ___ ___ ___ ___	___ ___ ___ ___ ___ ___ ___ ___ ___ ___
MEDICATIONS/ LINES	___ D/C Hep-Lock, if changed to PO antibiotics ___ Restart Venous Access Device if continued IV antibiotics or home infusion indicated ___ Oral antibiotics ___ Oral analgesics PRN ___ Hypoglycemic agent, if Diabetic	___ ___ ___ ___ ___ ___
NUTRITION	___ Diet as tolerated ___ Diabetic diet, if indicated	___ ___
ACTIVITY/ MOBILITY	___ Ambulate in room with assistive device PRN ___ ___ ___	___ ___ ___ ___

PATIENT/FAMILY EDUCATION	___ Review DC instructions re: Wound/skin care,
	     medications, physical activity and evaluate
	     understanding
	 ___ Continue Skin Care teaching
	 ___ Complete MPEPs give copy...
		___
		 ___
		 ___
		 ___
		 ___

PSYCHO-SOCIAL	___ Follow-up needs: ___ specify _____ ___ _____	___ ___ ___
DISCHARGE PLANNING	___ Arrange for follow-up appointments & referrals ___ Continue plans for outpatient parenteral antibiotics ___ Refer to Outpatient Diabetic classes and ___ Weight Control classes PRN	___ ___ ___ ___

This Plan of Care and guidelines do not purport to reflect all relevant medical considerations and are not intended to replace clinical judgment. REVISED 6/10/96, Approved by Pharmacy & Therapeutics Committee 8/96, Medical Records Committee 8/96, Executive Committee 9/96

DRG277.DOC

CHAPTER 13

Optic and Auditory Systems

■ OPTIC SYSTEM ASSESSMENT
(Fig. 13-1)

▇ SUBJECTIVE DATA

Blurred or double vision
Sudden loss of vision
Light, flashes, rainbows, floaters, or halos seen
Decreased or absent vision
Decreased night or peripheral vision
Glare at night and in bright light
Objects held too near or far
Needs stronger light to see
Collides with unfamiliar objects
Eye fatigue and strain
Sense of pressure or pulling within the eye
Tenderness or pain: sudden or gradual onset
Eyes water, itch, and burn
Dryness of eyes
Increased tearing
Trauma to head, face, or eyes
Inability to see in bright light
Headache
Squinting
Frequent falls
Clumsiness
Photophobia

▇ OBJECTIVE DATA

General appearance
Age of patient (see Gerontologic Considerations box)
Vital signs: elevated blood pressure (BP), temperature (T), pulse (P), or respiratory rate (R)
Pupil: equal, round, reacts to light and accommodation
Wears glasses, contact lenses, or eye patch
Position of reading material
Conjunctiva
   Conjunctivitis
   Drainage
     Amount
     Type
Rubbing eyes
Amount of dependence or independence
Visual acuity
   Distant vision (20/20)
   Near vision
   Peripheral vision

Exophthalmos
Eyelids
   Ability to close eyelid(s)
   Ability to blink
   Changes: edema, ptosis, redness, eversion, inversion
Abnormal eye movement
Opaqueness of eyeball
Increased tearing
Head tilts to improve vision
Squinting
Medication, eyedrops used
Bulging of one or both eyes
Allergies
Strabismus
Nystagmus
Scleral edema, infection, jaundice
Chalazion
Foreign body
Laceration, contusion
Enucleation

▇ PERTINENT BACKGROUND INFORMATION

CONCURRENT DISEASES OR CONDITIONS
Multiple sclerosis
Diabetes mellitus
Hypothyroidism
Hyperthyroidism
Sinus problems
Hypertension
Cerebral-associated diseases, trauma, or tumors
Sexually transmitted diseases
Myasthenia gravis
Glaucoma
Cataract
Retinal detachment
Autoimmune diseases
Arthritis, rheumatism
Stroke, aneurysm

PREVIOUS SURGERY OR ILLNESS
Eye surgery or treatments
Head or face trauma
Oxygen therapy as newborn
Coma

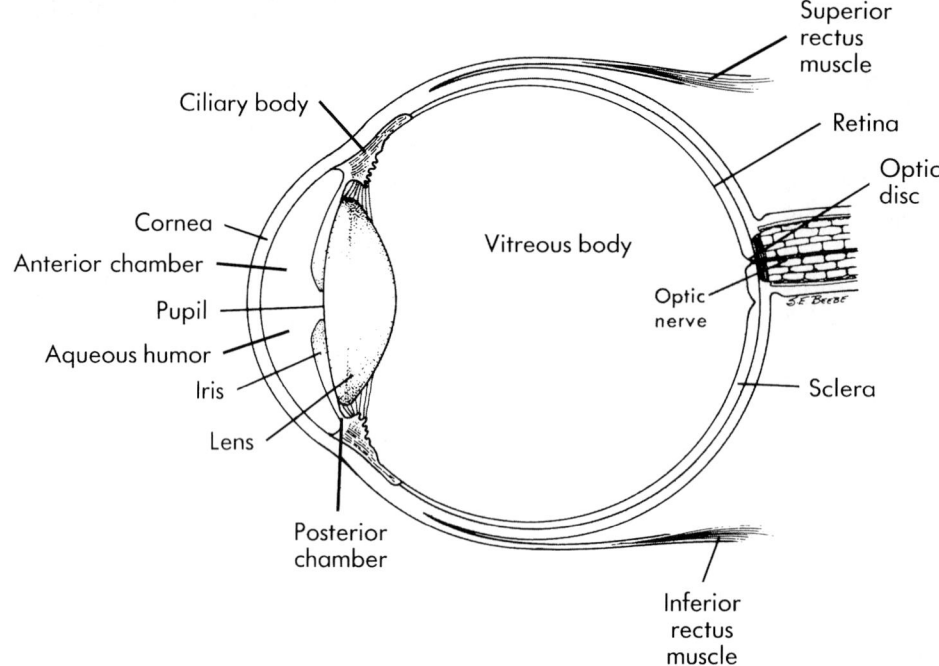

Fig. 13-1 The eye.

Gerontologic Considerations

- Multiple changes in vision that normally occur with aging include the following:
  - Changes in accommodation, resulting in increased difficulty focusing on close objects (presbyopia), which leads to difficulty reading or doing other close work
  - Decreased color perception and discrimination, particularly with shades of blue, green, and violet
  - Poor adaptation to changes in light, resulting in "night blindness" and increased sensitivity to glare
  - Alterations in depth perception, leading to increased risk of falls
  - Decreased secretion of tears, resulting in complaints of dryness or pruritus, which leads to a high risk for irritation of the cornea
  - Increased incidence of moving particles or "floaters" that interfere with visual tasks
- Older adults experience an increased incidence of eye disorders including cataracts, retinal detachment, macular degeneration, and glaucoma.

Modified from Christensen BL, Kockrow EO: Foundations of nursing, ed 3, St Louis, 1998, Mosby.

Hypertension
Substance abuse
Macular degeneration

FAMILY HISTORY
Glaucoma
Diabetes mellitus
Cataracts
Retinitis pigmentosa

SOCIAL HISTORY
Hazardous job or recreation
Safety precautions taken
Alcohol or drug abuse
Sexually transmitted diseases

MEDICATION HISTORY
Antibiotics
Antiemetics
Miotics
Acetazolamide
Mydriatics
Beta blockers
Epinephrine derivatives
Steroids (systemic, topical)
Antilipidemic agents
Hydroxychloroquine sulfate (Plaquenil)

DIAGNOSTIC TESTS
Visual fields and acuity
    Snellen chart
Biopsy and cultures
Magnetic resonance imaging (MRI)
Computed tomography (CT) scan
X-ray studies of orbit and skull
Ophthalmoscopic evaluation: direct, indirect
Slit-lamp examination
Pupil dilation
Tonometry
Flurescein angiography, stain
Ultrasonography
Gonioscopy
Brain scan
Ultrasound
Electroretinogram (ERG)

Color vision test
Refraction
Microscopic procedures and examination
Conjunctival scrapings

■ VISUALLY IMPAIRED PATIENT

The loss of visual acuity that encompasses partial or low vision to that of total blindness (Table 13-1)

ASSESSMENT
SUBJECTIVE AND OBJECTIVE DATA
Status of impairment
    Temporary (eye patch, shield)
    Permanent
Duration of impairment
Degree of visual loss
Degree of acceptance of impairment
Cause of visual impairment: diabetes, stroke, aneurysms, brain tumor, trauma, glaucoma
Condition of eyes: drainage, crusting, redness, pain, edema, squinting, abnormal eye movements, rubbing, opacities, bulging of one or both eyes
Difference in size of pupils
Variations in ability to perform activities of daily living (ADLs)

MULTIDISCIPLINARY MANAGEMENT
PATIENT PROBLEMS—NURSING DIAGNOSES/INTERVENTIONS

▼Sensory/perceptual alterations: visual related to altered sensory reception or transmission secondary to impairment

Familiarize patient with surroundings *to promote confidence*
Place all utensils and personal articles within easy reach and maintain consistent placement
Use patient's senses of touch and smell during orientation
Describe location of doors, windows, furniture, bathroom, and other patients
Establish effective lines of communication *to ensure understanding*
    Always identify self when approaching or touching patient
    Call patient by name
    Explain purpose of visit and visit often, especially at night
    Use visual aids: magnifying glasses, large print
Encourage and assist patient with independence *to encourage self-care activities:* explain position of food on tray and prepare food as necessary; use clock sequence (e.g., plate at 6 o'clock, fruit at 10 o'clock, milk at 1 o'clock); assist only as needed
Initiate grooming procedures as tolerated
Explain position of articles and place in same position each time
Withdraw assistance gradually

Table 13-1	Categories of Visual Impairment	
Category	Visual Acuity (with Optimum Correction)	Visual Field Radius
LOW VISION STATUS		
1	20/70	Not defined
2	20/70 to 20/200	Not defined
BLINDNESS STATUS		
3	Able to count fingers at 3 m; 20/200 to 20/400	Radius reduced to 5-10 degrees regardless of visual acuity status
4	Able to count fingers at 1 m; 20/400 to 20/1200 (5/300)	Radius reduced to 5-10 degrees regardless of visual acuity status
5	No light perception	—

From Thompson JM et al: Mosby's clinical nursing, ed 4, St Louis, 1997, Mosby.

Expected Outcomes
Performs self-care within limits of impairment
Communicates effectively using learned skills

▼Risk for injury/trauma related to sensory dysfunction secondary to visual impairment

Maintain safe environment *to prevent accidents, injuries*
    Place side rails up while patient is in bed
    Keep bed in locked, low position
    Place call bell and needed articles within easy reach
    Maintain environment as described (e.g., furniture, footstools, IV poles, wastebaskets)
    Keep doors fully open or closed
Flag chart and bed, indicating degree, type of visual impairment, and eye affected *to provide continuity of care*
Encourage patient to call nurse before ambulating; assist by standing on affected side, with patient's hand resting on your arm at elbow
Walk slowly and slightly ahead of patient
Allow patient to trace progress by running dorsal aspect of free hand along the wall
Describe surroundings and warn of impediments in advance
Instruct patient to avoid use of sharp items such as razors, scissors, and glass without supervision

Expected Outcomes
Demonstrates ability to perform activities in a safe manner
Verbalizes understanding of needed limitations

▼Anxiety related to threat to or change in role or health status secondary to degree of visual impairment

Assess level of anxiety and normal coping mechanisms *to provide a basis for assistance*

Encourage and allow time for verbalization of feelings

Explain daily plan of care and procedures *to reduce anxiety level*

Ensure privacy and assure patient that privacy is being provided

Allow as much independence as safety permits

Provide reassurance by being available and answering all questions

Provide time for use of relaxation measures

Encourage visitors and communication with significant others

Assist family members, staff, and visitors to use vocal and touch approach

Identify and reinforce use of adaptive coping mechanisms *to improve self-esteem*

Present a calm, caring attitude

Provide diversional activities *to reduce attention on anxiety*

Expected Outcomes

Identifies causative factors of anxiety

Accepts limitations and seeks ways to use remaining sight

Seeks assistance appropriately

▼Body image disturbance related to visual impairment

Discuss with patient and significant others alternatives in managing ADLs: dressing, bathing, grooming

Assess past coping mechanisms that have been successful

Allow time for patient to verbalize feelings *to reduce frustration*

Demonstrate acceptance of these feelings

Provide quiet, encouraging environment

Assist with and teach new skills as needed

Discuss and set small, realistic goals *to increase self-confidence*

Encourage patient to make as many decisions as possible about daily routines *to increase sense of autonomy and control*

Provide praise and encouragement

Promote support by significant other

Encourage involvement with others *to avoid isolation*

Assist patient in discussing and accepting altered visual acuity

Encourage independence as tolerated

Encourage use of other senses: touch, smell, hearing

Expected Outcomes

Demonstrates adaptive responses to altered body image

Expresses awareness of change and progresses toward acceptance

Additional Nursing Diagnoses to Consider

Self-esteem disturbance related to visual loss

Family coping: potential for growth related to acceptance of visual loss

Risk for injury at home related to loss of vision

PATIENT/FAMILY TEACHING

Reinforce safety precautions related to furniture placement, sharp objects and corners, scatter rugs, objects on floor

Reinforce physician's explanation of disease, disease process, and need to notify physician of any changes in condition

Assist patient and/or significant other in managing ADLs

Promote self-care within limits of visual impairment *to maximize independence*

Demonstrate procedure for instillation of eyedrops or ointments as prescribed

Refer to home health care agency and/or organizations for the visually impaired*

Contact state agency for the blind at time of discharge

Maintain regular outpatient care visits with physician

DISCHARGE/HOME CARE PLANNING

See Home care considerations for the visually impaired patient (p. 735)

■ ACUTE GLAUCOMA: ADULT ONSET

acute (closed-angle) glaucoma: Disease characterized by suddenly impaired vision resulting from intraocular pressure caused by imbalance in production and excretion of aqueous humor; if left untreated may cause optic nerve degeneration, visual field loss, and total blindness

ASSESSMENT

SUBJECTIVE DATA

Rapid onset of severe pain in eye(s)

Blurred vision

Headache

Rainbows in artificial light

Halos around lights

Nausea

Excessive tearing

OBJECTIVE DATA

Vomiting

Dilated pupil(s)

DIAGNOSTIC TESTS

Tonometry

Gonioscopy

Visual fields

Visual acuity

Ophthalmoscopy

Tonography

Fundoscopy

POTENTIAL COMPLICATIONS

Infection

Increased intraocular pressure (IOP)

Increased visual impairment

Blindness if untreated

American Foundation for the Blind, 11 Penn Plaza, Suite 300, New York, NY 10001

MULTIDISCIPLINARY MANAGEMENT
THERAPEUTIC MANAGEMENT
Miotic beta-blocker eyedrops
Carbonic anhydrase inhibitors
Hyperosmotic agents
Antiemetics
Analgesics
Laser iridotomy
Iridectomy

PATIENT PROBLEMS—NURSING DIAGNOSES/INTERVENTIONS

▼Pain related to increased intraocular pressure (IOP)

Assess type, intensity, and location of pain; be alert for signs of increased IOP
Use pain rating scale to determine analgesia dose
Maintain bed rest in quiet, darkened room with head elevated 30 degrees or in position of comfort
Administer analgesics and diuretics: assess for effectiveness, side effects; avoid morphine, which may cause nausea and vomiting
Avoid nausea and vomiting, which increase IOP: administer antiemetics as needed
Administer osmotics, carbonic anhydrase inhibitors *to decrease aqueous production*
Assess visual acuity
Administer back rubs, position changes *to promote comfort*

Expected Outcomes
Demonstrates knowledge of pain control measures
Experiences and demonstrates periods of uninterrupted sleep
Exhibits decreased IOP

▼Anxiety related to altered health status and decreased visual acuity

Assess anxiety level
Discuss previous coping methods *to provide a basis for counseling*
Encourage verbalization of anxieties
Maintain calm environment
Provide emotional support
Answer questions honestly
Explain all procedures
Reinforce physician's explanation of disease process and surgery if indicated
Visit frequently, especially at night
Explain nursing care plan
Discuss visual limitations as needed
Place all needed articles within reach and strive to keep them in same place at all times *to provide continuity of care*
Reassure that assistance with ADLs will be available
Assist and teach relaxation techniques: deep breathing, meditation, imagery

Keep patient informed of progress and planned medical and surgical interventions
Provide information and support for possible laser iridotomy (see Eye surgery, p. 739)

Expected Outcomes
Demonstrates adaptive coping measures to reduce anxiety
Expresses understanding of disease process

PATIENT/FAMILY TEACHING
Teach eyedrop instillation procedure to patient and significant other(s)
Discuss possible side effects
Interactions of eye medications with those prescribed for other diseases such as hypertension, diabetes, chronic obstructive pulmonary disease (COPD)
Timoptic: hypotension, bradycardia, bronchospasm
Miotics: blurred vision, diarrhea
Acetazolamide (Diamox): hyperkalemia, confusion, impotence
Always count drops and do not miss a dose
Keep extra bottles of drops in case of loss or breakage
Stress that drops will be needed over extended period
Discuss name, dose, and administration times of medications
Emphasize need to wear and carry medical alert bracelet and card
Stress importance of never taking medication containing atropine or any over-the-counter medications without consulting physician
Discuss symptoms of IOP to report to physician
Severe pain in eye(s)
Blurred vision
Headache
Halos or rainbows
Nausea, vomiting
Review factors that increase IOP and should be avoided:
Constrictive clothing
Constipation (straining)
Exertion or heavy lifting
Bending at waist
Sneezing or coughing
Nausea, vomiting
Refer to agencies for visually impaired
Explain importance of follow-up care with physician

DISCHARGE/HOME CARE PLANNING
See Home care considerations for the visually impaired patient (p. 735)

■ DIABETIC RETINOPATHY
Diabetic retinopathy is a vascular disorder resulting from juvenile or adult-onset diabetes; it is one of the leading causes of blindness and is related to the degree of control of diabetes in the early years of the disease

ASSESSMENT

SUBJECTIVE DATA

Sudden loss of vision (partial or complete)
Blurred vision
Absence of pain
Complaints of glare
Red shower over eyes or floaters seen

OBJECTIVE DATA

Decreased visual acuity
Opaqueness of eyeball

DIAGNOSTIC TESTS

Indirect ophthalmoscopy
Slit-lamp examination
Fluorescein angiography

POTENTIAL COMPLICATIONS

Vitreous hemorrhage
Retinal detachment
Increased visual impairment
Blindness if left untreated

MULTIDISCIPLINARY MANAGEMENT

THERAPEUTIC MANAGEMENT

Careful monitoring and control of diabetes
Photocoagulation (laser therapy)
Vitrectomy
    Cycloplegic agents
    Topical antibiotics/steroid agents
    Analgesics

PATIENT PROBLEMS—NURSING DIAGNOSES/INTERVENTIONS

▼ Sensory/perceptual alteration (visual) related to gradual loss of vision

Assess visual acuity
Review ADLs that are affected as a result of vision loss
Assess patient's family and support system to provide assistance in dealing with visual loss
Review with patient and family safety measures to use in home and community
Be aware of patient's guilt feelings about lack of self care
    Clear up any misconceptions patient has regarding blaming self for present conditions of vision loss
Offer support and comfort
Devise strategies for carrying out ADL with patient *to maximize patient independence*
Give realistic encouragement for maintenance of independence

Expected Outcomes

Communicates effectively using learned skills
Performs self-care within limits of impairment
Aware of safety measures to use in home and community related to visual changes or loss

▼ Anxiety related to threat of further visual loss

Assess patient's level of anxiety
Assess for present visual acuity, other physical problems, knowledge of condition and available support system
Inform patient of diabetes, hypertension, and their effects on present and future visual dysfunction *to reduce anxiety*
Be realistic in describing health status assessment and prognosis to patient and family
Offer continuing support and comfort to patient and family

Expected Outcomes

Fully informed regarding present visual status and prognosis
Able to draw on effective support system to aid in self-care

Additional Nursing Diagnoses to Consider

Risk for injury related to self-care and safety threatened by diminished vision
Knowledge deficit related to self-care and monitoring of diabetes mellitus

PATIENT/FAMILY TEACHING

Discuss with patient and family the need for careful monitoring and control of diabetes
Discuss importance of not smoking
Maintain patient's awareness of the diabetic sate and self-care needs
Stress importance of keeping high blood pressure under control
Stress the importance of regular visual examinations—*at least annually*
Discuss symptoms to report to physician
    Sudden loss of vision (usually unilateral; loss may be within seconds or persist over a day or two)
    Blurred or double vision
    Increased in floaters or persistent floaters
    Flashes of light
    Sharp pain/pressure in or around eyes
Discuss the importance of reporting any changes in vision status, especially peripheral vision
    Running into large objects
    "Blind" spots on either side of central vision
    Changes in ability to differentiate colors
Explain that visual changes may be very gradual (over many years)
Reassure patient realistically to help patient continue an independent lifestyle and to develop ways to adapt to diminishing vision
Refer to agencies for visually impaired

DISCHARGE/HOME CARE PLANNING

See Discharge/home care planning for the visually impaired patient (p. 735)

■ EYE SURGERY

cataract removal with or without intraocular lens transplant: *Surgical removal of a lens that has become opaque because of senile degenerative changes, trauma, or systemic disease (diabetes) or a congenitally opaque lens; an intraocular lens may be implanted simultaneously as an alternative to wearing cataract glasses or contact lenses postoperatively*

   corneal transplant: *Surgical procedure to replace a damaged cornea with a healthy, clear donor cornea of equal size*

   scleral buckling, retinal cryopexy, photocoagulation: *Surgical repair of a detached retina*

   enucleation: *Surgical removal of a blind, painful eye globe while maintaining orbital integrity for insertion of a prosthesis*

   iridectomy, laser iridectomy, trabeculectomy, goniotomy: *Surgical incision to release accumulated pressure caused by glaucoma by creating a channel for drainage of the aqueous humor*

   vitrectomy: *Surgical removal of all or part of vitreous humor that has become clouded with blood or fibrous membrane as a result of diabetes, intraocular foreign body, or hemorrhage. Saline is infused to replace the vitreous; gas, air, or silicone oil may be injected into the eye to keep the retina in place*

   NOTE: *Patients with retinal detachment may need special positioning in bed, patching of the eye, and restrictions on activity to prevent further or complete detachment*

DIAGNOSTIC TESTS

Complete blood count (CBC), prothrombin
   time/International Normalized Ratio (PT/INR)
Ophthalmoscopy
Slit-lamp examination
Visual fields
Tonometry, tonography
Gonioscopy

PREOPERATIVE ASSESSMENT AND TEACHING

Reinforce physician's explanation of surgical procedure
   to ensure patient is informed
Encourage and allow time for verbalization of fears and
   anxieties
Answer all questions with honesty, empathy, and
   understanding to increase patient's confidence and
   knowledge
Explain postoperative nursing care plan and availability of
   staff to reduce anxiety
Assess present degree of sight and assist as needed
Provide a safe environment; orient patient to room floor
   plan, placement of call bell, personal articles
Explain surgical preparation of eye according to hospital
   policy and physician's order *to involve patient and
   decrease fear*
Discuss preoperative and postoperative indications
Stress importance of wearing eye patch/shield
   postoperatively

Discuss with patient and teach not to bend, strain, lift
   heavy objects (more than 5 lb) postoperatively
Discuss importance of trying not to cough, sneeze, or
   vomit postoperatively
Advise patient not to touch or rub eyes *to prevent
   trauma or infection*
Explain that all eye makeup is removed before surgery

POSTOPERATIVE ASSESSMENT
SUBJECTIVE DATA

Nausea
Sudden, severe eye pain

OBJECTIVE DATA

Vomiting
Placement of eye bandage(s)
Restlessness
Position to be maintained while in bed

POTENTIAL COMPLICATIONS

Hemorrhage
Shock
Infection
Decreased visual acuity
Blindness

MULTIDISCIPLINARY MANAGEMENT
THERAPEUTIC MANAGEMENT

Medications
   Analgesics
   Antiemetics
   Antibiotics
   Stool softeners
Eye shield or patch
Nothing by mouth (NPO) until fully reactive, increase to
   presurgery diet
Ambulation and activities
Dressing changes/warm or cold sterile compresses
Prescription glasses (clear, dark)

PATIENT PROBLEMS—NURSING DIAGNOSES/INTERVENTIONS

▼ Risk for infection related to invasive surgical procedure

Monitor dressing q2h for 4 hours, then q4h if present
Assess for drainage, bleeding, pain: report immediately
Maintain eye shield or patch *to increase protection*
Caution patients not to touch, squeeze, or rub eye
Monitor vital signs q4h until stable
Administer postoperative and antibiotic or steroid drops
   as ordered

Expected Outcomes

Temperature remains normal
Eye remains clean, with no purulent drainage

▼Risk for injury/trauma related to sensory dysfunction secondary to altered visual acuity

Assess visual acuity

Keep side rails up at all times

Assist with limited activities or bedrest as ordered

Plan all care with patient; explain daily routines *to increase confidence and reduce anxiety*

Announce yourself when entering room *to avoid startling patient*

Assist with and teach deep-breathing exercises; stress need to avoid coughing, which increases IOP

Keep patient's articles in same place at bedside

Place call bell within easy reach

Enucleation patients have clean, plastic conformer in eye socket *to retain eye shape*

Advise patient to avoid squeezing eyelids shut or touching eyes postoperatively

Give analgesics and antiemetics as ordered to prevent excessive restlessness, bumping head, sneezing, coughing, or vomiting *to avoid increased intraocular pressure*

Increase activities and ambulation when patient demonstrates ability to remain safe

Assist with ambulation as needed; stand on affected side *to provide visual support*

Teach self-care activities and assist as needed

Expected Outcomes

Demonstrates understanding of safety precautions

Notifies staff for assistance

▼Pain related to surgical procedure

Assess pain intensity using pain rating scale

Administer analgesics; assess pain to ensure that it is not caused by increased IOP or bleeding; monitor for effectiveness

Administer back care and position changes *to relieve discomfort*

Vitrectomy patients must spend 4 to 5 days on abdomen or sitting forward with unoperative side of head resting on a table if air has been injected; provide skin care for knees and elbows

Teach and assist with alternative pain relief measures *to decrease attention on discomfort*

Expected Outcomes

Reports a reduction of pain

Appears calm and relaxed

▼Sensory/perceptual alteration related to impaired vision

Visit frequently *to determine needs and allay anxiety*, especially at night

Identify yourself when entering room; touch patient upon approach and identify yourself to notify patient of your proximity

Encourage patient to express feelings and thoughts

Involve significant others in care and activities *to provide support and assistance*

Reduce noise, traffic in area

Provide balanced rest and activity

Encourage diversional activities *to decrease attention on anxiety*

Allow patient to wear glasses, if allowed, *to increase sensory perception*

Expected Outcomes

Accepts and copes appropriately with visual limitations

Uses remaining sight or other senses adequately

PATIENT/FAMILY TEACHING
GENERAL

Instruct patient and/or significant other in care of the eyes

Dressing changes using aseptic techniques

Stress need to clean eyelid

Use of eye patch or shield at night

Method of eyedrop instillation

Avoid eye makeup until consent is given by physician

Avoid rubbing, squeezing, or touching eye, or bumping eye

Use of eyeglasses as ordered; sunglasses to reduce glare

Keep an extra bottle of eyedrops in case of loss or breakage and while traveling

Instruct the patient to avoid sleeping on the operative side

Caution patient to avoid constipation, bending, vacuuming, straining, and lifting heavy objects (more than 5 lb)

Discuss with the patient the need to avoid strenuous activity for 4 to 6 weeks

Provide list of organizations for visually impaired (see p. 735)

Discuss home care with patient and family/significant other(s)

Arrange furniture for safety and convenience

Encourage self-care

Avoid being overprotective

Provide diversional activities: records, tapes, recorded books; television and reading if able

Know name of medication, dosage, time of administration, purpose, and side effects

Avoid using over-the-counter medications, eyedrops, or ointments without physician approval

Make and keep follow-up appointments with physician

Discuss symptoms to report to physician

Pain in eye

Redness

Drainage

Decreased visual acuity

Blurred, double vision

Floaters

Halos, sparks

Fever

Swelling

SPECIFIC
Cataract Removal
Without lens implant, using glasses: explain that glasses
  Usually magnify objects 25% to 30%
  Decrease peripheral vision
  Can cause visual disturbance if fit is incorrect
  Allow patient to focus; patient will be unable to focus without them
  Are temporary glasses and new ones will be prescribed in about 4 to 8 weeks
  Sometimes alter distance judgment
Without lens implant, using contact lenses: explain that contact lenses
  Will be fitted and worn after 4 to 8 weeks
  Allow patient to focus, but patient will need glasses for close vision
With intraocular lens implant: explain that lens implant
  Aids in focusing, but glasses will be fitted for close vision in 8 to 12 weeks
  Does not cause depth perception loss

Trabeculectomy, Laser Iridotomy
Discuss signs of increased IOP
  Severe eye pain
  Headache
  Nausea
  Increased tearing
  Halos, sparks
Explain importance of using glaucoma eye drops in unoperated eye
Explain that medications do not cure glaucoma but can control it
Advise to use nonaspirin pain medication to prevent bleeding

Scleral Buckling, Retinal Cryopexy
Discuss symptoms of further detachment
  Sudden loss of vision
  Severe pain
  Flashing light
  Progressive shadows
  Increased floaters
Explain that reading must be avoided for 1 week

Corneal Transplant, Keratoplasty
Discuss signs of graft rejection, which occur about 10 to 14 days postoperatively
  Pain
  Clouding
  Inflammation
  Drainage
  Decreased vision
Explain that sutures will remain in eye up to 1 year
Explain that functional vision will not return until sutures are removed

Enucleation
Conformer for eyeball may become dislodged; explain that this is of little consequence and it need not be reinserted

Discuss use of antibiotic drugs and need to wear eye shield until prosthesis is fitted (in about 10 to 14 days)
Explain that in 4 to 6 weeks after surgery, patient will receive ocular prosthesis
Review care of eye socket. Discuss care for, insertion of, and removal of artificial eye if used

Vitrectomy
Stress importance of continuing cycloplegic, antibiotic, and antiinflammatory eye drops for 4 to 6 weeks
Advise to wear dark glasses to reduce discomfort from photophobia
Explain that depth perception will be lost and 50% of peripheral vision will be lost on affected side
No reading will be permitted while operative side is patched, to prevent eye movement
Watching television is permitted
Explain that visual function will be restored to the extent that the retina is intact. Advise patient to review visual prognosis with physician
If gas or air bubble was injected, caution patient to get advice from physician regarding air travel while bubble is present

DISCHARGE/HOME CARE PLANNING
Assess and continue with patient/family education and monitor the following:
  Environmental/safety status
    Evaluate and discuss
      Lighting for ease in movement
      Turning head to visualize the other side
      Using up and down head movements to judge stairs and oncoming objects
      Difficulty with night vision
      Hand rails, carpet or nonskid treads on stairs
      Carpets and rugs secured to floor
      Presence of telephone and emergency numbers in large print
      Presence of Lifeline or Life Dial system for emergencies
      Living quarters free of clutter (no throw rugs, articles on floor or stairs, electrical cords)
      Furniture arrangement adequate to allow a clear pathway
      Presence of smoke detectors, fire extinguishers
      Nonslip strips in tub
      Medications for easy administration; labeled correctly and in large enough print for identification
      Ability to instill eyedrops correctly (see p. 743)
      Presence of medication box that can be filled for daily use
      Presence of clock with large digital numbers or one that chimes
      Use of watch with raised numbers
      Use of slippers, shoes in good repair with nonskid soles
      Use and availability of walker, cane
      Use of available support groups
      Presence of sharp objects, pointed corners

Safe placement of cleaning materials with all poisons clearly marked

Adjusted water temperature to prevent burns

Transportation available for shopping, errands, and medical appointments

Eye care status

Evaluate and discuss the following:

Dressing change procedure if indicated

Condition of the eye for signs of infections, redness, pain, drainage

Care, insertion, and removal of lenses if indicated

Procedure for instilling eyedrops/ointments

Medication for correct administration times

Side effects of medications and to report

Handwashing technique

Personal care and hygiene status

Evaluate and discuss the following:

Availability of a caregiver if needed

Ability to bathe self in tub or shower or with sponge bath, with or without assistance

Grooming ability (hair, nails, clothing selection, shaving, makeup) with or without assistance

Dressing self: able to select and put on clothes with or without assistance

Height of toilet seat for easy access on and off

Nutritional status

Evaluate and discuss the following:

Ability to prepare meals alone or with assistance

Adequate fluid intake

Selection of food to provide adequate nourishment

Weight to monitor adequate intake

Elimination status

Evaluate and discuss management of bowel elimination to prevent constipation with natural laxatives (bran, prunes) or psyllium

Emotional status

Evaluate and discuss the following:

Degree of acceptance attained

Feelings of anxiety, low self-esteem, depression (see p. 56)

Knowledge of outside support groups available

American Foundation for the Blind
11 Penn Plaza, Suite 300
New York, NY 10001
800-232-5463

National Eye Institute
National Institute of Health
Bldg. 31, Room 6A03
9000 Rockville Pike
Bethesda, MD 20892
301-496-2234

Lions Club International
300 22nd Street
Oak Brook, IL 60523
630-571-5466

Importance of maintaining social interaction with family and friends

Availability of communication devices such as recorded books, telephone, alarm clocks, doorbell, fire alarm attached to vibrating device

Knowledge of local groups providing braille instruction

■ CONTACT LENS REMOVAL

Occasionally, unconscious, paralyzed, disoriented, or elderly patients and patients with limited or restricted use of their arms may be wearing contact lenses; lenses must be removed to prevent eye damage

ASSESSMENT

OBSERVATIONS/FINDINGS

Level of consciousness (LOC), ability to cooperate

Presence of contact lenses in unconscious patient: shine flashlight into eye from outer canthus; lenses will appear around iris or slightly beyond

Type of lenses

Hard: covers iris, may be tinted

Soft: covers iris, may be tinted

Extended wear (1 week)

Disposable (1 week)

Scleral: covers iris and sclera

Small suction cup apparatus for removing contact lenses is often kept in emergency room

REMOVAL PROCEDURE

Wash hands thoroughly before procedure

Removal of hard lenses

Place forefinger at outer canthus of eye

Gently push finger up and then down

Do not use force

Lens will appear from under lid

Store in distilled water, keeping right and left lenses separate and containers marked

Removal of soft lenses

Place thumb and forefinger on lower and upper lid, respectively

Gently open eye

With other hand *gently* lift lens off iris, using thumb and forefinger

Store in normal saline solution, keeping right and left lenses separate and containers marked, or discard if disposable

Removal of scleral lenses

Place forefinger at edge of and parallel to lower lid

Gently press lid downward until lower edge of lens is visible

Continue gentle pressure, pulling lid toward ear

Lens will slide out from under lid

Store in distilled water, keeping right and left lenses separate and containers marked

Removal of all types of lenses using suction cup apparatus

Depress bulb between thumb and forefinger

Position cup over lens

Slowly release pressure on bulb

Lens will adhere to cup

Remove lenses and store in marked containers with appropriate solution

If lenses are not visible (eyes rolled back) or difficulty is experienced in removal procedure, notify ophthalmologist to remove lenses

■ INSTILLATION OF EYEDROPS/OINTMENTS

PREINSTILLATION ASSESSMENT

Assess patient's ability to hold eyes open and cooperate

Explain purpose of medication, procedure, and side effects

Perform medication assessment

Correct medication, patient, dosage, time, and eye

Check dropper for defects

Understand abbreviations

OD: right eye

OS: left eye

OU: both eyes

INSTILLATION PROCEDURE (FIG. 13-2)

Eyedrops are sterile, and any contamination of the dropper or squeeze bottle can cause infection

Always discard when contamination occurs

Position patient in chair with head tilted back or in dorsal recumbent position in bed

Wash hands before procedure

Draw medication into dropper (keep medication from going into bulb end) or open squeeze bottle of drops or tube of ointment

Gently pull down skin beneath lower lid with thumb and place forefinger above upper lid; put pressure on the cheekbone, not on soft tissue of eye

Instruct patient to look upward

Allow time between drops: patient will blink after each drop

Instill drops or dab ointment into pocket formation in center of lower lid; do not touch conjunctiva with dropper or tube

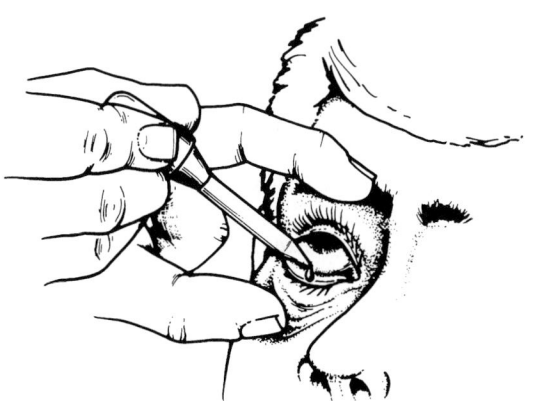

Fig. 13-2 Installation of eye drops.

Instruct patient to close eye gently and not to squeeze eye closed or rub it

Wipe off excess medication with tissue

Instruct patient to open and close eye slowly for a few minutes to distribute medication evenly

Wash hands after instilling medication

■ AUDITORY SYSTEM ASSESSMENT
(Fig. 13-3)

▐ SUBJECTIVE DATA

Earache (otalgia)

Headache

Decreased, absent hearing acuity in one or both ears

Sound distortion

Tinnitus

Feeling of fullness or blockage in ear

Own voice echoes

Popping noise when yawning or swallowing

Vertigo, dizziness, disequilibrium

Itching in ear

Heart pulsating in ear

Ear drainage

Dark

Red

Black

Clear

Yellow

Use of oils, cotton swabs, hairpins to clean ears

▐ OBJECTIVE DATA

General appearance

Vital signs: elevated BP, T, P, and R

Ability to hear; use of hearing aid

Ability to lip-read or use sign language

Delayed speech and language development (if small child)

Startle reflex

Tolerance of loud sounds

Type, color, and amount of ear drainage

Medication history (streptomycin, salicylates, quinine, gentamycin)

Allergies

Age (see Gerontologic Considerations box)

▐ PERTINENT BACKGROUND INFORMATION

CONCURRENT DISEASES OR CONDITIONS

Otitis media

Otosclerosis

Acoustic nerve tumor

Labyrinthitis

Ménière's, Graves' disease

Tinnitus

Cerebral tumors, contusion, diseases, fractures

Diabetes mellitus

Arteriosclerosis

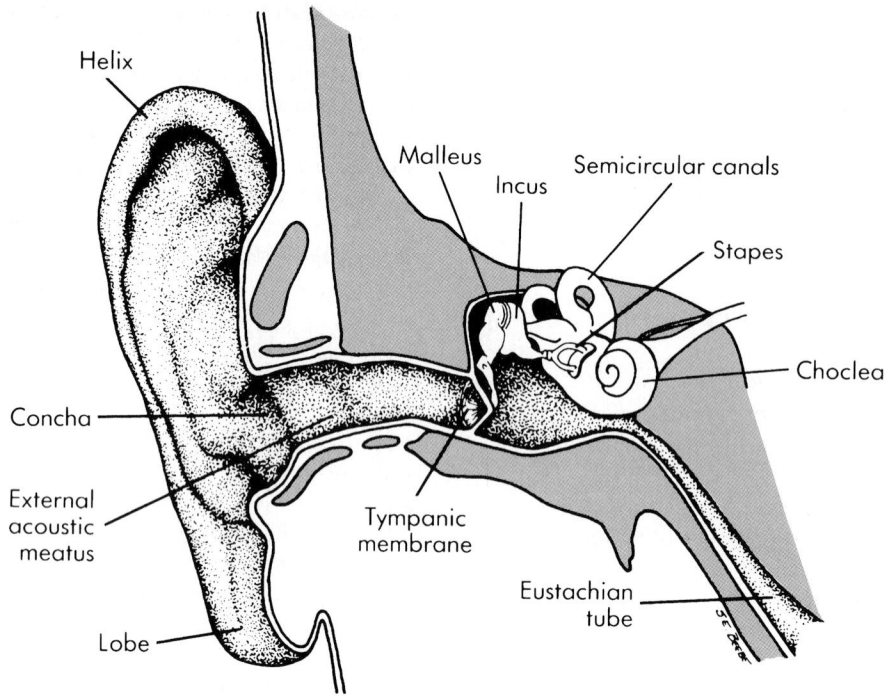

Fig. 13-3 The ear.

Gerontologic Considerations

- A third of all individuals over the age of 70 have significant hearing loss.
- Hearing loss in older adults is most often sensorineural and involves loss of the high frequencies. Hearing loss results in the distortion of speech, which can lead to failure to respond to directions or inappropriate behaviors often misinterpreted as disorientation.
- Hearing loss can lead to social isolation when the older adult is unable to understand and participate in normal conversation.

Modified from Christensen BL, Kockrow EO: Foundations of nursing, ed 3, St Louis, 1998, Mosby.

Hypertension
Hypotension
Mastoiditis
Bleeding disorders

PREVIOUS SURGERY OR ILLNESS
Stapes mobilization
Syphilis
Otitis media
Head trauma
Mastoidectomy

SOCIAL HISTORY
Sexually transmitted diseases
Recreational hazards: swimming, diving
Exposure to loud noises

Safety precautions taken
Use of tobacco, coffee, alcohol
Substance abuse

MEDICATION HISTORY
Antineoplastics
Diuretics
Narcotics
Narcotic antagonists
Ear drops
Antibiotics
Salicylates
Quinine

DIAGNOSTIC TESTS
Audiogram, audiometry, whisper test
Mastoid x-ray examination
Tuning fork test (Rinne)
Otologic examination to assess for cerumen buildup, foreign objects
"Lateralization" tuning fork test (Weber)
Pneumatic otoscopy
Tympanometry, acoustic reflex test
Caloric examination
Electronystagmography (ENG)
Electrocochleography
Tomogram
Cerebral arteriography
CT scan
MRI
Schwabach test

Platform posturography
Culture for pathogens
Lumbar puncture

■ HEARING-IMPAIRED PATIENT

The loss of hearing acuity that encompasses partial hearing loss to that of total deafness
Types of loss
   conduction: An interference of sound waves through auditory canal, eardrum, middle ear
   sensorineural: Injury or disease that affects the inner ear and nerve pathways to the brain
   mixed: Interference with conduction in all three areas: external, middle, and inner ear

ASSESSMENT
OBSERVATIONS/FINDINGS
Assess hearing acuity and communication skills
   Speaks loudly
   Inattentive
   Withdraws
Lip-reading or sign language
Hearing aid
Pad and pencil
Flash cards
Determine status and duration of impairment
Assess acceptance of impairment and skills learned
   Well adjusted
   Fear/anxiety
   Anger, hostility
Examine ears for drainage, crusts, cerumen accumulation, and deformities

MULTIDISCIPLINARY MANAGEMENT
PATIENT PROBLEMS—NURSING DIAGNOSES/INTERVENTIONS

▼Sensory/perceptual alteration related to hearing impairment

Assess level of hearing impairment
Reinforce physician's explanation of hearing impairment *to increase patient knowledge and feeling of security*
Assess and establish means of communication
   Lip-reading (speech reading)
      Speak slowly and enunciate well
      Do not exaggerate sounds
      Have only one person speak at a time
      Stand so patient can see your mouth clearly
      Speak in simple phrases first to determine expertise in the skill
      NOTE: Nurses with mustaches may be more difficult to understand
      Point to objects of conversation where appropriate

      Avoid chewing gum and shouting
      Rephrase statements if not understood initially
   Sign language
      Determine whether patient can communicate with pad and pencil, because most hospital personnel are not skilled in sign language
      Enlist cooperation of family/significant other in communication *to provide support*
   Hearing aid
      Assess patient's ability to use and care for appliance
      Make certain aid is in place and turned on before speaking
      Check for power level, battery, proper functioning
      Establish a pitch that is comfortable for patient
      Avoid shouting
      Stand so patient can see your face
   Pad and pencil
      Write messages clearly in short, simple phrases
      Develop a checklist of phrases most often used and instruct patient to check appropriate one(s)
      Allow time for patient to understand and answer

Expected Outcomes
Accepts limitations caused by hearing impairment
Demonstrates positive coping behaviors
Uses learned skills for communicating

▼Risk for injury/trauma related to hearing impairment

Maintain safe environment
   Locate bed so door is visible when possible
   Orient patient to surroundings; have call bell within reach
   Answer call light promptly
   Keep side rails up if appropriate
   Approach patient carefully if eyes are closed; a gentle touch on patient's arm will arouse but not startle
   Explain all procedures *to ensure understanding*
   Flag chart and bed indicating type of impairment and ear(s) involved *to provide continuity of care*

Expected Outcomes
Understands safety factors associated with hearing impairment
Demonstrates ability to perform activities in safe manner
Notifies staff for assistance

▼Anxiety related to hearing impairment

Maintain quiet, nonstressful environment
Assess level of anxiety *to provide baseline for counseling*
Encourage and allow time for verbalization of feelings
Explain nursing plan of care and involve patient in planning care *to reduce anxiety level*
Display confidence and a caring, nonjudgmental manner
Use pictures when explaining procedures or treatment
Encourage communication with significant other *to provide support*

Avoid using electronic nurse-patient intercommunication system if patient has partial hearing *because it can cause frustration*

Evaluate patient's ability to use other senses (sight and touch especially) *to aid in daily living*

Provide diversional activities: puzzles, cards, hobbies *to decrease attention on anxiety*

Expected Outcomes
Understands causes of anxiety
Demonstrates positive behaviors in coping with anxiety
Reports a reduction in anxiety level

PATIENT/FAMILY TEACHING
Reinforce physician's explanation of cause of impairment and prescribed treatment

Explain safety factors important in home environment

Discuss availability of hearing devices: amplifiers, flashing lights on telephones and door bells

Refer to local telephone company and/or hearing institute for assistance

Refer to local schools for classes on lip-reading and/or sign language

Instruct patient in care of hearing aid and to have extra battery available at all times

Demonstrate care of ear dressings and ear drop instillation if applicable

Encourage patient to make and keep follow-up appointments with physician

DISCHARGE/HOME CARE PLANNING
See Discharge/home care planning for the hearing-impaired patient (p. 749)

■ MÉNIÈRE'S DISEASE
A common disorder of the ear, both auditory and vestibular, that is thought to be caused by an alteration in the metabolism of the labyrinthine fluid of the vestibular system; this in turn causes the membrane of the labyrinth to dilate from the increased production of endolymph; severe attacks can be very disabling

ASSESSMENT
SUBJECTIVE DATA
Dizziness
Nausea, vomiting
Sweating
Abdominal pain
Blurred vision
Eyes sensitive to light
Roaring sensation in ears

OBJECTIVE DATA
Acute attack
  Rapid onset: recurrent deafness
  Tinnitus
  Incapacitating vertigo
  Diarrhea

Bradycardia
Disequilibrium: falls toward affected ear
Photophobia
Nystagmus
History of the following:
  Otitis media
  Arteriosclerosis
  Allergies
  Leukemia
  Tobacco, alcohol, caffeine abuse
Medication use
  Quinine
  Salicylates
  Streptomycin

DIAGNOSTIC TESTS
Audiologic testing
Audiometry
Electrocochleography
Electronystagmography
Audiogram
Caloric tests
X-ray examination of petrous bone

POTENTIAL COMPLICATIONS
Dehydration
Increased hearing impairment
Permanent disequilibrium, vertigo
Fractures from falling

MULTIDISCIPLINARY MANAGEMENT
THERAPEUTIC MANAGEMENT
Bed rest during acute attack
Low-sodium or neutral-ash diet
Restriction of salt and water intake
Diuretics: hydrochlorothiazide (Diuril), triamterene (Dyazide)
Vestibular depressants: diazepam (Valium), prochloperazine (Compazine), lorezepam (Ativan)
Adrenergic agents: meclizine (Antivert), epinephrine
Avoidance of tobacco, alcohol, caffeine, and high triglycerides
Surgical interventions: labyrinthectomy, vestibular neurectomy, endolymphatic decompression

PATIENT PROBLEMS—NURSING DIAGNOSES/INTERVENTIONS

▼ Sensory/perceptual alteration related to disequilibrium

Assess audiogram results
Assess patient's hearing acuity, which may be decreased
Flag chart and bed *to indicate impairment and provide continuity of care*
Stand so that patient can see your face
Speak slowly and enunciate carefully
Explain all procedures and nursing care plan *to promote confidence*

Maintain quiet environment *to alleviate confusion*
  Minimize activities in room
  Avoid bumping bed
Assist with personal care and activities as needed
Assist and teach patient to deep breathe q2h to 4h and
  turn on affected side when symptoms subside
Administer antianxiety agents

Expected Outcomes
Exhibits a more accepting manner
Appears more aware of surroundings

▼Risk for injury/trauma related to disequilibrium,
vertigo

Administer vestibular depressant
Maintain bed rest in position of comfort during acute
  attack *to prevent injury*
Keep side rails of bed up and bed in low position
Discourage smoking
Assess visual acuity because balance depends on it as
  well as the vestibular system
Instruct patient to call nurse before getting up
Ambulate as ordered
  Observe for vertigo, nausea, and nystagmus
  Provide unobstructed pathway *to prevent accidents*
  Assist with ambulation
  Increase distance as tolerated
Instruct patient to turn head slowly *to prevent*
  vertigo
Encourage use of walker, cane *to improve*
  equilibrium

Expected Outcomes
Expresses understanding of preventing injury
Uses devices to assist in ambulating

▼Risk for fluid volume imbalance (deficit) related to
fluid loss secondary to vomiting

Monitor intake and output for severe vomiting to form
  basis for fluid replacement
  Include emesis, diarrhea, urine
  Administer antiemetics *to reduce vomiting*
Monitor vital signs qid
Provide low-sodium diet as tolerated *to decrease*
  endolymph production
  Assist with eating
  Avoid caffeine
  Restrict fluid intake as ordered
Assess skin turgor, mucous membranes *to identify*
  dehydration
Monitor electrolytes *to assess for hypokalemia*

Expected Outcomes
Vital signs and electrolytes are within normal limits
Skin turgor is normal
Mucous membranes are moist
Appetite has improved

▼Anxiety related to change in health status

Assess level of anxiety *to assist in planning*
  interventions
Encourage and allow time for discussion of feelings
Explain plan of care and involve patient in care *to reduce*
  anxiety level
Provide diversional activities *to decrease attention on*
  anxiety
Discuss and teach stress management techniques, which
  may assist in reducing severe vertigo attacks
Reinforce physician's explanation of disease *to decrease*
  anxiety and increase knowledge

Expected Outcomes
Exhibits a more relaxed appearance
Discusses and practices relaxation techniques
Understands methods of dealing with vertigo

Additional Nursing Diagnoses to Consider
Body image disturbances related to acute
  vertigo/disequilibrium
Fear related to effects of vertigo

PATIENT/FAMILY TEACHING
Reinforce physician's explanation of disease process and
  procedures to follow when attacks occur
Explain that vertigo is usually first symptom; patient
  should immediately do the following:
  Take medication as ordered
  Lie or sit down when vertigo appears
  Not walk unassisted
  Notify physician of recurrence
  Stress to patient that progressive hearing loss may
    occur if treatment is not initiated or successful
Explain that tinnitus may always be present; advise
  patient to utilize background music, radio, or TV to
  overcome tinnitus
Discuss importance of leading a normal life when vertigo
  is absent
Explain importance of vestibular/balance exercise on a
  daily basis
Discuss importance of not driving when taking
  medication that slows reflexes
Assist patient and family to identify hazards in home
  environment and recommend modifications
Discuss importance of following low-sodium diet or
  neutral-ash diet as ordered
Warn patient to avoid ototoxic medications: salicylates,
  quinine, some diuretics, and aminoglycoside
  antibiotics
Instruct patient to avoid smoking, caffeine, alcohol
Explain importance of periodic audiologic examinations

DISCHARGE/HOME CARE PLANNING
See Home care considerations for the hearing-impaired
  patient (p. 749)

■ EAR SURGERIES

stapedectomy: *Surgical removal of all or part of the stapes footplate and creation of a patent oval window and pathway for sound transmission using natural or artificial materials, performed for otosclerosis*

myringotomy with tube insertion: *Surgical incision into the tympanic membrane to aspirate collected fluid and insertion of a ventilating tube to keep the pressure equal between the middle and outer ear, performed to correct serous otitis media*

tympanoplasty: *Surgical repair of tympanic membrane perforated or largely destroyed by infection, trauma, otosclerosis, stenosis, or necrosis of the middle ear; type performed depends on degree of perforation and destruction, as well as ossicular involvement and damage*

PREOPERATIVE ASSESSMENT/TEACHING

Assess hearing acuity in both ears *to provide basis for interventions*

Reinforce physician's explanation of procedure

Establish means of communication because hearing may be impaired

Encourage and allow time for verbalization of fears and anxieties

Explain postoperative patient care plan and availability of staff to reduce anxiety about procedure

Explain that hearing may not improve immediately

POSTOPERATIVE ASSESSMENT
SUBJECTIVE DATA

Restlessness resulting from decreased hearing

Location and character of pain

Excessive pain

Hearing acuity

Nausea

Headache

Vertigo

Altered taste

OBJECTIVE DATA

Vomiting

Character and amount of ear drainage

POTENTIAL COMPLICATIONS

Infection

Hemorrhage

Decreased hearing acuity

Tinnitus

Facial nerve paralysis

Perforation

MULTIDISCIPLINARY MANAGEMENT
THERAPEUTIC MANAGEMENT

Analgesics

Antiemetics

Antihistamines for nasal congestion

Antibiotics

Dressing change schedule

PATIENT PROBLEMS—NURSING DIAGNOSES/INTERVENTIONS

▼ Pain related to surgical procedure and position restriction

Maintain bed rest in quiet environment

Supine position with operative side up for prescribed length of time

    Keep side rails up *to promote slight position changes*

    Do not turn unless ordered

    Provide back rubs prn *to promote comfort and relaxation*

    Elevate head of bed when allowed *to provide comfort*

Assess pain intensity using a pain rating scale of 0 to 5

Administer analgesics and assess effectiveness of pain relief

Report excessive pain to physician; increasing pain may be a sign of bleeding

Avoid nose blowing and sneezing, which increase pain

Avoid vomiting by administering antiemetics

Expected Outcomes

Expresses satisfaction with pain relief measures

Appears calm and relaxed in position of comfort

▼ Risk for infection related to invasive surgical procedure

Monitor vital signs q4h, especially temperature

Monitor for signs of infection q4h

    Increased drainage/pain

    Fever

    Headache

    Administer antibiotics as prescribed

Keep outer ear plug clean and dry

Change ear plugs prn

Report excessive bleeding, drainage to physician

Maintain aseptic technique

Expected Outcomes

Patient is afebrile

Exhibits no purulent ear drainage

▼ Sensory/perceptual alteration related to hearing impairment

▼ Anxiety related to change in health status

Assess level of anxiety *to assist in planning interventions*

Encourage and allow time for discussion of feelings

Explain plan of care and involve patient in care *to reduce anxiety level*

Provide diversional activities *to decrease attention on anxiety*

Discuss and teach stress management techniques, which may assist in reducing severe vertigo attacks

Reinforce physician's explanation of disease *to decrease anxiety and increase knowledge*

Expected Outcomes
Exhibits a more relaxed appearance
Discusses and practices relaxation techniques
Understands methods of dealing with vertigo

Additional Nursing Diagnoses to Consider
Body image disturbances related to acute vertigo/disequilibrium
Fear related to effects of vertigo

PATIENT/FAMILY TEACHING
GENERAL
Explain importance of nutritious diet, fluid intake, rest, and activity
Avoid blowing nose, which could cause secretions to be forced up eustachian tube into middle ear
Discuss signs and symptoms to report to physician
  Elevated temperature
  Increased pain and/or ear drainage
  Decrease in hearing acuity
  Bleeding
  Dizziness
  Headache
  Stiff neck
Discuss medications: name, dosage, time of administration, purpose, and side effects
  Explain necessity for completing prescribed course of antibiotics
Avoid persons with upper respiratory tract infections (URIs) or cold symptoms
Avoid smoking
Encourage follow-up visits with physician

SPECIFIC
Stapedectomy
Instruct patient on ear care
  Change only outer ear plug prn
  Keep plug clean and dry
  Avoid nose blowing for 1 week
  Keep ear covered while outside
  Avoid sneezing; if unavoidable, open mouth wide to sneeze
  Wash hair only after 2 weeks
  No air travel or diving for 6 months
Plugs and packing are removed after 1 week

Tympanoplasty
Discuss precautions and restrictions in ear care
  Wear shower cap when bathing or place lamb's wool pledget in ear to protect ear from water
  Avoid blowing nose and sneeze through mouth
  Remove inner ear dressing only if prescribed by physician
  May swim or fly after healing has taken place
Explain that meclizine (Antivert) may be needed for about 1 month postoperatively to offset vertigo

Myringotomy With Tube Insertion
Discuss special precautions and restrictions
  Keep water out of ear
  Place petroleum jelly–covered cotton or lamb's wool pledget in ear before showering or shampooing
  Wear well-fitting ear plugs or a cap when swimming is allowed
  Do not dive, because it increases ear pressure
Explain that tube will come out naturally in 2 to 8 months, and there may be bloody drainage; if tube is dislodged earlier, instruct patient or parent(s) to notify physician
Demonstrate ear drop instillation, and instruct patient or parent(s) to complete prescribed course of oral or ear drop antibiotic therapy

DISCHARGE/HOME CARE PLANNING FOR THE HEARING-IMPAIRED PATIENT
Assess and continue with patient/family teaching and evaluate/discuss the following:

Communication Devices
Hearing aid(s)
Telephone receivers with amplifiers
Flashing lights for phones, doorbells, fire alarms, security systems
Vibration attachments for alarm clocks
Headsets for television, radio, stereo

Care of the Ear
Presence of drainage, pain, tenderness, fever
Importance of keeping ear clean and dry
Avoidance of showering/shampooing until permitted by physician
Use of ear plugs when swimming, showering
Procedure for instilling ear drops
Compliance with medication schedule

Understanding of Disease Process
Presence of support group to reduce fear, anxiety, and hopelessness
Knowledge of outside support groups to assist in decreasing feelings of low self-esteem, isolation, and depression
Presence of names, phone numbers of home health team
Knowledge of national support groups such as the following:
  Self Help for Hard of Hearing
    910 Woodmont Avenue
    Suite 1200
    Bethesda, MD 20814
  National Institute on Deafness and Other Communication Disorders
    NIDCD Information Clearinghouse
    1 Communication Avenue
    Bethesda, MD 20892-3456
    800-241-1044
    TDD 800-241-1055

American Tinnitus Association
P.O. Box 5
Portland, OR 97207
503-248-9985

BIBLIOGRAPHY

Beare PG, Myers JL: *Principles and practice of adult health nursing,* ed 2, St Louis, 1994, Mosby.

Brinkmann KL: Why can't your patient hear you? *RN* 54(1):46, 1991.

Cleveland PJ, Morris J: Ménière's disease, *RN* 53(8):28, 1990.

Canobbio MM: *Mosby's handbook of patient teaching,* St Louis, 1996, Mosby.

Doenges ME et al: *Nursing care plans: guidelines for planning and documenting patient care,* ed 3, Philadelphia, 1993, FA Davis.

Faucher D et al: Why some eye surgery patients are seeing dots, *Nursing '93* 23(2):41, 1993.

Kim MJ et al: *Pocket guide to nursing diagnoses,* ed 6, St Louis, 1995, Mosby.

Handbook of medical-surgical nursing, ed 2: Springhouse, Pa, 1998, Springhouse.

Illustrated handbook of nursing care: Springhouse, Pa, 1998, Springhouse.

Illustrated manual of nursing practice, ed 2: Springhouse, Pa, 1994, Springhouse.

Marelli TM: *Handbook of home health standards,* ed 3, St Louis, 1998, Mosby.

McCance KL, Huether SE: *Pathophysiology: the biological basis for disease in adults and children,* ed 2, St Louis, 1994, Mosby.

McFarland GK, McFarlane EA: *Nursing diagnosis and intervention: planning for patient care,* ed 2, St Louis, 1993, Mosby.

Nettina SM: *Lippincott manual of nursing practice,* ed 6, Philadelphia, 1996, Lippincott.

Rogers-Seidle FF: *Geriatric nursing care plans,* St Louis, 1991, Mosby.

Seigler BA, Schuring LT: *Ear, nose and throat disorders, Mosby's clinical series,* St Louis, 1993, Mosby.

Smith JF, Graham MD: Exercise helps these postop patients, *RN* 55(2):38, 1992.

Thompson JM et al: *Mosby's clinical nursing,* ed 4, St Louis, 1997, Mosby.

Webber-Jones J: Doomed to deafness? *Am J Nurs* 92(11):37, 1992.

BARNES

**CARE PATH
850
SCLERAL BUCKLE PROCEDURE**

SERVICE	PHYSICIAN	
PRIMARY NURSE	PRIMARY NURSE	**A-8**
DC DATE	ADM DATE	DATE OF SURGERY

PROBLEM NUMBER	PATIENT PROBLEMS / NURSING DIAGNOSES
#1	SENSORY ALTERATION
#2	LACK OF KNOWLEDGE
#3	POTENTIAL FOR INJURY
	*AS APPROPRIATE

PROB. NO.		PRE-ADM	DAY 1 DOS PRE-OP	DAY 1 DOS POST-OP
#1 **#2** **#3**	ASSESSMENT/MONITORING	Determine if pt. is diabetic	Preparation for surgery in SDS: **VS stable:** **If SBP > 190** **DBP > 100 notify MD** **If DBP > 110 call Anesthesia** **No arrhythmia** **Pulse 60-100** **No SOB** **Afebrile** Assess if pt. brought meds from home Assess: Normal ECG CXR = NAD **Lab values within Barnes guidelines** Assess NPO status	VS every 30" until at baseline then ×1 ×2 Evaluate degree of visual deficit Evaluate for fall program Evaluate effectiveness of pain control Evaluate symptoms of increased IOP (nausea, vomiting, uncontrolled pain) **Serosanguinous drainage less than half-dollar size**
	CONSULTS	Pvt. MD clearance		Social work as appropriate Diabetes Nurse specialist as appropriate.
#2	PROCEDURE/TEST	In SDS: ECG within 6 months if pt. over 40 yrs. CXR within 1 yr. if pt. over 50 yrs. HCT within 15 days SMA6 within 15 days (see anesthesia guidelines)		
	TREATMENT			
#1 **#2** **#3**	ACTIVITY		Bedrest with BRP	Bedrest with assistance

Continued

(2)

BARNES

CARE PATH
850
SCLERAL BUCKLE PROCEDURE

CNS	DIETARY	RT
HOME HEALTH	OT	OTHER
PT	SW	OTHER

A-8

PROBLEM NUMBER	PATIENT PROBLEMS / NURSING DIAGNOSES

DAY 2 POD 1	DAY 3 POD 2	D/C OUTCOMES	RESOURCE INFORMATION
VS ×1 ×2	VS ×1	**VS at baseline**	No bending with head below waist
			No straining
			No lifting over 20 #
Evaluate effectiveness of pain control	**Evaluate minimal or no eye pain**	**Minimal or no eye pain**	May remove patch on arrival home
Evaluate for increased IOP			Wear glasses during the day and eyeshield at bedtime
Evaluate bladder / bowel status	**Voiding without difficulty** **No constipation**	**Voiding adequately at baseline** **No straining**	Avoid getting soap in eyes when taking a tub bath or shower
Serous drainage less than size of a dime	**Minimal or no drainage**	**Minimal or no drainage**	Avoid direct sunlight
			Take a cough syrup for persistent coughing
			Do not hold back sneezes
		Discharge to home	If gas / air is injected in the eye, do not fly in an airplane until your doctor gives permission
		MD or clinic follow-up	
		7 - 10 days	Do not drive a car until after F / U appt. with MD
			Call Primary Nurse as needed.
Eye dressing change	Eye dressing change		
AM dilation Eye Exam	AM dilation Eye Exam		
BRP with assistance	Ad lib or as tolerated	**Return to baseline level of ADL**	
Chair ×1 ×2 ×3			

3

		PRE-ADM	DAY 1 DOS PRE-OP	DAY 1 DOS POST-OP
#1 #2	MEDS/IVS		SDS / OP / OR / Floor Nurse - Initiate dilation x1 x2 x3 x4 IV per Anesthesia	IVFs
#2	NUTRITION	Admitting Nursing: NPO after MN except meds as instructed by MD	NPO except Meds	Clear liquids
#1 #3	PATIENT/FAMILY EDUCATION	Admitting Nursing: Reinforce pt. to bring meds from home as instructed by MD Admitting arrival time	OR Nurses: Review dilating drops, OR procedures, retrobulbar injection	Floor Nurses: Explain call system Positioning per MD order Availability of analgesia / antiemetic Primary Nurse Role **Pt. able to demonstrate use of call system**
#1 #2 #3	DISCHARGE PLANNING		**Pt. / family verbalize understanding of Care Path. Plan of care has been mutually set with pt. / family.**	Nursing: Evaluate home care needs, transportation, support system
#1	PSYCHOSOCIAL / EMOTIONAL / SPIRITUAL NEEDS		Holding area: Give emotional support for surgery, i.e., reassurance - verbal & non-verbal (touch)	Nursing: Give emotional support for decreased vision. Encourage pt. to express feeling about visual loss Assess coping ability. Give reassurance - verbal & non-verbal
	SIGNATURES			

850

3100-53 (REV. 4/93)

Continued

DAY 2 POD 1	DAY 3 POD 2	D/C OUTCOMES	RESOURCE INFORMATION
D/C IV or change to Heplock Begin post-op eye gtts	D/C Heplock Post-op eye gtts	**Pt. / Care Provider able to administer eye drops**	
Regular diet	Regular diet	**Tolerating regular diet**	
Explain eye meds Teach eye drop instillation Pt. able to instill eye gtts independently Distribute teaching booklet & explain contents Teach cleansing of eye: soft, clean washcloth & tap water. Teach signs of infection: increase in redness, purulent drainage, increase in pain. Teach signs of increased eye pressure (see DOS post-op). Teach observance of any decrease in vision **Pt. able to verbalize eye cleansing, signs of infection, increased eye pressure, and understanding of visual testing.**	Instruct pt. to wear eye shield or glasses Teach eye drop schedule Reinforce teaching booklet instructions **Pt. verbalizes understanding of eye safety and medication schedule.**	**Pt. verbalizes Understanding Discharge Instructions**	
Nursing: Finalize home arrangements and transportation Call Social Worker if needed	D / C pt. with caregiver	**Discharge to home with caregiver to self-care.**	
Nursing: Continue emotional support			

3100-53 (REV. 4/93)

A-8

			VARIANCE		
DATE	**TIME**	**VARIANCE**	**ACTION PLAN**	**INITIALS**	

CHAPTER 14

Immune System

■ IMMUNE SYSTEM ASSESSMENT
(Fig. 14-1)

■ SUBJECTIVE DATA

Cardiopulmonary system
   Shortness of breath (SOB)
   Palpitations, chest pain
Central nervous system (CNS)
   Paresthesia
   Headache
   Photophobia
Gastrointestinal (GI) system
   Loss of appetite, anorexia
   Altered taste sensation
   Nausea, abdominal pain
   Rectal itching
Musculoskeletal system
   Fatigue, malaise
   Joint pain/stiffness, arthralgia
Ophthalmologic: ocular pain

■ OBJECTIVE DATA

Age, race
Gender, ethnic background
Weight loss
Cardiopulmonary system
   Hypertension/hypotension
   Jugular vein distension
   Pericarditis
   Cardiomegaly, dysrhythmia
   Edema
   Cough, dyspnea, wheezing
   Tachypnea, intercostal retractions
   Cyanosis
   Hemoptysis
   Lung infiltrates, hemorrhage
   Breath sounds; crackles
Central nervous system
   Dementia, personality changes, psychosis
   Depression
   Memory impairment
   Poor concentration, slowed thought processes
   Confusion
   Unsteady gait

Decreased hand coordination
Raynaud's disease
Neuritis
Peripheral nerve vasculitis; foot drop, wrist drop
Tremors
Seizures
Decreased animation
Withdrawal
Depression
Emotional lability
Psychosis
Nuchal rigidity
Altered level of consciousness (LOC)
Coma
Gastrointestinal system
   Difficulty chewing, swallowing
   Oral/esophageal lesions
   White/gray patches, dried patches may appear hairy
   Red to purple/brown lesions; may appear nodular, macular, plaquelike
   Gingivitis, parotitis
   Perioral/lips: red fissures, crusted, herpetic vesicles
   Vomiting
   Unintentional weight loss
   Abdominal cramping
   Change in bowel habits
   Diarrhea
   Constipation
   Rectal bleeding, fissures
   Peritonitis
Musculoskeletal system
   Weakness of extremities
   Swelling, warmth of joints
   Impaired joint function
   Joint effusions, deformities
   Muscle spasms, atrophy, contracture
   Subcutaneous nodules over pressure points
   Clubbing of fingers
Ophthalmologic system
   Dry eyes, sclera
   Cotton, wool exudate, lacrimation
   Bright subconjunctival masses
   Conjunctival infection
   Blurred vision
   Papilledema

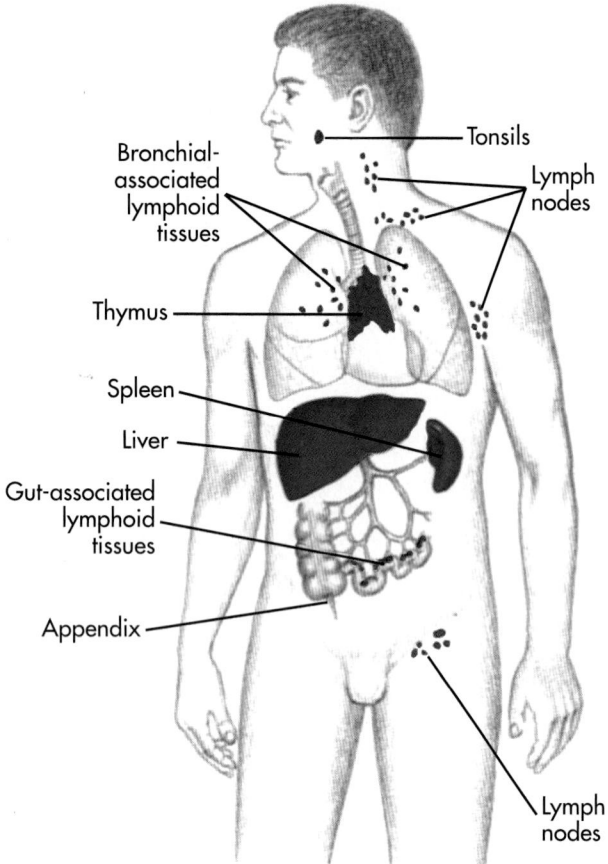

Fig. 14-1 Organization of immune system. Cellular constituents of immune system are derived from bone marrow stem cells. On maturation, these cells are released into peripheral blood and subsequently populate organized tissues of lymphoreticular system. *(From Thompson JM et al: Mosby's clinical nursing, ed 4, St Louis, 1997, Mosby.)*

Diplopia
Visual field deficits
Retinal cystoid bodies
Blindness
Ears, nose, throat status
    Nasal ulcerations
    Sensorineural hearing loss
Integumentary system
    Skin lesions: purple to brown
    Vasculitic skin lesions
    Skin vesicles
    Diaphoresis
    Rashes, hyperpigmentation
    Shiny, taut skin over joints
    Dryness
    Sensitivity to the sun
    Alopecia
    Delayed wound healing
    Lymphadenopathy
Hematologic system
    Hepatosplenomegaly
    Petechiae

    Purpura
    Easy bruising
    Elevated temperature (T)
Renal/genitourinary system
    Hematuria, hemorrhagic cystitis
    Urine casts
    Proteinuria
Comorbidities
    Anemia
    GI bleeding
    Renal calculi
    Renal failure
    Pericarditis
    Myocardial infarction (MI)
    Tenosynovitis
    Interstitial fibrosis, pneumonitis
    Pneumonia
    Cerebrovascular accident (CVA)
    Infection, diabetes from steroid use

Graft versus host disease (GVHD)
Retinopathy

 **PERTINENT BACKGROUND
INFORMATION**

MEDICAL HISTORY/RISK FACTORS
Hepatitis
Sexually transmitted diseases
Frequent viral illness
Amebiasis
Transfusion of blood products
Chemical exposure
Occupational risks
Chemotherapy
Radiation therapy
Radioactive iodine therapy
Family history

SOCIAL HISTORY
Exposure to contaminated needles, intravenous (IV) drug use
Multiple sex partners
Sexual preference
Work, productive activities
Stress factors, coping mechanisms
Previous losses, coping mechanisms
Self-concept
Conceptualization of illness
Support network
Living arrangements
Significant other/partner
Ability to perform activities of daily living (ADLs)
Transportation

DIAGNOSTIC TESTS
Hematologies
  Leukocyte count
  Lymphocyte count
  Complete blood cell count (CBC)
  Coagulation profile
  Erythrocyte sedimentation rate (ESR)
  Blood type and cross/screen
  Human leukocyte antigen (HLA) typing
B cell counts
Immunoglobulin quantification
  Kveim skin test
  Immunofluorescence assay
  $T_{4,8}$ cell count
  T helper/T suppressor ratio
  Serum immunoglobulin
  Antistreptolysin O (ASO) titer, rheumatoid factor
  Serum protein levels: IgG, IgA, IgM
  C-reactive protein
  Antinuclear antibodies
  Lupus erythematosus (LE) prep
  Antinuclear antibody

Antidouble-standard deoxyribonucleic acid (DNA)
    antibody
  Complement
Viral, serology studies
  Enzyme-linked immunosorbent assay (ELISA) for
      human immunodeficiency virus (HIV)
  Western blot test
  HBsAg, HBsAb
  Herpes zoster (HZ)
  Herpes simplex (HS)
  Cytomegalovirus (CMV)
  Epstein-Barr virus (EBV)
  Venereal Disease Research Laboratories (VDRL),
      fluorescent treponemal antibody absorption (FTA-A)
  Toxoplasmosis
Chemistries
  Lactate dehydrogenase (LDH)
  Alkaline phosphatase, aspartate transferase (AST),
      alanine aminotransferase (ALT)
  Bilirubin
  Serum cholesterol
  Serum iron, magnesium
  Electrolyte panel, blood urea nitrogen (BUN), creatinine
  Fasting blood sugar (FBS)
Cultures
  Sputum
  Spinal fluid
  Bone marrow
  Mucous membranes
  Blood
  Stool
Urine
  Urinalysis
  Creatinine clearance
X-rays
  Chest
  Sinus
  Joint
Imaging studies
Nuclear medicine: gallium scan
CT scan, MRI
Arthroscopy
Neurophysiology studies
  Stereotactic brain biopsy
  Electromyelography
  Nerve conduction studies
Cardiopulmonary studies
  Arterial blood gases (ABGs)
  Pulmonary function
  Electrocardiogram (ECG), echocardiogram
Biopsies
  Skin
  Kidney
  Lymph nodes
  Bronchial, open lung
Malabsorption studies
  Villi biopsy
  D-Xylose absorption test
  Decreased intestinal enzymes

■ ACQUIRED IMMUNODEFICIENCY SYNDROME (AIDS)

AIDS includes the final stages of a wide range of health problems caused by the human immunodeficiency virus (HIV) type I (Fig. 14-2); this virus attacks the cell-mediated immune system through invasion of CD4 cells, causing a major deficit in the system (Box 14-1); the infected person becomes vulnerable to opportunistic infections and cancers (Table 14-1). HIV is transmitted by exposure to infected blood/body fluids; the exposures that put people at risk include sexual contact with an infected partner, receptive anal intercourse, multiple sexual partners, anonymous sexual activity, IV drug use, contact with contaminated blood products or tissue through transfusion, transplant, or occupational risk, and infants exposed in utero by infected mothers

ASSESSMENT
SUBJECTIVE DATA
Cardiopulmonary system: SOB
Central nervous system
    Paresthesia
    Headache
    Photophobia

Ophthalmologic system
    Floaters
    Flashing lights in peripheral vision
Gastrointestinal system
    Loss of appetite
    Nausea
    Abdominal pain
    Rectal itching, pain
    Severe fatigue

OBJECTIVE DATA
Cardiopulmonary system
    Cough
    Dyspnea
    Wheezing
    Tachypnea
    Cyanosis
    Hemoptysis
    Intercostal retractions
Central nervous system
    AIDS dementia complex
        Memory impairment
        Poor concentration
        Slowed thought processes

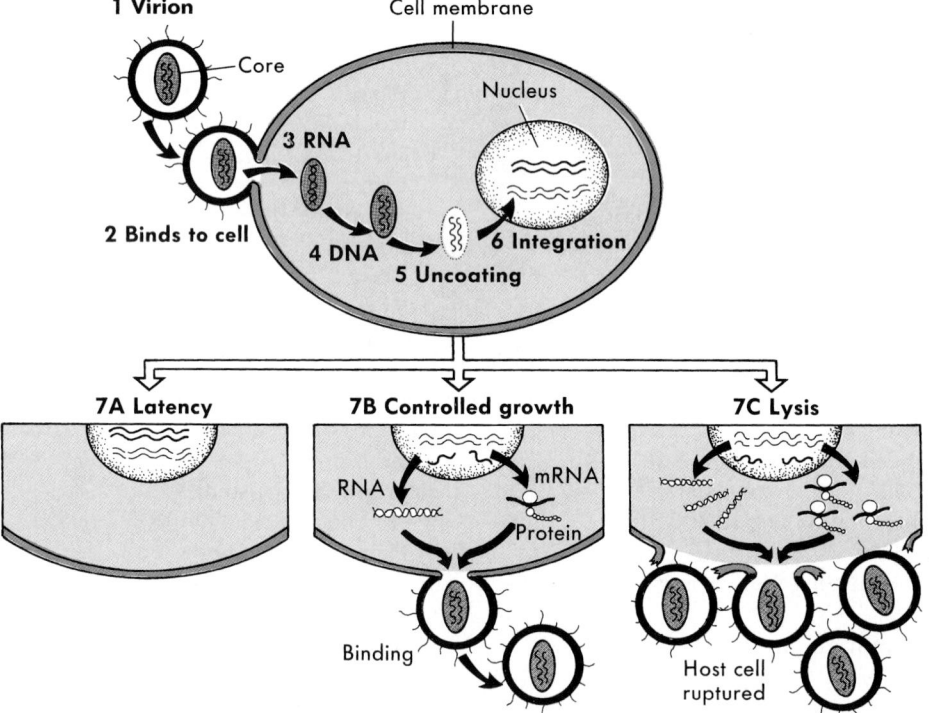

Fig. 14-2 Infection and cellular outcomes of the HIV. HIV infection begins *(1)* when a virion, or virus particle *(2)* binds to the outside of a susceptible cell and fuses with it, *(3)* injecting the core proteins and two strands of viral RNA. Uncoating occurs, during which the core proteins are removed and the viral RNA is released into the infected cell's cytoplasm. *(4)* The double-stranded DNA (provirus) migrates to the nucleus, *(5)* uncoats itself, and *(6)* is integrated into the cell's own DNA. The provirus then can do a couple of things: *(7A)* remain latent or *(7B)* activate cellular mechanisms to copy its genes into RNA, some of which is translated into viral proteins or ribosomes. The proteins and additional RNA then are assembled into new virions that bud from the cell. The process can take place slowly, sparing the host cell *(7B)*, or so rapidly that the cell is lysed or ruptured *(7C)*.
(From McCance KL, Huether SE: Pathophysiology: the biological basis for disease in adults and children, *ed 2, St Louis, 1994, Mosby.)*

Confusion
Unsteady gait
Weakness of extremities, especially lower
extremities
Decreased hand coordination
Tremors
Seizures
Decreased animation
Withdrawal
Depression
Emotional lability
Psychosis
Nuchal rigidity
Altered LOC
Coma
Ophthalmologic system
Cotton wool exudate, spots
Blurred vision
Papilledema
Diplopia
Visual field deficits
Retinal hemorrhage
Bright red subconjunctival masses
Blindness
Ear, nose, throat (ENT) status
Oral cavity and esophogeal lesions
White/gray patches, dried patches may appear hairy
Red to purple/brown lesions; may appear macular,
nodular, or plaque like

Gingivitis, bleeding
Perioral/lips: red fissures, crusted, herpetic vesicles
Integumentary system
Skin vesicles
Diaphoresis
Rashes
Skin lesions: purple to brown
Dryness
Delayed wound healing
Lymphadenopathy, nodes not fixed or hard
Gastrointestinal system
Difficulty chewing, swallowing
Vomiting
Unintentional weight loss, 10% in 1 to 2 months
Abdominal cramping
Intractable diarrhea
Rectal bleeding, fissures
Hematologic system
Splenomegaly
Petechiae
Purpura
Easy bruising
Night sweats
Elevated temperature

MEDICAL HISTORY

Hepatitis
Sexually transmitted diseases
Frequent viral illness
Amebiasis
Exposure to contaminated needles, IV drug use
Transfusion of blood/blood products
Females
Recurrent vaginal candidiasis
History of abnormal Pap test

SOCIAL HISTORY

Sexual practices: history of unprotected sex, exposure to
body fluids, multiple sex partners
Sex partner of IV drug user, hemophiliac, bisexual male
Sexual orientation
Substance use/abuse
Work, productive activities
Stress factors, coping mechanisms
Previous losses, coping mechanisms
Self-concept
Conceptualization of illness

DIAGNOSTIC TESTS

WBC: Leukocytopenia
Lymphocytopenia
Red blood cells (RBCs), hematocrit (Hct), hemoglobin
(Hgb): decreased
Platelets: thrombocytopenia
Immunologies
ELISA: reactive
Western blot assay or immunofluorescence assay:
positive

Box 14-1	**1993 CDC Classification for HIV Infections in Adults**

CATEGORY A

Asymptomatic; primary HIV or persistent lymphadenopathy

A1	CD4	T cell count $\geq$500/mm^3
A2	CD4	T cell count 200 to 499/mm^3
A3	CD4	T cell count <200/mm^3

CATEGORY B

Symptomatic; examples include candidiasis (oral, vulvo-vaginal), cervical dysplasia/cancer, diarrhea lasting longer than 1 month, herpes zoster, pelvic inflammatory disease, idiopathic thrombocytopenia

B1	CD4	T cell count $\geq$500/mm^3
B2	CD4	T cell count 200 to 499/mm^3
B3	CD4	T cell count <200/mm^3

CATEGORY C

AIDS indicators; examples include candidiasis (trachea, bronchi, lungs), cytomegalovirus (other than liver, spleen, nodes), lymphomas, Kaposi's sarcoma, *Mycobacterium, Pneumocystis carinii,* wasting syndrome, encephalopathy

C1	CD4	T cell count $\geq$500/mm^3
C2	CD4	T cell count 200 to 499/mm^3
C3	CD4	T cell count <200/mm^3

Table 14-1	Opportunistic Infections, Neoplasms, and Systems Involved in AIDS

Opportunistic Infections and Neoplasms	System Involved
OPPORTUNISTIC INFECTIONS	
Protozoal	
Pneumocystis carinii pneumonitis (PCP)	Pulmonary, cutaneous, ophthalmologic, neurologic
Cryptosporidiosis	Systemic, neurologic, gastrointestinal
Toxoplasmosis	Neurologic, systemic, ophthalmologic
Viruses	
Cytomegalovirus (CMV)	Systemic, neurologic, gastrointestinal, pulmonary, ophthalmologic
Herpes simplex I, II—disseminated	Neurologic, cutaneous, ophthalmologic, gastrointestinal
Epstein-Barr virus (EBV)	Systemic
Herpes zoster—multidermal	Neurologic, cutaneous, ophthalmologic
Progressive multifocal leukoencephalopathy (PML)	Neurologic
Hairy leukoplakia	Cutaneous, gastrointestinal
Fungi	
Candidiasis	Neurologic, cutaneous, pulmonary, ophthalmologic, gastrointestinal, vaginal
Cryptococcosis	Neurologic, systemic, pulmonary, cutaneous, ophthalmologic
Histoplasmosis	Pulmonary, systemic, cutaneous, neurologic, gastrointestinal
Coccidioidomycosis	Pulmonary, cutaneous, systemic, neurologic
Bacterial	
Mycobacterium avium—intracellular (MAI) infection	Neurologic, systemic, pulmonary, gastrointestinal, ophthalmologic
Mycobacterium tuberculosis infection	Neurologic, pulmonary, systemic, gastrointestinal
NEOPLASMS	
Kaposi's sarcoma (KS)	Neurologic, cutaneous, ophthalmologic, gastrointestinal, pulmonary
Lymphoma (p. 844)	Neurologic, systemic, gastrointestinal
OTHER ASSOCIATED INFECTIONS, CONDITIONS NOT CONSIDERED OPPORTUNISTIC	
Anemia	Hematologic, systemic
Aspergillosis	Pulmonary, ophthalmologic, systemic
Giardiasis	Gastrointestinal
Klebsiella pneumoniae infection	Pulmonary
Salmonellosis	Gastrointestinal, cutaneous, skeletal, systemic
Idiopathic thrombocytopenia purpura (ITP) (p. 206)	Hematologic, gastrointestinal, neurologic
Xerostomia	Gastrointestinal

HIV-1, ribonucleic acid (RNA) polymerase chain reaction (PCR): detectable
HIV culture: positive
T_4 cells: decreased
T_8 cells: increased
T helper/T suppressor ratio: inverted
Serum immunoglobulin: elevated
Chemistries
  Alkaline phosphatase: elevated
  Serum cholesterol: decreased
  Serum iron: decreased
  Electrolytes: imbalanced
  Liver function, amylase creatinine phosphokinase (CPK)

Cultures/serologies
  Sputum: *Pneumocystis carinii,* acid-fast bacillus (AFB), fungus, *Mycobacterium avium-intracellulare* (MAI)
  Spinal fluid: MAI, cryptococcal antigen, HIV, CMV
  Bone marrow: disseminated MAI, CMV
  Mucous membranes: candidiasis, herpes, CMV
  Blood: cryptococcal antigen, toxoplasmosis Ab, MAI, CMV, DNA, polymerase chain reaction, HIV-1, RNA, PCR
  Stool: ova and parasites, cryptosporidiosis, microsporidiosis, bacterial
Imaging studies, nuclear medicine
  Chest x-ray: interstitial infiltrates, pulmonary KS; granulomatous disease

Gallium lung scan: positive
Bronchoscopy: biopsy positive
CT scan/MRI: positive for toxoplasmosis lesions, HIV progressive multifocal leukoencephalopathy (PML) infections
Stereotactic brain biopsy: differentiate intracranial lesions
Neurophysiology studies
Electromyelography
Nerve conduction studies: slowed
Cardiopulmonary studies
ABGs
Pulmonary function

POTENTIAL COMPLICATIONS
Pneumocystis carinii
Candidiasis
Cryptococcosis
Cryptosporidiosis
AIDS dementia complex (HIV encephalopathy)
Distal sensory polyneuropathy

MULTIDISCIPLINARY MANAGEMENT
THERAPEUTIC MANAGEMENT
Chest physiotherapy: postural drainage
Nutrition/diet
High-caloric, high-protein diet
Total parenteral nutrition (TPN)
Appetite stimulants
Parenteral therapy
Medications
Antiretroviral therapy
Zidovudine (AZT, Retrovir), Didanosine (ddl, Videx), Zalcitabine (ddC, HIVID), stavudine (D4T, Zerit)
Lamivudine (Epivir)
Antiretroviral protease inhibitors
Saquinavir (Invirase)
Indinavir (Crixivan)
Nelfinavir (Viracept)
Retonavir (Norvir)
Chemotherapy
Antiemetics
Antidiarrheals
Antivirals
Antifungals
Biologic modifiers
Sulfonamides
Antipyretics
Analgesics
Radiotherapy

PATIENT PROBLEMS—NURSING DIAGNOSES/INTERVENTIONS

▼Impaired gas exchange related to alveolar-capillary membrane changes secondary to opportunistic pulmonary infections

Assess respiratory status, monitoring rate, depth, work of breathing and breath sounds q4h and prn *to* determine changes from baseline that may indicate infection
Monitor ABGs, pulse oximetry as ordered; *changes may indicate onset/progression of pulmonary infection*
Administer oxygen therapy as ordered *to maintain optimal oxygen level*
Suction airways prn *to remove secretions if patient is unable to do so*
Obtain sputum specimen for culture *to determine infective agent and appropriate therapy*
Provide chest physiotherapy and postural drainage as needed *to remove secretions, which increase bacterial growth*
Assist patient to turn, cough, and deep breathe q2h and prn *to assist in secretion removal, which promotes better oxygenation*
Position patient in high-Fowler's position, *which provides for optimal respiratory excursion*
Assist patient with relaxation exercises *to decrease rapid, shallow breathing*
Evaluate ADLs in relationship to oxygen demands, assist patient prn *to conserve energy*

Expected Outcomes
Exhibits no signs/symptoms of acute respiratory distress, or signs/symptoms are recognized and treated immediately

▼Risk for infection related to suppressed immune system

Screen personnel and visitors for symptoms of infection *to reduce patient's exposure to foreign pathogens*
Use strict sterile technique for all invasive procedures *to prevent pathogen infiltration*
Monitor sites of invasive lines, tubes, drains for signs of infection q8h; *tissue response to pathogen infiltration*
Check body fluids for alteration in color, odor, consistency, *which may indicate infection*
Ensure excellent personal hygiene is maintained, especially after bowel movements *to prevent infection*
Provide uninterrupted periods of sleep and rest *to provide energy to combat invading pathogens*
Ensure required fluid/nutrient intake, supplement with total oral nutrition products prn, institute calorie count as needed *to provide adequate nutrition*
Record intake and output *to ensure balance*
Monitor vital signs, especially temperature and breath sounds; *fever is hallmark of infection; increased BP, pulse may indicate sepsis*
Monitor CBC, white blood cell (WBC) count results per physician order *so increased WBC count, indicative of infection, can be reported and treated promptly*
Maintain skin integrity: *intact skin may prevent entry of microorganisms*
Encourage clearance of pulmonary secretions; turn, cough, deep breathe q2h; perform chest percussion and drainage prn; encourage use of incentive spirometer *to remove secretions, which enhance growth of pathogens*

Maintain intact mucous membranes; scrupulous oral care using soft instruments prn *to prevent a port of entry for pathogens*

Expected Outcomes
Exhibits improvement, resolution of current infections, and/or new infections do not develop

▼Altered thought processes related to memory deficits/problems secondary to AIDS dementia complex

Assess for disruptions in thinking processes, time management, task orientation, memory, changes in attention span, labile emotions daily: *changes may indicate cerebral involvement*

Assist patient to explore appropriateness of goal setting for the present and future

Assess LOC and orientation q8h and prn *to determine early changes*

Develop a supportive, therapeutic nurse/patient relationship *to promote trust*

Reorient to person, place, time prn

Call patient by name, identify self, and state purpose when entering the room *to prevent distortions of interpretation*

Speak directly to patient, avoid vague comments and conversations not addressing the patient *to decrease multiple stimuli, which may confuse patient*

Be clear and direct when providing instructions, give one direction at a time, break complex tasks into simple steps *to promote feelings of accomplishment*

Redirect misinterpretations of stimuli to reality-centered discussions

Assist patient to clarify thoughts and feelings, learn to recognize reactions to automatic thoughts

Assess environment and attempt to decrease stimuli that the patient may misinterpret

Teach patient how to make more appropriate self-evaluations by examining consistency of thoughts

Adjust lighting to prevent shadows, use night light *to prevent visual distortions*

Make familiar objects, pictures, clock, and correctly dated calendar visible to patient *to assist in maintaining orientation*

Provide radio, TV, newspapers as patient wishes

Develop and maintain with patient a consistent daily schedule; post schedule for patient *to promote routine, reality-based behavior*

Encourage significant others to visit often *to assist in maintaining orientation*

Maintain consistent arrangement of room *to protect patient from injury*

Use soft restraints or jacket restraint only as needed and when patient is alone *to prevent injury*

Encourage acceptance of responsibility for actions

Plan care with patient *to encourage self-control,* encourage patient to make choices as appropriate

Give positive reinforcement for participation in self-care; teach patient to reward self in concrete ways

In collaboration with physician, refer for neuropsychiatric or psychosocial evaluation

Expected Outcomes
Actively participates in ADLs to extent possible based on physical limitations

Maintains reality orientation, communicates clearly with others

Participates in developing plan of care, ordering meals, making other choices as appropriate

Expresses delusional thoughts less frequently

▼Pain related to physical disability secondary to neoplasm and/or involvement of multiple organ systems

Assess nature, intensity, location, duration, and precipitating and alleviating factors; use consistent pain rating scale *to determine baseline and deviations that indicate intervention is needed*

Assess nonverbal signs of pain particular to patient *so that early signs can be noted and treatment started*

Obtain information from patient regarding past pain experiences and methods used for relief

Control environmental factors that may increase perception of pain: temperature, noise, lighting

Assist patient to achieve positions *that promote comfort*

Assist patient to achieve state of minimal physical tension through techniques such as relaxation, music, visualization, diversion *to decrease need for medication*

Provide a restful environment with opportunities to rest during the day and uninterrupted periods of sleep at night

In collaboration with physician, provide analgesic medications as required, observing for therapeutic and side effects

Discuss noninvasive pain relief measures: relaxation, cutaneous stimulation, distraction, hot/cold therapy

Expected Outcomes
Verbalizes decrease in or relief of pain

Able to incorporate existing pain while participating in daily activities

▼Diarrhea related to infectious process, gastrointestinal infection, chemotherapy

Assess usual patterns of elimination: quantity, frequency, color, consistency, presence of overt/occult blood, undigested food

Assess current use of laxatives/antidiarrheals, *which may cause/interfere with current condition*

Evaluate hydration and electrolyte status; maintain record of intake and output, measuring liquid stools *to determine fluid deficit*

Assess abdomen: bowel sounds, distension, softness/firmness

Assess for flatus, cramping

Weigh patient daily (same time, scale, and clothing)

Adjust diet to eliminate foods inducing bowel irritation; offer frequent, small meals

Provide protein and electrolyte supplements, total oral or parenteral nutrition

Provide fluids at least in equal amount to output *to maintain balance*

In collaboration with dietitian and patient, maintain calorie count and select nondiarrheic foods

In collaboration with physician, administer antidiarrheals, antiinfective agents

Expected Outcomes

Frequency and quantity of abdominal pain, cramping, and diarrheal stools per day are decreased

Weight is maintained or increased if appropriate

Able to identify foods to consume/avoid *to prevent exacerbation*

▼Altered nutrition: less than body requirements related to reduced food intake, malabsorption, anorexia, vomiting, diarrhea, stomatitis

Assess nutritional status daily: weight, electrolytes, total protein, serum albumin, Hgb, skin turgor, muscle mass *to determine fluid deficit and weight loss*

Determine amount and types of foods patient likes and is able to tolerate *to increase intake*

Provide for oral hygiene before and after meals *to enhance comfort and sense of taste*

Administer anesthetics to oral mucosa before meals as needed *to promote comfort*

Offer high-calorie, high-protein diet with variation in taste, texture, and presentation of foods *to stimulate appetite*

In collaboration with physician, provide oral and parenteral nutritional supplements *to supply required nutrients and calories*

Serve frequent, light meals and nutritional, high-calorie snacks; *small amounts more easily tolerated*

Assist patient to eat if fatigue is a factor

Present meals in an attractive, pleasing manner

Provide a pleasant atmosphere *to increase desire to eat:* encourage significant others to join patient for meals, remove bedpans/urinals from area, maintain well-ventilated room, serve food as soon as it arrives, remove tray as soon as patient finishes eating

In collaboration with clinical dietitian: calculate number of calories and nutrients *needed to maintain/gain weight and support metabolic needs*

Encourage family to bring favorite foods from home *to enhance patient's appetite*

In collaboration with physician, administer antiemetics before meals as needed

Expected Outcome

Weight is maintained within 10% of baseline

▼Altered oral mucous membranes related to opportunistic infections

Assess oral mucous membranes q8h to 12h for color, moisture, texture, presence of lesions *to determine baseline and, thereafter, changes indicative of infection*

Assess ease of swallowing *to note any difficulties that may lead to aspiration*

Obtain cultures of lesions per physician order *to determine infective pathogen*

Provide oral hygiene q2h while awake: use instruments appropriate for condition of mucous membranes; avoid abrasives, alcohol-containing mouthwash, and lemon glycerin swabs, *which may cause irritation and a port of entry for infective agents*

Perform oral hygiene as soon as possible after eating *to remove food particles, which enhance growth of pathogens*

Use baking soda, antifungal medications, topical anesthetics per physician order

Apply water-soluble lubricant to lips q2h *to maintain hydration*

Provide foods that are nonirritating to mucous membranes, easily chewed

Avoid very sweet, spicy, acidic foods, *which may cause irritation to membranes*

Provide foods at neutral temperature or per patient tolerance

If patient is unable to assist in oral hygiene: irrigate mouth with soft rubber catheter, use soft utensil to remove debris

Discourage smoking and alcohol use, *which increase dehydration of membranes*

Expected Outcomes

Able to take oral nutrition

Oral mucous membranes intact; lesions healing

▼Risk for impaired skin integrity related to malnutrition, immobility, opportunistic infection

Assess skin condition q8h; pay close attention to axilla, skin folds, groin and perineal area, heels, scapula, back of head, dependent extremities, sacral area, mucous membranes *for irritation or breaks*

Note condition of skin related to temperature, moisture, color, texture, lesions

Assist with bathing as necessary, use mild soaps, rinse and dry well *to prevent sites of moisture, which enhance skin irritation and bacterial growth*

Do not leave skin moist with lotions; avoid deodorants, cologne

If patient is diaphoretic, rinse and dry skin well, keep clothing and bedding dry

Keep linen wrinkle free, avoid pressure from linen on feet, use foot cradle prn *to prevent areas of pressure*

Lift patient when turning; avoid sliding on sheets, *which may cause shearing of skin*

Prevent pressure on bony prominences using pillows, air therapy beds prn *to promote circulation to all areas*

Encourage small shifts in position q30min and turn at least q2h *to decrease pressure points*

Increase active mobility *to increase circulation;* encourage walking and sitting in chair, avoid chair sitting in one position for longer than 30 minutes

Provide for perianal care after each elimination *to prevent irritation and/or promote healing*

Avoid intramuscular (IM) injections and multiple venipunctures *to eliminate/decrease sites of invasion*

Expected Outcomes

Skin and mucous membranes remain intact

Current skin breakdown is healing

▼Bleeding related to thrombocytopenia*

Assess neurologic status q8h: *changes may indicate intracranial bleeding*

Observe urine and stools for obvious blood, test for occult blood per physician order

Assess skin and mucous membranes for extension/new sites of ecchymosis, hematoma q8h

Use smallest gauge needles possible, perform finger sticks (or draw from central line when possible), consolidate blood draws *to decrease number of invasive sites and lower risk of bleeding*

Apply manual pressure for 5 minutes to all puncture sites; do not disturb clots/scabs *to prevent fresh, unobserved bleeding*

Avoid rectal temperature, medications, *which may inadvertently break mucosa, providing a bleeding site*

Use nonabrasive soaps, soft brushes, soft washcloths and towels *to maintain skin integrity*

Assist with ambulation as needed to avoid bumps and falls, *which provide sites of internal bleeding*

Avoid constipation

Transfuse blood products per physician order

Expected Outcomes

Skin and mucous membranes remain intact, without bruising/hematoma

Hgb, Hct remain stable

▼Fatigue related to chronic disease process

Assess causative/contributing factors; identify activities that are difficult for patient and use excessive energy

Coordinate activities *to provide for undisturbed periods of rest and sleep*

Perform active/passive range of motion (ROM) exercises qid, collaborate with physical therapy to determine most therapeutic exercises *to decrease energy expenditure*

Determine whether patient becomes posturally hypotensive; change positions gradually *to prevent injury*

Monitor for hypotension and tachycardia, *which indicate increased expenditure of energy*

Not a NANDA-approved diagnosis.

Gauge amount and intensity of activity tolerated by monitoring patient's subjective complaints of fatigue and changes in vital signs

Assist patient to identify strengths, abilities, interests; assist in development of realistic goals progressing from simple to complex *to conserve energy*

Encourage patient to participate in self-care to tolerance; assist as needed to avoid exhaustion; assist to identify energy patterns and schedule activities appropriately

Teach energy conservation techniques, use of assistive devices

Place patient on falls-prevention protocol

Collaborate with physical therapist to design measures *to maintain activity and independence*

Expected Outcomes

Participates in self-care to tolerance

Ability to be active increases; patient states a feeling of increased energy

▼Anticipatory grieving related to lifestyle changes, decreased physical abilities, changes in physical appearance, life-threatening prognosis

Be sensitive to changes patient is experiencing; encourage patient to express feelings, frustrations, anger, hopes *to begin work of grieving process*

Provide a therapeutic environment conducive to open discussion; actively listen, perceive nonverbal cues; be patient and empathetic *to facilitate trust*

Encourage questions and provide information freely as patient expresses the desire for knowledge about disease, treatments, and prognosis *to ease fear of the unknown*

Support adaptive behaviors that suggest progression and resolution of the grieving process

Set limits on maladaptive coping behaviors if they interfere with patient's well-being

Provide opportunities for private, uninterrupted time with significant others

Assist in identifying ways to adapt lifestyle as condition changes *to enhance participation and feelings of control*

Provide information regarding support groups, including electronic access groups, for patient and significant others

Collaborate with other professionals (social worker, clergy, psychologist, psychiatrist) *to provide support and facilitate grieving process*

Provide reference for financial assistance, answers to questions regarding medical insurance

Provide information to assist patient in completing advanced directives or similar document *to ensure patient's wishes are known to significant others and care providers*

Expected Outcomes

Progresses through stages of the grieving process and moves toward acceptance

Demonstrates effective coping mechanisms

Participates in decisions about own future

▼Altered sexuality patterns related to limitation imposed by symptoms (fatigue, decreased libido, impotence), fear of rejection by partner, fear of spreading infection to partner

Determine knowledge level about AIDS and attitude about AIDS in relation to sexuality

Clarify uncertainties, misconceptions if present *to ensure relationships are maintained within safe boundaries*

Provide opportunities for expression of concerns, fears *to decrease feelings of isolation*

Be nonjudgmental, aware of how own discomfort level and personal attitude may affect ability to be therapeutic

Provide private time and encourage patient to discuss concerns and feelings with sex partner including imagined responses, fear of rejection *so that unspoken fears do not interfere with relationship*

Provide information about alternative methods for sexual expression while avoiding activities that permit exchange of body fluids, feces, or blood between partners *to prevent transmission of causative agents*

Instruct patient and partner in safer sex guidelines (Box 14-2)

Expected Outcomes

Makes informed statements concerning alternative modes of sexual expression

Identifies safer sex practices

Openly discusses concerns and makes plans for safer sexual activities with sex partner

▼Social isolation related to social stigma of AIDS and fear of infecting others

Determine patient's support systems, significant others, family, social groups; encourage patient to continue interactions

Encourage expression of feelings of aloneness, rejection, isolation if present

Be nonjudgmental; listen openly and accept feelings being expressed

Reinforce with patient and visitors that AIDS is not communicated through casual contact such as holding hands, hugging *so that touching and usual contacts with others continue*

Assist patient to maintain contact with others via telephone, letters

Encourage visitors to return frequently

Spend time with patient when not required to perform caregiving tasks *to increase feelings of self-worth*

Avoid unnecessary use of barrier techniques that convey fear of caregiver contamination

Assist patient in assessing self-worth, achievements positively

Arrange with significant others to bring personal mementos, pictures, favorite videos, books, tapes, surprises such as flowers, balloons

---

Box 14-2	**Safer Sex Guidelines**

SAFER SEX PRACTICES/PATIENT EDUCATION

Inform previous and present partners (and those with whom you share needles) of their possible exposure to HIV; if partner is female and pregnant, immediate referral for medical evaluation is advised

If female, avoid pregnancy

Selectively choose partners, know partners' sexual histories; limit partners, preferably to one person

Avoid oral-genital contact

Avoid sexual intercourse, especially those practices that may injure tissue, such as anal intercourse

Modify practices so that body fluids, blood, and feces are not exchanged

LOW-RISK SEX PRACTICES

Vaginal penetration

    Instruct in proper selection and application of latex condoms

    Use latex condoms from start to finish to protect from body fluid exchange (natural skin condoms allow the passage of HIV)

    Apply spermicide with nonoxol-9 inside and outside of the condom for added protection in the event of condom breakage

    Use water-soluble lubricant to decrease friction on mucous membranes (oil-based lubricants may cause the condom to break)

French (wet) kissing

    Controversial because HIV is found in saliva, but no instance of transmission via this route is reported; avoid kissing if either partner has mouth sores

Mutual masturbation

    Use latex gloves to guard against possible exposure through cuts on hands

UNSAFE SEX PRACTICES

Vaginal, anal, or oral intercourse without a condom or latex barrier (dental dams)

Unprotected penetration of vagina or anus with fingers or hands

Blood contact of any kind

Sharing sex toys or needles

Provide patient and significant others with information about support groups

Expected Outcomes

Maintains healthy, supportive interpersonal relationships with significant others

Verbalizes sense of belonging and feelings of being loved and supported

Additional Nursing Diagnoses to Consider

Risk for caregiver role strain

Ineffective individual coping

PATIENT/FAMILY TEACHING

Explain the following:

Chest physiotherapy and postural drainage

Importance of turning, coughing, deep breathing

Pursed-lip or diaphragmatic breathing

Oxygen administration

Use of walking aids

Universal precautions and handwashing, especially after using bathroom and before preparing food

Importance of maintaining clean home environment

How to handle and store foods to minimize bacterial count

Disposal of infectious wastes in secured bags

Washing of soiled linen separately using 1% bleach solution

Safe disposal of needles in impervious containers

Not to clean litter boxes, bird cages, fish tanks to avoid exposure to toxoplasmosis

Never to donate blood or semen

Importance of avoiding persons who may be infectious, persons who have been recently vaccinated, and crowds

Care of skin and mucous membranes, oral hygiene

Relaxation techniques, stress management; maintain balance between activity and rest

Diet choices that increase caloric intake without irritating oral cavity or bowel

Safer sex practices (see Box 14-2)

Changes in condition, signs/symptoms of opportunistic infections that need to be reported to physician

Procedure of taking oral/axillary temperature and when to notify physician of elevation

Administration and side effects of medications

Care of central line, flushing, and medication administration

Avoid use of alcohol, tobacco, recreational drugs

Importance of receiving ongoing outpatient care

Importance of obtaining flu vaccines

Importance of informing all care providers of HIV infection

Reasons for wearing medical alert ID band; how to obtain band

DISCHARGE/HOME CARE PLANNING

Explain that condition/layout of home, safe arrangement of furniture and other household items, and adequate lighting are necessary to prevent accidental injury

Discuss storage of dressing change supplies; oxygen equipment; walking aid; puncture-proof container for needles, gloves, masks; clean linens

Discuss safe disposal and/or cleaning of sharp objects and other blood or body-fluid contaminated items

Assess assistance available for shopping, cleaning, transportation; arrange providers as needed

Arrange for durable medical equipment as required

Facilitate hospice care if condition requires

■ BONE MARROW TRANSPLANT (BMT)

A treatment approach that results in the replenishing of depleted bone marrow cell reserves; care is divided into four phases: pretransplant (preparation), conditioning, transplant, and posttransplant (Table 14-2); there are three sources of donor marrow: **allogenic** *is most common and the treatment of choice for patients with aplastic anemia under 50 years of age for which an identical HLA donor can be found*

allogenic grafts: *May also be used for severe immunodeficiency disorders, acute and chronic leukemia, and multiple myeloma*

autologous transplants: *Peripheral blood stem cell transplant is being used to treat Hodgkin's and non-Hodgkin's lymphoma; acute leukemia; lymphoma; responsive solid tumors; neuroblastoma; tumors of the breast, ovaries, and testes; small cell lung cancers. In an autologous transplant the patient donates his or her own marrow during disease remission. Syngeneic marrow comes from an identical twin, which eliminates the problems of rejection and graft versus host disease (GVHD)*

▌ PREPARATION PHASE

ASSESSMENT

NOTE: May be asymptomatic if in remission

SUBJECTIVE DATA

SOB

Chronic fatigue

Pain in joints and bones

OBJECTIVE DATA

Anemia

Easy bruising

Tendency to bleed

Petechiae

Maculopapular rash

Fever

Weakness

DIAGNOSTIC TESTS

Bone marrow studies

Blood type and screen

CBC with differential

Complete RBC type

Platelet count

FBS

AST, ALT

Bilirubin, direct and total

Alkaline phosphatase

BUN

Creatinine

Urinalysis

Quantitative immunoglobin

HAA, HAV

HBsAG, HBsAB, HBcAB

Magnesium

Table 14-2	**Typical Bone Marrow Transplant Schedule**
Day	**Scheduled Activity**

PREPARATION PHASE

−10 to −8	Admission
	Consents
	Bone marrow aspiration
	Lumbar puncture with intrathecal methotrexate instillation (acute leukemia)
	Administration of nonabsorbable antibiotics
	Laboratory tests
	Begin low-bacteria diet
−7	Insertion of double-lumen right atrial catheter
	Dosimetry
	Begin teaching self-care procedures and activity requirements

CONDITIONING PHASE

−6	Insertion of three-way urinary catheter
	Leukemia: high-dose cytarabine (ARA-C) or cyclophosphamide administered
	Aplastic anemia: high-dose cyclophosphamide administered
	Lymphoma: Etoposide (Vp16)
	Neuroblastoma: cisplatin; Vp16, melphalan
	Force fluids: 4000 to 4500 ml for adults; 3000 ml/m² for children
−5	Continue high-dose chemotherapy and increased fluid intake
−4	Three-way urinary catheter discontinued if no bleeding after completion of high-dose chemotherapy
−3	Total-body irradiation (divided dose) (ordered for leukemia; may be ordered for aplastic anemia)
−2	Total-body irradiation (divided dose)
	Begin cyclosporine
−1	Total-body irradiation (divided dose)
	Immunoglobin (given day 1 and every other week thereafter)
	Donor admitted for preoperative workup

TRANSPLANT

0	Marrow, aspirated from donor, is infused to establish graft
	If autologous transplant, granulating colony stimulating factor (GCSF) is infused 3 hr after marrow infusion

POSTTRANSPLANT

+1 to +30	Observe for engraftment, reactions to total-body irradiation, and complications of transplanted marrow; supportive therapy: blood products, TPN, antibiotics, pain management

Total protein
Toxoplasmosis titer
Viral studies
    HZ
    Herpes simplex virus HS
    CMV
    HIV
    EBV
    VDRL
Cardiopulmonary studies
    Chest x-ray
    Echocardiogram
    ECG
    Pulmonary function tests
Microbiology studies: surveillance cultures on admission
    and weekly

MULTIDISCIPLINARY MANAGEMENT
THERAPEUTIC MANAGEMENT

Informed consents
Central venous catheter insertion
Medications
    Intrathecal methotrexate (for acute leukemia)
    Nonabsorbable antibiotics
    Allopurinol (except aplastic anemia)
    Bactrim
    Fluconazole (if previous fungal infections)
Dosimetry
Low-bacteria diet
Consults
    Dietary
    Physical and occupational therapy
    Pharmacology

PATIENT PROBLEM—NURSING DIAGNOSIS/INTERVENTIONS

▼Knowledge deficit related to procedures, preparation schedule, daily routines, and patient's expected participation

Explore with patient and significant other(s) their understanding of the BMT procedure and related other procedures involved; clarify misunderstandings, answer questions, request physician to clarify as needed *to increase decision-making ability*

Request consults from other disciplines as needed *to assist patient's understanding,* introduce caregivers from other disciplines who will be involved with patient *so they are familiar to patient*

Explain sequence of events for each phase *to decrease fear of the unknown and increase compliance*

Explain expected care and participation by patient *to increase compliance*

Explain importance of participation in self-care and maintaining exercise and activity levels throughout hospital stay

Teach patient and have patient return demonstrate handwashing techniques, mouth care, skin care, perineal care, use of incentive spirometer

Explain intake and output measurement; provide measurement tools and list of volumes of various containers; have patient record on bedside record sheet

Explain and demonstrate assessments that will be done and their frequency: inspection of oral cavity, skin, and perineal status; respiratory, cardiac, GI, and neurologic assessments, testing for occult blood in stool and urine

Discuss activity level patient will be expected to maintain: shower and bathroom activities, ambulation and active ROM exercises, use of exercycle

Promote interest in diversionary activities: TV watching, reading, computer/video games, handicrafts, puzzles; consult occupational therapy *to assess patient abilities and interests and provide challenging activities*

Explain all procedures before their occurrence, expected sensations during, patient participation in, and expected duration of procedures

Collaborate with clinical dietitian *to educate patient regarding low-bacteria diet:* only sterile water for drinking/ice cubes, list of permitted foods, not to leave food at bedside, food from home must be approved and cooked the same day it is eaten

Collaborate with clinical pharmacist to explain medication regimen, actions, benefits, and potential side effects

Expected Outcome

Patient and significant other verbalize understanding of BMT and related procedures, medication administration, diet, and self-care

CONDITIONING PHASE

First phase of the clinical course; involves treatment of patient with a pretransplant conditioning regimen; for patients with leukemia, high-dose cytarabine (Ara-C) or cyclophosphamide and total body irradiation (TBI) have become standard; for patients with aplastic anemia, high-dose cyclophosphamide is given with or without TBI; for patients with lymphomas, etoposide and TBI; and for patients with neuroblastoma, cisplatin, etoposide, melphalan, and TBI

ASSESSMENT (RELATED TO SIDE EFFECTS OF DRUGS AND TBI)
SUBJECTIVE DATA
Nausea
Anorexia

OBJECTIVE DATA
Stomatitis/mucositis
Diarrhea
Pancytopenia
Hemorrhagic cystitis
Sensorineural hearing loss
Azotemia, renal tubular dysfunction
Hypocalcemia, hypomagnesia
Hypotension
Fever
Alopecia
Syndrome of inappropriate antidiuretic hormone (SIADH)
Vomiting
Anorexia
Parotid gland swelling
Erythema
Decreased saliva and tears
Tumor lysis syndrome: hyperkalemia, hyperphosphatemia, hyperuricemia, hypocalcemia
Venoocclusive disease: liver toxicity
Pulmonary complications: idiopathic pneumonia syndrome (IPS)
Psychosocial
Response to treatments
Relationships and support systems
Coping mechanisms
Understanding of disease and treatment

DIAGNOSTIC TESTS
CBC, platelet count
RBC, PT/INR, activated partial thromboplastin time (APTT)
Electrolytes, calcium, BUN, creatinine, triglycerides
Liver function tests, AST, ALT, bilirubin, alkaline phosphatase
CMV cultures: urine, blood
Urinalysis
Cardiopulmonary tests: ECG (weekly)

MULTIDISCIPLINARY MANAGEMENT
THERAPEUTIC MANAGEMENT
Parenteral fluids and nutrition, TPN
Irradiated blood products
High-dose cyclophosphamide
Cyclosporin
Antiemetics
Antipyretics
Antibiotics
Antidiarrheals
Diuretics
Daily weights
Accurate intake and output measurement
Protective environment
Bladder irrigation, three-way Foley catheter
TBI (1000 rad over 3 days), or ARA-C and fractionated TBI
Cardiac monitoring during TBI and cyclophosphamide

PATIENT PROBLEMS—NURSING DIAGNOSES/INTERVENTIONS

▼ Knowledge deficit (lack of exposure) regarding sequence of events during TBI procedure

Explain/reinforce physician's information regarding procedure *to decrease fears*
Patient will be alone in room but will be able to communicate with personnel
Patient will be visually monitored and cardiac monitored at all times during procedure
Nurse will remain in radiology department and be available to speak to patient, provide support and comfort prn
Patient must remain positioned without moving during procedure
Patient must wear mask and will be placed in protective isolation following the procedure

Expected Outcomes
Patient and significant other verbalize understanding of procedure and degree of patient cooperation required
Participates as directed during the procedure

▼ Potential for hemorrhagic cystitis related to effects of TBI and cyclophosphamide*

Ensure adequate hydration and diuresis 24 hours before and during and 24 to 48 hours after administration of cyclophosphamide *to prevent/lessen effects of medication on bladder*
Force fluids to 4000 to 5000 ml/day (unless contraindicated); enlist patient to make choices of fluids, offer small amounts frequently *so required volume can be taken*

---

*Not a NANDA-approved diagnosis.

Administer parenteral fluids per physician order, usually at rapid rates (200 ml/hr) for several hours before, during, and after chemotherapy administration *to decrease concentration of medication*
Insert and maintain indwelling Foley catheter (three-way for irrigation) *to keep bladder empty, thereby decreasing chance of bleeding;* using strict aseptic technique *to prevent introduction of pathogens*
Perform bladder irrigation per physician order; accurately record intake and output *so imbalance can be noted and treated promptly*
Test urine for occult blood q2h to 4h *to determine effects of medication on bladder*

Expected Outcome
Signs/symptoms of hemorrhagic cystitis do not develop or are recognized and treated without delay

▼ Altered nutrition: less than body requirements related to nausea/vomiting, anorexia, parotid gland swelling

Assess amount and type of foods and liquids tolerated and desired; sweet and highly seasoned foods usually are not well tolerated
Assess and eliminate predisposing factors when possible: unpleasant odors, perfumes, body positioning, disturbing sights/sounds *to decrease noxious stimuli*
Arrange for quiet rest periods before meals *to conserve energy for eating*
Arrange for visitors to join patient for meals; may bring favorite (approved) foods from home; *food tolerated better in a social setting*
Ensure patient's room is well ventilated and odors controlled; remove trash, bedpans; remove food tray as soon as meal is finished *to prevent delayed responses to negative stimuli*
Provide foods that may be served cold or at room temperature *to assist in odor control*
Encourage patient to control nausea through relaxation, rhythmic breathing, imagery exercises
Have patient remain sitting for 30 minutes after meals *to prevent fullness and bloating*
Provide clear liquid diet: juices, carbonated beverages, ice pops *to reduce nausea*
Supplement diet with high-protein, total oral nutrition drinks *to reduce volume required to maintain nutrient level*
Remind patient to eat slowly and chew well
Assist patient in or administer oral care before meals; administer topical anesthetics to oral cavity as needed per physician order *to increase comfort*
In collaboration with clinical dietitian, maintain calorie count and develop meal plans *to meet caloric and nutritional needs* while incorporating patient preferences: BMT patients require 33 to 38 kcal/kg and 1.5 g protein/kg
Weigh patient daily (same time, scale, and clothing)

Administer TPN per physician order *to provide required nutrients and fluids to support metabolic needs*

Expected Outcomes

Maintains body weight within 5% of baseline

Nausea is controlled, allowing patient to take sufficient calories, nutrients, fluids orally

▼ **Risk for infection related to suppressed immune system**

Protective environment to be maintained at all times (protocols will vary among centers): caregivers and visitors must wash hands with antibacterial scrub and don mask and gloves before entering patient room *to prevent/decrease introduction of organisms*

Doors to patient's room to remain closed

No infectious caregivers or visitors to enter room

Patient must wear mask if necessary to leave room

All items entering room are to be sterile or cleaned with bactericidal solution

No flowers or plants to be taken to room *(they harbor infective agents)*

Tap water used for bathing only, never drinking

Instruct visitors in use of protective gear, not to use patient's equipment or bathroom *to prevent transmission of microorganisms*

In collaboration with environmental services: ensure all patient equipment, furniture, fixtures are cleaned with bactericidal solution daily; remove trash, soiled linen from room immediately *to decrease exposure to potentially harmful microorganisms*

Maintain low-bacteria diet and caution in handling and preparation of foods: wash hands before and ensure clean utensils used in food preparation; serve foods at proper temperature; wash thick-skinned fruits in alcohol and peel before serving; dispose of uneaten foods outside patient room; sterile water only for drinking and food preparation

Observe for signs/symptoms of infection: redness, swelling, pain, elevated temperature, changes in breath sounds, cough, sputum, reports of sore throat or burning on urination, urinary frequency/character of urine, *which may indicate early onset infection*

Assess skin condition, paying particular attention to skin folds and orifices, *which provide ideal environment for growth of infective microorganisms*

Use central venous catheter for blood draws and medication administration; ensure perianal care is performed after each elimination; prevent constipation/diarrhea; keep patient and linen clean and dry; encourage mobility and position shifts at least q2h *to maintain skin integrity, which provides a barrier to microorganisms*

Pay particular attention to central venous line insertion site for signs of infection; remind physician of catheter schedule change at intervals required by type of catheter; use strict sterile technique whenever manipulating catheter or changing dressing

Perform daily IV tubing changes; do not allow blood to pool and dry in connections or ports, *which creates a medium for growth of microorganisms*

Avoid urinary catheterization; if necessary, use strict sterile technique when manipulating catheter and providing catheter care

Encourage pulmonary exercises, use of incentive spirometer q1h while awake

Assess condition of oral mucous membranes q8h; assist patient to provide scrupulous oral hygiene before and after meals and q4h *to maintain integrity*

Ensure adequate intake of calories and nutrients and promote uninterrupted periods of rest and sleep *to provide energy for body defenses*

Expected Outcome

Exhibits no signs/symptoms of infection

▼ **Anxiety/fear related to treatment protocols, physical responses to conditioning regimen, and uncertain prognosis**

Assess level of anxiety/fear patient possesses; collaborating with social worker, clergy, significant others in assessment process may be helpful

Provide an environment conducive to open discussion; encourage patient to ventilate feelings, worries, fears; *validation of feelings increases self-awareness*

Continue to provide information and clarify misunderstandings regarding disease and course of treatment; be clear and consistent in responses

Visit frequently when not required to perform tasks; reassure patient that he or she will not be alone *to enhance feelings of trust*

Assist patient in using relaxation methods *to cope with new and unsettling situations*

Use touch and positive body language *to decrease anxious feelings*

Encourage continued relationships and frequent visits from significant other(s) *to provide support to patient*

Expected Outcomes

Verbalizes decreasing anxiety/fears

Demonstrates decreasing overt signs of anxiety/fear

▼ **Body image disturbance related to changes in physical appearance and abilities**

Discuss with patient perceptions of changes and effects on lifestyle and relationships *to provide an opportunity to begin self-assessment*

Provide an atmosphere of open discussion and allow for genuine expression of feelings regarding changes that are occurring *to facilitate acceptance and trust*

Give correct information about expected positive changes following conclusion of treatment: regrowth of hair, weight gain *to encourage hope*

Assess patient's desire and ability to participate in self-grooming; assist patient as needed

Compliment patient on strengths, successful completion of difficult procedures/tasks, physical appearance, *which assist patient to recognize positive accomplishments*

Assist patient to find ways of improving physical appearance: clothing, hats, scarves, hair pieces, makeup, grooming *to enhance self-concept*

Consult social services, psychiatry services as needed *to assist patient to work through acceptance of changes*

Expected Outcomes

Verbalizes feelings about losses and effects on lifestyle and relationships and demonstrates positive coping skills and interest in personal appearance

▌ TRANSPLANT PHASE

Phase in which histocompatible donor bone marrow or peripheral blood stem cells (PBSC) is infused to establish a graft and reinstate production of normal blood cellular components; autologous transplant: patient's marrow that was previously harvested, preserved with dimethyl sulfoxide (DMSO), and frozen is thawed and infused; allogenic and syngeneic transplant: marrow is obtained from donor and immediately infused

ASSESSMENT
SUBJECTIVE DATA

Chest pain
SOB
Taste of garlic/oyster

OBJECTIVE DATA

Reaction to white cells in marrow: chills, fever, hives
Bacterial contamination of marrow: hypotension, fever, shaking chills
Pulmonary overload: tachypnea, dyspnea, crackles, hypertension
Pulmonary emboli: tachycardia, ECG changes
Hematuria: pink or red urine, heme positive (12 to 24 hours postinfusion)
Garlic or oyster smell from patient
BUN/creatinine elevations (lasts for 24 to 48 hours postinfusion)

MULTIDISCIPLINARY MANAGEMENT
THERAPEUTIC MANAGEMENT

Administer marrow
    Autologous/PBSC marrow
        Premedicate patient with diphenhydramine, acetaminophen, and hydrocortisone
        Thaw 50-ml bags of marrow one at a time in basin of warm water
        Draw contents of bag into syringe and inject quickly into central venous catheter, through running normal saline (NS) IV infusion
    Allogenic, synergetic marrow
        Premedicate patient with diphenhydramine, hydrocortisone, and acetaminophen; administer

marrow via IV infusion over no more than 4 hours through central venous catheter

POTENTIAL PATIENT PROBLEM/INTERVENTION

▼Fluid overload, allergic reaction, pulmonary emboli related to infusion of bone marrow

Keep epinephrine, diphenhydramine, hydrocortisone at bedside
Assess patient q5min during the infusion, then q15min × 2, then q30min × 4 *to observe early, subtle changes indicative of overload*
Have nitroglycerine and oxygen available at bedside in case of chest pain, SOB
Remain with patient during infusion *to offer support and reassurance*

Expected Outcome

Exhibits no adverse reactions, or reactions are recognized early and treated promptly

▌ POSTTRANSPLANT/ENGRAFTMENT PHASE

The period after infusion of bone marrow is a critical time in which many problems can occur; the degree that the patient is affected may depend on the underlying disease and clinical status before transplant

ASSESSMENT
SUBJECTIVE DATA

Photophobia, eye pain
Blurred vision
Taste distortion
Nausea, anorexia
Pruritus

OBJECTIVE DATA

Skin and mucous membranes
    Petechiae
    Diffuse maculopapular rash; may be first sign of graft vs. host disease
    Bruising
    Breaks, lesions
    Hyperpigmentation; onset 2 to 3 weeks after TBI
    Jaundice
    Perianal erythema, excoriation
    Abscess
Stomatitis: oral cavity
    Irritation, swelling
    Erythema, ulcerations
    Leukoplakia
    Secretions: color, amount, consistency
    Herpes infection
Lymph nodes (cervical, axillary, groin): size, tenderness, pain
Nutritional status
    Anorexia
    Vomiting
    Weight loss

Parotitis: onset 4 to 24 hours posttransplant; resolved in 24 to 72 hours
  Diarrhea: frequency, color, consistency, occult blood, gross bleeding
Urine: color, amount, odor, hematuria, occult blood, presence of sugar
Breath sounds
  Crackles, diminished
  Rate, depth, pattern of respirations
  Cough, character, frequency
  Sputum color, character, frequency
Venoocclusive disease (VOD)
  Sudden weight gain
  Right upper quadrant (RUQ) pain
  Jaundice
  Hepatomegaly
Cardiovascular system
  Apical rate, rhythm
  Dependent edema
Ophthalmologic system: photophobia, abnormal tear secretion
Activity level: fatigue
Comorbidities
  Infections, hemorrhage
  GVHD (Box 14-3)

DIAGNOSTIC TESTS
Same as conditioning phase, increased frequency of testing (p. 770)

MULTIDISCIPLINARY MANAGEMENT
THERAPEUTIC MANAGEMENT
TPN
IV fluids/electrolytes
Blood products
Pain management
Low-bacteria diet
Daily weights (same time, scale, and clothing)
Accurate measurement of intake and output
Maintain protective environment
Incentive spirometer, oxygen therapy, support of respirations
Medications
  Antibiotics
  Antivirals
  Antipyretics
  Antidiarrheal
  Antiemetics
  Antifungals

POTENTIAL PATIENT PROBLEM/INTERVENTIONS

▼Bleeding related to thrombocytopenia
To determine early and/or subtle signs of bleeding
  Assess neurologic status q8h
  Inspect condition of oral cavity and gums q4h
  Inspect skin q8h for bruising, petechiae, swelling
  Inspect joints q8h for swelling, decreased mobility

Box 14-3 Graft Versus Host Disease (GVHD)

Acute condition usually appears 2 weeks to 3 months after transplant; new bone marrow cells recognize their environment as foreign and try to destroy their new host

Chronic condition appears 3 months to 1 year after transplant; caused by autoreactive T cells and autoantigens

Manifestations
  Skin
    Maculopapular rash
    Erythroderma
    Exfoliative dermatitis
    Bulbous formation
    Desquamation
    Hair loss
    Jaundice
  Gastrointestinal system
    Denuding
    Abdominal pain
    Ileus
  Hepatomegaly/splenomegaly
  Muscle wasting
  Emaciation
  Increased susceptibility to infection
  Pneumonitis
  Hemolytic anemia
  Bone marrow aplasia
  Lymphatic depletion
  Death

Inspect nasal cavity q8h; discourage vigorous nose blowing
Assess abdomen q8h for distension, firmness, tenderness, *which may indicate GI bleeding*
Test emesis, stool, and urine for occult blood
Use central venous catheter for blood draws and administration of medications *to decrease incidence of bleeding caused by multiple punctures*
Avoid skin punctures
Avoid use of rough towels and washcloths, razors, restraints, tight clothing, *which may cause irritation and subsequent bleeding*
Maintain clutter-free environment; use a night light *to prevent bumping into objects and falling*
Administer gentle oral hygiene; to *maintain integrity of oral mucosa do not use a toothbrush*
Monitor results of CBC, platelet, PT/INR, APTT as ordered per physician *to note changes indicative of bleeding*
Administer platelet, other blood products per physician order
Administer H_2 blockers and antacids per physician order
Administer stool softeners prn *to prevent constipation*

Expected Outcome
Occult/frank bleeding is prevented or detected and treated immediately

Table 14-3	Proposed Clinical Stage of Graft Versus Host Disease According to Organ System		
Stage	**Skin**	**Liver**	**Intestinal Tract**
+	Maculopapular rash over 25% of body surface	Bilirubin 2-3 mg/dl	Greater than 500 ml diarrhea/day
++	Maculopapular rash over 25% to 50% of of body surface	Bilirubin 3-6 mg/dl	Greater than 1000 ml diarrhea/day
+++	Generalized erythroderma	Bilirubin 6-15 mg/dl	Greater than 1500 ml diarrhea/day
++++	Generalized erythroderma with bulbous formation and desquamation	Bilirubin >15 mg/dl	Severe abdominal pain with or without ileus

From Thomas ED: Reprinted by permission of New Engl J Med *292:896, 1975, Massachusetts Medical Society.*

PATIENT PROBLEMS—NURSING DIAGNOSES/INTERVENTIONS

▼ Altered oral mucous membrane related to infection or conditioning/transplant regimen

Encourage patient to seek needed dental care before BMT *so oral mucosa and teeth are in optimal condition*

Inspect oral mucous membranes q4h *so therapy can be started promptly when changes are noted*

Assist patient/provide oral care q4h while awake, as well as before and after meals and q4h at night to *keep mouth free of irritating particles and decrease bacteria count*

Use soft sponge cleaners or gauze

Rinse mouth frequently with nonalcohol mouthwash, sterile water

If patient wears dentures: assess for proper fit *to prevent irritation;* keep dentures scrupulously clean; remove dentures and rinse mouth often; dental consult as needed

Keep mouth moist: provide appealing, tepid liquids for sipping, ice chips, flavored ice pops; use water-soluble ointment for lips, artificial saliva

Administer topical anesthetic, antihistamine, antacid mixture as ordered

Administer antifungal medications as ordered

If patient is unable to open mouth for oral care, irrigate mouth with sterile saline/water solution, allowing to drain into emesis basin *to remove irritating particles and enhance healing*

Consult with clinical dietitian *to provide soft foods that are nonirritating*

Use straws or cups because *hard utensils may be irritating and cause discomfort and breaks in mucosa*

Expected Outcomes
Oral mucous membranes remain intact
Healing of disrupted membranes is progressive

▼ Risk for impaired skin integrity related to conditioning/treatment regimen and/or graft versus host disease (Tables 14-3 and 14-4)

Table 14-4	Overall Clinical Grading of Severity of Graft Versus Host Disease	
Grade	**Degree of Organ Involvement**	
I	+ to ++ skin rash; no gut involvement; no liver involvement; no decrease in clinical performance	
II	+ to +++ skin rash; + gut involvement or + liver involvement (or both); mild decrease in clinical performance	
III	++ to +++ skin rash; ++ to +++ gut involvement or ++ to ++++ liver involvement (or both); marked decrease in clinical performance	
IV	Similar to grade III with ++ to ++++ organ involvement and extreme decrease in clinical performance	

From Thomas ED: Reprinted by permission of New Engl J Med *292:896, 1975, Massachusetts Medical Society.*

Assess skin q8h: focus on trunk, palms, soles of feet, ears for maculopapular erythematous rash *so that early changes can be noted and therapy instituted*

Shower/bathe daily and as needed to keep skin clean and dry; pat dry, do not rub *to avoid irritation/abrasions*

Do not leave skin moist with lotions; avoid perfumes, deodorants, *which may cause allergic reactions*

Keep bed dry and linen wrinkle free *to prevent areas of decreased circulation leading to skin disruption;* use sterile linen and gowns

Use foot cradle, air fluid therapy bed as needed *to maintain circulation to all skin areas*

Turn, sit up in chair, ambulate q2h as tolerated; encourage small shifts in position q30min while in bed

Assist patient to perform perineal care after each elimination *to maintain skin integrity*

Maintain a safe environment and assist patient *to avoid bumps, cuts, scratches*

Instruct patient to avoid scratching

Keep nails short and cut straight across

Protect feet with slippers, shoes when out of bed

Avoid wearing jewelry *because moisture and bacteria can collect underneath, certain metals can irritate, rough edges may scratch*

Assess condition of all invasive sites q8h; maintain strict sterile techniques when changing dressings

Expected Outcomes
Skin integrity is maintained
Disrupted skin heals progressively

▼Diarrhea related to conditioning/treatment regimen, graft versus host disease

Observe stools for frequency, amount, consistency, presence of gross/occult blood
Measure liquid stool for inclusion in intake and output calculations
Maintain food diary: eliminate foods that increase/stimulate bowel motility
Cooked foods may be better tolerated than raw fruits and vegetables; omit hot, spicy foods, *which may irritate bowel or enhance peristalsis;* decrease amount of dairy products in diet *to decrease bloated feeling or allergic response*
Encourage foods that decrease bowel motility: rice, bananas
Administer antidiarrheal medications per physician order

Expected Outcome
Frequency of stools decreases, consistency becomes more solid

▼Impaired gas exchange related to complications of radiation/chemotherapy, bone marrow transplant

Assess respiratory status q4h to 8h: rhythm, rate, depth, breath sounds, use of accessory muscles, *which indicates decreased function*
Monitor results of ABGs per physician order
Report cough, fever, tachycardia, dyspnea, increased respirations/distress at rest or with activity
Position patient for maximum chest excursion and comfort of respiration: upright supported by pillows or leaning on overbed table
Encourage coughing and deep breathing, use of incentive spirometer q2h while awake *to facilitate movement/removal of secretions*
Suction airways as needed if patient is unable to clear with coughing
Provide oxygen therapy and support ventilation per physician order
Administer medications per physician order

Expected Outcome
Exhibits breathing patterns that support adequate respiration and gas exchange

▼Risk for fluid volume excess related to venoocclusive disease of the liver

Assess volume status
    Weigh patient daily (same time, scale, and clothing): *sudden weight gain may indicate liver congestion*
    Measure abdominal girth and palpate right upper quadrant q8h to 12h: *increasing girth/tenderness may indicate liver congestion, ascites*
    Record accurate intake and output; *positive balance may indicate volume overload*
    Assess lung sounds for crackles, wheezes, *which may indicate pulmonary congestion*
    Maintain fluid, sodium restrictions as indicated
    Monitor results of bilirubin and AST/ALT: *elevated values may indicate compromised liver function*

Expected Outcomes
Intake and output are balanced
Signs/symptoms of volume overload/compromised liver function do not develop or are recognized and treated promptly

▼Fatigue related to interrupted sleep patterns, inadequate nutrition, anemia, emotional distress, effects of radiation/chemotherapy

Cluster activities, schedule treatments/tests purposefully *to provide uninterrupted periods of sleep and rest*
Assist patient as needed with meal preparation and consumption, personal hygiene, and daily activities *to conserve energy for required activities*
Assess response to activity; alter sequence or amount of assistance provided if not tolerated
Increase activities slowly and only as tolerated; encourage patient to remain involved in physical activities to tolerance

Expected Outcome
Able to participate in daily activities with increasing independence and decreased fatigue

Additional Nursing Diagnoses to Consider
Ineffective individual coping related to prolonged disease, uncertain prognosis, multiple life changes, inadequate support systems
Sexuality patterns, altered: impotence, sterility related to disease process, effects of treatment regimen
Pain from oral mucositis related to infection, treatment regimen

PATIENT/FAMILY TEACHING
Review procedure discussing measures for preventing complications
Self-care procedures: demonstrate and explain rationale, observe return demonstrations for the following:
    Care and flushing of central venous access device
    Administration of IV medication via central line; use of IV pump
    Oral mucous membrane assessment and hygiene
    Skin assessment, skin care, perianal care

Handwashing
Use of incentive spirometer
Measurement of intake and output
Occult blood testing of urine and stool
Methods for taking and recording body temperature
Low-bacteria diet
Instruct in assessment and prevention of the following potential/actual complications
Activity intolerance
Importance of planned rest periods throughout the day and uninterrupted sleep at night
Plan activities for after rest periods
Increase activities to tolerance; seek assistance with ADLs as needed
Importance of changing positions slowly; use of assistive devices as needed
Maintaining a diet high in iron (to combat anemia)
Bleeding
Have emergency telephone numbers on hand; how to reach paramedics, physician
Location of nearest emergency room
Notification of all medical/dental personnel of posttransplant status and medications currently taking
Maintain a safe, clutter-free environment
Avoid over-the-counter medications without consulting physician
Avoid sharp objects; use electric razor
Avoid harsh nose blowing; demonstrate methods for applying pressure for nose bleeding
Infection
Avoid persons who may be infectious, recently vaccinated; avoid crowds
Avoid multiple sex partners
Wash hands before and after eating and toileting
Prevent skin injury, wear protective garments when gardening, cleaning
Avoid overexposure to sun: wear hats, sunscreen
Avoid going barefoot; cut nails straight across
Performing oral hygiene before and after meals and sleep
Avoid drinking fountains
Stomatitis
Explain importance of maintaining oral hygiene routine in morning, before and after meals, and at bedtime
Discuss equipment to use to avoid irritation; avoid alcohol-containing mouthwashes
Teach importance of avoiding irritating foods, controlling temperature and texture to tolerance
Diarrhea
Discuss importance of maintaining fluid intake at least equal to output
Avoid diet high in fiber, roughage; other foods to avoid per individual patient tolerance
Explain importance of taking prescribed medications for diarrhea, avoiding over-the-counter medications

Box 14-4	Temperatures (°F) for Food Safety
165° to 195°	This temperature kills most harmful bacteria
140° to 150°	Minimum temperature at which to cook foods to kill bacteria
45° to 140°	Danger zone for food safeness; rapid bacterial growth
34° to 45°	Cold or chill food storage; slow bacterial growth
0° to −10°	Frozen food storage

Diet
Explain need to maintain low-bacteria diet
Discuss need to supplement diet with total parenteral/oral nutrition
Teach procedures for handling, storing, and cooking foods for safe consumption (Box 14-4)

DISCHARGE/HOME CARE PLANNING

Explain how to prepare environment to receive patient: must be clean and dust free; all surfaces and furniture must be washed/vacuumed; environment should be clutter free
Remove living flowers and plants
Pets should be boarded elsewhere for the first 100 days
Explain necessity of daily cleaning and damp dusting (avoid dry dusting)
Store health care equipment and supplies in clean area
Change towels and washcloths at least daily
Change bed linens at least twice per week
Clean and dry kitchen utensils immediately after use
Empty trash immediately
Continuing health care
Explain importance of keeping appointments for laboratory, diagnostic work and physician providers
Provide information regarding community resources, support groups, home care agencies, durable medical equipment suppliers
Teach names, actions, side effects, potential adverse reactions of medications to report to physician

■ RHEUMATOID ARTHRITIS

A chronic, systemic, inflammatory disease of unknown etiology that is characterized by an inflammatory reaction in the synovial membrane and leads to destruction of joint cartilage and subsequent deformities; the disease may also affect the pulmonary, cardiac, central nervous, integumentary, and reticuloendothelial systems; rheumatoid arthritis occurs more frequently in women and the incidence increases with advancing age

ASSESSMENT
SUBJECTIVE DATA
Fatigue, malaise

Sleep disturbances

Paresthesia of hands and feet

Joint pain, morning stiffness, over 1 hour after periods of
rest

OBJECTIVE DATA
Involved joints: swelling, pain, warmth, redness, impaired
function, effusions, deformities

Shiny, taut skin over affected joints

Low-grade fever

Muscular weakness, spasms, atrophy, contractions

Subcutaneous nodules over pressure points

Vasculitic skin lesions

Vasculitis of peripheral nerves; wrist drop, foot drop

Weight loss

Dry eyes, sclera

Anemia

Tenosynovitis

Keratoconjunctivitis (Sjögren's syndrome)

DIAGNOSTIC TESTS
Serum studies

    CBC: Hgb, Hct decreased; WBC elevated

    ESR: elevated

    ASO titer, rheumatoid factor: positive

    C-reactive protein: positive during acute phase

    Antinuclear antibodies: positive

Radiography

    Soft tissue swelling, bone erosion, joint space
        narrowing, osteoporosis, cartilage destruction

Arthroscopy with synovial fluid analysis

MULTIDISCIPLINARY MANAGEMENT
THERAPEUTIC MANAGEMENT
Medications

    Disease modifying antirheumatic drugs (DMARDS)

        Antimalarials: hydroxychoroquine

        Gold

        Sulfasalazine

        Penicillamine

    Nonsteroidal antiinflammatory drugs (NSAIDs)

        Ibuprofen, naproxen

    Immunosuppression

        Methotrexate

        Azathioprine

        Cyclophsophamide

    Corticosteroids

    Cytokine and cytokine inhibitors

    Investigative agents: Cox-II–specific inhibitors

    Antidepressants, tranquilizers, antipyretics

Surgery

    Joint replacement

    Reconstructive surgery

    Synovectomy

    Arthrodesis

    Arthroplasty

Physical therapy

    Warm moist heat

    Whirlpool

    Paraffin glove

Orthotic devices: splints, braces

Passive/active ROM to joints

Activity level: rest during acute flares

Diet: well-balanced; low-calorie for weight control

PATIENT PROBLEMS—NURSING DIAGNOSES/INTERVENTIONS

▼ Chronic pain related to physical disability secondary to joint inflammation, swelling

Assess location, intensity of pain using consistent pain
rating scale *to determine tolerance and symptoms for
which intervention should occur*

Use firm mattress, bedboard, footboard as appropriate *to
provide support*

Maintain proper alignment of joints *to increase comfort*

    Extend joints as tolerated

    Avoid external rotation of joints; use supports as
        necessary

    Avoid neck flexion; use thin pillow

Apply splints, braces, traction *to immobilize/support joint*

Handle affected limbs gently, providing support above
and below joint *to avoid jarring, jerky movements,
which increase pain*

Monitor effectiveness of treatments: heat/cold, paraffin,
whirlpool

Administer skin care and gentle rubs *to enhance feeling
of comfort*

Use sheepskin, foam, water, air mattress, elbow and heel
guards

Administer analgesic, antiinflammatory medications *to
relieve inflammation*

Observe response to medications in terms of pain relief
and for potential adverse reactions

Discuss and assist patient to use alternative methods of
pain relief

Expected Outcomes

States pain level is tolerable and is able to incorporate
existing pain into lifestyle and self-care activities

▼ Self-care deficit: feeding, grooming, toileting, bathing, dressing related to musculoskeletal impairment and impaired physical mobility

Assess current level of functioning; assist patient with
task analysis of daily activities *to determine priorities*

Administer pain medications before activities

Assist with activities as needed; coach patient through
daily activities *to simplify task, conserve energy, and
increase use of assistive devices*

Consult with physical/occupational therapist *to provide
assistive devices: reachers, elevated seats, extended
shoe horn, large-grip spoons, walking aids*

Set goals with patient: encourage short-term, easily
achieved goals

Be patient; allow sufficient time for patient to complete
tasks *to enhance compliance and independence*

Expected Outcomes

Able to incorporate current level of functioning into
performing independent ADLs

Uses assistive devices to increase independence

Additional Nursing Diagnoses to Consider

Impaired physical mobility related to progressive joint
disease

Body image disturbance related to altered appearance
and function

Fatigue related to sleep disturbances, chronic illness

PATIENT/FAMILY TEACHING

Discuss disease process, contributing factors, signs and
symptoms to report

Discuss self-care management during periods of flare-up

Importance of maintaining prescribed exercise, activity,
rest program

Discuss proper joint alignment and use of supports

Discuss diet management, stress importance of avoiding
undue weight gain

Demonstrate use of assistive devices and walking aids

Review allowances and limitations with respect to
occupation, recreational activities

Review medication administration and potential side
effects, especially means to avoid potential GI effects

Importance of follow-up care with physician, laboratory
tests, and physical therapist

DISCHARGE/HOME CARE PLANNING

Assess home for potentially dangerous situations: loose
rugs, cluttered furniture, inadequate lighting, many
steps, smooth bathtub bottom, dangling cords

Assess assistance available for physical needs, shopping,
cleaning, transportation; arrange providers as required

Ensure provision of ADLs and walking aids to take home;
contact durable medical equipment provider

Discuss importance of regular exercise program such as
walking, swimming

Discuss importance of alternating activities with rest
periods

Discuss pain management: applying heat or cold to
painful joint for temporary relief

Discuss importance of maintaining good body alignment
to reduce pain

Extend joints as tolerated

Avoid use of pillow under knee

Avoid flexion of neck

■ SARCOIDOSIS

A multisystem granulomatous disorder of unknown etiology affecting any organs, but lungs (most common), eyes, and joints may be involved; in most cases the process re- *solves spontaneously without residual effects; 10% become chronic conditions, staged according to international standards, based on chest x-ray findings, fatal in 10% of cases; most common in young adults (ages 20 to 40) and African Americans*

ASSESSMENT
SUBJECTIVE DATA

Anorexia

Fatigue, malaise

SOB, dyspnea on exertion (DOE)

Palpitations

Mild to severe chest pain (rare)

Ocular pain

Joint pain

OBJECTIVE DATA

Fever, night sweats

Weight loss

Respiratory

    Dyspnea

    Cough: usually nonproductive but may be
incapacitating, paroxysms may lead to vomiting

    Clubbing of fingers

    Hypoxemia

    Lung sounds: diffuse crackles or at the bases

Ophthalmologic

    Blurred vision, lacrimation

    Photophobia

    Conjunctival infection

    Uveitis, iritis

    Sjögren's syndrome

    Dry eye

    Blindness (rare)

Musculoskeletal

    Arthralgias

    Arthritis (symmetric, migratory)

Integumentary system

    Skin nodules on face, neck, extremities

    Erythema nodosum

    Bone cysts in hands, feet

    Nasal mucosa lesions, alopecia

Parotid, cervical lymphadenopathy, splenomegaly,
hepatomegaly

Cardiovascular system

    Dysrhythmia, conduction defects

    Pericarditis

    Papillary dysfunction

Nervous system: peripheral neuropathy

DIAGNOSTIC TESTS

Kveim skin test (intradermal injection of sarcoid tissue
suspension): positive in 3 to 6 weeks

CBC

Serum protein levels

    C-reactive protein: elevated

    Polyclonal hypergamma globulin: decreased

    IgG, IgA, IgM: may be elevated

ESR: elevated

Angiotensin-converting enzyme level: may be elevated
Pulmonary tests
  Transbronchial biopsy
  Open lung biopsy
  Bronchoalveolar lavage
Biopsies: skin, conjunctiva, lip
Chest x-ray; bilateral hilar lymphadenopathy with/without diffuse infiltrates and pulmonary fibrosis
Pulmonary function tests: normal to decreased vital capacity and expiratory flow volumes, decreased compliance
Imaging/nuclear medicine tests
  Gallium-67 scan of lungs
Optic: tests for visual acuity; slit-lamp test
Urine: elevated 24-hour calcium level
ABGs: hypoxemia

POTENTIAL COMPLICATIONS
Respiratory failure
Parenchymal bleeding
Congestive heart failure

MULTIDISCIPLINARY MANAGEMENT
THERAPEUTIC MANAGEMENT
Dictated by development of symptoms/involvement of organ systems; none may be necessary
Medications
  Glucocorticosteroids
  Indomethacin
  Optic agents: methylcellulose eyedrops
  NSAIDs
Serial chest x-rays and pulmonary function testing
Serial optic studies
Physical therapy consultation: chest physiotherapy— breathing exercises, percussion, and postural drainage
Oxygen therapy
Supportive/definitive treatment for arthritis

PATIENT PROBLEMS—NURSING DIAGNOSES/INTERVENTIONS

▼ Impaired gas exchange related to alveolar- capillary membrane changes secondary to pul- monary fibrosis, parenchymal lesions, or infection

Assess respiratory status: observe for coughing, adventitious sounds, dyspnea, abnormal rate, rhythm *indicative of changed function*
Obtain sputum specimen for culture *to identify presence of infection;* observe sputum for changes in color, character
Assist patient to use energy conservation techniques
Assist patient to use pursed lip breathing and positioning *to facilitate ease of breathing*
Monitor results of pulmonary function tests for changes from baseline
Administer oxygen therapy, breathing treatments per physician order

Expected Outcomes
Maintains adequate gas exchange
ABGs within baseline
Lung sounds, pulmonary function tests within normal limits

▼ Chronic pain related to disease-induced arthral- gia and ocular discomfort

Assess pain: location, onset, duration, precipitating and alleviating factors *to determine best method to use to enhance comfort*
Use consistent (0 to 10) pain rating scale
Assess nonverbal signs of pain
Assist patient to identify and achieve comfortable positions
Assist patient to achieve state of minimal physical tension through relaxation
In collaboration with physician, provide analgesic medications as required, observing for therapeutic results and side effects

Expected Outcomes
Verbalizes decrease/relief of pain
Incorporates pain into performance of daily activities
Facial expressions and body positioning are relaxed

Additional Nursing Diagnoses to Consider
Risk for body image disturbance related to perceived/actual physical changes of illness
Risk for decreased cardiac output related to dysrhythmias, heart failure

PATIENT/FAMILY TEACHING
Explain disease process, contributing factors, and treatment
Explain management of lung disease: administration of oxygen and nebulized medications, chest physiotherapy, positioning, breathing exercises, avoiding persons who smoke
Review signs and symptoms to report to physician: SOB, red/watery eyes, dizziness, chest pain, swollen joints, unusual fatigue, fever
Explain medication administration side effects: need to take steroids with food, antacids; do not take over-the- counter medications without consulting physician
Teach aseptic technique for administering eye drops to avoid contamination
Encourage patient to pace activities, avoid overexertion, especially during "flare up"
Advise on diet choices to provide balanced nutrition within restrictions
Discuss importance of continued medical follow-up every 2 to 3 months while disease is active
Discuss importance of not smoking and avoiding second-hand smoke
Avoid exposure to lung irritating substances such as dust, chemicals

For women: discuss importance of planning all pregnancies

DISCHARGE/HOME CARE PLANNING

Assess patient support system and ability to provide assistance for physical needs, cooking, cleaning, shopping, and transportation as needed; arrange home care providers as necessary

Assess sufficient, clean space available to store medical equipment and supplies; arrange for durable medical equipment provider as necessary

■ SYSTEMIC LUPUS ERYTHEMATOSUS (SLE)

A chronic autoimmune inflammatory disease of the connective tissues that produces biochemical and structural changes in skin, joints, and muscles, usually with multiple organ involvement; SLE is characterized by antibody formation against itself (autoantibody); women are affected nine times more than men

ASSESSMENT
SUBJECTIVE DATA
Malaise

Anorexia

Nausea

Abdominal pain

Headache

Photophobia

OBJECTIVE DATA
Fever, weakness

Hemolytic anemia

Thrombocytopenia

Gastrointestinal system

  Vomiting, diarrhea, weight loss

  Hepatosplenomegaly

Genitourinary system

  Hematuria

  Cellular casts*

  Proteinuria*

Cardiovascular system

  Hypertension, cardiomegaly, edema

  Pericarditis, murmurs

  ECG changes, dysrhythmia

Renal system: azotemia, hypoproteinuria

Neurovascular system

  Neuritis, seizures*

  Raynaud's phenomenon

  Vasculitis; necrosis of small arteries

Musculoskeletal system

  Nondeforming arthritis

  Joint warmth and swelling

Integumentary system

  Sensitivity to sun*

Rash/erythema, "butterfly" over cheeks and bridge of nose*

  Partial alopecia*

  Oral/nasal ulcerations*

Respiratory system

  Pleuritis

  Parenchymal lung infiltrates

  Pulmonary hemorrhage

Ophthalmologic system

  Retinal cystoid bodies

  Conjunctivitis

  Diplopia

Personality changes

Depression

Psychosis

Hemolytic anemia*

DIAGNOSTIC TESTS
Serum studies

  LE prep: positive

  Antinuclear antibody (ANA): positive

  Anti-DNA antibody: positive

  Fluorescent treponemal antibody absorption (FTA-ABS): negative

  Complement (C3 and C4): decreased during flares

  CBC: thrombocytopenia, leukopenia

  C-reactive protein: positive

  ESR: elevated

  Coagulation profile: prolonged prothrombin time (PT), partial thromboplastin time (PTT)

  Rheumatoid factor: positive

Synovial fluid analysis

False-positive serology*

Urine studies: proteinuria, protein casts

Chest x-ray, CT scans

Skin and kidney biopsy

POTENTIAL COMPLICATIONS
Steroid-induced infections

Renal failure

Pneumonia

MULTIDISCIPLINARY MANAGEMENT
THERAPEUTIC MANAGEMENT
Medications

  NSAIDS

  Corticosteroids

  Immunosuppressive or cytotoxic agents

  Antiinfective agents

  Antihypertensives

  Analgesics

  Antipyretics

  Antibiotics

Plasmapheresis

Joint arthroplasty or replacement

Four or more of these findings support the diagnosis of SLE.

Four or more of these findings support the diagnosis of SLE.

Diet: salt restriction, low fat
Dialysis

POTENTIAL PATIENT PROBLEM/INTERVENTIONS

▼Renal, cardiac, and neurologic system dysfunction related to tissue destruction from deposition of immune complexes and antibodies

Assess renal status: monitor for presence of edema, nausea, hematuria, hypertension
  Accurately record intake and output
  Monitor results of urinalysis and kidney function studies
Assess neurologic status: observe for changes in level of consciousness (LOC), judgment, mental acuity, speech, personality changes
Assess cardiac status: monitor vital signs, hemodynamic status, cardiac rhythm, presence of edema, jugular vein distention

Expected Outcome
Changes in renal, cardiac, and/or neurologic function are detected early, and treatment is initiated

PATIENT PROBLEMS—NURSING DIAGNOSES/INTERVENTIONS

▼Impaired gas exchange related to alveolar-capillary membrane changes secondary to pulmonary fibrosis

Assess respiratory system: observe for dyspnea, cyanosis, diminished breath sounds, coarse/fine crackles, tachypnea, bradypnea *to detect changes in pulmonary function*
Elevate head of bed for ease of respiration
Administer oxygen therapy as indicated
Encourage turning, controlled coughing, deep breathing *to clear lungs and airways*
Administer pulmonary medications as ordered: bronchodilators, steroids
Obtain sputum cultures as ordered *to determine presence of infective agents*
Maintain adequate hydration *to facilitate movement of secretions*

Expected Outcomes
Exhibits no signs of respiratory distress:
  Breath sounds normal
  Respiratory rate within normal limits
  Verbalizes no dyspnea

▼Altered nutrition: less than body requirements related to fatigue, nausea, anorexia

Assess nutritional status, maintain calorie count; monitor serum protein and albumin levels

Consult with dietitian *to develop meal plans that incorporate caloric requirements and restrictions based on organ system involvement*
Provide frequent, small meals, *which are more easily tolerated;* provide supplements as indicated
Provide an environment conducive to pleasant eating: provide oral care before meals, remove bedpans/urinals, have patient sit up in chair for meals; assist patient to eat as necessary
Weigh patient daily (same time, scale, and clothing); compare with ideal body weight *to determine increase or decrease*

Expected Outcomes
Consumes and retains 80% to 90% of each meal
Weight is maintained within 2% of patient's ideal body weight

▼Impaired physical mobility related to muscle weakness, fatigue, and joint involvement

Coordinate activities *to provide for undisturbed periods of rest and sleep*
Assess degree of physical limitation: fatigue, muscle weakness, joint pain, and swelling *to develop activity/exercise plan of care*
Evaluate pain and effectiveness of current exercise regimen
Administer analgesics as needed before activity *to increase comfort*
Set goals with patient *to gradually increase activity tolerance*
Perform active/passive ROM exercises qid *to maintain joint integrity;* collaborate with physical therapist *to determine appropriate activities*
Provide assistive devices as needed *to support/immobilize joints*
Maintain proper alignment of joints *to increase comfort;* avoid neck flexion, use thin pillow
Use firm mattress, bedboard, footboard as indicated *to provide support*
Encourage patient to participate in activities to tolerance; promote a positive attitude; assist as needed *to prevent exhaustion*
Set activity goals with patient; help patient identify progress made

Expected Outcomes
Participates in prescribed exercise program
Performs ADLs at optimal level
Verbalizes a feeling of increased energy

▼Risk for infection, related to altered immune system, immunosuppressive medications, multiple organ system dysfunction

Assess for signs, symptoms of infectious process: chills, fever, malaise, increased fatigue

Monitor results of laboratory tests: CBC, WBC differential, ESR, C-reactive protein, urinalysis, cultures

Obtain culture of drainage from any site: sputum, urine, blood as indicated

Assist patient to maintain personal hygiene *to decrease environment conducive to growth of infective microorganisms*

Assess level of risk for hospital-acquired infections: skin breaks, use of invasive procedures

Restrict visitors, caregivers who may be infectious

Provide for optimal nutrition and fluid intake *to enhance body defense mechanisms*

Avoid multiple injection sites

Use strict sterile technique for all invasive procedures

Administer antibiotics and other antiinfectives per order

Expected Outcome
Exhibits no signs of infection

Additional Nursing Diagnoses to Consider
Impaired skin integrity, related to inflammation, infection secondary to altered immune system

Body image disturbance related to perceived/actual change in physical appearance and abilities

PATIENT/FAMILY TEACHING
Assess level of understanding

Discuss nature and course of disease process, precipitating factors (psychologic or physical stress, abrupt cessation of drugs, photosensitivity) and treatment

Discuss and teach to monitor for organ involvement

Review medications, discussing names, dosage, time of administration, and side effects

Discuss importance of need to avoid penicillin, sulfa, phenytoin, oral contraceptives

Review signs/symptoms of flare-up to reported to physician: fever, chills, excessive fatigue, muscle weakness, increased joint pain, chest pain

Explain importance of continuing follow-up care

Discuss need to wear medical alert identification band

Teach importance of notifying all caregivers of diagnosis

For women: discuss importance of planning all pregnancies; refer to gynecologist for evaluation and prescription of contraceptive

DISCHARGE/HOME CARE PLANNING
Assess patient's ability to provide for own self-care and daily living needs; arrange for home care providers as needed

Discuss importance of skin care and protection from the sun: use SPF 15 sunblock and large-brimmed hats, avoid sunbathing

Discuss approved cosmetic/makeup coverups available at department stores

Provide instruction for daily skin care: keep skin dry and clean, avoid use of hot water, use unscented lotions

Discuss importance of balanced nutrition and hydration

Discuss importance of protecting against infections: avoid large crowds, infected individuals

Discuss importance of pacing activities; avoid overexertion, allow regular rest periods; increase rest periods during episodes of flare-ups

Encourage regular exercise to maintain weight, perform range of motion exercises of joints to maintain overall sense of wellness

Discuss activity allowances and limitations; encourage use of assistive devices such as splints, walkers as indicated

Refer to community resources and national support services:

Lupus Foundation of America
1300 Piccard Drive, Suite 200
Rockville, MD 20850-4303
800-558-0121/301-670-9292

BIBLIOGRAPHY
Anastasi JK, Rivera J: Understanding prophylactic therapy for HIV infections, *Am J Nurs* 94(2):36, 1994.

Anastasi JK, Lee VS: HIV wasting: how to stop the cycle, *Am J Nurs* 94(6):18, 1994.

Ackley BJ, Ladwig GB: *Nursing diagnosis handbook: a guide to planning care,* ed 3, St Louis, 1997, Mosby.

Atal M et al: Prevention of gram-positive infections after bone marrow transplantation by systemic vancomycin: a prospective, randomized trial, *J Clin Oncol* 9:865, 1991.

Beare PG, Myers JL: *Adult health nursing,* ed 3, St Louis, 1998, Mosby.

Belcher A: *Cancer nursing,* St Louis, 1992, Mosby.

Bradley-Springer L: Nutritional support in HIV infection: a multilevel analysis, *IMAGE J Nurs Sch* 23(3):155, 1991.

Canobbio M: *Mosby's handbook of patient teaching,* St Louis, 1996, Mosby.

Concensus Conference: Activity of sarcoidosis, Third WASOG Meeting, *Eur Respir J* 7:624, 1994.

Crouch R: Current concepts in autologous bone marrow transplantation, *Semin Oncol Nurs* 10(1):12, 1994.

El-Sadr et al: *Evaluation and management of early HIV infection: clinical practice guideline,* Washington, DC, US Department of Health and Human Resources.

Ezzone et al: Survey of oral hygiene regimens among bone marrow transplant centers, *Oncol Nurs Forum* 20(9):1375, 1993.

Fauci AS, Braunwalt E, et al: *Harrison's principles of internal medicine,* ed 14, New York, 1998, McGraw-Hill.

Franco, Gould: Allogenic bone marrow transplantation, *Semin Oncol Nurs* 10(1):3, 1994.

Grimes D et al: *Infectious diseases,* St Louis, 1991, Mosby.

Keithley JK et al: Nutritional alterations in persons with HIV infection, *IMAGE J Nurs Sch* 24(3):183, 1992.

Kim MJ et al: *Pocket guide to nursing diagnoses,* ed 7, St Louis, 1997, Mosby.

Lader: HIV infections of the central nervous system, *Nurs Clin North Am* 28(4):838, 1993.

LeMone P: Analysis of a human phenomenon: self-concept, *Nurs Diagn* 2(3):126, 1991.

Lisati P, Zwolski K: Understanding the devastation of AIDS, *Am J Nurs* 97(7):27, 1997.

Mack CH: Assessment of the autologous bone marrow transplant patient according to Orem's self care model, *Cancer Nurs* 15(6):429, 1992.

McCance KL, Huether SE: *Pathophysiology: the biological basis for disease in adults and children,* ed 3, St Louis, 1998, Mosby.

McCorkle R, GM et al: *Cancer nursing: a comprehensive textbook,* ed 2, Philadelphia, 1996, WB Saunders.

McFarland GK, McFarlane EA: *Nursing diagnosis and intervention: planning for patient care,* ed 3, St Louis, 1997, Mosby.

Mehmert PPA, Delaney CW: Validating impaired physical mobility, *Nurs Diagn* 2(4):143, 1991.

Miller-Blair, Robbins: Rheumatoid arthritis: new science, new treatment, *Geriatrics* 48(6):28, 1993.

Mudge-Grout C: *Immunologic disorders,* St Louis, 1992, Mosby.

Muma et al: *HIV manual for health care professionals,* Norwalk, Conn, 1994, Appleton & Lange.

Nokes et al: Development of an HIV assessment tool, *IMAGE J Nurs Sch* 26(2):133, 1994.

Ouellet LL, Rush KL: A synthesis of selected literature on mobility: a basis for studying impaired mobility, *Nurs Diagn* 3(2):72, 1992.

Roitt IM et al: *Immunology,* ed 5, St Louis, 1998, Mosby.

Singla et al: The role of nutrition support and megesterol therapy in reversing malnutrition in AIDS, *AIDS Patient Care* 7(3):132, 1993.

Sparks SM: Exploring electronic support groups, *Am J Nurs* 12:62, 1992.

Thompson J et al: *Mosby's clinical nursing,* ed 4, St Louis, 1997, Mosby.

Wjcik D: Advances in bone marrow transplantation, *Semin Oncol Nurs* 10(1):3, 1994

Zepp: The "potential for injury" and the risk for falls in patients with HIV disease, *AIDS Patient Care* 7(5):249, 1993.

USC UNIVERSITY HOSPITAL

1500 San Pablo
Los Angeles, CA 90033

MULTIDISCIPLINARY PLAN

NAME _____
ALLERGIES _____
MR# _____

ADMIT DATE _____

DIAGNOSIS HIV with Severe Diarrhea ± Fever
SURGERY _____

DISCHARGE OUTCOMES	DRG 490 ALOS 8.4
PHYSIOLOGICAL	Bowel function: diarrhea controlled with treatment of causative organism. Fluid/electrolyte within normal limits. Adequate nutritional intake as evidenced by maintenance of weight and labs within normal limits.
COGNITIVE	Verbalizes medical follow-up plan, and signs and symptoms to report to health care team. Verbalizes modes of transmission of HIV, universal precautions, high and low risk behaviors.
PSYCHOLOGICAL	Anxiety/fear controlled as evidenced by ability to participate in medical decisions/care. Demonstrates methods to manage fear/anxiety. Knowledgeable about available community support.

DISCIPLINE	PRE-OP/ PRE-ADMIT	D.O.S. DATE ___ DAY 1	P.O.#1 DATE ___ DAY 2	P.O.#2 DATE ___ DAY 3	P.O.#3 DATE ___ DAY 4	P.O.#4 DATE ___ DAY 5	P.O.#5 DATE ___ DAY 6
LOCATION		Med/Surg	Med/Surg	Med/Surg	Med/Surg	Med/Surg	Med/Surg
LABS		CBC, Chem 20 Blood culture Stool culture, O & P. AFB, C. difficile	Chem 7 CBC Stool for O & P	Chem 7 Stool for O & P	Chem 7 CBC		CBC
CARDIO-PULMONARY							
IMAGING/ NUCLEAR MEDICINE		CXR Verify with MD any bowel preparations.	Verify with MD any bowel preparations.	Verify with MD any bowel preparations.	Verify with MD any bowel preparations.	Verify with MD any bowel preparations.	Verify with MD any bowel preparations.
SOCIAL SERVICES D/C PLAN REHAB. SERVICES		Assess home situation, and psychological response to illness. Provide support prn.	D/C planning. Home health as indicated.	Continued psychosocial support.		Reassess D/C plan.	
PHARMACY		• K⁺, electrolyte replacement • IV fluid replacement Antidiarrheals unless salmonellosis. Antibiotic therapy as indicated for identified pathogen.	Electrolyte replacement. IV fluid replacement. Antidiarrheals.				
DIETARY/ NUTRITION		DAT. If n/v clear, advance as tolerated.	NPO status as indicated for testing; otherwise, advance diet. Dietitian/consult.	NPO status as indicated for testing; otherwise, advance diet.	Begin calorie count x3 days	Nutritional supplement as indicated.	

Used by permission of USC University Hospital, Los Angeles, California.

Continued

USC UNIVERSITY HOSPITAL

1500 San Pablo
Los Angeles, CA 90033

MULTIDISCIPLINARY PLAN

NAME _____
ALLERGIES _____
MR# _____

DIAGNOSIS HIV with Severe Diarrhea ± Fever

SURGERY _____

DISCHARGE OUTCOMES	DRG 490 ALOS 8.4
PHYSIOLOGICAL	Bowel function: diarrhea controlled with treatment of causative organism. Fluid/electrolyte within normal limits. Adequate nutritional intake as evidenced by maintenance of weight and labs within normal limits.
COGNITIVE	Verbalizes medical follow-up plan & signs and symptoms to report to health care team. Verbalizes modes of transmission of HIV, universal precautions, high and low risk behaviors.
PSYCHOLOGICAL	Anxiety/fear controlled as evidenced by ability to participate in medical decisions/care. Demonstrates methods to manage fear/anxiety. Knowledgeable about available community support.

DISCIPLINE	PRE-OP/ PRE-ADMIT	P.O.#6 DATE	DAY 7	P.O.#7 DATE	DAY 8	P.O.#8 DATE	DAY 9	P.O.#9 DATE	DAY 10	P.O.#10 DATE	DAY 11	P.O.#11 DATE	DAY 12
LOCATION													
LABS													
CARDIO-PULMONARY													
IMAGING/ NUCLEAR MEDICINE													
SOCIAL SERVICES D/C PLAN REHAB. SERVICES			Home health plan established as indicated.										
PHARMACY													
DIETARY/ NUTRITION	Diet as tolerated.												

PATIENT NAME: _____   MEDICAL RECORD # _____

MULTIDISCIPLINARY PLAN

DISCIPLINE	PRE-OP/ PRE-ADMIT	D.O.S. DATE ___ / DAY 1	P.O. #1 DATE ___	DAY 2 / P.O. #2 DATE ___	DAY 3 / P.O. #3 DATE ___	DAY 4 / P.O. #4 DATE ___	DAY 5 / P.O. #5 DATE ___	DAY 6
PATIENT ACTIVITY		Up ad lib, as tolerated. Daily wt before breakfast.		Up ad lib, as tolerated. Daily wt before breakfast.	Up ad lib, as tolerated. Daily wt before breakfast.	Daily wt before breakfast.	Daily wt before breakfast.	Daily wt before breakfast.
EDUCATION	Hospital orientation. Preprocedure instructions.	Preprocedure instructions. Medication education.		Preprocedure instructions.	Preprocedure instructions.	Preprocedure instructions. Nutritional education prn.	Side effects of medication.	

COLLABORATIVE PROBLEMS

	DATE				DC DATE INIT			DATE				DC DATE INIT

1. Alteration in elimination: diarrhea R/T infection or medication.
2. Skin integrity, impaired, R/T diarrhea, malnutrition, immobility.
3. Potential/actual for infection, R/T immunodeficiency.
4. Alteration in comfort, pain.
5. Fluid/electrolyte imbalance, potential.
6. Anxiety/fear.
7. Potential for injury R/T drug administration (liver/renal toxicities).
8. Alteration in nutrition, < body requirements.
9. Alteration in coping R/T diagnosis/ prognosis.
10. Knowledge deficit R/T disease, transmission, medications, &/or follow-up plan.

KEY

1. To initiate a problem or intervention, document under corresponding date.
2. Document outcomes under appropriate date for achieving the goal.
3. To discontinue an intervention, or resolve a patient problem, highlight date and initial.

SBFT = small bowel follow through

OUTCOMES

2. No skin breakdown, or implementation of skin care program.
3. No infection throughout hospitalization, or infection managed with no evidence of systemic infection.
4. Pain controlled at a level "3 on 1-10 scale.
6. Verbalizes anxiety/fear.

1. Diarrhea diminished.
7. No injury R/T drug administration.
5. Fluid/electrolytes improved - approaching normal limits.

4. Continued pain control at level "3 on 1-10 scale.
6. Anxiety diminished. Verbalizes understanding of anxiety & demonstrates methods to manage.

2. Skin integrity maintained, or improved skin integrity.
5. Fluids/electrolytes within normal limits.

1. Diarrhea controlled.

9. Identified appropriate resources to seek prn.
7. Verbalizes signs & symptoms of side effects of meds. Knowledgeable about S/S to report to medical team.
8. Optimal nutritional status is maintained. Albumin/ protein within normal limits.

Continued

PATIENT NAME: _____   MEDICAL RECORD # _____

MULTIDISCIPLINARY PLAN

DISCIPLINE	PRE-OP/ PRE-ADMIT	P.O.#6 DATE	DAY 7	P.O.#7 DATE	DAY 8	P.O.#8 DATE	DAY 9	P.O.#9 DATE	DAY 10	P.O.#10 DATE	DAY 11	P.O.#11 DATE	DAY 12
PATIENT ACTIVITY		Up ad lib.											
EDUCATION		Disease process methods to prevent transmission. Pt risk reduction. Risk factors for infection.											

KEY

1. To initiate a problem or intervention, document under corresponding date.

2. Document outcomes under appropriate date for achieving the goal.

3. To discontinue an intervention, or resolve a patient problem, highlight date and initial.

SBFT = small bowel follow through

COLLABORATIVE PROBLEMS

DATE	COLLABORATIVE PROBLEMS	DC DATE INIT	DATE	COLLABORATIVE PROBLEMS	DC DATE INIT
	2. Skin integrity, impaired R/T diarrhea, malnutrition, immobility.				
	3. Potential for infection R/T immunodeficiency.				
	8. Alteration in nutrition " body requirements.				

OUTCOMES

2. Skin intact, no breakdown.

3. No infection/infection resolving with normal VS & no evidence of systemic infection.

8. Nutritional intake supports healing/maintenance of wt.

10. Verbalizes modes of transmission, precautions, high/low risk behaviors.

1. Frequency of stools are within normal limits for patient.

10. Self administration of po meds. Able to verbalize need to maintain treatment/med plan. Verbalizes when to consult medical/health care team.

PLAN OF CARE DISCUSSED WITH	D.O.S. DAY 1 DATE___	P.O.#1 DAY 2 DATE___	P.O.#2 DAY 3 DATE___	P.O.#3 DAY 4 DATE___	P.O.#4 DAY 5 DATE___	P.O.#5 DAY 6 DATE___	
INTERVENTIONS							
DATE INIT SO/P	Assess risk factors: • recent travel • antibiotic exposure	Continued assessment/management of elimination, infection, skin integrity, fluid & electrolyte & pain problems.					
	• seafood exposure • gay male • common source outbreak, i.e., food poisoning	Encourage participation as much as possible. Monitor for s/sx of adverse effects from meds:			Pace care/rest activities to provide for as much independence as possible.	Explain disease process, methods to prevent transmission.	
CASE MANAGER:	Assess elimination pattern, quality, quantity, frequency.	• nausea/vomiting, diarrhea, bone marrow suppression			Consult P.T./O.T. prn.	Discuss need to follow safe sex guidelines.	
CONSULTING MD:	presence of blood. Strict I/O. Monitor VS for hypovolemia.	• renal/liver toxicity • anorexia/rash		Education regarding support available in the community.		Discuss pt risk reduction. Maintenance of home environment.	
___	Monitor labs, & s/sx of fluid/electrolyte imbalance.	Assess nutritional status, height, wt, total protein/albumin.		support & MSW consult. Assist pt/family to use social network for support, assistance in care.		Adequate nutritional intake.	
SOCIAL SERVICE:	Assess skin, monitoring perianal skin condition & provide skin care to prevent breakdown.	Consult Dietary prn. Provide small frequent high caloric meals as tolerated/desired.		Discuss possible areas of conflict that may arise.	Teach pt about prescribed meds, indications for use, side effects.		
ANOINTING OF THE SICK DATE: ___	Monitor for s/sx of septicemia temp>101, <98 wbc/bacteria in urine & blood culture.	Allow for adequate rest & assist with ADLs prn. Monitor tolerance to visitors/phones.		When appropriate, encourage pt to document preferences regarding decision		Avoidance of people with infection.	
	Institute measures to prevent exposure to known sources of infection.			maker/advance directive. Continued nutritional support.		Prevention of injury. Mgmt of activity/rest.	
	Assess pain level, characteristics. Medicate as ordered.					Avoidance of high risk behaviors (i.e., use of ETOH, tobacco, recreational drugs).	
	Enteric precautions. Assess level of anxiety:					Teach reduction of risk factors for infection:	
	• provide opportunities to express feeling.					• malnutrition • exposure to infectious sources or invasive procedure	
	• MSW consult prn.						
	Maintain immediate environment to allow for self-control.					Avoidance of frequent venipuncture.	

MULTIDISCIPLINARY PLAN UPDATE					
DATE	SIGNATURES	DATE	SIGNATURES	DATE	SIGNATURES

USC UNIVERSITY HOSPITAL

1500 San Pablo
Los Angeles, CA 90033

MULTIDISCIPLINARY PLAN

DIAGNOSIS HIV with Fever of Unknown Origin	NAME _____
SURGERY _____	ALLERGIES _____
DRG 490 ALOS 8.4 ADMIT DATE:	MR# _____

DISCHARGE OUTCOMES

PHYSIOLOGICAL — Physiological symptoms controlled with treatment of causative organism. Vital signs within normal limits. Adequate nutritional intake as evidenced by maintenance of weight, and laboratory tests within normal limits.

COGNITIVE — Patient/significant other verbalizes medical follow-up plan, signs and symptoms to report to healthcare team. Verbalizes modes of transmission of infection of HIV, universal precautions, high- and low-risk behaviors.

PSYCHOLOGICAL — Anxiety/fear controlled as evidenced by ability to participate in medical decisions/care. Demonstrates methods to manage fear/anxiety. Knowledgeable about available community support.

DISCIPLINE	PRE-OP/ PRE-ADMIT	DOS DATE ___ DAY 1	PO#1 DATE ___ DAY 2	PO#2 DATE ___ DAY 3	PO#3 DATE ___ DAY 4	PO#4 DATE ___ DAY 5	PO#5 DATE ___ DAY 6
LOCATION		Med/Surg	Med/Surg	Med/Surg	Med/Surg	Med/Surg	Med/Surg
LABS		CBC, Chem 20, U/A. If abnormal U/A, urine for C/S. Blood culture[1] for conventional bacteria, mycobacteria, viral (CMV). Blood cryptococcal Ag. Histoplasmosis Ag, coccidiomycosis[2].	If CBC indicates cytopenias, bone marrow bx.	Sputum for AFB. If chest x-ray positive, and cough, LDH abnormal, induce sputum for PCP and AFB.	If blood cryptococcal Ag. positive, lumbar puncture. If abnormal liver function studies, hepatitis serology, liver biopsy.		
CARDIO-PULMONARY							
IMAGING/ NUCLEAR MEDICINE		Chest x-ray. Sinus x-ray if respiratory symptoms.		Absence of focal findings, CT of chest, head, and abdomen.		Abnormal lymph adenopathy, consider biopsy. If skin lesion, biopsy.	
SOCIAL SERVICES D/C PLAN REHAB. SERVICES		Assess home situation and psychological response to illness. Provide support prn.	Assess support system. Discharge planning. Home health as indicated.			Reassess DC plan.	
PHARMACY		PPD and anergy screen. IV fluid replacement. If FUO and clinical findings consistent with pneumonia, PCP, empiric therapy. Suspect bacterial findings, broad spectrum antibiotics.					
DIETARY/ NUTRITION		DAT. Dietary consult prn.	NPO status as indicated for testing; otherwise, advance diet.				

PATIENT NAME _____

MEDICAL RECORD # _____

page 2 of 4

MULTIDISCIPLINARY PLAN

DISCIPLINE	PRE-OP/ PRE-ADMIT	DOS DATE	DAY 1	PO#1 DAY 2 DATE	PO#2 DAY 3 DATE	PO#3 DAY 4 DATE	PO#4 DAY 5 DATE	PO#5 DAY 6 DATE
PATIENT ACTIVITY		Up ad lib, as tolerated.		Up ad lib, as tolerated. Daily weight before breakfast.	Daily weight before breakfast.	Daily weight before breakfast.	Daily weight before breakfast.	Daily weight before breakfast.
EDUCATION		Hospital orientation. Preprocedure instructions. Medical treatment plan.		Preprocedure instructions. Medication education.	Preprocedure instructions.	Preprocedure instructions. Nutritional education.	Side effects of medication.	

	DATE	COLLABORATIVE PROBLEMS	DC DATE INIT	DATE	COLLABORATIVE PROBLEMS	DC DATE INIT
KEY 1. To initiate a problem or intervention, document under corresponding date. 2. Document outcomes under appropriate date for achieving the goal. 3. To discontinue an intervention or resolve a patient problem highlight date and initial.		1. Hyperthermia.			7. Alteration in coping related to diagnosis/prognosis.	
		2. Fluid/electrolyte imbalance, potential.			8. Knowledge deficit related to disease, transmission, medications, and/or follow-up plan.	
		3. Potential/actual for infection, R/T immunodeficiency.				
		4. Alteration in comfort, pain.				
		5. Anxiety/fear.				
		6. Potential for injury R/T drug administration (liver/renal toxicities).				

OUTCOMES

1. Patient will maintain/regain near normal body temperature.	5. Anxiety diminished. Verbalizes understanding of anxiety and demonstrates methods of manage.	4. Continued pain control less than or equal to 3 on 1-10 scale.		7. Identified appropriate resources to seek prn.	
2. Fluid/electrolyte balanced throughout hospitalization.		2. Fluids, electrolytes within normal limits.		8. Verbalizes signs and symptoms of side effects of meds. Knowledgeable about S/E to report to medical team.	
3. No infection throughout hospitalization, or infection managed with no evidence of systemic infection.					
4. Pain controlled at a level ≤3 on 1-10 scale.					
5. Verbalizes anxiety/fears.					
6. No injury related to drug administration					

Continued

PATIENT NAME _____

MEDICAL RECORD # _____

page 3 of 4

MULTIDISCIPLINARY PLAN

DISCIPLINE	PRE-OP/ PRE-ADMIT	PO#6 DAY 7	PO#7 DATE	DAY 8	PO#8 DATE	DAY 9	PO#9 DATE	DAY 10	PO#10 DAY 11 DATE	DAY 11	PO#11 DAY 12 DATE
PATIENT ACTIVITY		Up ad lib.									
EDUCATION		Disease process methods to prevent transmission. Patient risk reduction. Risk factors for infection.									

COLLABORATIVE PROBLEMS

DATE		DC DATE / INIT	DATE				DC DATE / INIT
	3. Infection, actual.						
	4. Alteration in comfort.						
	8. Knowledge deficit R/T to disease, transmission, medications, &/or follow-up plan.						

KEY

1. To initiate a problem or intervention, document under corresponding date.
2. Document outcomes under appro-date for achieving the goal.
3. To discontinue an intervention or resolve a patient problem highlight, date, and initial.

OUTCOMES

3. Infection managed throughout hospitalization.	
4. Pain control ≤3 on scale of 1-10.	
8. Pt verbalizes medical follow-up plan, s/sx to report to team, modes of transmission of infection, & preventative interventions.	

	DOS DAY 1 DATE ___	PO#1 DAY 2 DATE ___	PO#2 DAY 3 DATE ___	PO#3 DAY 4 DATE ___	PO#4 DAY 5 DATE ___	PO#5 DAY 6 DATE ___
PLAN OF CARE DISCUSSED WITH						
DATE INIT SO/P	**INTERVENTIONS** — Continued assessment/management of elimination, infection, skin integrity, fluid & electrolyte, & pain problems.					
	Confirm fever. Question if temperature log maintained. Thorough med hx to R/O cause.					Explain disease process, methods to prevent transmission.
	Obtain recent travel hx. Implement cooling measures. Avoid inducing shivering/chills.	Encourage participation as much as possible		Create private/supportive environment for pt family. Explore pt/family perceptions.	Pace care/rest activities to provide for as much independence as possible.	Discuss need to follow safe sex guidelines.
	Provide ↑ nutritional/fluid intake. Strict I & O.	Monitor for s/sx of adverse effects from meds:		Promote strengths & appropriate coping mechanisms providing	Consult P.T./O.T. prn.	
CASE MANAGER:	Monitor for signs & symptoms of fluid electrolyte imbalance. Monitor temperature q 4'.	• nausea/vomiting, diarrhea, bone marrow suppression • renal/liver toxicity		support & MSW consult. Assist pt/family to use social network for support assistance in care.	Education regarding support available in the community.	Discuss pt risk reduction. Maintenance of home environment.
CONSULTING MD:	Assess pain level, characteristics Medicate as ordered.	• anorexia/rash		Discuss possible areas of conflict that may arise.	Teach pt about prescribed meds, indications for use, side effects.	Adequate nutritional intake.
SOCIAL SERVICE:	Monitor for s/sx of septicemia temp >101 or <98 WBC/bacteria in urine & blood cultures.	Assess nutritional status, height, wt, total protein/albumin.		When appropriate, encourage pt to document preferences regarding decision		Avoidance of people with infection.
ANOINTING OF THE SICK DATE:	Institute measures to prevent exposure to known sources of infection.	Consult dietary prn. Provide small, frequent high-calorie meals as tolerated/desired.		maker/advance directive. Continued nutritional support.		Prevention of injury. Management of activity/rest.
	Assess level of anxiety • provide opportunities to express feelings	Allow for adequate rest & assist with ADLs prn. Monitor tolerance to visitors/phones.		Lumbar Puncture • maintain activity as specified • hand carry all specimens to laboratory		Avoidance of high-risk behaviors (i.e., use of ETOH, tobacco, recreational drugs).
	• MSW consult prn	Assess psychological response to illness.				Teach reduction of risk factors for infection:
	Maintain immediate environment to allow for self-control	Bone Marrow Biopsy • monitor site for hematoma, bleeding • maintain activity as specified • hand carry all specimens to laboratory				• malnutrition • exposure to infectious sources or invasive procedures
						Avoidance of frequent venipuncture.

MULTIDISCIPLINARY PLAN UPDATE

SIGNATURES	DATE	SIGNATURES	DATE	SIGNATURES	DATE	SIGNATURES

CHAPTER 15

Cancer

■ ASSESSMENT

Cancer diagnosis is based on physical and psychosocial assessment, including laboratory data, radiologic studies, biopsies, and surgical procedures. Classifications of tumor, lymph node involvement, and metastasis are used to determine the stage of the malignant condition (Box 15-1 and Tables 15-1 and 15-2). The performance ability of the patient is evaluated and may be used to determine the type and length of treatment (Table 15-3)

▨ CURRENT CONDITION

General appearance
   Posture
   Body movements
   Hygiene
General survey of mental status
   Orientation
   Attention span
   Speech
Behavior/mannerisms
Chief complaint
Vital signs (VS)
Weight and height
Patient's concerns
Patient's problems or needs
Patient's knowledge of the following:
   Disease process
   Treatment
   Outcome

▨ PHYSICAL ASSESSMENT

Hematologic system
   Monitor complete blood cell count (CBC),
      hemoglobin (Hgb), platelet count
   Bleeding/hemorrhage
      Petechiae
      Unexplained bruises or ecchymoses
      Hematomas
      Bleeding from any body orifice
      Prolonged oozing of blood from intramuscular
        (IM) or intravenous (IV) sites
   Change in vital signs
   Change in neurologic status (headache,
      disorientation)
   Pad count high for menstruating females

Anemia
   Palpitations, chest pain on exertion
   Dyspnea
   Dizziness, syncope
   Fatigue, weakness
   Glossitis, anorexia, indigestion
   Insomnia, hypersensitivity to cold
Infection(s), present and past
   Temperature (T)
   White blood cell count (WBC), including
      differential
   Skin and mucous membrane integrity
      Skin folds (axillae, buttocks, perineum)
      Body cavities (mouth, vagina, rectum)
      Venous access sites
      Surgical wounds
   Respiratory tract
   Genitourinary system
   Eyes
      Conjunctivitis, iritis
      Infection of eyelid or lacrimal gland
Pain
   Type
      Acute
      Chronic
   Location, circumstances of onset
   Intensity, quality
   Activities that increase pain: eating, separation from
      significant other
   Effects on patient and family
   Relief measures
      Medication
      Distraction, meditation, relaxation, exercises
      Imagery; psychosocial and/or spiritual counseling
      Variables affecting response
         Anxiety/fear
         Ethnic/cultural background
         Past experiences with pain management
         Meaning of pain (recurrence of disease, death)
         Perceptions of pain therapy (fear of addictions)
Skin
   Color: pallor, duskiness, jaundice
   Integrity
      Breaks, lesions, ulcers
      Petechiae, bruises, erythema, ecchymosis

Box 15-1	**TNM Classifications***

PRIMARY TUMOR

T_X: Minimal requirements to assess the primary tumor cannot be met

T_0: No evidence of primary tumor

T_{IS}: Carcinoma in situ

T_1, T_2, T_3, T_4: Progressive increase in tumor size or involvement

N: Regional lymph nodes

  N_0: No evidence of regional nodal involvement

  N_1, N_2, N_3, N_4: Increasing degree of demonstrable abnormality of regional lymph nodes

M: Distant metastasis

  M_0: Indicates absence

  M_+: Indicates presence

HISTOPATHOLOGY

G_1: Well-differentiated grade

G_2: Moderately well-differentiated grade

G_3 and G_4: Poorly to very poorly differentiated grade

RESIDUAL TUMOR

R_0: No residual tumor

R_1: Microscopic residual tumor

R_2: Macroscopic residual tumor

STAGING METHOD

cTNM: Staging determined by clinical noninvasive physical examination, laboratory, and radiographic studies

sTNM: Staging information based on surgical procedures, biopsies, and histopathologic analysis

pTNM: Staging determined by correlation of clinical, pathologic, and residual tumor findings

*T, *Primary tumor;* N, *regional lymph nodes;* M, *metastasis by vascular dissemination.*

Table 15-1	**Cancer Staging Using TNM* Classifications**

Stage	T	N	M	Survival	Comments
I	1	0	0	70%-90%	Mass limited to organ of origin; nodes not involved; operable and resectable
II	2	1	0	50%±	Local spread to surrounding tissue; nodal involvement suspected or proved; operable but without certainty of total resection
III	3	2	0	20%±	Extensive primary tumor with fixation to deeper structures; nodes involved; operable but not resectable
IV	4	3	+	<5%	Distant metastases; inoperable

*T, *Primary tumor;* N, *regional lymph nodes;* M, *metastasis by vascular dissemination.*

Temperature
  Local and systemic
  Feeling of warmth and/or cold
Hydration: turgor, edema, perspiration
Hair: distribution, alopecia
Nails: color, texture, clubbing
Eyes, ears, nose, throat
Pupil size and response
Color
Sclera
Cataract formation
Nose: bleeding, drainage, crusting
Mouth, tongue, lips
  Color, moisture; presence of lesions on palate, tongue, buccal mucosa, inner surface of lips, and oral pharynx
  Color, amount, and consistency of saliva
  Condition of teeth
    Dental caries, rough edges
    Plaque, dental fit

  Mobility of tongue
  Ability to chew and taste
  Breath odor
Parotid gland: size, tenderness, pain
Lymph nodes
  Neck, axilla, groin
  Size, tenderness, pain
  Thyroid size
Gastrointestinal (GI) system
Appetite
Food and fluid intake
  Type, consistency, amount
  Frequency, preferences
Nausea, vomiting
  Frequency, character
  Color, amount
  Factors affecting occurrence
    Anticipation
    Activities, treatments, time of day
    Other associated factors
  Relief measures used; variables affecting response

Table 15-2	**Classification of Tumors**	
Tissue of Origin	**Benign**	**Malignant**
Epithelium: surface skin and mucous membranes	Papilloma Polyp	Squamous cell or epidermoid carcinoma Basal cell carcinoma
Glands	Adenoma Cystadenoma	Adenocarcinoma
Connective tissue		
Embryonic fibrous tissue	Myxoma	Myxosarcoma
Fibrous tissue	Fibroma	Fibrosarcoma
Cartilage	Chondroma	Chondrosarcoma
Bone	Osteoma	Osteosarcoma
Fat	Lipoma	Liposarcoma
Synovial membrane	Synovioma	Synovial sarcoma
Blood vessels	Hemangioma	Hemangiosarcoma
Lymph vessels	Lymphangioma	Lymphangiosarcoma
Muscle tissue		
Smooth muscle	Leiomyoma	Leiomyosarcoma
Striated muscle	Rhabdomyoma	Rhabdomyosarcoma
Hematopoietic tissue		
Lymphoid tissue		Malignant lymphoma Non–Hodgkin's lymphoma Lymphocytic leukemia
Granulocytic tissue		Myelocytic leukemia
Erythrocytic tissue		Erythroleukemia
Plasma cells		Multiple myeloma
Nerve cells		
Glial cells	Glioma	Glioblastoma (astrocytoma) Spongioblastoma
Meninges	Meningioma	Meningeal sarcoma
Nerve cells	Neuroma; ganglioneuroma	Neurogenic sarcoma
Neuroectoderm	Nevus	Neuroblastoma
Fibers	Neurofibroma	Neurofibrosarcoma
Retina		Retinoblastoma
Adrenal medulla	Pheochromocytoma	Pheochromocytoma
Nerve sheaths	Neurilemmoma	Neurilemmal sarcoma
Tumors of more than one tissue		
Breast	Fibroadenoma	Cystosarcoma phyllodes
Embryonic kidney		Nephroblastoma (Wilms')
Multipotent cells	Teratoma	
Uterus		Mixed mesodermal
Miscellaneous		
Melanoblasts	Pigmented nevus	Malignant melanoma Melanocarcinoma
Placenta	Hydatidiform mole	Choriocarcinoma (chorionepithelioma)
Ovary	Granulosa–theca cell tumor	Carcinoma
Testes	Interstitial cell tumor	Seminoma (spermatocytic) Carcinoma (embryonal)
Thymus	Thymoma	Thymoma

Table 15-3	**Host Performance Status***		
Status		**ECOG/Zubrod**	**Karnofsky (%)**
H0: Normal activity		0	90-100
H1: Symptomatic and ambulatory; cares for self		1	70-80
H2: Ambulatory more than 50% of time; occasionally needs assistance		2	50-60
H3: Ambulatory less than 50% of time; requires special nursing and/or medical assistance		3	30-40
H4: Bedridden; may need hospitalization		4	10-20

From American Joint Committee on Cancer, Manual for staging of cancer, ed 3, 1988.
*The host performance status is determined at the time of classification; the condition of the patient does not enter into determination of stage but may be a factor in deciding type and time of treatment. Host performance status may also be used as a predictive factor in survival evaluation of cancer patients.

 Gerontologic Considerations

- There are more cases of cancer among older adults than people of any other age-group.
- The incidence of cancer increases with aging, possibly as a result of decreased effectiveness of the immune system and changes in deoxyribonucleic acid (DNA).
- The types of cancers seen in older adults are prostate, lung, breast, and colorectal cancer. Cancers of the skin, urinary bladder, vagina, and vulva are seen primarily in older adults. Chronic lymphocytic leukemia and multiple myeloma are seen more frequently in older adults than in younger people.
- Many of the early signs and symptoms of cancer may be misdiagnosed as normal changes of aging. The importance of routine medical screening and self-examination should be stressed to the aging adult.
- Because of fear or past experience, older persons may adopt a fatalistic frame of mind after hearing the diagnosis of cancer. Use of the terms *tumor* or *growth* may be more acceptable.
- The type of treatment for cancer should be based on the individual's wishes and overall state of health. The patient, their family members, and significant others should be presented with all options so that informed decisions regarding treatment can be made.

Modified from Christensen BL, Kockrow EO: Foundations of nursing, *ed 3, St Louis, 1998, Mosby.*

Abdomen
   Distention
   Bowel sounds
      Present: type, frequency, character
      Absent
   Rigid, flaccid, tender
Spleen and liver: size, tenderness, pain
Stool
   Normal pattern: frequency (time of last stool), amount, color, consistency

Aids to normal elimination
   Dietary (food and fluid)
   Medications (laxatives)
   Enemas
Method of elimination: toilet, commode, bedpan
Artificial orifices: colostomy, ileostomy
Method of care for excretions from artificial orifices
Pain related to defecation
Presence of blood (on surface or mixed throughout)
Mucus, pus
Level of mobility/immobility
Stress
Diarrhea/constipation
   Frequency, amount
   Consistency, color
   Bleeding, occult bleeding
   Flatulence
   Associated factors
   Medications
   Relief measures, methods of coping

Genitourinary system
Urine, urination
   Usual pattern
   Frequency, amount
   Color, odor, specific gravity
   Presence of usual constituents
   Character, bleeding
   Any urgency felt
   Effort in starting and stopping
   Pain, burning, itching
   Nocturia
   Incontinence
   Retention
   Method of urine elimination (void, in-and-out catheter, Foley, urinary diversion)
   Care measures, methods of coping
Fluid intake
Medications (diuretics)
History of urinary tract infection (UTI)

Respiratory system

Respiratory rate: depth and character of breathing

Type of airway

Patency of airway

Breath sounds (normal, adventitious, increased, decreased)

Color of skin and mucous membranes

Chest size and shape

Chest excursion and symmetry

Position of trachea

Shortness of breath (SOB) on exertion

Use of accessory muscles

Nasal flaring, pursed-lip breathing, clubbing of extremities

Cough: ability, frequency, depth, force, productivity

Sputum: color, amount, odor, consistency, time of day produced

Audible grunting, snoring, stridor

Frequency of suctioning

Present level and tolerance of activity

History of the following:

Smoking, pulmonary infection, pulmonary diseases, exposure to air pollutants

Chemotherapy (bleomycin), radiation therapy to thorax

Laboratory tests: blood gas, sputum, blood cultures, WBC

Diagnostic studies: chest x-ray examination, pulmonary function tests

Cardiovascular system

Heart rate (HR), blood pressure (BP)

Heart sounds

Peripheral pulses: rate, rhythm, volume

Skin color, dryness/moistness

Decreased cardiac output

Tachycardia

Electrocardiogram (ECG) changes

Dyspnea on exertion, exercise intolerance

Rales, wheezing, cough

Edema: location, type

Neurologic system

Sensorium (awake, alert, lethargic, stuporous, comatose)

Orientation to time, person, place, and situation

Ability to follow commands

Memory (recent, remote)

Attentiveness, distractibility

Language spoken, clarity, appropriateness

Ability to read and write

Motor response

Voluntary, involuntary

Gait, balance, paralysis, weakness

Reflex response: pupil, gag, cough, Babinski sign, deep tendon reflex

Tics, trembling, seizures

Pain

Rate pain using pain scale

Location, onset, duration, type

Precipitating factors, relief measures

Sensations: tingling, numbness, leg cramps

Foot drop, wrist drop, hand grip

Sensory

Visual

Auditory

Olfactory

Taste

Tactile

Safety measures used

PERTINENT BACKGROUND INFORMATION

Sleep/rest

Usual pattern; hours of sleep at night

Difficulties

Number and duration of daily naps

Use of sleep aids: name, dosage of drug, frequency of use, length of time used

Symptoms that may affect sleep: pain, anxiety, night sweats

Signs and symptoms of sleep disturbance: irritability, anxiety, loss of train of thought

Care measures

Sexuality

Sexual history

Current practices, reproductive history

Impact of therapies on sexuality/sexual function; reaction of partner to illness

Expressions of affection

Methods of coping

Social

Support system; most significant other

Role function

Housing/living arrangement

Presence of dependent, independent behaviors

Spirituality: beliefs, faith, concerns

Activities of daily living (ADLs)

Lifestyle (active, sedentary); exercise tolerance

Degree of immobility

Household assistance

Employment, leisure/hobbies

Other activities and concerns

Home environment

Caregiver, facilities, and equipment available for meeting care needs

Pets

Concerns

Teaching needs

During hospitalization

Self-care

Previous conditions

Acute or chronic diseases or conditions

Surgery

Radiation therapy

Chemotherapy

Biologic response modifiers

Trauma

Physical

Emotional

PSYCHOSOCIAL ASSESSMENT

PREDIAGNOSTIC PERIOD (DETERMINATION OF FEELINGS AND PRIOR KNOWLEDGE)

Awareness of signs and symptoms; length of time known

Delay in seeking treatment; threats to the following:
  Independence
  Group belongingness
  Influence on others
  Adaptive functioning
  Preexisting stability
  Decision-making ability
  Cherished values
  Desired roles
  Limitless future
  Control over destiny

Information about treatment
  Knowledge deficits
  Level of understanding
  Misconceptions and myths
  Ethnic/cultural beliefs

Knowledge of resources

DIAGNOSTIC PERIOD

Fears of outcome

Perceptions of threat

Significance of studies

Information about cancer and body functions
  Factual
  Deficits
  Misconceptions
    Myths
    Fantasies

Knowledge and level of understanding
  Diagnostic tests and examinations
  Schedule of tests and examinations
  Reasons for studies and preparation
  Role of patient in studies
  Physical effect of studies; expected symptoms and responses

Continuously validate patient's understanding and perceptions

Coping methods of patient, significant other, or family
  Daily activities
  Use of work and leisure activities
  Relationships
  Methods of communication
    Ability to disclose: open with family, peers, counselors, and/or medical and nursing staff
    Inability to communicate; awareness of significance

Behavioral responses
  Anxiety
    Apprehensive expectation
    Fear and worry about negative outcome
  Vigilance and scanning
    Hyperattentiveness
    Distractibility
    Concentration problems

    Impatience
    Feeling "on edge"
  Motor tension
    Jumpiness
    Restlessness
    Inability to relax
    Insomnia
    Strained facies
    Easily startled
  Autonomic hyperactivity
    Tachycardia
    Tachypnea
    Dry mouth
    Sweating
    Cold, clammy hands
    Upset stomach
    Nightmares

CONFIRMATION OF DIAGNOSIS

Knowledge of results and meaning of diagnostic studies
  X-ray examinations
  Imaging
    Computed tomography (CT) scans
    Magnetic resonance imaging (MRI)
    Positron emission tomography (PET) scan
    Ultrasound examinations
  Isotope studies
  Endoscopy
  Cytology
  Laboratory data
  Biopsy

Meaning of illness
  Perceived threat to the following:
    Independence
    Job and economic security
    Career goals
    Relationships
    Integrity of body
    Body functions
    Recreational activities
    Sexual attractiveness and functioning
    Intimacy
  Fears of disfigurement and pain
  Secondary gains: alteration in behavior
    Acting out
    Demands for attention
    Controlling behaviors
  Methods for handling past crises

Availability of knowledgeable and supportive resources
  Family
  Significant others
  Co-workers
  Social contacts
  Religious counsel
  Community

Behavioral responses
  Shock/denial
    Rejection of reality
    Increased perspiration

Pallor
Faintness
Nausea
Anorexia
Insomnia
Confusion
Difficulty in concentrating
Difficulty in working
Anger
   Impatience
   Bitterness
   Jealousy
   Helplessness
   Increased awareness
   Limited attention span
   Uncooperative behavior
   Attention-seeking behavior
   Loud talking
   Vulgar language
   Multiple complaints
Guilt/punishment
   Underlying reasons
   Misconceptions about cancer: seen as unclean,
      contagious
   Diagnosis attributed to something person did or did
      not do
Hopelessness (p. 58)
   Quiet
   Withdrawn
   Melancholy
   Older appearance
   Poor posture
   Gait: slow, dragging
   Decreased respiration
Bargaining
   Depression
   Exhaustion
   Attempts to avoid reality
   Self-questioning
   SOB
   Feelings of weakness
Panic attack
   Dyspnea
   Palpitations
   Chest pain
   Feelings of choking or smothering
   Dizziness
   Feelings of unreality
   Tingling of hands and/or feet
   Hot and cold flashes
   Sweating
   Faintness
   Trembling or shaking
   Fear of dying, "going crazy," or doing something
      uncontrollable during an attack
Be aware of importance of need to initiate appropriate
   interventions rapidly when the following are observed:
   Agitation
   Uncharacteristic, unexplained, extreme behavior

Unrealistic perceptions and expectations
Feelings of the following:
   Worthlessness
   Extreme guilt
   Suicide
Inappropriate resistance to treatment
Use of controversial treatments (e.g., laetrile,
   megavitamins, mechanical devices, miracle drugs,
   psychic surgeons, Hoxsey and Krebiozen potions)
Acceptance
   Contemplativeness
   Serenity
   Talks about condition

TREATMENT PHASE
Adequate information for informed decision making
   Options for the following:
      Types of surgery
      Radiotherapy
      Chemotherapy
      Biologic response modifiers
      Palliative care
   Risks, benefits, and complications for each type of
      treatment
   Results of current research: unpredictable outcome
   Prognosis associated with each therapy
Level of understanding of chosen therapy
   Preparation
   Associated physical changes
   Complications
   Local and systemic effects
Reactions to treatment
   Follows directions
   Alterations in ADLs
Expresses needs for the following:
   Hope associated with cure
      Future pleasurable experiences
      Ability to reach some goals
      Others being available for support
      Idea that life has meaning
   Honesty
      Answers questions
      No protection from the truth
      Not withholding information
   Information about the following:
      Treatment; side or toxic effects
      Special procedures or treatments
      Changes in expected outcomes
      Expected patient participation
      Availability and support of resources
      Whether patient can share what he or she has
         learned about care
Expresses feelings or conveys
   Anger
   Fear
   Sadness
   Helplessness
   Dependency
   Powerlessness

PREPARATION FOR DISCHARGE

Knowledge of continuing care
Methods for dealing with pain
  Increase or decrease in functioning
  Complications of treatment as disease progresses
  Special procedures
  Psychologic needs
Daily activity allowances
Signs and symptoms of recurrence or progression
Need for follow-up care
Support groups and counselors: specific information and contact person (e.g., wellness community)
Emergency care instructions

RECURRENCE

Expresses fears of the following:
  Increased dependency
  Increased weakness
  Increased immobility
  Isolation
  Disintegration of relationships
Communicates need for the following:
  Being told death is close
  Information about practical things to do before death
  Discussing pain, pain relief measures, and fear of loss of control
  Discussion of beliefs
Ability to continue treatment

ADVANCED OR TERMINAL CONDITION

Knowledge of present diagnosis and prognosis
Symptom-control methods; patient and family participation
Responsibilities
  Relationships
  Completion of unfinished business
Ability to discuss fears of the following:
  Inability to continue with life's activities and relationships
  Being abandoned
Hospice: alternative methods of care
Meaning of death
  Shameful
  Peaceful
Disengagement
  Life's business finished
  Good-byes said
  Psychologic withdrawal
  Few interactions

■ ACUTE LEUKEMIA

Uncontrolled proliferation of leukocytes and their precursors in the bone marrow with infiltration of lymph nodes, spleen, liver, and other body organs

acute lymphocytic (lymphoblastic) leukemia (ALL): *Lymphoblasts proliferate in bone marrow and lymph nodes and invade other tissues; primarily a disease of childhood*

acute myelocytic (myelogenous) leukemia (AML): *Proliferation of myeloblast (immature polymorphonuclear leukocytes); occurs in all age groups but is more common in adults age 60 years and older; also called acute granulocytic leukemia (AGL), acute nonlymphocytic leukemia (ANLL) and myeloid leukemia*

ASSESSMENT

SUBJECTIVE DATA

Easily fatigued
Malaise
Irritability
Headache
Abdominal discomfort, nausea
Dysphagia
Anorexia
Palpitations
SOB
Bone/joint pain

OBJECTIVE DATA

Elevated temperature
Syncope
Pallor
Petechiae
Easy bruising, ecchymosis
Purpura
Gingival hypertrophy, bleeding, periodontal infections
Oropharyngeal lesions, stomatitis
Epistaxis
Upper respiratory tract infection (URI)
UTI, uric acid nephropathy
Wound infection: may appear dark red or dark without pus
Esophagitis
Weight loss
Perirectal abscess
Hepatosplenomegaly
Hypotension
Tachycardia
Cough
Mediastinal mass with tenderness
Enlarged lymph nodes

MEDICAL HISTORY

Exposure to ionizing radiation
  Work environment
  Prenatal
  Treatment of preexisting cancer
Genetic factors
  Bloom's syndrome
  Trisomy 21 (Down syndrome; 15 to 20 times the risk)
  Trisomy G (Klinefelter's syndrome)
  Fanconi syndrome
  Philadelphia chromosome present
  Ataxia telangiectasis
  Family history of hematologic disorder
Chemical exposure
  Benzene

Phenylbutazone
Arsenic
Medications
    Chloramphenicol
    Alkylating chemotherapeutic agents
Immunodeficiency
Viral exposure

DIAGNOSTIC TESTS
WBC
  Low or elevated, with "left shift"
  Excessively elevated (T cell ALL)
  Blasts
  Lymphocytes (ALL)
  Auer rods (AML)
  Phi bodies (AML)
Reticulocytopenia
  Normochromic (AML)
  Normocytic
CBC: anemia
Platelet count: thrombocytopenia
Chemistries
  Serum uric acid: elevated
  Serum copper: elevated
  Serum zinc: decreased
Urine uric acid: elevated
Hypergammaglobulinemia (AML)
Bone marrow: proliferation of blast cells, karyotypic analysis

POTENTIAL COMPLICATIONS
Acute infection
Severe anemia
Hemorrhage
Organ failure

MULTIDISCIPLINARY MANAGEMENT
PREVENTION/DETECTION TEACHING
Teach importance of limiting exposure time to radiation sources, especially in young children; use proper shields and positioning during necessary x-ray examinations
Explain importance of limiting exposure to toxic chemicals; use proper protective devices during unavoidable exposure
Discuss importance of regular, periodic physical examinations: palpation of lymph nodes, inspection of skin and mucous membranes, palpation of bones and joints, screening laboratory testing
Explain importance of reporting suspect signs and symptoms to physician

THERAPEUTIC MANAGEMENT
Chemotherapy *to induce remission* (see Table 15-8, p. 864)
Maintenance chemotherapy
Fluid, parenteral nutritional support
Antibiotics

Total body irradiation (TBI) (see Transplant preparation, p. 770)
Transfusion of blood components
Bone marrow transplant (see p. 768)
Pain management, patient-controlled analgesia (PCA)
Hypnotics
Social services, support group

PATIENT PROBLEMS—NURSING DIAGNOSES/INTERVENTIONS

▼ Risk for infection related to suppressed immune system

Screen personnel and visitors for symptoms of infection
Use strict sterile technique for all invasive procedures
Monitor sites of invasive lines, tubes, drains for signs of infection q8h
Check body fluids for alteration in color, odor, consistency
Ensure excellent personal hygiene is maintained, especially after bowel movements
Provide uninterrupted periods of sleep and rest
Begin stress management counseling
Avoid chilling; provide socks, extra blankets; keep bed and clothing dry
Ensure required fluid, nutrient intake; supplement with total oral nutrition products prn, institute calorie count prn *to ensure optimum metabolic state to avoid infection*
Record intake and output
Monitor vital signs, especially temperature, q4h and prn
Monitor CBC, WBC results per physician order
Administer antibiotics, sulfa-type medications, and other antiinfectives as ordered
Maintain skin integrity *to prevent entry of microorganisms*
Auscultate breath sounds q8h
Encourage clearance of pulmonary secretions: turn, cough, deep breathe q2h; perform chest percussion and drainage as needed; encourage use of incentive spirometer qh
Maintain intact mucous membranes; perform scrupulous oral care using soft instruments q4h and prn
Provide high-calorie, high-protein, high–vitamin C and E diet

Expected Outcomes
Exhibits improvement, resolution of current infections
New infections are not developed
Patient/significant other verbalizes knowledge of infection prevention

▼ Altered nutrition: less than body requirements related to reduced food intake, malabsorption, anorexia, vomiting, diarrhea, stomatitis

Assess nutritional status daily: weight, electrolytes, total protein, serum albumin, Hgb, skin turgor, muscle mass

Determine amount and types of foods patient likes and is
able to tolerate

Provide oral hygiene before and after meals

Administer anesthetics to oral mucosa before meals prn

Offer high-calorie, high-protein diet with variation in
taste, texture, and presentation of foods

In collaboration with physician, provide oral and
parenteral nutritional supplements

Serve frequent, light meals and nutritional, high-calorie
snacks

Assist patient to eat if fatigue is a factor

Present meals in an attractive, pleasing manner

Provide a pleasant atmosphere *to increase desire to eat:*
encourage significant others to join patient for meals,
remove bedpans/urinals from area, maintain
well-ventilated room, serve food as soon as it arrives,
remove tray as soon as patient finishes eating

In collaboration with clinical dietitian: calculate number
of calories and nutrients needed *to maintain/gain
weight and support metabolic needs*

Maintain calorie count

Encourage family to bring patient's favorite foods from home

In collaboration with physician, administer antiemetics
before meals prn

Expected Outcome
Weight is maintained within 10% of baseline

▼Chronic pain related to involvement of multiple
organ systems

Assess nature, intensity, location, duration, and
precipitating and alleviating factors

Use consistent pain rating scale *to assess level of pain*

Assess nonverbal signs of pain

Obtain information from patient regarding past pain
experiences and methods used for relief

Control environmental factors that may increase
perception of pain: temperature, noise, lighting

Assist patient to achieve comfortable positions *to
minimize pain*

Assist patient to achieve state of minimal physical tension
through techniques such as relaxation, music,
visualization, diversion

Provide a restful environment with opportunities to rest
during the day and uninterrupted periods of sleep at
night *to diminish perception of pain caused by
fatigue*

In collaboration with physician, provide analgesic
medications as required, observing for therapeutic and
side effects

Discuss noninvasive pain relief measures: relaxation,
cutaneous stimulation, distraction, hot/cold therapy

Reduce/eliminate factors that precipitate or increase the
pain experience

Expected Outcomes
Verbalizes decrease in or relief of pain
Incorporates existing pain while participating in daily
activities

▼Fatigue related to chronic disease process

Assess causative/contributing factors; identify activities
that are difficult for patient

Coordinate activities to *provide for undisturbed periods
of rest and sleep*

Perform active/passive ROM exercises qid; collaborate
with physical therapy *to determine most therapeutic
exercises*

Determine whether patient becomes posturally
hypotensive; change positions gradually; monitor for
hypotension and tachycardia

Gauge amount and intensity of activity tolerated by
monitoring patient's subjective complaints of fatigue,
as well as changes in vital signs

Assist patient to identify strengths, abilities, interests;
assist in development of realistic goals to progress
from simple to complex

Encourage patient to participate in own care to
tolerance; assist as needed *to avoid exhaustion;* assist
to identify energy patterns and schedule activities
appropriately

Teach energy conservation techniques, use of assistive
devices *to minimize fatigue*

Monitor nutritional intake to ensure adequate energy
resources

Monitor sleep/rest patterns

Limit environmental stimuli

Place patient on fall-prevention protocol

Collaborate with physical therapist to design measures *to
maintain activity and independence*

Administer filtered, leukocyte-poor red blood cells (RBCs)
when ordered

Expected Outcomes
Participates in own care to tolerance
Ability to be active increases
States feeling of increased energy

▼Potential for bleeding related to thrombocytopenia*

Monitor vital signs q4h and prn; assess for tachycardia
and hypotension; avoid rectal temperature

Determine neurologic status q8h to 12h, assess for
changing level of consciousness (LOC), changing
affect, confusion

Assess skin and mucous membranes q8h for increased
bruising, bleeding

Observe all urine and stool for gross bleeding; check
for occult blood every shift

Maintain integrity of central line; use Leur-Lok
connections on all IV tubing

Monitor laboratory results: assess for trends in CBC,
platelet count, coagulation studies

Use pull sheet to turn patient *to prevent shearing of
tissues and skin trauma*

Not a NANDA-approved diagnosis.

Use pillows for support of pressure points; avoid excess pressure

Avoid restrictive clothing and bed linen; use bed cradle

Use dental care products appropriate for condition of oral cavity

Use electric razor *to prevent razor cuts*

Avoid vigorous nose blowing

Prevent trauma to decrease risk of bleeding

Avoid invasive procedures (IM, subcutaneous injections) when possible

Use smallest-gauge needles possible

Apply manual pressure for 5 to 10 uninterrupted minutes after any skin puncture *to prevent bruising or hematoma formation*

Provide safe environment: lighting, placement of furniture, well-fitting slippers *to prevent falls*

Prevent constipation; administer stool softeners per physician order

Avoid vomiting; administer antiemetics per physician order

Administer blood components per physician order: platelets are usually ordered at fast rate of infusion and immediately before any invasive procedure for maximal therapeutic effectiveness

Administer vasopressors and corticosteroids per physician order

Expected Outcome

Reduction of stimuli that may induce bleeding

No signs or symptoms of active bleeding occur

▼Anticipatory grieving related to lifestyle changes, decreased physical abilities, changes in physical appearance, life-threatening prognosis

Be sensitive to changes patient is experiencing; encourage patient to express feelings, frustrations, anger, hopes

Provide a therapeutic environment conducive to open discussion: actively listen, tune in to nonverbal cues, be patient and empathetic

Encourage questions and provide information freely as patient expresses the desire for knowledge about the disease, treatments, and prognosis

Set limits on maladaptive coping behaviors if they interfere with patient's well-being

Support adaptive behaviors that suggest progression and resolution of the grieving process

Rehearse techniques needed to cope with upcoming event or crisis

Provide opportunities for private, uninterrupted time with significant others

Assist in identifying ways to adapt lifestyle as condition changes

Provide information regarding support groups for patient and significant others

Collaborate with other professionals (social worker, clergy, psychologist, psychiatrist) *to provide support and facilitate grieving process*

Provide reference for financial assistance, answers to questions regarding medical insurance

Provide information to assist patient in completing advanced directives or similar document to ensure patient wishes are known to significant others and care providers

Expected Outcomes

Progresses through stages of the grieving process and moves toward acceptance

Demonstrates effective coping mechanisms; participates in decisions about own future

PATIENT/FAMILY TEACHING
POSTDIAGNOSIS

Disease process

Provide information about disease and treatment

Discuss symptoms of recurrence or progression of disease to report to physician

Demonstrate how to examine skin and mucous membranes

Emphasize importance of maintaining follow-up appointments for treatment and examinations

Complications

Demonstrate how to check for occult blood in urine and stool

Discuss accident/injury prevention

Avoid restrictive clothing and bed linen

Maintain clutter-free environment

Use assistive devices for ambulation and ADLs as required by condition

Assist patient to select dental hygiene devices and techniques of oral hygiene appropriate for condition of oral mucous membranes and gums

Avoid sports and activities that may result in accidental injury

Handle equipment and sharp objects with care

Discuss prevention of constipation, diet, medications

Infection

Discuss signs and symptoms of infection to report to physician: elevated temperature, sore throat, flulike symptoms, coughing, burning on urination, infected cuts, lesions that do not heal quickly

Discuss infection-prevention measures: maintain clean environment, avoid handling pets and their equipment, avoid persons with infections and large crowds, practice handwashing techniques (all members of household), routine personal hygiene including perianal care after each elimination

Activity

Discuss importance of maintaining balance between activity and rest

Assist to identify activities that can be performed by family/friends

Discuss use of assistive devices as necessary

Discuss importance of assuming activity to tolerance, avoiding fatigue

Assist to identify realistic activity goals

Nutrition
Consult with clinical dietitian to develop a meal plan, containing necessary calories and fluids, which is consistent with patient's physical condition and considers patient's preferences
Demonstrate administration and management of parenteral nutrition
Anxiety/fear
Explain importance of maintaining open communication with significant others
Teach recognition of early symptoms of depression, maladaptive anxiety/fear
Discuss problem-solving and coping techniques that patient is comfortable practicing
Discuss sources of psychologic, financial, spiritual assistance
Medications
Discuss administration, expected therapeutic effects, side effects, and potential adverse reactions of prescribed medication; prepare written instructions
Discuss side/adverse effects that must be reported to physician
Demonstrate use of IV therapy equipment: infusion pump, tubing and connections, storage and handling of medication bags
Need to avoid over-the-counter medications without consulting physician

DISCHARGE/HOME CARE PLANNING
Assess ability of patient to provide for physical care needs and ADLs; arrange home care providers as necessary
Evaluate ability of patient to administer own parenteral nutrition and medications; teach significant other(s) to assist or provide care; arrange for home health nurse as needed
Provide sufficient, clean space and refrigeration for storage of supplies and medications
Assess availability of transportation to follow-up appointments; assist with arrangements as needed
Arrange for durable medical equipment: assistive devices, hospital bed, raised commode, IV infusion pump as needed
Assist patient to contact community groups for ongoing psychologic/emotional support

■ CANCER OF THE BONE (OSTEOSARCOMA)
Rapidly growing malignant bone tumor of unknown etiology occurring most often in the long bones of young people; 50% arising from around the knees; secondary malignant tumors of the bone metastasize from other primary sites

ASSESSMENT
SUBJECTIVE DATA
Pain over affected area of extremity, especially at night
Anorexia
Fatigue

OBJECTIVE DATA
Limited use of extremity
Weight loss
Localized swelling with or without trauma
Increased skin temperature over affected area
Elevated temperature
Fracture
Spinal cord compression

RISK FACTORS
May coincide with adolescent growth spurt
Radiation exposure
Survivors of cancer treatment
Heredity

DIAGNOSTIC TESTS
Serum calcium: decreased
Urine calcium: increased
Alkaline, acid phosphatase: elevated
Imaging/nuclear medicine studies
Radiographs of affected bones
Bone scan
Bone biopsy
CT scan, MRI
PET scan

MULTIDISCIPLINARY MANAGEMENT
THERAPEUTIC MANAGEMENT
Antineoplastic agents, systemic chemotherapy
Radiation therapy
Pain management
Surgical intervention and endoprosthesis
Potential complications
Respiratory metastasis
Pathologic fractures
Infection at surgical site
Physical therapy consultation
Bone allograft
Social services; support group

PATIENT PROBLEMS—NURSING DIAGNOSES/INTERVENTIONS

▼Pain related to progression of disease process

Assess location, intensity of pain using consistent pain rating scale
Use firm mattress, bedboard, footboard as appropriate
Maintain proper alignment of extremities
Extend extremities as tolerated
Avoid external rotation of joints; use supports as necessary
Avoid neck flexion; use thin pillow
Apply splints, braces, traction to immobilize/support per physician order
Avoid jarring, jerky movements *to prevent potentiation of pain*
Handle affected limbs gently, providing support above and below joint

Administer skin care

Administer analgesic, antiinflammatory medications per physician order

Observe response to medications in terms of pain relief and adverse reactions

Discuss alternative methods of pain relief

Expected Outcomes

States pain level is tolerable

Incorporates existing pain into lifestyle and self-care activities

▼Impaired physical mobility, related to swelling, pain in affected limb, fracture, immobilization device

Provide for bed rest with limb properly aligned, using assistive devices as needed: splint, sand bags, pillows

Physical therapy consultation to assess activity tolerance, need for assistive devices

Use sheepskin, pressure-reducing mattress, elbow and heel guards *to prevent pressure ulcers caused by impaired mobility*

Encourage activity, self-care to tolerance using assistive devices as required

Expected Outcomes

Participates in activities to tolerance

Demonstrates ability to correctly use assistive devices

▼Anticipatory grieving related to lifestyle changes, decreased physical abilities, changes in physical appearance, life-threatening prognosis

Be sensitive to changes patient is experiencing; encourage patient to express feelings, frustrations, anger, hopes

Provide a therapeutic environment conducive to open discussion: actively listen, perceive nonverbal cues, be patient and empathetic *to support grief process*

Encourage questions and provide information freely as patient expresses the desire for knowledge about the disease, treatments, and prognosis

Set limits on maladaptive coping behaviors if they interfere with patient's well-being

Support adaptive behaviors that suggest progression and resolution of the grieving process

Rehearse techniques needed to cope with upcoming event or crisis

Provide opportunities for private, uninterrupted time with significant others

Assist in identifying ways to adapt lifestyle as condition changes

Provide information regarding support groups for patient and significant others *to deal with grief*

Collaborate with other professionals (social worker, clergy, psychologist, psychiatrist) *to provide support and facilitate grieving process*

Provide reference for financial assistance, answers to questions regarding medical insurance

Provide information to assist patient in completing advance directives or similar document *to ensure patient wishes are known to significant others and care providers*

Expected Outcomes

Progresses through stages of the grieving process and moves toward acceptance

Demonstrates effective coping mechanisms; participates in decisions about own future

Additional Nursing Diagnosis to Consider

Altered nutrition: less than body requirements related to anorexia, fatigue

PATIENT/FAMILY TEACHING

Reinforce physician explanations related to treatment plan, surgical intervention, rehabilitation

Explain chemotherapy/radiation therapy regimen: expected therapeutic effects, side effects, and potential adverse reactions

Explain management of side and adverse effects

Provide information regarding signs and symptoms to report to physician

Discuss importance of following therapy schedule as instructed by physical therapist

Explain importance of taking medication as prescribed

Advise on importance of keeping follow-up appointments with care providers

DISCHARGE/HOME CARE PLANNING

Evaluate availability of assistance and ability to provide physical care and home care; arrange home health provider as needed

Assess physical layout: stairs, distance between rooms, arrangement of furniture that may be hazardous; access ability for wheelchair if required

Exhibits ability to provide for durable medical equipment and assistive devices as needed; arranges for provider as needed

■ CANCER OF THE BREAST/ SURGICAL INTERVENTION

Breast cancer is the leading cancer and the second cause of cancer deaths among women in the United States; the most common form is invasive ductal; the incidence of breast cancer increases with increasing age; surgical intervention may include removal of the entire breast, axillary lymph nodes, and all fat, fascia, and adjacent tissues (modified radical mastectomy); excision and removal of tumor (lumpectomy); excision of tumor and wide margin of healthy tissue (partial mastectomy); removal of one quarter of the breast (quadrantectomy)

ASSESSMENT
SUBJECTIVE DATA

Postoperative pain

Bone pain caused by metastasis

OBJECTIVE DATA

Detection

    Palpable lump: usually painless, upper outer
        quadrant

    Nipple discharge, retraction

    Dimpling of skin

    Edema (peau d'orange)

    Erythema

    Change in contour of breast

    Axillary adenopathy

    Metastasis: pleural effusions

Postoperative

    Incision site; skin graft site; nipple graft site: redness,
        edema, drainage

    Wound drains

RISK FACTORS

Female: 99% incidence

Age: more than 40 years of age, increased incidence

Upper socioeconomic status: increased incidence

Nulliparous or first parity after age 30 to 35 years

Family history of breast cancer: mother, sister, maternal
    aunt, grandmother

Positive genetic pattern

Personal history of breast cancer, other cancers

Adverse hormonal milieu

    Early menarche

    Late menopause

    Thyroid disorders

    Diabetes

Lowered immunologic competence

    Thymic atrophy

    Decreased thymus-dependent (T) lymphocytes

    Exposure to excessive radiation

    Use of chemotherapy

    Use of immunosuppressives

Obesity, high intake of fat

Chronic psychologic stress

Physical inactivity

DIAGNOSTIC TESTS

Surgical biopsy

    Estrogen, progestin receptors

    CA 15-3

    Sentinal node examination

    S-phase index

    Ploidy

Image-directed needle biopsy

Imaging/nuclear medicine studies: mammography, biopsy,
    guided wire biopsy

POTENTIAL COMPLICATIONS: POSTOPERATIVE

Infection

Hemorrhage, shock

Pneumonia

Brachial plexus damage: contracture, shortening of
    muscles

Metastatic disease; bone, lung, liver, skin, brain

MULTIDISCIPLINARY MANAGEMENT
PREVENTION/DETECTION TEACHING

Emphasize that prognosis for most breast cancers is more
    favorable when cancer is detected early

Discuss importance of monthly breast self-examinations
    (most women discover own disease)

Premenopausal: perform 1 week after menses begin

Postmenopausal: same time each month (for ease of
    remembrance)

Techniques for self-examination

    Visually examine breasts in front of mirror (Fig. 15-1)
        (examine with arms at side, arms above and behind
        head, palms of hands on hips); notice differences in
        size, shape, anything unusual

    While standing: raise one arm over head and examine
        opposite breast, repeating for other breast; repeat
        examination while lying on back with pillow under
        same shoulder as arm over head, repeating for other
        breast

Methods of examination (all equally effective)

    Wedge method (Fig. 15-2): using flat surface of three
        middle fingers, press gently in straight line from
        outer edges toward nipple; repeat in parallel lines
        around breast until all tissue is examined; squeeze
        nipple

    Circular method (Fig. 15-3): using flat surface of three
        middle fingers, press gently in small circular
        motions around the breast, working from outer to
        inner aspect of breast until all tissue is examined;
        squeeze nipple

    Vertical strip method (Fig. 15-4): using flat surface of
        three middle fingers, press gently from top outer
        edge down to the bottom, continuing up and down
        until you reach the inner aspect of the breast and
        have examined all tissue; squeeze nipple

Discuss importance of breast examination by professional
    caregiver: every 3 years for women less than 40 years
    of age, every year for women more than 40 years of age

Explain importance of routine mammography: baseline at
    age 35 to 40 years; every 1 to 2 years for women age
    40 to 49; every year for women more than 49 years of
    age; earlier/more frequent mammography for women
    with positive family/personal history

Discuss importance of low-fat, high-fiber diet to reduce
    endogenous estrogen

Explain need for weight control, reduction

THERAPEUTIC MANAGEMENT

Surgical intervention: breast conserving, mastectomy

Postoperative physical therapy

Breast reconstruction; prosthesis

Social services, support group

Chemotherapy

Radiation therapy: brachytherapy, teletherapy

Estrogen, androgen, progestin therapy

Reach to recovery program

Hormonal therapy

Peripheral stem cell transplant (bone marrow transplant
    [BMT])

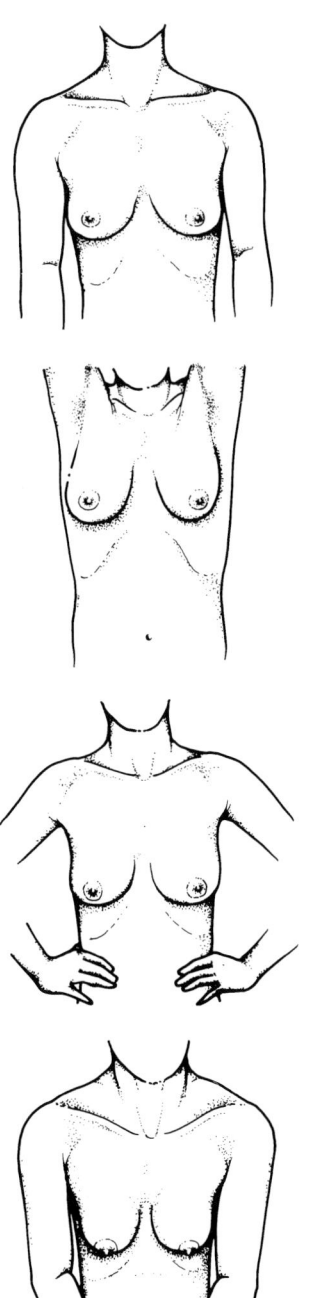

Fig. 15-1 Breast self-examination. Visual inspection.

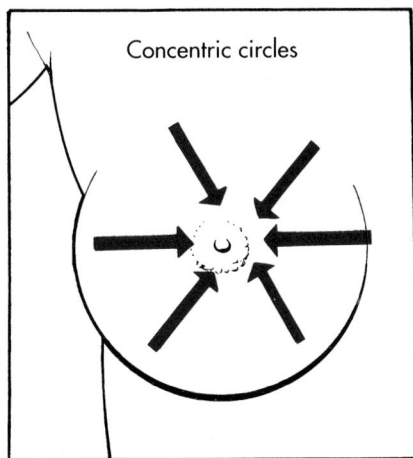

Fig. 15-2 Wedge section.
(From Belcher AE: Mosby's clinical nursing series: cancer nursing, *St Louis, 1992, Mosby.)*

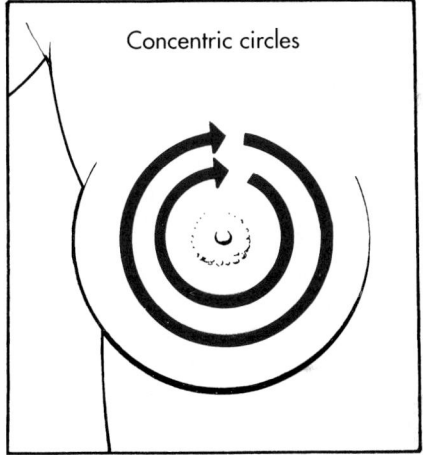

Fig. 15-3 Concentric circles.
(From Belcher AE: Mosby's clinical nursing series: cancer nursing, *St Louis, 1992, Mosby.)*

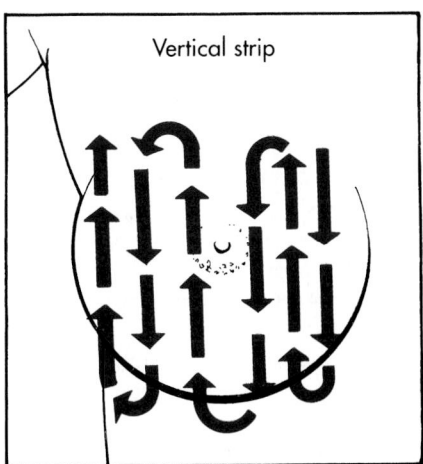

Fig. 15-4 Vertical strip.
(From Belcher AE: Mosby's clinical nursing series: cancer nursing, *St Louis, 1992, Mosby.)*

PATIENT PROBLEMS—NURSING DIAGNOSES/INTERVENTIONS
See perioperative care

▼ Anticipatory grieving, related to lifestyle changes, decreased physical abilities, changes in physical appearance, life-threatening prognosis

Be sensitive to changes patient is experiencing; encourage patient to express feelings, frustrations, anger, hopes

Provide a therapeutic environment conducive to open discussion: actively listen, perceive nonverbal cues, be patient and empathetic

Encourage questions and provide information freely as patient expresses the desire for knowledge about the disease, treatments, and prognosis

Set limits on maladaptive coping behaviors if they interfere with patient's well-being

Decision making should involve the patient to the extent desired by the patient

Support adaptive behaviors that suggest progression and resolution of the grieving process

Provide opportunities for private, uninterrupted time with significant other(s)

Assist in identifying ways to adapt lifestyle as condition changes

Provide information regarding support groups for patient and significant others *to deal with grief*

Collaborate with other professionals (social worker, clergy, psychologist, psychiatrist) to provide support and facilitate grieving process

Provide reference for financial assistance, answers to questions regarding medical insurance

Provide information to assist patient in completing advance directive or similar document to ensure patient wishes are known to significant others and care providers

Expected Outcomes

Progresses through stages of the grieving process and moves toward acceptance

Demonstrates effective coping mechanisms; participates in decisions about own future

▼Risk for infection, related to surgical procedure, depressed immune system from radiation therapy, chemotherapy

During nadir of chemotherapy, limit visitors and crowd exposure *to decrease chances of infection*

Use strict sterile technique for all invasive procedures

Monitor venous access device for signs of infection

Check body fluids for alteration in color, odor, consistency

Ensure excellent personal hygiene is maintained, especially after bowel movements

Provide uninterrupted periods of sleep and rest *to increase resistance to infection*

Ensure required fluid/nutrient intake; supplement with total oral nutrition products prn; institute calorie count prn

Monitor vital signs, especially temperature, q4h and prn *to assess for fever*

Monitor CBC, WBC results per physician order

Administer antibiotics, sulfa-type medications, and other antiinfectives as ordered

Maintain skin integrity *to prevent entry of microorganisms*

Auscultate breath sounds q8h *to assess for signs of pulmonary congestion/infection*

Encourage clearance of pulmonary secretions: turn, cough, deep breathe q2h; encourage use of incentive spirometer qh

Provide high-carbohydrate, high-protein, low-fat diet *to prevent increased body fat and weight*

Maintain weight within 10% of baseline

Expected Outcomes

Exhibits no signs of infection

▼Potential for lymphedema of affected arm and hand*

Avoid administering parenteral fluids, drawing blood from affected arm

Alternate lying on back and unaffected side

Take BP on unaffected arm only

Check color, sensation, motion in fingers and hand on affected side q1h to 8h as indicated postsurgery

Collaborate with physical therapist to plan exercise regimen and instruct in wrist, hand, elbow, arm exercises

Monitor edema in affected arm: measure upper arm and forearm

Expected Outcome

Functioning of affected arm and hand is maintained

PATIENT/FAMILY TEACHING

Postdiagnosis, postoperative

Instruct patient in precautions for affected arm/breast

Exercise to tolerance; slowly resume housekeeping activities; stop at point of pain

No blood drawing, IV therapy, or injections in affected arm

No BP taken on affected arm

Incision and chest wall may feel numb; avoid accidental injury

Instruct patient to carry handbag on unaffected shoulder or side

Avoid pressure on affected chest wall, arm: sleeping, sexual positions

Report increase in size of arm (sleeves fit tighter)

Gradually increase extent of daily exercise of affected arm and hand; encourage use of affected arm/hand to perform simple care activities; wash face, brush teeth, eating

Discuss types of prostheses, reconstruction (if not performed at time of mastectomy)

Care of incision, signs and symptoms to report to physician

Medication/radiation therapy/chemotherapy regimen: expected therapeutic effects, side effects, potential adverse reactions

*Not a NANDA-approved diagnosis.

DISCHARGE/HOME CARE PLANNING

Discuss sources for obtaining prostheses

Teach about availability of assistance for ADLs; arrange home health provider as needed

Discuss availability of transportation to follow-up appointments with care providers; assist with arrangements as necessary

Inform about resources for support groups

Discuss importance of continuing interaction with others

■ CANCER OF THE CERVIX

Although rates have dramatically decreased over the last 50 years, cancer of the cervix remains the sixth most common cancer among women in the United States; cancer of the cervix is largely influenced by lifestyle factors

ASSESSMENT
SUBJECTIVE DATA

Pelvic pain (late symptom)

Loss of appetite (late symptom)

OBJECTIVE DATA

Unexplained vaginal spotting/bleeding

Postcoital bleeding, postdouche bleeding

Vaginal discharge: watery, purulent, mucoid

Late symptoms

Irritation

Vulvitis

Yellow, foul-smelling vaginal discharge

Urinary symptoms, leakage of urine or feces from vagina

Weight loss

RISK FACTORS

Immunosuppression

Low socioeconomic status: increased incidence

First coitus at early age: within 1 year of menarche

Multiple sex partners

Frequent genital infections; viral exposure

Mismanaged parturition

Nonbarrier contraception

Chronic vaginal douching

Human papillomavirus

Cigarette smoking

DIAGNOSTIC TESTS

CBC

Culposcopy, biopsy

CT scan, MRI

Lymphangiography, needle aspiration

Cytologic smear (pap)

MULTIDISCIPLINARY MANAGEMENT
PREVENTION/DETECTION TEACHING

Explain importance of maintaining an accurate menstrual cycle history: frequency, length, amount, color

Maintain good gynecologic hygiene

Avoid frequent douching

Delay beginning sexual activity, especially during teen years, limit partners, use condoms

Discuss need for regular, periodic gynecologic examinations including pap test and bimanual examination

The American College of Surgeons, American College of Obstetrics and of Gynecologists, and American Medical Association recommend first examination at age 18 or onset of sexual activity, followed by two annual examinations; if these three examinations are normal, the frequency may decrease as determined by the personal physician

Self-visualization examination

Skin excoriation, ulcers

Lumps, leukoplakia

Narrowing of introitus, atrophy

THERAPEUTIC MANAGEMENT

Surgical intervention

Conization

Cryotherapy, laser ablation

Hysterectomy (p. 672)

Loop electrosurgical excision procedure

Radiation therapy

Chemotherapy: advanced disease

PATIENT PROBLEMS—NURSING DIAGNOSES/INTERVENTIONS

See Chapter 11 for surgical interventions (e.g., Hysterectomy, p. 672)

■ CANCER OF THE ESOPHAGUS

The most common esophageal carcinoma is of the squamous cell or adenocarcinoma type; generally developing in the middle or lower third of the esophagus, this cancer is usually fatal because the condition is advanced before symptoms appear; the highest incidence is in males between the ages of 50 and 70 years

ASSESSMENT
SUBJECTIVE DATA

Difficulty swallowing

Early: when swallowing hard, solid food

Later: constantly when swallowing saliva

Vague epigastric discomfort

Vague feeling of fullness after eating

Loss of appetite, early satiety

Substernal pain, pyrosis (heartburn)

General malaise

OBJECTIVE DATA

Hoarseness, coughing

Glossopharyngeal neuralgia

Foul-smelling breath

Hiccups

Esophageal obstruction
   Sialism
   Nocturnal aspiration
   Regurgitation of saliva and food
Weight loss, dehydration
Increased salivation and mucus formation
Eructation
Hepatomegaly
Diaphragmatic paralysis (from phrenic nerve
   involvement)
Cervical/supraclavicular lymphadenopathy
Hematemesis, melena
Iron deficiency anemia
Superior vena cava syndrome

RISK FACTORS

Heavy smoking
Chronic, excessive alcohol intake
Drinking and eating very hot, spicy foods; smoked meats
Exposure to foods containing nitrites and nitrates
Nutritional deficiency: riboflavin, vitamins A, E, C and
   niacin, zinc
Diet high in nitrosamine
History of head and neck tumors, strictures, peptic ulcer
   disease
Environmental
   Water pollution
   Petroleum products
Chronic irritation, reflux disease, Barrett's esophagus
Achalasia
Scleroderma

DIAGNOSTIC TESTS

CBC
Complete chemistry panel
Liver function tests
Imaging/nuclear medicine studies
   Chest radiograph
   Barium studies of the GI tract
   CT scan/MRI
Cardiopulmonary studies
   Bronchoscopy
   ECG
Endoscopy with biopsy and cytology

POTENTIAL COMPLICATIONS

Malnutrition, anemia
Fluid and electrolyte imbalance
Aspiration pneumonia
Infection
Metastasis to other organs
Hemorrhage

MULTIDISCIPLINARY MANAGEMENT
THERAPEUTIC MANAGEMENT

Pain management
Chemotherapeutic agents
Radiation therapy
Insertion of plastic (Celestin) tubes to maintain nutrition
Esophageal surgery (p. 309)

Gastrostomy tube insertion
Dietition consultation
Social services, support groups
Speech and occupational therapy
Dilation, stenting
Photocoagulation

PATIENT PROBLEMS—NURSING DIAGNOSES/INTERVENTIONS

▼Altered nutrition: less than body requirements
related to anorexia, dysphagia, surgical intervention, radiation therapy, chemotherapy

Assess nutritional status daily: weight, electrolytes, total
   protein, serum albumin, Hgb, skin turgor, muscle mass
   *to evaluate response to plan of care and make
   needed changes*
Consult speech therapy *to assess patient's ability to
   masticate and swallow*
Determine amount and types of foods patient likes and is
   able to tolerate
Provide for oral hygiene before and after meals
Administer anesthetics to oral mucosa before meals prn
Offer high-calorie, high-protein diet with variation in
   taste, texture, and presentation of foods *to enhance
   appetite*
In collaboration with physician, provide oral and
   parenteral nutritional supplements
Serve frequent, light meals and nutritional, high-calorie
   snacks
Assist patient to eat if fatigue is a factor
Present meals in an attractive, pleasing manner
Provide a pleasant atmosphere *to increase desire to eat:*
   encourage significant others to join patient for meals,
   remove bedpans/urinals from area, maintain
   well-ventilated room, serve food as soon as it arrives,
   remove tray as soon as patient finishes eating
In collaboration with clinical dietitian: calculate number
   of calories and nutrients needed *to maintain/gain
   weight and support metabolic needs*
Maintain calorie count
Encourage family to bring patient's favorite foods from
   home
In collaboration with physician, administer antiemetics
   before meals prn

Expected Outcome
Weight is maintained within 10% of baseline

▼Pain related to progressive disease process, surgical intervention

Assess nature, intensity, location, duration, and
   precipitating and alleviating factors *to establish
   baseline and evaluate responses to plan of care*
Use consistent pain rating scale
Assess nonverbal signs of pain
Obtain information from patient regarding past pain
   experiences and methods used for relief

Control environmental factors that may increase perception of pain: temperature, noise, lighting

Assist patient to achieve comfortable positions

Assist patient to reach state of minimal physical tension through techniques such as relaxation, music, visualization, diversion

Provide a restful environment with opportunities to rest during the day and uninterrupted periods of sleep at night

In collaboration with physician, provide analgesic medications as required, observing for therapeutic and side effects

Discuss and institute noninvasive pain relief measures: relaxation, cutaneous stimulation, distraction, hot/cold therapy

Expected Outcomes

Verbalizes decrease in or relief of pain

Incorporates existing pain while participating in daily activities

▼Anticipatory grieving, related to lifestyle changes, decreased physical abilities, changes in physical appearance, life-threatening prognosis

Be sensitive to changes patient is experiencing; encourage patient to express feelings, frustrations, anger, hopes

Provide a therapeutic environment conducive to open discussion: actively listen, perceive nonverbal cues, be patient and empathetic *to support grief process*

Encourage questions and provide information freely as patient expresses the desire for knowledge about the disease, treatments, and prognosis

Set limits on maladaptive coping behaviors if they interfere with patient's well-being

Support adaptive behaviors that suggest progression and resolution of the grieving process

Provide opportunities for private, uninterrupted time with significant other(s)

Assist in identifying ways to adapt lifestyle as condition changes

Provide information regarding support groups for patient and significant other(s)

Collaborate with other professionals (social worker, clergy, psychologist, psychiatrist) *to provide support and facilitate grieving process*

Provide reference for financial assistance, answers to questions regarding medical insurance

Provide information to assist patient in completing advance directive or similar document to ensure patient wishes are known to significant others and care providers

Expected Outcomes

Progresses through stages of the grieving process and moves toward acceptance

Demonstrates effective coping mechanisms; participates in decisions about own future

▼Ineffective airway clearance, related to esophageal obstruction

Maintain elevated upper body at 30 to 45 degrees *to facilitate respiratory excursion*

Avoid supine positions, hyperflexing knees *to prevent circulatory compromise*

Consult with occupational or speech therapist *to assess swallowing ability and develop plan of care*

Instruct patient in use of tonsil tip suction; have suction available within patient's reach

Suction patient as needed

Provide emesis basin and tissues for expectoration

Expected Outcome

Patent airway is maintained

PATIENT/FAMILY TEACHING

Reinforce physician's explanation of disease and treatment plan

In collaboration with clinical dietitian, speech therapist, and occupational therapist instruct patient regarding diet required, tolerated

Gastrostomy tube management: assessment of placement, tube feedings, flushing, checking for residual

Care of Celestin tube

Elevating head at all times

Swallowing only small amounts

Method for clearing obstruction

Methods for pain management

Discuss importance of maintaining follow-up appointments with care providers, radiation, chemotherapy appointments

Explain medication regimen, side effects, potential adverse reactions

Discuss signs and symptoms to report to physician

DISCHARGE/HOME CARE PLANNING

Discuss transportation to care provider visits

Ensure assistance with ADLs: shopping, cooking, cleaning as needed

Teach about durable medical equipment provider for suction equipment and supplies

Discuss importance of clean, sufficient space for storing equipment and supplies, care and maintenance of supplies

Discuss importance of ongoing outpatient care, continued interaction with others who are supportive

■ CANCER OF THE HEAD AND NECK

The most common site of head and neck cancer is the larynx; other sites include the oral cavity, pharynx; 90% or more is due to lifestyle or environmental risk factors that are significantly preventable; the origin of cancer of the head and neck is most commonly squamous cell carcinoma; these cancers are more likely to present with regional lymphatic metastasis at the time of diagnosis

ASSESSMENT
SUBJECTIVE DATA
Earache

Sore throat lasting longer than 2 weeks

Pain

OBJECTIVE DATA
Oral cavity: leukoplakia, erythroplasia, other lesions may appear infiltrating, ulcerative, exophytic

Chronic, nonhealing, often painless sores: lips, eyelids, external ear and canal, scalp

Submaxillary, parotid, sublingual glands positive for swelling, adenopathy

Regional lymph nodes may be enlarged, firm, nonmobile, overlying skin may be discolored

Thyroid may be enlarged

Loss of structure/support of external nose, nasal discharge, smell changes, loss of nasal patency

Altered voice tone: hoarseness, cough

Hemoptysis

Glossitis

Dysphagia

Visual changes

Hearing loss

Taste changes

DIAGNOSTIC TESTS
Nasolaryngoscope

CT scan

Endoscopy

Needle aspiration, biopsy

RISK FACTORS
Epstein-Barr virus

Tobacco use: cigarettes, cigars, snuff, chewing tobacco, pipe

Chronic moderate to heavy use of alcohol

Chronic intake of extremely hot or cold liquids

Exposure to nickel, wood dust, hydrocarbon gases, asbestos, mustard gas, radiation, uranium, syphilis, herpes simplex, Epstein-Barr virus

Chronic inflammatory disease; chronic irritation to oral mucosa from poorly fitting dentures, malocclusion of teeth, poor hygiene

Premalignant lesions: erythroplasia, leukoplakia

THERAPEUTIC MANAGEMENT
Surgical intervention

Chemotherapy

Radiation therapy

Brachytherapy

Biologic response modifiers

Chemoradiotherapy

PREVENTION/DETECTION
Explain importance of avoiding tobacco and heavy alcohol use

Discuss importance of proper oral hygiene and routine, preventive dental visits, properly fitting dentures

Teach avoidance of chemical and other carcinogens

Teach about protection from excess exposure to the sun

Discuss maintaining healthy, well-balanced diet

Explain community support groups for quitting smoking and alcohol use counseling

■ LARYNGECTOMY: RADICAL NECK DISSECTION
Removal of larynx and surrounding neck tissue to treat a cancerous condition; a permanent tracheal stoma is created

ASSESSMENT
PREOPERATIVE
SUBJECTIVE DATA
Pain in "Adam's apple" radiates to ear

Anxiety/fear

OBJECTIVE DATA
Tachypnea

Dysphagia

Hemoptysis

Stridor

Hoarseness

Enlarged cervical nodes

Cough

Behavioral manifestations of fear, anxiety, panic, denial, anger

POSTOPERATIVE
SUBJECTIVE DATA
Fear of suffocation

Pain at surgical site

OBJECTIVE DATA
Hemorrhage

Airway obstruction: restlessness, tachycardia, use of accessory muscles of respiration, tachypnea, noisy respirations, wheezing, stridor, pallor, cyanosis

Atelectasis

Dehydration

Sputum: amount, character

Incision site: discoloration, swelling, drainage, sloughing of tissue, condition of stoma

Wound drains: amount, character of drainage

Body temperature elevation

Behavioral manifestations of helplessness, fear, anxiety, anger, frustration

DIAGNOSTIC TESTS
CBC

Type and cross/screen

Electrolytes

Blood chemistries

Epstein-Barr virus antibody titer

Imaging/nuclear medicine studies

    Chest x-ray

    Skull and neck x-rays

    Bone scan

    CT scan, MRI

Cardiopulmonary studies
  ABGs
  Baseline pulmonary function tests
  ECG
Fiberoptic endoscopy studies
Biopsy of suspect lesions

POTENTIAL COMPLICATIONS
Pneumonia
Respiratory failure
Metastasis
Cardiac erosion
Pneumothorax
Shock
Tracheoesophageal fistula

MULTIDISCIPLINARY MANAGEMENT
THERAPEUTIC MANAGEMENT
Radiation therapy
Mechanical support of ventilation, oxygen therapy
Nasogastric tube
Dietitian consultation
Nutritional support, total parenteral nutrition (TPN),
  gastrostomy tube feedings
Parenteral therapy, fluids, medications
Speech therapy
Respiratory therapy
Social services, support groups

PATIENT PROBLEMS—NURSING DIAGNOSES/INTERVENTIONS

▼ Impaired skin integrity, related to radiation therapy

Assess skin completely q8h
Skin care guidelines
  Avoid bath or shower until ordered by physician
  Do not wash skin in area being irradiated until ordered
    by physician *to prevent removal of landmarks*
  Do not remove skin markings between treatments
  Avoid use of any products (soap, lotion, deodorants,
    cosmetics) without checking with physician/nurse
  Avoid tight garments to *prevent rubbing and skin
    irritation*
  Avoid extremes of temperature
  Dry desquamation: use cornstarch sparingly
  Moist desquamation: use water/saline to keep clean
    and moist (slow healing)
  Expose skin to air when possible
  Cover broken areas with hydrocolloid dressing; use
    stretch-type tubular dressing to hold in place

Expected Outcome
Skin remains intact and/or impaired skin progressively
  heals

▼ Anticipatory grieving, related to lifestyle changes,
decreased physical abilities, changes in physical
appearance, life-threatening prognosis

Be sensitive to changes patient is experiencing;
  encourage patient to express feelings, frustrations,
  anger, hopes *to begin work of grieving process*
Provide a therapeutic environment conducive to open
  discussion: actively listen, perceive nonverbal cues, be
  patient and empathetic *to facilitate trust*
Encourage questions and provide information freely as
  patient expresses the desire for knowledge about the
  disease, treatments, and prognosis *to ease the fear of
  the unknown*
Set limits on maladaptive coping behaviors if they
  interfere with patient's well-being
Support adaptive behaviors that suggest progression and
  resolution of the grieving process
Provide opportunities for private, uninterrupted time
  with significant others
Assist in identifying ways to adapt lifestyle as condition
  changes *to enhance participation and feelings of
  control*
Provide information regarding support groups for patient
  and significant other(s)
Collaborate with other professionals (social worker,
  clergy, psychologist, psychiatrist) *to provide support
  and facilitate grieving process*
Provide reference for financial assistance, answers to
  questions regarding medical insurance
Provide information to assist patient in completing
  advance directive or similar document to ensure
  patient wishes are known to significant others and
  care providers

Expected Outcomes
Progresses through stages of the grieving process and
  moves toward acceptance
Demonstrates effective coping mechanisms; participates
  in decisions about own future

▼ Altered nutrition: less than body requirements related to dysphagia, radiation therapy, chemotherapy, perceived changes in taste and smell of foods, disinterest in eating

Assess nutritional status daily: weight, electrolytes, total
  protein, serum albumin, Hgb, skin turgor, muscle mass
  *to evaluate response to plan of care and make
  needed changes*
Consult speech therapist to assess patient's ability to
  masticate and swallow
Determine amount and types of foods patient likes and is
  able to tolerate
Provide for oral hygiene before and after meals
Administer anesthetics to oral mucosa before
  meals prn
Offer high-calorie, high-protein diet with variation in
  taste, texture, and presentation of foods
In collaboration with physician, provide oral and
  parenteral nutritional supplements
Serve frequent, light meals and nutritional, high-calorie
  snacks
Assist patient to eat if fatigue is a factor

Provide a pleasant atmosphere *to increase desire to eat:* encourage significant others to join patient for meals, remove bedpans/urinals from area, maintain well-ventilated room, serve food as soon as it arrives, remove tray as soon as patient finishes eating

In collaboration with clinical dietitian: calculate number of calories and nutrients needed *to maintain/gain weight and support metabolic needs*

Maintain calorie count

Encourage family to bring favorite foods from home

In collaboration with physician, administer antiemetics before meals prn

Expected Outcome
Weight is maintained within 10% of baseline

▼Ineffective airway clearance, related to removal of laryngeal structures, newly created tracheostomy, altered ability to cough and swallow

Assess surgical site around laryngectomy, tracheostomy tube for bleeding and/or excess secretions

Assess respiratory pattern: rate, depth, quality

Auscultate breath sounds for crackles, wheezes

Assess amount of oropharyngeal secretions; have suction readily available within patient's reach

Maintain patient in upright position *to facilitate respiratory excursion*

Apply humidification to tracheostomy per physician order

Suction tracheostomy and mouth prn to keep clear of secretions; use sterile technique

If on ventilator support, hyperoxygenate and/or hyperventilate before suctioning (hospital protocols will vary) *to prevent depletion of oxygen*

Perform tracheostomy care q8h and prn; replace disposable inner cannula with each cleaning *to decrease exposure to pathogens*

Avoid occluding tracheostomy tube when positioning patient or changing bed linens

Maintain manual resuscitator bag at bedside; maintain extra laryngectomy tube of same size and type at bedside *for emergency use*

Assist patient to turn, cough, deep breathe q2h

Expected Outcome
Secretions are effectively cleared, and patent airway is maintained

▼Risk for impaired skin integrity, related to exposure to tracheostomy secretions

Assess surgical area for signs of wound infection q8h: redness, purulent drainage, edema of tissues, condition of suture lines

Clean skin around stoma q8h and prn *to maintain cleanliness*

Wash with hydrogen peroxide and rinse with saline; pat dry

Place sterile, preslit 4 × 4 gauge around stoma; change prn *to keep stoma clean and dry*

Change laryngectomy tube holder during stoma care and as needed *to keep holder clean and dry*

Ensure laryngectomy holder is snug but not tight around patient's neck *to prevent skin irritation*

Elevate head of bed 45 to 60 degrees *to promote respiratory excursion*

Prevent forward flexion of neck; place small towel under shoulders as needed; remove pillows if necessary

Assess and record output from drains; examine area around drains for signs/symptoms of infection

Expected Outcomes
Integrity of surgical incisions and skin around incisions is maintained

Surgical wounds begin to heal without signs or symptoms of infection

▼Impaired verbal communication, related to laryngectomy

Provide patient with immediate means of communication; have call light within reach; arrange signs and signals that call for immediate attention

Have paper/pencil, communication board, Magic Slate* available for written messages

Read written messages aloud *to confirm meaning with patient*

Avoid asking questions that require *yes* or *no* answers

Be patient; wait for patient to complete message before assuming answer or course of action to take

If call light is answered at nurses' station, ensure patient is not asked questions that cannot be answered simply

Encourage patient to express fears, frustrations related to inability to speak

Encourage and teach visitors to use assistive devices *to communicate with patient*

Collaborate with speech therapy in development of plan of care, assess ability to use artificial larynx

Expected Outcomes
Patient/caregivers develop an effective communication system

Able to communicate thoughts/ideas, needs, desires to staff and visitors

PATIENT/FAMILY TEACHING
PREOPERATIVE
Reinforce physician's explanation of disease and treatment plan

Demonstrate/explain laryngectomy tube care and suctioning

Explain purpose and location of tubes/drains and their care; gastrostomy tube feedings

Western Publishing Co., Inc., Racine, Wis.

Develop a communication system to use postoperatively that incorporates patient's level of ability to read and write and primary language

Schedule visit from speech therapist to explain postoperative course

Provide opportunities for patient to attend support groups or visits from persons who have had similar experiences

POSTOPERATIVE

Explain importance of maintaining sufficient caloric and fluid intake even though food may not taste or smell appetizing

Review hygiene activities: when showering, direct spray under neck, wear shield over stoma, avoid getting soap into stoma, do not use aerosol sprays around stoma

When shaving the face: shield stoma to prevent small hairs from entering; use electric razor to prevent shaving lather from entering stoma site

Explain need to keep stoma lightly covered at all times, avoid tight-fitting necklines, natural fiber scarves, neck jewelry

Discuss importance of covering stoma when coughing

DISCHARGE/HOME CARE PLANNING

Teach laryngectomy and stoma care: inner cannula care, removing and replacing outer cannula, suctioning, dressing changes, cleaning stoma, and changing holder

Ensure understanding of medications, diet, administration of tube feedings, signs and symptoms to report to physician

Teach about care of surgical incisions

Refer to community support groups: American Cancer Society; Lost Cord/New Voice Club

Explain importance of clean area to store dressing and suction supplies; care and maintenance of supplies

Establish contact with durable medical equipment agency to supply suction equipment

Make available handheld mirror

Make available paper and pencil or alternative communication devices

Discuss importance of avoiding persons with URIs, smoky environments

Emphasize importance of ongoing outpatient care, continued communication with others who are supportive

■ CANCER OF THE INTESTINE/ COLORECTAL CANCER

Cancer of the small intestine is uncommon; when it occurs it is usually found in the lower duodenum and lower ileum; mortality is high; early signs and symptoms are usually absent

Cancer of the large intestine is a slow-growing malignancy most frequently found in the cecum, lower ascending and sigmoid colon; prognosis is optimistic; early signs and symptoms are usually absent

Table 15-4	Duke's Classification of Colorectal Cancer	
Stage	Involvement	5-Year Survival
A	Mucosa and subcutaneous tissues	81.2%
B	All layers of bowel wall and may invade adjacent structures	64%
C	Regional lymph node invasion	27%
D	Metastasis to distal organs and structures	14.3%

Colorectal cancer most frequently occurs in the fifth decade of life and if treated early has an 80% to 90% survival rate (Table 15-4)

ASSESSMENT
SUBJECTIVE DATA
Nausea
Loss of appetite
Upper abdominal pain, cramps
Generalized weakness
Feeling of incomplete evacuation

OBJECTIVE DATA
Abdominal pain
Change in bowel habits
Alternating constipation and diarrhea
Jaundice
Right colon involvement
  Anemia
  GI bleeding
  Weight loss
Sigmoid colon
  Obstruction
  Blood per rectum
Left colon involvement
  Mucus in stool
  Constipation
  Decreased-caliber stools
  Blood or blood mixed with stool
  Vomiting
Rectum
  Rectal bleeding
  Mucosal diarrhea
  Tenesmus

RISK FACTORS
Obesity
Smoking
Alcohol abuse
More than 40 years of age
High-fat, low-fiber diet
Familial polyps, Gardner's syndrome, adenomatous polyps, villous adenomas, colon cancer

Ulcerative colitis, Crohn's disease, Pentz-Jegher's syndrome

Previous colon cancer, first-degree relative with colorectal cancer

History of breast, ovarian, uterine cancer

Physical inactivity

DIAGNOSTIC TESTS

Digital rectal examination

CBC

Electrolyte panel

Coagulation panel

Occult blood testing

Serum tumor markers, carcinoembryonic antigen (CEA)

Imaging/nuclear medicine studies

    Upper/lower GI series

    Duodenoscopy with biopsy

    Abdominal series

    Barium contrast studies

    Sigmoidoscopy/colonoscopy with biopsy

POTENTIAL COMPLICATIONS

Fluid and electrolyte imbalance

Anemia

Intestinal obstruction

Bowel abscess, fistula

Metastatic disease

MULTIDISCIPLINARY MANAGEMENT
PREVENTION/DETECTION TEACHING

Explain risk factors

Discuss regular, periodic rectal examinations and occult blood testing after age 40

Teach importance of sigmoidoscopy/colonoscopy at age 50; then every 2 to 3 years if negative

Advise on low-fat diet including fresh cruciferous vegetables, fruits, fiber

Drink eight glasses of water per day

Exercise regularly

Stress need to report abnormal stools to physician

Teach about home occult blood testing annually after age 50

Provide written information on detection measures

THERAPEUTIC MANAGEMENT

Collaborate with clinical dietitian to plan diet consistent with condition

Parenteral fluids, nutrition

Nasogastric/intestinal decompression/aspiration

Pain management

Chemotherapeutic agents (see Table 15-8, p. 864)

Radiation therapy, immunotherapy

Surgical intervention (bowel resection, ostomy, abdominoperineal resection)

Wound, Ostomy, Continence/ET Nurse

Social services; support groups enterostomal therapy

PATIENT PROBLEMS—NURSING DIAGNOSES/INTERVENTIONS

▼ Altered nutrition: less than body requirements related to dysfunctional bowel, nausea, vomiting, diarrhea

Assess nutritional status daily: weight, electrolytes, total protein, serum albumin, Hgb, skin turgor, muscle mass

Determine amount and types of foods patient likes and is able to tolerate

Provide for oral hygiene before and after meals

Administer anesthetics to oral mucosa before meals prn

Offer high-calorie, high-protein diet with variation in taste, texture, and presentation of foods *to enhance appetite*

In collaboration with physician, provide oral and parenteral nutritional supplements

Serve frequent, light meals and nutritional, high-calorie snacks

Assist patient to eat if fatigue is a factor

Present meals in an attractive, pleasing manner

Provide a pleasant atmosphere *to increase desire to eat:* encourage significant others to join patient for meals, remove bedpans/urinals from area, maintain well-ventilated room, serve food as soon as it arrives, remove tray as soon as patient finishes eating

In collaboration with clinical dietitian: calculate number of calories and nutrients needed *to maintain/gain weight and support metabolic needs*

Maintain calorie count

Encourage family to bring patient's favorite foods from home

In collaboration with physician, administer antiemetics before meals prn

Expected Outcome

Maintains weight within 10% of baseline

▼ Pain related to progression of disease process

Assess nature, intensity, location, duration, and precipitating and alleviating factors

Use consistent pain rating scale

Assess nonverbal signs of pain

Obtain information from patient regarding past pain experiences and methods used for relief

Control environmental factors that may increase perception of pain: temperature, noise, lighting

Assist patient to achieve comfortable positions

Assist patient to achieve state of minimal physical tension through techniques such as relaxation, music, visualization, diversion

Provide a restful environment with opportunities to rest during the day and uninterrupted periods of sleep at night

In collaboration with physician, provide analgesic medications as required, observing for therapeutic and side effects

Discuss and institute noninvasive pain relief measures: relaxation, cutaneous stimulation, distraction, hot/cold therapy

Expected Outcomes
Verbalizes decrease in or relief of pain
Incorporates existing pain while participating in daily activities

▼Anticipatory grieving related to poor prognosis

Be sensitive to changes patient is experiencing; encourage patient to express feelings, frustrations, anger, hopes *to begin work of grieving process*
Provide a therapeutic environment conducive to open discussion: actively listen, perceive nonverbal cues, be patient and empathetic *to facilitate trust*
Encourage questions and provide information freely as patient expresses the desire for knowledge about the disease, treatments, and prognosis *to ease fear of the unknown*
Set limits on maladaptive coping behaviors if they interfere with patient's well-being
Support adaptive behaviors that suggest progression and resolution of the grieving process
Provide opportunities for private, uninterrupted time with significant other(s)
Assist in identifying ways to adapt lifestyle as condition changes *to enhance participation and feelings of control*
Provide information regarding support groups for patient and significant other(s)
Collaborate with other professionals (social worker, clergy, psychologist, psychiatrist) *to provide support and facilitate grieving process*
Provide reference for financial assistance, answers to questions regarding medical insurance
Provide information to assist patient in completing advanced directive or similar document *to ensure patient wishes are known to significant others and care providers*

Expected Outcomes
Progresses through stages of the grieving process and moves toward acceptance
Demonstrates effective coping mechanisms; participates in decisions about own future

▼Diarrhea or constipation related to diseased gastrointestinal tract, malabsorption, effects of chemotherapy, radiation therapy

Assess usual pattern of elimination and changes experienced
Assess stools for consistency, color, character, presence of occult/gross blood
Auscultate for bowel sounds and measure abdominal girth q8h

Consult with clinical dietitian and physician *to develop nutrition plan consistent with patient condition and tolerance*
Ensure intake is equal to output; include diarrhea in output measurement
Check patient for impaction if no or minimal hard bowel movements
Administer medications: stool softeners, antidiarrheals

Expected Outcome
Elimination pattern is maintained within parameters of disease process

PATIENT/FAMILY TEACHING
Reinforce physician's explanation of disease and treatment plan
Diet management and/or parenteral IV nutrition administration
Advise on activity/rest patterns and their importance
Discuss medications, actions, side effects, potential adverse reactions
Explain radiation, chemotherapy regimen; management of side effects
Discuss importance of follow-up visits with care providers

DISCHARGE/HOME CARE PLANNING
Assess patient's ability to care for self and support systems available in the home
Arrange for home care providers as needed to assist with physical and home management needs: shopping, cooking, cleaning
Assess availability of transportation to ensure ability to keep appointments
Ensure adequate, clean storage space for medical supplies; care and maintenance of supplies
Explain importance of ongoing outpatient care, continued interaction with others who are supportive

■ CANCER OF THE KIDNEY AND BLADDER
Transitional cell carcinomas make up 93% of all bladder cancers; the highest incidence occurs among white men more than 65 years of age; primary renal carcinoma is rare, accounting for 2% of all adult malignancies; most often found in the renal parenchyma, the metastasis rate is high and the prognosis is poor; the incidence of renal carcinoma increases with age

ASSESSMENT
SUBJECTIVE DATA
Burning, pain on urination
Urgency
Back pain
Fatigue

OBJECTIVE DATA

Hypertension
Gross, painless hematuria; may be intermittent
Microhematuria
Frequency of urination
Weight loss
Anemia
Fever, night sweats
Paraneoplastic syndrome associated with renal cancer
    Hypercalcemia
    Hypertension
    Polycythemia

RISK FACTORS

Smoking
Age: 50 to 70 years
Exposure to carcinogens through skin or vapor
    Aniline dye; rubber and cable industry
    Beta-napthylamine
    4-Amino diphenyl
    Tobacco tar
    Benzidine
Exposure to pelvic irradiation
Chronic UTIs
Chronic bacterial cystitis with calculi: strictures,
    diverticulae, paralytic stasis
Chronic intake of analgesics containing phenacetin
Potential risks
    Coffee drinking
    High use of sodium, saccharin, cyclamates
    Urine stasis

DIAGNOSTIC TESTS

Urinalysis
Urine cytology
Complete chemistry panel
Imaging/nuclear medicine studies
    Intravenous pyelogram (IVP)
    Retrograde pyelography
    Nephrotomography
    Ultrasonography
    CT scan, MRI to detect lymph node metastases
    Renal arteriogram
Cystoscopy
Biopsy

MULTIDISCIPLINARY MANAGEMENT
PREVENTION/DETECTION TEACHING

Ensure patient and family understand risk factors and the
    importance of providing detailed occupational history:
    type and length of exposure, protective measures
    taken to reduce risk of exposure
Explain need to continue use of protective equipment as
    needed in work setting
Discuss importance of reporting suspicious signs and
    symptoms to physician
Explain need for periodic physical examinations: rectal
    and pelvic examinations, cystoscopy, and cytology

THERAPEUTIC MANAGEMENT

Cystectomy and continent reservoir
Transurethral resection
Local resection
Nephrectomy, p. 651
Chemotherapy (see Table 15-8, p. 864)
Radiotherapy, p. 855
Intravesical chemotherapy
Social services

PATIENT PROBLEM—NURSING DIAGNOSIS/INTERVENTIONS

See type of therapeutic management for patient care

■ CANCER OF THE LIVER

Malignant tumor most frequently caused by metastatic disease lesions in other organs; primary lesions are rare and may be asymptomatic

ASSESSMENT
SUBJECTIVE DATA

General weakness
Loss of appetite
Fatigue
Nausea
Abdominal fullness, discomfort
Abdominal pain when coughing or deep breathing
Referred pain to back, scapular, and shoulder area

OBJECTIVE DATA

Progressive weight loss
Increased flatulence
Light-colored, bulky stools; stools containing fat
Diarrhea, melena
Low-grade fever
Dehydration
Anemia
Electrolyte imbalance
Jaundice
Edema, ascites

RISK FACTORS

Chronic hepatitis B and C
Cirrhosis of the liver

DIAGNOSTIC TESTS

Prothrombin time/Internationalized Normal Ratio
    (PT/INR): increased
Erythrocyte sedimentation rate (ESR): elevated
Bleeding, clotting times: prolonged
CBC; WBC: leukocytosis
Fasting blood sugar (FBS)
Liver function studies: lactate dehydrogenase (LDH),
    alanine aminotransferase (ALT), aspartate
    aminotransferase (AST)
Alkaline phosphatase: elevated
Serum albumin: decreased
Urinalysis

In collaboration with clinical dietitian: calculate number of calories and nutrients needed *to maintain/gain weight, support metabolic needs, and maintain blood glucose within limits*

Maintain calorie count

Encourage family to bring patient's favorite foods from home

In collaboration with physician, administer antiemetics before meals prn

Expected Outcome

Maintains weight within 10% of baseline

▼Anticipatory grieving related to changes in physical functioning and poor prognosis

Be sensitive to changes patient is experiencing; encourage patient to express feelings, frustrations, anger, hopes *to begin work of grieving process*

Provide a therapeutic environment conducive to open discussion: actively listen, perceive nonverbal cues, be patient and empathetic *to facilitate trust*

Encourage questions and provide information freely as patient expresses the desire for knowledge about the disease, treatments, and prognosis *to ease fear of the unknown*

Set limits on maladaptive coping behaviors if they interfere with patient's well-being

Support adaptive behaviors that suggest progression and resolution of the grieving process

Provide opportunities for private, uninterrupted time with significant other(s)

Assist in identifying ways to adapt lifestyle as condition changes *to enhance participation and feelings of control*

Provide information regarding support groups for patient and significant others

Collaborate with other professionals (social worker, clergy, psychologist, psychiatrist) *to provide support and facilitate grieving process;*

Provide reference for financial assistance, answers to questions regarding medical insurance

Provide information to assist patient in completing advance directive or similar document *to ensure patient wishes are known to significant others and care providers*

Expected Outcomes

Progresses through stages of the grieving process and moves toward acceptance

Demonstrates effective coping mechanisms; participates in decisions about own future

▼Risk for fluid volume deficit related to NPO status, diarrhea, altered glucose metabolism

Administer parenteral fluids, electrolytes, and nutrition per physician order

Calculate intake and output; measure diarrhea and nasogastric aspirate and include in output measurement

Administer insulin per physician order

Monitor vital signs for signs of dehydration: tachycardia, hypotension, orthostatic hypotension

Expected Outcome

Intake and output are balanced

Remains hydrated

▼Potential for altered glucose metabolism, ascites, bleeding, jaundice related to impaired liver function*

Monitor results of blood glucose, bilirubin, coagulation, CBC, albumin per physician order

Monitor gastric aspirate and stools for gross/occult blood

Perform capillary blood glucose measurements and administer insulin per physician order

Monitor skin and sclera for signs of jaundice

Monitor lower extremities for edema and tenderness

Auscultate abdomen for bowel sounds and measure abdominal girth q8h

Monitor mental status, acuity q8h

Administer medications per physician order

Expected Outcome

Potential complications are avoided or are recognized and treated promptly

PATIENT/FAMILY TEACHING

Provide information about diagnosis and treatment plan

Explain chemotherapy/radiation therapy schedule; expected effects of treatment, side effects, potential adverse reactions

Explain symptomatic care of side and adverse effects

Contact clinical dietitian to assist in planning a therapeutic diet consistent with patient's physical condition and preferences

Contact certified diabetes educator to assist in structuring education related to insulin administration, capillary blood glucose testing, diet, and activity

Discuss medications: administration, therapeutic actions, side effects, potential adverse reactions

Explain importance of reporting changes in condition to physician: weight gain, increase in abdominal girth, jaundice, bleeding from any site, increased pain, hematemesis, tarry/bloody stools, peripheral edema, dyspnea

Discuss importance of follow-up visits with care providers

Not a NANDA-approved diagnosis.

DISCHARGE/HOME CARE PLANNING

Advise where to purchase a capillary blood glucose monitor and supplies for self-testing of capillary blood sugar

Teach importance of refrigerating insulin

Plan for a safe, secure area in which to keep new and used insulin needles/syringes

Discuss patient's and/or family's ability to care for patient and home; obtain home care providers as needed for physical needs: shopping, cooking, cleaning

Plan for transportation to follow-up visits with care providers

▮ PANCREATIC SURGERY

pancreatic duodenectomy (Whipple's procedure): Radical procedure for cancer of the head of the pancreas; the proximal head of the pancreas, adjoining duodenum, distal part of the stomach, and distal portion of the common bile duct are resected, and an anastomosis of the jejunum to the pancreatic duct, common bile duct, and stomach is performed (Fig. 15-5)

total pancreatectomy: Alternative procedure for cancer of the head of the pancreas; the pancreas and the spleen are removed, as well as the nearby lymph nodes; the jejunal stump is closed, and a proximal choledochojejunostomy and distal gastrojejunostomy or duodenojejunostomy is performed; pancreatic function is lost

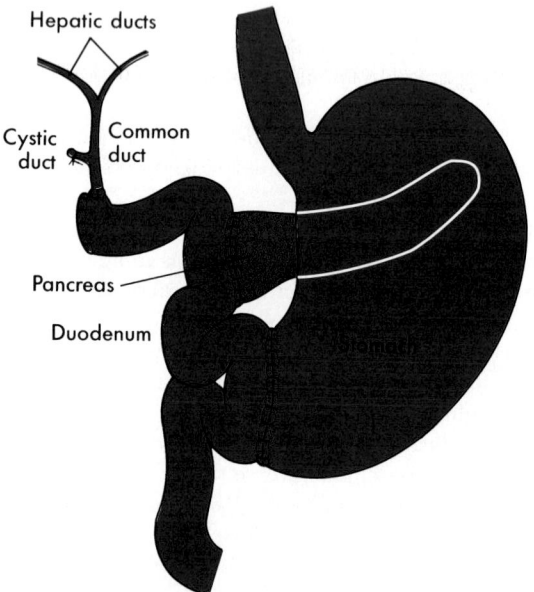

Fig. 15-5 Whipple's procedure, or radical pancreas resection, entails resection of proximal pancreas, adjoining duodenum, distal portion of stomach, and distal segment of common bile duct. Anastomosis of pancreatic duct, common bile duct and stomach to jejunum is done.

(From Beare PG, Myers JL: Adult health nursing, ed 3, St Louis, 1998, Mosby.)

PREOPERATIVE ASSESSMENT AND CARE

Assess respiratory, circulatory, and neurologic status; take baseline vital signs; observe for abdominal distention and peripheral edema

Assess nutritional status and history of substance abuse

Provide nourishing diet as tolerated

Administer parenteral fluids, TPN, and/or blood transfusions as ordered

Insert nasogastric tube and/or indwelling urethral catheter as ordered

Provide emotional support and reinforce physician's explanation of surgical procedure; clarify misconceptions

Administer vitamin K, salt-poor albumin, and antibiotics as ordered

Explain and teach about possibility of insulin and pancreatic enzyme therapy postoperatively

POSTOPERATIVE ASSESSMENT

SUBJECTIVE DATA

Location and character of pain

Nausea

OBJECTIVE DATA

Hypotension, with or without orthostatic changes

Patency of nasogastric tube

Character and amount of the following:

    Gastric drainage

    Wound drainage

    Urine output

    Bile drainage if T tube is in place

Type of parenteral therapy equipment

    Central venous pressure (CVP) line

    TPN line

Tachycardia

Splinting of respirations

Decreased breath sounds

Vomiting

Abdominal distention

DIAGNOSTIC TESTS

Electrolytes, PT/INR, FBS, Hgb, hematocrit (Hct)

Arterial blood gases (ABGs), pH, serum albumin

Serum and urine osmolalities

POTENTIAL COMPLICATIONS

Oliguria

Dehydration

Electrolyte imbalance

Decreased serum albumin levels

Increased PT/INR

Hyperglycemia

Hypoglycemia

Atelectasis

Pneumonia

Elevated temperature

Jaundice

Subdiaphragmatic abscess, intraperitoneal infection

Immunoserologic assay
Serum tumor markers
Stools for steatorrhea
Imaging/nuclear medicine studies
  Chest x-ray
  Abdominal ultrasound
  CT scan, MRI
  Hepatic scintiscan
  Hepatic angiography
Liver biopsy
Paracentesis cytology
Serum alpha-fetoprotein (AFP)

POTENTIAL COMPLICATIONS
Hypoglycemia
Hepatomegaly/splenomegaly, hepatorenal failure
Hematemesis, GI bleeding
Portal hypertension
Jaundice
Ascites
Peripheral edema
Respiratory distress
Change in mental status, hepatic coma

MULTIDISCIPLINARY MANAGEMENT
  THERAPEUTIC MANAGEMENT
Pain management
Antiemetics, antacids
Diuretics
Corticosteroids
Nutritional consult
  Therapeutic diet, parenteral nutrition
Parenteral therapy: fluids, electrolytes, vitamins, albumin
Nasogastric aspiration, irrigation if bleeding
Urethral catheter
Percutaneous hepatic arterial catheter for chemotherapy and chemoembolization (alcohol injection)
Hepatic resection
Liver transplant
Social services

PATIENT PROBLEMS—NURSING DIAGNOSES/INTERVENTIONS

▼Pain related to progression of disease process

Assess nature, intensity, location, duration, and precipitating and alleviating factors
Use consistent pain rating scale *to determine baseline and deviations that indicate intervention is needed*
Assess nonverbal signs of pain
Obtain information from patient regarding past pain experiences and methods used for relief
Control environmental factors that may increase perception of pain: temperature, noise, lighting
Assist patient to achieve comfortable positions
Assist patient to achieve state of minimal physical tension through techniques such as relaxation, music,

visualization, diversion *to decrease need for medication*
Provide a restful environment with opportunities to rest during the day and uninterrupted periods of sleep at night
In collaboration with physician, provide analgesic medications as required, observing for therapeutic and side effects
Discuss and institute noninvasive pain relief measures: relaxation, cutaneous stimulation, distraction, hot/cold therapy

Expected Outcomes
Verbalizes decrease in or relief of pain
Incorporates existing pain while participating in daily activities

▼Altered nutrition: less than body requirements related to anorexia, malnutrition, fatigue

Assess nutritional status daily: weight, electrolytes, total protein, serum albumin, Hgb, skin turgor, muscle mass
Determine amount and types of foods patient likes and is able to tolerate
Provide for oral hygiene before and after meals
Administer anesthetics to oral mucosa before meals prn
Offer high-calorie, high-carbohydrate diet with variation in taste, texture, and presentation of foods *to enhance appetite*
In collaboration with physician, provide oral and parenteral nutritional supplements
Serve frequent, light meals and nutritional, high-calorie snacks
Assist patient to eat if fatigue is a factor
Present meals in an attractive, pleasing manner
Provide a pleasant atmosphere *to increase desire to eat:* encourage significant other(s) to join patient for meals, remove bedpans/urinals from area, maintain well-ventilated room, serve food as soon as it arrives, remove tray as soon as patient finishes eating
In collaboration with clinical dietitian: calculate number of calories and nutrients needed *to maintain/gain weight and support metabolic needs*
Maintain calorie count
Encourage family to bring patient's favorite foods from home
In collaboration with physician, administer antiemetics before meals prn

Expected Outcome
Weight is maintained within 10% of baseline

▼Anticipatory grieving related to changes in physical functioning and poor prognosis

Be sensitive to changes patient is experiencing; encourage patient to express feelings, frustrations, anger, hopes *to begin work of grieving process*

Monitor indwelling urethral catheter and/or T tube and closed gravity drainage system if applicable
Monitor urine output qh; report output of <50 ml/hr to physician *because urine volume decreases in hypovolemia*
Monitor urine for sugar and acetone q4h
Calculate intake and output q8h; report discrepancies and collaborate with physician to correct
Monitor vital signs qh until stable; report hypotension to physician
Encourage frequent movement of legs *to promote venous return*
Monitor electrolytes, glucose, and albumin levels
Monitor urine specific gravity; *>1.030 indicates hypovolemia*
Auscultate abdomen for bowel sounds q4h
Assess effectiveness, side effects of diuretics

Expected Outcomes
Vital signs are stable
Intake and output are balanced
Laboratory studies are within normal limits
Skin turgor is good

▼Altered protection related to abnormal blood profile resulting from coagulation abnormalities and/or bleeding

Monitor incision and dressing q2h for bleeding or drainage; reinforce and change dressing as necessary
Monitor character and color of gastric aspirate and bile drainage for blood
Observe skin, sclera, and urine for jaundice
Provide measures to reduce itching and scratching if present
Monitor PT/INR and liver function levels
Monitor temperature for elevation q4h
Monitor Hgb and Hct

Expected Outcomes
Laboratory values within normal limits
Shows no evidence of bleeding or jaundice

▼Risk for infection, related to inadequate primary defenses

Maintain aseptic technique
Change dressings; observe for signs of infection (redness, swelling, tenderness) and healing process
Monitor temperature q4h, more frequently if elevated
Administer and assess effectiveness of antibiotics and antipyretics
Collect urine specimen for culture/sensitivity when indwelling catheter is removed; initiate voiding measures when needed
Monitor breath sounds, signs of cough, sputum *to assess for pneumonia, atelectasis*

Expected Outcomes

Remains afebrile

Wound is healing adequately

Surrounding tissue is clear, dry, and intact

Lungs are clear

Urine shows no evidence of infection

▼ Pain related to surgical intervention

Assess type, intensity, and location of pain; use pain rating scale

Administer analgesics before pain becomes severe and before treatments

Collaborate with physician about PCA (p. 40)

Assess for effectiveness of pain relief measures

Change position frequently; administer back rubs *to promote comfort and relieve fatigue*

Discuss and teach alternative pain relief techniques: imaging, relaxation, deep breathing

Provide skin care and oral hygiene q4h *to relieve dryness and increase comfort*

Perform passive or assist with and teach active range-of-motion (ROM) exercises q4h

Ambulate with assistance when tolerated *to aid in decreasing gas discomfort*

Provide diversional activities *to reduce attention on pain*

Expected Outcomes

States that pain is decreasing

Appears relaxed

Demonstrates use of alternate pain relief measures

▼ Altered nutrition: less than body requirements related to malnutrition preoperatively, NPO status, and/or anorexia

Continue with TPN as indicated

Auscultate abdomen for return of bowel sounds

Collaborate with physician, nutritionist/registered dietitian and provide water and other clear liquids in small amounts after removal of nasogastric tube; monitor tolerance; progress to soft diet or diabetic diet as tolerated; provide small, frequent meals; measure intake

Administer and assess for effectiveness, side effects of insulin and pancreatic enzymes

Monitor serum glucose

Clamp T tube when ordered and observe for signs of pain, distention, and nausea (see p. 362)

Weigh patient daily (same time, scale, and clothing)

Monitor color, consistency, frequency of stools

Use stool softeners to prevent constipation; discourage straining

Expected Outcomes

Tolerates prescribed diet/TPN

Demonstrates progressive weight gain

Presents serum glucose within normal limits

PATIENT/FAMILY TEACHING

Provide and review written dietary instructions for regular or diabetic diet as needed

Demonstrate insulin administration (p. 431) and blood testing procedures (p. 433)

Discuss signs of hypoglycemia and hyperglycemia (p. 438)

Demonstrate care of T tube if applicable (p. 362)

Discuss medications: name, schedule, dosage, purpose, and side effects; explain importance of taking only medicines prescribed by physician and need to use narcotics discriminately

Explain incisional care and signs of wound infection: pain, redness, swelling, discharge

Provide information about outside sources available for substance abuse rehabilitation

Demonstrate management of TPN if applicable (p. 24)

Discuss use of stool softeners, natural laxatives to prevent constipation

Discuss symptoms to report to physician

   Increased abdominal pain, distention

   Fever, jaundice

   Nausea, vomiting

   Gastric bleeding, tarry stools

   Mucosal bleeding

   Hypoglycemia/hyperglycemia

Encourage follow-up visits with physician

DISCHARGE/HOME CARE PLANNING

Provide information on what supplies and equipment are required and to purchase them

Refer to social medicine for assistance with home care, meal planning, transportation

Demonstrate wound care and observe return demonstration for aseptic technique

Provide names, phone numbers of home health care team members

Evaluate home surroundings for comfort, safety requirements

Encourage patient to seek professional assistance with substance abuse if indicated

■ CANCER OF THE STOMACH

Carcinoma most frequently occurring in the pyloric segment and along the lesser curvature of the stomach; there are no early, definitive signs of the disease process

ASSESSMENT

SUBJECTIVE DATA

Feeling of fullness after eating, early satiety

Indigestion

Belching

Epigastric pain or discomfort after eating

Loss of appetite

Malaise, fatigue

PATIENT PROBLEMS—NURSING DIAGNOSES/INTERVENTIONS

▼ Pain related to progression of disease process

Assess nature, intensity, location, duration, and precipitating and alleviating factors

Use consistent pain rating scale *to determine baseline and deviations that indicate intervention is needed*

Assess nonverbal signs of pain particular to patient

Obtain information from patient regarding past pain experiences and methods used for relief

Control environmental factors that may increase perception of pain: temperature, noise, lighting

Assist patient to achieve comfortable positions

Assist patient to achieve state of minimal physical tension through techniques such as relaxation, music, visualization, diversion *to decrease need for medication*

Provide a restful environment with opportunities to rest during the day and uninterrupted periods of sleep at night

In collaboration with physician, provide analgesic medications as required, observing for therapeutic and side effects

Discuss and institute noninvasive pain relief measures; relaxation, cutaneous stimulation, distraction, hot/cold therapy

Expected Outcomes

Verbalizes decrease in/relief of pain

Able to incorporate existing pain while participating in daily activities

▼ Altered nutrition: less than body requirements related to anorexia, insulin secretion disorder, nausea, diarrhea, fatigue

Assess nutritional status daily: weight, electrolytes, total protein, serum albumin, Hgb, skin turgor, muscle mass

Determine amount and types of foods patient likes and is able to tolerate

Provide for oral hygiene before and after meals

Administer anesthetics to oral mucosa before meals prn

Offer high-calorie, high-protein diet with variation in taste, texture, and presentation of foods *to enhance appetite*

In collaboration with physician, provide oral and parenteral nutritional supplements

Serve frequent, light meals and nutritional, high-calorie snacks

Assist patient to eat if fatigue is a factor

Present meals in an attractive, pleasing manner

Provide a pleasant atmosphere *to increase desire to eat:* encourage significant other(s) to join patient for meals, remove bedpans/urinals from area, maintain well-ventilated room, serve food as soon as it arrives, remove tray as soon as patient finishes eating

General weakness

Dizziness (vertigo, syncope)

Nausea

OBJECTIVE DATA

Dysphagia

Weight loss

Pallor

Vomiting

Occult blood in stool

RISK FACTORS

Chronic excessive alcohol intake

Drinking and eating very hot, spicy foods, meats cured
   with nitrates/nitrites

Exposure to foods containing nitrates, nitrites

Nutritional deficiency: limited intake of vitamins A, C, E,
   and dairy products

Peptic ulcer disease

Exposure to asbestos, coal, rubber, timber, nickel

Family history

   Pernicious anemia

   Gastric polyps

   Gastritis

   Alchlorhydria

   Gastric cancer

DIAGNOSTIC TESTS

CBC, Hct

Plasma tumor markers

Stool for occult blood

Gastric content analysis

Imaging studies

   Upper GI series

   Endoscopy with biopsy and cytology

   Chest radiography

   CT scan

   Ultrasound

   Endoscopic ultrasound

POTENTIAL COMPLICATIONS

Malnutrition

Fluid and electrolyte imbalance

Hematemesis

Pyloric obstruction

Enlarged axillary, supraclavicular lymph nodes

Epigastric mass

Recurrent phlebitis

Metastasis to the liver

MULTIDISCIPLINARY MANAGEMENT
THERAPEUTIC MANAGEMENT

Pain management

Parenteral fluids, TPN

Radiation therapy

Chemotherapy (see Table 15-8, p. 864)

Surgery: gastric resection, gastrectomy

Clinical dietitian consult

Social services, support group

PATIENT PROBLEMS—NURSING DIAGNOSES/INTERVENTIONS

▼Altered nutrition: less than body requirements
   related to dysphagia, anorexia, nausea, vomiting

Assess nutritional status daily: weight, electrolytes, total
   protein, serum albumin, Hgb, skin turgor, muscle
   mass

Consult occupational therapist *to assess patient's ability
   to masticate and swallow*

Determine amount and types of foods patient likes and is
   able to tolerate

Provide for oral hygiene before and after meals

Administer anesthetics to oral mucosa before meals prn

Offer high-calorie, high-protein diet with variation in
   taste, texture, and presentation of foods *to enhance
   appetite*

In collaboration with physician, provide oral and
   parenteral nutritional supplements

Serve frequent, light meals and nutritional, high-calorie
   snacks

Assist patient to eat if fatigue is a factor

Present meals in an attractive, pleasing manner

Provide a pleasant atmosphere *to increase desire
   to eat:* encourage significant other(s) to join patient
   for meals, remove bedpans/urinals from area,
   maintain well-ventilated room, serve food as soon
   as it arrives, remove tray as soon as patient finishes
   eating

In collaboration with clinical dietitian: calculate number
   of calories and nutrients needed *to maintain/gain
   weight and support metabolic needs*

Maintain calorie count

Encourage family to bring patient's favorite foods from
   home

In collaboration with physician, administer antiemetics
   before meals prn

Expected Outcome

Maintains weight within 10% of baseline

▼Pain related to progression of disease process

Assess nature, intensity, location, duration, and
   precipitating and alleviating factors

Use consistent pain rating scale *to determine baseline
   and deviations that indicate intervention is
   needed*

Assess nonverbal signs of pain particular to patient *so
   that early signs can be noted and treatment
   started*

Obtain information from patient regarding past pain
   experiences and methods used for relief

Control environmental factors that may increase
   perception of pain: temperature, noise, lighting

Assist patient to achieve comfortable positions

Assist patient to achieve state of minimal physical tension
   through techniques such as relaxation, music,

visualization, diversion *to decrease need for medication*

Provide a restful environment with opportunities to rest during the day and uninterrupted periods of sleep at night

In collaboration with physician provide analgesic medications as required, observing for therapeutic and side effects

Discuss and institute noninvasive pain relief measures: relaxation, cutaneous stimulation, distraction, hot/cold therapy

Expected Outcomes

Verbalizes decrease in or relief of pain

Incorporates existing pain while participating in daily activities

▼Anticipatory grieving, related to lifestyle changes, decreased physical abilities, changes in physical appearance, life-threatening prognosis

Be sensitive to changes patient is experiencing; encourage patient to express feelings, frustrations, anger, hopes *to begin work of grieving process*

Provide a therapeutic environment conducive to open discussion: actively listen, perceive nonverbal cues, be patient and empathetic *to facilitate trust*

Encourage questions and provide information freely as patient expresses the desire for knowledge about the disease, treatments, and prognosis *to ease fear of the unknown*

Set limits on maladaptive coping behaviors if they interfere with patient's well-being

Support adaptive behaviors that suggest progression and resolution of the grieving process

Provide opportunities for private, uninterrupted time with significant other(s)

Assist in identifying ways to adapt lifestyle as condition changes *to enhance participation and feelings of control*

Provide information regarding support groups for patient and significant other(s)

Collaborate with other professionals (social worker, clergy, psychologist, psychiatrist) *to provide support and facilitate grieving process*

Provide reference for financial assistance, answers to questions regarding medical insurance

Provide information to assist patient in completing advanced directive or similar document *to ensure patient wishes are known to significant others and care providers*

Expected Outcomes

Progresses through stages of the grieving process and moves toward acceptance

Demonstrates effective coping mechanisms; participates in decisions about own future

PATIENT/FAMILY TEACHING

Reinforce physician's explanation of disease and treatment plan

In collaboration with clinical dietitian explain nutrition plan consistent with patient's condition, provide written instructions and menu plans

Discuss management of dumping syndrome

Identify with patient support systems, community resources, and support groups

Discuss medication regimen, actions, side effects, and potential adverse reactions to report to physician

Explain importance of keeping follow-up appointments with care providers and diagnostic, therapeutic visits

DISCHARGE/HOME CARE PLANNING

Assess patient's ability for self-care; contact home health agency for support as needed

Assess transportation needs to maintain follow-up care

Assess ability to shop, cook, clean; arrange assistance as needed

Discuss importance of ongoing outpatient care, continued interaction with others who are supportive

■ CANCER OF THE PROSTATE

Cancer of the prostate represents the most common malignancy in the United States, accounting for 41% of all newly diagnosed cancer in men; median age at diagnosis is 72, with the incidence rate increasing each decade after age 50; incidence rate is nearly twice that of the population in black men and the death rate is almost 3 times greater

Treatment can include prostatectomy, radiation, hormone therapy, cryotherapy, and chemotherapy

ASSESSMENT
SUBJECTIVE DATA

Early signs
    Urinary hesitancy
    Dysuria
    Urgency
    Straining to start stream
Later signs
    Hematuria
    Chronic urinary retention with dribbling
    Bone and neuritic pain
    Weight loss, lethargy
    Low back pain

OBJECTIVE DATA

Prostatic hypertrophy
Decreased strength of stream
Hematuria
Bladder distention
Foul smelling urine
Decreased urinary output

Table 15-5	**Prostate Cancer Staging Systems**	
Whitmore-Jewett	Description	AJCC
A	*Incidental finding of carcinoma on examination of prostate tissue after prostatectomy or transurethral resection*	T1
A$_1$	Histologically well- or moderately well–differentiated tumor or tumor consisting of <5% of resected specimen	T1a
A$_2$	Histologically poorly differentiated or anaplastic tumor or tumor consisting of >5% of resected specimen	T1b
B	*Clinically palpable tumor confined to prostate*	T2
B$_1$	Focal ≤1.5 cm	T2a
B$_2$	Diffuse >1.5, cm ≥ two foci	T2b
C	*Extension beyond prostate capsule to seminal vesicles or contiguous tissue*	T3
D	*Metastatic tumor*	N-M
D$_1$	Regional nodal involvement	M1 to M3
D$_2$	Metastasis to any of the following: Bone Lymph nodes above aortic bifurcation Other organ(s)	M

From Otto, SE: Oncology nursing, *ed 3, St Louis, 1999, Mosby.*

RISK FACTORS

Advancing age: usually over 50 years
Male relative with prostate cancer
African-American men
Post vasectomy

DIAGNOSTIC TESTS

Digital rectal exam (DRE)
Imaging
    Transrectal ultrasonography
    MRI
    CT scan
Biopsy
Prostate cancer staging systems (Whitmore-Jewett and American Joint Commission on Cancer [AJCC]) (Table 15-5)
Biologic markers
    Prostate-specific antigen (PSA) level
    AFP and human chorionic gonadotropin (HCG)
Acid/alkaline phosphatase

POTENTIAL COMPLICATIONS

Hemorrhage, shock
Wound infection
Metastasis

MULTIDISCIPLINARY MANAGEMENT
PREVENTION/DETECTION TEACHING

Instruct regarding time frames for periodic examination by health care provider including DRE at age 40
Discuss signs and symptoms to report to physician
Explain importance of not ignoring symptoms

THERAPEUTIC MANAGEMENT

Prostatectomy (p. 633)
Bilateral orchiectomy
Hormonal therapy
    Estrogens (diethylstilbestrol [DES]), leutinizing hormone–releasing hormone (LHRH) analogues, progestational agents, antiandrogens (flutamide [Eulexin, Casodex])
Ketoconazole
Aminoglutethimide
Radiation; external beam radiotherapy, brachytherapy (interstitial implantation of radioisotopes)
Chemotherapy (see Table 15-8, p. 864)
Cryotherapy
Sexual counseling
Social services

PATIENT PROBLEMS—NURSING DIAGNOSIS/INTERVENTIONS

▼ Sexual dysfunction related to potential erectile dysfunction

Support readiness to discuss sexual concerns; use open-ended statements and questions
Encourage spouse/caregiver to discuss concerns with patient
Confer with social services and give appropriate referral information to patient and significant other

Expected Outcome

Expresses feelings and discusses sexuality with health care provider and significant other

Refer to applicable therapeutic management for other nursing diagnoses, care, teaching, and home care considerations
Prostatectomy, p. 633
Orchiectomy, p. 832
Rediation, p. 855
Chemotherapy, p. 862

■ CANCER OF THE TESTICLE/ORCHIECTOMY

Cancer of the testicle is the most common cancer in males age 15 to 35 years; however, testicular cancers occur in men of all ages. 50% of testicular cancers occur in men close to the age of 40 years. The incidence is four times greater in whites than blacks; 97% of the cancers are germ cell, which carries a 3-year survival rate of 96% when detected and treated in its early stages

Surgical removal of the testis is most commonly performed in the presence of testicular cancer via an inguinal incision; for more advanced nonseminomatous germ cell cancer, a retroperitoneal lymph node dissection may be necessary

ASSESSMENT
SUBJECTIVE DATA
Detection
"Dragging" pain in lower back and abdomen
Malaise
Diffuse pain/discomfort in testes

Postoperative
Pain at operative site
Anxiety; fear

OBJECTIVE DATA
Detection
Testicular mass, palpable hardness
Testicular swelling, thickness
Scrotal edema, discoloration
Weight loss
Gynecomastia, nipple pigmentation
Elevated temperature

Postoperative
Hemorrhage
Swelling at operative site
Discoloration at operative site
Condition of suture line
Wound drains: amount, character of drainage
Body temperature elevation
Pulmonary status
Hydration status
Behavioral signs of pain, fear, anxiety, anger, frustration

RISK FACTORS
Age: 15 to 40 years
Cryptorchism (undescended testis)

Previously atrophic testes
Childhood hernia and other genitourinary anomalies
Trauma
Orchitis, especially mumps
Family history of testicular cancer: father, brother
Klinefelter's syndrome
Exposure in utero to diethystilbesterol (DES)

DIAGNOSTIC TESTS
AFP and HCG for tumor markers
Urine for "pregnancy" test
Plasma tumor markers
Imaging/nuclear medicine studies
    Intravenous urography (IVU)
    CT scan
    Radionuclide study
    Testicular ultrasound
Lymphangiogram

POTENTIAL COMPLICATIONS
Hemorrhage, shock
Wound infection
Atelectasis, pneumonia
Metastasis; radical lymph node dissection

MULTIDISCIPLINARY MANAGEMENT
PREVENTION/DETECTION TEACHING
Instruct regarding time frame for periodic examination by health care provider
Discuss signs and symptoms to report to physician
Explain importance and technique for performing testicular self-examination (beginning at age 15 or before if family history) (Fig. 15-6)
    Technique: perform after warm shower/bath with relaxed scrotal skin
    In standing position
        Place middle and index fingers below one testis with thumb on top
        Gently roll testis between thumb and finger
            Normal findings: rubbery, spongy, smooth, no lumps
            Abnormal findings: hard, painless nodule, usually on lateral or anterior surface
        Hold one testicle in palm of hand, then the other; note weight differences

THERAPEUTIC MANAGEMENT
Radiation therapy for seminomatous germ cell tumor
Chemotherapy (see Table 15-8, p. 864)
Bone marrow transplant
Surgical intervention
Postoperative management (lymph node dissection)
NPO until bowel sounds are active
Nasogastric tube: *most patients experience postoperative ileus*
Parenteral fluids until liquids are tolerated
Routine postoperative vital signs
Analgesics, antibiotics

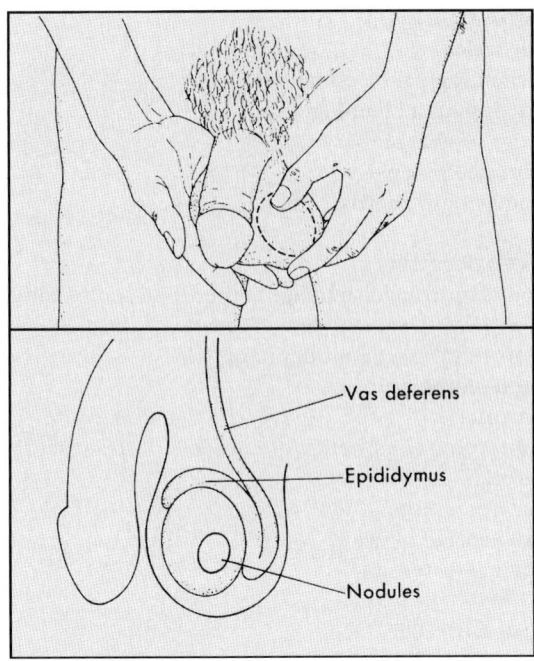

Fig. 15-6 Testicular self-examination.

Scrotal support
Sexual counseling
Social services, support group

PATIENT PROBLEMS—NURSING DIAGNOSES/INTERVENTIONS

▼Pain related to scrotal swelling, surgical intervention

Assess nature, intensity, location, duration, and
    precipitating and alleviating factors
Use consistent pain rating scale *to determine baseline
    and deviations that indicate intervention is needed*
Assess nonverbal signs of pain particular to patient *so
    that early signs can be noted and treatment started*
Obtain information from patient regarding past pain
    experiences and methods used for relief
Control environmental factors that may increase
    perception of pain: temperature, noise, lighting
Assist patient to achieve comfortable positions
Provide topical cooling and scrotal support measures
Assist patient to achieve state of minimal physical tension
    through techniques such as relaxation, music,
    visualization, diversion *to decrease need for
    medication*
Provide a restful environment with opportunities to rest
    during the day and uninterrupted periods of sleep at
    night
In collaboration with physician provide analgesic
    medications as required, observing for therapeutic and
    side effects
Discuss and institute noninvasive pain relief measures:
    relaxation, cutaneous stimulation, distraction

Expected Outcomes
Verbalizes decrease in or relief of pain
Incorporates existing pain while participating in daily
    activities

▼Anticipatory grieving related to lifestyle changes,
decreased physical abilities, changes in physical
appearance, life-threatening prognosis

Be sensitive to changes patient is experiencing;
    encourage patient to express feelings, frustrations,
    anger, hopes *to begin work of grieving process*
Provide a therapeutic environment conducive to open
    discussion: actively listen, perceive nonverbal cues, be
    patient and empathetic *to facilitate trust*
Encourage questions and provide information freely as
    patient expresses the desire for knowledge about the
    disease, treatments, and prognosis *to ease fear of the
    unknown*
Set limits on maladaptive coping behaviors if they
    interfere with patient's well-being
Support adaptive behaviors that suggest progression and
    resolution of the grieving process
Provide opportunities for private, uninterrupted time
    with significant other(s)
Assist in identifying ways to adapt lifestyle as condition
    changes *to enhance participation and feelings of
    control*
Provide information regarding support groups for patient
    and significant other(s)
Collaborate with other professionals (social worker,
    clergy, psychologist, psychiatrist) *to provide support
    and facilitate grieving process*
Provide reference for financial assistance, answers to
    questions regarding medical insurance

Expected Outcomes
Progresses through stages of the grieving process and
    moves toward acceptance
Demonstrates effective coping mechanisms; participates
    in decisions about own future

▼Risk for infection related to suppressed immune
system

Screen personnel and visitors for symptoms of infection
Use strict sterile technique for all invasive procedures
Monitor sites of invasive lines/tubes/drains for signs of
    infection q8h
Check body fluids for alteration in color, odor, consistency
Ensure excellent personal hygiene is maintained,
    especially after bowel movements
Provide uninterrupted periods of sleep and rest
Ensure required fluid/nutrient intake, supplement with
    total oral nutrition products prn, institute calorie count
    prn *to maintain weight within 10% of baseline*
Record intake and output
Monitor vital signs, especially temperature, q4h and prn
Monitor CBC, WBC results per physician order

Administer antibiotics, sulfa-type medications, and other antiinfectives as ordered

Maintain skin integrity *to prevent entry of microorganisms*

Auscultate breath sounds q8h

Encourage clearance of pulmonary secretions: turn, cough, deep breathe q2h; use incentive spirometer qh

Maintain intact mucous membranes: scrupulous oral care using soft instruments q4h and prn

Expected Outcomes

Improvement, resolution of current infections

New infections do not develop

▼Acute urinary retention related to scrotal swelling

Measure urine output every void; assess abdomen for bladder distension

Request patient to inform nurse of bladder fullness and inability to void

Promote measures to facilitate bladder emptying

Ensure privacy, comfortable position for voiding

Run tap water, flush toilet

Place hands in warm water, running water

Pour warm water over penis

Apply heat to suprapubic area

Assist patient to use relaxation techniques

Crede bladder

Stroke inner aspect of thigh with ice

Catheterize patient per physician order

Expected Outcomes

Able to empty bladder without use of indwelling catheter

Bladder distension and urinary retention are prevented

PATIENT/FAMILY TEACHING
Postdiagnosis, postoperative

Avoid constipation

Care of surgical incision

Avoid heavy lifting/straining until cleared by physician

Report signs and symptoms to physician: incision pain, redness, swelling, drainage, elevated temperature

Medication/chemotherapy/radiation therapy regimen: expected therapeutic effects, side effects, potential adverse reactions; management of side and/or adverse effects

Need to resume usual daily routine as soon as possible

■ CANCER OF THE UTERUS/ RADICAL HYSTERECTOMY

ASSESSMENT
SUBJECTIVE DATA
Detection

Lower abdominal and back pain (late disease)

Postoperative

Pain at surgical site

OBJECTIVE DATA
Detection

Abnormal vaginal bleeding

Postmenopausal bleeding

Purulent discharge

Endometrial polyps

Enlarged, boggy uterus

Postoperative

Vaginal hemorrhage, drainage (other than serous); foul odor

Incision: redness, edema, drainage

Elevated temperature

Tachycardia

Amount, color, consistency of contents of surgical drains

Hematuria

Urinary retention

Vaginal leakage of urine

Abdominal distension

RISK FACTORS

Age: over 50 years

Menstrual irregularities

Infertility, anovulation

Nulliparous

Late menopause

Long-term, nonconjugated estrogen use

Obesity, hypertension

Diabetes

Adenomatous hyperplasia

DIAGNOSTIC TESTS

Endometrial biopsy or fractional dilation and curettage (D & C)

Laparotomy with sampling of peritoneal fluid or washings

POTENTIAL COMPLICATIONS

Hemorrhage

UTI

Constipation, paralytic ileus

Pneumonia

Thrombophlebitis

Pulmonary embolus

Wound infection

Ureteral fistula

Ureter ligation

Metastatic disease: low back pain; decreased urine output

Lymphocyst

MULTIDISCIPLINARY MANAGEMENT
PREVENTION/DETECTION TEACHING

Discuss importance of maintaining accurate menstrual cycle history

Frequency, length

Amount, color

Explain importance of routine pelvic examinations

THERAPEUTIC MANAGEMENT

Radiation therapy

Chemotherapy (see Table 15-8, p. 864)

Surgical intervention
Sexual counseling
Social services; support group

PATIENT PROBLEMS—NURSING DIAGNOSES/INTERVENTIONS

▼ Anticipatory grieving related to lifestyle changes, decreased physical abilities, changes in physical appearance, life-threatening prognosis

Be sensitive to changes patient is experiencing; encourage patient to express feelings, frustrations, anger, hopes *to begin work of grieving process*

Provide a therapeutic environment conducive to open discussion: actively listen, perceive nonverbal cues, be patient and empathetic *to facilitate trust*

Encourage questions and provide information freely as patient expresses the desire for knowledge about the disease, treatments, and prognosis *to ease fear of the unknown*

Set limits on maladaptive coping behaviors if they interfere with patient's well-being

Support adaptive behaviors that suggest progression and resolution of the grieving process

Provide opportunities for private, uninterrupted time with significant other(s)

Assist in identifying ways to adapt lifestyle as condition changes *to enhance participation and feelings of control*

Provide information regarding support groups for patient and significant other(s)

Collaborate with other professionals (social worker, clergy, psychologist, psychiatrist) *to provide support and facilitate grieving process*

Provide reference for financial assistance, answers to questions regarding medical insurance

Provide information to assist patient in completing advance directive or similar document *to ensure patient wishes are known to significant others and care providers*

Expected Outcomes

Progresses through stages of the grieving process and moves toward acceptance

Demonstrates effective coping mechanisms; participates in decisions about own future

▼ Pain related to progression of disease process, surgical intervention

Assess nature, intensity, location, duration, and precipitating and alleviating factors

Use consistent pain rating scale *to determine baseline and deviations that indicate intervention is needed*

Assess nonverbal signs of pain particular to patient *so that early signs can be noted and treatment started*

Obtain information from patient regarding past pain experiences and methods used for relief

Control environmental factors that may increase perception of pain: temperature, noise, lighting

Assist patient to achieve comfortable positions

Assist patient to achieve state of minimal physical tension through techniques such as relaxation, music, visualization, diversion *to decrease need for medication*

Provide a restful environment with opportunities to rest during the day and uninterrupted periods of sleep at night

In collaboration with physician provide analgesic medications as required, observing for therapeutic and side effects

Discuss and institute noninvasive pain relief measures: relaxation, cutaneous stimulation, distraction, hot/cold therapy

Expected Outcomes

Verbalizes decrease in or relief of pain

Incorporates existing pain while participating in daily activities

PATIENT/FAMILY TEACHING
Postoperative

Avoid constipation; use stool softeners, laxatives per physician order

Teach care of suprapubic or indwelling ureteral catheter if patient will be discharged with catheter in place

Teach clean, intermittent, self-catheterization as required

Discuss restrictions: no intercourse, tampons, douching, tub baths for 4 to 6 weeks as indicated by physician

Avoid prolonged sitting, jarring activities, driving, heavy lifting, vacuuming for 6 weeks as indicated by physician

Discuss symptoms to report to physician: elevated temperature, vaginal bleeding, abdominal cramps, difficulty urinating, change in bowel habits

Discuss that remaining vagina will stretch with sexual intercourse, and normal relations will be possible

DISCHARGE/HOME CARE PLANNING

Discuss community resource/support groups for women with cancer/hysterectomy; sexual counseling

Plan for sufficient, clean space to store medical supplies as required

Assess ability to provide for physical and daily living needs: arrange home health provider as needed

Assess transportation availability to follow-up appointments; assist with arrangement as necessary

Reinforce need to continue relationships with supportive people

■ CANCER OF UTERUS/ PELVIC EXENTERATION

total exenteration: Removal of all reproductive organs and adjacent tissues; radical hysterectomy, pelvic node dissection, cystectomy with formation of urinary conduit, vaginectomy, and resection of the rectum with colostomy

anterior exenteration: Excludes rectal resection with colostomy

posterior exenteration: Excludes cystectomy with urinary conduit

POSTOPERATIVE ASSESSMENT
SUBJECTIVE DATA
Pain (may describe level and location)

OBJECTIVE DATA
Incision site: redness, edema, drainage
Colostomy, ileostomy, urinary diversion
    Condition of stoma and surrounding skin
    Amount, color, character of output
Elevated temperature
Vital signs: tachycardia, hypotension
Lower extremity edema
Character of popliteal/pedal pulses
Intake and output balance

POTENTIAL COMPLICATIONS
First 48 hours: hemorrhage
Days 2 to 4: infection
Days 5 to 21: urinary or GI fistula
Shock
Fluid/electrolyte imbalance
Paralytic ileus
Thrombophlebitis
Pulmonary embolus
Pneumonia
Sepsis

MULTIDISCIPLINARY MANAGEMENT
THERAPEUTIC MANAGEMENT
Pain management; PCA pump
Parenteral therapy/nutrition
Administration of blood/blood components
Management of ostomies
Sexual counseling
Wound, Ostomy, Continence/ET Nurse consult
Social services, support group

PATIENT PROBLEMS—NURSING DIAGNOSES/INTERVENTIONS

▼Anticipatory grieving related to lifestyle changes, decreased physical abilities, changes in physical appearance, life-threatening prognosis

Be sensitive to changes patient is experiencing; encourage patient to express feelings, frustrations, anger, hopes *to begin work of grieving process*
Provide a therapeutic environment conducive to open discussion: actively listen, perceive nonverbal cues, be patient and empathetic *to facilitate trust*
Encourage questions and provide information freely as patient expresses the desire for knowledge about the disease, treatments, and prognosis *to ease fear of the unknown*

Set limits on maladaptive coping behaviors if they interfere with patient's well-being
Support adaptive behaviors that suggest progression and resolution of the grieving process
Provide opportunities for private, uninterrupted time with significant other(s)
Assist in identifying ways to adapt lifestyle as condition changes *to enhance participation and feelings of control*
Provide information regarding support groups for patient and significant other(s)
Collaborate with other professionals (social worker, clergy, psychologist, psychiatrist) *to provide support and facilitate grieving process*
Provide reference for financial assistance, answers to questions regarding medical insurance
Provide information to assist patient in completing advanced directive or similar document *to ensure patient wishes are known to significant others and care providers*

Expected Outcomes
Progresses through stages of the grieving process and moves toward acceptance
Demonstrates effective coping mechanisms; participates in decisions about own future

▼Pain related to disease process and surgical intervention

Assess nature, intensity, location, duration, and precipitating and alleviating factors
Use consistent pain rating scale *to determine baseline and deviations that indicate intervention is needed*
Assess nonverbal signs of pain particular to patient *so that early signs can be noted and treatment started*
Obtain information from patient regarding past pain experiences and methods used for relief
Control environmental factors that may increase perception of pain: temperature, noise, lighting
Assist patient to achieve comfortable positions
Assist patient to achieve state of minimal physical tension through techniques such as relaxation, music, visualization, diversion *to decrease need for medication*
Provide a restful environment with opportunities to rest during the day and uninterrupted periods of sleep at night
In collaboration with physician provide analgesic medications as required, observing for therapeutic and side effects
Discuss and institute noninvasive pain relief measures: relaxation, cutaneous stimulation, distraction, hot/cold therapy

Expected Outcomes
Verbalizes decrease in or relief of pain
Incorporates existing pain while participating in daily activities

Additional Nursing Diagnoses to Consider

Body image disturbance related to changes in physical appearance and functioning

Altered sexuality patterns, related to physical changes associated with surgical procedure, limitations imposed by symptoms (fatigue, decreased libido)

PATIENT/FAMILY TEACHING

Preoperative

Consult with enterostomal therapist to explain ostomy/urinary diversion that will be created: demonstrate with model devices that will be used to hold output, location on abdomen

Discuss purpose of different drains and tubes that may be in place postoperatively

Discuss patient concerns related to sexuality, possible vaginal reconstruction

If patient desires, facilitate visit from patient who has recovered from similar surgery

Postoperative

Teach and have patient return demonstrate care of colostomy and urinary diversion and surgical wounds

Discuss perineal care, importance of sitz baths bid and prn

Explain signs and symptoms to report to physician
Unusual odor, drainage
Fresh bleeding
Unusual pain
Elevated temperature
URI

Discuss importance of balance between rest and activity; avoid prolonged sitting

Consult with clinical dietitian to plan high-protein, high-carbohydrate meals consistent with physical condition and preferences

Administer parenteral nutrition as required

Explain medications: administration, expected therapeutic effects, potential side effects, and potential adverse reactions

Manage side/adverse effects

DISCHARGE/HOME CARE PLANNING

Arrange home health nurse for continued support and teaching related to ostomy care and parenteral nutrition administration

Assess patient's and/or family's ability to provide physical care and ability to provide for daily living needs; arrange home health provider prn

Assess transportation availability to follow-up appointments; assist with arrangements prn

Plan for sufficient, clean space for storage of medical supplies

Assist patient to access support community groups for women with cancer, persons with ostomies, sexual counseling

■ CHORIOCARCINOMA

Highly malignant neoplasm derived from chorionic epithelium; may develop after a hydatidiform mole, miscarriage, or full-term delivery

ASSESSMENT

OBSERVATIONS/FINDINGS

Amenorrhea
Profuse and/or intermittent vaginal bleeding
Malodorous vaginal discharge between menses
Cough
Hemoptysis
Headache
Irritability
Nausea, vomiting
Hypertension
Tachypnea
Orthopnea
Vaginal or vulvar lesion
Anemia
Sepsis
Cachexia
Weight loss
Positive pregnancy test

DIAGNOSTIC TESTS

Rising HCG titer
Ultrasonography

POTENTIAL COMPLICATIONS

Metastasis (lung, kidney, central nervous system [CNS], liver)

MULTIDISCIPLINARY MANAGEMENT

THERAPEUTIC MANAGEMENT

Total abdominal hysterectomy and bilateral salpingo-oophorectomy (TAH-BSO)

Antineoplastic chemotherapy (methotrexate, actinomycin D, cytoxan)

Contraception

Social services, counseling

PATIENT PROBLEMS—NURSING DIAGNOSES/INTERVENTIONS

See Total abdominal hysterectomy/Bilateral salpingo-oophorectomy (TAH-BSO) (p. 672)
See Chemotherapy (p. 862 and Table 15-8, p. 864)

■ OVARIAN CANCER

Accounts for 4% of female cancers. Epithelial cell is the most common histologic type (70%) and is most often seen in women aged 70 and above; germ cell type is seen in women ages 10 to 25 years

ASSESSMENT

RISK FACTORS

Upper socioeconomic status
Hormonal factors
　Nulliparous

Older at first parity
Reduced fertility
Infertility
Exogenous therapy
Exposure to carcinogens
　Radiation
　Asbestos
History of breast cancer
Family history of breast, colon, or ovarian cancer
History of the following:
　Pentz-Jeghers syndrome
　Mucocutaneous pigmentation
　Intestinal polyps

SUBJECTIVE DATA
Dyspepsia
Vague abdominal discomfort
Pelvic pressure
Urinary frequency

OBJECTIVE DATA
Change in abdominal girth, distention
Bilateral or unilateral, irregular, immobile ovarian mass
Palpable ovaries after menopause
Adnexal thickening: postmenopausal or nulliparous women
Constipation, obstipation
Nausea, early satiety
Advanced disease
　Weight loss
　Pleural/abdominal effusions
　Bowel obstruction
　Anemia
　Malnutrition

DIAGNOSTIC TESTS
Tumor markers; HCG, AFP
Ultrasound
Serum CA-125

MULTIDISCIPLINARY MANAGEMENT
PREVENTION/DETECTION TEACHING
Oral contraceptives decrease risk
Breast feeding decreases risk
Genetic counseling if first-degree relative with ovarian
　cancer
Ensure that patient and significant other know and
　understand the following:
　Risk factors
　Importance of maintaining accurate menstrual cycle
　　history
　　Frequency
　　Length of menses
　　Amount
　　Color
　Need for regular, periodic gynecologic examinations
Annual pelvic examination
Signs and symptoms to report to physician
Early detection is rare (no early symptoms)

THERAPEUTIC MANAGEMENT
See specific surgery
　Chemotherapy, p. 862
　　Table 15-8, p. 864
　Radiotherapy, p. 855
　Surgical intervention (TAH/BSO)
Social services

PATIENT PROBLEMS—NURSING DIAGNOSIS/INTERVENTIONS
See type of therapeutic management for patient care

■ CANCER OF THE VULVA/VULVECTOMY
Cancer of the vulva is an uncommon tumor, accounting for 5% of all gynecologic tumors; 86% of these tumors are squamous cell; surgical intervention may include skinning vulvectomy with skin graft (excision of the upper layers of the vulva and placement of a skin graft from the buttocks or thigh), vulvectomy with lymphadenectomy, excision of the vulva (labia majora/minora, clitoris, surrounding tissue) and pelvic lymph nodes

ASSESSMENT
SUBJECTIVE DATA
Itching/skin irritation; pain in the vulvar area

OBJECTIVE DATA
Mass, lesion, lump on vulva
Postoperative
　Condition of incision, graft site
　Lower extremities for edema, pulses (pedal, popliteal)
　Constipation or impaction
　Anemia

RISK FACTORS
Age: 70 years and older
Obesity
Hypertension
Smoking
Diabetes
Early menopause
Cervical cancer
Multiple sexual partners or single partner who has had
　multiple partners
Sexually transmitted diseases
Long-term pruritus
Immunosuppression

DIAGNOSTIC TESTS
Biopsy of lesions

POTENTIAL COMPLICATIONS
Wound breakdown/graft failure
Lymphedema
UTI
Metastatic disease

MULTIDISCIPLINARY MANAGEMENT

PREVENTION/DETECTION TEACHING

Need for regular, periodic gynecologic examinations

Importance of maintaining good gynecologic hygiene

Need for periodic self-examination

THERAPEUTIC MANAGEMENT

Electrocautery, cryosurgery

Laser treatment

Radiation therapy
   External beam
   Internal implant

Chemotherapy

Surgical intervention
   Wide local incision
   Simple/radical vulvectomy with pelvic
      lymphadenectomy, groin node dissection
   Skinning vulvectomy

Psychologic support

Social services

Sexual counseling

Consult with Wound, Ostomy, Continence/ET Nurse

Dietitian consultation

PATIENT PROBLEMS—NURSING DIAGNOSES/INTERVENTIONS

▼Pain related to progression of disease process

Assess nature, intensity, location, duration, and
   precipitating and alleviating factors

Use consistent pain rating scale *to determine baseline
   and deviations that indicate intervention is needed*

Assess nonverbal signs of pain particular to patient *so
   that early signs can be noted and treatment started*

Obtain information from patient regarding past pain
   experiences and methods used for relief

Control environmental factors that may increase
   perception of pain: temperature, noise, lighting

Assist patient to achieve comfortable positions

Assist patient to achieve state of minimal physical tension
   through techniques such as relaxation, music,
   visualization, diversion *to decrease need for
   medication*

Provide a restful environment with opportunities to rest
   during the day and uninterrupted periods of sleep at
   night

In collaboration with physician provide analgesic
   medications as required, observing for therapeutic and
   side effects

Discuss and institute noninvasive pain relief measures:
   relaxation, cutaneous stimulation, distraction, hot/cold
   therapy

Expected Outcomes

Verbalizes decrease in or relief of pain

Incorporates existing pain while participating in daily
   activities

▼Anticipatory grieving related to lifestyle changes,
decreased physical abilities, changes in physical
appearance, life threatening prognosis

Be sensitive to changes patient is experiencing;
   encourage patient to express feelings, frustrations,
   anger, hopes *to begin work of grieving process*

Provide a therapeutic environment conducive to open
   discussion: actively listen, perceive nonverbal cues, be
   patient and empathetic *to facilitate trust*

Encourage questions and provide information freely as
   patient expresses the desire for knowledge about the
   disease, treatments, and prognosis *to ease fear of the
   unknown*

Set limits on maladaptive coping behaviors if they
   interfere with patient's well-being

Support adaptive behaviors that suggest progression and
   resolution of the grieving process

Provide opportunities for private, uninterrupted time
   with significant other(s)

Assist in identifying ways to adapt lifestyle as condition
   changes *to enhance participation and feelings of
   control*

Provide information regarding support groups for patient
   and significant other(s)

Collaborate with other professionals (social worker,
   clergy, psychologist, psychiatrist) *to provide support
   and facilitate grieving process*

Provide reference for financial assistance, answers to
   questions regarding medical insurance

Provide information to assist patient in completing
   advance directive or similar document *to ensure
   patient wishes are known to significant others and
   care providers*

Expected Outcomes

Progresses through stages of the grieving process and
   moves toward acceptance

Demonstrates effective coping mechanisms; participates
   in decisions about own future

▼Risk for impaired tissue integrity (wound break-
down/graft failure) related to stress on operative
site

Provide overhead trapeze to *lift and move (do not slide)
   to prevent shearing of skin*

Maintain bed rest with head of bed elevated 30 to 45
   degrees

Provide pressure-relief mattress

Provide bed cradle

Instruct patient not to cross legs

Avoid chair sitting *to prevent ischemic pressure areas on
   buttocks*

Place pillows between knees while positioned on side

Maintain indwelling urinary catheter

Provide wound care and dressing changes per physician
   order (dressing may remain in place for several days)

Use sitz bath or whirlpool per physician order *to stimulate circulation and provide comfort*

Avoid straining at stool; provide stool softeners, laxatives per physician order *to prevent development of anal fissures and bleeding associated with constipation*

Assess amount and character of drainage from wound drains; inform physician if amount increases or character changes

Change dressings immediately if soiled with stool/urine

Expected Outcome
Wound remains clean and dry; healing begins

▼Sexual dysfunction related to progressive disease process/surgical intervention

Establish therapeutic, open communication with patient and significant other

Begin with least sensitive issues and proceed to more sensitive

Discuss patient's and significant other's perception of illness and restrictions on sexuality

Discuss necessary modifications to sexual activity, encourage patient and significant other to identify satisfactory alternatives

Provide access to sexual counseling for patient and significant other

Reassure that desire for sexuality, current and new practices are healthy, as appropriate

Use humor and encourage patient to use humor *to relieve anxiety or embarrassment*

Expected Outcome
Patient and significant other focus on need to make adjustments in sexual practices resulting in enhanced coping and satisfying intimate relationship

PATIENT/FAMILY TEACHING
Postoperative
Instruct patient in wound care
  Irrigation and dressing changes
  Sitz baths
Discuss signs and symptoms to report to care provider
  Unusual odor
  Fresh bleeding
  Perineal pain
  Elevated temperature
  Increased swelling of operative site/groin
  Frequency, urgency, burning on urination
Instruct patient to elevate legs periodically, avoid prolonged chair sitting, do not cross legs
Avoid constipation; collaborate with clinical dietitian to plan diet high in protein for wound healing that is nonconstipating
Avoid heavy lifting
Resume sexual activity according to physician guidelines
Discuss options to intercourse
Explain that fertility is not affected (if no metastasis)

Explain medication/radiation/chemotherapy regimen; expected therapeutic effects, side effects, potential adverse reactions

Discuss management of side effects

DISCHARGE/HOME CARE PLANNING
Discuss community resource/support groups for women with cancer; sexual counseling

Assess ability to provide for physical and daily living needs; arrange home health provider as needed

Assess transportation availability to follow-up appointments with care providers; assist with arrangements as necessary

Assess physical space available to store medical supplies

■ HODGKIN'S DISEASE
Malignant disorder characterized by painless enlargement of lymphoid tissue; usually one lymph node is affected initially, but other nodes and the spleen become involved throughout the lymphatic system (Fig. 15-7). Peak age at diagnosis is in mid 20s, with a second peak after age 50

ASSESSMENT
SUBJECTIVE DATA
Fatigue
Malaise, lethargy
Loss of appetite
Bone pain

OBJECTIVE DATA
Enlarged nodes (Table 15-6)
  Initially: supraclavicular and cervical
  Firm, rubbery nodes become hard with sclerosing
  Vary from nontender without skin changes to tender with skin changes
  Cervical node enlargement: venous occlusion, neck edema, airway obstruction
  Mediastinal adenopathy: dyspnea, cough
  Inguinal: dysuria, frequency, lumbar discomfort
Pruritus: generalized and severe, infrequent
Temperature: alternating afebrile and febrile periods
Night sweats
Jaundice
Edema of face and neck
  Weight loss
  Splenomegaly, hepatomegaly

RISK FACTORS
Familial, identical twin with Hodgkin's disease
Men: higher incidence
White
Age: under 45, over 70
High socioeconomic status
No or few siblings
History of the following:
  Infectious mononucleosis
  Immunodeficiency syndrome

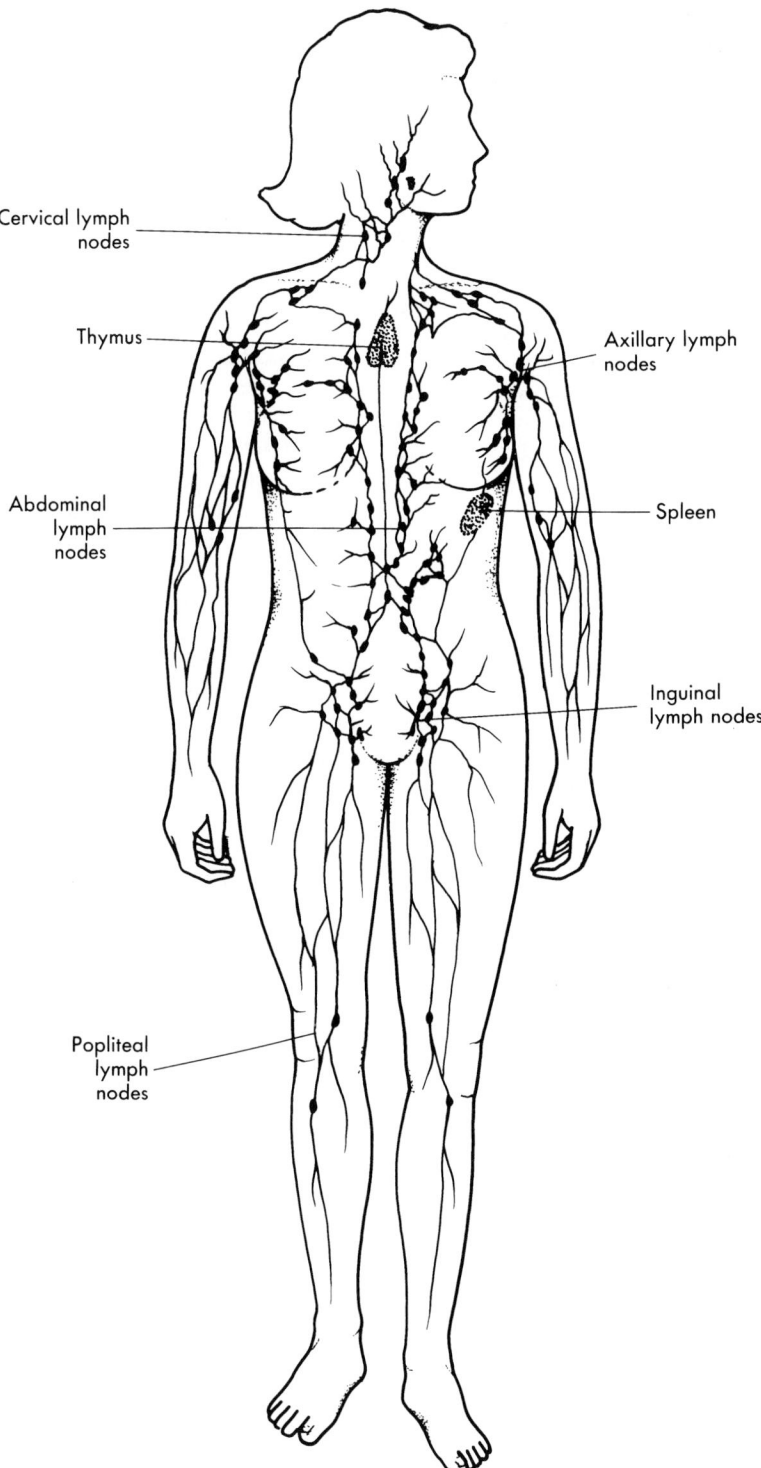

Cervical lymph
nodes

Thymus

Abdominal
lymph
nodes

Popliteal
lymph
nodes

Axillary lymph
nodes

Spleen

Inguinal
lymph nodes

Fig. 15-7 Lymphatic system.

Table 15-6	Staging of Hodgkin's Disease

Stage	Definition
Stage I	Involvement of a single lymph node region or of a single extralymphatic organ or site
Stage II	Involvement of two or more lymph node regions on the same side of the diaphragm
Stage III	Involvement of lymph node regions on both sides of the diaphragm
Stage IV	Disseminated involvement of one or more extralymphatic organs or tissues

From Otto SE: Oncology nursing, *ed 3, St Louis, 1999, Mosby.*

Epstein-Barr virus
Herpesvirus-6
Cytomegalovirus (CMV)

DIAGNOSTIC TESTS
Normocytic, normochromic anemia
WBC with differential (may include any of the following)
    Neutrophilia
    Monocytosis
    Eosinophilia
    Lymphocytopenia
Abnormal ESR: increased alkaline phosphatase (bone involvement)
Lymph node biopsy
    Reed-Sternberg cells
    Nodular fibrosis
    Lymphangiography
    Necrosis
Chest x-rays and CT scan
Gallium scan
MRI
Abdominal CT scan
Bone scan, bone marrow biopsy
Laparotomy, peritoneoscopy
PET scan

POTENTIAL COMPLICATIONS
Respiratory distress
Infections
Fractures

MULTIDISCIPLINARY MANAGEMENT
PREVENTION/DETECTION TEACHING
Discuss importance of reporting suspect symptoms to physician
Explain importance of scheduling periodic physical examinations to include screening laboratory tests and imaging studies as indicated

THERAPEUTIC MANAGEMENT
Radiation therapy
Chemotherapy (see Table 15-8, p. 864)
Social services, support groups
Autologous bone marrow reinfusion
Clinical Dietitian consultation

PATIENT PROBLEMS—NURSING DIAGNOSES/INTERVENTIONS

▼ Impaired skin integrity related to malnutrition, immobility, opportunistic infection related to cellular immunity (herpes, mumps, varicella, CMV)

Assess skin condition q8h: pay particular attention to axilla, skin folds, groin and perineal area, heels, scapula, back of head, dependent extremities, sacral area, mucous membranes
Note condition of skin related to temperature, moisture, color, texture, lesions
Assist with bathing prn; use mild soaps, rinse and dry well
Do not leave skin moist with lotions; avoid deodorants, cologne *to prevent chemical irritation of skin*
If patient is diaphoretic, rinse and dry skin well; keep clothing and bedding dry
Keep linen wrinkle free; avoid pressure from linen on feet; use foot cradle prn
Lift patient when turning, avoid sliding on sheets *to prevent shearing of skin*
Prevent pressure on bony prominence using pillows, air therapy beds prn
Encourage small shifts in position q30min and turn at least q2h *to promote circulation and prevent pressure ulcers*
Increase active mobility; encourage walking and sitting in chair; avoid chair sitting for longer than 30 minutes in one position
Provide for perianal care after each elimination
Avoid IM injections and multiple venipuncture

Expected Outcomes
Skin and mucous membranes remain intact
Current breakdown is healing

▼ Fatigue related to chronic disease process

Assess causative/contributing factors; identify activities that are difficult for patient
Coordinate activities *to provide for undisturbed periods of rest and sleep*
Perform active/passive ROM exercises qid; collaborate with physical therapist to determine most therapeutic exercises
Determine whether patient becomes posturally hypotensive; change positions gradually; monitor for hypotension and tachycardia
Gauge amount and intensity of activity tolerated by monitoring patient's subjective complaints of fatigue, as well as changes in vital signs
Assist patient to identify strengths, abilities, interests; assist in development of realistic goals to progress from simple to complex tasks
Encourage patient to participate in own care to tolerance; assist as needed *to prevent exhaustion;* assist patient to identify energy patterns and schedule activities appropriately

Teach energy conservation techniques, use of assistive devices

Place patient on fall-prevention protocol

Collaborate with physical therapist to design measures *to maintain activity and independence*

Expected Outcomes
Participates in self-care to tolerance

Ability to be active increases

States a feeling of increased energy

▼Altered nutrition: less than body requirements related to reduced food intake, malabsorption, anorexia, vomiting, diarrhea, stomatitis

Assess nutritional status daily: weight, electrolytes, total protein, serum albumin, Hgb, skin turgor, muscle mass

In collaboration with physician administer antiemetics, usually on routine schedule *to prevent severe nausea and vomiting caused by medication therapy*

Determine amount and types of foods patient likes and is able to tolerate

Provide for oral hygiene before and after meals

Administer anesthetics to oral mucosa before meals prn

Offer high-calorie, high-protein diet with variation in taste, texture, and presentation of foods

In collaboration with physician, provide oral and parenteral nutritional supplements

Serve frequent, light meals and nutritional, high-calorie snacks

Assist patient to eat if fatigue is a factor

Present meals in an attractive, pleasing manner

Provide a pleasant atmosphere *to increase desire to eat:* encourage significant other(s) to join patient for meals, remove bedpans/urinals from area, maintain well-ventilated room, serve food as soon as it arrives, remove tray as soon as patient finishes eating

In collaboration with clinical dietitian: calculate number of calories and nutrients needed *to maintain/gain weight and support metabolic needs*

Maintain calorie count

Encourage family to bring patient's favorite foods from home

Expected Outcome
Maintains weight within 10% of baseline

▼Pain related to involvement of multiple organ systems

Assess nature, intensity, location, duration, and precipitating and alleviating factors

Use consistent pain rating scale *to determine baseline and deviations that indicate intervention is needed*

Assess nonverbal signs of pain particular to patient *so that early signs can be noted and treatment started*

Obtain information from patient regarding past pain experiences and methods used for relief

Control environmental factors that may increase perception of pain: temperature, noise, lighting

Assist patient to achieve comfortable positions

Assist patient to achieve state of minimal physical tension through techniques such as relaxation, music, visualization, diversion *to decrease need for medication*

Provide a restful environment with opportunities to rest during the day and uninterrupted periods of sleep at night

In collaboration with physician provide analgesic medications as required, observing for therapeutic and side effects

Discuss and initiate noninvasive pain relief measures: relaxation, cutaneous stimulation, distraction, hot/cold therapy

Expected Outcomes
Verbalizes decrease in or relief of pain

Incorporates existing pain while participating in daily activities

▼Risk for infection related to suppressed immune system

Screen personnel and visitors for symptoms of infection

Use strict sterile technique for all invasive procedures *to prevent nosocomial infection*

Monitor sites of invasive lines/tubes/drains for signs of infection q8h

Check body fluids for alteration in color, odor, consistency

Ensure excellent personal hygiene is maintained, especially after bowel movements

Ensure required fluid/nutrient intake; provide high-calorie, high-protein diet; supplement with total oral nutrition products prn, institute calorie count prn

Record intake and output

Monitor vital signs, especially temperature, q4h and prn

Monitor CBC, WBC results per physician order

Administer antibiotics, sulfa-type medications, and other antiinfectives as ordered

Maintain skin integrity *to prevent entry of microorganisms*

Auscultate breath sounds q8h

Encourage clearance of pulmonary secretions: turn, cough, deep breathe q2h; perform chest percussion and drainage prn; use incentive spirometer qh

Maintain intact mucous membranes; scrupulous oral care using soft instruments q4h and prn

Expected Outcomes
Current infections are improved, resolved

New infections are not developed

▼Ineffective airway clearance related to edema and/or enlarged mediastinal lymph nodes

Assess respiratory effort, pattern, breath sounds q4h and prn

Assist patient to achieve comfortable position; sitting position usually decreases work of breathing

Administer oxygen therapy per physician order

Assess patient's response to activity; assist as needed *to prevent respiratory distress*

Position patient *to minimize respiratory effort and maximize quality of ventilation*

Keep emergency airway equipment at bedside

Expected Outcome

Effective breathing pattern is sustained

Additional Nursing Diagnosis to Consider

Altered urinary elimination, related to uremia caused by tumor lysis syndrome and increased uric acid

PATIENT/FAMILY TEACHING
Postdiagnosis

Discuss symptoms of recurrence/progression to report to physician

Discuss importance of keeping follow-up appointments with care providers

Explain medications: therapeutic effects, potential side effects, potential adverse reactions

Explain management of potential side/adverse effects

Infection

Discuss importance of reporting signs and symptoms of infection: cold or influenza symptoms, coughing, dysuria, lesions that do not heal quickly, infected cuts

Explain need to maintain skin integrity: avoid excess scratching, perform careful skin care, observe for skin changes

Discuss need to maintain clean environment; avoid handling pets; avoid persons with infections and large crowds; perform routine handwashing and personal hygiene

Respiratory distress

Discuss early signs of respiratory distress to report

Increasing cough

Hoarse voice

Decreased activity tolerance

Change in breathing pattern

Nutrition

Collaborate with clinical dietitian to plan meals and instruct patient in selecting foods appropriate to patient's physical condition and considering the patient's preferences

Instruct patient to weigh weekly and report loss ≥5%

Activities and comfort

Explain importance of involvement in routine activity as soon as physical condition permits

Discuss need to balance activity and rest periods

Explain skin care measures to decrease itching

Explore pain relief measures acceptable and successful for the patient

Anxiety/fear

Explain importance of maintaining open communication with significant other

Teach recognition of early symptoms of depression, maladaptive anxiety/fear

Discuss problem-solving, coping strategies that patient is comfortable practicing

Discuss sources of psychologic, financial, spiritual assistance

DISCHARGE/HOME CARE PLANNING

Plan for sufficient, clean space to store supplies and medications

Emphasize need to have emergency plans and phone numbers available for periods of acute distress

Explore availability of weighing scale

Assess ability of patient to provide for physical needs and daily living needs; arrange home health providers as necessary

Assess availability of transportation to follow-up appointments; assist with arrangements as needed

Assist patient to contact community groups for ongoing psychologic/emotional support

■ MALIGNANT LYMPHOMA

Refers to a grouping of neoplasms originating in lymphoid tissue, which are classified by degree and differentiation of cellular content involving either T or B cell lymphocytes; grouping includes non–Hodgkin's lymphomas and lymphosarcoma; etiology is unknown, but a viral source is suspected; it can occur in all age groups and is more common in men, whites, and people of Jewish ancestry

ASSESSMENT
SUBJECTIVE DATA

Fatigue

Malaise

Pressure symptoms in area of involvement

GI: difficulty swallowing, loss of appetite, nausea

Retroperitoneal: abdominal, low back pain

CNS: numbness, weakness, nerve pain, headache

OBJECTIVE DATA

Enlarged lymph nodes

Cervical and supraclavicular

Nontender, rubbery, movable, size fluctuations

Enlarged tonsils/adenoids

Oropharyngeal and mediastinal mass

Weight loss

Elevated temperature

Susceptibility to infections related to type of immunity affected

Vomiting

Constipation

RISK FACTORS

Acquired immunodeficiency syndrome (AIDS) related

Epstein-Barr virus

DIAGNOSTIC TESTS

WBC differential

Abnormal-appearing lymphocytes (early disease)

Lymphocytes with monoclonal surface immunoglobulin (Ig) (early disease)

Blood chemistries
  Serum calcium: elevated
  Serum copper: elevated
  LDH: elevated
  Serum albumin: hypoalbuminemia or
    hypergammaglobulinemia (late disease)
Antiglobulin (Coombs): positive
Bone marrow: disease infiltration
Monoclonal Ig spikes

POTENTIAL COMPLICATIONS
Pleural effusions
Paralysis

MULTIDISCIPLINARY MANAGEMENT
THERAPEUTIC MANAGEMENT
Staging procedures
  Biopsies for histologic evaluation
    Lymph nodes
    Tonsils
    Liver
    Bone marrow
    Bowel
    Tissue removed during laparotomy
  Lumbar puncture
  Chest x-ray
  CT scans
    Liver, spleen
    Abdomen
    Bone
    MRI
    Gallium scan
Radiation therapy
Chemotherapy (see Table 15-8, p. 864)
Allogenic bone marrow transplant
Social services, support group

PATIENT PROBLEMS—NURSING
DIAGNOSES/INTERVENTIONS
See Hodgkin's disease (p. 840)

■ MULTIPLE MYELOMA
*Malignant disorder in which immature plasma cells
proliferate in the bone marrow and form osteocyte tumors of the skeleton; initially, the pelvis, spine, and ribs
are involved; other bones, the lymph nodes, spleen, liver,
and kidneys are affected later; occurs primarily in males
50 to 70 years of age; diagnosis is often made in late
stages, so prognosis is often poor*

ASSESSMENT
SUBJECTIVE DATA
Bone pain
  Predominantly severe back pain on movement
  Ribs
  Extremities
Fatigue
Weakness

OBJECTIVE DATA
Firm, nontender masses over areas of skeletal
  involvement
Skeletal deformities
Pathologic fractures
Shortened stature: 5 inches or more (resulting from
  compression fractures)
Renal: hypercalcemia (renal calculi)
Bleeding tendency
Classic triad
  Increased bone marrow plasma cells
  Lytic bone lesions
  Serum/urine monoclonal immunoglobulins

DIAGNOSTIC TESTS
Hgb: decreased
RBCs: decreased
ESR: elevated
Serum calcium: elevated
Total protein: elevated
Plasma cells: 3%
Lymphocytes: 40% to 50%
Urine: proteinuria, Bence-Jones protein, hypercalciuria
Immunoelectrophoresis: positive IgM or IgG
Platelet count: decreased
Imaging studies
  Skeletal survey
    Diffuse osteoporosis
    Osteolytic lesions
  Intravenous pyelogram (IVP), renal involvement
  MRI
Bone marrow: abnormal increase in immature plasma
  cells

POTENTIAL COMPLICATIONS
Spinal cord compression
Nephrocalcinosis
Acute renal failure
Bleeding problems
Infections

MULTIDISCIPLINARY MANAGEMENT
THERAPEUTIC MANAGEMENT
Pain management
Parenteral fluids
Laminectomy
Radiation therapy
Chemotherapy (see Table 15-8, p. 864)
Interferon
Social services, support

PATIENT PROBLEMS—NURSING
DIAGNOSES/INTERVENTIONS

▼Pain related to involvement of multiple organ
  systems

Assess nature, intensity, location, duration, and
  precipitating and alleviating factors

Use consistent pain rating scale *to determine baseline and deviations that indicate intervention is needed*

Assess nonverbal signs of pain particular to patient *so that early signs can be noted and treatment started*

Obtain information from patient regarding past pain experiences and methods used for relief

Control environmental factors that may increase perception of pain: temperature, noise, lighting

Assist patient to achieve comfortable positions

Assist patient to achieve state of minimal physical tension through techniques such as relaxation, music, visualization, diversion *to decrease need for medication*

Provide a restful environment with opportunities to rest during the day and uninterrupted periods of sleep at night

In collaboration with physician provide analgesic medications as required, observing for therapeutic and side effects

Discuss and institute noninvasive pain relief measures: relaxation, cutaneous stimulation, distraction, hot/cold therapy

Expected Outcomes

Verbalizes decrease in or relief of pain

Incorporates existing pain while participating in daily activities

▼ Risk for infection related to suppressed immune system

Screen personnel and visitors for symptoms of infection

Use strict sterile technique for all invasive procedures

Monitor sites of invasive lines/tubes/drains *for signs of infection* q8h

Check body fluids for alteration in color, odor, consistency indicative of an infectious process

Ensure excellent personal hygiene is maintained, especially after bowel movements

Provide uninterrupted periods of sleep and rest

Ensure required fluid/nutrient intake, provide high-calorie, high-protein diet; supplement with total oral nutrition products prn, institute calorie count prn

Monitor vital signs, especially temperature, q4h and prn *to assess for fever*

Monitor CBC, WBC results per physician order *to assess degree of infection*

Administer antibiotics, sulfa-type medications, and other antiinfectives as ordered

Maintain skin integrity *to prevent entry of microorganisms*

Auscultate breath sounds q8h

Encourage clearance of pulmonary secretions; turn, cough, deep breathe q2h; perform chest percussion and drainage prn; use incentive spirometer qh

Maintain intact mucous membranes; scrupulous oral care using soft instruments q4h and prn

Expected Outcomes

Current infections are improved or resolved

New infections are not developed

▼ Potential for bleeding related to thrombocytopenia*

Assess all systems for signs of bleeding q8h

Assess for systemic signs of bleeding: hypotension, tachycardia, pallor

Monitor results of CBC, coagulation studies, platelet counts as ordered by physician

Avoid invasive procedures when possible *to reduce potential for bleeding*

Use smallest-gauge needles possible

Hold pressure on all invasive sites for 5 to 10 uninterrupted minutes *to prevent bruising/extravasation of blood in subcutaneous tissue*

Avoid constipation; administer stool softeners prn

Avoid rectal medications, taking rectal temperature

Change positions frequently and take measures to avoid pressure points

Use oral care appliances appropriate for condition of mouth *to prevent trauma to mucous membranes*

Expected Outcome

No signs or symptoms of active bleeding occur

▼ Impaired physical mobility related to bone lesions, pathologic fractures

Collaborate with physical therapist to assist with mobility/ambulation as required to support patient; use assistive devices as required

Allow patient to proceed at own pace; encourage patient to be mobile to tolerance

Use pain management techniques/medications before and during activity

Arrange furniture, equipment, personal items for ease of patient maneuvering

If spine is involved take precautions to support it before activity; use brace as required

Expected Outcomes

Increases periods of activity; uses assistive devices appropriately

Demonstrates spine precautions and ability to don and doff brace

Additional Nursing Diagnosis to Consider

Neurologic problems, paralysis, renal insufficiency, constipation related to spinal cord compression

Not a NANDA-approved diagnosis.

PATIENT/FAMILY TEACHING

Disease process and treatment

Discuss symptoms of progression of disease to report to physician

Discuss medication therapeutic actions, side effects, and potential adverse reactions to report to physician

Discuss management of side and adverse effects of medications

Explain importance of keeping follow-up appointments with caregivers

Mobility

Teach use, application of assistive devices

Collaborate with physical therapist to plan progressive daily activity to tolerance

Teach spine precautions *to prevent further degeneration*

Discuss measures *to provide support and decrease musculoskeletal stress while on bed rest*

Pain management

Assist in selection of nonpharmacologic methods of pain management that offer greatest relief

Teach proper administration and timing of pain medications

Emphasize need to have planned rest and sleep periods alternating with activity

Renal dysfunction

Discuss need to be observant regarding amount of fluid intake in relation to urine output; discuss need to inform physician if intake/output relationship is unbalanced

Discuss need for daily weighing and reporting significant (≥5%) gains or losses

Importance of low-calcium diet

Potential for bleeding

Teach detection methods for occult blood in urine and stool

Explain need to avoid over-the-counter, aspirin-containing medications

Instruct in injury prevention: furniture layout, nonskid rugs, clutter-free environment

Assist patient to select appropriate oral care appliances

Explain importance of avoiding activities that may result in accidental injury

Discuss handling tools and kitchen appliances with care

Discuss methods to prevent constipation

Infection

Discuss signs and symptoms of infection to report to physician

Explain importance of avoiding persons with infections or recently vaccinated

Explain importance of avoiding large crowds, common drinking fountains

Discuss importance of maintaining excellent personal hygiene; teach handwashing techniques

Explain importance of avoiding skin disruption; use electric razor, wear gloves when gardening or doing housework

Avoid going barefoot

Instruct on importance of maintaining clean household environment and proper food handling

Anxiety/fear

Explain importance of maintaining open communication with significant other(s)

Teach recognition of early signs of depression, maladaptive anxiety/fear

Discuss problem-solving, coping strategies that patient will be comfortable performing

Discuss sources of psychologic, spiritual, financial assistance

DISCHARGE/HOME CARE PLANNING

Plan for sufficient, clean space to store supplies and medications

Emphasize need to have emergency phone numbers available

Discuss availability of weighing scale

Assess availability of transportation to follow-up appointments; assist with arrangements prn

Assess ability of patient to provide for physical and home care needs; arrange home health providers prn

Arrange for durable medical equipment service prn

Assist patient to contact community groups for ongoing psychologic/emotional support

ONCOLOGIC EMERGENCIES

An oncologic emergency arises from tumor progression or metastasis and can cause irreversible morbidity or death if not promptly recognized and treated

■ HEMATOLOGIC EMERGENCIES

Tumor progression may cause hemorrhage via blood vessel erosion or through coagulation abnormalities such as disseminated intravascular coagulation (DIC)

HEMORRHAGE

OBSERVATIONS

Acute hemorrhage, most commonly from the following:

Nose

Bronchus

Stomach

Colon

Carotid artery

Vagina

ASSOCIATED CONDITIONS/FACTORS

Cancer

Stomach

Esophageal

Gynecologic

Head and neck

Colorectal

Leukemia
Lymphoma
Multiple myeloma
Chemotherapy treatment 10 days before
Platelet count <20,000

INTERVENTIONS

Assess for bleeding; monitor vital signs and mental status; check mouth, nose, rectum, vagina, and skin; check stools and urine for occult blood
Monitor laboratory data
Notify physician of suspected or frank bleeding
Apply direct pressure for carotid artery hemorrhage
Depending on bleeding site, prepare for the following:
    Packing: nose, rectum, or vagina
    Occlusion balloon catheter: bronchus
    Iced saline lavage: stomach
    Iced saline enemas: colon/rectum
Monitor vital signs q15min; decrease frequency as hemorrhage is controlled
Measure and document amount of blood loss; measure and record intake and output
Maintain calm atmosphere
Support patient and significant other psychologically
Monitor IV fluids and blood products, platelets or fresh-frozen plasma
Prepare patient for surgery or laser surgery when ordered

DISSEMINATED INTRAVASCULAR COAGULATION (DIC)

Condition associated with infection and sepsis; presence of simultaneous coagulation and bleeding

OBSERVATIONS

May be hemorrhagic or thrombotic
Clot formation with serous drainage around clot
Increased bleeding from sites of invasive procedures
Ecchymotic extensions
Systemic bleeding to hemorrhage
Thromboemboli in any system
Hypotension
Tachycardia
Cool, pale, clammy skin
SOB
Loss of consciousness
Hemoptysis
Scleral hemorrhage

ASSOCIATED CONDITIONS/FACTORS

Cancer
    Pancreas
    Stomach
    Colon
    Lung
    Prostate
Leukemia
Metastases
Sepsis
Infection
Hepatic failure

INTERVENTIONS

Monitor vital signs q15min
Assess all body systems for presence of bleeding or thromboemboli and evidence of adequate tissue perfusion
Monitor sites of bleeding; apply pressure
Monitor continuous heparin infusion, IV fluids, and administration of blood products and medications (e.g., vasopressors, antidysrhythmics)
Measure and record intake and output; report deficits
See p. 211 for detailed care

■ CARDIOVASCULAR EMERGENCIES

▌ SUPERIOR VENA CAVA SYNDROME (SVCS)

Mechanical obstruction of the SVC from compression caused by tumor progression or enlarged mediastinal lymph nodes, from intraluminal occlusion caused by some sarcomas, lung cancer, Hodgkin's disease, or lymphomas or from thrombosis caused by central line devices

OBSERVATIONS

Prominent neck and chest veins
Telangiectasia, upper thorax
Facial plethora
Edema of face, neck, upper thorax, upper extremities
Jugular vein distention
Headache, unrelieved
Dizziness
Visual disturbances
Feeling of facial fullness
Dysphagia
Dyspnea
Cough
Hoarseness
Chest pain
Respiratory distress
Altered LOC
Horner syndrome: one-sided drooping of eye with pupil constriction and conjunctivitis with loss of sweating on same side of forehead
Enlarged heart on x-ray examination
CT scan confirmation, MRI

ASSOCIATED CONDITIONS/FACTORS

Lung cancer
Hodgkin's disease
Non-Hodgkin's lymphomas
Breast, thymus, testicular, and head and neck carcinomas (metastases)
Chemotherapy via indwelling central line devices
Radiation-induced fibrosis

INTERVENTIONS

Assess head, neck, upper thorax, and upper extremities for signs of SVCS
Assess mental status, LOC, respiratory status, vision, and voice for changes indicative of SVCS

Report findings indicative of SVCS

Position patient *to reduce edema*

  Semi-Fowler's to high-Fowler's position

  Elevate upper extremities on pillows; overbed table may increase comfort

  Perform passive ROM exercises q4h

Place venous access devices in lower extremities when ordered

Provide skin care for face, eye care to prevent infection and breakdown

Initiate oral hygiene measures

Prevent pressure or trauma to face, thorax, and upper extremities

  Wear lose-fitting bedclothes

  Avoid jewelry

  Reduce bending, stooping, lying down

  Monitor oxygen administration equipment carefully

  Avoid venous punctures for fluid or laboratory studies

  Place identification band on lower extremity

  Avoid Valsalva maneuver, lifting, or bending

  Provide easily chewed foods or full liquid diet

  Assist with oral and hygiene measures and diet *to decrease oxygen demand*

Focus on treatment of underlying disease, radiation/chemotherapy, thrombolysis, stent placement

Provide information about radiation or chemotherapy as appropriate when scheduled *to reduce anxiety*

Maintain calm, quiet atmosphere

Answer questions and provide information *to reduce anxiety for patient and significant other(s)*

Assess effectiveness of medications administered and observe for toxic or side effects (e.g., chemotherapeutics, anticoagulants, oxygen therapy, steroids)

Maintain accurate intake and output

▌CARDIAC TAMPONADE

Cardiac tamponade may be caused by pericardial effusions related to metastatic spread of malignant cells or bleeding from coagulopathies such as DIC; also may result from constrictive pericarditis caused by radiation to mediastinum

OBSERVATIONS

Beck's triad

  Decreased BP with narrow pulse pressure

  Increased CVP

  Muffled heart sounds

Pulsus paradoxus: 20 mm Hg or more variation

Kussmaul's sign

Tachycardia

Precordial dullness on percussion

Peripheral constriction; cold, clammy

Tachypnea

Pale

Diaphoretic

Dyspnea, cough

Chest pain

Anxiety, apprehension, feeling of doom

Low-voltage ECG, electrical alternans

Enlarged heart on x-ray examination

Weak point of maximal impulse (PMI)

Effusion on echocardiogram

Jugular vein distention

Ascites, hepatomegaly

Peripheral edema

Pulmonary congestion

Constriction of pericardial sac

  Audible knock at heart apex

  Friction rub

Shock

Cardiac arrest

ASSOCIATED CONDITIONS/FACTORS

Metastases from the following:

  Lung

  Breast

  Lymphomas

  Leukemias

  Melanomas

  Sarcomas

  Stomach

  Ovaries

  Kidney

Radiation therapy

INTERVENTIONS

Assess for signs of cardiac tamponade

  Auscultate heart and breath sounds

  Assess carotid, radial, femoral, and pedal pulses

  Assess vital signs; calculate pulse pressure and presence of pulsus paradoxus

  Monitor respiratory status and continuous ECG

  Assess mental status and LOC

Report signs of cardiac tamponade immediately

Prepare to assist with emergency pericardiocentesis or immediate transfer to intensive care unit (ICU) or operating room (OR)

  Observe for dysrhythmias during and after procedure

  Auscultate breath sounds for possible pneumothorax

  Ensure venous access for fluid requirements

  Have airway intubation and suction equipment available

Support patient psychologically

  Explain need for frequent assessment and monitoring

  Provide information about emergency procedures, detailing steps as they are taken

  Remain calm; answer questions clearly

Monitor effect of oxygen therapy

Restrict activities to reduce oxygen demand; assist with positioning, toileting

Position patient to increase venous return

Provide information about further treatments, sclerosing agents, chemotherapy, radiation therapy, or pericardial windows

Oxygen therapy

Pericardiocentesis

  See p. 111 for further care

■ METABOLIC EMERGENCIES

 ### SYNDROME OF INAPPROPRIATE ANTIDIURETIC HORMONE (SIADH)

Ectopic production of a substance similar to antidiuretic hormone (ADH) by a tumor or stimulation of the posterior pituitary gland to produce ADH by the tumor; or by specific drugs; this causes water intoxication and dilutional hyponatremia, which, if unrecognized and treated, may lead to congestive heart failure

OBSERVATIONS

Lethargy
Weakness
Irritability
Confusion
Seizures
Nausea, vomiting
Anorexia
Sudden weight gain, usually without edema
Decreased urine output without change in intake
Congestive heart failure (CHF)
Serum sodium <135 mEq/L
Serum osmolality <280 mOsm/kg H_2O
Urine osmolality >1200 mOsm/kg H_2O
Urine sodium >20 mEq/L
Elevated blood urea nitrogen (BUN)

ASSOCIATED CONDITIONS/FACTORS

Small cell lung cancer
Lymphoma
Pancreatic cancer
Prostatic cancer
Chemotherapeutic agents
    Vincristine
    Cyclophosphamide
Infections; viral/bacterial pneumonia
Increased intracranial pressure (ICP)

INTERVENTIONS

Assess for fluid retention and dilutional hyponatremia
Monitor intake and output
Weigh patient daily (same time, scale, and clothing)
Assess neurologic and mental status
Evaluate laboratory values for electrolytes
Auscultate lungs for breath sounds
Report adverse signs immediately
In collaboration with physician, restrict fluids to 500 to 1000 ml/24 hours
Assess effectiveness of parenteral hypertonic saline solution and diuretics administered: monitor for signs of hypokalemia and hypomagnesemia (p. 26)
Provide safety measures (e.g., bed in low position with side rails up, call light within reach); assist with ambulation; assist with hygiene and diet *to prevent injury*
Maintain seizure precautions
Provide calm, nonstressful environment
Teach patient and significant other signs of SIADH to report

■ HYPERCALCEMIA

Elevated calcium levels result from resorption of calcium from the bones, which results from bone destruction by metastases of the skeleton; prostaglandins, leukocyte cytokines, and ectopic production of a substance similar to parathyroid stimulates release of calcium from the bones; this may result in a gradual or sudden onset of renal failure

OBSERVATIONS

Polyuria
Nocturia
Polydipsia
Lethargy
Confusion
Disorientation
Bradycardia, atrial and ventricular dysrhythmias, short QT interval
Fatigue
Muscle weakness
Hypotonia
Loss of deep tendon reflexes
Dehydration
Nausea, vomiting
Anorexia
Elevated serum calcium
Serum albumin may be decreased with serum calcium within normal limits
Bone pain
Constipation
Seizures

ASSOCIATED CONDITIONS/FACTORS

Cancer
    Breast
    Lung, squamous cell
    Thyroid
    Kidney
    Ovarian
    Esophageal
    Parotid
    Head and neck
    Ewing's sarcoma
    Melanoma
    Multiple myeloma
    Leukemia
    Lymphoma
Immobility
Skeletal metastases
Medications
    Thiazide diuretics
    Lithium

INTERVENTIONS

Assess for signs and symptoms of hypercalcemia
    LOC and mental status
    Muscle reflexes and activity tolerance
    Nutritional status
    Intake and output
    Daily weight (same time, scale, and clothing)

Vital signs
Skin turgor
Electrolyte values and albumin levels, Ca^{++} levels
Assess effectiveness of parenteral saline, medications
  administered (e.g., plicamycin, calcitonin or
  phosphates or diphosphonates) that inhibit calcium
  resorption, and diuretics (e.g., furosemide)
Encourage fluids to 2500 ml/day
Monitor diet intake of oxalates *to bind dietary calcium*
Teach and assist with ROM exercises if on bed rest;
  increase activity and exercise as tolerated *to decrease
  further calcium resorption from bones;* use rocking
  chair if mobility is limited
Provide safety measures when needed *to prevent injury*
  Bed in low position with side rails up
  Assist with ambulation or provide assistive devices
  Call light and articles required by patient within reach;
    nightlight available
Assist with diet and hygiene measures
Teach signs and symptoms of hypercalcemia that patient
  and/or significant other should report to care giver
  before discharge

◼ HYPOGLYCEMIA/HYPERGLYCEMIA

*Abnormal blood sugar levels can occur in nondiabetic
patients with cancer as a result of certain therapies, TPN,
or primary tumors of pancreas*

OBSERVATIONS
See Diabetes (p. 426); Hyperglycemia (p. 438)

ASSOCIATED CONDITIONS/FACTORS
Glucocorticosteroid therapy may cause hyperglycemia in
  patients with the following:
  Lymphomas
  Leukemias
  Radiation therapy to reduce swelling
  Cerebral metastases to reduce edema
TPN with high glucose concentration may cause
  hyperglycemia
Primary beta-islet cell tumors or insulinomas may cause
  hyperglycemia through stimulation or oversecretion of
  insulin
Severe malnutrition

INTERVENTIONS
See Diabetes (p. 426); Hyperglycemia (p. 436)

◼ TUMOR LYSIS SYNDROME

*This emergency occurs with the rapid release of
intracellular components, potassium, phosphorus, and
uric acid as a result of rapid tumor cell necrosis
induced by chemotherapy or radiation; the combined
electrolyte disturbances may result in renal failure and
cardiac arrest*

OBSERVATIONS
Oliguria
Anuria

Flank pain
Urine crystals
Hematuria
Cardiac dysrhythmias
  Bradycardia
  Ventricular tachycardia
  Prolonged P-R and Q-T intervals
  Depressed ST segment
  Tall peaked T waves
  Widened QRS complex
Muscular cramps; tetany
Positive Chvostek's and Trousseau's signs
Confusion
Elevated
  Serum uric acid
  BUN
  Serum creatinine
  Serum phosphate
  Serum potassium
Decreased serum calcium
Anemia

ASSOCIATED CONDITIONS/FACTORS
Non-Hodgkin's lymphomas
Leukemia
Small cell lung cancer
Breast cancer
Neuroendocrine cancers
After chemotherapy, radiation, surgical tumor debulking

INTERVENTIONS
Assess cardiac status
  Apical pulse: rate, rhythm; BP
  Monitor for cardiac dysrhythmias and signs of CHF
  Evaluate potassium and calcium levels
Assess neuromuscular status
  Monitor for carpopedal spasms, presence of Chvostek's
    and Trousseau's signs, seizure activity, or
    confusion
  Evaluate calcium and phosphate levels
Assess renal status: monitor intake and output, daily
  weight, urine pH, uric acid, BUN, and creatinine
  levels
Assess effectiveness of parenteral fluids with sodium
  bicarbonate, calcium supplements, allopurinol,
  phosphate binders, and diuretics when
  administered
Monitor dietary intake
  Restrict foods with potassium
  Encourage sodium intake if allowed
Provide safety measures, assist with ADLs, and reorient if
  confusion is present *to prevent injury*
Maintain seizure precautions: padded side rails and airway
  at bedside
Instruct patient to avoid pressure on motor nerves *to
  decrease spasms,* (e.g., no knee hyperflexion or
  crossing of legs)
See CHF (p. 112) if symptoms observed
Prepare for peritoneal or hemodialysis when necessary
  (pp. 648 and 645)

◼ NEUROLOGIC EMERGENCY

◼ SPINAL CORD COMPRESSION

This emergent situation occurs as a result of tumor growth or spread of metastases to the vertebral body with growth into the epidural space; usually develops rapidly and can cause permanent neurologic deficits such as paraplegia

OBSERVATIONS

Pain
- Neck, back, and lumbar
  - Increases with motion; Valsalva's maneuver, supine position, coughing, and sneezing; intense, localized, and persistent
  - Radicular root: increases with movement; related to distribution of segmental dermatome
  - Medullary: diffuse, referred, bilateral pain with shooting or burning in peripheral area; not increased with Valsalva's maneuver

Muscular weakness
- Gait and balance disturbances
- Foot drop
- Paralysis

Increased tendon reflexes; positive Babinski sign
Sensory changes, ascend from feet up
- Paresthesia
- Numbness, tingling
- Loss of sensation
- Coolness in affected area
- Sexual dysfunction

Loss of bowel and bladder control

ASSOCIATED CONDITIONS/FACTORS

Spinal cord tumors
Vertebral metastases from the following:
- Lung
- Breast
- Lymphoma
- Multiple myeloma
- Prostate

INTERVENTIONS

Assess pain: location, type, duration, radiation effects on movement or position change; use pain rating scale
Assess neuromuscular function and sensation; monitor tendon reflexes
Assess bowel sounds and bladder distention
Report changes immediately to prevent irreversible loss of function
Maintain bed rest at first appearance of signs of cord compression
Turn and reposition using log-roll method and sufficient personnel to prevent injury
Administer corticosteroids on time; assess effectiveness in reducing cord inflammation when ordered
Prepare patient for surgical decompression or radiotherapy (p. 855) when necessary
See Laminectomy (p. 467) and paraplegia (p. 585)

◼ PULMONARY EMERGENCIES

◼ PLEURAL EFFUSIONS

Tumor progression or metastasis causes increased capillary permeability, obstruction of lymphatics, decreased reabsorption of pleural fluid; or obstruction of pulmonary veins causes increased hydrostatic pressure

OBSERVATIONS

Dyspnea
Cough
Tachypnea
Decreased or absent breath sounds
Pleuritic chest pain
Tachycardia
Asymmetric bulging of intercostal space
Dullness on percussion over fluid field
Decreased fremitus
Confirmation with chest x-ray studies, pleural fluid cell count/cytology
Restricted chest wall expansion on the affected side

ASSOCIATED CONDITIONS/FACTORS

Lymphomas
Lung cancer
Breast cancer
Leukemia
Mesothelioma
Ovarian cancer
Infection
Tuberculosis
Cisplatin, cyclophosphamide, ifosfamide chemotherapy

INTERVENTIONS

Auscultate chest for heart and lung sounds
Assess respiratory effort, rate, and rhythm and use of accessory muscles
Monitor vital signs; skin color, temperature, and moisture; neck vein distention; intake and output
Assess chest pain: location, character, onset, intensity
Report adverse findings to physician
Position patient for comfort and maximal respiratory excursion; usually semi-Fowler's to high-Fowler's position preferred
Teach and assist patient to turn, cough, and deep breathe q2h and use incentive spirometer qh
Prepare emergency equipment for respiratory depression before thoracentesis
Premedicate when ordered
Explain thoracentesis procedure and assist prn *to increase psychologic comfort*
Monitor vital signs and breath sounds; check for bleeding or leakage q15min for 1 hour, then qh for 2 hours after thoracentesis
Rotate patient position to all four sides if sclerosing agent instilled
NOTE: Chest tube may be clamped for defined period if in place; unclamp at specified time
Provide oxygen therapy and humidification when indicated

Explain and prepare for surgical procedures
(pleuroperitoneal shunt, pleurectomy, sclerotherapy) if
effusion is unrelieved

▓ PULMONARY OBSTRUCTION

*Tumor progression causes airway obstruction; prompt
intervention can prevent lung collapse beyond the obstruction*

OBSERVATIONS

Dyspnea, severe
Progressive stridor on inhalation, exhalation, or both
Inability to speak
Use of accessory muscles
Nasal flaring
Asymmetric chest excursion
Decreased tactile fremitus
Decreased or absent breath sounds
Rapid onset of anxiety

ASSOCIATED CONDITIONS/FACTORS

Primary lung tumors

INTERVENTIONS

Assess breathing pattern, effort, respiratory rate, presence
of stridor and speech, character of secretions, and
breath sounds q4h; report changes indicating
obstruction immediately
Maintain pharyngeal and/or endotracheal airway,
tracheostomy tray, and resuscitation equipment at
bedside
NOTE: Tracheobronchial stents and positive-pressure
devices may be used as temporary measures to
prevent compression, or a tracheostomy may be
required until underlying cause is treated with
radioactive or laser therapy
Be prepared to administer oxygen therapy
Position patient for maximal chest excursion with least
amount of effort
Provide suction for secretions patient is unable to handle
Maintain a calm atmosphere; stay with patient during
times of increased anxiety and quietly coach patient in
methods for breathing easier, as well as relaxation
techniques
Encourage fluids to 2000 to 2500 ml/day
See Care of patient with tracheostomy (p. 278)

▓ RENAL EMERGENCY

▓ RENAL OBSTRUCTIONS OR FAILURE

*Tumor progression can lead to obstruction of flow
through ureters, bladder outlet obstruction, ureteral obstruction, or renal failure caused by a solid tumor*

OBSERVATIONS

Urinary output <30 ml/hr
Anuria
Palpable bladder
Dysuria

Frequency
Hesitancy
Urgency
Incontinence, aware or unaware
Nocturia
Retention
Hematuria
Acute renal failure (p. 641)

ASSOCIATED CONDITIONS/FACTORS

Cancer of the following:
  Bladder
  Rectum
  Prostate
  Cervix
  Edometrium
  Ovary
  Lymphoma
  Hodgkin's lymphoma

INTERVENTIONS

Measure and record intake and output; report output
<30 ml/hr
Assess character, color, and odor of urine
Assess bladder level with decreasing output; report
distention
Insert indwelling catheter and connect to closed gravity
drainage as ordered
Prepare patient for surgery for obstructions
  Stents may be placed for solid tumor obstructions
    while radiation or chemotherapy is initiated
  Urinary diversion may be created for obstructions not
    responsive to other therapies (p. 623)
Monitor for signs of renal failure (p. 641); restrict fluids as
ordered
Assess urinary elimination pattern, using voiding diary to
determine type of incontinence or retention
  See Incontinence for nursing diagnoses and
    interventions (p. 616)
  See Urinary retention (p. 612)

■ SEPSIS AND SEPTIC SHOCK

*Sepsis occurs in response to a disseminated infection,
usually a gram-negative bacteria that releases endotoxins into the bloodstream; endotoxins release endogenous
pyrogens, causing fever and local damage to endothelial
lining of capillaries, activate clotting factor XII, and the
complement system, which may result in bleeding (DIC);
multiplying bacteria cause release of kinens, which enhance vasodilation; shock occurs from a generalized severe reduction in tissue perfusion caused by inadequate
circulating blood volume, resulting in cellular hypoxia
and decreased cardiac output*

OBSERVATIONS

Initial
  Irritability, restlessness, confusion
  Fever
  Chills

Warm, dry skin
Red, flushed face
Cardinal signs of infection may be absent if
   neutropenia <1000; may present with initial
   symptoms of the following:
   Change in LOC
   Decreased BP
   Decreased urine output
Tachycardia, tachypnea
Weak peripheral pulse

Slow refill of capillary nail bed
Oliguria: <50 ml/hr
Glycosuria
Excessive thirst
Muscular weakness
Decreased BP
Mental confusion
Increasing severity
   Decreased cardiac output, circulatory volume, and
      tissue perfusion

Table 15-7 Infections in Cancer Patients

Pathogen	Sources	Common Sites	Presentation
BACTERIA			
Pseudomonas	Multiple	Wounds	Purulence
		GI	Enterocolitis
		GU	UTI
		Lung	Pneumonia
Klebsiella	Multiple	Lung	Pneumonia
Escherichia coli	Multiple	GI	Enterocolitis
		GU	UTI
		Bone	Osteomyelitis
		Wounds	Purulence
		Blood	Sepsis
Staphylococcus	Multiple	Lung	Pneumonia
		Bone	Osteomyelitis
		GI	Enterocolitis
		CNS	Meningitis
		Wounds	Purulence
VIRUSES			
Herpes simplex type 1	Oral secretions	UGI	Stomatitis, esophagitis
		Skin	Eczema
		CNS	Encephalitis
Cytomegalovirus	Normal flora, blood products	Lung	Pneumonia
		CNS	Encephalitis
		Eye	Retinitis
Varicella zoster	Person-to-person transmission	Skin	Shingles
FUNGI			
Candida	Normal flora	GI	Thrush, esophagitis
		Lung	Pneumonia
		GU	UTI, vaginitis
Cryptococcus	Soil, pigeon feces	Lung	Pneumonia
		CNS	Meningitis
Aspergillus	Air, building materials, pigeon feces	Lung	Bronchopneumonia
PROTOZOA			
Pneumocystis carinii	Normal flora, person-to-person transmission	Lung	Pneumonia
Toxoplasma gondii	Oocytes in cat feces, inadequately cooked meat, blood products	Disseminated	Chills, fever, diaphoresis, encephalitis, pericarditis

Dry, cool skin progressing to cold, clammy skin
Peripheral edema
Oliguria progressing to anuria
Weak, rapid HR
Hypotension
Hyperventilation progressing to slow, shallow
   respirations and respiratory failure
Greater alterations in LOC
Blood culture
Chest x-ray for infiltrates
CBC for WBC changes ABGs for metabolic acidosis
PT/INR/partial thromboplastin time (PTT)
   prolonged

ASSOCIATED CONDITIONS/FACTORS
Preexisting neutropenia secondary to treatment or
   disease
Sources of infection (Table 15-7)

INTERVENTIONS
Assess vital signs, breath sounds, and cardiac status;
   hypothermia may be precursor to sepsis
Monitor for skin and oral infections, URI, UTI, vaginal
   discharge, and perirectal abscess
Assess mental status and change in LOC
Assess for changes in GI system and elimination
Obtain cultures of suspected areas of infection and blood,
   throat, urine
Monitor laboratory values, especially absolute neutrophil
   count and culture reports
Report earliest signs of infection for prompt
   treatment
Initiate antibiotics and parenteral fluids as soon as
   ordered *to begin sepsis treatment and restore*
   volume
Measure intake and output
Institute measures *to prevent infection* (p. 885)
Assess for signs of bleeding; report if present; see DIC
   (p. 211)
Provide cooling measures for temperature >103.5° F
   (39.8° C): warm to tepid bath; wet towels covering
   body with ice applications in axilla; use cooling
   blanket if ineffective; administer antipyretics
Provide warmth for hypothermic patients; avoid bathing;
   cover with warmed blankets
Observe for signs and symptoms of late shock
Monitor blood gas values
Provide oxygen therapy for decreased arterial oxygen
   content when ordered
Assess effectiveness of IV sodium bicarbonate when
   administered for metabolic acidosis
Place patient in supine or reverse Trendelenburg's
   position *to improve cardiac output*
Maintain bed rest *to conserve energy* and observe for
   signs of CHF
Turn q1h to 2h; use pillows to position edematous
   extremities; provide skin care

CANCER THERAPY

■ SURGERY
*This modality has been the diagnostic and therapeu-
tic treatment of choice over the years and is performed
for various reasons*
   biopsy: *To determine a definite diagnosis and/or to
establish presence of a tumor or metastasis*
   staging: *To determine the type and extent of the carcinoma and treatment indicated*
   resections
      curative: *To remove tumor/organ and sufficient
surrounding tissue to ensure a cure*
      palliative: *To reduce or eliminate disease or treat-
ment related symptoms without trying to cure; to prolong
or improve the quality of life*
      reconstruction: *To restore and regain an improved
cosmetic appearance or body function*
   *Comprehensive preoperative teaching has been found
to be a critical part of this type of therapy, as well as meticulous postoperative care and teaching; the education of
the patient and significant other begins on admission
and continues until discharge, which ensures maximal
recovery and rehabilitation*

■ RADIOTHERAPY
*Use of therapeutic radiation for the purpose of curing,
controlling, or palliating neoplastic disease; may be used
alone or in combination with surgery or chemotherapy*
   teletherapy: *The external beam administration of
electrons, protons, or neutrons at the target tissue via a
super voltage device*
   brachytherapy: *The administration of radiation internally via sealed or unsealed sources*
   ***stereotactic external beam irradiation (gamma
knife):*** *High-dose treatment with a three-dimensional
distribution beam*
   radiolabeled antibodies: *Systemic injection of radioactive materials coupled with tumor-specific antibodies*

▌TELETHERAPY

ASSESSMENT
NOTE: Symptoms will vary depending on the site being
   irradiated; intensity of symptoms will also vary

SUBJECTIVE DATA
Common side effects
   Fatigue
   Loss of appetite
   Complaints of skin irritation
Head/neck radiotherapy
   Loss/altered taste
   Decreased appetite/anorexia

Gastrointestinal tract radiotherapy
  Nausea
  Cramping
  Abdominal bloated feeling
  Rectal discomfort
Brain radiotherapy
  Headache
  Irritability
Genitourinary radiotherapy
  Frequent urination
  Infrequent or loss of menses
  Erectile dysfunction
Cardiorespiratory response
  SOB

OBJECTIVE DATA

Skin changes at radiation site
  Increased sensitivity
  Erythema
  Edema
  Desquamation (dry or moist)
  Fibrosis, atrophy (delayed effects)
Head/neck
  Dry mouth, dental cavities
  Pharyngitis
  Mucositis, oral infections
Gastrointestinal tract
  Xerostomia
  Esophagitis
  Diarrhea
  Weight loss
Brain irradiation
  Increased ICP
  Sensory perceptual changes
  Hair loss, changes in texture, color
Genitourinary
  Vaginal stenosis
  Ovarian failure
  Cystitis
  Hematuria
  Changes in urinary elimination pattern
Cardiorespiratory response
  Tachycardia
  Pericarditis, myocarditis
  Pneumonia

DIAGNOSTIC TESTS

CBC: decreased Hgb
Leukocyte count: decreased to pancytopenia (usually receiving chemotherapy also)
Thrombocyte count: decreased
Electrolytes

POTENTIAL LONG-TERM COMPLICATIONS

Lymphedema
Bone marrow suppression
Myelopathy, chronic
Brachial plexopathy
Pulmonary fibrosis

Osteoadinonecrosis
Teleangectasia
Bladder/bowel obstruction
Sterility
Malignancies
Paresthesias

MULTIDISCIPLINARY MANAGEMENT
THERAPEUTIC MANAGEMENT

Clinical dietitian for nutrition counseling
Artificial saliva
Antiemetics, antifungals, antidiarrheals
Viscous lidocaine, topical antacids
Parenteral/nasogastric fluids, nutrition
Urinary anesthesia
Antibiotics
Pain management
Skin care therapist consultation
Blood component administration

PATIENT PROBLEMS—NURSING DIAGNOSES/INTERVENTIONS

▼ Fatigue related to effects of radiation therapy

Assess causative/contributing factors; identify activities that are difficult for patient *to plan appropriate assistance*

Coordinate activities to provide for undisturbed periods of rest and sleep *to increase energy level*

Perform active/passive ROM exercises qid; collaborate with physical therapist to determine most therapeutic exercises *to maintain muscle tone*

Determine whether patient becomes posturally hypotensive; change positions gradually; monitor for hypotension and tachycardia *to prevent accidents and decrease fear of movement*

Gauge amount and intensity of activity tolerated by monitoring patient's subjective complaints of fatigue, as well as changes in vital signs *so activity can be increased as patient's tolerance increases*

Assist patient to identify strengths, abilities, interests; assist in development of realistic goals progressing from simple to complex *to enhance feelings of accomplishment*

Encourage patient to participate in own care to tolerance; assist as needed *to prevent exhaustion;* assist to identify energy patterns and schedule activities when energy level is highest

Teach use of assistive devices *to conserve energy*

Place patient on fall-prevention protocol *to prevent injury*

Collaborate with physical therapist to design measures/activities *to maintain independence*

Expected Outcomes

Participates in own care to tolerance
Ability to be active increases
States a feeling of increased energy

▼Risk for fluid volume deficit related to nausea, vomiting, or diarrhea

Monitor intake and output balance q8h to 12h
Inspect skin turgor and mucous membranes for hydration
Weigh patient daily (same time, scale, and clothing)
Monitor results of electrolytes, blood sugar, Hct as ordered *to determine adequacy of treatment plan*
Maintain oral/parenteral intake of fluids *consistent with fluid volume status; push for deficit; restrict for excess*
Offer and assist with oral care *to promote comfort*

Expected Outcomes
Intake and output are balanced

▼Impaired skin integrity related to effects of external beam radiotherapy

Assess affected skin areas q8h
Skin care guidelines
   Do not remove skin markings; do not replace if removed, notify radiation oncologist
   Wash skin in area being irradiated with lukewarm water avoiding soaps, which may dry or irritate
   Avoid use of any skin care products (topical medications, lotions, deodorants, cosmetics), especially those containing alcohol or scent *to prevent irritation*
   Avoid tight garments *to prevent rubbing*
   Avoid extremes of temperature
   Dry desquamation: use cornstarch sparingly
   Moist desquamation: use water/saline to keep clean and moist (slow healing, may require days without radiation treatment)
   Expose skin to air *to promote healing* when possible; avoid direct sunlight
   Do not shave affected areas *to avoid cuts or abrasions*
   Cover broken areas with hydrocolloid dressing, using stretch-type tubular dressing to hold in place; avoid bandages, tape, which will irritate skin and cause injury when removed

Expected Outcome
Skin remains intact and/or impaired skin progressively heals

Additional Nursing Diagnoses to Consider
Altered urinary/bowel elimination, related to effects of radiation
Altered sexuality patterns, related to fatigue, sterility
Risk for infection, related to suppression of bone marrow
Alteration in nutrition, less than body requirements, related to nausea and vomiting

PATIENT/FAMILY TEACHING
Explain radiation therapy procedures and pretreatment, posttreatment events
Explain need for time, distance, and shielding precautions
Explain need to avoid persons with infections, especially URIs
Discuss symptoms of infection to report to physician
   Cold, flu, elevated temperature
   Diarrhea and frequency of or burning on urination
   Reddened, painful skin areas
   Mouth redness, swelling, ulceration, bleeding, increased salivation
Emphasize importance of maintaining nutritious diet and fluid intake to 3000 ml/day unless contraindicated
   Take six to eight small meals daily
   Avoid eating immediately before or after treatment
Explain that radiation effects continue for 10 to 14 days after last treatment; tell patient signs of healing will not be seen until 18 to 21 days after last treatment
Explain need for daily oral hygiene—in the morning, after meals, and at bedtime—to keep mouth fresh and clean
Discuss the following symptoms to report to physician
   Mucositis (p. 890)
   Nausea and vomiting (p. 889)
   Inability to eat
   Increasing headache or tiredness
   Severe diarrhea (p. 892)
   Increasing redness, swelling, pain, or pruritus at site of therapy
Emphasize importance of follow-up outpatient care
Teach name of medication, dosage, time of administration, purpose, and side effects
Explain need to avoid taking over-the-counter medications without physician approval

DISCHARGE/HOME CARE PLANNING
Assess ability to provide for own physical care and daily living needs; arrange home health providers as needed
Assess availability of transportation to follow-up appointments; assist with arrangements as necessary
Plan for sufficient, clean storage space for medical supplies

■ BRACHYTHERAPY
Used to deliver large amounts of radiation to a specific site using radioactive implants

ASSESSMENT
NOTE: Symptoms will vary depending on isotope used, dosage, and target tissue; intensity of symptoms will also vary.

HEAD AND NECK IMPLANTS (SEALED SOURCES OF CESIUM-137, IRIDIUM-192) (FIG. 15-8)
SUBJECTIVE DATA
Painful swallowing
Painful speaking
Decreased appetite/anorexia
Fatigue

OBJECTIVE DATA
Dry mouth/stomatitis
Oral infections

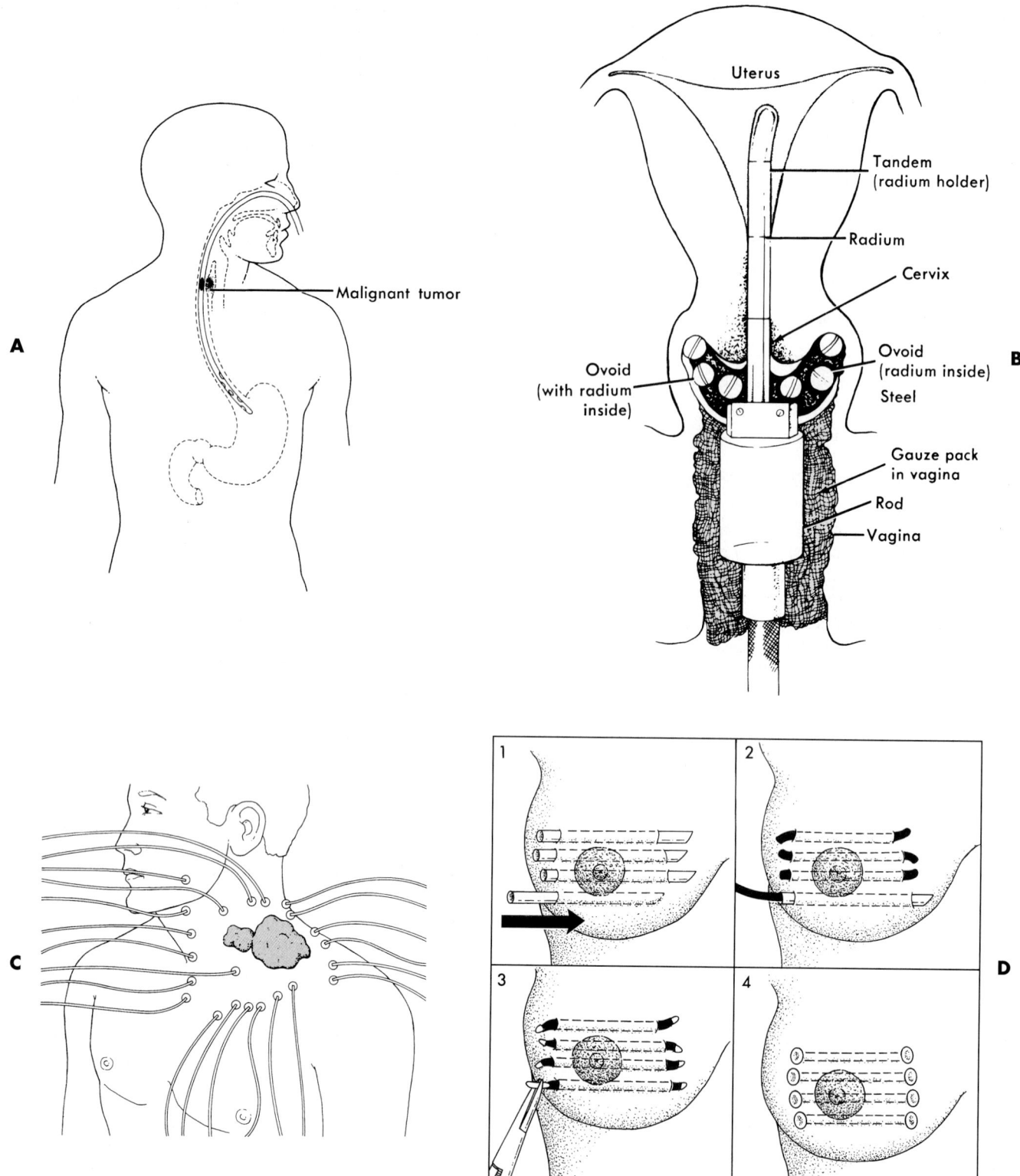

Fig. 15-8 Examples of internal radiation therapy. **A,** Radium bougie in place for patient with cancer of the esophagus; note that radium is placed next to the tumor. **B,** Radium treatment of cancer of the cervix via application with tandem and ovoids. **C,** Iridium seeds implanted for left neck mass. **D,** Iridium seeds implanted for breast cancer.
(A and B From Marino LB: Cancer nursing, *St Louis, 1981, Mosby; C and D from Beare PG, Myers JL:* Principles and practice of adult health nursing, *ed 2, St Louis, 1994, Mosby.)*

Xerostomia
Thick oral secretions
Erythema/dry desquamation at implant site
Weight loss
Alopecia

POTENTIAL COMPLICATIONS
Erosion/bleeding at implant site
Obstructed airway

GYNECOLOGIC IMPLANTS (SEALED SOURCES OF CESIUM-137, IRIDIUM-192) (SEE FIG. 15-8)
SUBJECTIVE DATA
Fatigue
Nausea
Abdominal cramping/feeling of fullness
Low back pain
Urge to void
Dysuria

OBJECTIVE DATA
Diarrhea/constipation
Cystitis
Vaginal fibrosis/shortening
Vaginal dryness

POTENTIAL COMPLICATIONS
Vaginal erosion/bleeding/infection
Vaginal stenosis

PROSTATE IMPLANTS (IODINE-125 SEEDS, GOLD-198 SEEDS)
SUBJECTIVE DATA
Fatigue
Difficult urination

OBJECTIVE DATA
Hematuria
Loss of seeds

THYROID IMPLANTS (UNSEALED SOURCE OF IODINE-131)
SUBJECTIVE DATA
Fatigue
Pain/tenderness in area of thyroid gland

BREAST IMPLANTS (SEALED SOURCE OF IRIDIUM-192) (SEE FIG. 15-8)
SUBJECTIVE DATA
Fatigue
Pain at implant site

OBJECTIVE DATA
Erythema at implant site

DIAGNOSTIC TESTS
CBC
Electrolytes
Urinalysis

MULTIDISCIPLINARY MANAGEMENT
THERAPEUTIC MANAGEMENT
Head and neck implants
    Head of bed to remain elevated 45 degrees
    Clinical dietitian/speech therapist consultation for swallowing and food consistency tolerance
    Nasogastric tube/parenteral nutrition
Gynecologic implants
    Bed rest/supine position/head of bed lower than 15 degrees
    Foley catheter management
    Antidiarrheals *to prevent bowel movement*
    Clinical dietitian consultation for low-fiber diet *to prevent bowel movement*
    Antiembolic stockings, alternating pressure device
Prostate implants
    Foley catheter management prn
    Strain all urine for lost seeds

PATIENT PROBLEMS—NURSING DIAGNOSES/INTERVENTIONS

▼Anxiety related to limited social contact with others

Reassure that nurse will come quickly if patient calls
Visit frequently for brief periods from the doorway *to reassure patient that assistance is and will be available when needed* (per guidance of radiotherapy MD) (Boxes 15-2 and 15-3)
Provide diversional activities patient enjoys
Encourage significant other(s) (excluding children and pregnant women) to visit for short periods *to decrease*

Box 15-2	**Physical Environment Considerations**

Prepare room before patient arrives
Radiation safety officer to select appropriate room
Label door and chart with radiation precaution signs (Fig. 15-9)
Place lead shields in room *or* mark appropriate distance from bed on the floor with tape (lead aprons are not sufficient)
Protect floor from spills with impermeable covering
Place isolation linen and trash hampers in the room
Order disposable meal trays and utensils
Arrange needed items within patient's easy reach
Encourage self-care
Ensure call light is within easy reach
Place long-handled forceps and lead container in room
All trash, linen must remain in room for entire length of stay
Dispose of all waste in toilet and flush three times
Room remains sealed until cleared by radiation safety officer

feelings of abandonment (per guidance of radiotherapy MD) (see Box 15-3)
Encourage telephone contact with family and friends

Expected Outcome
Expresses/demonstrates calm manner and adaptive coping

Box 15-3	**Precautions for Caregivers and Visitors**

No pregnant staff or visitors
Visit frequently from the doorway
No children under the age of 18
Rotate nurse assignments daily
Wear gloves in room at all times
Stay at least 6 feet away from patient for indirect care
Work from opposite side from implant when giving direct care
Be efficient when providing care
Wear lead aprons; remain behind lead shields as directed
Minimize time spent close to patient
Use time efficiently
Use telephone/intercom to check on/reassure patient frequently
Wear radiation film badge as directed
Handle radiation-contaminated objects with forceps
Transport any specimens to the laboratory in labeled lead containers

▼ Impaired skin integrity (breast) related to effects of brachytherapy implants

Assess affected skin areas q8h
Skin care guidelines
Wash skin in area being irradiated with lukewarm water, avoiding soaps that cause irritation
Avoid use of any skin care products (topical medications, lotions, deodorants, cosmetics) *to prevent increased drying*
Avoid tight garments *to prevent rubbing*
Avoid extremes of temperature *to prevent damage to highly sensitive skin*
Dry desquamation: use cornstarch sparingly
Expose skin to air when possible; avoid direct sunlight
Cover broken areas with hydrocolloid dressing, using stretch-type tubular dressing to hold in place; avoid bandages, tape, which can tear skin when removed

Expected Outcome
Skin remains intact and/or impaired skin progressively heals

▼ Fatigue related to effects of brachytherapy

Identify activities that are difficult for patient and plan for assistance
Coordinate activities *to provide for undisturbed periods of rest and sleep*

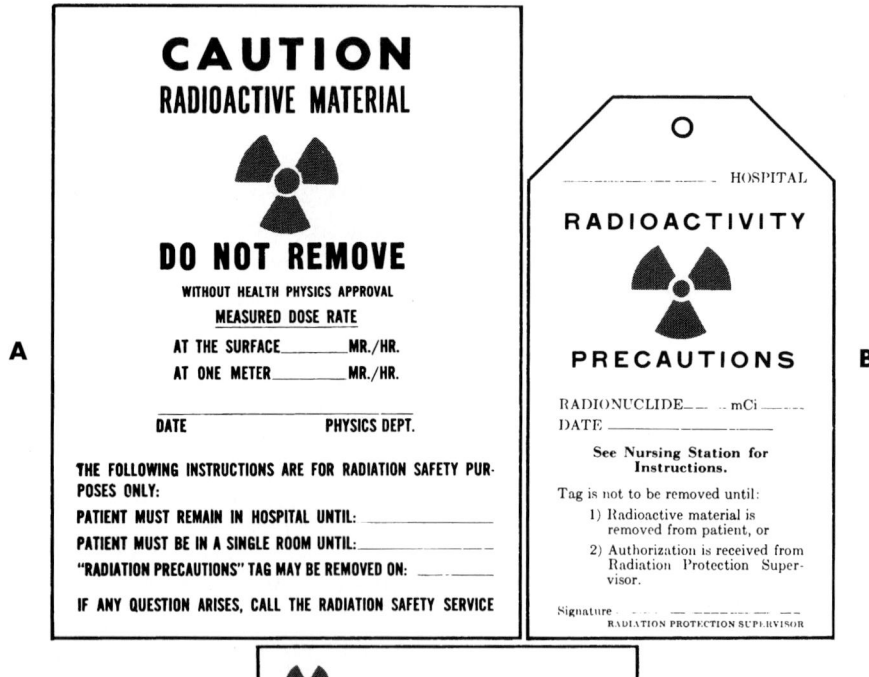

Fig. 15-9 Radiation precaution tags. **A,** Tag placed on patient chart. **B,** Tag placed at foot of patient's bed or attached to door of patient's room. **C,** Tag placed in a wristband on patient.
(From National Council on Radiation Protection and Measurement: Precautions in the management of patients who have received therapeutic amounts of radionuclides, rep no 37, Washington, DC, 1970, The Council.)

Perform active/passive ROM exercises qid; collaborate with physical therapist to determine most therapeutic exercises *to promote increased muscle tone*

Determine whether patient becomes posturally hypotensive; change positions gradually *to avoid injury and reduce fear of moving alone*

Monitor for hypotension and tachycardia *so schedule can be adjusted to meet patient's energy level*

Gauge amount and intensity of activity tolerated by monitoring patient's subjective complaints of fatigue, as well as changes in vital signs

Place patient on fall-prevention protocol *to prevent injury*

Expected Outcomes
Participates in own care to tolerance
Ability to be active increases
States a feeling of increased energy

▼Ineffective airway clearance related to head and neck brachytherapy implant

Maintain elevated upper body at 45 degrees
Avoid supine positions, *which decrease respiratory excursion*
Do not hyperflex knees, *which may increase pressure on diaphragm, preventing adequate inspiration*
Consult with occupational therapist *to assess swallowing ability and develop plan of care to enhance communication*
Instruct patient in use of tonsil tip suction; have suction available within patient's reach so it can be used readily *to decrease fear of choking*
Suction patient as needed *to promote comfort*
Provide emesis basin and tissues for expectoration
Provide oral hygiene *to enhance comfort*

Expected Outcome
Patent airway is maintained

▼Altered oral mucous membranes related to effects of brachytherapy of head and neck regions

Encourage patient to seek dental care before brachytherapy *to ensure optimum condition of membranes*
Inspect oral mucous membranes q4h *to determine changes that need care*
Assist patient/provide oral care q4h while awake, as well as before and after meals and q4h at night
Use soft sponge cleaners or gauze *to prevent breaks in mucosa*
Rinse mouth frequently with nonalcohol mouthwash, sterile water *to keep mouth free of irritating particles and decrease bacteria count*
If patient wears dentures: assess for proper fit, keep dentures scrupulously clean, remove dentures and rinse mouth often, dental consultation prn
Keep mouth moist *to enhance comfort;* provide appealing, tepid liquids for sipping, ice chips, flavored

ice pops; use water-soluble ointment for lips and artificial saliva
If patient is unable to open mouth for oral care, irrigate mouth with sterile saline/water solution, allowing to drain into emesis basin *to remove debris, which can cause bacterial multiplication*
Consult with clinical dietitian to provide mechanically soft foods that are nonirritating
Use straws or cups *to prevent irritation and discomfort*

Expected Outcome
Oral mucous membranes remain intact

▼Altered urinary elimination related to effects of brachytherapy implants (gynecologic/prostate)

Assess pattern of urination; monitor for burning, frequency, hesitancy, retention, incontinence
Monitor for signs of UTI
Force fluids unless contraindicated; monitor for urine output equal to intake
Administer urinary antiseptics per physician order *to reduce inflammation*
Care for and maintain Foley catheter prn *to prevent infection*
Use voiding measures (see p. 13) *to promote voiding when Foley catheter is removed*

Expected Outcomes
Usual pattern of urinary elimination is maintained; signs of UTI are not present

PATIENT/FAMILY TEACHING
Explain that patient is not a source of danger from radioactivity to family or others if precautions are followed
Discuss importance of continued activity balanced with periods of rest *to enhance well-being*
Stress importance of continuing follow-up care with physician
Gynecologic implants
Discuss methods *to eliminate constipation prn*
Instruct patient to notify physician of vaginal bleeding (slight spotting is expected)
Discuss signs and symptoms of UTI to report
Instruct patient to use water-soluble lubricant during intercourse (when physician approves resumed sexual activity)
Instruct patient in use of vaginal dilator prn
Prostate implants
Instruct patient to strain all urine for dislodged seeds
Instruct in safe retrieval of seeds with tweezers and foil, need to return to radiation therapy physician
Instruct patient to report changes in urine elimination pattern and/or hematuria
Instruct patient to wear condoms during sexual activity
Head and neck implants
Instruct patient to report increased difficulty swallowing or controlling secretions to physician

DISCHARGE/HOME CARE PLANNING

Patient is no longer a source of radiation exposure once discharged; however, if seeds are implanted, pregnant women and young children should stay several feet away for first 2 months

Assess patient's ability to provide for own physical and daily living needs; arrange home health providers prn

Assess availability of transportation to follow-up appointments; assist with arrangements as necessary

■ CHEMOTHERAPY

chemotherapy: *Systemic cancer treatment using drugs that affect the cell cycle (Fig. 15-10) to treat cancer; useful when there is disseminated disease or when there is a high risk of recurrence in the body; can be curative, can prolong life, or can be palliative; is often used as an adjuvant to surgery and/or radiation therapy*

ASSESSMENT

OBSERVATIONS/FINDINGS

Adverse side effects and system toxicities related to specific drugs and individual patient responses

Ability and desire to learn

Barriers to learning: fatigue, denial

Knowledge of plan of care; diagnosis, treatment, expectations of results, patient's perception of his or her role

Attitude related to chemotherapy

Psychosocial response based on patient's coping mechanisms, support system, previous experience with chemotherapy, and amount of information received about disease process

Obtain baseline assessment before beginning chemotherapy and continue throughout treatment period (see Assessment, p. 795)

DIAGNOSTIC TESTS

Specific to each medication and expected responses

POTENTIAL COMPLICATIONS

Side effects and toxicities specific to each medication (see Table 15-8, p. 864)

Common problems

Bone marrow suppression

Cutaneous manifestations

GI dysfunction

Respiratory dysfunction

Renal dysfunction

Cardiac dysfunction

Sexual and reproductive dysfunction

Electrolyte/chemical imbalance

Musculoskeletal dysfunction

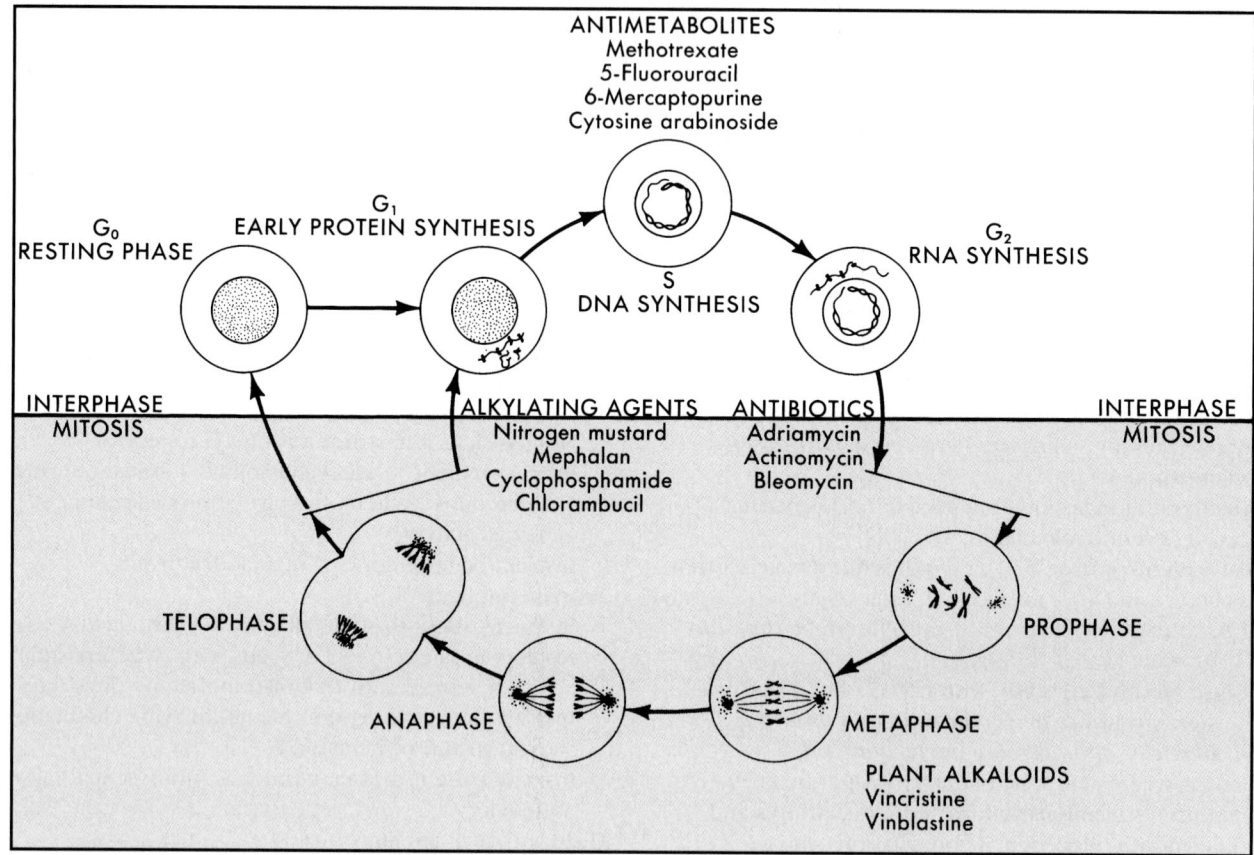

Fig. 15-10   The cell cycle. Drugs are identified by the location at which they exert their effect. *(From Beare PG, Myers JL: Adult health nursing, ed 3, St Louis, 1998, Mosby.)*

MULTIDISCIPLINARY MANAGEMENT
THERAPEUTIC MANAGEMENT
Antineoplastic medications according to protocol or standard regimen

Serial monitoring of results of diagnostic studies

Symptom-specific medications: antiemetics, antidiarrheals, oral anesthetics, antibiotics

Pain management

Parenteral fluids and nutrition

PATIENT PROBLEM—NURSING DIAGNOSIS/INTERVENTIONS
See specific condition and/or specific symptomatic care

Additional Nursing Diagnoses to Consider
Anxiety/fear related to therapeutic interventions and uncertain outcome

Altered nutrition: less than body requirements related to nausea, vomiting, anorexia, fatigue, stomatitis, decreased food intake

Risk for fluid volume deficit related to nausea, vomiting, diarrhea

Body image disturbance related to changes in physical appearance and ability to function

Fatigue related to effects of chemotherapy and chronic illness

PATIENT/FAMILY TEACHING
With help of audiovisual aids, explain how drugs work and expected therapeutic effects of chemotherapy treatment

Provide patient and/or significant other(s) with written material regarding name of drug, action of drug, and potential side effects

Explain method, frequency, and duration of administration of each drug

Provide verbal and written material regarding management of side effects/toxicity

Instruct patient regarding early side effects, such as nausea and vomiting, and side effects that will be delayed such as myelosuppression

Discuss side effects that are reversible

Instruct patient regarding side effects to report to physician

Give written information on how and where to reach health care personnel if necessary

Involve significant other(s) in care planning as much as possible

DISCHARGE/HOME CARE PLANNING
Assess patient's ability to provide for own physical and daily living needs; arrange home health providers as needed

Assess availability of transportation to follow-up appointments; assist with arrangements as needed

Facilitate patient joining a community support group for continuing psychosocial and emotional counseling and support

Plan for sufficient, clean space for storage of medical supplies

Arrange for durable medical equipment as needed

ADMINISTRATION OF CHEMOTHERAPEUTIC DRUGS
See Table 15-8

Verify patient's identification

Review patient's allergy history

Determine patient's history in regard to liver, pulmonary, cardiac, and/or renal disease

Assess patient's ability and motivation to learn

Assess patient's perceived ability to manage and cope with expected side effects

Assess learning needs and concerns; answer questions appropriately

Review educational materials (films, pamphlets) with patient and family

Check physician's order for drug dose, route, rate, and time of administration

Verify that informed consent has been given

Review laboratory data with knowledge of acceptable parameters

Review immediate and long-term side effects of drugs

Calculate dosage, double-check calculation, and ascertain whether dosage is within normal administration range

Know amount and type of diluent to use for reconstitution (mix in biologic safety hood and observe safety precautions [p. 881])

Verify drug dosage with another nurse, pharmacist, or physician

Correctly label drug with patient's name, dose, and route of administration

Wear personal protective equipment

Administer antiemetic 30 minutes before administration of chemotherapy if indicated

Dispose of all used supplies in approved leak and puncture-resistant containers located outside patient area

Have emergency medications and antidote readily available for adverse reaction

SITE SELECTION AND STARTING IV
Select site for venipuncture with regard to previous trauma to arm (blood drawing or lymphatic resection) and drug to be given (vesicant versus nonvesicant); begin at distal portion of extremity

Avoid use of preexisting IV for vesicant drugs

Avoid use of antecubital space, hand, wrist for vesicants and irritants

Avoid use of lower extremities and areas over joints

Wash hands

Site selection, sequence of administration of 2 or more drugs, and site of IV catheter are controversial; always follow guidelines of facility's policy and procedures

Avoid multiple sticks; test patency of IV—blood backflows easily

Stabilize arm or hand; use pillow or board if necessary

Text continued on p. 878

Table 15-8	**Chemotherapeutic Drugs**

Medication	Dosage	Routes of Administration	Side Effects and Toxicities*
ALKYLATING AGENTS			

Busulfan (Myleran)	4-8 mg/day (initially); 1-3 mg/day (maintenance); given according to protocol	PO	Myelosuppression
			Low doses
			  Granulocytopenia
			  Platelets, lymphoid elements spared
			Hyperpigmentation
			High doses: leukopenia
			Delayed-refractory: pancytopenia
			Long-term therapy: pulmonary fibrosis (rare)
			Venooclusive disease with high dose

Carboplatin (Paraplatin)	360 mg/m² q4wk IV
	Should not be administered until neutrophils are >2000 and platelets >100,000
		IV
		Intraarterial
		Intraperitoneal
			Myelosuppression
			  Leukopenia
			  Thrombocytopenia
			  Anemia
			Nausea and vomiting

Chlorambucil (Leukeran)	0.1-0.2 mg/kg; given according to protocol
	2 mg/day maintenance
		PO	Myelosuppression: leukopenia
			Nausea and vomiting, mild
			Amenorrhea
			Depressed spermatogenesis
			Long-term therapy
			  Alveolar dysplasia
			  Pulmonary fibrosis
			  Nausea and vomiting
			  Metallic taste
			  Sinus burning

Cisplatin (Platinol)	80-120 mg/m²; given according to protocol Higher doses may be mixed in hypertonic saline solution to prevent nephrotoxicity	IV Intraarterial Intraperitoneal	Anaphylaxis Nephrotoxicity Ototoxicity Severe nausea and vomiting Hypomagnesemia

Cyclophosphamide (Cytoxan, Endoxana, CTX)	40-50 mg/kg; given according to protocol
	1-5 mg/kg/day (oral)
		PO
		IV
		Intraperitoneal
			Myelosuppression
			  Leukopenia
			  Thrombocytopenia may occur
			Common with high doses
			  Stomatitis
			  Alopecia
			  Hemorrhagic cystitis
			Amenorrhea, dose-limiting
			Testicular atrophy, dose-limiting

*See Symptomatic care in chemotherapy, p. 884

Table 15-8	**Chemotherapeutic Drugs—cont'd**		

Nadir	Recovery after Nadir (Days)	Indications	Administration and Nursing Implications
10-12 days	42-50	Chronic myelogenous leukemia Preparation for BMT	Oral tablets may be taken any time of the day
11-30 days 1-10 yr	24-54		
21-30 days	28-30	Ovarian cancer	Assess baseline BP, P, T, R Give by continuous IV infusion Monitor input and output Give antiemetics as ordered and indicated Be prepared to treat anaphylaxis Have life-support equipment and medications available
14-28 days	28-42	Chronic lymphocytic leukemia, ovarian cancer, Hodgkin's and non-Hodgkin's lymphoma	Give oral medication as ordered; no specific directions
18-25 days	39	Testicular and ovarian cancer; squamous cell carcinoma; lung, head, and neck cancer	Assess baseline BP, P, T, R Give by continuous IV infusion Force fluids to 3000 ml/day and give parenteral therapy as ordered 12-24 hr before drug administration Monitor intake and output Mannitol may be ordered with or after administration Ensure output of 100-150 ml/hr before giving medication Give antiemetics as ordered and indicated Be prepared to treat anaphylaxis Have life-support equipment and medications available *High-dose*—investigational Parenteral hydration and bladder irrigation may be ordered
8-14 days	18-25	Non-Hodgkin's lymphoma, sarcoma, breast, lung, and ovarian cancer; acute and chronic lymphocytic leukemia	Give IV push over 3-5 min through side port of patent IV Give oral doses with or immediately after meals Administer antiemetic before therapy and as indicated Force fluids to 3000 ml/day before administration and 48 hr after

Continued

Table 15-8   **Chemotherapeutic Drugs—cont'd**

Medication	Dosage	Routes of Administration	Side Effects and Toxicities*
ALKYLATING AGENTS—CONT'D			
Dacarbazine (DTIC)	2-150 mg/kg daily for 5-10 days, repeated every 3-4 wk	IV	Nausea, vomiting Anorexia Diarrhea (rare) Stomatitis Leukopenia Thrombocytopenia Flulike symptoms Alopecia Facial flushing Paresthesias Neurotoxicity
Estramustine	10-16 mg/kg per day in divided doses	PO	Cardiotoxicity GI toxicity Night sweats Breast changes Painful, tearing eyes Anxiety Lethargy

Ifosfamide (Ifex)	1000-2000 mg/m^2/day for 5 days q4wk	IV	Myelosuppression
			  Leukopenia
			  Less thrombocytopenia
			Hematuria—hemorrhagic cystitis
			Alopecia
			CNS toxicity

Mechlorethamine (nitrogen mustard, HN$_2$)	IV: 10-16 mg/m^2/course
	Intracavity: 0.2-0.4 mg/kg
	Topical: 0.01%
		IV, intracavitary, intralesional
		Topical
			Myelosuppression, dose-limiting
			  Lymphocytopenia, dose-limiting
			  Thrombocytopenia
			  Granulocytopenia (leukocytopenia)
			Nausea and vomiting, severe onset 1-2 hr, lasting 8 hr
			Diarrhea
			Skin rash
			Amenorrhea
			Impaired spermatogenesis
			Vesicant; pain and tissue necrosis if extravasated

Melphalan (Alkeran)	PO: 0.25 mg/kg/day for daily dosage; 0.1-0.15 mg/kg for interval dosage; given according to protocol
	IV: 16 mg/m^2 at 2-wk intervals for four doses
		PO
		Intraperitoneal (investigational)
		IV
			Myelosuppression
			  Leukopenia
			  Thrombocytopenia
			High-dose therapy: nausea and vomiting
			Long-term therapy
			  Acute leukemia
			  Alopecia
			  Dermatitis
			  Stomatitis

Thio-tepa (triethylene-thiophosphoramide)	IV: 0.3-0.4 mg/kg/day
	Bladder instillation: 60-mg instillations/60 ml
		IV, intracavitary, bladder instillation	Myelosuppression
			  Leukopenia
			  Thrombocytopenia

Table 15-8 **Chemotherapeutic Drugs—cont'd**

Nadir	Recovery after Nadir (Days)	Indications	Administration and Nursing Implications
24 hr to several wk			Check output; if falling, notify physician for parenteral therapy orders IV hydration and bladder irrigation usually ordered when high doses given Give within 15 to 30 min after reconstitution
2-4 weeks		Melanoma, Hodgkin's (soft tissue sarcoma, leiomyosarcoma, fibrosarcoma, rhabdomyosarcoma, neuroblastoma)	Causes severe pain at injection site, use hot packs Avoid infiltration
None		Prostate	Take 1 hr before or 2 hr after meals with water, avoid milk products and calcium-rich foods Store in refrigerator
8-14 days	18-25	Testicular cancer	Give IV over a minimum of 30 min Force fluids to 3000 ml/day before administration and 48 hr after Protector such as MESNA should also be used to prevent hemorrhagic cystitis
7-15 days Within 24 hr 6-8 days	28 10-20 Several days	Hodgkin's disease, non-Hodgkin's lymphomas, lung cancer, malignant pleural effusions	Give IV push through side port of patent IV; check blood backflow before instilling each ml; flush line with 30 ml IV fluid before each blood check; flush line after administration; monitor for extravasation; give antidote as ordered Administer antiemetic before therapy and then as indicated Tell patient a metallic taste may be experienced just after drug injection Inform patient that veins may become discolored Reposition patient q15min ×4 after intracavitary instillation
10-12 days	42-50	Breast, ovarian, and testicular cancer, myeloma, melanoma	Give oral doses 2 hr after meals
5-30 days	21-28	Papillary bladder tumors, malignant serous effusions	Give IV push over 2-3 min through side port of patent IV

Continued

Table 15-8	**Chemotherapeutic Drugs—cont'd**

Medication	Dosage	Routes of Administration	Side Effects and Toxicities*
ALKYLATING AGENTS—CONT'D			
Thio-tepa (triethylene-thiophosphoramide) —cont'd	Given according to protocol; dosage reduced with hepatic or renal dysfunction		Anemia Mild 　Local pain 　Nausea, vomiting 　Dizziness 　Headache
NITROSOUREAS			
Carmustine (BCNU)	IV: 150 mg/m^2 or up to 200 mg/m^2; given according to protocol Intraarterial: 100-200 mg/m^2	IV Intraarterial	Myelosuppression, dose-limiting 　Leukopenia 　Thrombocytopenia Immediate 　Burning pain at IV site 　Facial flushing 　Severe nausea and vomiting: onset 2 hr lasting 4-6 hr Long-term therapy: pulmonary fibrosis
Lomustine (CCNU)	100-130 mg/m^2; given according to protocol	PO	Myelosuppression, dose-limiting 　Thrombocytopenia 　Leukopenia Nausea, vomiting; onset 2-4 hr Anorexia Diarrhea
Semustin (investigational) (methyl CCNU)	125-200 mg/m^2; given according to protocol; dosage reduced with liver dysfunction and impaired marrow function	PO	Myelosuppression, dose-limiting 　May be cumulative 　Thrombocytopenia 　Leukopenia 　Erythrocytopenia Nausea and vomiting; onset 4-6 hr
Streptozocin (Zanosar)	1.0-1.5 g/m^2/wk; 500 mg-1.0 g/m^2/day; given according to protocol	IV Intraarterial	Severe nausea and vomiting Nephrotoxicity, dose-limiting Mild hepatotoxicity Immediate burning pain at IV site; decreases after 15-20 min of infusion
ANTIMETABOLITES			
Cytarabine (Ara-C, Cytosar)	1-3 mg/kg/day given according to protocol; dosage reduced with severe hepatic dysfunction	IV, intrathecal SC Intraperitoneal	Myelosuppression, dose-limiting 　Leukopenia 　Thrombocytopenia Nausea and vomiting especially with rapid infusion Stomatitis High dose: flulike syndrome

868

Table 15-8   **Chemotherapeutic Drugs—cont'd**

Nadir	Recovery after Nadir (Days)	Indications	Administration and Nursing Implications
5-30 days —cont'd		Formerly breast and ovarian cancer and Hodgkin's lymphoma	Reposition patient q15min ×4 after intracavitary administration Bladder instillation is retained for 2 hr; reposition patient q15min during this period
4-6 wk 3-5 wk	7-14	Multiple myeloma, Hodgkin's disease, non-Hodgkin's lymphoma; brain tumor, colorectal adenocarcinoma; gastric adenocarcinoma, melanoma, hepatoma	Give IV small volume for 15-45 min Apply ice pack at IV site Teach patient to report pain to staff immediately Flush vein before and after administration Administer antiemetics before administration and as ordered after
40-50 days 26-34 days 28-42 days	60 6-10 9-14 24 hr	Palliative: brain tumors, Hodgkin's disease, lung cancer, colorectal adenocarcinoma	Protect oral drug from heat and moisture Teach patient to take on an empty stomach; avoid alcohol after dose
28-63 days 21-35 days 28-42 days	82-89 6-8 hr	GI cancer, brain cancer, Hodgkin's disease, non-Hodgkin's lymphoma	Teach patient to take on an empty stomach (may lessen nausea and vomiting), observe patient preference Absorbed in 30-60 min if stomach is empty
7-14 days	—	Pancreatic islet cell tumors, non–beta cell pancreatic tumors: stomach, carcinoid, colon	Give IV push through side port of patent IV; check blood backflow before instilling each ml; flush line with 30 ml IV fluid before each blood check; flush line after administration; monitor for extravasation (p. 880), give antidote if extravasation occurs Administer antiemetics before therapy and then as indicated Tell patient burning sensation may be experienced; slow infusion to decrease burning Force fluids to 3000 ml/day, unless contraindicated, to ensure adequate urine output Observe for hypoglycemia reactions immediately after administration Have glucose 50% available
12-14 days	22-24	Acute lymphocytic leukemia, acute granulocytic leukemia	Give IV push over 3-5 min through side port of patent IV; may be given as a continuous infusion Keep patient flat 4-6 hr after intrathecal administration

Continued

| Table 15-8 | **Chemotherapeutic Drugs—cont'd** | | |

Medication	Dosage	Routes of Administration	Side Effects and Toxicities*
ANTIMETABOLITES—CONT'D			
Floxuridine (FUDR)	0.1-0.6 mg/kg per day for 1-6 wk	Intraarterial	Nausea, vomiting Diarrhea Cramps Anorexia Stomatisis Enteritis Local erythema GI hemorrhage Leukopenia Anemia CNS toxicity
Fludarabine (Fludara)	25-30 mg/m^2 per day for 5 days, repeated every 28 days	IV	CNS toxicity Pulmonary toxicity Nausea, vomiting Diarrhea Genitourinary symptoms Dermatitis Fever Tumor lysis syndrome

5-Fluorouracil (5-FU, fluorouracil)	12 mg/kg/day, not to exceed 800 mg/day; given according to protocol
	Maintenance dosage: 6-15 mg/kg; given according to protocol; dosage adjusted with liver or kidney dysfunction
		Topical
		IV
			Myelosuppression, dose-limiting
			  Leukopenia (granulocytes)
			  Thrombocytopenia
			Nausea and vomiting
			Alopecia
			Neurotoxicity
			Diarrhea
			Stomatitis

Hydroxyurea (Hydrea)	80 mg/kg every 3 days or 20-30 mg/kg every day	PO	Leukopenia Thrombocytopenia Anemia

Mercaptopurine (Purinethol, 6-mercaptopurine)	2.5-5 mg/kg/day; given PO according to protocol; dosage reduced one third to one fourth with allopurinol	PO
		IV
			Myelosuppression
			  Thrombocytopenia, mild
			  Leukopenia, mild
			Mild nausea and vomiting
			Cumulative hyperbilirubinemia

Methotrexate (MTX, amethopterin)	2.5-5 mg PO daily
	50-70 mg/m^2 IV (low dose)
	100-150 mg/m^2 IV (high dose)
	IM 15-30 mg daily for 5-day course
	Given according to protocol
		PO
		Intrathecal
		Intraarterial
		IV
		IM
			Myelosuppression
			  Leukopenia
			  Thrombocytopenia
			  Anemia
			    Hgb effect
			    Reticulocytes
			Nausea and vomiting
			Anorexia
			Mucositis
			Hepatoxicity
			Dermatitis
			Alopecia
			Increased ICP
			Nephrotoxicity

Table 15-8 | **Chemotherapeutic Drugs—cont'd**

Nadir	Recovery after Nadir (Days)	Indications	Administration and Nursing Implications
7-14 days	When discontinued	Adenocarcinoma of the GI tract with metastasis to the liver	Patient must be in hospital for initial course, maintain good nutritional status
3-32 days	5-7 wk	Chronic lymphocytic leukemia, acute leukemias, other lymphoid malignancies (many solid tumor types)	Well hydrated; observe for CNS toxicity, wear gloves when handling
7-14 days	16-24	Breast cancer, oral lesions, gastric tumors, and colorectal cancer; topically—basal cell carcinomas	Give IV push over 3-5 min through side port of patent IV using two-syringe technique; flush line after therapy Tell patient to expect vein discoloration
7-21 days	Rapid	Melanoma, chronic granulocytic leukemia, ovarian (head and neck, chronic lymphocytic leukemia)	May empty contents of capsule into water for easier swallowing (avoid contact with powder)
7-14 days 12-21 days 11-23 days	14-21	Acute lymphocytic leukemia, chronic granulocytic leukemia	Give oral dose daily

7-14 days
4-7 days
5 days
 	
6-13 days
2-7 days
	14-21	Acute lymphoblastic and myeloblastic leukemia, trophoblastic tumors, osteogenic sarcoma, epidermoid cancer of head and neck, multiple myeloma, lung, breast, and ovarian cancer	Ensure that patient knows not to take *any* medication before checking with physician when taking methotrexate PO
			Check patency of IV before administration; flush IV after administration
			High-dose (investigational)
			  Force fluids to 3000-4000 ml/day to ensure high-volume output
			  Check creatinine results with increased dosage, sodium bicarbonate may be ordered to maintain urine pH 7.0
			  Administer citrovorum (leucovorin) rescue factor on time as ordered
			  After intrathecal administration keep patient flat 4-6 hr
			  Never give with salicylates, sulfonamide, phenytoin, *p*-aminobenzoic acid (PABA), alcohol, warfarin, amphotericin B

Continued

Table 15-8 **Chemotherapeutic Drugs—cont'd**

Medication	Dosage	Routes of Administration	Side Effects and Toxicities*
ANTIMETABOLITES—CONT'D			
Mercaptopurine (6-MP)	2.5-5 mg/kg per day until remission, then 1.5-2.5 mg/kg per day maintenance	PO	Leukopenia Anemia Thrombocytopenia Hepatotoxicity Nausea, vomiting Fever Headache Weakness
Thioguanine (6-thioguanine)	2-3 mg/kg/day; given according to protocol; dosage reduced with liver or kidney dysfunction	PO IV	Leukopenia Thrombocytopenia Anemia
VINCA ALKALOIDS			

Etoposide	75-200 mg/m^2/day × 3; given according to protocol	IV
		PO
			Myelosuppression; dose-limiting
			  Leukopenia
			  Thrombocytopenia
			  Mild nausea and vomiting
			  Alopecia
			  Severe hypotension with rapid infusion

Teniposide (VM-26)	100 mg/m^2/wk, 45-50 mg/m^2/day; given according to protocol; dosage reduced with prior irradiation/chemotherapy	IV
		Intravesicular
			Myelosuppression, dose-limiting
			  Leukopenia
			  Thrombocytopenia
			Hypotension especially with rapid infusion
			Rare anaphylaxis

Vinblastine sulfate (Velban)	0.1-0.4 mg/kg/wk; given according to protocol; dosage decreased with liver disease and neurologic problems	IV	Leukopenia, dose-limiting Thrombocytopenia, mild Mild nausea and vomiting Alopecia, mild Mucositis Constipation Ileus Abdominal pain Long-term therapy: neurotoxicity
Vincristine sulfate (Oncovin)	1-2 mg/m^2—adult; given according to protocol; dosage decreased with liver disease	IV	Myelosuppression, unusual Neurotoxicity, dose-limiting Peripheral neuropathy, dose-limiting Constipation Ileus Alopecia

Vindesine (Eldesine)	2-4 mg/m^2; given according to protocol; dosage decreased with impaired liver function	IV	Neutropenia, dose-limiting
			Thrombocytopenia
			Leukopenia
			Neurotoxicity, dose-limiting at low doses
			  Alopecia
			  Constipation
			  Paralytic ileus

Table 15-8	**Chemotherapeutic Drugs—cont'd**		

Nadir	Recovery after Nadir (Days)	Indications	Administration and Nursing Implications
7-14 days	When discontinued	Leukemias	Monitor oral dosing regimen
14-28 days	—	Acute granulocytic and lymphocytic leukemia	Give total oral dose at one time between meals
16 days	20-22	Leukemia, lung cancer, lymphoma, testicular cancer	Give through side port of patent IV over at least 30 min to avoid severe hypotension Take baseline BP before therapy then 15 min into administration and at conclusion
3-14 days	28	Hodgkin's disease, non-Hodgkin's lymphoma, malignant pleural effusions, bladder cancer, CNS cancer	Give IV infusion in volume 5 times medication volume; over at least 45-min period through patent IV Take baseline BP before therapy then 15 min into administration and at conclusion Flush line after administration
4-10 days	7-14	Breast and testicular cancer, choriocarcinoma, Hodgkin's disease, and lymphoma	Give IV push through side port of freely running IV; check blood backflow before instilling each ml; flush line with 30 ml IV fluid before each blood check; flush line after administration Monitor closely for extravasation Give antidote as ordered Avoid eye contact Experimentally given by IV infusion over 24-hr period; monitor site closely Administer stool softeners and laxatives as ordered
4-5 days	7	Acute lymphocytic leukemia, breast cancer, sarcomas, Hodgkin's disease, neuroblastoma, non-Hodgkin's lymphoma, small cell lung carcinoma	Ensure patent IV; give IV push over 3-5 min through side port; check blood backflow before instilling each ml; flush line with 30 ml IV fluid before each blood check Monitor for extravasation Give antidote if extravasation occurs Administer stool softeners and laxatives as ordered
5-10 days 5-10 days	15-28	Acute leukemia, lung cancer, esophageal cancer, melanoma	Give IV push over 3-5 min through side port of newly inserted patent IV; flush tubing with 50-100 ml after administration; monitor for extravasation Administer stool softeners and laxatives as ordered

Continued

873

Table 15-8 | **Chemotherapeutic Drugs—cont'd**

Medication	Dosage	Routes of Administration	Side Effects and Toxicities*
VINCA ALKALOIDS—CONT'D			
Vinorelbine (Navelbine)	30 mg/m^2 per week	IV infusion	Granulocytopenia Leukopenia Thrombocytopenia Anemia Neurotoxicity Alopecia Nausea, vomiting Fatigue
Bleomycin sulfate (Blenoxane, "Bleo")	10-30 U/m^2 given according to protocol; dosage decreased with renal failure; test dose may be ordered Total cumulative lifetime dose not to exceed 400 U	IV Intrapleural Intraarterial IM SC	Anaphylaxis Elevated temperature with or without chills Hypotension Pulmonary toxicity Mild nausea and vomiting, dose-limiting Cutaneous reactions Alopecia

Dactinomycin (actinomycin D, Cosmegen)	0.5 mg/day for adult; 0.015-0.5 mg/kg for children; both given according to protocol	IV	Myelosuppression
			  Thrombocytopenia
			  Leukocytopenia
			  Anemia
			Nausea and vomiting, onset 1-2 hr, lasting several days
			Mucositis
			Alopecia
			Skin changes, especially irradiated areas

Daunorubicin (Daunomycin, rubidomycin)	30-60 mg/m^2; given according to protocol; dosage reduced with impaired renal or liver function	IV	Myelosuppression; dose-limiting Nausea and vomiting Alopecia
Doxorubicin (Adriamycin)	60-70 mg/m^2 single dose; given according to protocol; dosage decreased with hepatic dysfunction Total cumulative lifetime dose not to exceed 450-550 mg/m^2	IV Intraarterial Intraperitoneal	Myelosuppression: leukopenia, dose-limiting Nausea and vomiting, onset 3-4 hr Stomatitis Marked alopecia Reactivation of irradiated skin areas Cardiotoxicity, dose-limiting
Idarubicin HCl (Idamycin)	12 mg/m^3/day × 3 (usually with Ara-C); 100 mg/m^2/day × 7 or 25 mg/m^2 IV bolus, then 200 mg/m^2/day × 5	IV	Severe myelosuppression Nausea, vomiting, abdominal pain Severe diarrhea Mucositis Alopecia

| Table 15-8 | **Chemotherapeutic Drugs—cont'd** |

Nadir	Recovery after Nadir (Days)	Indications	Administration and Nursing Implications
7-10 days	7-14 days	Lung	Vesicant precautions Administer IV over 6-10 minutes
—	—	Squamous cell carcinoma, Hodgkin's disease, non-Hodgkin's lymphoma, mycosis fungoides, lung cancer, testicular cancer, malignant effusions	Give IV push or IV infusion as ordered after obtaining baseline Be prepared to treat anaphylaxis; have life-support equipment and medications available Take BP, T q4h during infusion Assess breath sounds and respiratory function Teach patient to report signs of respiratory difficulty immediately to staff Reposition patient q15min ×4 when administering intracavitary doses
14-21 days	22-25	Choriocarcinoma, Wilms' tumor, sarcoma, testicular cancer	Give IV push through side port of patent IV; check blood backflow before instilling each ml, flush line with 30 ml IV fluid before each blood check; flush line after administration Monitor for extravasation; give antidote if extravasation occurs Establish oral and skin hygiene care before therapy Administer antiemetic before administration and as indicated and ordered
7-14 days	21	Acute lymphocytic leukemia; acute granulocytic leukemia; neuroblastoma	Administer IV push through side port of patent IV Monitor closely for extravasation; give antidote as ordered Tell patient that urine will be colored red
10-14 days	21-24	Acute leukemia, Hodgkin's disease, non-Hodgkin's lymphoma, sarcomas, Wilms' tumor, ovarian, breast, lung, thyroid, and bladder cancer	Give IV push through side port of patent IV; check blood backflow before instilling each ml; flush line with 30 ml IV fluid before each blood check; monitor carefully to prevent extravasation that may cause severe ulceration; flush line after administration with 50-100 ml solution Teach patient to report *any sensation* during administration to staff Give antiemetics before administration and as indicated after Assess cardiac status before administration Institute oral hygiene care before administration
—	—	Leukemia	Give IV push over 10-15 min through side port of free-flowing IV Check blood backflow before instilling each ml; monitor continuous IV closely; flush line

Continued

Table 15-8	Chemotherapeutic Drugs—cont'd

Medication	Dosage	Routes of Administration	Side Effects and Toxicities*
VINCA ALKALOIDS—CONT'D			
Idarubicin HCl (Idamycin)— cont'd	continuous IV; dosage reduced with impaired renal or liver function		Rash: palms, soles of feet Dysrhythmias

Mitomycin (Mutamycin, Mitomycin C)	10-20 mg/m² dose; given according to protocol	IV
		Intraarterial
		Intravesicular
			Myelosuppression cumulative
			  Leukopenia
			    Thrombocytopenia: erythrocytopenia
			Nausea and vomiting, onset 1-2 hr, lasting 6-8 hr
			Stomatitis
			Alopecia
			Purple bands on nails
			Mild nephrotoxicity

Plicamycin† (Mithracin)	0.025-0.050 mg/kg; given according to protocol	IV	Myelosuppression
			  Thrombocytopenia
			    Decreased clotting factors
			    Mild leukopenia
			Nausea and vomiting
			Diarrhea
			Stomatitis
			Neurotoxicity
			Dermatologic reactions
			Nephrotoxicity
			Hepatotoxicity

MISCELLANEOUS			
Aminoglutethimide (Cytadren)	250 mg bid for 2 weeks then 250 mg qid; given according to protocol	PO	Lethargy, somnolence, malaise Dizziness, fever Adrenal/thyroid insufficiency Myelosuppression
Amsacrine (AMSA)	75 mg/m²/day; 120 mg/m²/wk; given according to protocol; dosage reduced with hepatic dysfunctions	IV	Myelosuppression: leukopenia, dose-limiting Neurotoxicity (cerebellar dysfunction, grand mal seizures) Conjunctivitis: nausea and vomiting, mild mucositis Dermatologic toxicity Cardiac dysrhythmias Phlebitis
Asparaginase (Elspar, L-Asparaginase)	10,000-40,000 IU/m²/day, q2-3wk; given according to protocol Skin test may be ordered before administration	IV IM	Anaphylaxis Mild nausea and vomiting Neurotoxicity Hepatotoxicity Pancreatitis Hyperosmolar, nonketotic hyperglycemia
Hexamethylmelamine (Atrelamine)	260 mg/m²/day for 14-21 days	PO	Nausea, vomiting, abdominal cramps Diarrhea Myelosuppression Peripheral neuropathy Alopecia

†Used to treat hypercalcemia, not an antitumor agent.

Table 15-8	**Chemotherapeutic Drugs—cont'd**		

Nadir	Recovery after Nadir (Days)	Indications	Administration and Nursing Implications
			Monitor for extravasation; give antidote and follow policy if occurs Assess cardiac status before and during administration
28-42 days	42-56	Cancer of stomach and pancreas	Give IV push over 3-5 min through side port of patent IV; check blood backflow before instilling each ml; flush line with 30 ml IV fluid before each blood check; flush line after administration Monitor closely for extravasation; give antidote if extravasation occurs Administer antiemetics before administration and then as indicated Institute oral hygiene care before therapy Observe for skin changes at IV site or distal to site for 6 wk
14 days	21-28	Hypercalcemia in malignancy	Give in small volume IV over 30-45 min through side port of patent IV; may be ordered as IV infusion given over 4-6 hr for hypercalcemia Observe for extravasation; give antidote as ordered
4-8 wk	—	Breast cancer	Postural hypotension Given in conjunction with high-dose hydrocortisone to reduce severity to adverse reactions
10 days	21-25	Acute myeloblastic leukemia, lymphoma, sarcoma, lung and breast cancer	Give within 30-60 min of preparation Dilute only in D_5W, never use saline Administer through side port of patent IV Administer corticosteroid eye medication as ordered Tell patient skin may have yellow-orange tinge
—	—	Acute lymphocytic leukemia	Give IV push over 3-5 min through side port of patent IV Assess baseline BP, P, T, R before administration Be prepared to treat anaphylaxis; have life-support equipment readily available
3-4 wk	42	Ovarian cancer Small cell/non–small cell lung cancer	Take 2 hr after meals, at bedtime MAO inhibitor interaction

Continued

Table 15-8	Chemotherapeutic Drugs—cont'd		
Medication	**Dosage**	**Routes of Administration**	**Side Effects and Toxicities***
VINEA ALKALOIDS—CONT'D			
Mitotane (Lysodren)	2-6 g/day; given according to protocol	PO	Nausea, vomiting Rash Adrenal insufficiency Visual disturbances Myelosuppression Keratoconjunctivitis Prolonged bleeding times
Paclitaxel (Taxol)	135-200 mg/m² over 24 hr	IV	Cardiotoxicity Dyspnea Urticaria Facial flushing Rash Hypotension Phlebitis Myelosuppression Neurotoxicity Alopecia Stomatitis Diarrhea
Pentostatin (Covidarabine, DCF)	4 mg/m² every other wk; given according to protocol	IV	Hyperuricemia Neurotoxicity Keratoconjunctivitis
Procarbazine (Matulane)	50-200 mg/day; given according to protocol	PO	Myelosuppression, dose-limiting Thrombocytopenia Leukopenia Anemia

BMT, Bone marrow transplant; ICP, intracranial pressure; IV, intravenous; MAO, monoamine oxidase; TPR, total peripheral resistance.

Ensure patient's comfort

Instruct patient to notify nurse immediately of adverse effects

INTERVENTIONS FOR SPECIFIC TYPES OF DRUGS
Nonvesicants

Can be given by IV bolus through side arm of free-flowing IV containing no additives, by continuous IV drip through a peripheral vein, or by two-syringe technique, with one syringe containing 10 ml of normal saline to test vein before drug administration and to flush vein following injection of drug

When administering through side arm of IV by bolus, check for blood backflow by pinching IV tubing and quickly releasing, before administration of drug, at halfway mark, and at end of administration; before removing needle from injection port, place 4 × 4 with alcohol swab beneath injection port to catch drop

When giving drug by continuous infusion, ensure vein patency throughout infusion period; before removing needle from injection port, place 4 × 4 and alcohol swab beneath injection port to catch drop (prevent spill)

Irritants

Drugs that are capable of producing pain at the IV site or along the vein, with or without inflammatory reaction; never give direct IVP

Can be given by infusion over 30 to 60 minutes depending on dosage

Check for blood backflow before administration and ensure vein patency throughout infusion period; apply ice pack prophylactically at infusion site to prevent discomfort

Vesicants

Drugs that are capable of causing blister formation and tissue destruction; never give direct IVP

See Extravasation (p. 880)

When given peripherally, avoid sites where damage to underlying tendons or nerves are more likely to occur

Can be safely administered through side arm of newly inserted, free-flowing peripheral IV containing no additives

Check for blood backflow before instillation of each milliliter (as described for nonvesicants)

Table 15-8	**Chemotherapeutic Drugs—cont'd**			
Nadir	**Recovery after Nadir (Days)**	**Indications**		**Administration and Nursing Implications**
—	—	Adrenocortical carcinoma		Glucocorticoid, mineralocorticoid therapy may be required Avoid use of alcohol
7-10 days	15-21	Ovarian cancer Lung cancer, non–small cell cancer		Cardiac monitor during administration Give via polyethelene tubing Premedicate for allergic reaction Irritant
—	—	Hairy cell leukemia		May give with allopurinal
25-36 days	36-50	Hodgkin's disease and non-Hodgkin's lymphomas, malignant melanoma, lung and brain cancer		Avoid use of alcohol, sympathomimetic drugs, trycyclic antidepressants, CNS depressants, and heavy intake of dark beer, cheese, bananas

These drugs are not given as continuous infusions except through a well-established central venous access device

When administering by central venous device, obtain blood backflow before instillation of chemotherapeutic drug (see Care of patient with central venous catheter, p. 34)

Use mechanical or electrical controller for continuous chemotherapy infusion

Keep IV site and as much of limb as possible visible
    Avoid obstructing view of site and vein with tape
    Keep clothing well above site; remove clothing from arm when possible

GENERAL INTERVENTIONS

Monitor for allergic reaction: anaphylaxis and extravasation (p. 880) on initiation, continuously during infusion, and then q4h to 8h for 24 hours

Manage pain as indicated and ordered; adjust flow rate of irritating medication to patient tolerance if possible

Know and observe for side or toxic effects and complications during administration, then for 24 to 48 hours; be aware of nadir of drugs ordered

Differentiate between effect of drug and reaction to disease when possible

Infuse parenteral fluids after drug administration to flush tubing, needle, and vein

Apply pressure over site for 3 to 4 minutes following removal of needle

Document medication, site, and responses or untoward effects of interventions

SPECIFIC ALTERNATIVE ADMINISTRATION ROUTES
INTRATHECAL

Assist physician to place lumbar catheter

Observe strict aseptic technique during insertion of catheter and administration of chemotherapy

Use sterile isotonic diluent without preservatives *to prevent/minimize neurotoxic reactions*

Instruct patient to lie flat for 2 to 4 hours after administration of chemotherapy

Assess for signs of changing neurologic status: sleepiness, headache, changing LOC

Monitor for signs of cerebral spinal fluid leak around insertion site

Medications to be administered by MD or may be infused via reservoir or implanted pump

INTRAVENTRICULAR

Assist physician to insert infusion reservoir

Observe strict aseptic technique during insertion and administration of chemotherapy

Ensure that the volume of CSF removed is equal to the volume of chemotherapy infused

Infusion rate not to exceed 2 ml/min

Assess for signs of changing neurologic status

Assess for signs of infection/bleeding in withdrawn CSF: purulence, color change

Assess for signs of CSF leak around insertion site

INTRAARTERIAL

Typically given through implanted pump reservoir into one of several arteries depending on site to be treated

Instruct patient to avoid hot baths/saunas, high altitude, *which may increase rate of pump*

Instruct patient to avoid contact sports/activities

Drugs are administered via infusion pump in heparinized solution

REGIONAL PERFUSION

Intraarterial infusion into an isolated extremity using tourniquets *to limit systemic absorption*

Performed in the operating room under general anesthesia

Assess for signs and symptoms of deep vein thrombosis, sensorineural changes in affected extremity

INTRAPERITONEAL

Administration directly into the peritoneal cavity

Chemotherapy is mixed in a large volume (1 to 2 L) for maximal distribution

Administration is usually done via Tenckoff catheter or an abdominal implanted port

Warm solution to body temperature before administration

Encourage position changes during dwell time for maximal distribution of solution

Drain solution as ordered

Assess patient for signs of nausea/abdominal pain, peritonitis, respiratory distress

Maintain careful intake and output measurement

Monitor abdominal girth

INTRACAVITARY

Administration of chemotherapy into a specific body space

Usually excess fluid in the space is removed before administration of chemotherapy

Ensure free flow of solution during administration; aspirate frequently throughout administration

Turn patient side to side q15min ×4; then q2h to 4h to ensure maximum distribution throughout the cavity

INTRAVESICAL (URINARY BLADDER)

Avoid fluids 4 hours before administration

Administration via Foley catheter; 2-hour dwell time during which patient may not void

Assess for dysuria, hematuria

INTRAPLEURAL

Administration via chest tube; tube clamped for 2 to 6 hours after administration

Discontinue chest tube when drainage is <50 ml/24 hr

Assess for respiratory status and onset of chest pain

INTRAPERICARDIAL

Administered via pericardial catheter with ECG guidance

Assess for ECG changes, onset of chest pain

▮ EXTRAVASATION

Escape of agents from a vein into the tissue; escape of certain antineoplastic agents can cause necrosis of local tissue; care must be taken when giving these agents (see Administration of chemotherapeutic drugs, p. 862); vesicant drugs cause pain and tissue necrosis if they infiltrate; irritants can cause aching, tightness, phlebitis at the injection site. A flare is a red, blotchy reaction without pain, along the line of the vein

ASSESSMENT
OBSERVATIONS/FINDINGS

Venipuncture site
  During infusion
    Burning
    Pain
    Swelling
    Induration
    Erythema
    Significant change in IV flow rate
    No blood return or questionable blood return (blood return is obtained, but patient questions or complains of pain—drug escape could be above injection site)
  Postinfusion
    Ulceration
    Desquamation
    Necrosis
    Phlebitis
      Pain
      Increased temperature
      Redness
      Swelling
  Predisposing factors
    Sclerotic vascular disease
    Multiple venipunctures

MULTIDISCIPLINARY MANAGEMENT
THERAPEUTIC MANAGEMENT

Institute extravasation protocol/standard regimen for specific drug
  Sodium thiosulfate
  Sodium bicarbonate
  Hydrocortisone
  Hyaluronidase
  Dimethyl sulfoxide (DMSO)
  Warm/cold compresses

Consult with Wound, Ostomy Continence/ET Nurse for skin integrity problem as indicated

▼ Risk for impaired tissue integrity, related to extravasation of chemotherapeutic agents

Take measures to prevent extravasation

Administer vesicant medication through a freshly inserted IV site with a good blood return

Select large veins in region with large amount of soft tissue *to avoid possible involvement of tendons should IV infiltrate*

Check medication dosage and dilution carefully *to avoid error*

Administer at rate ordered; monitor closely *to decrease immediate side/toxic effects*

Monitor IV site continuously during infusion *to observe first sign of extravasation*

Instruct patient to notify staff immediately if burning sensation is felt at site or IV slows or stops

After infusing medication, infuse neutral solution through IV line as ordered *to remove traces of drug*

Observe for possible clinical signs of extravasation: pain, burning, swelling, no blood return or questionable blood return

Observe for possible clinical signs of tissue necrosis: erythema, induration, tenderness, pain, eventual ulceration with tissue breakdown

Anticipate and be prepared to initiate protocol/standard regimen for specific drug immediately for any occurrence of extravasation

Avoid direct pressure to site of extravasation *to prevent spread of drug to surrounding tissue*

Mechlorethamine (mustargen, nitrogen mustard)

Aspirate residual drug from existing IV line

Administer ⅙ molar solution of sodium thiosulfate through existing IV line and into surrounding subcutaneous tissues *to neutralize drug effects*

Repeat dosing over next several hours (no dose limit established)

Apply topical cooling measures for 20 minutes qh for the next 24 hours

Elevate and rest extremity

Dactinomycin (actinomycin D, Cosmegen); plicamycin (mithramycin, Mithracin), danorubicin (Daunomycin), doxorubicin (Adriamycin), streptozocin (Zanosar), amsacrine

Discontinue IV

Apply topical cooling measures for 24 hours

Elevate and rest extremity

Vinblastine (Velban), vincristine (Oncovin), vindesine, teniposide, etoposide

Discontinue IV

Infiltrate subcutaneous tissues with 1 to 6 ml hyalurondase; repeat over next several hours *to neutralize drug effects*

Apply topical warming measures for 24 h *to increase absorption*

Elevate and rest extremity

Carbustine

Administer 2 to 6 ml of 1:1 solution of sodium bicarbonate and sterile normal saline into existing IV line and into subcutaneous tissues; may repeat *to neutralize drug effects*

Total dose not to exceed 10 ml of solution

Topical cooling measures for next 24 hours

Elevate and rest extremity

Expected Outcome

Extravasation of chemotherapeutic agents is prevented and/or recognized and treated immediately

■ SAFETY IN HANDLING CANCER CHEMOTHERAPY AGENTS

Only pharmacists, physicians, and nurses with special training should prepare chemotherapeutic agents for administration (Table 15-9)

Preparation of cytotoxic agents should be performed in a Class II biologic safety cabinet (hood)

Transport parenteral drugs in plastic cover to prevent spillage and contamination

All equipment and unused drug(s) should be treated as hazardous waste and disposed of according to facility's policy and procedure: place linen in double bag marked "Caution, Chemotherapy"; instruct personnel to observe precautions in handling; wash twice

Personnel who are planning to become or who may be pregnant may request reassignment

Avoid eating, drinking, smoking, and using cosmetics while preparing and/or administering drug

Wash hands thoroughly before putting on gloves and after gloves are removed

Wear disposable cover gowns with closed front and cuffed, long sleeves and latex gloves throughout preparation, administration, and disposal period when handling medication or equipment *to protect self in case of accidental spills*

Wear protective garment and gloves when handling patient excreta during administration and for 48 hours following administration

Syringes and IV sets with Leur-Lok fitting should be used whenever possible *to prevent spillage*

When priming IV line and removing needle from injection port, place alcohol swab and 4 × 4 beneath site *to collect small spills;* discard in hazardous waste container

Occupational Safety and Health Administration (OSHA) recommends drug administration sets should be attached and primed within a hood before the drug is added to the fluid

Wipe up spills immediately; contain spills by gently covering them with disposable absorbent material *to prevent aerosolization* (wear gown, mask, eye wear, double gloves); place absorbent material in double plastic bag marked "Hazardous Waste" *to prevent accidental spill*

Table 15-9	Hazards Associated With Chemotherapeutic Drugs		
Medication	**Route**	**Hazard**	**Precaution and Action**
ALKYLATING AGENTS			
Cyclophosphamide (Cytoxan)	IV, PO	Teratogenic and carcinogenic; skin irritation is rare	Wear protective gloves; flush spills with large amounts of water
Mechlorethamine hydrochloride (Mustargen, nitrogen mustard)	IV, intracavitary, topical, intralesional	Strong vesicant, nasal irritant, highly toxic	Wear protective gloves; protect eyes; wash skin with large amounts of water, sodium carbonate (3%), or isotonic solution of sodium thiosulfate (2.5%); wash eyes with large amounts of water; irrigate with sodium thiosulfate in isotonic solution (contact physician)
Ifosfamide (Ifex)	IV	Teratogenic and carcinogenic; skin irritation is rare	Wear protective gloves; flush spills with large amounts of water
ANTIMETABOLITES			
Cytarabine (Ara-C, Cytosar)	IV, SC, IM, intrathecal	Teratogenic; not absorbed through intact skin	Wear protective gloves; wash spills with water
5-Fluorouracil (Fluoroplex, Fluorouracil, Adrucil)	IV, PO, topical	Minor inflammatory reaction if skin is broken	Flush spills with large amounts of water
Methotrexate (Mexate, Amethopterin MTX)	IV, IM, intrathecal	Teratogenic, carcinogenic skin irritant	Wear protective gloves; wash spills with water; apply nonmedicated cream for stinging; for systemic absorption of significant quantity notify physician; give folinic acid (leucovorin calcium)
ANTIBIOTICS			
Dactinomycin (Cosmegen, actinomycin D)	IV	Teratogenic; corrosive to soft tissues	Wear protective gloves; protect eyes; rinse spillage in running water for 10 min; rinse with buffered phosphate solution
Bleomycin (Blenoxane)	IV, IM, SC intraarterial, intratumoral, intracavitary	Cytostatic: local, toxic, or allergic reaction	Wear protective gloves; wash spills thoroughly with water
Daunomycin (Cerubidin, Daunorubicin, DNR)	IV	Skin and mucous membrane irritant	Wear protective gloves; wash spills immediately with water or isotonic saline
Doxorubicin (Adriamycin)	IV	Potential teratogenic; suspected carcinogenic skin irritant, but not absorbed into bloodstream	Wear protective gloves; wash spills immediately with large amounts of water

Table 15-9	Hazards Associated With Chemotherapeutic Drugs—cont'd		
Medication	**Route**	**Hazard**	**Precaution and Action**
ANTIBIOTICS			
Plicamycin (mith-racin)	IV	Rare skin irritation	Wash spills with water
Mitomycin (Mito-mycin C, Muta-mycin)		Teratogenic; suspected carcinogenic skin irritant	Wear protective gloves; wash spills thoroughly and immediately with large quantities of water; irrigate contaminated eyes with large amounts of water; notify physician
PODOPHYLLOTOXINS			
Etoposide (VP-16)	IV	Suspected teratogenic and carcinogenic irritants	Wear protective gloves; wash spills with large amounts of water
Teniposide (VM-26)			
VINCA ALKALOIDS			
Vinblastine (Vel-ban)	IV	Suspected teratogenic skin irritant	Wear protective gloves; wash spills thoroughly and immediately with large amounts of water
Vincristine (On-covin)	IV	Suspected teratogenic skin irritant	Wear protective gloves; wash skin with large amounts of water
Vindesine	IV	Suspected teratogenic skin irritant; may produce corneal ulcers	Wear protective gloves; protect eyes; wash areas with large amounts of water
MISCELLANEOUS			
Asparaginase (L-Asparaginase)	IV, IM	Potentially teratogenic	
Azathioprine (Imuran)	IV (investiga-tional)	Potentially teratogenic, suspected carcinogenic skin irritant	Wear protective gloves; protect eyes; wash spills with water immediately
Cisplatin (Pla-tinol)	IV	Suspected teratogen and carcinogen; skin reaction in sensitive patients	Wear protective gloves; rinse spills thoroughly with water
Dacarbazine (DTIC)	IV	Teratogenic, carcinogenic irritant to skin and mucous membranes	Wear protective gloves; wash spills with soap and water immediately; irrigate eyes with water
Carboplatin (Para-platin)	IV	Suspected teratogen and carcinogen; skin reaction in sensitive patients	Wear protective gloves; rinse spills thoroughly with water

SYMPTOMATIC CARE IN CHEMOTHERAPY

■ HEMATOLOGIC MYELOSUPPRESSION

Inhibition of bone marrow activity resulting in decreased production of blood cells and platelets caused by the effects of chemotherapy, the disease state, or radiation therapy; the majority of chemotherapeutic agents produce some degree of myelosuppression; because the blood count nadirs (the point of lowest drop in blood count) produced by most chemotherapeutic agents can be predicted, the schedule of drug delivery is designed to coincide with the recovery of the bone marrow; the nurse must be aware of the nadir for each chemotherapeutic drug

■ LEUKOPENIA

Temporary reduction in the total number of circulating WBCs; because the life span of the leukocyte is very brief (6 to 8 hours), leukopenias occur frequently in patients receiving chemotherapy, placing them at risk for infections; neutropenia is a good indication of a patient's ability to fight infection, as is the absolute neutrophil count (ANC), which is calculated by multiplying the total WBC count by the percentage of neutrophils in the differential:

$$ANC = WBC \times \% \text{ Neutrophils (mm}^3\text{)}$$
$$(\% \text{ Bands} + \% \text{ Segs} = \text{Neutrophils})$$

When ANC is <1000 cells/mm³, patient is at risk of infection; opportunistic endogenous organisms can cause systemic and severe infections; severe neutropenia is often defined as <500 neutrophils/mm³

ASSESSMENT

SUBJECTIVE DATA
Dyspnea on exertion
Chest pain
Sore throat
Perineal discomfort, pain
Rectal tenderness
Dysuria, urgency

OBJECTIVE DATA
Elevated temperature if not masked by corticosteroids or antiinflammatory drugs
Any sudden rise or fall of temperature of even 1° F
Elevated temperature of 100.4° F (38.3° C) lasting 24 hours or longer, not associated with blood products or drugs
Elevated temperature may be caused by other factors such as atelectasis, tumor, or response of disease process
Sudden rise and fall in neutrophils may be indicative of infection
In neutropenic patients, inflammatory response (redness, heat, edema, pus formation, pain) may be diminished or absent

Respiratory system
  Cough, sputum production, change in color of sputum
  Changes in breath sounds (wheezes, rales, rhonchi)
  Colds and flu
Skin and mucous membranes
  Skin breaks, puncture sites
  Redness
  Swelling
  Drainage
  Ulceration
  Flushed skin
  Diaphoresis
Oral cavity
  Fissures
  Redness
  Swelling
  Ulceration
  White, cream-colored lesions
Perineum
  Excoriation
Rectum
  Fissures
  Abscess
Genitourinary system
  Frequency
  Neurogenic bladder: monitor residual urine; check urine for clarity and odor
  Vaginal discharge
  Prostate enlargement
Eye or ear drainage
Confusion, mental status changes
Malaise, lethargy

DIAGNOSTIC TESTS
WBC
Differential values
  Granulocytes
    Comprise 56% to 75% of total WBC
    Responsible for fighting bacterial and fungal infection
    Life of 6 to 7 hours
    Type: neutrophils, eosinophils, basophils
  Lymphocytes
    Comprise 20% to 40% of total WBC
    Responsible for immune defenses
    B lymphocytes: humoral immunity
    T lymphocytes: cell-mediated immunity
  Monocytes
    Comprise 2% to 8% of total WBC
    Defense against bacteria and fungi
Cultures: urine, sputum, blood
Urinalysis
Chest x-ray
Pulmonary function studies

POTENTIAL COMPLICATIONS
Septicemia

MULTIDISCIPLINARY MANAGEMENT

THERAPEUTIC MANAGEMENT

Treatment based on results of cultures

Antibiotics

Antifungals

IV gamma globulin

Antiviral therapy

Granulocyte colony-stimulating factors (G-CSF)

PATIENT PROBLEM—NURSING DIAGNOSIS/INTERVENTIONS

▼Risk for infection, related to depressed immune system

Check results of WBC and differential *to ensure that they are within acceptable limits;* calculate ANG

Assess patient for increasing myelosuppression; nursing management will depend on severity of condition

Assess skin and mucous membranes for signs and symptoms of infection; give special attention to skin folds and body cavities

Assess respiratory and genitourinary tract for evidence of infection

Document findings and interventions

Instruct patient and/or significant other(s) that WBC count may decrease following most chemotherapy; WBC count usually recovers before next dose; however, recovery may be delayed, and an occasional dose of chemotherapy may be rescheduled

Teach patient *to guard against infection* by the following:

Maintaining meticulous total body hygiene including perineal care

Avoiding crowds and persons with infections

Maintaining good nutrition and fluid intake

Practicing good oral hygiene after meals

Getting adequate rest and exercise

Reporting signs and symptoms of infection to health care personnel immediately

Place patient in noninfectious environment if ANC is $<1000/mm^3$ or as ordered; private room is recommended

Use physical means *to reduce exposure to microbes*

Instruct and ensure that personnel and visitors follow handwashing procedure with povidone-iodine before entering room

No one with an infectious condition (e.g., cold, flu, skin rash,) may enter room

Staff assigned to care for patient with neutropenia must not be assigned to care for patients who have infections, if possible

Care for neutropenic patient first and take precautions to avoid transferring any infectious agents to neutropenic patient

Keep room clean

Avoid any trash in room and bathroom

Remove food and examination trays immediately after use

Maintain furniture, fixtures, floor, and equipment free of dust and spills

Ensure that allied health personnel (e.g., laboratory technicians) do not bring into patient's room equipment that has been in other areas of hospital

If patient requires transportation, avoid using elevator with potentially infectious passengers present; mask for patient may be required

Maintain skin integrity

Avoid IM injections

Observe IV or central line site q4h

Change dressing daily if nonporous type is used, using aseptic technique

Change IV tubing and bottles daily

Avoid infiltrations that necessitate restarting IV; position IV site *to prevent stress and movement at site of insertion*

Consolidate laboratory work; clean skin with povidone-iodine scrub before puncture

Assess previous puncture sites q8h

Assess and record condition of oral cavity q8h

Teach or assist with oral hygiene measures in morning, after food ingestion, at bedtime, and q2h to 4h when patient is awake at night

Administer antifungal and antiviral medication as ordered

Assess and record condition of perineum daily

Initiate and teach perineal care to be performed after each bowel movement

Prevent constipation (p. 893) and diarrhea (p. 892)

Administer medications as ordered

Avoid use of enemas and suppositories

Monitor and record vital signs q4h; take temperature more frequently if trend is beginning; report any change in temperature immediately

Institute comfort and cooling measures as indicated by condition

Change linen and clothing *to keep patient dry*

Avoid chilling, *which may increase temperature elevation*

Administer antipyretics as ordered

Mechanical cooling blanket may be ordered

Monitor intake and output; report urinary frequency, burning, or changes in character of urine

Use voiding measures when indicated *to avoid catheterization*

If catheterization is necessary

Use strict aseptic technique for insertion

Perform catheter care q8h to 12h

Obtain cultures as ordered (e.g., blood, urine, sputum, skin, drainage)

Assess and record respiratory status q4h; report changes in breath sounds, cough, and sputum; increases in respiratory rate; or presence of sore throat immediately

Assist and teach patient to turn, cough, and deep breathe q2h *to remove secretions and prevent site for growth of microorganisms*

Administer oxygen if ordered

Encourage mobility q8h

Turn and position immobile patient q2h *to prevent pressure sores*

Pressure reduction mattress

Provide mild antibacterial soaps and soft cloths and towels for skin hygiene, daily and prn

Administer IV antibiotics as ordered

Monitor laboratory data daily; report changes that indicate infection

Administer gamma globulin as ordered

   Monitor for anaphylactic reaction, phlebitis, nausea, back or abdominal pain, and chills

   Minimize side effects by initiating comfort measures, use of blankets, decreasing rate of infusion and premedicating with acetaminophen (Tylenol) as ordered

Administer colony-stimulating factors (CSFs) as ordered; assess for headache; institute interventions

Instruct patient about low-bacteria diet

Instruct about need to remove flowers and plants from environment during neutropenic phase

Expected Outcome

Exhibits no signs and symptoms of infection or signs and symptoms of infection are recognized early and treated quickly

PATIENT/FAMILY TEACHING

Discuss signs and symptoms of infection to report to physician or nurse

Emphasize importance of avoiding persons who may be infectious or have potentially contagious conditions

Explain need to avoid persons who have been recently vaccinated

Explain need to maintain safe sex practices

Explain need to wash hands after using bathroom, before eating, and before and after performing any procedures

Emphasize importance of preventing injury to skin
   Use electric razors
   Handle knives and sharp objects carefully
   Wear protective gloves when gardening and when using strong household cleaning solutions
   Wear broad-brimmed hat and sunscreen when in sun
   Avoid going barefoot
   Wear warm clothing and boots in cold weather
   Avoid cutting cuticles, corns, or calluses
   Wear padded gloves when using oven

Explain need to perform oral hygiene periodically throughout the day

Emphasize importance of daily hygiene including perineal and rectal care

Emphasize importance of fluid intake of 3000 ml/day unless contraindicated; explain need to avoid using common drinking fountain

Explain need to maintain clean home environment and handle food properly

Caution patient to avoid contact with pets or other animals during neutropenic phase

Teach name of medication, dosage, time of administration, purpose, and side effects

Explain need to tell all health care personnel, especially dentists, about need *to prevent infections*

Emphasize importance of follow-up outpatient care

Ensure that patient and significant other(s) demonstrate the following:
   Method for taking and recording temperature
   Procedure for caring for very small cuts or breaks in skin

DISCHARGE/HOME CARE PLANNING

Assess patient's ability to obtain needed protective gear such as gloves, hats, sunglasses, electric razor, dental care items; assist in procurement as needed

Assess patient's ability to provide for own physical care needs and daily living needs: cooking, housekeeping, shopping, laundry; arrange home health providers as needed

◼ THROMBOCYTOPENIA

Reduction in the number of circulating platelets caused by the effect of the tumor or destruction of bone marrow during chemotherapy and/or radiation therapy; plate-lets circulate for about 10 days before removal from circulation

ASSESSMENT
SUBJECTIVE DATA

Abdominal pain

Blurred vision

Headache

OBJECTIVE DATA

Mental status changes

Signs and symptoms of increased ICP

Petechiae, easy bruising

Bleeding gums, nose
   Purpura
   Hypermenorrhea
   Blood in emesis, urine, stool; tarry stools
   Prolonged bleeding from invasive procedures
   Vaginal, rectal bleeding

DIAGNOSTIC TESTS

CBC

Platelet count

ABO, Rh, HLA compatibility

MULTIDISCIPLINARY MANAGEMENT
THERAPEUTIC MANAGEMENT

Bleeding precautions

Stool softeners

Blood component transfusion

Safety measures

POTENTIAL PATIENT PROBLEM/INTERVENTIONS

▼ Bleeding related to thrombocytopenia

Monitor platelet count and coagulation studies

Anticipate time of nadir after chemotherapy (time that patient is most vulnerable to bleed)

Identify drugs and/or other factors to avoid that may lower platelet count and predispose patient to bleeding

Assess and report any signs and symptoms of bleeding

Inspect gums and oral cavity for bleeding q8h

Inspect skin q8h for increased bruising, petechiae, ecchymosis, and swelling

Inspect and palpate joints q8h for increased size and decreased mobility

Assess sensorium and neurologic status q8h

Inspect nasal cavity at least once q8h

If epistaxis occurs

Have patient sit at 90-degree angle

Apply pressure to nose

Place ice pack at back of neck

If nasal bleeding is not controlled in 10 to 15 minutes

Notify physician

Administer platelet transfusion immediately when ordered by physician

Institute safety measures as platelet count decreases below 50,000/mm^3

Avoid needle sticks when possible

Consolidate laboratory work; apply pressure to site for 5 minutes and observe site q15min for at least 1 hour

Avoid IM injections, aspirin, aspirin-containing products, and NSAIDs

Do not take rectal temperature or administer medications rectally; avoid enemas

Avoid bladder catheterization when possible

Take BP only when necessary and pump cuff only as high as necessary

Avoid use of the following:

Rough towels and washcloths

Razors

Restraints

Tight clothing

Maintain clutter-free environment

Provide night-light *to prevent bumping into objects or falling*

Administer careful oral hygiene *to prevent mucosal breaks*

Use toothettes or gauze pads

Avoid use of dental floss or toothpicks

Encourage use of mouth rinse q2h to 4h

Half saline and half water

Half saline and half hydrogen peroxide followed by saline rinse

Inspect IV or central line site q20 min to 30 minutes for hematoma or oozing

Maintain pressure at site for 5 minutes when IV is discontinued

Inspect q15 min ×4

Administer antacids as ordered

Test stool for blood after each bowel movement

Test urine for blood each time patient voids

Administer stool softeners as ordered *to prevent bleeding from constipation*

Avoid vaginal douches

Use lubricant during intercourse to avoid trauma

Expected Outcomes

Has no bleeding due to preventable causes

PATIENT/FAMILY TEACHING

Explain relationship between platelets and bleeding risk

Teach patient signs and symptoms of bleeding to be reported to physician in any of the following areas

Skin

Oral

Nasal

Rectal

GI tract

Vagina

Cerebral

Urinary tract

Discuss emergency plan to follow if spontaneous hemorrhage occurs at home

Have emergency numbers available

Call paramedics

Go to nearest emergency area

Emphasize importance of telling dentist and other medical personnel about chemotherapy and low platelet count

Emphasize importance of maintaining safe, clutter-free environment

Explain need to apply pressure at blood withdrawal site after laboratory work is completed

Emphasize importance of avoiding over-the-counter medications, especially those containing acetylsalicylic acid (i.e., aspirin), without consulting physician

Caution patient to avoid use of sharp objects when possible

Use electric razor

Use caution when handling knives or other equipment

Explain need to avoid harsh coughing, blowing of nose, straining, and strenuous exercise

If cough persists, notify physician

Take cough medication as ordered

Emphasize importance of follow-up outpatient care

Routine laboratory appointments

Return physician and nurse appointments

Ensure that patient and significant other(s) demonstrate the following:

Method for applying pressure to bleeding site

Apply dressing or clean material directly over site

Apply pressure for 5 minutes

Apply ice in covered plastic bag over site once bleeding stops

Check site for further bleeding q15 min for 1 hour

Method for testing stool and urine for occult blood

DISCHARGE/HOME CARE PLANNING

Discuss importance of having emergency telephone numbers immediately accessible; know nearest emergency care facility

Assist patient in obtaining medical alert identification: bracelet, necklace

Assess patient's ability to safely provide for own physical care and daily living needs; arrange home health providers as needed

Plan for sufficient, clean storage space for medical supplies: occult blood testing products, emergency dressing supplies

▮ ANEMIA

Temporary reduction in the number of circulating RBCs and the level of Hgb caused by destruction of cells during chemotherapy, leading to tissue hypoxia from impaired oxygen-carrying capacity

ASSESSMENT

SUBJECTIVE DATA

Headache, dizziness
Fatigue, irritability
Difficulty concentrating
Dyspnea
Palpitations
Feeling cold

OBJECTIVE DATA

Pallor
Syncope
Loss of color in nails and palms of hands
Tachycardia
Low blood pressure

DIAGNOSTIC TESTS

Decreased Hgb and Hct (dehydration may raise Hgb/Hct); if precipitous drop in Hgb, may be caused by hemorrhaging
CBC and platelet count
Reticulocyte count
ABO, Rh compatibility
Mean cell volume (MCV)
Mean cell hemoglobin (MCH)
Mean cell hemoglobin concentration (MCHC)
Bone marrow aspirate
Total iron-binding capacity (TIBC)

POTENTIAL COMPLICATIONS

Tissue hypoxia

MULTIDISCIPLINARY MANAGEMENT

THERAPEUTIC MANAGEMENT

IV fluid therapy
Serial ECG or telemetry monitoring
Blood product transfusion
Erythropoetin administration

PATIENT PROBLEM—NURSING DIAGNOSIS/INTERVENTIONS

▼ Fatigue related to anemia

Note signs and symptoms of fatigue, SOB, tachycardia on exertion, and/or dizziness
Adjust ADLs *to match energy level*
Monitor laboratory data
  Hgb, Hct
  MCV, MCH, MCHC, reticulocyte count
Anticipate time of nadir after chemotherapy (see Table 15-8)
Provide adequate periods of rest and sleep *to improve energy level*
  Plan nursing activities *to avoid interrupting sleep*
  Provide activity-free periods throughout the day for rest
  Schedule examinations and tests carefully
Conserve patient's energy for desired activities
  Assist with meal preparation
  Keep needed items within reach
  Assist with hygiene measures
  Plan activities after rest periods
Gradually increase activity under supervision as problem resolves
Keep patient warm *to avoid expending energy to create body warmth*
  Encourage use of warm robes, socks, and clothing
  Provide extra blankets; cotton sheets are often more comfortable
Assess systems for signs indicating anemia
  CNS: irritability, headache, dizziness
  Skin: pallor, petechiae, purpura, jaundice
  Nailbeds: pallor, blanching
  Mucous membranes: pallor, petechiae
  Bones: tenderness over ribs and sternum
  Take and record vital signs q8h
  Assess respiratory and cardiac status q8h; report tachycardia, irregular cardiac sounds, and presence of wheezes or rales
Place patient at 60-degree angle *to facilitate breathing;* position with pillows if indicated
Administer oxygen therapy as ordered
Assess extremities, abdomen, and sacrum for presence of edema; report positive findings
Observe safety precautions: instruct patient to sit at side of bed before getting up; change position slowly *to avoid positional hypotension*
Provide nutritious diet high in iron
Administer blood components when ordered (p. 216); one unit of blood will usually raise Hgb 1 g/dl (and hematocrit by 3%)

Expected Outcome

Demonstrates a progressive increase in activity tolerance while maintaining physiologic response within acceptable range

PATIENT/FAMILY TEACHING

Teach patient about the relationship between Hgb and availability of oxygen as required for normal tissue function

Teach signs and symptoms of anemia to report to physician

Emphasize importance of eating foods high in protein, vitamins, and minerals, which are necessary for RBC production

Explain need to include foods high in iron, vitamin B_{12}, and folic acid

Arrange for dietitian to teach patient and significant other foods to include in diet

Discuss methods to conserve energy
Planned rest periods
Adequate rest
Activities planned after rest periods
Assisting with ADLs
Keeping needed items within reach

Explain need to change position slowly; use appliances (e.g., walker bars) for movement if indicated

Emphasize importance of continuing to perform ADLs and other desired activities to tolerance

Emphasize importance of follow-up care

Emphasize importance of preventing secondary problems related to tissue hypoxia: infection, tissue breakdown, and/or blood loss

DISCHARGE/HOME CARE PLANNING

Assess patient's ability to provide for nutritious diet; arrange for home health provider, Meals-on-Wheels prn

Assess patient's ability to provide for own physical and daily living needs; arrange for home health provider prn

Assess patient's need for assistive devices; arrange for durable medical equipment prn

■ GASTROINTESTINAL

▌ NAUSEA, VOMITING, AND ANOREXIA

Caused by physiologic changes resulting from cancer, the toxicities of radiation therapy or chemotherapy, and/or psychologic expectation

ASSESSMENT
SUBJECTIVE DATA
Nausea
Anorexia
Abdominal pain

OBJECTIVE DATA
Time of onset of nausea and vomiting before or after chemotherapy administration or radiation therapy
Duration
Severity
Possible cause
Anticipation
Foods

Bowel obstruction
Other medications
Brain metastasis
Vomitus: amount, frequency, character, color
Nutritional status: weight loss, decreased food/fluid intake
Dehydration
Dry mucous membranes and skin
Poor skin turgor
Sunken, soft eyeballs
Concentrated urine; decreased output
Antiemetics: type, frequency, and method of administration

DIAGNOSTIC TESTS
Electrolytes
CBC
Serum transferrin

POTENTIAL COMPLICATIONS
Severe dehydration
Electrolyte imbalance
Malnutrition

MULTIDISCIPLINARY MANAGEMENT
THERAPEUTIC MANAGEMENT
Parenteral fluids/nutrition
Antiemetics
Sedatives/hypnotics
Relaxation/hypnosis therapy

PATIENT PROBLEM—NURSING DIAGNOSIS/INTERVENTIONS

▼Altered nutrition: less than body requirements related to nausea/vomiting, anorexia, decreased food intake

General
Remove food trays as soon as patient has eaten *to reduce negative stimuli*
Be aware that flowers and scents may be noxious
Instruct personnel and visitors to avoid wearing colognes and perfumes or smoking, which may be noxious to patient
Provide oral hygiene materials *to enhance appetite*
Keep dentifrice and mouth rinse pleasing to patient within reach
Encourage and assist with dental and oral care before and after meals and especially after vomiting

Nausea and Vomiting
Instruct patient and/or significant other about drugs that are known to cause severe emetic action such as cisplatin and nitrogen mustard
Instruct patient and/or significant other about measures used to minimize side effects
Assess history of nausea and vomiting
Assess for known or probable preexisting disease states such as diabetes or hypercalcemia

Administer antiemetics before administration of agents and q4h to 6h for 24 hours rather than prn *to maintain good control of nausea*

Administer antihistamines or barbiturates combined with an antiemetic as ordered *to decrease stimulation of the vomiting center in the brain*

If metoclopramide (Reglan) is given, assess for extrapyramidal side effects; keep diphenhydramine (Benadryl) available *to counteract side effects*

Lorazepam (Ativan) may be given as an amnesic during chemotherapy administration *to help control nausea and vomiting*

Provide safety measures when administering these medications *to prevent physical injury*

Give chemotherapy in late afternoon or at night when possible *so a nutritious meal can be taken without anticipating nausea*

Continually evaluate effectiveness of antiemetics *to help patient find the most effective combinations of drugs*

Teach patient and/or significant other methods *to prevent nausea and vomiting*

Small, frequent meals

Small dietary intake before treatment

Avoidance of greasy or spicy foods

Rest periods before and after meals

Quiet, restful environment

Monitor laboratory values, CBC, electrolytes

Monitor vital signs

Maintain chart of onset of symptoms, reaction to varying dosage of medication, and frequency of administration *to determine best interventions*

Monitor intake and output *to assure adequate hydration*

Administer IV replacement fluids as ordered

Weigh patient daily (same time, scale, and clothing)

Experiment with several methods *to reduce or alleviate nausea and/or vomiting before or after chemotherapy*

Withhold food and fluids for 4 to 6 hours

Eat a light, bland meal

Take only fluids for 4 to 6 hours if nausea is severe

Eat dry salty foods

Assist patient with belching air swallowed during feeding

Avoid motions conducive to nausea (rapid or frequent change of position)

Use other methods *to prevent onset or reduce severity of symptoms*

Animated conversation

Absorbing projects or activities

Relaxation methods

Rhythmic breathing exercises

Imagery experiences

Self-hypnosis

Behavior modification techniques

Music therapy

Place patient in well-ventilated room *to control odors*

Room should be away from food preparation area and soiled linen and waste product storage

Remove trash frequently

Empty and remove emesis basin, bedpans, and urinals immediately after use

Anorexia

Plan appetizing meals based on patient's preference *to enhance nutrition*

Serve food attractively arranged and at proper temperature

Eat in a social environment

Avoid liquids with meals

Provide foods high in carbohydrates to promote earlier emptying of stomach

Cool foods that are bland, soft, and odorless may be tolerated more easily

Sweet foods are often preferred

Add calories and nutrients by adding supplements to food (e.g., high-protein supplements, dry milk products)

Encourage patient to chew food well to ensure easier digestion

Breakfast is usually best tolerated; eat ⅓ of daily calories at this time

Expected Outcome

Maintains stable weight or increases weight and improves caloric and nutritional value of food ingested

PATIENT/FAMILY TEACHING

Teach method and rationale of all aspects of ongoing care to be implemented at home

Emphasize importance of maintaining adequate food and fluid intake

Emphasize importance of reporting the following to physician or nurse

Continuous vomiting for 24 hours without food or fluid intake

Signs and symptoms of dehydration

Feeling of extreme stomach fullness and/or abdominal pain relieved by vomiting

DISCHARGE/HOME CARE PLANNING

Assess patient's ability to obtain, store, and prepare nutritious meals; arrange for home health provider or have foods brought to patient as needed

Assist patient to develop relationships with community support groups for continuing nutritional and psychologic counseling and support

▌STOMATITIS/MUCOSITIS

stomatitis: *Temporary inflammatory response of the oral mucosa to the cytotoxic effects of chemotherapy and/or radiation; may progress to ulcerative bleeding and secondary infection*

mucositis: *Temporary inflammatory response of mucous membrane*

ASSESSMENT

SUBJECTIVE DATA

Buccal mucosa pain

Change in taste and sensation

Inability to take food and/or fluids

OBJECTIVE DATA
Buccal mucosa
General erythema
Swelling
Bleeding
Ulceration
Infected lesions
Candida albicans: soft whitish patches; may be
localized or extensive
Herpes simplex: painful clusters of vesicles or
ulceration
Gram positive: dry, brownish yellow, circular, raised
eruptions
Gram negative: creamy white, raised, moist,
nonpurulent painful ulcer
Lips
Red fissures at corners of mouth
Edema
Surface abnormalities on palpation
Ability to chew and swallow
Hydration status

DIAGNOSTIC TESTS
CBC, platelet count
Cultures of oral cavity

POTENTIAL COMPLICATIONS
Infection
Malnutrition
Dehydration
Electrolyte imbalance

MULTIDISCIPLINARY MANAGEMENT
THERAPEUTIC MANAGEMENT
Consult with clinical dietitian to plan diet with needed
calories and nutrients that patient is able to chew and
swallow
Antibacterial agents
Antifungal agents
Antiviral agents
Analgesics; topical and systemic
Consult with Wound, Ostomy, Continence/ET Nurse as
indicated

PATIENT PROBLEMS—NURSING
DIAGNOSES/INTERVENTIONS

▼Altered oral mucous membranes, related to effects
of chemotherapy

Establish oral hygiene regimen at initiation of
chemotherapy
Assess oral cavity daily with tongue blade and light,
noting color, moisture, and presence of lesions
Note color, amount, and consistency of saliva
Institute prophylactic oral hygiene regimen before, within
30 minutes after each meal, and q2h to 4h during
waking hours *to reduce foreign flora*
Brush teeth with soft-bristled toothbrush and
nonabrasive toothpaste

Use foam stick moistened with mouthwash to remove
debris from mucosa if unable to tolerate brush or if
platelet count is greatly decreased
Use mouthwashes with no alcohol content
Remove dentures and bridges and cleanse following
oral hygiene regimen
Keep mucosa moist by frequent fluid intake and eating
soft, moist food; suggest saliva substitute *to
maintain moisture*
Obtain order for mild analgesia if pain is present
Assess history of alcohol use, smoking, radiation therapy,
and previous and current treatment with
chemotherapy
Teach patient about oral complications of chemotherapy,
how to examine mouth, and complete oral care

Expected Outcome
Oral mucosa remains clean and intact or lesions heal
progressively

▼Impaired tissue integrity related to stomatitis,
pharyngitis/esophagitis, and/or rectal or vaginal
mucositis related to effects of chemotherapy

Stomatitis
NOTE: Stomatitis generally occurs 5 to 7 days after
chemotherapy and persists for up to 10 days
If mild stomatitis occurs
Culture oral cavity
Assess oral cavity q8h
Encourage oral hygiene regimen q2h during waking
hours and q6h during the night *to reduce
microorganism count*
Brush teeth with soft-bristled toothbrush and
nonabrasive toothpaste q4h
Use dilute nonalcohol mouthwash or normal saline:
swish, gargle, and expectorate
¼ tsp salt, pinch of baking soda and 8 oz of water:
swish, gargle, and expectorate 4 times daily
Use toothette or cotton-tipped applicator to remove
mucus and debris
Apply lip lubricant q2h during waking hours
Assess need for use of antifungal or antibacterial
agents
Topical anesthetics such as viscous lidocaine (Xylocaine)
or Orabase may be used before meals and oral care for
discomfort
Use mild analgesic q3h to 4h
Encourage bland diet high in protein *to promote
healing*
Encourage fluid to 2000 ml/day; avoid citrus juices
If severe stomatitis occurs
Request order for culture for oral cavity *to determine
causative organism*
Assess oral cavity q8h
If patient has difficulty in eating and maintaining fluid
intake, parenteral nutrition may be necessary
If oral hygiene is difficult because of pain in oral cavity,
encourage patient to rinse with 1 tsp viscous lidocaine
15 minutes before oral hygiene

If patient is unable to brush or rinse, irrigate mouth with syringe or soft rubber catheter using salt, soda, and water mixture q3h to 4h

If oral candidiasis is present, instruct patient to swish and swallow an oral suspension of nystatin (Mycostatin)

Teach patient how to examine mouth and perform oral care

Pharyngitis/esophagitis
Assess for difficulty in swallowing and for infection

Antacids may be helpful

Obtain physician's order for Sucralfate

Rectal or vaginal mucositis
Eat low-residue, easily digested foods

Antidiarrheal medications

Instruct female patients to report any pain, ulceration, or bleeding of mucous membrane lining perineum or vagina

Instruct patient to include perineal washing with mild soap and water after voiding; pat dry

Instruct patient to use sitz baths *to increase comfort*

Caution patient to avoid douches *to avoid further irritation*

Discuss need to avoid sexual activity while symptomatic

Instruct male patient to report signs and symptoms involving perineum

Expected Outcome
Affected tissues heal progressively

▌ DIARRHEA
Passage of frequent stools of a soft or liquid consistency with or without discomfort caused by effects of chemotherapy on epithelium

ASSESSMENT
SUBJECTIVE DATA
Abdominal cramping

Feeling of fullness, bloating

OBJECTIVE DATA
Frequent stools
  Watery
  Bloody
  Containing mucus
  Tarry
Dehydration
  Dry mucous membranes
  Poor skin turgor
  Decreased urine output

DIAGNOSTIC TESTS
CBC

Electrolytes

Stool cultures

POTENTIAL COMPLICATIONS
Electrolyte imbalance

Dehydration

Malnutrition

GI bleeding

MULTIDISCIPLINARY MANAGEMENT
THERAPEUTIC MANAGEMENT
Parenteral fluids/nutrition

Antidiarrheals

Antispasmodics

Collaborate with clinical dietitian to plan meals with sufficient caloric and nutritional values that assist in controlling or do not promote diarrhea

Consult with Wound, Ostomy Continence/ET Nurse as indicated

PATIENT PROBLEM—NURSING DIAGNOSIS/INTERVENTIONS

▼ Diarrhea related to chemotherapy effects on GI mucosa

Assess usual pattern of elimination including use of laxatives

Determine other probable causes of diarrhea such as inappropriate diet, treatment side effects, infection, stress, or disease progression

Evaluate hydration and electrolyte status
  Monitor intake and output, weight, and electrolytes
  Assess frequency, character, and volume of stool
  Assess abdomen, including bowel sounds; note distention, cramping, or flatus
  Assess perineal/perianal region for skin status

Adjust diet as appropriate; include bananas and cheese; avoid hot liquids, coffee, fresh fruits, and prune juice

Include foods high in potassium to prevent weakness when laboratory values indicate a low potassium level

Encourage increased fluid intake of 3000 ml/day if not contraindicated; suggest liquids, such as sports drinks, grape juice, and fruit drinks, that contain electrolytes

Administer medications, such as Kaopectate or difenoxin (Lomotil) as ordered, *to control diarrhea*

Observe and report early signs of constipation

Establish protocol for care of perineal area
  Gently clean area with water and mild soap after each stool; dry thoroughly and inspect for breakdown
  Apply ointments as indicated
  Use sitz baths as indicated *to increase comfort*
  Use skin barrier as needed *to promote healing*

Check and record all stools for the following:
  Frequency
  Amount
  Consistency
  Presence of blood, overt or occult

Perform perineal care if patient is unable

Apply topical medication to perineum as ordered *to promote healing*

Assess and record status of perineal area at least q8h; q4h if frequency of stools increases

Weigh patient daily (same time, scale, and clothing)

Consult with physician *to determine possibility of interrupting treatment until diarrhea is controlled*

Assess for edema; third spacing of fluids may occur from protein deficiency and electrolyte imbalances

Expected Outcome
Healthy bowel elimination pattern is achieved

PATIENT/FAMILY TEACHING
Teach patient to perform perineal care after each defecation
    Use mild soap and water
    Wash with soft cloths, front to back for women
    Dry by gentle patting with soft toweling
    Wash and dry hands well
Teach patient to test stool for blood once daily
Discuss signs and symptoms of diarrhea that must be reported to physician
Emphasize importance of maintaining oral fluid intake of 3000 ml/day unless contraindicated
Explain need to avoid diet high in fiber and roughage
Explain need to take prescribed medication during episodes of diarrhea
Explain need to avoid over-the-counter medications without physician or nurse consultation

DISCHARGE/HOME CARE PLANNING
Assess patient's ability to obtain and store occult blood testing supplies
Assess patient's ability to provide foods for and prepare therapeutic diet; arrange for home health provider or have foods brought to patient as needed
Assess need for assistance with personal hygiene

CONSTIPATION
Passage of irregular, infrequent, hard feces; may be caused by disease process, chemotherapy, or other factors

ASSESSMENT
SUBJECTIVE DATA
Rectal fullness, pressure
Difficult, painful stool evacuation

OBJECTIVE DATA
Frequency less than usual pattern
Stool
    Hard, dry
    Red-streaked
Absence of bowel sounds

DIAGNOSTIC TESTS
Depend on suspected cause

POTENTIAL COMPLICATION
Ileus

MULTIDISCIPLINARY MANAGEMENT
THERAPEUTIC MANAGEMENT
Stool softeners
Hydration: oral or parenteral
Laxatives or enemas if not contraindicated by the condition of the rectal mucosa

Collaborate with clinical dietitian to develop therapeutic meal plans that do not promote constipation
Consult with Wound, Ostomy, Continence/ET Nurse as indicated

PATIENT PROBLEM—NURSING DIAGNOSIS/INTERVENTIONS

▼Constipation related to effects of chemotherapy on the GI tract

Assess usual pattern of elimination, including use of laxatives *to establish baseline*
Identify factors that could alter usual pattern of elimination, such as immobility, chemotherapeutic drugs, opiate/narcotic analgesics, low-fiber diet, or inadequate fluid intake
Assess for presence of associated signs and symptoms such as flatus, distention, or discomfort
Assess for fecal impaction
Evaluate and record time and character of bowel elimination daily
Auscultate abdomen for bowel sounds q8h *to determine presence of ileus*
Administer enema type, amount, and solution as ordered; digital removal of feces may be necessary—follow hospital policy and procedure
If no spontaneous stool occurs within 24 hours after enema, administer stool softener, laxative, or suppository as ordered
Monitor intake and output *to ensure balance*
Force fluids to 3000 ml/day unless contraindicated
Maintain diet high in fiber and bulk
Encourage ambulation and exercise to tolerance
Perform ROM exercises q4h to 8h if patient is immobile
Provide privacy when needed
    Assist with ambulation to bathroom
    Screen patient in bed
    Do not schedule appointments or examinations at time of patient's usual evacuation
Perform perineal care after bowel movement
Assess condition of perineum daily
Apply medication to rectal area as ordered

Expected Outcome
Easily evacuates soft, formed stool

PATIENT/FAMILY TEACHING
Emphasize importance of noting daily bowel function and consistency of stool
Discuss/demonstrate methods to enhance daily bowel movements
    Take stool softener and laxative prn
    Maintain fluid level at 3000 ml/24 hr unless contraindicated
    Eat diet high in fiber
    Administer enema on advice of MD/RN
Explain need to report to physician if these methods fail
Explain need to avoid over-the-counter medications without consulting physician

DISCHARGE/HOME CARE PLANNING

Assess patient's ability to obtain and prepare sufficient
    fluids and foods necessary for therapeutic diet; arrange
    home health providers or have foods/fluids brought to
    patient as needed
Assess patient's ability to care for personal hygiene needs

■ INTEGUMENTARY

■ DERMATOLOGIC

hypersensitivity reactions: *Reactions to antineoplastic agents; can be very serious and/or life threatening,
particularly if an anaphylactic reaction occurs; drugs
most often associated with an anaphylactoid reaction include asparaginase, cisplatin (infrequent), and bleomycin*

hyperpyrexia: *Associated with bleomycin, especially
in patients with lymphoma*

erythema (Adria flaré): *Associated with doxorubicin; the flare usually results when the drug is too concentrated or if the patient has very sensitive skin*

ASSESSMENT
SUBJECTIVE DATA

Abdominal cramping (associated with hypersensitivity
    reaction)
Pruritus
Photosensitivity

OBJECTIVE DATA

Urticaria
Angioedema
Bronchospasm
Hypotension
Hyperpigmentation
Maculopapular rash
Vesicle formation
Acne
Thinning of skin and striae
Petechiae
Ecchymosis
Hives
Desquamation
Jaundice
Nail changes
    Horizontal or longitudinal banding
    Thickening of nail bed
Radiation "recall" phenomena
Blue discoloration of veins
Hyperpyrexia
    High fever
Erythema (Adria flaré)
    Redness (diffuse or streak above the vein)
    Urticaria

MULTIDISCIPLINARY MANAGEMENT
THERAPEUTIC MANAGEMENT

General
    Test doses of chemotherapy may be recommended
    Diphenhydramine (Benadryl)

Epinephrine
Parenteral corticosteroids
Hyperpyrexia
    Acetaminophen
    Fluid intake
Erythema (Adria flaré)
    Ice pack to affected area

PATIENT PROBLEM—NURSING DIAGNOSIS/INTERVENTIONS

▼ Risk for impaired skin integrity related to effects of
chemotherapy

Review patient's allergy history
Monitor vital signs and mental status
Observe patient throughout administration of drug *to
    note first signs of hypersensitivity*
Ensure that appropriate drugs and equipment are
    immediately available for possible emergency use; in
    the event of an anaphylactoid reaction, have the
    following available
    Diphenhydramine (Benadryl)
    Epinephrine
    Oxygen
    Airway
    Suction equipment
Be fully aware of facility procedure to follow in the event
    of such a reaction
For Adria flaré
    At first signs of itching or redness, reduce the speed
        and concentration of drug given (e.g., if giving 1 ml,
        reduce to ½ ml); flush vein well and continue
        administering drug at half dosage; if erythema and
        urticaria occur, stop IV and apply ice pack; start
        fresh IV and administer remainder of drug
        observing for repeated reaction
For hyperpyrexia
    Give acetaminophen q4h as ordered *to reduce
        temperature and increase comfort*
    Push oral fluids *to reduce temperature*
Advise patient to report adverse reactions immediately
Assess skin condition q8h, especially axillary and breast
    folds, groin, perirectal area, and dependent extremities
Assist with daily bath
    Use antibacterial soaps and soft cloths
    Rinse and dry well
    Avoid using lotions and powders, do not leave skin
        moist
Keep linens dry and wrinkle free *to prevent skin
    irritation*

Expected Outcome
Skin integrity is maintained

PATIENT/FAMILY TEACHING
Teach and assist with perianal care after each elimination
    Use soft towels or cloths
    Ensure that area is kept dry
    Advise patient to wear cotton clothing and underwear

Teach handwashing technique to be used after
elimination and prn

Caution patient to avoid bumps, bruising, cuts, and
scratches

Explain importance of skin care to patient

Caution patient to avoid use of sharp objects (e.g.,
razors, cuticle scissors)

Explain need to always wear slippers or shoes when
out of bed

Caution patient to avoid tight or constricting clothing

Caution patient to avoid use of rings and watches
when possible; moisture and bacteria collect
underneath, and sharp edges can cause scratches or
cuts

Avoid IM injections when possible

Central line may be ordered and inserted to avoid
multiple IV injections—perform daily central line care
if inserted

Consolidate laboratory work; use fingersticks when
possible; cleanse skin with povidone-iodine before
venipuncture

DISCHARGE/HOME CARE PLANNING
Ensure patient has access to and storage space for needed
skin care supplies

Assess patient's ability to provide self-care; arrange home
health provider as needed

ALOPECIA
Temporary loss of body hair as a result of chemotherapeutic agents that interact with cells that are in the anaphase of cell cycle (85% to 90% of total scalp hair cells at any one time); hair loss in area of radiotherapy; dose-dependent antineoplastics associated with alopecia include cyclophosphamide, doxorubicin, and vinblastine; antineoplastics associated with thinning rather than total hair loss include bleomycin, vincristine, 5-FU, and etoposide

ASSESSMENT
SUBJECTIVE DATA
Unhappy with appearance

Refuses to see visitors

OBJECTIVE DATA
Hair loss

Scalp especially affected early

Long-term therapy

Axilla

Extremities

Pubis

Alterations in body image

MULTIDISCIPLINARY MANAGEMENT
THERAPEUTIC MANAGEMENT
Consult with services related to wigs, caps, scarves

Social services, support group

PATIENT PROBLEM—NURSING DIAGNOSIS/INTERVENTIONS

▼Risk for impaired skin integrity, resulting in hair loss related to effects of chemotherapy

Establish therapeutic nurse-patient relationship

Inform patient in advance about impending hair loss *so patient can plan for measures that will enhance appearance and feelings of well-being;* hair loss varies among individuals

Have patient obtain wigs, scarves, hats, or caps before hair loss begins *so patient can become familiar with use*

Explain to patient when to expect hair loss

Begins about 10 days after scalp is irradiated

Usually begins 10–21 days after beginning chemotherapy

Stress temporary nature of hair loss *to alleviate concern*

Complete regrowth is usual after chemotherapy is completed

Regrowth may begin during treatment

Tell patient to expect alterations in texture and color *(physiology of hair follicle is changed by drugs)*

Assess patient's perception of effect of hair loss on lifestyle

Short hairstyles may be preferred

Beginning hair loss may not be readily noticeable

Patient comfort may be increased by a short hairstyle when maximal amount of hair is falling out

Stress importance of periodic rather than continuous use of wigs *to allow scalp to "breathe"*

Assist with gentle scalp care during susceptible period

Wash hair with pH-balanced shampoo

Expose hair and scalp to air as much as possible *to maintain skin tone and integrity*

Keep head covered when exposed to sun to prevent sunburn

Expected Outcome
Emotional response to hair loss is minimized

PATIENT/FAMILY TEACHING
Ensure that patient and significant other(s) know and understand the following:

Need to discuss feelings related to perceptions of hair loss

Importance of gentle hair and scalp care

Need to expose scalp to air as much as possible

Hair loss will be temporary throughout course of treatment

Avoiding use of hair dryer, curling iron, dyes, color rinses, permanents, and bleaches until such time as indicated by condition of scalp, hair, and physician's direction

DISCHARGE/HOME CARE PLANNING
Assist patient to contact community support groups for ongoing psychologic counseling and support

Assess patient's ability to provide for own hair and scalp care; arrange home health provider as needed

■ CARDIOTOXICITY

Cardiac damage caused by toxicity of antineoplastic medications (Table 15-10)

ASSESSMENT
OBSERVATIONS/FINDINGS
Tachycardia
Extrasystoles
ST-T wave changes
Transient ECG changes
Neck vein distention
SOB
Edema
Gallop heart rhythm
Predisposing factors
    Previous radiation therapy near heart
    Aortic stenosis
    Uncontrolled hypertension
    Distended neck veins
    Gallop heart rhythm
    Ankle edema

DIAGNOSTIC TESTS
Verify baseline cardiac status before administration
ECG
Cardiac enzymes
Chest x-ray examination
Echocardiogram
Radionuclide angiography
Percutaneous endomyocardial biopsy

POTENTIAL COMPLICATIONS
CHF
Cardiomyopathy
Dysrhythmia

MULTIDISCIPLINARY MANAGEMENT
THERAPEUTIC MANAGEMENT
Serial ECG monitoring
Oxygen therapy
Cardiac medications

POTENTIAL PATIENT PROBLEM/INTERVENTIONS

▼ Cardiotoxicity related to effects of chemotherapy

Monitor pulse rate and rhythm
Note significant variation in vital signs, skin color, temperature sensorium, decreased urine output, and dyspnea, *which indicate toxicity*
Be aware that weekly low-dose injection of doxorubicin and continuous infusions may be associated with less cardiotoxicity
Be aware that by the time cardiac toxicity is clinically detectable, it is often irreversible and debilitating
Be aware of agents that place patient at risk for cardiotoxicity such as doxorubicin (adult total cumulative dose not to exceed 450 to 550 mg/m^2) and daunorubicin (total cumulative dose is 550 mg/m^2); see Heart failure (p. 112)

Expected Outcome
Signs and symptoms of cardiotoxicity are recognized and treatment is initiated promptly

■ PULMONARY TOXICITY

Respiratory difficulties, temporary or chronic, related to chemotherapeutic toxicities; chemotherapeutic drugs

ASSESSMENT
SUBJECTIVE DATA
Headache
Malaise
SOB

Table 15-10	Major System Toxicity and Associated Chemotherapeutic Agents	
Toxicity	**Chemotherapeutic Agent**
Cardiac toxicity	Chlorambucil, cyclophosphamides, daunorubicin, doxorubicin, mitoxantrone, high-dose ifosfamide
Hepatic toxicity	Asparaginase, busulfan, carmustine, chlorambucil, cytarabine, doxorubicin, lomustine, mercaptopurine, methotrexate, mithramycin, streptozocin
Neurotoxicity	Ifosfamide, vinblastine, vincristine; high peak plasma levels of etoposimide, 5-fluorouracil; high dose or intrathecal administration of cytarbine, cisplatin, methotrexate
Ototoxicity	Cisplatin
Pulmonary toxicity	Bleomycin, busulfan, carmustine
Renal toxicity	Cisplatin, cyclophosphomide, ifosfamide, methotrexate, mithramycin, streptozocin, thioplex
Reproductive system toxicity	Busulfan, chlorambucil, cyclophosphadine, mechlorethamine, flutamide, leuprolide, tamoxifen, goserelin

Modified from Otto SE: Oncology nursing, *ed 3, St Louis, 1997, Mosby.*

OBJECTIVE DATA

Toxicities associated with bleomycin include pneumonitis and interstitial fibrosis

Persons over 70 years of age who receive total cumulative dose >400 to 500 units are at greatest risk

Fine, crackling basilar rales

Dyspnea at rest, hypoxemia

Tachypnea, fever

Pneumonia (noninfectious)

Pulmonary edema

Pulmonary fibrosis

Predisposing factors

Preexisting pulmonary disease

Radiation therapy

Pulmonary conditions: infection, edema, emboli

Dry, hacking cough

History of smoking

DIAGNOSTIC TESTS

Verify baseline pulmonary status before administration

Pulmonary function tests

ABGs

Chest x-ray

MULTIDISCIPLINARY MANAGEMENT
THERAPEUTIC MANAGEMENT

Steroids

Antimicrobials

Bronchodilators

Oxygen therapy

Respiratory therapy consult

POTENTIAL PATIENT PROBLEM/INTERVENTIONS

▼Pulmonary toxicity related to the effects of chemotherapy

Be aware that once pulmonary changes are clinically detected, the disease course is often progressive

Observe for SOB *for possible early detection*

Auscultate chest for breath sounds q4h during course of chemotherapy; report abnormal breath sounds immediately

Check BP, P, R, and T q4h; report temperature of 100.4° F (38° C) or above

Monitor pulmonary function tests as ordered

Teach and assist patient to turn, cough, and deep breathe q4h *to maintain adequate respirations*

Administer oxygen cautiously when ordered; high-dose oxygen may increase reaction, especially that caused by bleomycin

Force fluids to 3000 ml/day unless contraindicated

Administer IV fluid therapy as ordered

Measure intake and output q8h *to monitor for balance*

Administer medications as ordered: corticosteroids, bronchodilators, antimicrobials

Teach necessity of raising secretions and expectorating versus swallowing

Assist with nebulizer treatments and respiratory physiotherapy

See Adult respiratory distress syndrome (ARDS) (p. 270)

Expected Outcome

Pulmonary toxicity is minimized, or signs and symptoms of pulmonary toxicity are recognized and treated promptly

■ RENAL

▮ NEPHROTOXICITY

Dysfunction in any part of the renal system in the presence of chemotherapeutic agents that are excreted through the kidneys or act on the lining of the renal system

ASSESSMENT
SUBJECTIVE DATA

Muscle weakness

Nausea

Headache

Dysuria, frequency, urgency

OBJECTIVE DATA

Hematuria (mild to severe), proteinuria

Oliguria, anuria

Neuromuscular irritability

Tremors, personality change

Elevated uric acid

Hyperkalemia, hyperphosphatemia

Hypocalcemia, hypomagnesemia

Hyponatremia

Elevated BUN, serum creatinine, and creatinine clearance

Hypertension, vomiting

DIAGNOSTIC TESTS

Verify baseline renal function before administration

Electrolytes

BUN, uric acid, calcium, magnesium

Serum creatinine

Creatinine clearance

Cystoscopy

MULTIDISCIPLINARY MANAGEMENT
THERAPEUTIC MANAGEMENT

IV fluid (titrate according to output)

Measure intake and output

Medications

Bicarbonate

Allopurinol

Antihypertensives

Osmotic diuretics

Antiemetics

POTENTIAL PATIENT PROBLEM/INTERVENTIONS

▼Nephrotoxicity related to effects of chemotherapy

Ensure adequate hydration and diuresis 24 hours before, during, and 24 to 48 hours after medication administration

Force fluids to 3000 to 4000 ml/day unless contraindicated

Enlist patient's assistance *to maintain hydration*
  Provide fluids of choice and temperature
  Dietary restrictions of protein, potassium, and sodium may be necessary
  Offering small amounts frequently makes taking fluids less of a chore
  Serve attractively

Use antacids *to alleviate gastric distress*

Use antiemetics *for control of nausea*

Administer IV fluids as ordered: usually dextrose in saline with electrolytes; often ordered at 200 ml/hr for 5 to 6 hours before, during, and after chemotherapy infusion

Measure intake and output; report discrepancies and output of less than 120 ml/hr

Test urine for occult bleeding q8h during chemotherapy infusion; slow infusion and report overt hemorrhaging to physician

Monitor vital signs *so early changes can be noted and therapy started*

Administer antihypertensive drugs as ordered *to control elevated BP*

Test urine pH as ordered

Administer sodium bicarbonate as ordered *to maintain urine pH of 7*

Expected Outcome

Nephrotoxic effects of chemotherapy are minimized; signs and symptoms of nephrotoxicity are recognized and treated promptly

PATIENT/FAMILY TEACHING

Explain need to measure intake and output

Emphasize importance of maintaining fluid intake to 3000 to 4000 ml/day

Discuss signs and symptoms of nephrotoxicity to report to physician

Teach name of medication, dosage, frequency, and toxic or side effects to report to physician

Emphasize importance of follow-up outpatient care

Emphasize importance of taking antihypertensive drugs when ordered

▌ HEMORRHAGIC CYSTITIS

Dose-related chemical cystitis caused by toxic effects of cyclophosphamide's or ifosfamide's metabolite on bladder mucosa

ASSESSMENT
OBSERVATIONS/FINDINGS
Urinary frequency
Loss of bladder tone
Occult or gross hematuria

DIAGNOSTIC TESTS
Urinalysis
CBC
Cystoscopy

MULTIDISCIPLINARY MANAGEMENT
THERAPEUTIC MANAGEMENT
Parenteral fluids
Bladder irrigation
Antiemetics
Sedatives

POTENTIAL PATIENT PROBLEM/INTERVENTIONS

▼Hemorrhagic cystitis related to the effects of chemotherapy

Encourage high fluid intake to 3000 ml/day (if not contraindicated) before and 48 hours following drug administration *to maintain high urine output and drug dilution*

Encourage frequent voiding q3h to 4h; bladder should be emptied before bedtime and when patient is awake at night *to decrease irritation of bladder by stasis of high concentrations of drug in urine*

Observe and report signs and symptoms of cystitis
  Test urine for hematuria (dipstick)
  Monitor output closely; report decrease in urine *(may be indicative of SIADH secondary to drug)*

Administer cyclophosphamide early in the day *to prevent urine from pooling in bladder overnight*

Indwelling catheter may be ordered

Through-and-through bladder irrigation may be ordered *to decrease drug concentrations in urine*

Administer antiemetics and sedatives as needed

Teach exercises to regain bladder tone

Expected Outcome

Hemorrhagic cystitis does not occur or signs and symptoms of hemorrhagic cystitis are recognized and treated promptly

▌ NEUROTOXICITY

Damage to myelin sheath, paralysis of autonomic nerves, or CNS damage caused by effects of chemotherapeutic medications; antineoplastic agents typically associated with neurotoxicity are the vinca (plant) alkaloids: vincristine, vinblastine, and vindesine

ASSESSMENT
SUBJECTIVE DATA
Fatigue

Tingling, paresthesia

Muscle aches/pains

Jaw pain

Hoarseness

Hallucinations

Depression

Arachnoiditis (in relation to intrathecal administration)

 Back pain

 Dizziness, headache

OBJECTIVE DATA
Tremors

Muscle weakness

 Difficulty in heel walking

 Inability to get out of chair

Foot-drop

Ptosis

Hyporeflexia to loss of deep tendon reflexes

Ataxia

Hemiplegia

Slurred speech

Hoarseness

Irritability

Seizures

Somnolence

Personality change

Coma

Arachnoiditis (in relation to intrathecal administration)

 Fever

 Stiff neck

 Vomiting

Ototoxicity

Constipation and colicky pain

Ileus

Urinary retention

DIAGNOSTIC TESTS
Neurologic examination

Neuroradiology studies

MULTIDISCIPLINARY MANAGEMENT
THERAPEUTIC MANAGEMENT
Medications specific to symptoms

Stool softeners, laxatives

Physical therapy

POTENTIAL PATIENT PROBLEM/INTERVENTIONS

▼Neurotoxicity related to effects of chemotherapy

Assess for weakness/numbness of arms, hands, legs, and feet *(early signs of toxicity)*

Assess for hoarseness and jaw pain

Assess for abdominal cramping, constipation, and paralytic ileus

Perform neurologic assessment before administration of medication *for baseline information* then q4h to 8h after infusion is completed; report changes to physician immediately

Assess ability to perform ADLs

Evaluate for discomfort or pain associated with movement

Assess pain, cardiac, respiratory, and elimination status

Provide safe, uncluttered environment *to prevent falls*

Instruct patient to sit on side of bed, stand, and then begin to walk *to prevent postural hypotension;* provide walking aids as indicated

Instruct patient to report numbness and tingling or other signs of toxicity immediately

Assure patient and significant other that changes are usually reversible when medication is stopped; discuss specifics with physician—motor weakness may take many months to resolve

Provide environment and time conducive to discussing concerns and fears

Assess color and temperature of extremities, especially hands

Assess for CNS toxicity if methotrexate or cytarabine is given intrathecally; have patient lie flat for at least 1 hour following instillation of drug

Expected Outcome
Neurotoxicity effects are minimized

PATIENT PROBLEM—NURSING DIAGNOSIS/INTERVENTION

▼Constipation related to neurotoxic effects of chemotherapy

Auscultate abdomen for bowel sounds q4h to 8h

Check and record daily bowel elimination *(constipation and colicky pain that develop within 2 days of drug administration are early manifestations of toxicity)*

Administer stool softeners and laxatives prophylactically

Encourage fluid to 3000 ml/day unless contraindicated *to enhance motility*

Encourage diet high in fiber *to stimulate peristalsis*

Measure intake and output

Administer enemas as ordered

Encourage mobility as tolerated

Expected Outcome
Normal bowel motility is achieved and maintained

■ HEPATOTOXICITY
Dysfunction of the liver induced by chemotherapeutic medications, other hepatotoxic drugs, or preexisting hepatic conditions; because the hepatocytes are not rapidly dividing cells, they are less affected by many drugs; antineoplastic agents associated with hepatic toxicity include nitrosoureas, methotrexate, 6-mercaptopurine (6-MP),

cytosine arabinoside, mithramycin, asparaginase, and interferon

ASSESSMENT
SUBJECTIVE DATA
Lethargy, weakness
Abdominal tenderness
RUQ pain
Anorexia
Digestive discomfort

OBJECTIVE DATA
Pruritus
Jaundice
Dark urine
Sweet or sour odor of urine and breath
Clay-colored stools
Bleeding tendency
    Purpura
    Epistaxis
    Melena
Ascites
Generalized edema
Palmar erythema
Spider angiomas
Irritability
Apathy
Memory defects
Asterixis
Coma
Associated factors, preexisting or concurrent
    Viral hepatitis
    Abdominal radiotherapy
    Hepatic metastasis
    Hepatotoxic drugs
    Transfusion of blood products
    GVHD (p. 774)

DIAGNOSTIC TESTS
Elevated
    Serum transaminase
    Bilirubin
    Alkaline phosphatase
    Cholesterol
    Fibrinogen
Decreased
    Hepatic clotting factors
    Albumin
Liver function tests
Blood clotting test, CBC
Liver biopsy
Radiologic examinations

POTENTIAL COMPLICATIONS
Cirrhosis
Ascites
Hepatomegaly

MULTIDISCIPLINARY MANAGEMENT
THERAPEUTIC MANAGEMENT
Parenteral fluids/nutrition
Blood product transfusion
Nasogastric tube

PATIENT PROBLEMS—NURSING DIAGNOSES/INTERVENTIONS

▼ Risk for impaired skin integrity related to pruritus

Assess skin condition q8h
Bathe patient daily; use soothing baths (e.g., use cornstarch or oil) *to relieve itching*
Maintain skin hydration by application of lotion after bath and bid, adding bath oil to water (if not contraindicated by skin condition)
Teach distraction, relaxation, and imagery *to prevent scratching*
Administer skin care as needed *to decrease itching;* antihistamine drugs may be ordered
Keep nails short *to prevent scratching skin*
Encourage fluids to 3000 to 4000 ml/24 hr unless contraindicated; fluids may be limited in presence of edema

Expected Outcomes
States pruritus is diminished
Skin remains intact

▼ Potential for bleeding related to altered clotting mechanisms*

Assess sensorium q2h to 4h
Report changes of increased lethargy; *sign of potential bleeding*
Avoid use of drugs such as narcotics and barbiturates that cause CNS depression
Observe for signs of bleeding: hematemesis, melena, petechiae
Assess for abdominal distention; measure abdominal girth; *increasing girth may indicate abdominal bleeding*
Assess bowel sounds
Monitor vital signs and laboratory studies
If nasogastric tube is being used, maintain patency
    Provide oral care; keep nostrils clean and lubricated
    Maintain proper position of tube *to prevent irritation*
    Place in semi-Fowler's position unless contraindicated
Report changes in color, bleeding, and edema to physician *for changes in treatment plan*
Report changes in color of urine and stool that indicate bleeding

Not a NANDA-approved diagnosis.

Institute safety measures *to decrease bleeding tendency*
    Avoid IM injections
    Consolidate laboratory work
    Use fingersticks when possible
    Apply pressure at puncture or IV site for 5 minutes after procedure has been completed; check site q15 min ×4
    Carefully place furniture, equipment, and personal items *to prevent injuries from falls or bumping into objects*
    Administer gentle oral hygiene using toothettes or swabs
    Avoid use of harsh soaps and rough towels and cloths
    Test urine and stool for occult bleeding

Expected Outcomes
Preventable bleeding episodes are avoided
Signs and symptoms of bleeding are recognized and treated immediately

■ REPRODUCTIVE SYSTEM DYSFUNCTION
Testicular or ovarian dysfunction or sexual dysfunction caused by adverse effects of chemotherapeutic drugs (e.g., nitrogen mustard, cyclophosphamide, chlorambucil)

ASSESSMENT
OBSERVATIONS/FINDINGS
Reduction of spermatocytes
Irregular menses
Amenorrhea
Menopausal symptoms: hot flushes, insomnia, irritability, dyspareunia, vaginal dryness
Impotence
Loss of libido

DIAGNOSTIC TESTS
Serum follicle-stimulating hormone (FSH) level
Sperm count

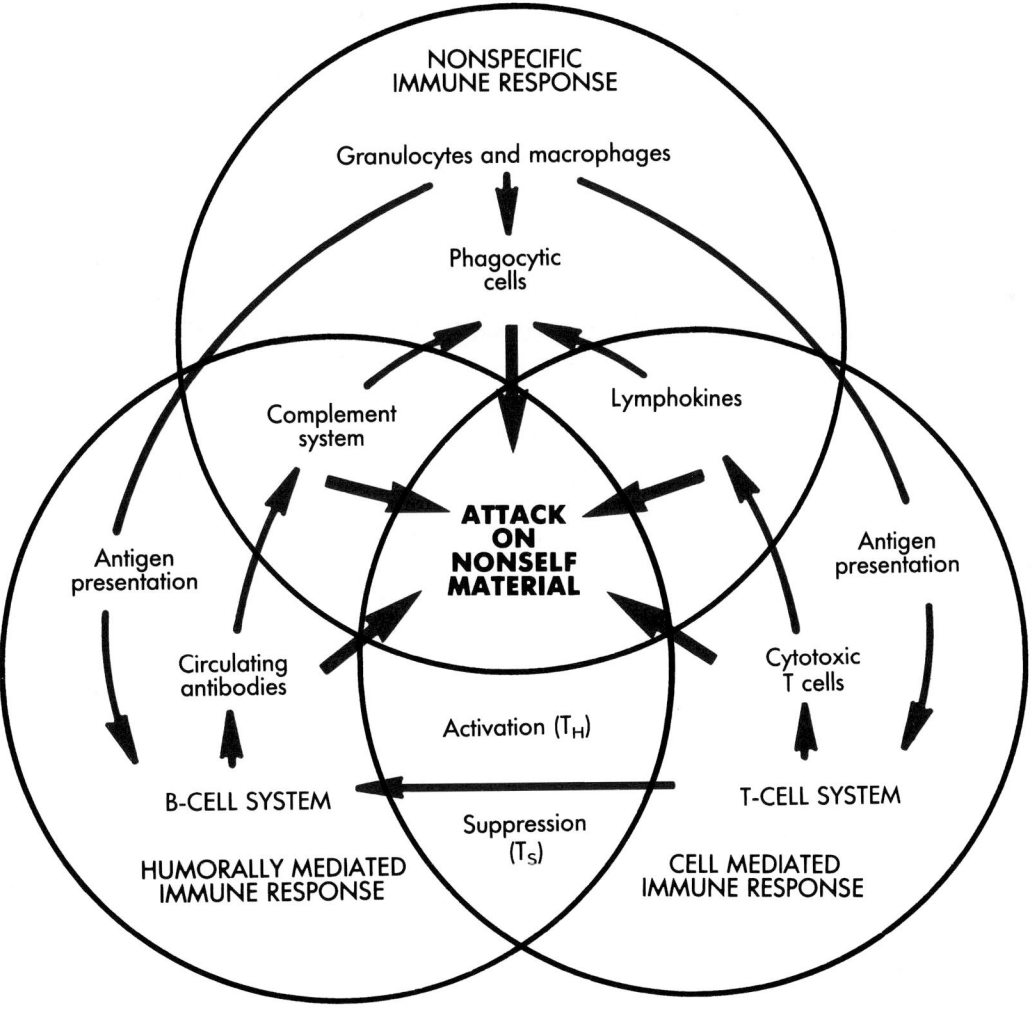

Fig. 15-11 Interrelationship of nonspecific, humorally mediated, and cell mediated immune response systems. *(From Phipps WJ et al: Medical-surgical nursing: concepts and clinical practice, ed 5, St Louis, 1995, Mosby.)*

POTENTIAL COMPLICATION
Temporary or permanent sterility
Teratogenic effects

MULTIDISCIPLINARY MANAGEMENT
   THERAPEUTIC MANAGEMENT
Estrogens (menopausal symptoms) (not in breast cancer)
Birth control practices for 2 years after chemotherapy

   PATIENT PROBLEM—NURSING DIAGNOSIS/INTERVENTIONS

▼Altered sexuality patterns, related to effects of chemotherapy on the reproductive system

Obtain brief sexual history including sexual practices, sex education and attitude, and effects of disease and treatment on sexual function

Advise male patients regarding sperm banking before chemotherapy administration if appropriate

Provide contraceptive information to patients before they initiate chemotherapy if appropriate

Initiate discussion related to infertility

Encourage ventilation of feelings

Evaluate patient's and/or partner's coping skills and response to infertility

Instruct patient that infertility may be temporary or permanent (dose related)

Inform patient that sexual drive and capability usually are not physically impaired as a result of chemotherapy

Advise that antifertility effects may be reversible in some cases after therapy is terminated

Refer patient for counseling if appropriate

Expected Outcome
Achieves satisfying sexual role functioning

BIOLOGIC RESPONSE MODIFIERS

This cancer therapy is based on the theory that if the immune system recognizes tumor cells as foreign, it will mobilize and destroy them. Through research, biologic and chemical agents produced by the body, biologic response modifiers (BRMs) have been discovered. A BRM is any soluble substance capable of altering (or modulating) the immune system with either a stimulatory or a suppressive effect (Fig. 15-11). BRMs can affect the host-tumor response in three ways: (1) by modulating the individual's immune response to the tumor; (2) by direct antitumor activity, killing or suppressing growth; (3) by altering other biologic activities that indirectly affect the tumor, such as interfering with tumor cell's ability to survive or metastasize, promoting cell maturation, or interfering with transformation of normal cells into cancer cells (Table 15-11)

Table 15-11	**Biologic Response Modifiers (Under Investigation)**			
Agent	**Route of Administration**	**Indications Under Investigation**	**Side/Toxic Effects**	**Administration and Nursing Indications**
Calmette-Guérin bacillus BCG Live	Scarification, intra-dermal by tine technique or heat gun	Superficial or subcutaneous melanoma	Local, inflammatory response that increases with treatment to ulceration with eschar formation Pruritus Enlarged painful nodes, malaise, mild fever	Anesthesize area Clean skin with acetone and allow to dry Choose site that is flat and near major lymph nodes to increase absorption and that is covered by clothing that does not bind Keep areas clean and dry Apply nonmedicated, hypoallergenic cream to previous sites when needed
	Intravesical (bladder) Retain for 2 hr	Bladder (FDA approved)	Bladder irritation, infection, chills, fever, cough, frequency, dysuria, hematuria	Before treatment Bladder culture Have patient limit fluids for 12 hr Void before administration

Table 15-11	**Biologic Response Modifiers *(Under Investigation)*—cont'd**			
Agent	**Route of Administration**	**Indications Under Investigation**	**Side/Toxic Effects**	**Administration and Nursing Indications**
				With first and each subsequent voiding for 6 hr add bleach equal to amount voided, close cover of toilet and flush Rehydrate patient Report fever, cough, chills to physician immediately for antibiotic therapy
	Intralesional	Cutaneous melanoma	Inflammatory reaction in 4 hr; fever, myalgia, nausea, vomiting for 2-3 days	
			Hypersensitivity reaction can occur: fever, chills, intravascular coagulation abnormalities, hypotension, and oliguria	Have antihistamines, corticosteroids, and emergency equipment available
			Disseminated BCG infection: persistent fever, weight loss, malaise, nausea, and vomiting	Patients with strongly positive tuberculin reaction may need diphenhydramine (Benadryl) before and after intratumor therapy
			Temporary, reversible hepatic dysfunction	Antipyretics usually control symptoms; isoniazid may be ordered
Interferons exhibit broad antiviral, antiproliferative, and immunodulatory activity	IM, IV (bolus, short-term infusion, a continuous infusion), SC intravesical, intrathecal, or intralesional	Hairy cell leukemia non-Hodgkin's lymphoma, Kaposi's sarcoma, renal cell carcinoma, malignant melanoma, multiple myeloma untreated, chronic granulocytic leukemia, mycosis fungoides, superficial bladder (intravesical), ovarian (intraperitoneal). Clinical trials for rhinovirus	Flulike symptoms; fever (100.4°-104° F [38°-40° C]) 2-4 hr after injection; malaise, chills, headache, and low-grade fever may last to 20 hr after first dose	Reconstitute according to manufacturer's directions
			Chronic fatigue, irritability, impatience, low motivation, depression; sense of doom, and paranoia with high doses	Premedicate with acetominophen, then q3-4h after *Avoid* aspirin, NSAIDs and steroids (may hinder effectiveness) Morphine may be ordered for severe chilling (rigor) lasting more than 10 min
			Nausea, altered taste, early satiety, anorexia, arthostatic hypertension; cardiovascular symptoms with history of problems	Instruct patient to plan rest periods; may need to alter work habits Provide nutritional counseling Encourage fluid intake
			Transient pancytopenia	Avoid sudden position changes

*FDA approved.

Continued

Table 15-11	Biologic Response Modifiers *(Under Investigation)*—cont'd			
Agent	**Route of Administration**	**Indications Under Investigation**	**Side/Toxic Effects**	**Administration and Nursing Indications**
			Proteinuria with preexisting renal disease Leukopenia Neutropenia Thrombocytopenia Anemia	Evening administration may diminish side effects
Thymosin fraction V	IM, SC	Small cell lung cancer, squamous cell carcinoma of head and neck	Allergic reaction, systemic itching	Antipruritics may be administered to relieve itching
Interleukin-2* (IL-2) Aldesleutin Adoptive immuno-therapy	IV bolus, continuous IV infusion, intra-hepatic infusion, peritoneal infusion	Advanced cancer in which standard therapy is ineffective (renal cell melanoma, colon, etc.) FDA approved for kidney and renal cancer	Symptoms are usually dose related and usually reverse in 8-21 days after IL-2 Disorientation, combativeness, psychosis, anxiety Oliguria, proteinuria, elevated creatinine and BUN Anemia, thrombocytopenia Elevated bilirubin, AST, ALT, LDH Erythematous rash, pruritus, desquamation Nausea, vomiting, mucositis, decreased appetite, diarrhea Hypotension Capillary leak syndrome	Assess baseline status of affected systems To be administered in hospital Provide safety measures, explanations and reorient Monitor intake and output; test urine for protein; monitor laboratory values Monitor for bleeding; evaluate daily laboratory values; test stool, urine, and vomitus for blood; avoid rectal manipulation and IM injections Monitor laboratory values Benadryl may be given prophylactically; assess skin daily; use water-based lotion; avoid harsh products; pat skin dry Monitor dietary intake; prophylactic antiemetic usually given; antidiarrheal given as necessary; see Mucositis (p. 890), and Nausea and vomiting (p. 889) Monitor vital signs qh during infusion then q4h; albumin, dopamine, or phenylephrine may be ordered

*FDA approved.

Table 15-11	Biologic Response Modifiers *(Under Investigation)*—cont'd				
Agent	**Route of Administration**	**Indications Under Investigation**	**Side/Toxic Effects**	**Administration and Nursing Indications**
			Weight gain, peripheral edema, ascites, dysrhythmias, dyspnea, pulmonary edema	Monitor intake and output; weigh daily; measure abdominal girth with ascites; elevate extremities with edema; monitor O_2 saturation
			Fever	Acetominophen given prophylactically Monitor temperature qh during infusion and for 24 hr Provide cooling measures prn
			Chills	Meperidine may be ordered for chills or rigor
			Flulike symptoms	Rest; acetaminophen q4h
IL-2 and LAK* Adoptive immunotherapy	IL-2 given for 3 days; collect leukocytes through lymphopheresis (for 4 to 5 days); separated lymphocytes incubated with IL-2; prepared LAK cells are infused after test dose for 3 days; IL-2 infused also and for several days after LAK infusion	Melanoma, nodular lymphomas, renal cell cancer, colorectal cancer	Fever Headache Chills Nausea	Acetaminophen usually given Meperidine administered for chills or rigor Antiemetics manage nausea
			High dosages: peripheral edema, ascites, or interstitial infiltrates	Vasopressors, diuretics, and careful fluid replacement may be required
			Thrombocytopenia	May require RBC transfusion Monitor for bleeding
			Mental status changes: confusion, paranoia, hallucinations, severe disorientation	Provide safety measures, reorient continuously; haloperidol may be required
Lymphotoxin effects delayed hypersensitivity; allow higher doses of chemotherapy and radiotherapy	Intralesional injection in accessible tumors	Melanoma, bladder, and prostate cancer	—	—

*LAK, Lymphokine-activated killer cells.

Continued

Table 15-11	**Biologic Response Modifiers *(Under Investigation)*—cont'd**			
Agent	**Route of Administration**	**Indications Under Investigation**	**Side/Toxic Effects**	**Administration and Nursing Indications**
Monoclonal antibodies Biologic tracers that react with one specific part of the antigen's surface (an epitome) Serve as carriers of antitoxin drugs, toxins, radioisotopes, or other biologic response modifiers to tumor cells	IV by infusion pump	Lymphoma, lymphocytic leukemia, T-cell leukemia, cutaneous T-cell lymphoma, gastric and colon cancer and melanoma	Fever, chills, headache, flushing, urticaria, rash Bronchospasm, dyspnea, hypotension, tachycardia, anaphylactic reaction	Diphenhydramine usually controls mild allergic response Assess patient q15min first hr; then q30min Infusion stopped; saline; epinephrine, hydrocortisone, and diphenhydramine may be ordered; monitor vital signs; keep resuscitation equipment nearby
Tumor cell vaccines Provide active, specific immune stimulation	Intradermal	—	Fever, chills, headache, malaise Hepatitis	Acetominophen usually relieves symptoms
Colony-stimulating factors (CSF)				
G-CSF (granulocyte (CSF) (filgrastim)	IV, short or continuous infusion; SC	Bone marrow destruction: iatrogenically induced: antiviral therapy in AIDS, cancer	Fever, myalgias, bone pain, fatigue	Acetaminophen usually controls symptoms
GM-CSF (granulocyte-macrophage CSF) (sargramostim)		Chemotherapy and bone marrow transplant	Anorexia Pericardial, pleural effusions	Monitor vital signs, intake, output and assess heart and breath sounds; report negative findings
Increase the production of granulocytes and monocytes by stimulating stem cell and precursor cell replication and maturation		Intrinsic states: myelodysplasia, congenital cyclic neutropenia, aplastic anemia, hairy cell leukemia		

Table 15-11	Biologic Response Modifiers *(Under Investigation)*—cont'd			
Agent	**Route of Administration**	**Indications Under Investigation**	**Side/Toxic Effects**	**Administration and Nursing Indications**
Erythropoietin Increases the production of RBC	SC	Anemias: End-stage renal disease Associated with antineoplastic chemotherapy and AZT	Fever, fatigue rare	Follow manufacturer's directions Rotate sites of injection Acetaminophen usually controls symptoms
Tumor necrosis factor (TNF) has the capability of destroying malignant cells but not normal cells; activation of cells of the immune system has also been reported	IM, IV, bolus, short-term infusion	Metastatic melanoma, advanced renal cancer, others being studied		Agitation of the biologic or rapid expulsion from a syringe may result in denaturing the molecules
			Pain, erythema at injection site	Rotate IM injection sites to reduce irritation; apply cold or warm compresses; acetaminophen may increase comfort
			Fever, chills, fatigue, headache	Premedicate with acetaminophen, then continue q4h as needed Encourage and monitor fluid intake during febrile episodes
			Hypotension	Monitor vital signs with BP lying and standing Report negative findings

BIBLIOGRAPHY

Ackley BJ, Ladwig GB: *Nursing diagnosis handbook: a guide to planning care,* ed 3, St Louis, 1997, Mosby.

Badger JM: Calming the anxious patient, *Am J Nurs* 94(5):46, 1994.

Baker C: Factors associated with rehabilitation in head and neck cancer, *Cancer Nurs* 15(6):395, 1992.

Bangerter M: New diagnostic imaging procedures in Hodgkin's disease, *Ann Oncol 7 Suppl* 4:55-59, 1996

Barse PM, Masny A: Adjuvant therapy and breast cancer treatment, *Am J Nurs Suppl,* 1998, pp 21-25.

Bartlett NL: Treatment of aggressive histology lymphoma, *Curr Opin Oncol* 9(5):413-419, 1997.

Beare PG, Myers JL: *Adult health nursing,* ed 3, St Louis, 1998, Mosby.

Beenken SW, Maddox WA, Urist MM: Workup of a patient with a mass in the neck, *Adv Surg* 28:371-383, 1995.

Belcher AE: *Blood disorders,* St Louis, 1992, Mosby.

Belcher AE: *Cancer nursing,* St Louis, 1992, Mosby.

Berman A et al: Cancer chemotherapy: intravenous administration, *Cancer Nurs* 16(2):145, 1993.

Boccadoro M, Pileri A: Diagnosis, prognosis, and standard treatment of multiple myeloma, *Hematol Oncol Clin North Am* 11(1):111-131, 1997.

Bohony J: Common IV complications and what to do about them, *Am J Nurs* 93(10):48, 1993.

Bosl GJ, Motzer RJ: Testicular germ-cell cancer, *New Engl J Med* 337(4):242-253, 1997.

Brack D et al: Testicular cancer, *Semin Oncol Nurs* 9(4):224, 1993.

Brown KK: Critical interventions in septic shock, *Am J Nurs* 94(10):20, 1994.

Brown KK: Septic shock: how to stop the deadly cascade, *Am J Nurs* 94(9):20, 1994.

Buccheri G, Ferringo D, Tamburini M: Karnofsky and ECOG performance status scoring in lung cancer: a prospective, longitudinal study of 536 patients from a single institution, *Eur J Cancer* 32A(7):1135-1141, 1996.

Carpenito JC: *Nursing diagnosis application to clinical practice,* ed 5, Philadelphia, 1993, JB Lippincott.

Cavanagh D, Hoffman MS: Controversies in the management of vulvar carcinoma, *Br J Obstet and Gynaecol* 103(4):293-300, 1996.

Chisholm LC et al: Cancer chemotherapy: alternative administration routes, *Cancer Nurs* 16(3):237, 1993.

Chisholm MA, Mulloy AL, Taylor AT: Acute management of cancer related hypercalcemia, *Ann Pharmacother* 30(5):507-513, 1996.

Collier J, Sherman M: Screening for hepatocellular carcinoma, *Hepatology* 27(1):273-278, 1998.

Davis M: Renal cell carcinoma, *Semin Oncol Nurs* 9(4):267, 1993.

DeMeester TR: Esophageal carcinoma: current controversies, *Semin Surg Oncol* 13(4):217-233, 1997.

Evans JD, Morton DG, Neoptolemos JP: Chronic pancreatitis and pancreatic carcinoma, *Postgrad Med J* 73(863):543-548, 1997.

Ferris DG: Office procedures: colposcopy, primary care, *Clin Office Pract* 24(2):241-267, 1997.

Forastiere AA, Heitmiller RF, Kleinberg L: Multimodality therapy for esophageal cancer, *Chest* 112(4 suppl):195S-200S, 1997.

Furlong TG: Neurologic complications of immunosuppressive cancer therapy, *Oncol Nurs Forum* 20(9):1337, 1993.

Gajewski W, Legare RD: Ovarian cancer, *Surg Oncol Clin North Am* 7(2):317-333, 1998.

Gore RM: Esophageal cancer: clinical and pathologic features, *Radiol Clin North Am* 35(2):243-263, 1997.

Hagemeister FB: Hodgkin's disease: the next decade, *Leukemia and Lymphoma* 21(1-2):53-61, 1996.

Halvorsen JA Jr, Yee J, McCormick VO: Diagnosis and staging of gastric cancer, *Semin Oncol* 23(3):325-335, 1996.

Helberg JL: Patients' status at home care discharge, *IMAGE J Nurs Sch* 25(2):93, 1993.

Hennessey B, Fitzgerald A, Graham D: Venous air embolism: keeping your patient out of danger, *Am J Nurs* 93(11):54, 1993.

Henriques I et al: Feasibility of Karnofsky performance status (KPS) as a prognostic indicator factor of survival in advanced terminal cancer patients, *Proc Annu Mtg Am Soc Clin Oncol* 15:A1825, 1996.

Hoebler I, Irwin M: Gastrointestinal tract cancer: current knowledge, medical treatment and nursing management, *Oncol Nurs Forum* 19(9):1403, 1992.

Hohenberger P, Hunerbein M: Detection and management of advanced gastric cancer, *Ann Oncol* 7(2):197-203, 1996.

Hossan E, Stregal A: Carcinoma of the bladder, *Semin Oncol Nurs* 9(4):252, 1993.

Hudson MM, Donaldson SS: Hodgkin's disease, *Pediatr Clin North Am* 44(4):891-906, 1997.

Johnson JR: Caring for the woman who's had a mastectomy, *Am J Nurs* 94(5):25, 1994.

Kim MJ et al: *Pocket guide to nursing diagnoses,* ed 7, St Louis, 1997, Mosby.

Kiningham RB: Physical activity and the primary prevention of cancer, *Prim Care: Clin Office Pract* 25(2):515-536, 1998.

Kurtz A: Disseminated intravascular coagulation with leukemia patients, *Cancer Nursing* 16(6):456-463, 1993.

Kwok LW, Longo DL: Lymphomas, *Cancer Chemother Biol Resp Modifiers* 16:376-440, 1996.

Lam S et al: Detection and localization of early lung cancer by imaging techniques, *Chest* 103(1):12S, 1993.

LeMone P: Analysis of a human phenomenon: self-concept, *Nurs Diagn* 2(3):126, 1991.

Lester J, Fulton JS: Breast cancer: advances in diagnosis and surgical treatment, *Am J Nurs Suppl* 98:8-11, 1998.

Levy W: Chemotherapy agents, I, *Cancer Nurs* 16(4):321, 1993.

Lieberman D: How to screen for colon cancer, *Annu Rev Med* 49:163-172, 1998.

Lorigan PC et al: Tumor lysis syndrome: case report and review of the literature, *Ann Oncol* 7(6):631-636, 1996.

Lowenberg B: Treatment of acute myelogenous leukaemia, *J Int Med Suppl* 740:17-22, 1997.

Lynes AC: Percutaneous hepatic arterial chemotherapy and chemoembolization, *Cancer Nurs* 16(4):283, 1993.

Maffezzini M et al: Bladder cancer, *Crit Rev Oncol Hematol* 27(2):151-153, 1998.

Martini N: The current state of the art in treating stage IIIA (N2) lung cancer, *Ann Oncol* 9(3):243-245, 1998.

Maxwell E: Carcinoma of the prostate, *Semin Oncol Nurs* 9(4):237, 1993.

McCance KL, Huether SE: *Pathophysiology: the biological basis for disease in adults and children,* ed 3, St Louis, 1998, Mosby.

McClosky JC: *Nursing interventions classification,* ed 3, St Louis, 2000, Mosby.

McEvilly JM, Dow KH: Treating metastatic breast cancer: principles and current practice, *Am J Nurs Suppl* 98:26-29, 1998.

McEwen DR et al: Managing patients with pancreatic cancer, *AORN J* 64(5):716-735, 1996.

McFarland GK, McFarlane EA: *Nursing diagnosis and intervention planning for patient care,* ed 3, St Louis, 1997, Mosby.

Mehmert PPA, Delaney CW: Validating impaired physical mobility, *Nurs Diagn* 2(4):143, 1991.

Meyers PA, Gorlick R: Osteosarcoma, *Pediatr Clin North Am* 44(4):973-989, 1997.

Micromedex on-line drug evaluation monographs: August, 1998, Micromedex, Inc.

Minsky BD et al: Treatment systems guidelines for primary rectal cancer from 1996 Patterns of Care study, *Int J Radiation Oncol, Biol, Physics* 41(1):21-27, 1998.

Morrison CS et al: Sexual behavior and cancer prevention, *Cancer Causes and Control Suppl* 1:521-525, 1997.

Niehoff ML: Epidemiology and early detection of prostate cancer in the primary setting, *J Am Acad Physic Assist* 7(3):147, 1994.

Nieweg R et al: Nursing care for oral complications associated with chemotherapy, *Cancer Nurs* 15(5):313, 1992.

Norris J: Nursing intervention for self-esteem disturbances, *Nurs Diagn* 3(2):48, 1992.

O'Callaghan A, Mead GM: Testicular cancer, *Postgrad Med J* 73(862) 481-486, 1997.

Oken MM: Multiple myeloma: prognosis and standard treatment, *Cancer Investig* 15(1):57-64, 1997.

Ouellet LL, Rush KL: A synthesis of selected literature on mobility: a basis for studying impaired mobility, *Nurs Diagn* 3(2):72, 1992.

Otto SE: *Chemotherapy quick reference,* ed 2, St Louis, 1997, Mosby.

Otto SE: *Oncology nursing,* ed 3, St Louis, 1997, Mosby.

Pack R: Descriptive epidemiology of genitourinary cancers, *Semin Oncol Nurs* 9(4):218, 1993.

Petrovich Z et al: Management of carcinoma of the bladder, *Am J Clin Oncol* 21(3):217-222, 1998.

Pickett M: Determinants of anticipatory nausea and anticipatory vomiting in adults receiving cancer chemotherapy, *Cancer Nurs* 14(6):334, 1991.

Quint-Kasner S: Chemotherapy agents, II, *Cancer Nurs* 16(5):398, 1993.

Radziewicz RM, Schneider SM: Using diversional activity to enhance coping, *Cancer Nurs* 15(4):293, 1992.

Regine WF, John WJ, Mohiuddin M: Current and emerging treatments for pancreatic cancer, *Drugs and Aging* 11(4):285-295, 1997.

Rose PG: Cervical cancer, *Emerg Med* 25(4):133, 1993.

Sahn SA: Pleural diseases related to metastatic malignancies, *Eur Respir J* 10(8):1907-1913, 1997.

Samet JM: The epidemiology of lung cancer, *Chest* 103(1):20S, 1993.

Scott-Conner CE, Christie DW: Cancer staging using the American Joint Committee on Cancer TMN System, *J Am Coll Surg* 181(2):182-188, 1995.

Shah JP, Lydatt W: Treatment of cancer of the head and neck, *CA Cancer J Clin* 45(6):352-368, 1995.

Skalla KA, Lacosse C: Patient education for fatigue, *Oncol Nurs Forum* 19(10):1537, 1992.

Sloan DA, McGrath PC, Kenady DE: Current considerations in multimodality therapy of head and neck cancer, *Clin Plastic Surg* 22(1):9-19, 1995.

Small EJ: Prostate cancer: who to screen and what the results mean, *Geriatrics* 48(12):28, 1993.

Smith DB, Babaian RJ: The effects of treatment for cancer on male fertility and sexuality, *Cancer Nurs* 15(4):271, 1992.

Sparks SM: Exploring electronic support groups, *Am J Nurs* 92(12):62, 1992.

Stock PS: Pap smears: still a reliable screening tool for cervical cancer, *Postgrad Med* 101(4):207-208, 211-214, 1997.

Stewart IE: Superior vena cava syndrome: an oncologic complication, *Sem Oncol Nurs* 12(4):312-317, 1996.

Stomper PC: Breast cancer, *Emerg Med* 25(4):113, 1993.

Sweeney CJ, Sandler AB: Treatment of advanced (stages III and IV) non-small-cell lung cancer, *Curr Prob Cancer* 22(2):85-132, 1998.

Thompson JM et al: *Mosby's clinical nursing,* ed 4, St Louis, 1997, Mosby.

Uaje C, Kahsen K, Parish L: Oncology emergencies, *Crit Care Nurs Quart* 18(4):26-34, 1996.

Veno-Sharp MB, Mrozek-Orlowski M: Breast cancer options: getting through the treatment, *Am J Nurs Suppl,* 1998, pp 12-16.

Veridiano NP: Vaginal and vulvar cancer, *Emerg Med* 25(4): 149, 1993.

Watson PG: The optimal functioning plan: a key element in cancer rehabilitation, *Cancer Nurs* 15(40):254, 1992.

Whelan JS: Osteosarcoma, *Eur J Cancer* 33(10):1611-1618, 1997.

Winchester DP, Cox JD: Standards for diagnosis and management of invasive breast carcinoma. American College of Radiology, American College of Surgeons, College of American Pathologists, Society of Surgical Oncology, *CA Cancer J Clin* 48(2):83-107, 1998.

Winchester DP, Strom EA: Standards for diagnosis and management of ductal carcinoma in situ (DCIS) of the breast. American College of Radiology, American College of Surgeons, College of American Pathologists, Society of Surgical Oncology, *CA Cancer J Clin* 48(2):108-128, 1998.

Woodtli MA, Van Ort S: Nursing diagnoses and functional health patterns in patients receiving radiation therapy: cancer of the head and neck, *Nurs Diagn* 2(4):171, 1991.

Yeaw EMJ: How position affects oxygenation: good lung down? *Am J Nurs* 92(3):27, 1992.

Youngblood M et al: A comparison of two methods of assessing cancer therapy related symptoms, *Cancer Nurs* 17(1):37, 1994.

1

BARNES

CARE PATH® 540
TOTAL MASTECTOMY WITH MALIGNANCY WITHOUT CC

SERVICE		PHYSICIAN	
PRIMARY NURSE		PRIMARY NURSE	

DC DATE	ADM DATE	DATE OF SURGERY	A-8

Problem Number	PATIENT PROBLEMS/NURSING DIAGNOSES
#1	ALTERATION IN COMFORT
#2	ALTERATION IN COPING
#3	ALTERATION IN SELF-CONCEPT
#4	LACK OF KNOWLEDGE

#	1, 2	2, 3	1	1, 3	1
	ASSESSMENT/MONITORING	CONSULTS	PROCEDURES/TEST	TREATMENT	ACTIVITY
DAY 1 DOS	VS q 4 hrs. x1 x2 x3 x4 x5 x6 I & O Pain Control Dressing/JP patency and drainage Ability to void Circulation Emotional response/family coping	Social Work		JP to bulb suction Incentive Spirometer/TCDB Avoid trauma to extremity	Up with assist to bathroom in PM
DAY 2 POD 1	VS q 8 hrs. if stable x1 x2 x3 I & O Pain Control Dressing/JP patency and drainage **Voiding without difficulty** Circulation Emotional response/family coping	Social Work visit Reach to Recovery		JP to bulb suction **Uses Incentive Spirometer independently** Avoid trauma to extremity	Up as tolerated with assist if needed
	SIGNATURE	INIT.	SIGNATURE	INIT.	SIGNATURE	INIT.

540

2

BARNES

**CARE PATH® 540
TOTAL MASTECTOMY WITH
MALIGNANCY WITHOUT CC**

CNS	DIETARY	RT	
HOME HEALTH	OT	OTHER	
PT	SW	OTHER	**A-8**

Problem Number	PATIENT PROBLEMS/NURSING DIAGNOSES

	1	**3, 4**	**2, 3, 4**	**, 3**		**INITIALS**	
MEDS / IVS	**NUTRITION**	**PATIENT/FAMILY EDUCATION**	**DISCHARGE PLANNING**	**PSYCHOSOCIAL/ EMOTIONAL/ SPIRITUAL NEEDS**		**(SEE KEY AT BOTTOM)**	
IVF IM analgesics Antibiotic if ordered	Clear liquid. Advance as tolerated to diet as prior to admission	Nursing: Pain control Positioning/mobility TCDB Incentive Spirometer Diet IV JP Primary Nursing	**Pt./family verbalizes understanding of Care Path.** **Plan of care has been mutually set with pt./family.**				
DC IVF when tolerating PO well DC IM analgesics Start oral analgesics **Pain controlled with oral analgesics**	**Tolerating diet as prior to admission**	Social Work: Assess resource needs Initiate education re: dx, prosthesis, support groups Nursing: Arm protection S/S infection BSE	Social Work: Complete high risk screening	Social Work: Assess counseling needs Initiate support Nursing: Therapeutic emotional care			

SIGNATURE	INIT.	SIGNATURE	INIT.	SIGNATURE	INIT.

Continued

#	1, 2	2, 3	1	1, 3	1
	ASSESSMENT / MONITORING	**CONSULTS**	**PROCEDURES / TEST**	**TREATMENT**	**ACTIVITY**
DAY 3 POD 2	VS q 8 hrs. if stable x1 x2 x3 D/C I & O Except JP(s) Incision/JP patency and drainage Circulation Lab results Emotional response/ family coping	Social Work visit if needed Reach to Recovery visit	CBC **Hematocrit not decreased more than 25% from pre-op value.**	JP to bulb suction JP dressing change/ site care daily Avoid trauma to extremity	**Up ad lib**
DAY 4 POD 3	VS prior to discharge			DC Incentive Spirometer	
DISCHARGE	**No wound complications. Afebrile / VSS** **Circulation adequate.**	**Seen by Social Work** **Seen by Reach to Recovery**	**CBC stable**	**No pulmonary complications.** **JP sites clean**	**As prior to admission except restrictions to affected extremity**
	SIGNATURE	**INIT.**	**SIGNATURE**	**INIT.**	**SIGNATURE**	**INIT.**

MEDS/IVS	1 NUTRITION	3, 4 PATIENT/FAMILY EDUCATION	2, 3, 4 DISCHARGE PLANNING	2, 3 PSYCHOSOCIAL/ EMOTIONAL/ SPIRTUAL NEEDS	INITALS (SEE KEY AT BOTTOM)		
		Reach to Recovery: Peer counseling MD: Arm mobility Showering Follow-up Activity Nursing: JP care, emptying, measuring	Social Work Home care support referral if needed				
		MD: Reinforce instruction Nursing: Validate learning Review DC summary with pt. Review DC meds with pt. if prescribed					
IV site without signs of phlebitis		**Identifies support systems and resources.** **Able to verbalize/demonstrate:** **JP care/emptying and measuring** **Arm protection** **Activity/exercise** **S/Sx infection** **Importance of BSE** **MD follow-up**	**Home with appropriate level of care.**	**Verbalizes feelings R / T dx and surgery.**			
SIGNATURE	**INIT.**	**SIGNATURE**	**INIT.**	**SIGNATURE**			**INIT.**

page 1 of 6

USC UNIVERSITY HOSPITAL
1500 San Pablo
Los Angeles, CA 90033 ©1991

SIDE 1

MULTIDISCIPLINARY PLAN

NAME _____
ALLERGIES _____
ADMIT DATE _____

DIAGNOSIS _____ Glioma

SURGERY _____ CRANIOTOMY FOR RESECTION OF TUMOR

DRG 001   ALOS 14.7

DISCHARGE OUTCOMES

PHYSIOLOGICAL: ADLs will be met by self or c̄ assistance of others(s). Complications/injury will be prevented or minimized, discomfort relieved/controlled, and infectious process(es) resolving/absent.

COGNITIVE: Verbalizes disease process/prognosis and therapeutic regimen. Will be able to explain surgical care, verbalizes precautions to take for medication use, and state s/sx to report to the health care team.

PSYCHOLOGICAL: Verbalizes acceptance of potential lifestyle changes and incorporates them into ADLs. Able to verbalize fears/anxieties and demonstrate effective coping mechanisms. Able to participate in self-care decisions.

DISCIPLINE	PRE-OP/ PRE-ADMIT DATE	DAY 1 DATE	DOS DAY 2 DATE	POD #1 DAY 3 DATE	POD #2 DAY 4 DATE	POD #3 DAY 5 DATE	POD #4 DAY 6 DATE
LOCATION		MED/SURG	SURGERY/PAR/NSICU	NSICU→DOU	DOU	DOU→MED/SURG	MED/SURG
LABS		Chem 20 CBC PT PTT UA T & screen 2u PRBCS Antiepileptic drug levels	Chem 20 ⟩ on arrival CBC ⟩ to unit	Lytes WBC	Lytes WBC Antiepileptic drug levels		
CARDIO-PULMONARY		ECG: R/O Arrhythmia	Pulse oximetry O₂ 40% face mask I.S. q 1° W/A A-line	DC A-line DC face mask & pulse oximetry	Encourage I.S. q 1° W/A		
IMAGING/ NUCLEAR MEDICINE		CXR: 2 Views	MRI c̄/s̄ contrast in am pre-op				
SOCIAL SERVICES D/C PLAN REHAB. SERVICES		Social services consult		Assess need for OT/PT/ speech evaluation	Assess need for rehab evaluation	Assess need for home health evaluation	Ordered therapies to assess pt D/C needs
PHARMACY		S.L. Corticosteroids antiepileptics H₂ Antagonist	Antiepileptics IV/po IV fluids Corticosteroids IV/po H₂ Antagonist IV/po Antiemetic Analgesics Antibiotics x 24°	Convert IV to S.L. if tolerating po's	Taper corticosteroids		DC S.L. DC H₂ antagonist p̄ corticosteroids DC'ed
DIETARY/ NUTRITION		Regular diet NPO p̄ midnight	NPO: ice chips when fully awake	Advance diet as tolerated			Regular diet

Used by permission of USC University Hospital, Los Angeles, California.

MULTIDISCIPLINARY PLAN

PATIENT NAME: _____

DISCIPLINE	PRE-OP / PRE-ADMIT	DAY 1	DOS DAY 2	POD #1 DAY 3	POD #2 DAY 4	POD #3 DAY 5	POD #4 DAY 6
		DATE ___	DATE ___	DATE ___	DATE ___	DATE ___	DATE ___
PATIENT ACTIVITY		Ad lib	BR c̄ HOB ↑30° Leg squeezers (begun in OR)	OOB to chair	Ambulate c̄ assistance TID	DC leg squeezers Ambulate as much as tolerated	
EDUCATION		I.S. instruction CDB Teach reason for surgery, postop restrictions, & expected LOS Orient to room, unit, & hospital routine	Reorient to present unit Teach monitoring of dressing & drainage Discuss need for foley	DC foley I & O cath q 6° prn	Review disease process, prognosis, and understanding of therapeutic regimen during hospitalization		Teach s/sx to report to the health care team Instruct pt in care of surgical site Pharmacy to educate pt on D/C medications

COLLABORATIVE PROBLEMS

	DATE				DATE		D/C DATE INIT
❶ Anxiety/fear R/T surgery, change in health status, & terminal illness.					❼ Knowledge deficit R/T lack of exposure to hospital, misinterpretation of information received, or limitation of cognitive ability; discharge planning.		
❷ Potential for altered cerebral tissue perfusion R/T cerebral edema altering or interrupting cerebral blood flow.					❽ Denial R/T severity of diagnosis; terminal illness.		
❸ Potential for injury R/T seizure activity, weakness, paralysis, paresthesia.							
❹ Potential for impaired physical mobility R/T neuromuscular impairment & strength, perceptual/cognitive impairment, pain, or restriction in activity.							
❺ Potential for infection R/T suppressed inflammatory response, medication induced, or exposure to pathogens.							
❻ Alteration in comfort R/T headache &/or surgical procedure.							

OUTCOMES

							D/C DATE INIT
❶ Will acknowledge and discuss fears. Reports anxiety reduction to a manageable level.					❼ Able to correctly perform procedures necessary.		
❷ Maintains usual or improved level of consciousness and motor/sensory function.					❽ Continues to demonstrate healing free from infectious spread.		
❸ Seizures controlled, free from injury during hospitalization.					❾ Verbalizes pain control c̄ po medication.		
❹ Demonstrates timely healing free from infection. Afebrile.					❿ Verbalizes understanding of D/C plans.		
❺ Verbalizes pain control c̄ ordered medication. Able to sleep/rest.					⓫ Pt & S/O verbalize understanding of treatment plan and begin to show signs of acceptance.		
❻ Verbalizes understanding of condition/disease process.							
❼ Regains and maintains optimal physical mobility.							

KEY

❶ To initiate a problem or intervention, document under corresponding date.

❷ Document outcomes under appropriate date for achieving the goal.

❸ To discontinue an intervention or resolve a patient problem highlight, date, and initial.

Continued

	DAY 1	DOS DAY 2	POD #1 DAY 3	POD #2 DAY 4	POD #3 DAY 5	POD #4 DAY 6
PLAN OF CARE DISCUSSED WITH — INITIAL / S.O. / Pt. DATE		DATE ___	DATE ___	DATE ___	DATE ___	DATE ___

INTERVENTIONS

DAY 1	DOS — DAY 2	POD #1 — DAY 3	POD #2 — DAY 4	POD #3 — DAY 5	POD #4 — DAY 6
– Assess pt and/or S/O level of anxiety – Answer questions & explain all procedures before initiation – Clarify misunderstanding of info & involve pt & S/O in decision making, care planning & evaluation – Assess baseline neurological status	– Assess neurological status per MD order, report changes to MD – Strict I & O – Monitor temp per routine – Monitor respiratory status – Reposition frequently & encourage use of I.S. – Evaluate for s/sx of ↑ ICP: • decreased response to stimuli • changes in VS • restlessness • weakness/paralysis of extremities • changes in vision or pupillary changes • worsening of headache – If pt has headache, reduce bright lights & room noises if possible – Medicate for pain as ordered & assess pain relief – Note location, intensity & duration of pain – Provide info to pt & S/O in short segments – Discuss expected length of recovery – Assess pt ability to swallow before advancing diet	– Increase activity & participation in ADLs – Encourage S/O to assist c̄ – Assess for need of stool softener – Assess pt & S/O understanding of disease process, prognosis, & therapeutic regimen – Continue use of I.S. – Temperature elevation may indicate meningitis – Monitor for CSF leakage – Assess for factors that impair physical mobility: • pain/nausea • dislodging tubes • compromising surgical wound – Treat those items present above &/or educate pt prn – Assure pt that activity ordered will enhance rather than compromise healing process – Provide praise and encouragement for all efforts to ↑ mobility – Reinforce need for assistance when getting OOB – Provide pt c̄ safe environment; seizure precautions may be indicated – Assess respiratory status, neurological status & VS per unit routine p̄ transfer	– Reassess pt and/or S/O level of anxiety – Support planning of a realistic lifestyle p̄ hospitalization within limitations but fully using capabilities – Explore sources of support: • S/O • Clergy • Social worker – Encourage use of oral pain medications – Assess need for home health evaluation & outpatient therapies – Continue to monitor for CSF leakage	– DC leg squeezers once pt fully ambulatory – Reassess need for stool softener – Encourage increased activity – Allow pt time to adjust to illness – Solicit help from S/O's, clergy during denial	– Instruct in showering technique – Teach s/sx to report to health care team • changes in vision • elevated temperature • intense headache • drainage from surgical site – Teach pt how to care for surgical site: • avoid scrubbing • dab very dry • keep hair off of wound x 72° • avoid sun exposure • OK to shampoo hair p̄ staples out x 24° • keep clean & dry x 72° p̄ staples out – Instruct pt & S/O regarding discharge medications including name, purpose, route, dosage, frequency, time of administration, and side effects

Case Manager: ___

Consulting MD: ___

Social Service

Anointing of The Sick Date:

MULTIDISCIPLINARY PLAN UPDATE

DATE	SIGNATURES	DATE	SIGNATURES	DATE	SIGNATURES

page 4 of 6

DIAGNOSIS   Glioma

SURGERY   CRANIOTOMY FOR RESECTION OF TUMOR

USC UNIVERSITY HOSPITAL
1500 San Pablo
Los Angeles, CA 90033   ©1991
SIDE 2

MULTIDISCIPLINARY PLAN

NAME _____
ALLERGIES _____

ADMIT DATE _____

DISCHARGE OUTCOMES	DRG 001 ALOS 14.7
PHYSIOLOGICAL	ADLs will be met by self or c assistance of others(s). Complications/injury will be prevented or minimized, discomfort relieved/controlled, and infectious process(es) resolving/absent.
COGNITIVE	Verbalizes disease process/prognosis and therapeutic regimen. Will be able to explain surgical care, verbalize precautions to take for medication use, and state s/sx to report to the health care team.
PSYCHOLOGICAL	Verbalizes acceptance of potential lifestyle changes and incorporates them into ADLs. Able to verbalize fears/anxieties and demonstrate effective coping mechanisms. Able to participate in self-care decisions.

DISCIPLINE	PRE-OP/ PRE-ADMIT	POD #5 DAY 7 DATE___	POD #6 DAY 8 DATE___	POD #7 DAY 9 DATE___	POD #8 DAY 10 DATE___	POD #9 DAY 11 DATE___	POD #10 DAY 12 DATE___
LOCATION		MED/SURG → HOME					
LABS							
CARDIO- PULMONARY							
IMAGING/ NUCLEAR MEDICINE							
SOCIAL SERVICES D/C PLAN REHAB. SERVICES							
PHARMACY		DC c̄ po pain medica- tions & antiepileptic therapy					
DIETARY/ NUTRITION		Regular diet					

Continued

PATIENT NAME: _____

MULTIDISCIPLINARY PLAN

DISCIPLINE	PRE-OP/ PRE-ADMIT	POD #5 DAY 7 DATE ___	POD #6 DAY 8 DATE ___	POD #7 DAY 9 DATE ___	POD #8 DAY 10 DATE ___	POD #9 DAY 11 DATE ___	POD #10 DAY 12 DATE ___
PATIENT ACTIVITY		Ad lib					
EDUCATION		DC teaching: • staples to be removed 7-10 days post-op • shower instructions • staples may be wet • towel dry thoroughly p̄ showering					

COLLABORATIVE PROBLEMS

DATE	DATE
❼ Knowledge deficit R/T lack of exposure to hospital, misinterpretation of information received, or limitation of cognitive ability; discharge planning.	DC DATE ___ INIT ___

OUTCOMES

❼ Verbalizes understanding of D/C plans	

COLLABORATIVE PROBLEMS

	DC DATE ___ INIT ___

❶ To initiate a problem or intervention, document under corresponding date.

❷ Document outcomes under appropriate date for achieving the goal.

❸ To discontinue an intervention or resolve a patient problem highlight, date, and initial.

KEY

_____

PLAN OF CARE DISCUSSED WITH	POD #5 DAY 7 DATE ____	POD #6 DAY 8 DATE ____	POD #7 DAY 9 DATE ____	POD #8 DAY 10 DATE ____	POD #9 DAY 11 DATE ____	POD #10 DAY 12 DATE ____
DATE	INITIAL	S.O.	Pt.			

INTERVENTIONS

- Explain safety precautions to maintain at home; continue to monitor for CSF leak
- Reinforce those s/sx that need to be reported to the health care team
- Encourage tips for recovery:
  • return to normal social & physical activity
  • verbalization of concerns c̄ health care team
  • emphasize the importance of ongoing outpatient care & follow-up visits
- Review those medications pt will take at home

Case Manager: ____

Consulting MD: ____

Social Service ____

Anointing of The Sick
Date: ____

MULTIDISCIPLINARY PLAN UPDATE

DATE	SIGNATURES	DATE	SIGNATURES	DATE	SIGNATURES	DATE	SIGNATURES

HARTFORD HOSPITAL CRITICAL PATHWAY
ACUTE NONLYMPHOCYTIC LEUKEMIA

NAME:

LEGEND:

A=Accomplished: intervention/outcome reached

V=Variance: intervention/outcome not reached

NA=Non-applicable: intervention/outcome deemed not clinically applicable

X=Write "X" in accomplished column when variance has been addressed and outcome/intervention will not be accomplished

PATIENT CARE COORDINATOR: ____

ADMISSION DATE: ____ ADMISSION TIME: ____

DISCHARGE DATE: ____ DISCHARGE TIME: ____

PATIENT UNIT: ____

LOS: EXPECTED: ____ ACTUAL: ____

PATIENT STATUS: ____

PATHWAY COMPLETED: ____

PATHWAY NOT CLINICALLY APPLICABLE: ____

EXPIRED: ____

AMA: ____

TX NEW PATHWAY: ____

NAME: ____

CP040401

PRECHEMO

DATE: ____

	A	V
OUTCOMES		
1. Patient will be able to state: diagnosis, treatment & plan, length of hospitalization, effect of chemo, possible S/E, understanding of blood counts		
2. Patients psychosocial treatment plan will be identified based on HAD		
3. Patient will verbalize understanding of Hickman catheter		
4.		
5.		
6.		
CONSULT		
7. Dietitian		
8. Dentist		
9. Vascular surgeon		
10.		
ASSESSMENT		
11. Patient's physical status will be assessed for upcoming chemo.		
12.		
13.		
14.		
TESTS		
15. CBC with diff		
16. HLA typing		
17.		
18.		
NUTRITION		
19. Diet as tol.		
20.		

DAY 1

DATE: ____

	A	V
OUTCOMES		
50. Patients nutritional status will be assessed and plan in place		
51. Hickman cath will be in place		
52. Chemo initiated		
53. N/V scale 2 or less		
54. Patient will verbalize concerns R/T chemo hospitalization		
55.		
CONSULT		
56. ID when temp spikes		
57.		
58.		
59.		
ASSESSMENT		
60. Mouth, lungs, skin, rectum		
61. Level of N/V anxiety		
62. Hickman site		
63.		
TESTS		
64. CBC with diff		
65.		
66.		
67.		
NUTRITION		
68.		
69.		

This critical path was developed through the consensus of a multidisciplinary group and depicts the sequence and timing of those critical events which drive the achievement of progressive patient outcomes during an episode of illness. This is not meant to represent the only acceptable way to design the care for a given patient nor would all patients' needs necessarily be met by such a path, therefore the content may be tailored to meet the needs of the individual patient.

The contents of this document incorporate the Standards of Patient Care.

Used by permission of Hartford Hospital, Hartford, Conn.

NAME: _____

DATE: _____

MEDICAL RECORD #: _____

DATE: _____

PRECHEMO	A	V	DAY 1	A	V
MEDICATIONS			**MEDICATIONS**		
21. Allopurinol			70. Allopurinol		
22. Mouth care protocol			71. Mouth care protocol		
23.			72. Chemo		
24.			73.		
25.			74.		
26.			75.		
27.			76.		
28.			77. Premeds		
29.			78.		
30.			79.		
31.			80.		
32.			81.		
TREATMENT/INTERVENTION			**TREATMENT/INTERVENTION**		
33. Transfuse per protocol			82. Transfuse per protocol		
- if plalets < 10,000					
- if hct < 24					
34. Neutrapenic precautions when ANC < 500			83. Neutrapenic precautions		
35.			84. OR for hickman		
36.			85. Wt 2x/wk		
37.			86.		
MOBILITY/ACTIVITIES			**MOBILITY/ACTIVITIES**		
38. As tol			87. As tol		
39.			88.		
PSYCHOSOCIAL MANAGEMENT			**PSYCHOSOCIAL MANAGEMENT**		
40.			89. PS consultant F/U 2x/wk		
41.			90.		
EDUCATION			**EDUCATION**		
42.			91. Review of blood counts		
43.			92. Chemo teaching		
44.			93. Hickman teaching		
45.			94. ID hickman caregiver		
46.			95. Offer leukemia video		
DISCHARGE MANAGEMENT			**DISCHARGE MANAGEMENT**		
47.			96. Obtain info re:		
48.			Insurance coverage, preferred provider		
			97.		
OTHER			**OTHER**		
49.			98.		

Continued

HARTFORD HOSPITAL CRITICAL PATHWAY
ACUTE NONLYMPHOCYCTIC LEUKEMIA

PATIENT CARE COORDINATOR: _____ ADMISSION TIME: _____
ADMISSION DATE: _____   DISCHARGE TIME: _____
DISCHARGE DATE: _____
PATIENT UNIT: _____
LOS: EXPECTED: _____   ACTUAL: _____
PATIENT STATUS: _____

PATHWAY COMPLETED: _____
PATHWAY NOT
CLINICALLY APPLICABLE: _____
EXPIRED: _____
AMA: _____

TX NEW PATHWAY: NAME: _____
CP040401

PRIOR TO DISCHARGE

OUTCOMES	A	V
DATE: _____		
147. D/C arrangements in place including:		
- hickman supplies		
- Nsg agency referral		
- MD F/U		
- Plans for Out patient care in place		
- Peripheral blood and BM indicate remission		
- Patient verbalizes knowledge of disease and F/U		
- Patient/family member able to care for hickman and recognize, report complications of catheter.		
148.		
149.		
150.		
CONSULT		
151. Dietitian		
152.		
ASSESSMENT		
153.		
154.		
155.		
156.		
TESTS		
157. CBC		
158.		
NUTRITION		
159. Diet as tol		
160.		

DAY 2-7

OUTCOMES	DAY 2	DAY 3	DAY 4	DAY 5	DAY 6	DAY 7	V
	A	A	A	A	A	A	
DATE: _____							
99. S/E of chemo will be controlled							
100. - mouth and rectal membranes will remain intact and free from pain							
101. - patient will be able to identify methods to control anxiety							
102. N/V < 2							
103. Patient is able to identify foods that are easily tolerated							
104.							
CONSULT							
105.							
106.							
ASSESSMENT							
107. Mouth, lung, skin, rectum							
108. Level of N/V							
109. Anxiety							
110. Hickman site with dsg changes							
TESTS							
111. CBC							
112.							
NUTRITION							
113.							
114.							

NAME: _____   MEDICAL RECORD #: _____

DAY 2-7   DATE: _____

	DAY 2	DAY 3	DAY 4	DAY 5	DAY 6	DAY 7	
	A	A	A	A	A	A	V

MEDICATIONS
115. Allopurinol
116. Mouth care prot.
117. Chemos
118.
119.
120.
121.
122. Premeds
123.
124.
125.
126.

TREATMENT/INTERVENTION
127. Hickman care M-W-F
128. Transfuse per protocol
129. Neutropenic precautions
130.

MOBILITY/ACTIVITIES
131. As tol.
132.

PSYCHOSOCIAL MANAGEMENT
133.

EDUCATION
134.
135.
136.
137.

DISCHARGE MANAGEMENT
138.
139.
140.
141.
142.
143.
144.
145.

OTHER
146.

PRIOR TO DISCHARGE   DATE: _____

	A	V

MEDICATIONS
161.
162.
163.
164.
165.
166.
167.
168.
169.
170.
171.
172.

TREATMENT/INTERVENTION
173.
174.
175.
176.

MOBILITY/ACTIVITIES
177. Ambulate in hallway
178.

PSYCHOSOCIAL MANAGEMENT
179.

EDUCATION
180. Patient/significant other demonstrates care of hickman
181. Verbalizes S&S of infection, occlusion, rupture, leakage
182. Review all D/C teaching
183.

DISCHARGE MANAGEMENT
184. F/U appt. with M.D.
185. Contact DME co. for Hickman supplies
186. Contact agency if appropriate
187. Obtain payment for _____ if needed
188. Determine if patient will require outpatient transfusions
189. Determine if patient candidate for BMT - MD will arrange
190. Determine date for consolidation
191.

OTHER
192.

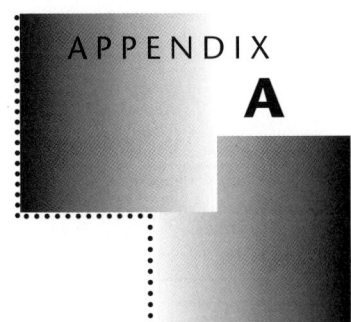

Combined Care Paths and Documentation Forms

With the increased use of flow charts, 24-hour documentation forms, preprinted care plans, and timeline-based plans of care or care paths, there have been some very successful attempts at avoiding duplication of documentation. This has been achieved by combining these formats to provide one chart form. These types of combination forms save time and money and serve to streamline documentation as well as provide a single guide for all nursing staff and other multidisciplinary healthcare providers to track and monitor the patient's progress.

The Total Hip Care Path: Inpatient Phase represents a combination of a care path and a multiple-day documentation tool. The Care Path for the Vaginal Delivery delineates the Standard of Care, The Standard of Practice, and the Physician's role and provides a documentation tool for the patient during the expected length of the patient's stay. In the Family Centered Maternity Unit, the Newborn documentation tools are included as part of the maternal packet since mother and baby are not separated during the hospital stay. These forms provide a comprehensive but efficient documentation system for the staff who can then focus more time on direct patient care and teaching and less time on direct care activities, namely inefficient documentation tools.

Panorama City Medical Center

TOTAL HIP CARE PATH: In-Patient Phase
☛ *This Care Path will be INDIVIDUALIZED for each patient.*

Instructions: Initial box when intervention is implemented. Mark box with ✕ if findings Not Within Normal Limits or intervention Not Implemented (then write documentation of the situation in the progress notes), or when Goal is Not Met. Mark box with ∅ if intervention is Not Applicable.

Addressograph

CARE PATH DAY PAGE 1	DAY 1 SURGERY DAY-ROOM #	N	D	E	DAY 2 ROOM #	N	D	E	DAY 3 ROOM #	N	D	E
Write date →	DATE				DATE				DATE			
● **TESTS**	X-ray _____ hip											
H/H post-op, then CBC Q AM ×3	H&H				CBC: H/H / Platelet				CBC: H/H / Platelet			
● **ASSESSMENT:**	Write time done →				Write time done →				Write time done →			
NEURO: •alert, awake •oriented ×3 •PERLA •no numbness	Assessed WNL				Assessed WNL				Assessed WNL			
CARDIO: •regular HR •peripheral pulses + •extremities warm •capillary refill 3-5 sec. •No calf tenderness •sensation intact •no edema	Assessed WNL				Assessed WNL				Assessed WNL			
RESP: •RR >10/regular •adequate depth •clear breath sounds •nailbeds pink	Assessed WNL				Assessed WNL				Assessed WNL			
GI: •bowel sounds + •no nausea/vomiting •no abd. distention •stool (character & #)	Assessed WNL				Assessed WNL				Assessed WNL			
GU: •clear urine •can empty bladder •no bladder distention	Assessed WNL				Assessed WNL				Assessed WNL			
SKIN: •warm, dry, intact •skin color good •no pressure ulcers to bony areas- esp. heels •IV site clear (write type, insertion date and site) •incision appearance - •surgical dressing - •drainage character -	Assessed WNL				Assessed WNL				Assessed WNL			
MUSCULOSKELETAL: •CSM intact_____ leg •proper alignment •no int./ext. hip rotation •able to do ROM	Assessed WNL				Assessed WNL				Assessed WNL			
PAIN: location and description (intensity in pain graph)	No Pain: WNL				No Pain: WNL				No Pain: WNL			
BEHAVIOR: •coping effectively •no multiple requests	Assessed WNL				Assessed WNL				Assessed WNL			
** RN Teamleader concurs with above assessments	11-7 / 7-3 / 3-11				11-7 / 7-3 / 3-11				11-7 / 7-3 / 3-11			
● **TREATMENTS**												
VS-Duramorph x24h	see pain graph/TPR				VS q4, then QID-see TPR				VS QID-see TPR			
SCD												
TEDS with heel cut off taken off/on BID												
Heel protectors												
Abduction pillow												
ROM to extremities												
Check drainage, I&O												
I/O cath or Foley									★			
Elevated toilet seat	Start with Stage III				★				★			
Fall protocol/Trapeze												
Drains	Autovac / Hemovac				Hemovac				DC Hemovac			
Therapeutic (write time) Positioning (L) (R) (S)												

Reproduced with permission of Kaiser Foundation Hospital, Center for Development, Education, and Research, Panorama City, Calif.

CARE PATH DAY	DAY 1				DAY 2				DAY 3			
PAGE 2	SURGERY: ROOM #				ROOM #				ROOM #			
Write date →	DATE	N	D	E	DATE	N	D	E	DATE	N	D	E
Transfuse ___/___ units if Hct < ____ / ____ %												
● HYGIENE: Bath	☐ Full ☐ Partial				☐ Full ☐ Partial				☐ Full ☐ Partial			
How accomplished?	☐ Self ☐ Assist				☐ Self ☐ Assist				☐ Self ☐ Assist			
● SAFETY												
Siderails ↑												
Bed Position - low												
Call light w/in reach												
ID band correct												
● MEDICATIONS												
IV therapy	see MAR				Heplock, if no PCA ... see MAR				Heplock, if no PCA ... see MAR			
Pain Medications	see MAR & pain graph				see MAR & pain graph				see MAR & pain graph			
Antibiotic IVPB	see				see MAR				see MAR			
Iron Meds	Medication				see MAR				see MAR			
Stool Softener	Administration				see MAR				see MAR			
Antiemetic Meds	Record				see MAR				see MAR			
Antipyretic Meds	(MAR)				see MAR				see MAR			
Anticoagulant Meds	*** start Enoxaparin day after surgery				see MAR				see MAR			
Restart Home Meds	Orders made				Continue home meds		see MAR		Continue home meds		see MAR	
● DIET: As ordered		B	L	D		B	L	D		B	L	D
Consumption (write %)												
Food taken per -	☐ Self ☐ Assist				☐ Self ☐ Assist				☐ Self ☐ Assist			
● PHYSICAL ACTIVITY	Bedrest				Stage 1 protocol- -isometric exercises, dangling at bedside				Stage II (if drain out) -exercises, dangling tranfers to chair			
Stage Protocol												
Weight bearing					WB _____				WB _____			
● TEACHING Patient Outcomes: 1=Needs reinforcement 2=Partial understanding 3=Complete understanding/skill. *Write rating in box.*												
Orient to unit routine								★				
Daily Plan of care	Review patient copy				Review patient copy							
Activity restriction												
Therapeutic position: hip flexion not > 75°												
Use of triflow, CDBE												
Use of SCD & TEDS												
Use of CPM, Trapeze												
Pain Mgt Meds/Rx												
Duramorph side effects								★				
● DISCHARGE PLANNING	Provide patient copy of care path				Order DME Refer to SNF Make HH referral							
● DAILY PATIENT GOALS	Normal vital signs				Proper position for bedside dangling				Safe transfer to chair			
	No resp. depression								Hip flexion not > 75°			
	Good pain control				Good pain control				Good pain control			
	No s/s of complications				No s/s of complications				No s/s of complications			
● InterDisciplinary Signatures. Review of Care Path done q shift by nursing					PT				PT			
	CM				CM				CM			
	11-7				11-7				11-7			
	7-3				7-3				7-3			
	3-11				3-11				3-11			

PAIN GRAPH. Patient's desired goal is _____ on 0-10 pain scale. Obtain pain rating before & after each intervention.

DATE		24	01	02	03	04	05	06	07	08	09	10	11	12	13	14	15	16	17	18	19	20	21	22	23
PAIN RATINGS Draw a dot inside the box or on the line for each pain rating.	10																								
	8																								
	6																								
	4																								
	2																								
	0																								
Respiratory Rate																									
Depth of Respiration ♣																									
Level of Arousal ☻																									
O₂ Saturation																									

See page 5 for Code Depth of Respiration and Level of Arousal

Continued

Panorama City Medical Center

Provider Initial & Date	STANDARDS OF CARE Outcomes	Target Date	STANDARDS OF PRACTICE Interventions
	Patient will be monitored for any side effects of intrathecal or epidural narcotics for early intervention; e.g. respiratory depression, itchiness, nausea or vomiting, urinary retention.	Care Path Day 1-2	**Anesthesia:** Initiate pre-printed MD order sheet & manage patient's pain × 24 hours. **Nursing:** Monitor RR, depth, level of arousal, O_2 Sat q 1 hr × 16 hrs, q 2 hrs ×2. Initiate Regional Narcotic protocol. Assess for any side effect & manage per MD orders. Notify Anesthesiologist as needed for pain mgt. × 24 hrs.
	Patient will verbalize relief or control of pain symptoms per patient's desired rating of _____ on 0-10 scale with the use of oral analgesics.	Care Path Day 3-4	**Ortho MD:** Initiate pre-printed post-op order sheet, PCA order sheet & other follow-up orders. Evaluate pain control daily. **Nursing:** Assess pain level using 0-10 scale before and after each intervention. Document on pain flow sheet. Use parenteral narcotics & offer regularly first 48 hours. Inform patient of need to report pain & rating. Change position q 2 hours; use pillows for support; relieve any pressure. Use distraction/diversional techniques. Notify surgeon for modifications in treatment plan, as needed.
	Patient will experience an absence of complication, e.g. a. hemorrhage	Care Path Day 1-5	**Nursing:** Monitor VS, note amount of bloody drainage from operative site q shift. Autotransfuse as indicated. Check H/H & platelet values daily. **Ortho MD:** Evaluate drainage output q shift and H/H & platelet values daily × 3.
	b. dislocation of prosthesis	Care Path Day 1-5	**Nursing:** Maintain therapeutic positioning q shift, to include use abduction pillow between legs at all times; maintain proper alignment; turn to unaffected side; avoid hip flexion greater than 75°. Activity restriction: avoid crossing legs; use raised toilet seat. Assess for s/s: extremity shortened, internal or external rotation, severe hip pain, unable to move leg. Notify MD. **Ortho MD:** Evaluate alignment daily & determine for any s/s.
	c. neurovascular compromise	Care Path Day 1-5	**Nursing:** Assess CSM (circulation, sensation, movement) q shift. Observe for edema or swelling. Encourage patient to do ROM q shift. **Ortho MD:** Determine neurovascular status of limb daily.
	d. deep vein thrombosis (DVT)	Care Path Day 1-5	**Nursing:** Use TEDS & SCD. Remove & reapply TEDS 2x/day- AM bath & HS. Assess pulses q shift, avoid pressure beneath knee. Assess lung status q shift. Administer anticoagulant Rx. **Ortho MD:** Order prophylactic anticoagulant medications. Check platelet status if on Enoxaparin (Lovenox) Rx. daily × 3.
	e. wound infeciton	Care Path Day 1-5	**Nursing:** Monitor VS q shift/ BID. Assess wound appearance & drainage q shift. Administer Antibiotic meds as ordered. **Ortho MD:** Check on wound appearance & other s/s daily.
	Patient will verbalize understanding of care & demonstrate patient care skills. Any Barriers to Learning? ☐ None ☐ Language ☐ Cultural/Religious Practices ☐ Emotional ☐ Desire/Motivation ☐ Limited Learning Ability ☐ Physical Limitation	Care Path Day 4	**Nursing:** Instruct patient on daily plan. Give patient copy of Care Path. Inform on need/purpose for triflow, SCD, TEDS, abduction pillow, pain meds, ROM exercises, activity restriction & therapeutic positioning. Reinforce PT instructions on exercises. Review "After Total Hip" booklet information prior to DC. If on Enoxaparin (Lovenox) Rx, start patient teaching on self-injection of anticoagulant on post-op day 3 in preparation for DC. Provide booklet. **PT:** Provide instrucitonsd on safe transfers and use of assistive device.
	Patient will ambulate and perform transfers safely with use of assistive device.	Care Path Day 4	**Nursing:** Use trapeze when in bed. Reinforce activities upon release by PT to Nursing. Encourage exercises while in bed. **PT:** Activity per stage protocol. Instruct and supervise patient on proper use of walker or crutches, and on safe transfers. Communicate with nursing on pre-medication of patient for pain prior to activity. Communicate daily with nursing on progress with patient activity.
	Patient will be discharged home safely with family and home health follow-up. Patient & care provider knowledgeable of care after DC.	Care Path Day 4-5	**Case Manager:** Assess DC needs preop & postop - DME, Home Health follow-up. Arrange for SNF transfer, if indicated. **Nursing:** Reinforce MD/PT instructions on activity, restrictions, medications, return appt., s/s to report to MD before DC. Ensure DC orders to include prophylactic anticoagulant Rx, if indicated.

NOTE: If patient develops any other problems, nursing or the department will initiate a plan of care for that specific problem and address the interventions and outcomes in the Progress Notes for Care Path Variances.

THR care Path 7/95

PAGE 4 *PAIN GRAPH: Patient's desired goal is _____ on 0-10 scale. Obtain pain rating before and after each intervention.*

DATE		24	01	02	03	04	05	06	07	08	09	10	11	12	13	14	15	16	17	18	19	20	21	22	23
PAIN RATINGS Draw a dot inside the box or on the line for each pain rating.	10																								
	8																								
	6																								
	4																								
	2																								
	0																								
Respiratory Rate																									
Depth of Respiration ♣																									
Level of Arousal ♥																									
O₂ Saturation																									

♣ Depth of Respiration: A=Adequate and Normal N=Not Adequate and Shallow

♥ Level of Arousal: 2=Patient awake 1=Patient frequently drowsy but easily aroused O-Patient somnolent & difficult to arouse S=Normal sleep, patient easily aroused.

DATE		24	01	02	03	04	05	06	07	08	09	10	11	12	13	14	15	16	17	18	19	20	21	22	23
PAIN RATINGS Draw a dot inside the box or on the line for each pain rating.	10																								
	8																								
	6																								
	4																								
	2																								
	0																								
Respiratory Rate																									
Level of Arousal ♥																									

DATE		24	01	02	03	04	05	06	07	08	09	10	11	12	13	14	15	16	17	18	19	20	21	22	23
PAIN RATINGS Draw a dot inside the box or on the line for each pain rating.	10																								
	8																								
	6																								
	4																								
	2																								
	0																								
Respiratory Rate																									
Level of Arousal ♥																									

DATE		24	01	02	03	04	05	06	07	08	09	10	11	12	13	14	15	16	17	18	19	20	21	22	23
PAIN RATINGS Draw a dot inside the box or on the line for each pain rating.	10																								
	8																								
	6																								
	4																								
	2																								
	0																								
Respiratory Rate																									
Level of Arousal ♥																									

DATE		24	01	02	03	04	05	06	07	08	09	10	11	12	13	14	15	16	17	18	19	20	21	22	23
PAIN RATINGS Draw a dot inside the box or on the line for each pain rating.	10																								
	8																								
	6																								
	4																								
	2																								
	0																								
Respiratory Rate																									
Level of Arousal ♥																									

Continued

Instructions: Initial box when intervention is Implemented. Mark box with × if findings Not Within Normal Limits or intervention Not Implemented (then write documentation of the situation in the progress notes), or when Goal is Not Met. Mark box with ⊘ if intervention is Not Applicable.

CARE PATH DAY PAGE 5	DAY 4 ROOM #				DAY 5 ROOM #				DAY 6 DISCHARGE - ROOM #			
Write date →	DATE	N	D	E	DATE	N	D	E	DATE	N	D	E
● TESTS	CBC: H/H				★				★			
CBC q AM ×3	Platelet				★				★			
● ASSESSMENT:	Write time done →				Write time done →				Write time done →			
NEURO: •alert, awake •oriented ×3 •PERLA •no numbness	Assessed WNL				Assessed WNL				Assessed WNL			
CARDIO: •regular HR •peripheral pulses + •extremities warm •capillary refill 3-5 sec. •no calf tenderness •sensation intact •no edema	Assessed WNL				Assessed WNL				Assessed WNL			
RESP: RR•>10/regular •adequate depth •clear breath sounds •nailbeds pink	Assessed WNL				Assessed WNL				Assessed WNL			
GI: •bowel sounds + •no nausea/vomiting •no abd. distention •stool (character & #)	Assessed WNL				Assessed WNL				Assessed WNL			
GU: •clear urine •can empty bladder •no bladder distention	Assessed WNL				Assessed WNL				Assessed WNL			
SKIN: •warm, dry, intact •skin color good •no pressure ulcers to bony areas- esp. heels •IV site clear (write type, insertion date and site) •incision appearance - •surgical dressing - •drain site appearance -	Assessed WNL				Assessed WNL				Assessed WNL			
MUSCULOSKELETAL •CSM intact ____ leg •proper alignment •no int./ext. hip rotation •able to do ROM	Assessed WNL				Assessed WNL				Assessed WNL			
PAIN: location and description (intensity in pain graph)	No Pain: WNL				No Pain: WNL				No Pain: WNL			
BEHAVIOR: •coping effectively •no multiple requests	Assessed WNL				Assessed WNL				Assessed WNL			
** RN Teamleader concurs with above assessments	11-7				11-7				11-7			
	7-3				7-3				7-3			
	3-11				3-11				3-11			
● TREATMENTS												
Vital signs BID	see TPR				see TPR				see TPR			
SCD												
TEDS with heel cut off taken off/on BID												
Heel protectors												
Abduction pillow												
ROM to extremities												
Check dressing												
I/O cath or Foley	★				★				★			
Elevated toilet seat												
Fall protocol/Trapeze												
Activity												
Therapeutic (write time) Positioning (L) (R) (S)												
● HYGIENE												
Bath	☐ Full ☐ Partial				☐ Full ☐ Partial				☐ Full ☐ Partial			
How accomplished?	☐ Self ☐ Assist				☐ Self ☐ Assist				☐ Self ☐ Assist			
● SAFETY												
Side rails ↑												
Bed position - low												

CARE PATH DAY	DAY 4				DAY 5				DAY 6			
PAGE 6	ROOM #				ROOM #				DISCHARGE - ROOM #			
Write date →	DATE	N	D	E	DATE	N	D	E	DATE	N	D	E
Call light w/in reach												
ID band correct												
● MEDICATIONS												
Pain Meds	IM or PO: see MAR & Pain Graph				PO meds: see MAR and graph				PO meds: see MAR and graph			
Iron Meds	see MAR				see MAR				see MAR			
Stool Softener	see MAR				see MAR				see MAR			
Antiemetic Meds	see MAR				see MAR				see MAR			
Anticoagulant Meds	see MAR				see MAR				see MAR			
Continue Home Med	see MAR				see MAR				see MAR			
● DIET: As ordered		B	L	D		B	L	D		B	L	D
Consumption (write %)												
Food taken per -	☐ Self ☐ Assist				☐ Self ☐ Assist				☐ Self ☐ Assist			
● PHYSICAL ACTIVITY												
Stage Protocol	Stage III: exercises, toilet transfers gait trng walker/crutches				Continue Stage III: -toilet transfers gait trng walker/crutches				Continue Stage III: -transfer skills and gait trng & exercises			
Weight bearing	WB				WB				WB			
Occupational therapy	OT to assess ADLs				★				★			
● TEACHING Patient Outcomes: 1=Needs reinforcement 2=Partial understanding 3=Complete understanding/skill. *Write rating in box.*												
Daily Plan of care												
Exercises												
Activity restriction: use abduction pillow												
Therapeutic position: hip flexion not > 75°												
Anticoagulant Rx: self-injection and s/s to report to MD	Use booklet and video											
DC instructions on meds, return appt., s/s to report to MD												
Review "After Total Hip" booklet info	"Recovering in the Hospital"				"Mastering Daily Activities & Going Home"				"Recovering At Home"			
● DISCHARGE PLANNING					Give info. for Home Heath follow-up Review home care plans				Provide equipment for home care			
●DAILY PATIENT GOALS	Ambulates with walker or crutches				Ambulates with walker or crutches				Ambulates safely with device, stairs PRN			
	Safe transfers				Safe transfers				Safe transfers			
	WB as instructed				WB as instructed				WB as instructed			
	No s/s of complications				No s/s: DVT, infection				No s/s: DVT, infection			
	Good pain control				Good pain control				Good pain control			
									Know self-care for DC			
● InterDisciplinary Signatures.	PT				PT				PT			
	CM				CM				CM			
	OT											
Review of Care Path done q shift by nursing	11-7				11-7				11-7			
	7-3				7-3				7-3			
	3-11				3-11				3-11			

ACUITY LEVEL: Patient acuity level on Care Path Day 1 (Surgery Day) and Care Path Days 2-5 is classified as 3. Acuity level on Day of Discharge is 2. Any variance from these acuity levels will be documented in the Progress Notes for Care Path Variances.

DOCUMENTATION GUIDELINES: Initialing box indicates that intervention was implemented and patient outcomes are within standards. If patient goes beyond (positive variance) or falls below (negative variance) expected daily outcomes or assessment findings are Not Within Normal Limits, or any item with a (★) symbol, nursing will document in the Progress Notes for Care Path Variances.

☞ All assigned nurses are responsible for updating, reviewing the care path, and evaluating the daily goals. Affix signature for each shift and use the end-of-shift reporting.

© FFS 1995 THR Care Path 7/95

KAISER PERMANENTE PANORAMA CITY
Vaginal Delivery

RN Initial	Standard of Care Outcomes	Zones	Standards of Practice Interventions	Physicians
	Patient will not have excessive Bleeding during hospitalization (no more than 2 pads/hour) (see discharge info sheet).	1,2 3	Check flow and fundus at least once per shift	MD/CNM initiate preprinted orders (Zone 1)
	Patient will void at least once during the first eight hours following delivery.	1	Measure output of first voiding and record. Encourage fluid intake between meals (Zones 1, 2, 3)	Initiate follow-up orders as needed (Zone 1, 2, 3).
	Patient will not develop redness and swelling or infection in perineal area during hospitalization.	1,2,3	Continuous use of ice or iced pad to perineum per MD order. Check perineal area to determine signs of infection on admission and discharge. Check temperature and lacertation repair on admission and at discharge.	Orders patient discharge and provides instructions (Zone 3).
	Patient will report minimal discomfort from pain on oral medication.	1,2,3	Instruct patient to report onset of pain ASAP. Assess pain and record. Give MD ordered pain medication PRN. Assess effectiveness of pain medication within 1 hour and record.	
	Patient will be able to demonstrate or verbalize knowledge and skill in self care and baby care by the time of discharge. Barriers to Learning (Check those that apply) ____None ____Culture ____Religious/Spiritual Practices ____Emotional Barriers ____Desire/Motivation ____Physical Limitation ____Limited Learning Ability	1,2,3	See Postpartum Patient/ Significant Other Education and Discharge Record.	
	Patient needs will be met despite inability to speak English.	1,2,3	Use Spanish speaking nurse or interpreter for communication. Utilize Guide for Parents (20 languages) as necessary. Encourage listening and viewing of Spanish tapes and CCTV. Utilize AT&T Language line as necessary.	

Reproduced with permission of Kaiser Foundation Hospital, Panorama City, Calif.

Catagories	Zone 1 (0-8hours)	Zone 2 (8-16 hours)	Zone 3 (16-24 hours)

Consults:
Social Service
 	
Home Heath
 	
Lactation
  Consultant
 	
Other:
	See Education and
	  Discharge Record
	
	See Progress Notes
	
	_____
		See Education and
		  Discharge Record
		
		See Progress Notes
		
		_____
			See Education and
			  Discharge Record
			See Education and
			  Discharge Record
			See Progress Notes
			
			_____

Teaching and Discharge Planning:	See Education and
	  Discharge Record
		See Education and
		  Discharge Record
			See Education and
			  Discharge Record

Bonding:
Enfold-Enface
Actively Care
  For Infant
Encourage
  Talking to
  Infant
	_____
	
	_____
	
	_____
		_____
		
		_____
			_____
			
			_____

Safety:
  Siderails
  Bed Position
  Call Bell
	Up Down
	Up Down
	Within Reach Yes No
		Up Down
		Up Down
		Within Reach Yes No
			Up Down
			Up Down
			Within Reach Yes No

Transfer Assessment

SKIN:
  Warm/Dry _____
Pink _____
Pale/Cool _____
*Other: _____

_____ _____

BREASTS:
Soft _____
NIPPLES:
  Inverted/Flat _____
*Other: _____

_____ _____

LOCHIA:
  Light _____
  Moderate _____
  Heavy _____

Edema Location Code
  F=Feet L=Legs H=Hands
  E=Eyelids G=Generalized

EPISIOTOMY/LACERATION:
Intact _____
Swelling _____
*Other: _____

_____ _____

CARDIOVASCULAR:
  Heart Sounds:
  Regular/*Irregular _____
  Edema _____
  Dizziness
*Other: _____

_____ _____

NEUROLOGICAL:
  Alert/Oriented _____
*Other: _____

_____ _____

Edema Code
  4=large,pitting 3=mod. large
  2=moderate 1=minimal
  TR=trace

ELIMINATION:
  Distended Bladder _____
*Other: _____

_____ _____

PSYCHOSOCIAL:
  Appropriate Affect _____
*Depressed _____
  Infant in NICU
*Other: _____

_____ _____

IV SITE:
  Location _____
  Condition _____
  Discontinued _____
IV Condition Code
P=Patent R=Reddened
E=Edematous
IV Location Code
R=Right L=Left
A=Arm H=Hand

Transfer Assessment: Time_____ _____ **RN/LVN**

*DOCUMENT STARRED ITEMS AND/OR VARIANCES

SHIFT	INITIAL	SIGNATURE	INITIAL	SIGNATURE
☽ ☽ ☽ NOCS				
☼☼☼ DAYS				
★ ★ ★ EVES				

Continued

KASIER PERMANENTE PANORAMA CITY
Date of Birth _____

Care Path: Catagories Time:	Newborn Record Zone 1 (0-8 hours)	Zone 2 (8-16 hours)	Zone 3 (16-24 hours)
Assessment: a. Vital Signs 　　Time: 　Temp 　Apical Pulse 　Respiratory Rate b. Activity 　Sleeping 　Awake 　Alert 　*Irritable 　*Lethargic 　*Jittery 　Mother/Inf. 　Interaction	Admission Assessment 　　See Back Time _____ _____ _____ _____ _____ _____ _____ _____ Refer to Newborn Discharge Instructions	See Progress Notes Time _____ _____ _____ _____ _____ _____	See Newborn Discharge Instructions See Newborn Discharge Instructions See Newborn Discharge Instructions
Treatments:	Bath: Time _____ Circ. Time _____ 　Vaseline _____ 　*Bleeding _____ Gomco　Mogen　Sheldon Warming Measures: 　Hat　Warmed Blanket 　Heat Lamp	Circ. Time _____ 　Vaseline _____ 　*Bleeding _____ Gomco　Mogen　Sheldon 　*Heat　Warmed Blanklet Heat Lamp	Circ. Time _____ 　Vaseline _____ 　*Bleeding _____ Gomco　Mogen　Sheldon
Medications: Time/Init. _____ Time/Init. _____	0.5cc HBV　IM　RAT　LAT Lot # _____ Other _____ _____	0.5cc HBV　IM　RAT　LAT Lot # _____	HBV Recorded in KIT Date _____　Initials _____
Tests: 　MD Exam 　Urine Tox 　Hct. 　Chemstrip 　Newborn Screen 　*Other:	Time _____ Time Sent: _____ Result: _____ Time: _____ Result: _____ Time: _____ Result: _____ Time: _____ Result: _____ Time: _____ _____	 *Result: _____ Time: _____ _____	 *Result: _____ Time: _____ See Discharge Instructions _____
Diet: 　　Time: Breast min.　R 　　　　　L Bottle cc. 　Other: Suck/Swallow *Emesis	Observed: Yes ____ No____	Observed: Yes ____ No____	Observed: Yes ____ No____
Elimination: 　　Time: Urine Stool: M/T			

RN Initial	Standards of Care Outcomes	Zones	Standards of Practice Interventions	Physicians
	Infant will successfully adapt to extrauterine life.	1	Observe and record skin color, activity, temperature, feeding and elimination at least once per shift.	Performs PE exam and verbalizes results to parent(s) Initiates pre-printed orders. (Zone 1)
	Infant will be in stable condition at time of discharge.	3	See above. Observe and record.	Initiates follow-up orders as needed. (Zone 1,2,3)
	Hypoglycemia will not occur during the transition period.	1	Obtain Chemstrips per MD order and document results. Notify MD if chemstrip less than 40 mg/dl and order stat blood sugar. Observe for signs of jitteriness and irritability.	
	Excessive circ bleeding will not occur during hospital stay.	1,2,3	Observe for bleeding from circ site. Apply pressure and notify OB MD for reasessment PRN.	
	Acceptance into the family unit with reciprocal interaction.	1,2,3	Observe and record parent/infant interaction.	

SKIN:		HEAD:		HEART:		EYES:	
Warm	___	Rounded	___	Regular Rhythm	___	Sclera Clear	___
Pink	___	Cephalhematoma	___	*Irreg. Rhythm	___	Discharge	___
*Pale	___	Molding	___	*Murmur	___	Edema	___
*Acrocyanosis	___	Caput	___	ABDOMEN:		Hemorrhage	___
*Dusky	___	Overriding		Soft/No Disten.	___	CHEST/LUNGS:	
*Plethoric	___	Sutures	___	*Distended	___	Breath Sounds	
*Jaundice	___	Fonts Flat/Soft	___	Bowel Sounds	___	Clear Bilat.	___
Good Turgor	___	*Fonts Bulging	___	EXTREMITIES:		*Abnormal	
Dry/Peeling	___	NEUROLOGICAL		Symet. Moves	___	BS	___
*Ecchymosis	___	REFLEXES:		Spontan. Moves	___	*Nasal Flaring	___
*Abrasions	___	Nml suck, root, cry	___	ANUS:		*Retractions	___
		Nml grasp & moro	___	Patent	___	*Grunting	___

Physical Assessment: Time _____   _____ **RN/LVN**

SECURITY: ID BAND # _____

ID Check/Shift: Days _____   **PM's** _____   **Nocs** _____

After Circ _____   **After PKU** _____   **Other** _____

***DOCUMENT STARRED ITEMS AND/OR VARIANCES**

SHIFT		INITIAL	SIGNATURE	INITIAL	SIGNATURE
☽☽☽	NOCS				
☼☼☼	DAYS				
★★★	EVES				

Continued

Date of Delivery: _____ **Gravida** _____ **Para** _____

Catagories Time:	Zone 1 (0-8 hours)	Zone 2 (8-16 hours)	Zone 3 (16-24 hours)
Assessment: a. V S : Time Temp. Pulse Resp. Rate BP b. Activity	Transfer Assessment Ambulate with assistance	See Progress Notes Up ad lib	See Education and Discharge Record Discharge
Treatments: Peri Care: a. peri bottle b. ice c. spray d. tucks / oint. Sitz Bath Catherize prn Fundus Check Location Firm Boggy / Massaged	_____ _____ _____ _____ _____ _____ cc. _____ _____ _____ _____	Self Care Self Care Self Care * _____ cc. _____ _____ _____ _____	Self Care Self Care Self Care _____ * _____ cc. _____ _____ _____ * _____
Medications: Pain Management	See MAR See PRN Medication Form	See MAR See PRN Medication Form	See MAR See PRN Medication Form
Tests: MD / CNM Visit H&H Drawn Type / RH Other: _____	Time _____ Time _____ Time _____ Time _____	Time _____ Time _____ Time _____ Time _____	Time _____ Time _____ Time _____ Time _____
Diet: Other: _____	Regular _____	Regular _____	Regular _____
Elimination: Voiding Encourage Fluid Intake Bowel Movement	First Voiding Measured ____ cc Time: _____ _____	*First Voiding Measured ____ cc Time: _____ _____	 See Eduaction and Discharge Record

Transfer Notes: Date_____ Time _____
    Transfer from Labor and Delivery via _____

    Patient oriented to: Room _____ Visiting Policy _____ Smoking _____

                Infant Security System _____ Blue Badge _____

                Patient understands: Yes_____ No _____

Medical History (Include Medications other than prenatal vitamins): _____
_____
_____

Discharge Planning Needs: (See Labor and Delivery Perinatal Record 2)
    Other: _____
Educational Needs: Knowledge related to self aand baby care.
    Other: _____

TIME	NURSING OBSERVATIONS

Glossary of Abbreviations

A/G	albumin-globulin ratio
ABGs	arterial blood gases
ACE	acetylcholinesterase
ACL	anterior cruciate ligament
ACTH	adrenocorticotropic hormone
ADH	antidiuretic hormone
ADL	activities of daily living
AFB	acid-fast bacillus
AFP	alpha-fetoprotein
AGL	acute granulocytic leukemia
AICD	automatic implantable cardioverter defibrillator
AIDS	acquired immune deficiency syndrome
AKA	above-knee amputation
ALL	acute lymphocytic leukemia
ALS	amyotrophic lateral sclerosis
ALT	alanine aminotransferase, alanine transaminase
AMC	arm muscle circumference
AMI	acute myocardial infarction
AML	acute myelocytic leukemia
ANA	antinuclear antibody
ANC	absolute neutrophil count
ANLL	acute nonlymphocytic leukemia
ANS	autonomic nervous system
APR	abdominal perineal resection
APTT	activated partial thromboplastin time
ARC	AIDS-related complex
ARDS	adult respiratory distress syndrome
ARF	acute renal failure
AST	aspartate aminotransferase, aspartate transaminase
ATN	acute tubular necrosis
ATP	antitachycardia pacing
AV	atrioventricular
AVM	arteriovenous malformation
BBB	bundle branch block
BCG	*Bacillus Calmette-Guerin*
bid	twice a day
BKA	below-knee amputation
BMI	body mass index
BMR	basal metabolic rate
BMT	bone marrow transplant
BP	blood pressure
BPH	benign prostatic hypertrophy
bpm	beats per minute
BRM	biologic response modifiers
BSA	body surface area
BSE	breast self-examination
BUN	blood urea nitrogen
C	Celsius
Ca/Ca2^{++}/Ca^{++}	calcium
CABG	coronary artery bypass graft
CAD	coronary artery disease
CAPD	continuous ambulatory peritoneal dialysis

CAT	computerized axial tomography
CAVH	continuous arteriovenous hemofiltration
CBC	complete blood count
CBF	cerebral blood flow
CBI	continuous bladder irrigation
CBV	cerebral blood volume
CCU	coronary care unit
CI	cardiac index
CO	cardiac output
CDC	Centers for Disease Control
CEA	continuous epidural anesthesia; carcinoembryonic antigen
CHD	congenital heart disease
CHF	congestive heart failure
CI	cardiac index
CK	creatine kinase
CMV	cytomegalovirus
CNS	central nervous system
CO$_2$	carbon dioxide
COLD	chronic obstructive lung disease
COPD	chronic obstructive pulmonary disease
CPAP	continuous positive airway pressure
CPG	carotid phonoangiogram
CPK	creatinine phosphokinase
CPK-MB	creatinine phosphokinase with MB isoenzymes
CPM	continuous passive motion
CPP	cerebral perfusion pressure
CRH	corticotropin-releasing hormone
CSF	cerebrospinal fluid; colony-stimulating factor
CST	contraction stress test
CT	computed tomography
CVA	cerebrovascular accident
CV	cardioversion
CVD	cardiovascular disease; cerebral vascular disease
CVP	central venous pressure
CVR	cerebravascular resistance
D&C	dilitation and curettage
DES	diethylstilbesterol
DEXA	dual energy x-ray absorptiometry
DI	diabetes insipidus
DIC	disseminated intravascular coagulation
DICC	disseminated intravascular coagulation, complex
DKA	diabetic ketoacidosis
DMSO	dimethyl sulfoxide
DNA	deoxyribonucleic acid
DOE	dyspnea on exertion
DRE	digital rectal exam
DSA	digital subtraction angiography
DTR	deep tendon reflexes
DVI	digital vascular imaging
DVT	deep vein thrombosis
EBV	Epstein-Barr virus

ECG, EKG	electrocardiogram		**HZ**	herpes zoster
ECMO	extracarporeal membrane oxygen		**IABP**	intraaortic balloon pump
EEG	electroencephalogram		**IB**	inclusion body
EF	ejection fraction		**IC**	inspiratory capacity
ELISA	enzyme-linked immunosorbent assay		**ICD**	implantable cardiodefibrillation
EMG	electromyelography		**ICH**	intracranial hemorrhage
EOM	extraocular movement		**ICOI**	intravenous continuous opioid infusion
ENG	electronystagmography		**ICP**	intracranial pressure
ENT	ear, nose, and throat		**ICU**	intensive care unit
EPO	erythropoetin		**IDDM**	insulin-dependent diabetes mellitus
EPS	electrophysiology study		**IF**	immunofluorescence
ERCP	endoscopic retrograde cholangiopancreatogram		**Ig**	immune globulin
ERT	estrogen replacement therapy		**IgG**	immune globulin G
ESR	erythrocyte sedimentation rate		**IgM**	immune globulin M
ESRD	end-stage renal disease		**IGT**	impaired glucose tolerance
EST	exercise stress test		**IM**	intramuscular
ESWL	extracorporeal shock wave lithotripsy		**INH**	isoniazid
ET	endotracheal, enterostomal therapy		**INR**	International Normalized Ratio
ETOH	ethylene hydroxide (alcohol)		**IOP**	intraocular pressure
F	Fahrenheit		**IPD**	intermittent peritoneal dialysis
FBS	fasting blood sugar		**IPPB**	intermittent positive-pressure breathing
FC	functional capacity		**IRV**	inspiratory reserve volume
FDA	U.S. Food and Drug Administration		**IRT**	infrared thermography
FDP	fibrin degradation products		**ITP**	idiopathic thrombocytopenic purpura
FEV	forced expiratory volume		**IU**	international unit
FFP	fresh frozen plasma		**IUD**	intrauterine device
FIo$_2$	fraction of inspired oxygen		**IV**	intravenous
FRC	functional residual capacity		**IVP**	intravenous pyelogram
FSH	follicle-stimulating hormone		**IVU**	intravenous urogram
FSP	fibrin split product		**kg**	kilogram
FTA-ABS	fluorescent treponemal antibody absorption		**KOH**	potassium hydroxide
FVC	forced vital capacity		**KS**	Kaposi's sarcoma
GBS	Guillain-Barré syndrome		**KUB**	kidney ureters bladder
G-CSF	granulocyte colony-stimulating factor		**LAK**	lymphokine-activated killer cells
GC	gonoccocus (gonorrhea)		**LAP**	left atrial pressure
GCS	Glasgow Coma Scale		**LATS**	long-acting thyroid hormone
GDM	gestational diabetes mellitus		**LDH**	lactic dehydrogenase
GERD	gastroesophogeal reflux disease		**LDL**	low-density lipoproteins
GFR	glomerular filtration rate		**LE prep**	lupus erythematosus prep
GH	growth hormone		**LEEP**	loop electrosurgical excision procedure
GI	gastrointestinal		**LES**	local excitatory state
GM-CSF	granulocyte-macrophage colony-stimulating factor		**LH**	luteinizing hormone
GN	glomerulonephritis		**LHRH**	luteinizing hormone–releasing hormone
GnRH	gonadotropin-releasing hormone		**LLQ**	left lower quadrant
GTT	glucose tolerance test		**LMP**	last menstrual period
GU	genitourinary		**LOC**	level of consciousness
GVHD	graft versus host disease		**LP**	lumbar puncture
H$_2$O	water		**LTH**	luteotropic hormone
HA	hepatitis A		**LTA**	laser thermal angioplasty
HAV	hepatitis A virus		**LUQ**	left upper quadrant
HB	hepatitis B		**LV**	left ventricle
HBV	hepatitis B virus		**LVH**	left ventricular hypertrophy
HCG	human chorionic gonadotropin		**MAI**	*Mycobacterium avium-intracellulare*
HCl	hydrochloric acid		**MCH**	mean cell hemoglobin
HCO$_3^-$	bicarbonate		**MCHC**	mean cell hemoglobin concentration
Hct	hematocrit		**MCV**	mean corpuscular volume
HCV	hepatitis C virus		**mEq**	milliequivalent
HDL	high-density lipoproteins		**mg**	milligram
Hgb	hemoglobin		**MI**	myocardial infarction
Hgb AS	sickle cell trait		**min**	minute
Hgb SS	sickle cell disease		**ml**	milliliter
HHNK	hyperosmolar hyperglycemic nonketotic (syndrome)		**mm**	millimeter
			MOD	multiple organ dysfunction
HIV	human immunodeficiency virus		**MPAP**	mean pulmonary artery pressure
HR	heart rate		**MRA**	magnetic resonance angiography
HS	herpes simplex		**MRI**	magnetic resonance imaging
hs	hour of sleep		**MSG**	monosodium glutamate
HUTT	head up–tilt table		**MUAC**	mid-upper arm circumference

MUGA	multiple-gated acquisition scan		RA	rheumatoid arthritis
NCV	nerve conduction velocity		RAH	right atrial hypertrophy
NG	nasogastric		RAIU	radioactive iodine uptake
ng	nanogram		RAP	right atrial pressure
NICU	neonatal intensive care unit		RBBB	right bundle branch block
NIDDM	non–insulin-dependent diabetes mellitus		RBC	red blood cell count
NPO	nothing by mouth		REM	reactive eye movements
NS	normal saline		RFA	radiofrequency ablation
NPI	nocturnal penile tumescence		RIA	radioimmune assay
NSAIDs	nonsteroidal antiinflammatory drugs		RLQ	right lower quadrant
NTG	nitroglycerine		RN	registered nurse
O_2	oxygen		RNA	ribonucleic acid
OR	operating room		ROM	range of motion; rupture of membranes
ORIF	open reduction with internal fixation		RPR	rapid plasma reagin
OSHA	Occupational Safety and Health Administration		RUQ	right upper quadrant
OTC	over-the-counter		RV	right ventricle, residual volume
P	pulse		RVF	right ventricular failure
PAC	premature atrial contraction		RVH	right ventricular hypertrophy
PACU	postanesthesia care unit		SA	signal averaging; status asthmaticus
PAP	pulmonary artery pressure		SAH	subarachnoid hemorrhage
PAS	p-aminosalicylic acid		SC	subcutaneous
PAWP	pulmonary artery wedge pressure		SCD	sequential compression device
PBC	packed blood cells		SCI	spinal cord injury
pc	after meals		SGOT	serum glutamic-oxaloacetic transaminase
PCA	patient-controlled analgesia		SGPT	serum glutamic-pyruvic transaminase
PCR	polymerase chain reaction		SIADH	syndrome of inappropriate antidiuretic hormone
PCWP	pulmonary capillary wedge pressure		SLE	systemic lupus erythematosus
PD	interpupillary distance		SLP	segmental limb systolic pressure
PE	pulmonary embolus		SMBG	self-monitoring blood glucose
PEEP	positive end-expiratory pressure		SNS	sympathetic nervous system
PEFR	peak expiratory flow rage		SOB	shortness of breath
PEG	percutaneous endoscopic gastrostomy		SPECT	single photon emission computed tomography
PES	programmed electrical stimulation		Spo_2	oxygenation saturation
PET	positron emission tomography		SQ	subcutaneous
PFT	pulmonary function test		stat	immediately
PICC	peripherally inserted central catheter		STD	sexually transmitted diseases
PID	pelvic inflammatory disease		SV	stroke volume
PIH	pregnancy-induced hypertension		SVC	superior vena cava
PKD	polycystic kidney disease		SVCS	superior vena cava syndrome
PME	polymorphonuclear eosinophil leukocytes; pelvic muscle exercises		SVI	stroke volume index
			SVR	systemic vascular resistance
PMI	point of maximal impulse		SVT	supraventricular tachycardia
PML	progressive multifocal leukoencephalopathy		T	temperature
PND	paroxysmal nocturnal dyspnea		T_3	triiodothyronine
po	by mouth		T_4	thyroxine
prn	as needed		TAH-BSO	total abdominal hysterectomy/bilateral salpingo-oopherectomy
PROM	premature rupture of membrane			
PSA	prostate specific antigen		TB	tuberculosis
PSP	phenolsulfonphthalein		TBI	total body irradiation
PSVT	paroxysmal supraventricular tachycardia		TBSA	total body surface area
PT	prothrombin time		TEE	tranesophageal echocardiogram
PTA	percutaneous transluminal angioplasty		TENS	transcutaneous electrical nerve stimulation
PTC	plasma thromboplastin component		TFT	thyroid function test
PTCA	percutaneous transluminal coronary angioplasty		TIA	transient ischemic attack
PTH	parathyroid hormone		TIBC	total iron-binding capacity
PLT	preterm labor		TLC	tender loving care; total lung capacity
PTT	partial thromboplastin time		TMJ	temporomandibular joint
PV	peripheral vascular; pulmonary valve		TORCH	toxoplasmosis, other, rubella, cytomegalovirus, herpes
PVC	premature ventricular contraction			
PVD	peripheral vascular disease		TPN	total parenteral nutrition
PVR	peripheral vascular resistance		TRH	thyrotopin-releasing hormone
PWP	pulmonary wedge pressure		TSF	triceps skinfold
PZA	pyrazinamide (antituberculin agent)		TSH	thyroid-stimulating hormone
q4h	every four hours		TTP	thrombotic thrombocytopenic purpura
qd	every day		TURP	transurethral resection of the prostate
qh, q2h, etc.	every hour, every 2 hours, etc.		TV	tidal volume
qod	every other day		URI	upper respiratory infection
R	respirations		UTI	urinary tract infection

VAD	ventricular assist device; venous access device	**VS**	vital signs
VC	vital capacity	**VT**	ventricular tachycardia
VDRL	Venereal Disease Research Laboratories	**WBC**	white blood cells
VF	ventricular fibrillation	**WNL**	within normal limits
VHD	valvular heart disease	**WOCN**	Wound, Ostomy, Continence Nurse
VMA	vanillylmandellic acid	**WPW**	Wolff-Parkinson-White syndrome
VNA	Visiting Nurses Association	**WWW**	World Wide Web
VOD	venoocclusive disease		

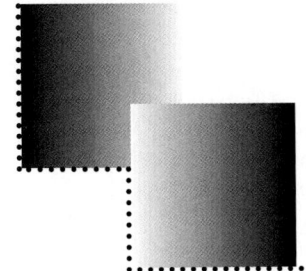

Index

NOTE: *t indicates table; f indicates figure.*

Testicle—cont'd
  self-examination of, 833*f*
  tumors in, 797*t*
Testosterone, production of, 402*t*
Tetraplegia, definition of, 547
Thallium-201 scintigraphy, angina pectoris diagnosed with, 92*t*
Theolair, bronchodilation with, 248*t*
Theophylline, bronchodilation with, 248*t*
Thermal burn, definition of, 718
Thigh, compartments and cross section of, 491*f*
Thioguanine, cancer treated with, 872*t*
Thio-tepa, cancer treated with, 866*t*
Third ventricle, diagram of, 514*f*
Thomas's splint, traction management and, 494*f*
Thoracentesis, 235-236
Thoracic spinal cord, injury to, 547
Thoracic vertebra, diagram of location of, 454*f*
Thoracotomy, 273-274
  chest tube and, 274
Thought process, altered, 55
Thrombocytopenia, 206-209
  acquired immunodeficiency syndrome and, 766
  chemotherapy and, 886-888
Thromboembolism, definition of, 77
Thrombolytic therapy, 156-157
Thrombophlebitis, definition of, 77
Thrombosis
  anticoagulant therapy for, 157-159
  therapy for, 156-157
Thumb, replantation of, 488-490
Thymosin fraction V, cancer treatment and, 904*t*
Thymus
  location of, 758*f*
  tumors in, 797*t*
Thyroid
  function and disorders of, 402*t*
  hormones affecting, 403
  radium implant in, 859
Thyroid crisis, 408-411
Thyroid storm, 408-411
Thyroidectomy, hyperthyroidism treated with, 441-443
Thyroid-stimulating hormone, production of, 401*t*
Thyrotoxicosis, 408-411
Thyrotropin-releasing hormone, production of, 401*t*
Thyroxine, production of, 402*t*
TIA; *see* Transient ischemic attack
Tibia, diagram of location of, 454*f*
Tissue, impaired integrity of, interventions for, 22-23
Tissue perfusion, altered
  polycythemia associated with, 204
  splenectomy and, 215
  thrombocytopenia and, 208
TNF; *see* Tumor necrosis factor
TNM classification, cancer assessment and, 796
Tocotransducer, care of mother on, 683
Tolazamide, diabetes treated with, 432*t*
Tolbutamide, diabetes treated with, 432*t*
Tolinase; *see* Tolazamide
Tonic neck reflex, 699*f*
Tonsils, location of, 758*f*

Torsades de point, 139-140
Torsus fracture, description of, 462
Total body irradiation, bone marrow transplant and, 770
Total hip replacement, care path for, 926-931
Total incontinence, 620
  definition of, 616
Toxic shock syndrome, 668-669
Toxoplasma gondii infection, cancer associated with, 854*t*
Toxoplasmosis, acquired immunodeficiency syndrome and, 762*t*
t-PA, precautions for administration of, 533
Trabeculectomy
  glaucoma treated with, 739
  patient education after, 741
Tracheostomy, 278-281
  suctioning, 237
Traction
  halo, neck immobilized with, 592
  management of, 494, 496*t*
Transcient ischemic attack, cerebral vascular disease associated with, 530
Transcultural patient care, 15-16
Transcutaneous electrical nerve stimulation, 42-43
Transcutaneous shock wave lithotripsy, urinary calculi treated with, 610*t*
Transhepatic biliary decompression catheter, 363
Transient ischemic attack, reversible ischemic neurologic deficit compared to, 532
Transurethral electrovaporization of prostate, 634*t*
Transurethral incision of prostate, 634*t*
Transurethral resection of prostate, 634*t*
Transverse fracture, description of, 462
Tridione; *see* Trimethadione
Triethylene-thiophosphoramide, cancer treated with, 866*t*
Triiodothyronine, production of, 402*t*
Trimethadione, seizure disorder controlled with, 527*t*
Troglitazone, diabetes treated with, 433*t*
TSH; *see* Thyroid-stimulating hormone
Tubal pregnancy, 670-672
Tuberculosis, pulmonary, 260-262
TUIP; *see* Transurethral incision of prostate
Tumor; *see also* Cancer
  brain, 540-543
  classification of, 797*t*
  osteocyte, 845
  resection of, care plan for, 914-919
  spinal cord, 541*t*-542*t*
Tumor cell vaccine, cancer treatment and, 905*t*
Tumor lysis syndrome, 851
Tumor necrosis factor, cancer treatment and, 907*t*
TURP; *see* Transurethral resection of prostate
Tympanic membrane, location of, 744*f*
Tympanoplasty
  definition of, 748
  patient education following, 749
Type 1 diabetes
  definition of, 427
  description of, 428*t*
Type 2 diabetes
  definition of, 427
  description of, 428*t*
  oral medications for, 432*t*-433*t*

Quick Reference Information

METRIC CONVERSIONS*

LENGTH
1 inch (in)	= 2.5 centimeters (cm)
1 foot (ft)	= 30 cm
1 yard (yd)	= 0.9 meters (m)
1 mile	= 1.6 kilometers (km)

MASS (WEIGHT)
1 ounce (oz)	= 28 grams (g)
1 pound (lb)	= 0.45 kilogram (kg)
1 short ton (2000 lb)	= 0.9 tonne

VOLUME
1 teaspoon (tsp)	= 5 milliliters (ml)
1 tablespoon (tbsp)	= 15 ml
1 fluid ounce (fl oz)	= 30 ml
1 cup	= 0.24 liters (L)
1 pint (pt)	= 0.47 L
1 quart (qt)	= 0.95 L
1 gallon (gal)	= 3.8 L

*Appropriate conversions to metric measures.

MASS EQUIVALENTS FOR MEDICATIONS (METRIC AND APOTHECARY SYSTEM)

APOTHECARY (GRAINS)	METRIC (MG)	METRIC (G)
1/200	0.3	0.0003
1/150	0.4	0.0004
1/100	0.6	0.0006
1/60	1	0.001
1/30	2	0.002
1/20	3	0.003
1/15	4	0.004
1/10	6	0.006
1/8	8	0.008
1/6	10	0.010
1/4	15	0.015
1/3	20	0.020
1/2*	30	0.030
3/4	50	0.050
1	60	0.060
1½	100	0.100
2	120	0.12
2½	150	0.15
3	200	0.2
4	250	0.25
5	300	0.3
7½	500	0.5
10	600	0.6
15	1000	1.0
30	2000	2.0

*From ½ to 5 grains; the following more accurate "approximate equivalents" are also acceptable.

¼ grain	= 16 mg	2½ grains	= 160 mg
½ grain	= 32 mg	3 grains	= 200 mg
1 grain	= 65 mg	4 grains	= 260 mg
1½ grains	= 100 mg	4 grains	= 260
2 grains	= 130 mg		